PATHOLOGY SIMPLIFIED
A Quick Review for Examination Preparation

PATHOLOGY SIMPLIFIED
A Quick Review for Examination Preparation

Harsh Mohan, MD FAMS FICPath FUICC
Former Professor and Head, Department of Pathology
Former Dean and Former Medical Superintendent
Government Medical College and Hospital
Sector-32, Chandigarh-160 031, INDIA
E-mail: *drharshmohan@gmail.com*

Ivan Damjanov, MD PhD dhc
Emeritus Professor of Pathology
The University of Kansas School of Medicine
Kansas City, Kansas-66160, USA
E-mail: *idamjano@kumc.edu*

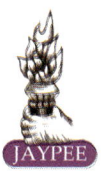

JAYPEE BROTHERS MEDICAL PUBLISHERS
The Health Sciences Publisher
New Delhi | London

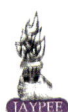 **Jaypee Brothers Medical Publishers (P) Ltd**

Headquarters

Jaypee Brothers Medical Publishers (P) Ltd
EMCA House, 23/23-B
Ansari Road, Daryaganj
New Delhi 110 002, India
Landline: +91-11-23272143, +91-11-23272703
+91-11-23282021, +91-11-23245672
Email: jaypee@jaypeebrothers.com

Corporate Office

Jaypee Brothers Medical Publishers (P) Ltd
4838/24, Ansari Road, Daryaganj
New Delhi 110 002, India
Phone: +91-11-43574357
Fax: +91-11-43574314
Email: jaypee@jaypeebrothers.com

Overseas Office

J.P. Medical Ltd
83 Victoria Street, London
SW1H 0HW (UK)
Phone: +44 20 3170 8910
Fax: +44 (0)20 3008 6180
Email: info@jpmedpub.com

Website: www.jaypeebrothers.com
Website: www.jaypeedigital.com

© 2022, Jaypee Brothers Medical Publishers

The views and opinions expressed in this book are solely those of the original contributor(s)/author(s) and do not necessarily represent those of editor(s) of the book.

All rights reserved. No part of this publication may be reproduced, stored or transmitted in any form or by any means, electronic, mechanical, photocopying, recording or otherwise, without the prior permission in writing of the publishers.

All brand names and product names used in this book are trade names, service marks, trademarks or registered trademarks of their respective owners. The publisher is not associated with any product or vendor mentioned in this book.

Medical knowledge and practice change constantly. This book is designed to provide accurate, authoritative information about the subject matter in question. However, readers are advised to check the most current information available on procedures included and check information from the manufacturer of each product to be administered, to verify the recommended dose, formula, method and duration of administration, adverse effects and contraindications. It is the responsibility of the practitioner to take all appropriate safety precautions. Neither the publisher nor the author(s)/editor(s) assume any liability for any injury and/or damage to persons or property arising from or related to use of material in this book.

This book is sold on the understanding that the publisher is not engaged in providing professional medical services. If such advice or services are required, the services of a competent medical professional should be sought.

Every effort has been made where necessary to contact holders of copyright to obtain permission to reproduce copyright material. If any have been inadvertently overlooked, the publisher will be pleased to make the necessary arrangements at the first opportunity.

Inquiries for bulk sales may be solicited at: jaypee@jaypeebrothers.com

Pathology Simplified: A Quick Review for Examination Preparation

First Edition: **2022**

ISBN: 978-93-5465-133-5

Printed at Rajkamal Electric Press, Kundli, Haryana.

Dedicated to

To my wife Praveen for being a pillar of my support always.
And my angelic and cute granddaughter Maya,
whose arrival has filled my life with limitless joy!

—HM

To Andrea, my wife of 50 plus years, who encouraged me
to take up this project despite my age.
And my granddaughter Olivia, who inspired me to persist
by telling me that she will study medicine.

—ID

Preface

Pathology, as a course for undergraduates and for those preparing for qualifying exams for further studies (such as postgraduate entrance exam in India PG-NEET, or the US medical licensing exam USMLE) is quite a complicated subject. Furthermore, as a basic medical science, pathology has been advancing at a rapid pace, and accordingly, the textbooks of pathology have become quite voluminous. With continuous addition of more and more of ancillary tools in laboratory medicine such as immunohistochemistry, genomics, proteomics and molecular methods, the field of its study has expanded exponentially. While only a few students in a class may choose pathology as their career, others may love it or hate it but they cannot avoid it! Basic knowledge of Pathology and its periodic updating will always remain an essential requirement for all practitioners of medicine.

Mastering knowledge of such a vast subject is quite a formidable task. For learning pathology, there are several comprehensive and fine textbooks available in the market; however, students overburdened with curricula or those in a hurry near exam, are confused and have several dilemmas on their minds which remain unresolved such as: What and how much is enough? How can I recall and reproduce what I learnt? How can I self-assess after I read and learnt a topic or a chapter?

Keeping these objectives in mind, both of us, with our experience in teaching, curricular design and implementation, realised that we must do something to help students master pathology in a shorter time. As a results of our best intentions, we present to you two years after it inception, our new Indo-US joint title 'Pathology Simplified: *A Quick Review for Examination Preparation*' in hybrid mode (as printed book and an online supplementary content).

Some of the *key features* which keep this book apart from other available books in the market are as follows:

Multiple choice questions and answers This Q&A user-friendly format of short questions and brief answers replicates the actual exams and contains many questions from previous exams, accompanied by succinct answers written in simple and easy-to-understand language.

Illustrations The book is profusely illustrated with over 500 labelled line-sketches of gross and microscopy of specimens/slides, schematic drawings and photographs. Some of these figures were also used for questions, to show the students that some questions on the forthcoming examination will be based on pictorial material.

Tables The book contains approximately 200 tables that include comparative features of closely resembling conditions, important classifications and listing of salient features.

Online learning resources The electronic supplement to the book includes approximately 1,200 high-yield questions (MCQs, clinicopathologic vignettes and figure-based questions), followed by corresponding answers and brief explanatory notes for the correct answers, as well as a full rationale for all other answer options.

Self-assessment The users have the facility for attempting online questions and knowing the score, followed by correct answers with explanatory notes.

In summary, we have prepared this compact but comprehensive and all-inclusive package which is made available to users at a reasonable cost. Our book is primarily targeted at recent medical school graduates to help them in preparing for the entrance exam for higher courses such as PG-NEET, or specialty training, or for medical licensing exams, like USMLE and similar exams in different countries. In essence, this book will help you revisit Pathology in shorter time that you studied earlier, and thus, assist you to prepare most efficiently for this most crucial exam of your career. You must know that these qualifying exams contain quite a bit of Pathology, since pathology is the basis of all clinical disciplines. Furthermore, undergraduate students who are in a 'hurry' to quickly study and prepare the subject to take their pathology exam will also find this book immensely useful.

ACKNOWLEDGEMENTS

In preparing this book, we have strived to be as accurate and as perfect as possible. In doing so, we have been greatly supported by the Production team at the M/s Jaypee Brothers Medical Publishers (P) Ltd. In particular, we appreciate sincere efforts by Mr Rajesh Sharma (Production Coordinator), Mr Deepak Saxena (Desktop Operator), and Mr Manoj Pahuja (Senior Graphic Designer), which are thankfully acknowledged. A special word of gratitude is due to Dr Madhu Choudhary, Publishing Head (Education) for this project, for coordination and in overseeing the entire project vigilantly and efficiently.

Our special thanks are due to Shri Jitendar P Vij (Group Chairman) and Mr Ankit Vij (Managing Director) of the M/s Jaypee Brothers Medical Publishers (P) Ltd, New Delhi, India, for their innovative ideas and efforts for getting the best final product at reasonable cost to the users.

Finally, in spite of our sincere effort to be as accurate as possible, an element of human error is still likely. We humbly request users to give their valuable suggestions, feedback or criticism, as that would help us improve and enhance the content further and carry out corrections, wherever required, at the earliest possible opportunity.

Harsh Mohan, MD FAMS FICPath FUICC
Ivan Damjanov, MD PhD dhc

Personal note by HM to ID It has been a wonderful experience for me working with and learning from the wisdom of my senior co-author Professor Ivan Damjanov. While he had been gracious in penning Foreword for my Textbook of Pathology since its 5th edition (2004) but it was a proud moment for me when he agreed to be a co-author for this project in a personal meeting in late-2018 in Philadelphia, PA, USA. He is not only such a hard-working and dedicated professional but a kind, warm-hearted and affable human being. Dear Ivan, I can never thank you enough for what I got to learn from you in the process!

Contents

SECTION I: GENERAL PATHOLOGY

Chapter 1: Introduction to Pathology — 1

Chapter 2: Molecular Cell Biology in Health and Ageing — 4

Chapter 3: Cellular Adaptations and Cell Injury — 19
- Cell Injury, Responses and Etiology   19
- Cellular Adaptations   20
- Pathogenesis of Cell Injury   27
- Morphology of Cell Injury   33
- Programmed Cell Death (Apoptosis)   40
- Intracellular Accumulations and Pigments   44

Chapter 4: Inflammation and Repair — 51
- Definition and General Features   51
- Acute Inflammatory Response   51
- Chemical Mediators of Inflammation   56
- Inflammatory Cells   62
- Acute Inflammation—Factors in Response, Morphologic Types, Effects and Outcome   64
- Chronic Inflammation—Types and General Features   67
- Common Granulomatous Diseases   69
- Tissue Repair   82

Chapter 5: Immunopathology Including Amyloidosis — 87
- Normal Immune System   87
- Major Histocompatibility Complex and Transplantation   91
- Immunodeficiency Diseases   94
- Hypersensitivity Reactions   102
- Autoimmune Diseases   106
- Amyloidosis   114

Chapter 6: Derangements of Homeostasis and Haemodynamic Disorders — 121
- Homeostasis   121
- Derangements of Body Water   122
- Disturbances of Electrolytes and pH of Blood   129
- Haemodynamic Derangements   130
- Obstructive Circulatory Disturbances   137

Chapter 7: Neoplasia — 148

- Nomenclature and Classification   148
- Characteristics of Tumours   150
- Epidemiology of Cancer   155
- Molecular Basis of Cancer   158
- Carcinogens and Carcinogenesis   166
- Clinical Aspects of Neoplasia   174

Chapter 8: Infectious Diseases — 180

- General Aspects   180
- Bacterial Diseases   181
- Fungal Diseases   184
- Viral Diseases   185
- Parasitic Diseases   189

Chapter 9: Environmental and Nutritional Diseases — 194

- Environmental Diseases   194
- Nutritional Diseases   199

Chapter 10: Genetic and Paediatric Diseases — 209

- Genetic Diseases   209
- Paediatric Diseases   218

SECTION II: HAEMATOPOIETIC SYSTEM AND LYMPHORETICULAR TISSUES

Chapter 11: Introduction to Haematopoietic System and Disorders of Erythroid Series — 221

- Bone Marrow and Haematopoiesis   221
- Erythropoiesis   224
- General Aspects of Anaemias   227
- Hypochromic Anaemias   230
- Megaloblastic Anaemias   235
- Haemolytic Anaemias and Anaemias of Blood Loss   238
- Aplastic Anaemia and Primary Bone Marrow Disorders   252

Chapter 12: Haemostatic System, Bleeding Disorders and Transfusion Medicine — 254

- Haemostatic System   254
- Bleeding Disorders   258
- Blood Transfusion   266

Chapter 13: White Blood Cells—Proliferations and Myeloid Neoplasms — 272

- White Blood Cells—Normal and Reactive Proliferations   272
- Haematolymphoid Malignancies—General Aspects   279
- Myeloid Neoplasms   281

Chapter 14: Lymphoid Cells of Blood and Lymphoreticular Tissues — 291

- Normal Lymph Nodes and Reactive Lymphadenitis   291
- Pathology of the Spleen   293
- Thymus   296
- Lymphoid and Histiocytic Neoplasms   297

SECTION III: SYSTEMIC PATHOLOGY

Chapter 15: Blood Vessels and Lymphatics — 317

Chapter 16: Heart — 338

Chapter 17: Respiratory System — 371
- Lungs   371
- Pleura   407

Chapter 18: Eye, ENT and Neck — 410
- Eye   410
- Ear   417
- Nose and Paranasal Sinuses   418
- Pharynx   419
- Larynx   420
- Neck   421

Chapter 19: Oral Cavity and Salivary Glands — 423
- Oral Soft Tissues   423
- Teeth and Periodontal Tissues   428
- Salivary Glands   432

Chapter 20: Gastrointestinal Tract — 436
- Oesophagus   436
- Stomach   440
- Small Intestine   453
- Appendix   468
- Large Intestine   470
- Peritoneum   478

Chapter 21: Liver, Biliary Tract and Exocrine Pancreas — 480
- Liver   480
- Biliary Tract   515
- Exocrine Pancreas   521

Chapter 22: Kidney and Lower Urinary Tract — 526
- Kidneys   526
- Lower Urinary Tract   564

Chapter 23: Male Genital System — 570
- Testis and Epididymis   570
- Penis   580
- Prostate   582

Chapter 24: Female Genital Tract — 588
- Vulva   588
- Vagina   590
- Cervix   591

- Uterus 595
- Ovary 600
- Placenta 609

Chapter 25: Breast 613

Chapter 26: Skin 625

Chapter 27: Endocrine System 641
- Basic Concept of Endocrines 641
- Pituitary Gland 642
- Adrenal Gland 645
- Thyroid Gland 651
- Parathyroid Glands 663
- Endocrine Pancreas 666

Chapter 28: Musculoskeletal System 675
- Bone and Cartilage 675
- Joints 687
- Skeletal Muscles 692

Chapter 29: Soft Tissue Tumours 695
- General Features 695
- Specific Types of Soft Tissue Tumours 699

Chapter 30: Nervous System 705
- Central Nervous System 705
- Peripheral Nervous System 729

APPENDIX

Chapter 31: Basic Diagnostic Cytopathology 735
- Overview 735
- Exfoliative Cytology 737
- Interventional Cytology 743

Index 747

CONTENTS AS PER COMPETENCY-BASED UNDERGRADUATE CURRICULUM FOR THE INDIAN MEDICAL GRADUATE (NATIONAL MEDICAL COMMISSION)*

Competencies (Outcomes) — Core (Must know) | Non-core (Desirable to know)
Assessment Methods — Written/Viva voce | Practical/Skill

SECTION I GENERAL PATHOLOGY

Chapter 1: Introduction to Pathology — 1

♦ Describe the role of a pathologist in diagnosis and management of disease (PA1.1)	Written/Viva voce
♦ Enumerate common definitions and terms used in pathology (PA1.2)	Written/Viva voce
♦ Describe the history and evolution of pathology (PA1.3)	Written/Viva voce

Chapter 2: Molecular Cell Biology in Health and Ageing — 4

♦ Describe and discuss the mechanisms of cellular ageing (PA2.7)	Written/Viva voce

Chapter 3: Cellular Adaptations and Cell Injury — 19

♦ Demonstrate knowledge of the causes, mechanisms, types and effects of cell injury and their clinical significance (PA2.1)	Written/Viva voce
♦ Describe the etiology of cell injury. Distinguish between reversible-irreversible injury: mechanisms; morphology of cell injury (PA2.2)	Written/Viva voce
♦ Intracellular accumulation of fats, proteins, carbohydrates, pigments (PA2.3)	Written/Viva voce
♦ Describe and discuss cell death—types, mechanisms, necrosis, apoptosis: basic as contrasted with necrosis, autolysis (PA2.4)	Written/Viva voce
♦ Describe and discuss pathologic calcifications, gangrene (PA2.5)	Written/Viva voce
♦ Describe and discuss cellular adaptations: atrophy, hypertrophy, hyperplasia, metaplasia, dysplasia (PA2.6)	Written/Viva voce
♦ Identify and describe various forms of cell injuries, their manifestations and consequences in gross and microscopic specimens (PA2.8)	Practical/Skill
♦ Describe and discuss the mechanisms of apoptosis (PA2.7)	Written/Viva voce

Chapter 4: Inflammation and Repair — 51

♦ Define and describe the general features of acute and chronic inflammation including stimuli, vascular and cellular events (PA4.1)	Written/Viva voce
♦ Enumerate and describe the mediators of acute inflammation (PA4.2)	Written/Viva voce
♦ Define and describe chronic inflammation including causes, types, non-specific and granulomatous; and enumerate examples of each (PA4.3)	Written/Viva voce
♦ Define and describe the etiology, types, pathogenesis, stages, morphology, microscopic appearance and complications of tuberculosis (PA26.4)	Written/Viva voce
♦ Describe the pathogenesis and pathology of tuberculous lymphadenitis (PA19.2)	Written/Viva voce
♦ Define and describe the pathogenesis and pathology of leprosy (PA10.3)	Written/Viva voce
♦ Define and describe the process of repair and regeneration including wound healing (PA5.1)	Written/Viva voce

---

* For readers from India

Competencies (Outcomes)	Core (Must know)	Non-core (Desirable to know)
Assessment Methods	Written/Viva voce	Practical/Skill

- ♦ Identify and describe the features of tuberculous lymphadenitis in a gross and microscopic specimen (PA19.3) — Practical/Skill
- ♦ Identify and describe acute and chronic inflammation in gross and microscopic specimens (PA4.4) — Practical/Skill
- ♦ Describe the etiology, pathophysiology, pathologic features and complications of syphilis on the cardiovascular system (PA27.10) — Written/Viva voce

Chapter 5: Immunopathology Including Amyloidosis — 87

- ♦ Describe the pathogenesis and pathology of amyloidosis (PA3.1) — Written/Viva voce
- ♦ Describe the principles and mechanisms involved in immunity (PA9.1) — Written/Viva voce
- ♦ Describe the mechanisms of hypersensitivity reactions (PA9.2) — Written/Viva voce
- ♦ Describe the HLA system and the immune principles involved in transplant and mechanism of transplant rejection (PA9.3) — Written/Viva voce
- ♦ Define autoimmunity. Enumerate autoimmune disorders (PA9.4) — Written/Viva voce
- ♦ Define and describe the pathogenesis of systemic lupus erythematosus (PA9.5) — Written/Viva voce
- ♦ Define and describe the pathogenesis and pathology of HIV and AIDS (PA9.6) — Written/Viva voce
- ♦ Define and describe the pathogenesis of other common autoimmune diseases (PA9.7) — Written/Viva voce
- ♦ Identify and describe amyloidosis in a pathology specimen (PA3.2) — Practical/Skill

Chapter 6: Derangements of Homeostasis and Haemodynamic Disorders — 121

- ♦ Define and describe oedema, its types, pathogenesis and clinical correlations (PA6.1) — Written/Viva voce
- ♦ Define and describe hyperaemia, congestion, haemorrhage (PA6.2) — Written/Viva voce
- ♦ Define and describe shock, its pathogenesis and its stages (PA6.3) — Written/Viva voce
- ♦ Define and describe normal haemostasis, and the etiopathogenesis and consequences of thrombosis (PA6.4) — Written/Viva voce
- ♦ Define and describe embolism, its causes and common types (PA6.5) — Written/Viva voce
- ♦ Define and describe ischaemia/infarction, its types, etiology, morphologic changes and clinical effects (PA6.6) — Written/Viva voce
- ♦ Identify and describe the gross and microscopic features of infarction in a pathologic specimen (PA6.7) — Practical/Skill

Chapter 7: Neoplasia — 148

- ♦ Define and classify neoplasia. Describe the characteristics of neoplasia including gross, microscopy, biologic behaviour and spread. Differentiate between benign and malignant neoplasms (PA7.1) — Written/Viva voce
- ♦ Describe the molecular basis of cancer (PA7.2) — Written/Viva voce
- ♦ Enumerate carcinogens and describe the process of carcinogenesis (PA7.3) — Written/Viva voce
- ♦ Describe the effects of tumour on the host including paraneoplastic syndrome (PA7.4) — Written/Viva voce
- ♦ Describe immunology and the immune response to cancer (PA7.5) — Written/Viva voce
- ♦ Identify, distinguish and describe common tumours of the skin (PA34.4) — Practical/Skill

Competencies (Outcomes)	Core (Must know)	Non-core (Desirable to know)
Assessment Methods	Written/Viva voce	Practical/Skill

Chapter 8: Infectious Diseases — 180

◆ Define and describe the pathogenesis and pathology of malaria (PA10.1)	Written/Viva voce
◆ Define and describe the pathogenesis and pathology of cysticercosis (PA10.2)	Written/Viva voce
◆ Define and describe the pathogenesis and pathology of common bacterial, viral, protozoal and helminthic diseases (PA10.4)	Written/Viva voce

Chapter 9: Environmental and Nutritional Diseases — 194

◆ Enumerate and describe the pathogenesis of disorders caused by air pollution, tobacco and alcohol (PA12.1)	Written/Viva voce
◆ Describe the pathogenesis of disorders caused by protein–calorie malnutrition and starvation (PA12.2)	Written/Viva voce
◆ Describe the pathogenesis of obesity and its consequences (PA12.3)	Written/Viva voce

Chapter 10: Genetic and Paediatric Diseases — 209

◆ Describe the pathogenesis and features of common cytogenetic abnormalities and mutations in childhood (PA11.1)	Written/Viva voce
◆ Describe the pathogenesis and pathology of tumours and tumour-like conditions in infancy and childhood (PA11.2)	Written/Viva voce
◆ Describe the pathogenesis of common storage disorders in infancy and childhood (PA11.3)	Written/Viva voce

SECTION II: HAEMATOPOIETIC SYSTEM AND LYMPHORETICULAR TISSUES

Chapter 11: Introduction to Haematopoietic System and Disorders of Erythroid Series — 221

◆ Describe haematopoiesis and extramedullary haematopoiesis (PA13.1)	Written/Viva voce
◆ Describe the role of anticoagulants in haematology (PA13.2)	Written/Viva voce
◆ Define and classify anaemias (PA13.3)	Written/Viva voce
◆ Enumerate and describe the investigation of anaemia (PA13.4)	Written/Viva voce
◆ Describe iron metabolism (PA14.1)	Written/Viva voce
◆ Describe the etiology, investigations and differential diagnosis of microcytic hypochromic anaemia ((PA14.2)	Written/Viva voce
◆ Describe the metabolism of vitamin B12, and the etiology and pathogenesis of B12 deficiency (PA15.1)	Written/Viva voce
◆ Describe laboratory investigations of macrocytic anaemia (PA15.2)	Written/Viva voce
◆ Identify and describe the peripheral blood picture of macrocytic anaemia (PA15.3)	Practical/Skill
◆ Define and classify haemolytic anaemias (PA16.1)	Written/Viva voce
◆ Describe the pathogenesis and clinical features and haematologic indices of haemolytic anaemia (PA16.2)	Written/Viva voce
◆ Describe the pathogenesis, features, haematologic indices and peripheral blood picture of sickle cell anaemia and thalassaemia (PA16.3)	Written/Viva voce

Competencies (Outcomes)	Core (Must know)	Non-core (Desirable to know)
Assessment Methods	Written/Viva voce	Practical/Skill

♦ Describe the etiology, pathogenesis, haematologic indices and peripheral blood picture of acquired haemolytic anaemia (PA16.4)	Written/Viva voce
♦ Describe the peripheral blood picture in different haemolytic anaemias (PA16.5)	Written/Viva voce
♦ Perform, identify and describe the peripheral blood picture in anaemias (PA13.5)	Practical/Skill
♦ Identify and describe the peripheral smear in microcytic anaemia (PA14.3)	Practical/Skill
♦ Prepare a peripheral blood smear and identify haemolytic anaemia from it (PA16.6)	Practical/Skill
♦ Enumerate the indications and describe the findings in bone marrow aspiration and biopsy (PA17.2)	Written/Viva voce
♦ Enumerate the differences; describe the etiology and distinguishing features of megaloblastic and non-megaloblastic macrocytic anaemia (PA15.4)	Written/Viva voce
♦ Enumerate the etiology, pathogenesis and findings in aplastic anaemia (PA17.1)	Written/Viva voce

Chapter 12: Haemostatic System, Bleeding Disorders and Transfusion Medicine 254

♦ Describe normal haemostasis (PA21.1)	Written/Viva voce
♦ Classify and describe the etiology, pathogenesis and pathology of vascular and platelet disorders including ITP and haemophilias (PA21.2)	Written/Viva voce
♦ Differentiate platelet from clotting disorders based on the clinical and haematologic features (PA21.3)	Written/Viva voce
♦ Define and describe disseminated intravascular coagulation, its laboratory findings and diagnosis of disseminated intravascular coagulation (PA21.4)	Written/Viva voce
♦ Define and describe laboratory findings and diagnosis of vitamin K deficiency (PA21.5)	Written/Viva voce
♦ Classify and describe blood group systems (ABO and Rh) (PA22.1)	Written/Viva voce
♦ Describe the correct technique to perform a cross match (PA16.7)	Written/Viva voce
♦ Enumerate the indications; describe the principles; enumerate and demonstrate the steps of compatibility testing (PA22.2)	Written/Viva voce
♦ Enumerate blood components and describe their clinical uses (PA22.4)	Written/Viva voce
♦ Enumerate and describe infections transmitted by blood transfusion (PA22.5)	Written/Viva voce
♦ Describe transfusion reactions and enumerate the steps in the investigation of a transfusion reaction (PA22.6)	Written/Viva voce
♦ Enumerate the indications and describe the principles and procedure of autologous transfusion (PA22.7)	Written/Viva voce

Chapter 13: White Blood Cells—Proliferations and Myeloid Neoplasms 272

♦ Enumerate and describe the causes of leucocytosis, leucopenia, lymphocytosis and leukaemoid reactions (PA18.1)	Written/Viva voce
♦ Describe the etiology, genetics, pathogenesis, classification, clinical and haematologic features of acute and chronic myeloid leukaemia (PA18.2)	Written/Viva voce

Chapter 14: Lymphoid Cells of Blood and Lymphoreticular Tissues 291

♦ Describe the etiology, genetics, pathogenesis, classification, clinical and haematologic features of acute and chronic lymphoid leukaemia (PA18.2)	Written/Viva voce
♦ Enumerate the causes and describe the differentiating features of lymphadenopathy (PA19.1)	Written/Viva voce

Competencies (Outcomes)	Core (Must know)	Non-core (Desirable to know)
Assessment Methods	Written/Viva voce	Practical/Skill

♦ Describe and discuss the pathogenesis, pathology and the differentiating features of Hodgkin and non-Hodgkin lymphoma (PA19.4)	Written/Viva voce
♦ Enumerate and differentiate the causes of splenomegaly (PA19.6)	Written/Viva voce
♦ Identify and describe the features of Hodgkin lymphoma in a gross and microscopic specimen (PA19.5)	Practical/Skill
♦ Identify and describe the gross specimen of an enlarged spleen (PA19.7)	Practical/Skill
♦ Describe the features of plasma cell myeloma (PA20.1)	Practical/Skill

SECTION III: SYSTEMIC PATHOLOGY

Chapter 15: Blood Vessels and Lymphatics — 317

♦ Distinguish arteriosclerosis from atherosclerosis. Describe the pathogenesis and pathology of various causes and types of arteriosclerosis (PA27.1)	Written/Viva voce
♦ Describe the etiology, dynamics, pathology, types and complications of aneurysms including aortic aneurysms (PA27.2)	Written/Viva voce

Chapter 16: Heart — 338

♦ Describe the etiology, types, stages, pathophysiology, pathology and complications of heart failure (PA27.3)	Written/Viva voce
♦ Describe the etiology, pathophysiology, pathology, gross and microscopic features, criteria and complications of rheumatic fever (PA27.4)	Written/Viva voce
♦ Describe the epidemiology, risk factors, etiology, pathophysiology, pathology, presentations, gross and microscopic features, diagnostic tests and complications of ischaemic heart disease (PA27.5)	Written/Viva voce
♦ Describe the etiology, pathophysiology, pathology, gross and microscopic features, diagnosis and complications of infective endocarditis (PA27.6)	Written/Viva voce
♦ Describe the etiology, pathophysiology, pathology, gross and microscopic features, diagnosis and complications of pericarditis and pericardial effusion (PA27.7)	Written/Viva voce
♦ Interpret abnormalities in cardiac function testing in acute coronary syndromes (PA27.8)	Practical/Skill
♦ Classify and describe the etiology, types, pathophysiology, pathology, gross and microscopic features, diagnosis and complications of cardiomyopathies (PA27.9)	Written/Viva voce
♦ Describe the etiology, pathophysiology, pathology features and complications of syphilis on the cardiovascular system (PA27.10)	Written/Viva voce

Chapter 17: Respiratory System — 371

♦ Define and describe the etiology, types, pathogenesis, stages, morphology and complications of pneumonia (PA26.1)	Written/Viva voce
♦ Describe the etiology, gross and microscopic appearance and complications of lung abscess (PA26.2)	Written/Viva voce
♦ Define and describe the etiology, types, pathogenesis, stages, morphology, complications and evaluation of obstructive airway disease (OAD) and bronchiectasis (PA26.3)	Written/Viva voce

| Competencies (Outcomes) | Core (Must know) | Non-core (Desirable to know) |
| Assessment Methods | Written/Viva voce | Practical/Skill |

♦ Define and describe the etiology, types, exposure, environmental influence, pathogenesis, stages, morphology, microscopic appearance and complications of occupational lung disease (PA26.5)	Written/Viva voce
♦ Define and describe the etiology, types, exposure, genetics, environmental influence, pathogenesis, stages, morphology, microscopic appearance, metastases and complications of tumours of the lung and pleura (PA26.6)	Written/Viva voce
♦ Define and describe the etiology, types, exposure, genetics, environmental influence, pathogenesis, morphology, microscopic appearance and complications of mesothelioma (PA26.6)	Written/Viva voce

Chapter 18: Eye, ENT and Neck 410

♦ Describe the etiology, genetics, pathogenesis, pathology, presentation, sequelae and complications of retinoblastoma (PA36.1)	Written/Viva voce

Chapter 19: Oral Cavity and Salivary Glands 423

♦ Describe the etiology, pathogenesis, pathology and clinical features of oral cancers (PA24.1)	Written/Viva voce

Chapter 20: Gastrointestinal Tract 436

♦ Describe the etiology, pathogenesis, pathology, microbiology, clinical and microscopic features of peptic ulcer disease (PA24.2)	Written/Viva voce
♦ Describe and identify the microscopic features of peptic ulcer (PA24.3)	Written/Viva voce
♦ Describe the etiology, pathogenesis and pathologic features of carcinoma of the stomach (PA24.4)	Written/Viva voce
♦ Describe the etiology, pathogenesis, pathologic and distinguishing features of inflammatory bowel disease (PA24.6)	Written/Viva voce
♦ Describe the etiology, pathogenesis, pathology and distinguishing features of carcinoma of the colon (PA24.7)	Written/Viva voce
♦ Describe the etiology, pathogenesis and pathologic features of tuberculosis of the intestine (PA24.5)	Written/Viva voce

Chapter 21: Liver, Biliary Tract and Exocrine Pancreas 480

♦ Describe bilirubin metabolism. Enumerate the etiology and pathogenesis of jaundice. Distinguish between direct and indirect hyperbilirubinaemia (PA25.1)	Written/Viva voce
♦ Describe the pathophysiology and pathologic changes seen in hepatic failure and their clinical manifestations, complications and consequences (PA25.2)	Written/Viva voce
♦ Describe the etiology and pathogenesis of viral and toxic hepatitis: distinguish the causes of hepatitis based on the clinical and laboratory features. Describe the pathology, complications and consequences of hepatitis (PA25.3)	Written/Viva voce
♦ Describe the pathophysiology, pathology and progression of alcoholic liver disease including cirrhosis (PA25.4)	Written/Viva voce
♦ Describe the etiology, pathogenesis and complications of portal hypertension (PA25.5)	Written/Viva voce
♦ Describe and interpret the abnormalities in a panel containing liver function tests (PA23.3)	Practical/Skill

| Competencies (Outcomes) | Core (Must know) | Non-core (Desirable to know) |
| Assessment Methods | Written/Viva voce | Practical/Skill |

- Interpret liver function and viral hepatitis serology panel. Distinguish obstructive from non-obstructive jaundice based on clinical features and liver function tests (PA25.6) — Practical/Skill
- Describe the etiology, pathogenesis, manifestations, laboratory and morphologic features, complications and metastases of pancreatic cancer (PA32.6) — Written/Viva voce

Chapter 22: Kidney and Lower Urinary Tract — 526

- Describe the normal histology of the kidney (PA28.1) — Written/Viva voce
- Define, classify and distinguish the clinical syndromes; describe the etiology, pathogenesis, pathology, morphology, clinical and laboratory and urinary findings, complications of renal failure (PA28.2) — Written/Viva voce
- Define and describe the etiology, precipitating factors, pathogenesis, pathology, laboratory and urinary findings, progression and complications of acute renal failure (PA28.3) — Written/Viva voce
- Define and describe the etiology, precipitating factors, pathogenesis, pathology, laboratory and urinary findings, progression and complications of chronic renal failure (PA28.4) — Written/Viva voce
- Define and classify glomerular diseases. Enumerate and describe the etiology, pathogenesis, mechanisms of glomerular injury, pathology, distinguishing features and clinical manifestations of glomerulonephritis (PA28.5) — Written/Viva voce
- Define and describe the etiology, pathogenesis, pathology, laboratory and urinary findings, progression and complications of IgA nephropathy (PA28.6) — Written/Viva voce
- Enumerate and describe the findings in glomerular manifestations of systemic disease (PA28.7) — Written/Viva voce
- Enumerate and classify diseases affecting the tubular interstitium (PA28.8) — Written/Viva voce
- Define and describe the etiology, pathogenesis, pathology, laboratory and urinary findings, progression and complications of acute tubular necrosis (PA28.9) — Written/Viva voce
- Describe the etiology, pathogenesis, pathology, laboratory findings, distinguishing features, progression and complications of acute and chronic pyelonephritis and reflux nephropathy (PA28.10) — Written/Viva voce
- Define, classify and describe the etiology, pathogenesis, pathology, laboratory and urinary findings, distinguishing features, progression and complications of vascular disease of the kidney (PA28.11) — Written/Viva voce
- Define, classify and describe the genetics, inheritance, etiology, pathogenesis, pathology, laboratory and urinary findings, distinguishing features, progression and complications of cystic disease of the kidney (PA28.12) — Written/Viva voce
- Define, classify and describe the etiology, pathogenesis, pathology, laboratory and urinary findings, distinguishing features, progression and complications of renal stone disease and obstructive uropathy (PA28.13) — Written/Viva voce
- Classify and describe the etiology, genetics, pathogenesis, pathology, presenting features, progression and spread of renal tumours (PA28.14) — Written/Viva voce
- Describe and interpret the abnormalities in a panel containing renal function tests (PA23.3) — Practical/Skill
- Describe the etiology, genetics, pathogenesis, pathology, presenting features and progression of thrombotic angiopathies (PA28.15) — Written/Viva voce
- Describe the etiology, genetics, pathogenesis, pathology, presenting features and progression of urothelial tumours PA28.16) — Written/Viva voce

Competencies (Outcomes) — Core (Must know) — Non-core (Desirable to know)
Assessment Methods — Written/Viva voce — Practical/Skill

Chapter 23: Male Genital System — 570

♦ Classify testicular tumours and describe the pathogenesis, pathology, presenting and distinguishing features, diagnostic tests, progression and spread of testicular tumours (PA29.1)	Written/Viva voce
♦ Describe the pathogenesis, pathology, presenting and distinguishing features, diagnostic tests, progression and spread of carcinoma of the penis (PA29.2)	Written/Viva voce
♦ Describe the pathogenesis, pathology, hormonal dependency, presenting and distinguishing features, urologic findings and diagnostic tests of benign prostatic hyperplasia (PA29.3)	Written/Viva voce
♦ Describe the pathogenesis, pathology, hormonal dependency, presenting and distinguishing features, diagnostic tests, progression and spread of carcinoma of the prostate (PA29.4)	Written/Viva voce
♦ Describe the etiology, pathogenesis, pathology and progression of prostatitis (PA29.5)	Written/Viva voce

Chapter 24: Female Genital Tract — 588

♦ Describe the epidemiology, pathogenesis, etiology, pathology, screening, diagnosis and progression of carcinoma of the cervix (PA30.1)	Written/Viva voce
♦ Describe the pathogenesis, etiology, pathology, diagnosis and progression and spread of carcinoma of the endometrium (PA30.2)	Written/Viva voce
♦ Describe the pathogenesis, etiology, pathology, diagnosis and progression of the leiomyoma and leiomyosarcoma (PA30.3)	Written/Viva voce
♦ Classify and describe the etiology, pathogenesis, pathology, clinical course, spread and complications of ovarian tumours (PA30.4)	Written/Viva voce
♦ Describe the etiology, pathogenesis, pathology, clinical course, spread and complications of gestational trophoblastic neoplasms (PA30.5)	Written/Viva voce
♦ Describe the etiology and morphologic features of cervicitis (PA30.6)	Written/Viva voce
♦ Describe the etiology, hormonal dependence, clinical features and morphology of endometriosis (PA30.7)	Written/Viva voce
♦ Describe the etiology and morphologic features of adenomyosis (PA30.8)	Written/Viva voce
♦ Describe the etiology, hormonal dependence and morphology of endometrial hyperplasia (PA30.9)	Written/Viva voce

Chapter 25: Breast — 613

♦ Classify and describe the types, etiology, pathogenesis, pathology and hormonal dependency of benign breast disease (PA31.1)	Written/Viva voce
♦ Classify and describe the epidemiology, pathogenesis, classification, morphology, prognostic factors, hormonal dependency, staging and spread of carcinoma of the breast (PA31.2)	Written/Viva voce
♦ Enumerate and describe the etiology, hormonal dependency and pathogenesis of gynaecomastia (PA31.4)	Written/Viva voce
♦ Describe and identify the morphologic and microscopic features of carcinoma of the breast (PA31.3)	Practical/Skill

Competencies (Outcomes)	Core (Must know)	Non-core (Desirable to know)
Assessment Methods	Written/Viva voce	Practical/Skill

Chapter 26: Skin — 625

- Describe the risk factors, pathogenesis, pathology and natural history of squamous cell carcinoma of the skin (PA34.1) — Written/Viva voce
- Describe the risk factors, pathogenesis, pathology and natural history of basal cell carcinoma of the skin (PA34.2) — Written/Viva voce
- Describe the distinguishing features between a naevus and melanoma. Describe the etiology, pathogenesis, risk factors morphology clinical features and metastases of melanoma (PA34.3) — Written/Viva voce
- Identify, distinguish and describe common tumours of the skin (PA34.4) — Practical/Skill

Chapter 27: Endocrine System — 641

- Enumerate, classify and describe the etiology, pathogenesis, pathology and iodine dependency of thyroid swellings (PA32.1) — Written/Viva voce
- Describe the etiology, iodine dependency, pathogenesis, manifestations, laboratory and imaging features, and course of thyrotoxicosis (PA32.2) — Written/Viva voce
- Describe the etiology, pathogenesis, manifestations, laboratory and imaging features and course of thyrotoxicosis/hypothyroidism (PA32.3) — Written/Viva voce
- Classify and describe the epidemiology, etiology, pathogenesis, pathology, clinical and laboratory features, complications and progression of diabetes mellitus (PA32.4) — Written/Viva voce
- Describe and interpret the abnormalities in a panel containing thyroid function tests (PA23.3) — Practical/Skill
- Describe the etiology, genetics, pathogenesis, manifestations, laboratory and morphologic features of hyperparathyroidism (PA32.5) — Written/Viva voce
- Describe the etiology, pathogenesis, manifestations, laboratory and morphologic features and complications of adrenal insufficiency (PA32.7) — Written/Viva voce
- Describe the etiology, pathogenesis, manifestations, laboratory and morphologic features and complications of Cushing syndrome (PA32.8) — Written/Viva voce
- Describe the etiology, pathogenesis, manifestations, laboratory and morphologic features of adrenal neoplasms (PA32.9) — Written/Viva voce

Chapter 28: Musculoskeletal System — 675

- Classify and describe the etiology, pathogenesis, manifestations, radiologic and morphologic features, and complications of osteomyelitis (PA33.1) — Written/Viva voce
- Classify and describe the etiology, pathogenesis, manifestations, radiologic and morphologic features, complications and metastases of bone tumours (PA33.2) — Written/Viva voce
- Classify and describe the etiology, pathogenesis, manifestations, radiologic and morphologic features, and complications of Paget disease of the bone (PA33.4) — Written/Viva voce
- Classify and describe the etiology, immunology, pathogenesis, manifestations, radiologic and laboratory features, diagnostic criteria and complications of rheumatoid arthritis (PA33.5) — Written/Viva voce

Chapter 29: Soft Tissue Tumours — 695

- Classify and describe the etiology, pathogenesis, manifestations, radiologic and morphologic features, complications and metastases of soft tissue tumours (PA33.3) — Written/Viva voce

Competencies (Outcomes)	Core (Must know)	Non-core (Desirable to know)
Assessment Methods	Written/Viva voce	Practical/Skill

Chapter 30: Nervous System — 705

♦ Describe the etiology, types and pathogenesis, differentiating features, and CSF findings in meningitis (PA35.1)	Written/Viva voce
♦ Classify and describe the etiology, genetics, pathogenesis, pathology, presentation, sequelae and complications of CNS tumours (PA35.2)	Written/Viva voce
♦ Identify the etiology of meningitis based on given CSF parameters (PA35.3)	Practical/Skill

APPENDIX

Basic Diagnostic Cytopathology — 735

♦ Describe the diagnostic role of cytology and its application in clinical care (PA8.1)	Written/Viva voce
♦ Describe the basis of exfoliative cytology including the technique and stains used (PA8.2)	Written/Viva voce/ Practical/Skill
♦ Describe abnormal findings in body fluids in various disease states (PA23.2)	Written/Viva voce
♦ Observe a diagnostic cytology and its staining and interpret the specimen (PA8.3)	Practical/Skill

SECTION I: GENERAL PATHOLOGY

CHAPTER 1

Introduction to Pathology

Q1. What is pathology?
Definition Pathology is scientific study of changes in the structure and function of body in disease. This is derived from two Greek words—*pathos* meaning suffering and *logos* meaning study. For medical students, study of pathology forms a vital bridge between preclinical studies and clinical medicine.

Q2. Define the common terms used in the study of diseases.
- *Patient* is the person affected by disease.
- *Lesions* (from Latin word for injury) are the characteristic changes in tissues and cells produced by disease in a person or an experimental animal.
- *Morphology* of lesions (from Greek word for shape or form), i.e. p*athologic changes* which are studied by gross (macroscopic) or microscopic examination of tissues.
- *Etiology (*from Greek word for cause*)* is the science and study of causes of the disease.
- *Pathogenesis* (from Greek word *genos* denoting birth) of diseases relates to the mechanisms by which the lesions develop or are produced.
- *Clinical findings* include detectable changes caused in patient's body by various diseases.
- *Symptoms* (from Greek word for what is happening) are subjective feelings or sensations elicited by disease, or patient's perception of the abnormalities caused by the disease.
- *Diagnosis* (from the Greek word for discerning or distinguishing) is recognition of a disease by distinguishing it from the normal (healthy) state; also the determination of the nature of a specific disease, distinguishing it from all others.

Q3. List the most important scientific disciplines that have promoted the practice of pathology.
Anatomic pathology that began with autopsies performed first by Italian physician-scientists in the middle ages; it is still studied and practiced in modern clinical medicine by pathologists, radiologists and surgeons, but also by specialists in other branches of medicine.
Microscopy that made possible the study of cells and tissues that led to histopathology which still forms the basis of modern pathology. Microscopy was supplemented by advances in staining, immunofluorescence microscopy, immunohistochemistry, and application of molecular biology to microscopy specimens.
Microbiology resulting in the discovery of various bacterial, viral and other pathogens, supplemented by major advances of pharmacology and therapeutics.
Genetics and molecular biology which are entering all branches of medicine at a rapid rate transforming the practice of pathology.

Q4. What is the role of pathologist in modern medicine?

The role of pathologist in a modern multidisciplinary medical team is complex and is best understood by listing the branches of pathology which include the following:

I. **Morphological branches**

i. **Surgical pathology** It deals with tissue and organs removed from living body by biopsy or surgical resection. Most of these specimens are fixed in formalin, embedded in paraffin and sectioned on a microtome to prepare histologic slides. These slides are stained with haematoxylin and eosin and examined under a microscope. Some slides are stained with special stains and some by immunohistochemical techniques.

ii. **Autopsy pathology** It deals with the examination of dead bodies and the organs that have been removed from them. Autopsy pathology provides feedback to clinicians about the nature of the disease that the patients harboured, allows one to evaluate the effects of treatment and also helps in evaluating the correctness of various diagnoses and the outcome of various therapeutic procedures (e.g. surgery). It also helps determine the cause of death.

iii. **Forensic pathology** It includes the study of organs, tissues, body fluids and cells obtained for medicolegal purposes during autopsy, by medical diagnostic procedures or at the site of crime and accidents. Forensic pathology techniques are used to determine the mode and cause of death and prepare an objective death report for both medico-legal purposes and epidemiologic report for public health purposes.

iv. **Cytopathology** It is based on the study of cells obtained by non-invasive approaches (e.g. exfoliative vaginal cytology for the diagnosis of cervical carcinoma or bronchial exfoliative cytology through the bronchoscope) or minimally invasive fine needle aspiration cytology (FNAC).

v. **Haematology** It deals with the study of blood and blood-forming organs. The samples are studied using microscopy, flow cytometry, cytogenetics, and various techniques of molecular biology.

II. **Non-morphological branches**

i. **Clinical biochemistry** It dealt with the analysis and study of various body fluids, including blood, urine, cerebrospinal fluid, semen, abnormal effusion, etc.

ii. **Microbiology** It includes the study of microbes. It is divided into several branches including bacteriology, virology, mycology, parasitology, etc.

iii. **Immunology** It deals with the study of immune system and it its disorders.

iv. **Medical genetics and cytogenetics** It studies the genetic basis of diseases, chromosomal abnormalities and mutations of various normal genes and their transmission and inheritance in populations.

v. **Molecular pathology** This discipline plays an important role in the diagnosis of hereditary and neoplastic diseases. Molecular biology techniques are used in other branches of pathology, such as haematology, microbiology or medical genetics. Non-medical uses of molecular biology techniques are in epidemiologic, population genetic, anthropological, archeological and many other branches of science.

Q5. How did pathology evolve over ages?

The progress of pathology can be divided into several historical periods as follows:

I. **Prehistoric times to the medieval period** This period is dominated by medical practitioners who had no scientific training, had rudimentary understanding of disease processes, and only limited diagnostic and therapeutic skills. Yet, this was the dawn of medicine as a profession and it produced luminaries such as:

- *Hippocrates*, a Greek physician, considered to be the 'father of medicine'. He dissociated medicine from magic and established the basis of formal medical education.
- *Celsus*, a Roman medical practitioner and writer, who was the first to describe the cardinal signs of inflammation ('*rubor et tumor, cum calore et dolore*').
- *Galen*, a Roman physician and medical author, whose books were used as a medical textbook all over Europe for more than a thousand year. He was the first to describe the crab-like growth of cancer.

II. **Period of human anatomy, beginning of histology and gross pathology** This period lasted from the Medieval times to the second half of 19th century.

- This period produced the first great anatomists such as *Vesalius*, who produced the first scientific atlas of the human body.
- The microscope, invented by van *Leeuwenhoek*, was applied to the study of human tissues by *Malpighi*, known as the father of histology.
- *Morgagni* performed more than 600 autopsies and wrote the first scientific book of anatomic pathology.
- Many other famous physicians, whose names are still known by the diseases they described lived during those days such as *Bright* (kidney disease), *Addison* (adrenal), or *Hodgkin* (lymphoma).

III. **Era of technology development and cellular pathology** This era extends from the mid-19th century to the first part of 20th century. Too many luminaries lived and worked during this period; thus just to mention a few:
- *Virchow*, who introduced the use of the microscope in the study of diseases and is the father of cellular pathology
- *Pasteur* the father of modern microbiology
- *Ehrlich* the father of immunology and chemical pathology
- *Koch* the discoverer of *Mycobacterium tuberculosis*
- *Landsteiner* whose discoveries made possible blood transfusion.

IV. **Era of modern pathology that we live in** This era is characterised by exponential growth of biomedical sciences and clinical medicine and the development of technology that has influenced all aspects of human life, and irrevocably changed the practice of pathology.

Chapter 1e Supplement: Online Content

Digital content of this chapter available with this book is meant for enhanced learning and self-assessment. In addition, it contains 07 Multiple Choice Questions (MCQs), which are followed by their answers along with explanatory notes of correct and incorrect answers.

CHAPTER 2

Molecular Cell Biology in Health and Ageing

Q1. Why are cells important for understanding pathology?

Cells are basic units of life and their integrity is essential for the maintenance of life and its propagation. Rudolf Virchow, the founder of modern pathology, first gave the concept that every cells is derived from another cells (in Latin 'omnis cellula ex cellula'), thus establishing the basis of cellular pathology.

Q2. How do cells form tissues?

Cells are integrated self-contained units which can function on their own like primitive single cell organisms protozoa. However, in the human organism, most cells are arranged into anatomic and functional units called tissues. To function within tissue, cells must integrate with other cells into organisational structures in which they maintain a functional and structural equilibrium with their environment, called **homeostasis**.

This homeostasis depends on the maintenance of the following key features:
- Cell's integrity
- Cellular internal milieu including intracellular fluid, hyaloplasm with organelles and the nucleus
- Network arrangement with other cells in the same tissue
- Extracellular fluid composition
- Structural and functional integrity of the extracellular matrix

Q3. What are the main vital components of the cell?

These are as under **(Fig. 2.1)**:
I. **Nucleus** Most cells cannot survive without a nucleus. The only exceptions are red blood cells and platelets, which do not have a nucleus, but still survive and function inside the body. Platelets and RBC cannot replicate.
II. **Cytoplasm with its organelles**
III. **Cell membrane** Rupture or loss of cell membrane is not compatible with life of the irreversibly damaged cell.

Q4. How is chromatin distributed in the nucleus?

In interphase nuclei, DNA is arranged as chromatin which is found in two forms:
Euchromatin Finely dispersed and lightly stained, corresponding to the metabolically active part of the genome.
Heterochromatin Condensed dark blue staining with haematoxylin, corresponding to the metabolically inert part of the genome.

Q5. What are the main components of human genome?

i. Human genetic material forming the genome is stored in the *deoxyribonucleic acid (DNA),* stored in double-helix chains wound spirally around an axis **(Fig. 2.2)**.

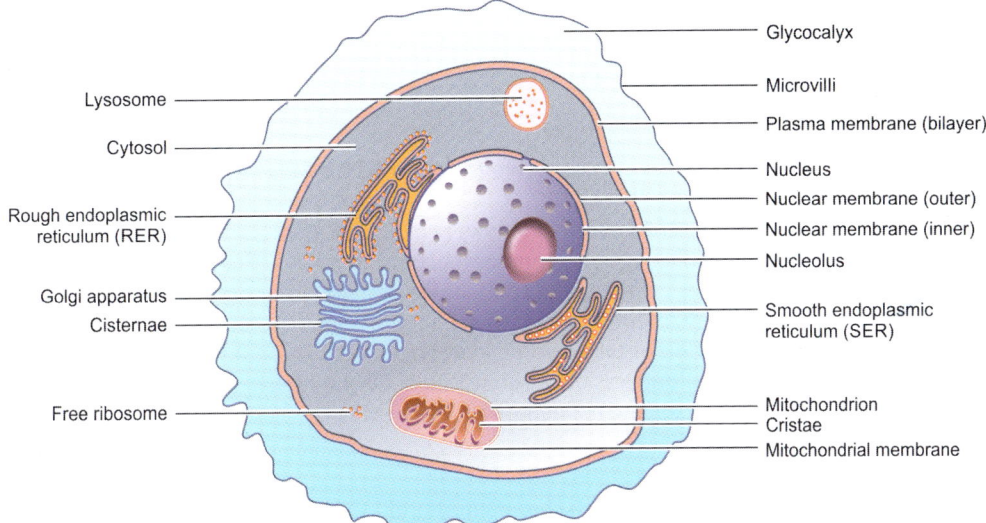

FIGURE 2.1: Basic structure of a typical human cell and its subcellular constituents dispersed in cytosol. It shows plasma membrane, membrane-enclosed nucleus and organelles, and cytoskeleton along with its protrusions as cilia.

ii. DNA is composed of 4 *nucleotide bases*: Two purines (adenine and guanine) and two pyrimidines (cytosine and guanine), mostly located in the nucleus and in very small amounts (1%) in the mitochondria (mtDNA).
iii. Functionally DNA is divided into *introns and exons*, i.e. coding and non-coding regions, including promoters, enhancers and other non-coding elements.
iv. About 50% of human genome consists of *transposones* ('jumping genes'), which played an important role in human evolution but are currently not fully understood.

Q6. What are chromosomes?

i. These are distinct nuclear structures composed of DNA and nuclear proteins *seen only during the mitosis*.
ii. Each species has a unique number of chromosomes (*euploid* for each species), which are all in identical duplicates except for the X and the Y chromosome.

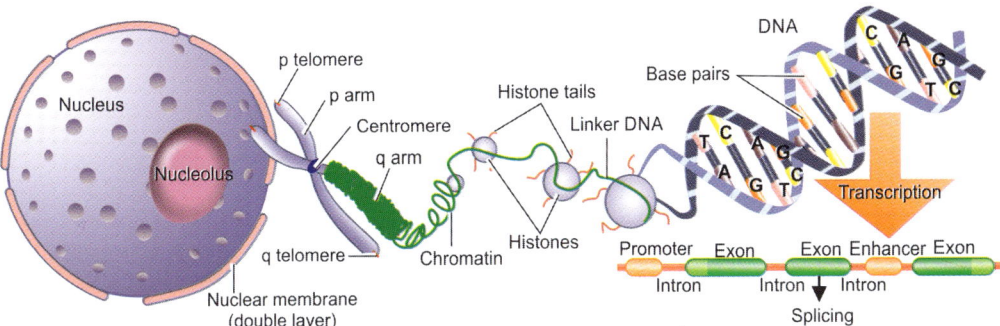

FIGURE 2.2: Structure and organisation of nuclear DNA from light microscopic view to molecular and biochemical level. The nucleus is enveloped by nuclear membrane and contains chromatin material having dispersed chromosomes. Each chromosome has X-shaped appearance and has paired chromatids (having short p arms and long q arms) connected in the middle at the centromere (which forms the locus for formation of kinetochores during metaphase) and has telomeres at the tips. Chromatin fibres have a central octameric histone core around which nucleosomes containing DNA are spirally wound and are connected via linker DNA forming a string. Nucleotide base pairs are located on the DNA as purines (A-G) and pyrimidines C-T). DNA has promoter region (which is non-coding region that initiates gene transcription) and enhancer region (which regulates gene expression) and other non-coding elements. During RNA splicing, introns (protein non-coding regions) are removed while exons (protein coding regions) are joined together to form a continuous coding chain and translated into protein while untranslated regions (UTR) having 3- and 5-ends are left behind.

iii. Normal cells that have duplicates of each chromosome are thus considered to be *diploid*.
iv. Diploid normal human cells have 46 chromosomes. Ovum and spermatozoa have only one set of 23 chromosomes and are termed *haploid*.

Q7. What are the principal parts of chromosomes?

i. **Chromatids** are filamentous parts of each chromosome forming its arms (*see* **Fig. 2.2**):
- Short arm (called *p arm* for petite)
- Long arm (*q arm,* named after the letter that follows p in the alphabet)

ii. **Centromere** is the point of junctions of chromosomal arms. Functions of centromere include:
- Subdivisions of chromosomes into long and short arms and maintenance of their structure.
- Provide the attachment point for the insertion of the mitotic spindle filaments during mitosis.

iii. **Telomere** is terminal part or 'tip' of each chromosome composed of repetitive nucleotide sequence allowing mitotic chromosomal duplication without loss of DNA material. **Telomerase** is a reverse transcriptase involved in the repair and maintenance of telomeres.

Q8. What are nucleosomes?

- Nucleosomes are the **basic units** of each chromatin strand.
- Composed of DNA wrapped around a positively-charged **histone octamer**.
- Nucleosomes are joined together with **linker DNA**.

Q9. What are the main functions of non-coding DNA?

Non-coding DNA accounts for 98% of the genome. Its main functions are as follows:
i. Transcription of messenger RNA (mRNA).
ii. Transcription of short and long non-coding RNAs (microRNA and lncRNAs).
iii. Provide binding of promoter and enhancer transcription factors.
iv. Provide location of transposons.
v. Form regions for genetic variations (polymorphism) of single nucleotides or their copy number.

Q10. How are genes modified epigenetically?

Epigenetic control of gene function means external activation or silencing of genes, involving their transcription and translation, without altering their DNA sequence. This process involves:
i. DNA methylation
ii. Histone modification that includes a) acetylation, b) methylation, c) phosphorylation, and d) ubiquitination
iii. Chromatin remodeling

Q11. What are the main features of plasma membranes?

i. Semipermeable membrane forming the external surface of the cell.
ii. Bilayered polarised complex structure, having an outer (exoplasmic) and inner (cytosolic) leaflet.
iii. Composed of proteins and lipids and, some of which may be glycosylated.
iv. Lipids are responsible for the flexibility of the membranes.
v. Proteins maintain the chemical environment of the cells and regulate the transport of molecules across the membranes.

Q12. What are the main lipids comprising the plasma membranes?

The principal lipids of the plasma membrane are as follows (**Fig. 2.3**):

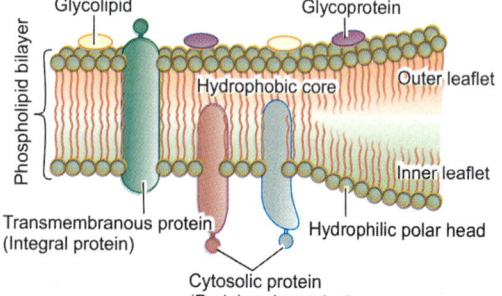

FIGURE 2.3: Schematic diagram of typical organisation of biomembrane and its constituents.

I. **Phospholipids** form the core of an outer and an inner leaflet each of which has a *hydrophilic outside* surface and a *hydrophobic inside* core.
- The best-known phospholipids of the plasma membrane are sphingomyelin, sphingosine, phosphocholine and ceramide.
- Positively charged phospholipids (e.g. sphyngomyelin) are found in the outer layer.
- Negatively charged and neutral phospholipids (e.g. phosphatidylinositol) are found in the inner layer.
- Phospholipids of the outer leaflet are prone to hydrolysis by phospholipases, which however, do not affect the phospholipids of the inner leaflet.

II. **Cholesterol** molecules are inserted between phospholipids, preventing tight packing of phospholipid molecules and, thus allowing bilayer fluidity.

III. **Glycolipids** are located in the exoplasmic outer leaflet where their carbohydrate chains form part of receptors and sensors, enabling cells to communicate with their environment.

Q13. What are the main functions of proteins in the cell membranes?

Proteins of the cell membranes can be classified as:
- **Integral proteins** which are transmembranous, extending through both phospholipid layers.
- **Peripheral membrane proteins**, located on the inner cytosolic membrane leaflet and primarily associated with specific protein-protein interactions.

Plasma membrane proteins have many functions. Most importantly they serve as:
i. Structural support proteins
ii. Cell membrane receptors facilitating the transfer of external signals
iii. Transport proteins and components of ionic channels
iv. Contact and adhesion molecules and sensors facilitating intercellular contacts and communications

Q14. What are the main functions of plasma membrane?

i. Protective role preserving the cell integrity and defending it against external injury
ii. Transport of nutrients into the cell and export of waste products of metabolism
iii. Preservation of the ionic composition of cytosol, its pH and osmotic pressure
iv. Mechanical anchoring surface to cytoskeletal fibres and thus maintaining cell shape

Membrane functions are carried out by three mechanisms **(Fig. 2.4)**:
- Passive diffusion of small and hydrophobic molecules
- Carrier-mediated by channel or carrier proteins
- Pinocytosis and receptor mediated transport (e.g. using clathrin and caveolin proteins)

Q15. What are the main functions of the cytoskeleton?

i. To maintain shape and provide mechanical support to the cell
ii. Intracytoplasmic structure and interrelationship of various organelles
iii. Overall mobility of the entire cell or its parts (e.g. chromosome during mitosis)
iv. Transmission of intercellular communication signals
v. Formation and function of specialised cell parts such as cilia and flagella

Q16. What are the most important cytoskeletal protein fibres?

Cytoskeleton is composed of filaments that are classified according to their diameter into three groups: microtubules, microfilaments, and intermediate filaments **(Fig. 2.5)**:

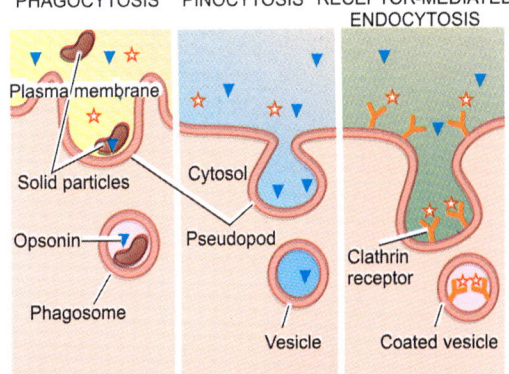

FIGURE 2.4: Three types of transport of material across the plasma membrane: phagocytosis (cell-eating of solid particulate material such as microbes), pinocytosis (cell-drinking) and receptor-mediated endocytosis (mediated by clathrin receptor).

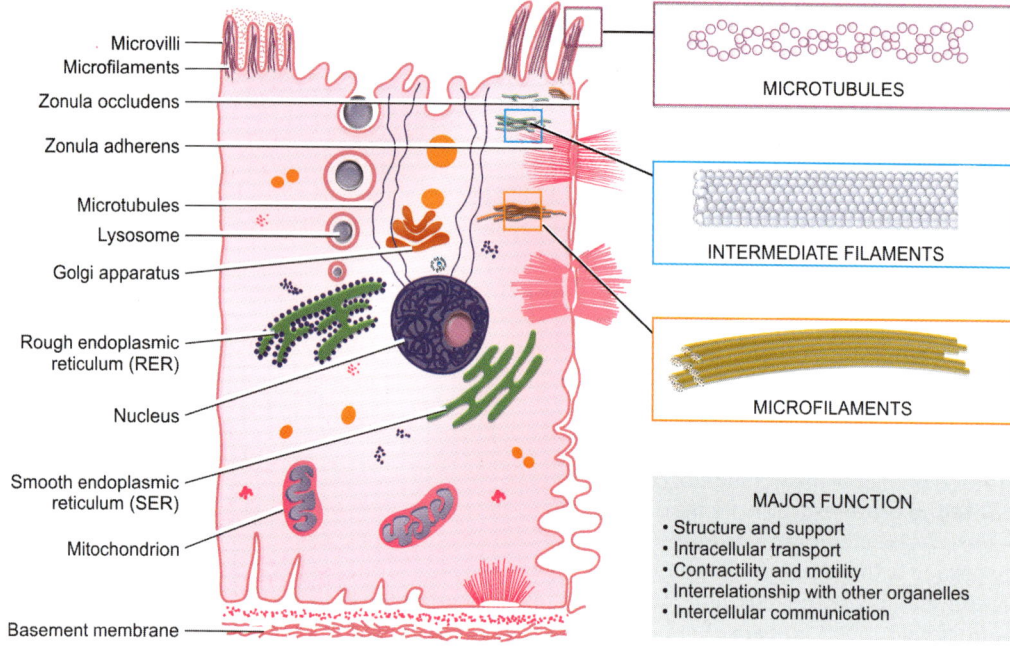

FIGURE 2.5: Organisation of cytoskeleton in the cell.

I. **Microtubules**
i. Hollow tubular fibrils, 25 nm in diameter.
ii. Composed of α-*tubulin* and β-*tubulin* (in all cells).
iii. Also contain two ATP powered motor proteins *kinesins* and *dyneins,* which pull cellular organelles toward cell membrane or the nucleus, respectively. Dyneins are also important for the movement of cilia in bronchi and the tail of the spermatozoa.
iv. Microtubules form the *mitotic spindle* and enable the *movement* of neutrophils as well as *phagocytosis* of bacteria.

II. **Microfilaments**
i. Measure 5–9 nm in diameter.
ii. Composed of *globular actin (G-actin)* and *filamentous actin (F-actin)* (in all cells).
iii. Intermediate filaments facilitate the intracytoplasmic movement of organelles.
iv. Provide structural support to cytoplasm.
v. G-actin is the most abundant cytosolic protein.

III. **Intermediate filaments**
i. 10 nm in diameter (i.e. intermediate between microfilaments and microtubules).
ii. Provide structural support and keep maintaining the shape of cells.
iii. *Biochemically heterogeneous,* depending on the cell type:
a. Cytokeratins: Epithelial cells
b. Desmin: Muscle cells
c. Vimentin: Mesenchymal cells
d. Glial fibrillary protein (GFAP): Glial cells
e. Neurofilament: Nerve cells
f. Lamins: Present in the nuclei of all cells

Q17. Briefly discuss the structure and function of mitochondria.

i. Bounded externally by *double layered membrane* that extends internally forming *cristae* **(Fig. 2.6)**.
ii. Unique organelle that may *divide and multiply* independent of cell division.
iii. Primary generator of *energy-rich ATP through oxidative phosphorylation.*
iv. Mitochnodria contain of signaling molecules and enzymes that are *important for apoptosis.*

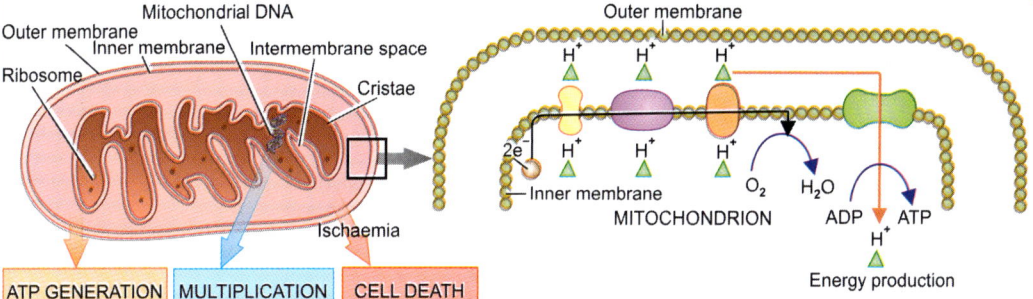

FIGURE 2.6: Mitochondrial morphology and basic pathway of energy generation.

v. *Mitochondrial DNA* (mDNA) accounts for 1% of the total DNA which is responsible for the mitochondrial *maternal inheritance* of a small number of genes and disease:
- mtDNA is circular, double-stranded, containing 100–1,000 copies per cell, forming 37 genes.
- mtDNA is polycistronic, i.e. forms mRNA that codes for many proteins.

Q18. Tabulate the contrasting features of nuclear and mitochondrial DNA.

Although most of the DNA is located in the nucleus of eukaryotic cells or nDNA (except in nerve and red cells), mitochondria contain a small amount of DNA in the mitochondrial matrix (about 1% of total DNA of a cell) called mtDNA which is increased in mitochondrial diseases. **Table 2.1** summarises the distinguishing features of nDNA and mtDNA.

TABLE 2.1 Contrasting features of nuclear DNA and mitochondrial DNA.

FEATURE	NUCLEAR DNA	MITOCHONDRIAL DNA
1. Location	Nucleus	Mitochondria
2. Membrane	Present in nucleus	Absent in mitochondria
3. Structure	Double-stranded, linear	Double-stranded, circular
4. Number of copies	Two copies per cell	100–1,000 copies per cell
5. Genome size	23 pairs ~20500 genes, ~3 billion base pairs	One chromosome 37 genes, ~16,000 base pairs
6. Inheritance	Equally from both parents; diseases may be inherited from both parents	Inherited from mother; diseases inherited maternally
7. Translation pattern	Follows universal codon pattern	Does not follow universal codon pattern
8. Transcription pattern	Monocistronic (i.e. codes for single protein)	Polycistronic (i.e. codes for many proteins)

Q19. What are the functions of rough endoplasmic reticulum (RER) and Golgi apparatus?

i. **RER** is composed of membrane-bound *cisterns* studded with ribosomes on their external surface.
ii. RER is the place where the *proteins for export are synthesised* by translation of ribosomal RNA.
iii. Synthesised proteins are folded and transferred into the **Golgi apparatus** where they are *glycosylated or phosphorylated* and then secreted outside of the cells **(Fig. 2.7)**.
iv. Golgi apparatus *transports* the synthesised proteins for export from the cell, or packages them into secretory vesicles, storage granules, or extrudes them into lysosomes for degradation.
v. Proteins that are *misfolded* in the cisterns of RER cannot be secreted and are transferred to **ubiquitin-proteasome system** for degradation and may be retained in the cytoplasm for long periods of time.
vi. Examples of such proteins for export are: albumin or α1-antitrypsin in liver cells, immunoglobulins in plasma cells, insulin in islet cells of pancreas.
NOTE: *Free ribosomes* in the cytoplasm are the site of synthesis of proteins for internal needs of the cells, e.g. cell growth, movement and replication.

Q20. What are the principal functions of the smooth endoplasmic reticulum (SER)?

i. SER is composed of *smooth tubules and vesicles* that do not have ribosome on their surface.
ii. Most prominent in liver cells, steroid hormone synthesising cells and skeletal muscle.

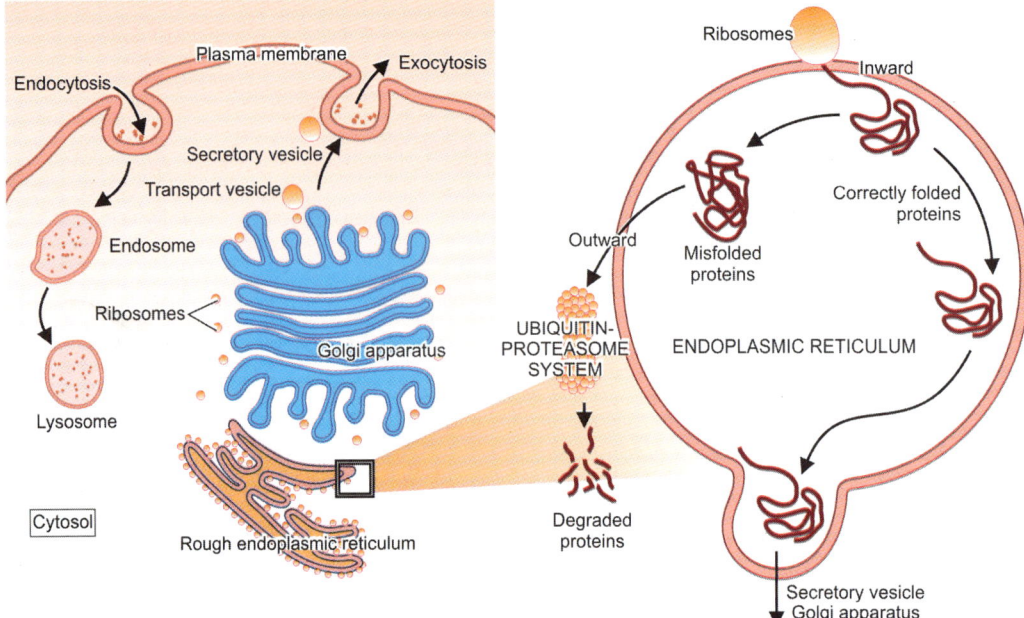

FIGURE 2.7: Composite intracellular endomembrane system of organelles comprised by endoplasmic reticulum (SER, RER), attached and free ribosomes, Golgi apparatus, lysosomes, peroxisomes and ubiquitin-proteasome system. All these organelles or systems are interconnected through biomembranes and with plasma membrane for transport and processing of synthesised products.

iii. *Transports* material from RER to Golgi apparatus.
iv. *Synthesis* of membrane phospholipids and carbohydrates.
v. *Catabolism* and neutralisation/detoxification of hormones, drugs and alcohol (in liver).
vi. Enzymatic synthesis of *steroid hormones* (in adrenal and gonads).
vii. *Sarcoplasmic reticulum* (a form of SER) is essential for the contraction of heart and skeletal striated muscle cells.

Q21. What are lysosomes and what are their functions?

i. Lysosomes are digestive/lytic vesicle and sacs.
ii. Filled with *hydrolytic enzymes* active at acid pH such as nucleases, proteases, lipases, phosphatases, glycosidases.
iii. Lysosomal vesicles *form by budding* from the Golgi apparatus or the invaginations of the plasma membrane.
iv. Their **main functions** are as follows:
a. Receptor mediated *endocytosis* and fluid phase *pinocytosis* leading to the formation of endosomes.
b. *Heterophagy,* i.e. phagocytosis of foreign particulate material and bacteria, leading to the formation of heterophagosomes.
c. *Autophagy* by which the cell digests its own organelles following cell injury, starvation or during senescence, leading to the formation of autophagosome.
d. Material that cannot be digested in autophagosome and heterophagosomes is excreted from the cell by *exocytosis*.
e. Material that is not exocytosed remains in the cytoplasm in the form of *residual bodies* and granules of brown lipid rich pigment *lipofuscin*.

Q22. What is extracellular matrix? Enumerate its major functions.

Extracellular matrix (ECM) is the material produced by the resident cells and filling the extracellular spaces. It consists of **interstitial matrix** and **basement membranes**. Its main functions are as follows:

i. *Provide structural support* to tissue, assuring its stiffness and elasticity
ii. *Segregate tissues* one from another
iii. *Regulate growth and differentiation* of cells by growth factors
iv. Control and mediate the flow of *communications* between cells or ECM molecules
v. Essential for *wound healing* and fibrosis
vi. Regulates, facilitates or impedes *tumour cell growth, invasion and metastasis*
vii. *Basement membranes* selectively filter macromolecules

Q23. What are the distinguishing features of two forms of extracellular matrix?

Interstitial ECM and basement membrane have different architecture and composition; **Table 2.2** summarises their salient differences.

TABLE 2.2 Contrasting features of two types of extracellular matrix.

FEATURE	INTERSTITIAL MATRIX	BASEMENT MEMBRANE MATRIX
1. Location	Interstitial spaces between cells e.g. ➢ Between connective tissue cells ➢ Between parenchymal cells of organs	➢ Under the epithelium in epithelium-lined tissues ➢ Under endothelium in vessels ➢ Glomerular basement membrane
2. Synthesising cells	Secreted by resident mesenchymal cells e.g. fibroblasts	Combined secretion of mesenchymal and epithelial/endothelial cells
3. Main functions	➢ Structural support ➢ Elasticity ➢ Growth and differentiation of cells ➢ Wound healing	➢ Structural support ➢ Elasticity ➢ As barrier to filtration of molecules
4. Composition	➢ Fibrillar collagens (type I most abundant; others type II, III, V) in connective tissue ➢ Non-fibrillar collagen: type IX in cartilage ➢ Elastin, fibrillin aggregates ➢ Proteoglycans aggrecan and hyaluronan ➢ Adhesive glycoprotein fibronectin	➢ Fibrillar collagens not present ➢ Non-fibrillar collagens: type IV as constituent, type VII for adherence to epithelium/endothelium ➢ Elastin, fibrillin aggregates ➢ Proteoglycans aggrecan and hyaluronan ➢ Adhesive glycoprotein laminin

Q24. What is the composition of extracellular matrix (ECM)?

There are three groups of substances comprising ECM **(Fig. 2.8)**:
i. *Fibrous structural proteins*: Collagens, elastin and fibrillin
ii. *Gel-like fluid*: Composed predominantly of proteoglycans, which serve as glue and also can bind and retain water)
iii. *Adhesive glycoproteins and adhesion receptors*: Fibronectin, laminin

Q25. How are collagens classified?

Collagens are divided in two groups:
I. **Fibrillar collagens:** Type I, II, III and V
II. **Nonfibrillar collagens:** Type IV (i.e. basement membrane), VII, and IX, and those belonging to the FACIT family (Fibril-Associated Collagen with Interrupted Triple Helices—collagens IX, XII and XIV).

Q26. What are the most important forms of collagen?

i. There are some *30 distinct forms of collagen*, labeled by Roman numerals from I onwards.
ii. Synthesis of collagens depends on enzyme *lysyl oxidase* (also known as protein-lysine 6-oxidase), which further depends upon adequate supply of vitamin C. That is why children with vitamin C deficiency have abnormal development of skeleton and patients with vitamin C deficiency have poor wound healing.
iii. **Collagen type I** accounts for 90% of all collagen. It is the main component of connective tissue, tendons, and bones.
- It is found in most organs.
- It has a triple helix structure which impart it tensile strength.

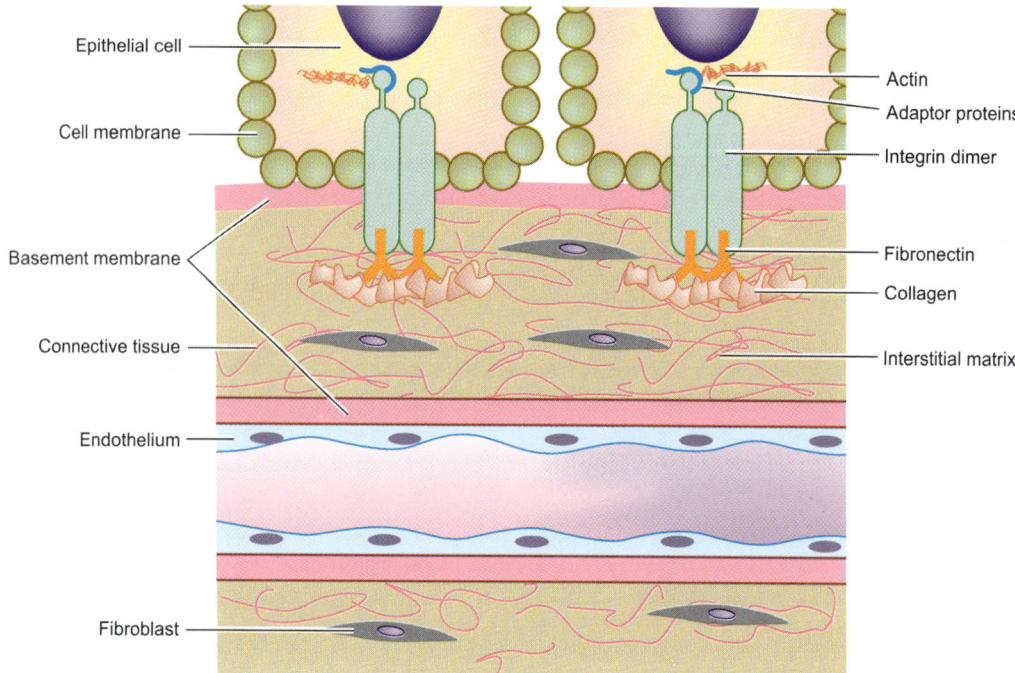

FIGURE 2.8: Schematic illustration depicting two types of extracellular matrix (interstitial and basement membrane) and its major components. The figure also includes interrelationship of ECM with cell adhesion molecules (integrin) and cytoskeleton.

iv. **Collagen type II**—forms the matrix of cartilage.
v. **Collagen type III**—abundant in hollow organs such as uterus and blood vessels is the first type of collagen laid down in healing of would.
vi. **Collagen type IV** is a nonfibrillar collagen found in basement membrane.

Q27. What are proteoglycans?

i. Proteoglycans form a family of hydrophilic ECM molecules that are composed of two components:
a. Carbohydrate polymer of disaccharide called *glycosaminoglycan (GAG)*
b. *Core proteins* linked to a hyaluronic acid polymer
ii. *Proteoglycans provide elasticity and* resistance to compressive forces.
iii. Various GAGs are found in specific tissues are:
a. Chondroitin sulphate—most abundant in cartilage joint, bone, cardiac valves
b. Keratan sulphate—cartilage, cornea
c. Hyaluronic acid—cartilage, synovial fluid, skin
d. Heparan sulphate
iv. Two important proteoglycans in the cartilage are:
a. *aggrecan* composed of chondroitin sulphate and keratan sulphate, and
b. *hyaluronan* composed of very long chains of hyaluronic acid and polymeric disaccharide representing the *largest soluble macromolecule* of proteoglycan variety.

Q28. What are the intercellular junctions that allow cells to communicate directly with one another?

I. **Occluding junction** (*zonula occludens*) Tight junctions just below the terminal margin of adjacent cells, typically in intestines. They are impermeable to large molecules and even ions.
II. **Adhering junction** (*zonula adherens*) Located just below the occluding zones and are permeable to small tracer molecules. They are in contact with cytoplasmic actin filaments.
III. **Desmosome** (*macula densa*) Adhesion plates between the adjacent cells, most prominently in squamous epithelia. Bundles of intermediate filaments (called *tonofilaments* in the epidermis) project from the cytosolic side of desmosomes into the cytoplasm.

V. **Gap junction** (*nexus*) Very narrow spaces between the lateral sides of cells in which the gap is filled with protein called *connexon*. Connexons form pores that allow the passage of small molecules from one cell to another, e.g. allowing rhythmic beating of the heart.

Q29. How do cells communicate one with another and with the extracellular matrix?

The cellular communications occur through three pathways as follows:
i. Adhesion receptors (ARs)
ii. Cell signaling
iii. Signal transduction and transcription
The cascade of intracellular events initiated by the signal protein acing on the plasma membrane receptor, ion channel or G-protein receptor is shown in **Figure 2.9**.

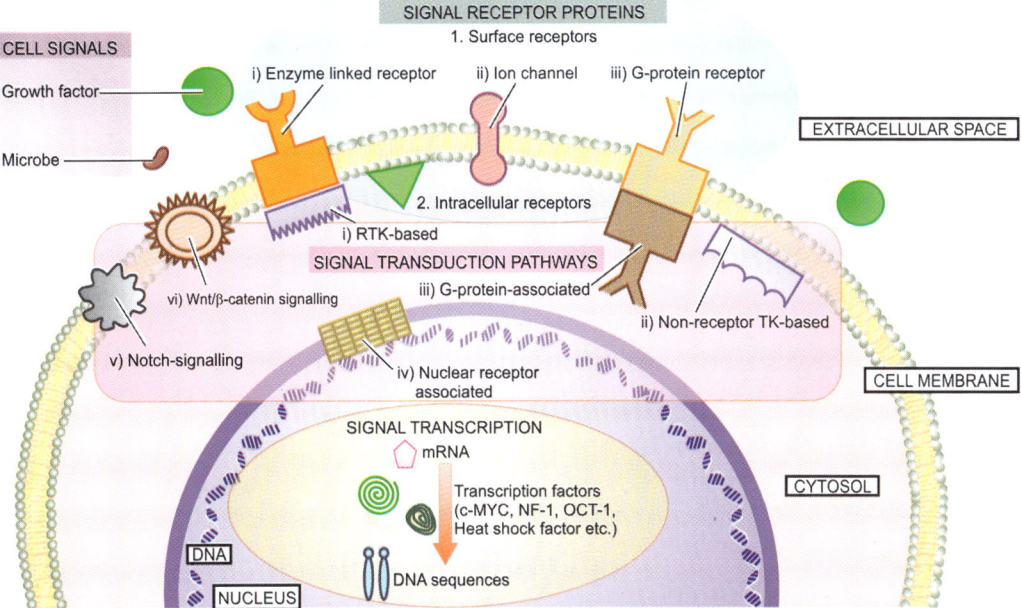

FIGURE 2.9: Schematic diagram showing molecular events how a cell signaling begins and the cell responds by a cascade of intracellular events, leading to transcription in the genome, thus altering the expression of existing genes (upstream or downstream), and controlling major cell functions (such as proliferation, differentiation, survival and apoptosis).
(RTK, receptor tyrosine kinase; TK, tyrosine kinase)

Q30. How do adhesion receptors function?

Adhesion receptors, also known as cell adhesion molecules (CAMs), hold cells together and also keep them tethered to extracellular matrix allowing transmembrane signaling. Thus, they act as glue and molecular sensors.

Q31. What are the basic features that all adhesion receptors have in common?

All adhesion receptors have the following common features:
i. They are integrated membrane molecules.
ii. All ARs have three regions: an extracellular, a transmembranous, and a cytosolic region.
iii. All ARs connect with cytoskeletal filaments directly, or through an adaptor protein in cytosolic portion.

Q32. How are adhesion receptors classified?

Based on their structure, ARs are subdivided into **four superfamilies** as under:
i. **Integrins** They bind the cells to ECM, most specifically basal lamina.

ii. **Cadherins** These calcium-dependent ARs keep specific cells together. Several cadherin types include: E-cadherin (epithelial), N-cadherin (neural), M-cadherin (muscle), and P-cadherin (placenta).
iii. **Selectins** Also called lectin, they bind to glycoproteins and glycolipids on cell surface. Three types of selectin are: P-selectin (platelet), E-selectin (endothelial cells), and L-selectin (leucocytes).
iv. **Immunoglobulin-like superfamily** These are expressed on the surface of most human cells. They bind through other CAMs and cytokines and include ICAM (intercellular adhesion molecule, also known as CD54), VCAM (vascular cell adhesion molecule), NCAM (neural cell adhesion molecule), and CD44 that binds to hyaluronic acid mediating leucocytes-endothelial interaction.

Q33. How are external signals transduced and transcribed in the target cell?

Following the binding of the biochemical signal molecule to the surface receptors of the target cells, a sequence of events is set in motion as follows:
- Amplification of signaling message
- Production of multiple intracellular signals to every bound receptor
- Generation of active transcription factors
- Entry of transcription factors into the nucleus that will alter gene expression

I. **Transduction** may take several pathways but the most prominent are:
i. Kinase activity associated pathways
ii. G-protein molecule-associated pathway
iii. Nuclear receptor-associated pathway
iv. Other protein ligand-associated pathways, such as
a. Notch signaling pathway
b. WNT/-catenin signaling pathway
The pathways involved vary depending on many variables.
II. **Transcription** The final outcome is the activation of the transcription factors and their binding to the DNA and the transcription which will influence or alter the expression of specific gene.

Q34. What are the principal stages of the cell cycle?

The cell cycles has two main stages, each of which has further specific phases **(Fig. 2.10)**:
I. **Interphase:** G1, S and G2 phases.
II. **Mitosis:** Prophase, prometaphase, metaphase, anaphase and telophase.
After the mitosis is completed, the cell may reenter a new mitosis or remain in a resting G0 phase.

Q35. How is mitosis internally controlled?

Mitosis is controlled at **checkpoints** that evaluate and monitor the condition of the cells prior to the next major event in the cell cycle. Four main checkpoints are located at different points of the mitotic cycle as follows (see **Fig. 2.10**):
- G1-S checkpoints (listed below as I and II)

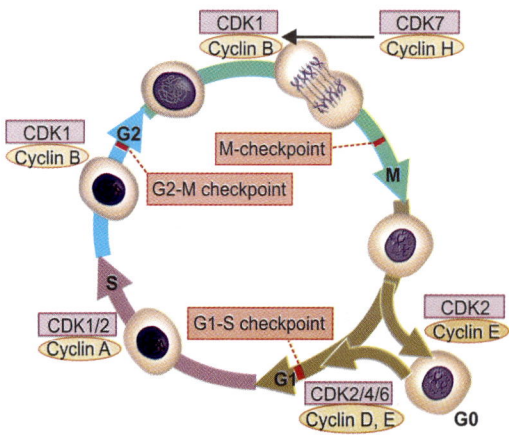

FIGURE 2.10: Cell cycle and its regulatory control. The figure shows major events in interphase (G1, S and G2 phases) and mitosis (prophase, prometaphase, metaphase, anaphase and telophase) with three main checkpoints (G1-S checkpoint, G2-M checkpoint, and mitotic spindle checkpoint). Regulatory control on the cell cycle is exerted by cyclins, CDKs and CDKIs by different molecules as shown.

- G2-M checkpoint (listed below as III)
- Mitotic spindle checkpoint (listed below as IV)

The distinct functions of these checkpoints are as follows:

I. **Cell size control** G1-S checkpoint is there to ensure that each daughter cell regulating the size of cell which needs to be commensurate with the amount of genetic and biosynthetic material available.

II. **DNA damage response** During the interphase, the cell repairs any DNA damage. The G1-S checkpoint is there to assure that any damage has been repaired. If it passes the restriction point in G1, it has committed itself to entering the mitosis.

III. **Appropriateness of DNA replication** At G2-M checkpoint, the cells with unrepaired DNA are not allowed to proceed for replicative polymerases and associated protein. This checkpoint prevents the entry of cells into mitosis if replication is not completed.

IV. **Mitotic spindle checkpoint** Also called M checkpoint since it is at the metaphase. It checks whether all chromatids are correctly attached to corresponding microtubule before the cell enters the anaphase.

Q36. What are the internal regulators of cell cycle checkpoints?

Cell cycle is internally regulated by activators (cyclins and cyclin-dependent kinases or CDK) and inhibitors (CDKI) **(Table 2.3)**.

It is important to note the following aspects of cell cycle regulation:
- Cyclins do not have enzymatic activity but act by activating CDKs.
- There are a family of more than 20 cyclins (A, B, C, etc.).
- CDKs form a family of a dozen phosphorylases (named CDK1, CDK2, etc.) whose activity is dependent on cyclins, to which they are paired in a specific manner. Some CDKs bind to more than one cyclin.
- CDK inhibitors (CDKI) may inhibit several CDKs but some of them act specifically on a single CDK. Two best known families of CDKI are: CDKN1 and CDKN2, each of which contains three inhibitors.

TABLE 2.3 Regulation of cell cycle phases and checkpoints.

CELL CYCLE PHASE	ASSOCIATED CYCLIN	CDK	CDK INHIBITORS
G1 Phase	E	CDK2	P16, p15, p18 (INK4 inhibitors)
G1-S checkpoint	D E	CDK-4, CDK6 CDK2	P21, p27, p57 (CDKN1 family)
S phase	A	CDK1, CDK2	P21, p27, p57 (CDKN1 family)
G2-M phase Mitotic spindle checkpoint	B	CDK1	P21, p27, p57 (CDKN1 family)

Q37. What are the most important negative regulatory proteins of the cell cycle?

- pRB-protein encoded by the retinoblastoma gene (**RB**). This protein inhibits protein synthesis necessary for the G1-S transition.
- p53-protein encoded by **TP53 gene**. This multifunctional protein acts in G1 phase halting the entry into the mitosis of cells with damaged DNA, triggering the repair. If the DNA damage cannot be repaired, the cell undergoes apoptosis.

Q38. What are the most important functions of extrinsic controls of the cell cycle?

The most important regulators are growth factors and growth factor receptors. They are multifactorial and thus have numerous functions including the following:

i. Recruiting cells from resting phase to cell cycle (i.e. G0 to G1)
ii. Preparation of cell organelles for mitosis
iii. Release the blocks for entry of the cell into mitosis
iv. Prevent apoptosis
v. Influence cell differentiation and movement
vi. Tissue repair and development of tumours

There are **many growth factors (GFs)** for example: epidermal growth factor (EGF), transforming growth factor (TGF- α and -β), platelet derived growth factor (PDGF), etc.
Growth factor receptors (GF-R) are transmembrane molecules on the cell surface, most of which have intrinsic tyrosine kinase activity, enabling phosphorylation.
The most important GFs and their corresponding receptors are listed in **Table 2.4**.

TABLE 2.4 Features and significance of major growth factors and their receptors.

GF AND GF-R	FEATURES	SIGNIFICANCE
1. EGF	➢ Produced by macrophages, epithelial cells	➢ Cell proliferation, differentiation and survival ➢ Tissue repair by epithelial regeneration and fibroblast proliferations
EGF-R	➢ EGFR1 (or ERB-B1) ➢ EGFR2 (or ERB-B2 or HER-2)	➢ Mutated in many cancers ➢ Overexpressed in breast cancer
2. TGF-α	➢ Produced by macrophages, epithelial cells	➢ Epithelial cell proliferation, differentiation and survival
EGF α -R	➢ Shares receptor for EGF	➢ Same as for EGF-R
3. TGF-β	➢ Produced by platelets, leucocytes, endothelial cells ➢ Secreted as precursor, activated by protease and metalloproteinases	➢ Blocks progress at G1 phase of cell cycle ➢ Stimulates production of collagen and other components of ECM ➢ Chemotactic for leucocytes ➢ Limits and terminates acute inflammation
TGFβ-R	➢ Exists in three isoforms: TGF-β1 (most common), TGFβ-2, TGF-β3 ➢ Type I and type II	➢ Has TK activity for cytoplasmic gene transcription by Smads (activation or inhibition)
4. PDGF	➢ Synthesised, released and stored in platelets ➢ Also produced by smooth muscle cells, macrophages, endothelial cells	➢ Growth of blood vessels ➢ Proliferation of mesenchymal cells ➢ Synthesis of ECM proteins
PDGFR-α and β	➢ PDGFR-α bind to PDGF homodimer and PDGFR-β to heterodimer	➢ has intrinsic TK activity
5. VEGF	➢ 5 members VEGF-A, VEGF-B, VEGF-C, VEGF-D and placental GF (PGF) ➢ Produced by mesenchymal cells	➢ VEGF-A is significant for angiogenesis (proliferation of endothelial cells from pre-existing ones) ➢ VEGF-B and PGF for embryonic vasculogenesis ➢ VEGF-C and D for lymphangiogenesis
VEGF-R	➢ Family of three: VEGFR-1, VEGFR-2 (most important) and VEGFR-3	➢ Tyrosine kinase activity
6. HGF (scatter factor)	➢ Secreted by mesenchymal cells	➢ Proliferation of various epithelial (including hepatocytes) and endothelial cells ➢ Cell migration
HGF-R	➢ Interacts with c-Met oncogene	➢ Has intrinsic TK activity ➢ Role in oncogenesis
7. FGF (a and b)	➢ Family of 23 cell signalling proteins ➢ Acidic (aFGF) and basic (bFGF) best characterised ➢ Secreted by macrophages, endothelial cells	➢ Role in granulation tissue formation ➢ Synthesis of ECM (especially heparan sulphate)
FGF-R	➢ Family of 4 members (FGFR-1, 2, 3, 4)	➢ Has intrinsic TK activity

(GF, growth factor; GF-R, growth factor-receptor; EGF, epidermal growth factor; EGF-R, EGF-receptor; TGF-α, transforming growth factor-α; TGF α-R, TGF α-receptor; TGF-β, transforming growth factor-β; TGFβ-R, TGFβ-receptor; PDGF, platelet-derived growth factor; PDGF-Rα and β, PDGF receptor α and β; HGF, hepatocyte growth factor; HGF-R, HGF-receptor; aFGF and bFGF, acidic and basic fibroblast growth factor; FGF-R, FGF receptor; VEGF, vascular endothelial growth factor; VEGF-R, VEGF-receptor).

Q39. What are the salient features of stem cells?

Definition Stem cells are primitive cells that have the capacity for self-renewal and also differentiation into other cell type.
Types Two types:
- *Embryonic stem cells* in embryos (harvested usually from umbilical cord blood)
- *Adult stem cells* (in adult organs)

Haematopoietic stem cells, bone marrow stromal cells and stem cells from umbilical cord blood have been the most widely used stem cells.

Q40. What are the main principles of stem cell therapy?

Three approaches have received most attention:
i. Direct injection of stem cells into the target tissue, or intravenously so that they could home in the desired location.
ii. Differentiation of stem cell in vitro followed by injection of differentiated cells into target sites.
iii. Stimulation of endogenous stem cells in situ by injecting differentiation inducing factors.

Q41. What are the main theories of ageing?

Changes at cellular and subcellular level linked with ageing are supported by the following theories **(Fig. 2.11)**:

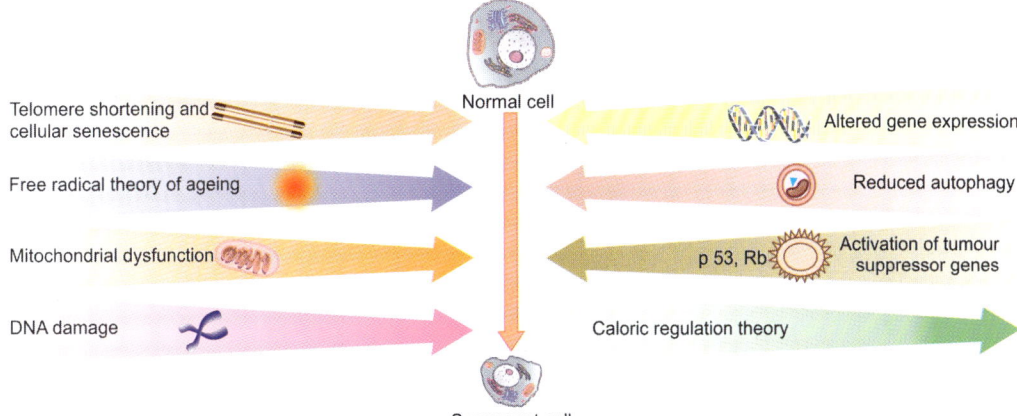

FIGURE 2.11: Schematic diagram shows various changes and mechanisms at cellular and subcellular level involved in ageing (shown in red) while factors associated with anti-ageing strategies are shown in green.

I. **Telomere shortening and cellular senescence** As the cells age, there is progressive shortening of telomeres accompanied by a loss of DNA base pairs during each mitosis. Body ages because it loses the capacity to renew lost cells. Somatic cells do not have telomerase (in contrast to germ cells which do have this repair enzyme) and, therefore, somatic cells age by telomerase shortening, which is irreversible.

II. **Free radical theory** This theory postulates that the body ages because of the accumulative damage caused by persistent oxidative stress. Antioxidants could theoretically retard the damage caused by free oxygen radicals.

III. **Mitochondrial dysfunction** With ageing, mitochondrial production of ATP diminishes and oxygen radical production will increase. Senescent cells contain fewer mitochondria and mitochondria show degenerative changes such as vacuolisation and megamitochondria.

IV. **DNA damage with defective DNA repair** Defective DNA repair is associated with premature ageing in Werner syndrome (*defective DNA helicase*), Bloom syndrome and ataxia telangiectasia (*defective genes encoding DNA repair enzymes*).

V. **Altered gene expression** Ageing is associated with reduced expression of many genes, reduced expression of microRNA, reduced methylation and histone acetylation. Supporting this theory are findings about *sirtuins,* a family of protein deacetylases, which promote longevity by inhibiting metabolic activity, reducing apoptosis stimulating protein folding, and reducing the harmful effects of oxygen radicals.

VI. **Reduced autophagy** With ageing, there is reduced removal of worn-out organelles, with accumulation of lipofuscin, tau proteins and β-amyloid.

VII. **Activation of tumour suppressor genes** For example, *Rb* and *Tp53* genes which promote apoptosis and senescence.

VIII. **Caloric regulation theory** This is based on the experimental data showing that in laboratory animals caloric restriction delays ageing. These effects are in part due to reduced release of hormones (growth hormone, insulin and insulin like growth factor 1).

Q42. What are the organ changes in ageing?

i. *Cardiovascular system:* Changes such as atherosclerosis, loss of elastic tissue in the wall of arteries with their dilatation, calcification of arterial walls, brown atrophy of the heart.
ii. *Nervous system*: Atrophy of gyri and dilatation of sulci and ventricles, Alzheimer disease, Parkinson disease.
iii. *Musculoskeletal system*: Degenerative joint disease, osteoporosis, loss of muscle mass and weakness of muscles.
iv. *Eyes*: Deterioration of vision, cataracts, macular degeneration.
v. *Hearing*: Loss of hearing, otosclerosis.
vi. *Immune system:* Reduced IgG response to antigenic stimulation, frequent and more severe infections.
vii. *Skin*: Laxity of skin, atrophy of epidermis.
viii. *Cancers*: Increased incidence; over 80% of cancers occur in the 50–80 years age group.

> **Chapter 2e Supplement: Online Content**
>
> *Digital content of this chapter available with this book is meant for enhanced learning and self-assessment. In addition, it contains 28 Multiple Choice Questions (MCQs), and 05 Clinicopathologic Vignettes; these are followed by their answers along with explanatory notes of correct and incorrect answers.*

CHAPTER 3

Cellular Adaptations and Cell Injury

CELL INJURY, RESPONSES AND ETIOLOGY

Q1. What is cell injury? What are the factors determining cellular responses?

Definition Cell injury is defined as the functional and morphological changes produced by stress due to the action of a variety of factors that alter the internal or external environment.

Cellular response and factors Cellular response to injury includes three forms of changes **(Fig. 3.1)**:

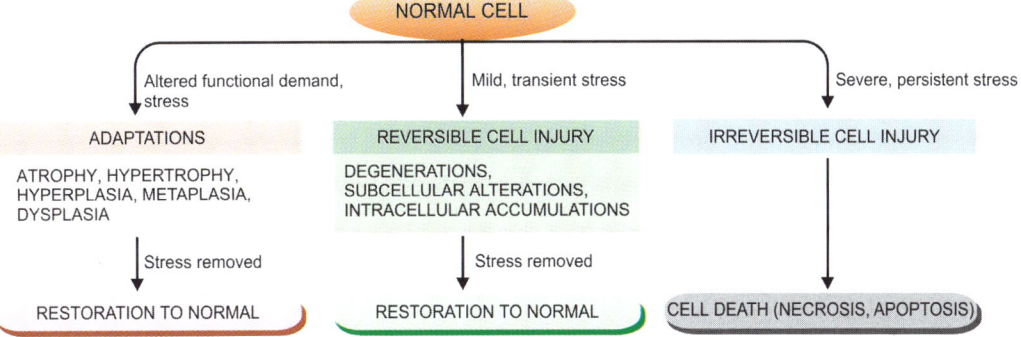

FIGURE 3.1: Cellular responses to cell injury.

i. *Cellular adaptations* in response to altered functional demand. The removal or cessation of the stress is followed by a reversal to the normal steady state.

ii. *Reversible cell injury* that follows typically a mild or moderate stress. It may be associated with *subcellular alterations* and *intracellular accumulations*.

iii. *Irreversible cell injury* which results in cell death related to the action of stress that is either of high intensity of long duration.

The cellular response depends on two sets of factors:
- *Host factors,* e.g. type of cells, nutritional status of the cell, etc.
- *External factors* pertaining to the injurious agent, i.e. its type, dose, duration.

Q2. What are the main causes (etiology) of cell injury?

Etiology (i.e. the science of the study of the causes) of diseases is based on two broad types of causes of cell injury: endogenous (genetic) and exogenous (acquired).

Acquired causes acting singly or in combination with one another, comprise the vast majority of human diseases. However, it should be noted that the body's response often depends on its genetic background, and thus exogenous and endogenous causes are always in a constant interaction.

For didactic purposes, we shall list here the most important acquired causes, whereas the genetic will be discussed in Chapter 10.

i. **Hypoxia** (deficiency of oxygen), the most common cause of cell injury in clinical medicine is most often related to *ischaemia* (inadequate blood supply). Cells need oxygen to generate energy and perform their essential function; without oxygen they will show signs of cell injury. Complete lack of oxygen is called *anoxia*. Some of the clinically important *causes of hypoxia* are:
- Thrombotic occlusion of an artery causing complete interruption of blood flow
- Hypoxaemia (subnormal oxygenation of RBCs, as in lung disease, or high altitude)
- Anaemia (deficiency of oxygen carrying RBCs)
- Carbon monoxide poisoning (due to binding of CO to haemoglobin which prevents binding of oxygen)
- Defective transport of RBCs in circulation due to heart-pump failure
- Increased demand for oxygen in tissues (exhaustion due to exercise, hyperthyroidism, high fever).

ii. **Physical agents**
- Mechanical impact (e.g. traffic accident)
- Bullet wound
- Thermal trauma, hot or cold
- Electricity
- Radiation
- Rapid change of atmospheric pressure

iii. **Chemicals and drugs**
- Chemical poisons (e.g. cyanide, arsenic, mercury)
- Strong acids and alkali
- Environmental pollutants
- Insecticides and pesticides
- Social agents such as alcohol and narcotic drugs
- Therapeutic drugs due to interaction with other drugs, or increased sensitivity of patient

iv. **Microbial agents** such as bacteria, viruses, fungi, protozoa, metazoa and other parasites.

v. **Immunologic causes** such as:
- Hypersensitivity reactions
- Allergies
- Autoimmune diseases

vi. **Nutritional derangements**

a. *Nutritional deficiencies* may pertain to total caloric intake of food or components of the food, e.g.:
- Starvations (lengthy deprivation of food)
- Marasmus and kwashiorkor (protein calorie deficiency)
- Vitamin deficiency
- Mineral deficiency (e.g. iron deficiency anaemia, iodine deficiency causing hypothyroidism)

b. *Nutritional excess* is a problem of affluent societies to be discussed later. Let us mention only that obesity is associated with an increased incidence of atherosclerosis, hypertension, steatohepatitis and diabetes, to mention a few.

vii. **Ageing** reduces capacity of cells to replicate and repair, and favours untimely cell death due to reduced compensatory defense mechanisms.

viii. **Psychogenic causes** include conditions such as anxiety, mental stress, overwork, frustration, psychiatric diseases such as schizophrenia, manic depressive disorder, etc.

ix. **Iatrogenic causes** related to physician's intervention, surgical operations and medical therapy, radiation therapy, errors of judgement and misdiagnosis.

x. **Idiopathic** ('of unknown causes'), are all those diseases for which we still do not know the causes.

■ CELLULAR ADAPTATIONS

Q3. What are the most important cellular adaptations? Briefly comment on their common features.

Definition Cellular adaptations are the adjustments which the cells make in response to stresses. These may be in response to physiologic needs (*physiologic adaptation*) or a response to non-lethal pathologic injury (*pathologic adaptation*).

Types The principal adaptations are: atrophy, hypertrophy, hyperplasia, metaplasia and dysplasia **(Fig. 3.2)**.

Etiology They may be related to:
- an *identifiable cause*; or
- of unknown etiology i.e. *idiopathic*.

Pathogenesis In principle, adaptations are *reversible,* and the cells return to the normal steady state after the withdrawal of the stimuli. *Important exceptions* to this rule are as follows:
- May appear irreversible because the reversal is slow and/or takes a long time (e.g. hyperplasia of the prostate in elderly men).
- Concomitant cell death (i.e. irreversible) may occur in an organ unable to regenerate (e.g. atrophy of the brain in Alzheimer disease).
- Progression to another form of adaptation; e.g. when metaplasia progresses to dysplasia and then to neoplasia (e.g. Barrett oesophagus).

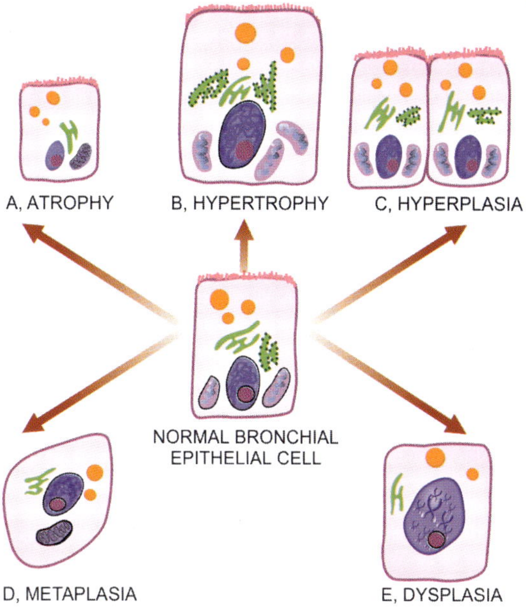

FIGURE 3.2: Adaptive disorders of growth.

Q4. What is atrophy?

Definition Reduction of the number and size of parenchymal cells of an organ or its part that were once normal. It needs to be differentiated from:
- *Hypoplasia,* i.e. a developmental disorder in which the organ remains small and never reaches its full size.
- *Aplasia,* i.e. failure of development of an organ which never develops beyond its foetal primordium, thus consisting of rudimentary remnants that persist instead of the organ.

Q5. What are the important forms of physiologic atrophy?

Most of these changes are age related:
i. Atrophy of lymphoid tissue with age
ii. Atrophy of thymus by the end of puberty
iii. Atrophy of ovary, uterus and vaginal epithelium after menopause
iv. Atrophy of testis in old age
v. Atrophy of brain in old age
vi. Senile osteoporosis and loss of muscle mass

Q6. What are the important forms of pathologic atrophy?

The *etiologic classification* of atrophy combined with clinical features recognises several distinct forms as follows:

i. **Starvation atrophy** due to nutritional caloric deficiency. First, it is marked by depletion of carbohydrates and fat stores, followed by protein catabolism.
Cachexia in cancer and severely ill patients is a subset of starvation atrophy marked by weight loss, general weakness, emaciation, anaemia and atrophy of many organs.

ii. **Ischaemic atrophy** Two best examples are:
a. Atrophy of the kidneys due to the atherosclerotic narrowing of the renal artery at its origin from the aorta.
b. Brain atrophy due to the atherosclerosis of cerebral arteries.

iii. **Disuse atrophy** Two best examples are:
a. Muscle atrophy in an extremity immobilised by plaster cast.
b. Atrophy of the jaw in an elderly edentulous person who does not masticate forcefully and thus, does not put pressure on the mandible bone.

iv. **Neuropathic atrophy** Skeletal muscles atrophy if they lose innervation through the motor neuron. Examples of such denervation atrophy are as follows:
a. Peripheral nerve transection
b. Spinal cord transection of the spinal motor pathways
c. Poliomyelitis, a viral disease that destroys the motor neurons in the anterior horn of the spinal cord
d. Amyotrophic lateral sclerosis which affect the upper and lower motor neurons.
v. **Endocrine atrophy** It occurs due to a lack of trophic hormones. Examples are:
a. Atrophy of thyroid, adrenals or gonads due to a lack of pituitary trophic hormones.
b. Atrophy of tissues that are hormone dependent, e.g. uterus atrophies after removal of the ovary or if the ovary stops secreting oestrogens after menopause.
c. Hypothyroidism affects the skin which atrophies and becomes oedematous (myxoedema).
vi. **Pressure atrophy** It is mostly due to compression by an expansile mass. Examples are:
a. Erosion of the spine bone due to compression of bone by a benign tumour of nerve roots.
b. Erosion of the skull by benign tumour of meninges (meningioma).
c. Erosion of sternum by an aneurysm of the ascending thoracic aorta.
vii. **Developmental disorders** Example of such an event is atrophy of the incompletely descended testis (cryptorchidism).
viii. **Idiopathic atrophy** Many forms of atrophy of old age are idiopathic, i.e. we still do not know their causes.

Q7. What are the pathologic features of atrophy?

Gross
i. *Reduced size of the organ:* The organs usually retain their normal shape but are much smaller in size than normal. Reduction in size is often accompanied by reduced function (e.g. weak muscles).
ii. *Brown appearance of parenchyma:* For example, brown atrophy of the heart and the testicle occurs due to the accumulation of lipofuscin ('brown pigment of ageing').
iii. *Diagnostic features:* Only a few organs show gross features that are indicative of atrophy.
a. *Brain atrophy* presents with narrowing of the gyri and widening of the sulci which are filled with cerebrospinal fluid (CSF). Lateral ventricles are dilated and contain increased amounts of CSF (*hydrocephalus ex vacuous*). Brain atrophy can be visualised by CT scan.
b. *Osteoporosis* is marked by thinning of trabeculae which can be seen by X-rays. Compression factures of spine are a common complication.

Microscopy
i. *Cells are smaller* and there may be a visible loss of cells and intercellular substance.
ii. *Autophagic vacuoles* and residual bodies filled with brown lipofuscin are increased in number.
iii. Atrophy and loss of cells may be *accompanied by interstitial fibrosis* or thickening and hyalinisation of basement membranes.

Molecular and ultrastructural features
i. *Reduced number* of certain organelles such as mitochondria, rough endoplasmic reticulum, as reflected in reduced basal metabolic rate, less energy production, and reduced protein synthesis.
ii. *Increased number* of autophagic vacuoles and lipofuscin granules, as well as ubiquitin-rich proteasomes, reflected in increased autophagocytosis and degradation of proteins.

Q8. What is hypertrophy? Briefly discuss its types, etiology and pathogenesis.

Definition Enlargement of parenchymal organs or their parts due to an enlargement of individual cells.
Classification It may be of two types:
i. *Physiologic,* e.g. uterine smooth muscle during pregnancy.
ii. *Pathologic,* e.g. cardiac left ventricular hypertrophy in hypertension.
Etiology Two types of hyperplasia are recognised:
i. *Hypertrophy with an identifiable cause,* such as ejection pressure forcing the contracting heart to work harder.
ii. *Idiopathic hypertrophy* if no direct cause can be identified, e.g. cardiac hypertrophy in congenital hypertrophic cardiomyopathy.

Pathogenesis Hypertrophy affects predominantly muscle cells, i.e. skeletal, cardiac and smooth muscle.
i. *Pure hypertrophy* occurs only in organs composed of non-dividing (post-mitotic) cells such as heart muscle and skeletal muscle.
ii. *Combined hypertrophy and hyperplasia* involve usually smooth muscle-rich organs, e.g. enlargement of urinary bladder due to prostatic obstruction.
NOTE: Parenchymal organs composed of labile or stable cells that can divide (e.g. kidneys, adrenals) may also undergo combined compensatory hypertrophy and hyperplasia.

Q9. What are the most common clinically important forms of hypertrophy?
I. Hypertrophy of cardiac muscle
i. Left ventricular hypertrophy in systemic arterial hypertension
ii. Left ventricular hypertrophy in aortic valve stenosis or insufficiency
iii. Left ventricular hypertrophy in mitral insufficiency
iv. Right ventricular hypertrophy in pulmonary hypertension and left ventricular failure
II. Hypertrophy of smooth muscles
i. Pyloric stenosis with hypertrophy of pyloric part of the stomach
ii. Achalasia of the oesophagus with hypertrophy of lower oesophageal sphincter
iii. Smooth muscle of the intestinal wall proximal to intestinal strictures
iv. Smooth muscle hypertrophy and hyperplasia in urinary bladder obstructed with hyperplastic prostate gland
v. Smooth muscle of renal muscular arteries in hypertension
III. Hypertrophy of skeletal muscle
Muscle in body-builders, athletes or manual labourers
IV. Compensatory hypertrophy
i. *Myocardium*: Individual cardiac myocyte hypertrophy next to an area of cell loss due to infarction.
ii. *Skeletal muscle*: Atrophy of some cells due to denervation may lead to hypertrophy of adjacent cells.
iii. *In paired organs*, such as kidneys or adrenals, removal of one organ may lead to hypertrophy of the remaining organ. It is usually associated with hyperplasia.

Q10. What are the pathologic features of hypertrophy?
Gross Increased size and weight of the affected organ.
Microscopy
i. Enlarged cell volume
ii. Increased amount of cytoplasm
iii. Enlarged nuclei with more DNA (hyperchromatic nuclei)
Molecular and ultrastructural features
i. Reactivation of *embryonic and foetal genes in cardiac myocytes* (e.g. cardiac α-actin, β-myoglobin)
ii. Increased number of *energy-producing organelles* (mitochondria) and activation of *respiratory enzymes* with increased and oxygen consumption.
iii. Increased activity of *signal transduction activity* and *transcription factor pathways* from the receptors on the cell membrane into the cytoplasm and nucleus.
iv. Increased synthesis of myofibrils-related *contraction proteins and growth factors*.

Q11. What is hyperplasia? Briefly discuss its types, etiology and pathogenesis.
Definition Enlargement of parenchymal organs or their component tissues due to an increased number of parenchymal cells.
Classification It may be of two types:
i. *Physiologic,* e.g. enlargement of breast or uterine smooth muscle during pregnancy.
ii. *Pathologic,* e.g. prostatic hyperplasia or endometrial hyperplasia.
Etiology It may be related to:
i. *An identifiable cause,* such as hormones causing endometrial hyperplasia, or
ii. *Idiopathic,* e.g. nodular hyperplasia of the liver.

Pathogenesis

i. Hyperplasia *involves only organs* composed of **labile cells** (e.g. epithelial cells of the skin or intestines, bone marrow or lymph nodes), or **stable cells** (e.g. parenchymal cells of the liver, kidney, adrenal, thyroid).
ii. It *does not* affect organs composed of **permanent cells** (e.g. heart cells, neurons, or skeletal muscle). Permanent cells cannot proliferate or enter mitosis!
iii. Proliferation of cells occurs due to **hormonal stimulation** (e.g. endometrial hyperplasia under the influence of oestrogen), or **growth factors** (e.g. liver regeneration after partial hepatectomy).
- Cells that are in G0 (resting phase of the cell cycle) enter mitosis and divide.
- The cells remain under the control of growth stimulating and inhibiting factors.
- Once the stimulation of growth is terminated, the cells stop proliferating.

Q12. What are the main forms of physiologic hyperplasia?

i. **Hormonal hyperplasia of pregnancy**
a. It is usually combined with hypertrophy.
b. It is under hormonal regulation.
c. It reverts to the normal steady state after pregnancy/lactational period.
d. It involves breasts and the uterus:
- *Breasts enlarge* at the end of the pregnancy in preparation for lactation and the glandular cells assume a lactating phenotype.
- *Uterine enlargement* involves predominantly the myometrium and to a lesser degree endometrium, which transforms into decidua.

ii. **Compensatory hyperplasia**
a. It usually involves paired organs, one of which is removed.
b. It may occur following removal of a part of an organ or increased demand for cells originating in that organ. The following are the best examples:
- *Enlargement of the kidney* following the removal of the kidney from the opposite side. It is usually accompanied by hypertrophy of tubular cells.
- Restoration to normal size of the *donor liver* following lobectomy done for liver transplantation of the resected part, or for the removal of a liver tumour.
- *Bone marrow hyperplasia* following massive bleeding or blood donation or haemolysis of RBCs. It is an effort of the body to restore the normal number or red blood cells in circulation.

Q13. What are the clinically most important forms of pathologic hyperplasia?

i. Endometrial hyperplasia following oestrogen excess.
ii. Usual ductal hyperplasia in the breast with fibrocystic changes.
iii. Benign prostatic hyperplasia in old age.
iv. Hyperplasia of the skin at the margin of non-healing ulcers.
v. Viral warts caused by human papilloma virus (HPV).
vi. Nodular hyperplasia of the thyroid (goitre).

Q14. Tabulate the contrasting features of hyperplasia and hypertrophy.

Salient distinguishing features between hypertrophy and hyperplasia are given in **Table 3.1**.

Q15. What is metaplasia and its types? Discuss salient features in its etiology and pathogenesis.

Definition Metaplasia is a reversible change of one type of mature differentiated epithelial or mesenchymal cells to another type of mature epithelial or mesenchymal cells.
- It evolves usually in response to chronic abnormal stimuli.
- It is assumed that the transformed cells are able to better counteract the adverse effects of the irritants.

Classification Metaplasia is always pathologic. There are two types of metaplasia: *epithelial and mesenchymal*.
- Epithelial metaplasia is more common and clinically more important.

TABLE 3.1 Differences between hypertrophy and hyperplasia.

FEATURE	HYPERTROPHY	HYPERPLASIA
1. *Definition*	Increase in the size of parenchymal cells; affects mainly muscles and may involve dividing as well as non-dividing cells; may coexist with hyperplasia	Increase in the number of parenchymal cells; involves only dividing cells; may coexist with hypertrophy
2. *Types and common examples*	*Physiologic hypertrophy, e.g.* i. Uterine myometrium in pregnancy ii. Hypertrophy of skeletal muscle in athletes *Pathologic hypertrophy, e.g.* i. Myocardial hypertrophy in hypertension, valvular deformities ii. Hypertrophy of smooth muscle in pyloric stenosis of stomach iii. Compensatory hypertrophy of contralateral organ after removal of kidney or adrenal on one side	*Physiologic hyperplasia, e.g.* i. Hormonal hyperplasia in breast and uterus during pregnancy ii. Compensatory hyperplasia following lobectomy of the liver or bone marrow after haemolysis or blood transfusion *Pathologic hyperplasia, e.g.* i. Endometrial hyperplasia due to oestrogen excess ii. Usual ductal hyperplasia in fibrocystic change of breast iii. Benign prostatic hyperplasia in old age iv. Hyperplasia of skin in viral warts, non-healing ulcers
3. *Morphology*	GA: Affected organ enlarged and heavy ME: Enlarged muscle fibres as well as nucleomegaly Ultrastructure: Increased synthesis of DNA and RNA	GA: Affected organ enlarged and heavy ME: Increased number of cells EM: Increased DNA, regular mitoses
4. *Molecular pathogenesis*	Increased protein synthesis by increased growth factors acting on cell surface and causing activation of signal transduction pathways	Increased proliferation of cells by increased growth factors acting on cell surface receptors and stimulating signal transduction pathways
5. *Natural history/ outcome*	Reversible on withdrawal of stimulus	May regress on removal of inciting stimulus; persistence of stimulus may lead to dysplasia or neoplasia

(GA, gross appearance; ME, microscopic examination; EM, electron microscopy).

- Metaplasia is always named by the terminally differentiated cells/tissues formed from the stem cells (e.g. squamous metaplasia when squamous cells are formed in a glandular epithelium).

Etiology The adverse stimuli causing metaplasia may be of three kinds:
i. Mechanical
ii. Chemical
iii. Viral

Pathogenesis and outcomes
i. Metaplasia occurs due to genetic re-programming of stem cells.
ii. The reprogrammed stem cells change their maturation pathway and differentiate into phenotypically different cells than those normally found in that anatomic site (e.g. squamous instead of glandular cells).
iii. The exact molecular mechanism of this cell reprogramming is not known.
iv. Metaplasia will persist as long as the adverse stimulation persists.
v. Upon cessation of stimulation, it may revert to normal tissue.
vi. In some cases, epithelial metaplasia may progress to dysplasia, and then even to neoplasia. Mesenchymal metaplasia is, however, never preneoplastic.

Q16. What are the clinically most important forms of epithelial metaplasia?

Two types: squamous and columnar.
I. **Squamous metaplasia**
i. *Bronchi:* Pseudostratified columnar ciliated → squamous epithelium, usually in heavy smokers under the influence of chemical irritant in tobacco smoke.
ii. *Endocervical uterine glands*: Simple columnar epithelium → squamous epithelium in older women.

iii. *Excretory ducts*: In several organs such as pancreas, bile ducts, salivary glands, or prostate. Columnar epithelium lining the ducts → squamous metaplasia due to mechanical irritation by intraductal stones.
iv. *Transitional epithelium*: Renal pelvis, ureter or bladder→ squamous metaplasia, if irritated by chronic infection and urinary stones.
v. *Vitamin A deficiency:* Corneal epithelium in xerophthalmia and the respiratory tract → squamous metaplasia.

II. **Columnar metaplasia**
i. *Barrett oesophagus*: Lower oesophageal squamous epithelium → into columnar intestinal like epithelium with mucin-containing goblet cells. It is encountered in gastro-oesophageal reflux and is related to the irritant effects of gastric digestive juices. It may progress to dysplasia and adenocarcinoma.
ii. *Intestinal metaplasia*: In chronic gastritis replacing the multilayered specialised normal gastric mucosa.
iii. *Mucinous columnar epithelium*: Replacing the ciliated pseudostratified epithelium of the bronchi in chronic bronchitis and bronchiectasis.

Q17. What are the common forms of mesenchymal metaplasia?

The most common form of mesenchymal metaplasia is osseous metaplasia. It is of limited clinical significance. It may occur in the fibrous tissues, cartilage or myxoid connective tissue:
i. Fibrous scars
ii. Foci of chronic inflammation
iii. Arterial wall of calcified medium-sized arteries (Mönckeberg's calcific media sclerosis)
iv. Myositis ossificans in soft tissue, often at the site of a haematoma
v. Cartilage of the larynx and trachea in elderly persons
vi. Fibrous stroma of some tumours

Q18. What is dysplasia? Briefly discuss its classification, etiology, pathogenesis and its morphologic features.

Definition Dysplasia is a disordered cellular development, often preceded or accompanied by metaplasia and/or hyperplasia. Therefore, it is also known as *atypical hyperplasia*.
• Dysplasia involves only epithelial cells.
• Dysplasia may regress, but it may also progress to neoplasia.
• It evolves usually in response to abnormal stimuli so that the transformed cells are able to withstand better the adverse effects of the irritant.

Classification Dysplasia is always pathologic.
• Dysplasia may be histologically graded as *mild, moderate or severe*.
• In the cervical epithelium dysplasia, it is also called *cervical intraepithelial neoplasia (CIN)* and graded mild as CIN1, moderate as CIN2, and severe as CIN3.
• Severe dysplasia is also known as carcinoma in situ.

Etiology Dysplasia occurs on the background of chronic inflammation and irritation. Two most important causes are as follows:
i. *Chemicals and carcinogens:* Inhaled in tobacco smoke acting on the bronchial epithelium, which usually first undergoes squamous metaplasia, and then progressing to dysplasia.
ii. *Human papilloma virus*: Acts on the cervical squamous epithelium of the uterus.

Pathogenesis and outcome
i. Chemicals and viruses induce permanent genetic changes in the epithelial cells.
ii. Genetically altered cells may progress to neoplasia, which retains the same 'neoplastic genetic imprint'.

Microscopy of cervical dysplasia The changes reflect disorderly proliferation of cells and lack of regular differentiation as the cells move from the basal to the superficial layer.
i. Increased number of cell layers in the epithelium that appears thicker than normal.
ii. Disorderly arrangement of cells from basal to surface layers.
iii. Loss of basal cell nuclear polarity which normally face toward the basal membrane.
iv. Cellular and nuclear pleomorphism.

v. Increased nuclear-cytoplasmic ratio.
vi. Nuclear hyperchromasia.
vii. Increased mitotic activity above the basal layer.

Q19. What are the differences between metaplasia and dysplasia?

The differences between metaplasia and dysplasia are given in **Table 3.2**.

TABLE 3.2 Differences between metaplasia and dysplasia.

FEATURE	METAPLASIA	DYSPLASIA
1. *Definition*	Change of an adult type of epithelial or mesenchymal cell to another type of adult epithelial or mesenchymal cell; often in response to inciting stimulus	Disordered cellular development, may be accompanied with hyperplasia or metaplasia; often in response to inciting stimulus
2. *Types and common examples*	*Squamous metaplasia*, e.g. bronchus, uterine cervix, calculi in ducts (in biliary passages, pancreas, salivary), renal pelvis, urinary bladder, xerophthalmia in vitamin A deficiency *Columnar metaplasia*, e.g. Barett's oesophagus, gastric ulcer, bronchial mucosa *Osseous metaplasia*, e.g. arteriosclerosis, myositis ossificans, cartilage in bronchus and larynx	Epithelial only, e.g. Uterine cervix (cervical intraepithelial neoplasia (CIN) Bronchus (squamous cell dysplasia, carcinoma in situ) Oral cavity (dysplasia, intraepithelial neoplasia) Oesophagus (squamous cell dysplasia, Barett columnar cell dysplasia)
3. *Morphology*	Mature cellular development from specialised to less well-specialised and resistant cells	Disorderly cellular developnent (increased layers, loss of polarity, pleomorphism, nuclear hyperchromasia, mitoses)
4. *Molecular pathogenesis*	Reprogramming of precursor stem cells triggered by exogenous stimuli to another pathway	Abnormal cell growth by mutations in genes as in neoplasia
5. *Natural history/ outcome*	Reversible on withdrawal of stimulus; persistence of stimuli may cause progression to dysplasia	Mild and moderate grades regress on removal of inciting stimulus; severe grade and persistence of stimuli may cause progression to carcinoma *in situ* and invasive cancer

PATHOGENESIS OF CELL INJURY

Q20. What are the general features that characterise most forms of cell injury by various agents?

General features of all forms of cell injury fall into following four categories:

I. **Factors pertaining to the etiologic agent and the host**
- Etiologic agents must be assessed with regard to their type, duration and severity of injury.
- The host's response will depend on the type, status and adaptability of its target cells.

II. **General underlying mechanisms**
These mechanisms include mitochondrial injury causing ATP depletion, cell membrane damage, release of oxygen-derived free radicals, reduced protein synthesis.

III. **Usual morphologic changes**
These changes include organelle pathology accompanied by biochemical changes that characterise reversible and irreversible cell injury, which may lead to cell death.

IV. **Functional implications and disease outcome**
Cellular injury leads to dysfunction of organs and the appearance of signs and symptoms of the disease that need to be evaluated by current clinical methods. The knowledge of clinical features of the disease will allow us to formulate the prognosis and decide on the treatment.

Q21. What is the sequence of events leading to ischaemia/hypoxia induced reversible and irreversible cell injury?

The pathogenesis of reversible and irreversible cell injury is illustrated in **Figure 3.3** and sequentially listed below. Key words are in bold letters as follows:

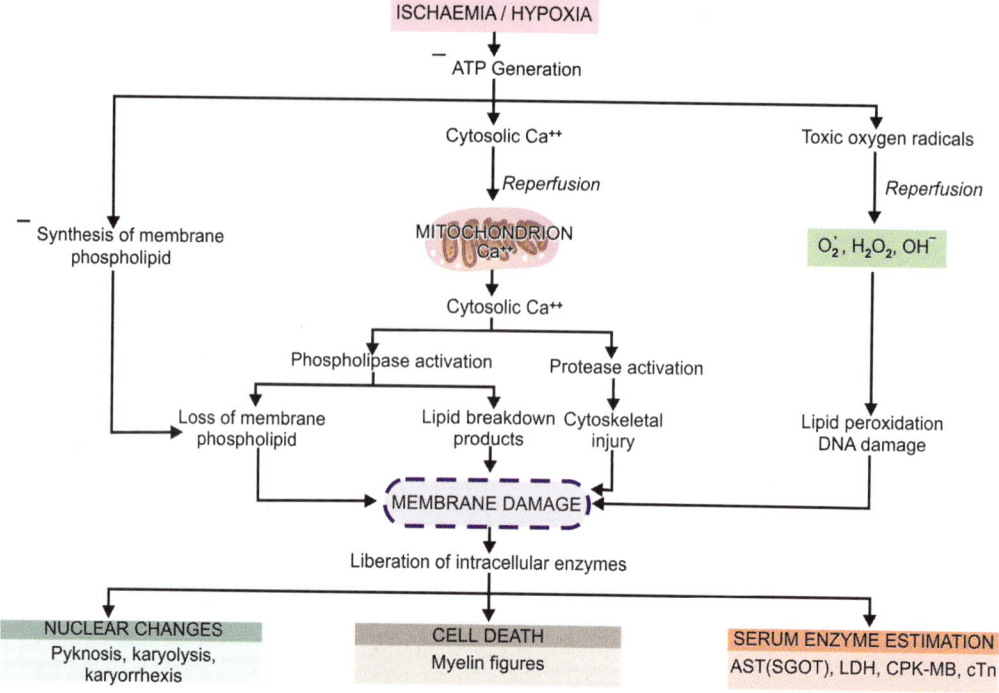

FIGURE 3.3: Sequence of events in the pathogenesis of reversible and irreversible cell injury caused by hypoxia/ischaemia. (AST, aspartate transaminase from the liver; LDH, lactic dehydrogenase from damaged cells; CPK-MB, MB fraction of creatine phosphokinase released from cardiac muscle; cTn, cardiac troponin from damaged myocardium).

i. Decreased generation of **ATP** due to inhibition of **oxidative phosphorylation.**
ii. **Anaerobic glycolytic oxidation** is activated through the action of hypoxia-inducible factor 1 **(HIF-1)** and serves as an alternative, but less efficient, energy generating pathway.
iii. Highly specialised cells, such as cardiac myocytes, neurons and proximal tubular cells of the kidney depend on aerobic generation of ATP and are most severely damaged.
iv. Rapid depletion of **glycogen stores** leads to **lactic acidosis** in the cytoplasm.
v. Cytoplasmic acidosis leads to **nuclear changes** and clumping of the chromatin.
vi. Lack of ATP damages the function of the ATP-dependent **cell membrane pump** (also known as **Na⁺/K⁺ ATPase**), which leads to a loss of cell membrane selective **semipermeability** and an influx of sodium and water into the cytoplasm resulting in hydropic swelling.
vii. **Influx of calcium** into the cytoplasm.
viii. Calcium ions act as 'secondary messengers' activating several lytic **enzymes** such as endonucleases, proteases, lipases, phosphatases, and glycosidases.
ix. Lipids liberated from phospholipids are oxidized into **lipoperoxides** which act as oxygen radicals, inducing more mitochondrial damage (**myelin figures**).
x. Cell membrane damage will allow the leakage of enzymes from the cytoplasm into the interstitial fluid (**aminotransferases** like **ALT, AST,** and **lactic dehydrogenase (LDH)**. Cell specific enzymes are released in some instances: **lipase and amylase** from pancreatic acinar cells, **creatin kinase-MB** fraction from cardiac myocytes. Proteins such as cardiac **troponins** are released from damaged cardiac myocytes.
xi. **Enzymes** released from severely damaged or dying cells enter circulating blood and thus, can be analysed in the **clinical laboratory**.
xii. Protease activation damages the **cytoskeleton.**
xiii. Acidity of the cytoplasm activates lysosomes and promotes **autophagocytosis** → residual bodies → increased exocytosis → **lipofuscin** accumulates.
xiv. Ischaemic reperfusion injury occurs due to flooding of the cytoplasm with oxygen which contributes to the formation of **oxygen derived free radicals** (also known as **reactive oxygen radicals, ROS**).

Q22. What are the various enzyme markers of cell death?

Common enzyme and cytoplasmic protein markers of cell injury and death are listed in **Table 3.3**.

Q23. What are the ultrastructural changes in the hypoxia-ischaemia induced cell injury?

The ultrastructural appearance of cell injury are listed below and presented in **Figure 3.4**. It should be noted that the differences between reversible and irreversible cell injury are mostly quantitative rather than qualitative, i.e. they differ one from another only in intensity and extent.

The only definitive signs of irreversible cell injury are the rupture of cell membrane and the nuclear changes associated with cell death (pyknosis, karyorrhexis, and karyolysis).

TABLE 3.3 Common enzyme markers of cell death.

ENZYME	DISEASE
1. Aspartate amino-transferase (AST, SGOT)	Diffuse liver cell necrosis, e.g. viral hepatitis, alcoholic liver disease Acute myocardial infarction
2. Alanine amino-transferase (ALT, SGPT)	More specific for diffuse liver cell damage than AST, e.g. viral hepatitis
3. Creatine kinase-MB (CK-MB)	Acute myocardial infarction, myocarditis Skeletal muscle injury
4. Lipase	More specific for acute pancreatitis
5. Amylase	Acute pancreatitis Sialadenitis
6. Lactic dehydrogenase (LDH)	Acute myocardial infarction Myocarditis Skeletal muscle injury
7. Cardiac troponin (CTn)	Specific for acute myocardial infarction

i. **Mitochondria** Swelling and formation of amorphous densities, followed by rupture of mitochondria with fragmentation. **Myelin figures** form from these membrane fragments.

ii. **Cell membrane** Formation of blebs and invaginations, which lead to cell swelling. Damaged cell membrane fragments and these short segments roll up to form myelin figures. Ultimately, the cell **membrane ruptures** (one of the signs of irreversible injury) and the cytoplasmic contents pour out into the intercellular spaces.

iii. **Rough endoplasmic reticulum and ribosomes** Cisterns of RER swell and become vesicular, while the ribosome on their outer surface disperse and detach ('**degranulation of RER**'). Ultimately, RER membranes are lysed and ribosomes disappear.

iv. **Lysosomes** They enlarge and are more numerous. Upon the uptake of damaged organelles into the inside of lysosomes, they transform into **autophagosomes**. Lytic enzymes inside the lysosomes (active at low pH and therefore called 'acid hydrolases') digest the autophagocytosed material and the undigested material is condensed into residual bodies. Residual bodies are initially extruded from the cytoplasm (**exocytosed**) but when the cell becomes energy deficient they remain in the cytoplasm as aggregates of **lipofuscin**. Ultimately, lysosomes rupture and release their hydrolytic enzymes contributing to the autolysis of the cytoplasm.

v. **Cytoskeleton** All three components of cytoskeleton (**microfilaments, intermediate filaments and microtubules**) are damaged through the action of proteases. Damaged cytoskeleton fibres form either aggregates or fragments.

Q24. What are the distinguishing features of reversible and irreversible cell injury?

Salient distinguishing features of reversible and irreversible cell injury are summed up in **Table 3.4**.

Q25. What are the main features of ischaemic-reperfusion cell injury?

- *Short-term ischaemia* of low intensity produces cellular changes that are usually reversible.
- *Long-lasting ischaemia* or high intensity cell injury will result in cell death.
- *Ischaemia of intermediate duration/intensity* will usually produce reversible cell injury, which may be intensified upon *reperfusion*, once the blood circulation is reestablished.

Ischaemia-reperfusion injury occurs due to its *three components:*

i. **Calcium overload** It occurs due to the higher concentration of calcium in blood than in the cytoplasm of injured cells and dysfunction of the calcium pump that is supposed to move the calcium out of the cytoplasm. Calcium accumulates in the mitochondria damaging their function, and also in the cytosol where it acts as a secondary messenger activating lytic enzymes.

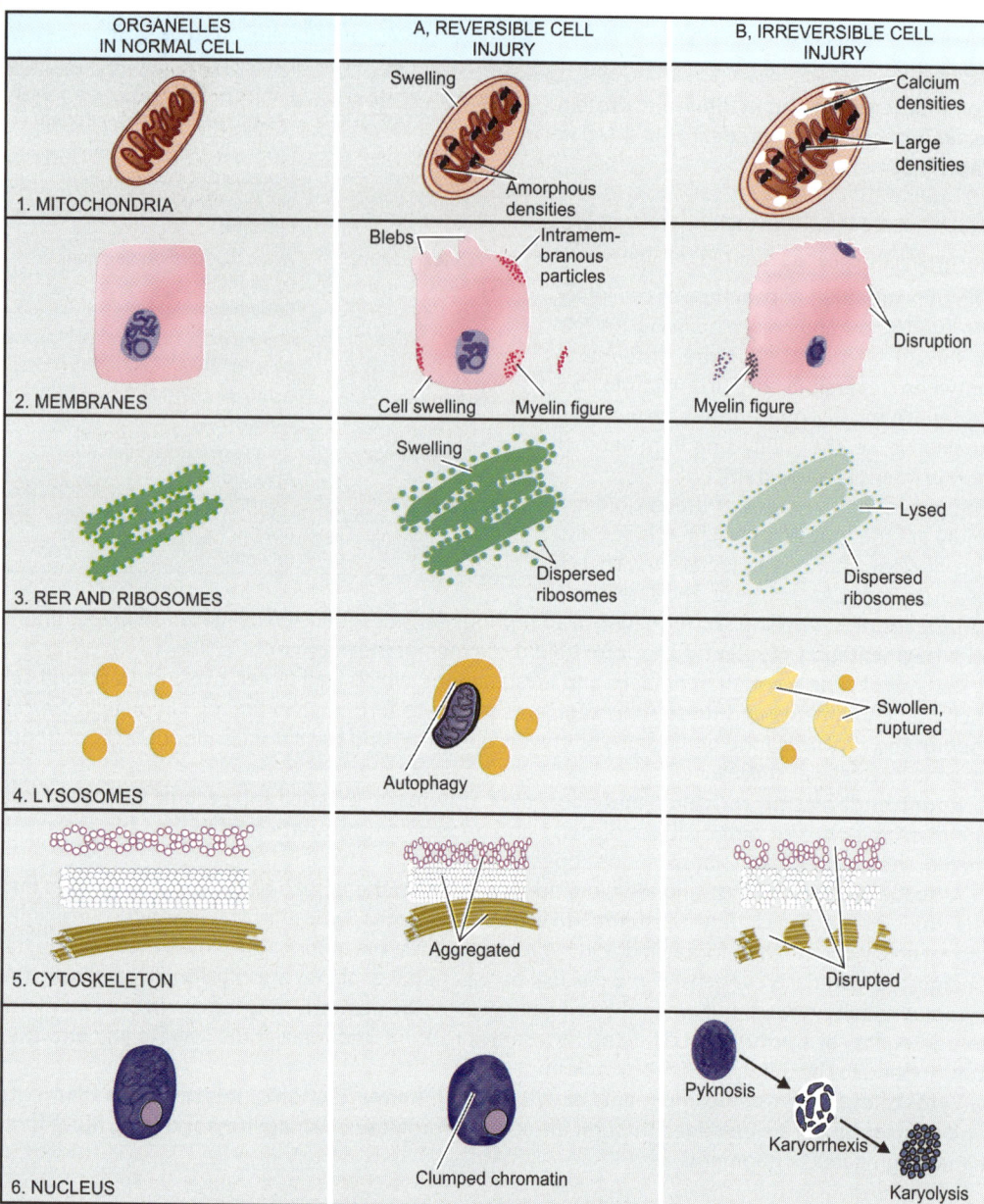

FIGURE 3.4: Ultrastructural changes during cell injury due to hypoxia-ischaemia.

ii. **Excessive generation of free radicals** These radicals (*superoxide oxygen or O^-_2; hydrogen peroxide or H_2O_2; and hydroxyl radical or OH^-*) are formed in small amounts within the mitochondrial inner membrane as intermediary products in the process of coupling O_2 to H_2O during oxidative phosphorylation and ATP production in the mitochondrial inner membrane. However, upon reperfusion, they are produced in excessive amounts and become toxic.

iii. **Acute inflammatory reaction** It is based on the chemotaxis of neutrophils to the ischaemic area.

Q26. What are oxygen free radicals and their types? Discuss the mechanism of their generation.

Definition Free radicals are reactive unstable compounds, that have an unpaired electron in their outer orbit and are, thus, labile and highly reactive, producing so called *oxidative stress*.

Types and generation of free radicals They include i) oxygen free radicals, ii) other free radicals (such as nitric oxide and halide reagents), and iii) exogenous free radicals.

TABLE 3.4 Distinguishing features of reversible and irreversible cell injury.

FEATURE	REVERSIBLE CELL INJURY	IRREVERSIBLE CELL INJURY
1. Definition	Exposure to injurious agent for short duration; its removal reverts the cell back to normal	Persistence of injurious agent; causes irreversible structural and functional damage to the cell
2. Biochemical and molecular mechanisms	➤ Decreased cellular ATP generation ➤ Intracellular lactic acidosis: nuclear clumping ➤ Damage to plasma membrane Na-K, Ca pumps: hydropic swelling ➤ Reduced protein synthesis: dispersal of ribosomes	➤ Continued cytosolic influx of calcium: mitochondrial damage ➤ Activated phospholipases: membrane damage ➤ Activated intracellular proteases: cytoskeletal damage ➤ Activated endonucleases: nuclear damage ➤ Liberation of lysosomal hydrolytic enzymes in blood
3. Morphology ➤ Cell membrane ➤ Endoplasmic reticulum ➤ Ribosomes ➤ Lysosomes ➤ Mitochondria ➤ Cytoskeleton ➤ Nuclear changes	➤ Blebs, intramembranous particles, myelin figures ➤ Swollen ➤ Dispersed ➤ Autophagy ➤ Swollen, amorphous densities ➤ Aggregated ➤ Clumped chromatin	➤ More prominent blebs, or disrupted membrane, myelin figures ➤ Swollen and lysed ➤ Dispersed and lysed ➤ Swollen and ruptured ➤ Swollen, large densities ➤ Disrupted ➤ Pyknosis, karyorrhexis, karyolysis

I. **Oxygen free radicals** are the most important free endogenous radicals. These include: *superoxide oxygen*, O_2^-; *hydrogen peroxide*, H_2O_2; and *hydroxyl radical*, OH^-) which are formed as byproducts of ATP production in the process that leads to transfer of four electrons and the formation of water (H_2O) from biradical oxygen (O_2) binding two hydrogen atoms (2H) **(Fig. 3.5)**:

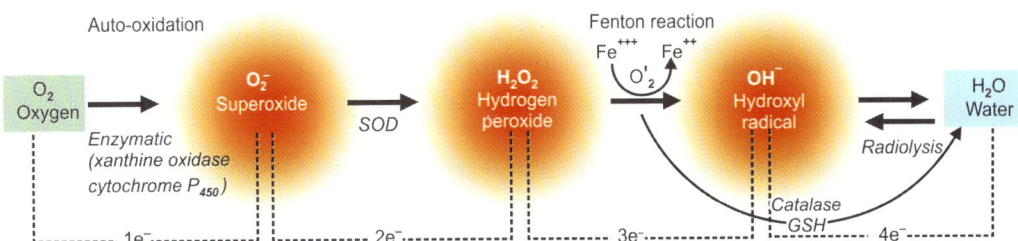

FIGURE 3.5: Mechanisms of generation of free radicals by four electron step reduction of oxygen. (SOD, superoxide dismutase; GSH, glutathione peroxidase).

i. *Superoxide* is formed by direct autooxidation of O_2 during mitochondrial electron transport. It may be produced enzymatically by *xanthine oxidase* and *cytochrome* P_{450} in the mitochondria or cytosol.

ii. *Hydrogen peroxide* is formed from superoxide by enzyme *superoxide dismutase*. It is further reduced to water by *catalase* (an enzyme found in peroxisomes) and glutathione peroxidase (found in cytosol and mitochondria).

iii. *Hydroxyl radical* is formed by two ways: by radiolysis of water and by the reaction of H_2O_2 with bivalent ferrous (Fe^{++}) ions in the Fenton reaction, which involves transition of ferric (Fe^{+++}) to ferrous (Fe^{++}) iron facilitated by O_2^-). Hydroxyl radical is the most toxic of all oxygen free radicals.

II. **Others free radicals** that are active in the body are as follows:

i. *Nitric oxide (NO)* is produced by various cells (endothelial cells, neurons, macrophages) as a chemical mediator of their action but also may act as free radical. It binds with superoxide to form *peroxynitrite (ONOO)*, a highly reactive free radical.

ii. *Halide reagents* contain chloride and are released in leucocytic phagocytic vacuoles with superoxide to form bactericidal *hypochlorous acid (HClO)*.

III. **Exogenous free radicals** enter the body inhaled as pollutants in the air or ingested in food and water.

Q27. How do free oxygen radicals damage cells?

Free oxygen radicals may damage essentially all cell components but, most importantly, their actions involve the following:

I. **Lipid peroxidation,** thus causing a damage of cell membrane and membrane bound organelles such as mitochondria, lysosomes and RER.

II. **Oxidative injury of proteins**, by cross-linking of labile amino acids and fragmenting the polypeptide chains. Protein components of cell membrane and organelles will be injured as well as cytoskeletal fibres and cytosolic enzymes.

III. **DNA damage** will cause single strand breaks and genetic mutations.

Q28. Enumerate various pathologic processes and diseases which are mediated by free oxygen radicals.

Free oxygen radicals play an important role in many pathologic processes including the following:
i. Ischaemic reperfusion injury following occlusion of the blood vessels or hypoperfusion of tissue during shock
ii. Ionising radiation by causing hydrolysis of water
iii. Toxicity of chemicals and drugs
iv. Chemical carcinogenesis
v. Cellular ageing
vi. Killing of microbial agents
vii. Inflammatory damage
viii. Destruction of tumour cells
ix. Atherosclerosis

Q29. How does the body defend itself from oxygen free radicals?

Antioxidants are endogenous and exogenous substances which inactivate the free radicals. These protective substances include the following:
- Vitamins E, A, and C (ascorbic acid).
- Sulfhydryl containing amino acids and proteins like cysteine and glutathione.
- Serum metal transport proteins, like ceruloplasmin and transferring.

Q30. What are stress proteins? How do they protect cells from injury?

Definition When cells are exposed to stress of any type, they can release protective agents or proteins which are called stress protein.

Types and actions There are two groups of stress-related proteins: *heat shock proteins (HSP)* and *ubiquitin* (so named due to its universal presence in the cells of the body):

I. **Heat shock proteins (HSP)** These are a variety of intracellular carrier proteins present in most cells of the body.
- Physiologically, HSP act as house-keeping proteins *('molecular chaperones')* and participate in protein folding, disaggregation of protein-protein complexes, and transport of proteins into various intracellular organelles (protein kinesis).
- They leak into the plasma under various stressful conditions in response to toxins, ischaemia, cancer, etc., thus called *stress proteins*.
- They have been found to *limit tissue necrosis* in ischaemia.
- Moderate protein aggregation in *amyloidosis*.

II. **Ubiquitin** Ubiquitin is a stress protein that directs effete and damaged proteins into proteasomes for degradation. It also regulates the synthesis of many proteins.

Q31. How do chemicals and toxins kill cells?

Chemicals and toxins kill cells by two mechanisms:

I. **Direct toxicity** Two examples are given:
i. *Cyanide* kills cells by poisoning mitochondrial cytochrome oxidase.
ii. *Mercury chloride* acts on disulfide bonds between amino acids or the proteins inhibiting many essential enzymes of the GI tract where it is absorbed, or kidney where it is excreted.

II. **Metabolic conversion** Conversion from a non-toxic compound to a toxin, or a weak toxin into more potent toxin. This occurs typically in the liver. Two examples are given:
i. *Carbon tetrachloride (CCl$_4$)*, an industrial toxin used for dry-cleaning industry, which is transformed into a toxic free radical (CCl$_3$) by liver cytochrome P$_{450}$ enzyme system.
ii. *Acetaminophen*, an analgesic drug, is transformed into a hepatotoxin, which is normally neutralised by glutathione peroxidase, until its concentration in blood and tissues exceeds the body's capacity to neutralise it.

Q32. How does ionising radiation kill cells?
i. Radiation-induced killing of cells results from the action *hydroxyl radical* formed during radiolysis of water. In proliferating cells, there is direct DNA damage and inhibition of DNA replication leading to *apoptosis* **(Fig. 3.6)**.
ii. Sublethal injury results in genetic damage and *mutations*.
iii. In nonproliferating cells (e.g. neurons), there is lethal cell membrane injury combined with inhibition of DNA synthesis which leads to *necrosis*.

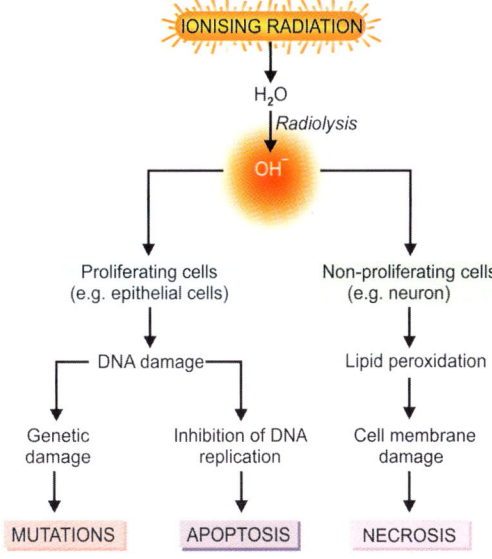

FIGURE 3.6: Mechanisms of cell injury by ionising radiation.

MORPHOLOGY OF CELL INJURY

Q33. Briefly discuss important morphologic forms of reversible cell injury (degenerations).

I. **Hydropic change** It is caused by an influx of fluid and sodium into the cytoplasm due to the failure of the Na$^+$/K$^+$ ATPase caused by a lack of energy rich ATP.
Microscopy **(Fig. 3.7)**
• The cytoplasm and even the nucleus appear pale.
• It is marked by the appearance of *cytoplasmic vacuoles*, which represent dilated RER and mitochondria.
• Swollen cells compress interstitial capillaries.
At biochemical level, there is also influx of calcium and efflux of potassium.
II. **Hyaline change** It refers to intracellular changes, i.e. *hyaline change of the entire cytoplasm*. Hyaline means 'glassy'.
Under the microscope, the entire cell cytoplasm appears glassy, homogeneous, and eosinophilic.

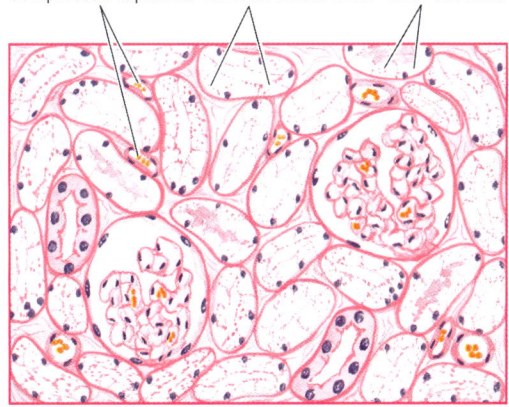

FIGURE 3.7: Hydropic change kidney. The tubular epithelial cells are distended with cytoplasmic vacuoles while the interstitial vasculature is compressed. The nuclei of affected tubules are pale.

In liver cells it is most often caused by chronic drug ingestion. For example,
i. *Hyaline droplets* are proteins, such as absorbed protein in proximal tubules in proteinuria. Protein droplets (staining red with eosin in routine histopathology slides are seen by light microcopy in liver cells in congenital α-1-antitripsin deficiency. By electron microscopy, these protein droplets are located within the cisterns of rough endoplasmic reticulum.
ii. *Mallory hyaline* is composed of aggregates of intermediate filaments in hepatocytes of chronic alcoholics.
iii. *Russell bodies* are droplets of immunoglobulin which begin accumulating in cisterns of rough endoplasmic reticulum but then expand and coalesce to the point, where the entire

cytoplasm is filled with a single large eosinophilic hyaline globule, pushing the nucleus to the periphery.

NOTE: *Intracellular hyaline should be distinguished from extracellular hyaline*, which is most often composed of condensed collagen fibres (e.g. in old scars) or basement membrane material (e.g. hyalinised glomeruli), or amyloid. The biochemical nature of the extracellular hyaline can be determined by special stains or biochemically.

III. **Mucoid change** It means mucus-like alterations.
- It is marked by accumulation of *mucin* (a glycoprotein, which is the main component of mucus) in the cytoplasm.
- Normally, mucin is present in mucus-secreting goblet cells of the bronchi or intestines.

Accumulation of mucin in epithelial cells occurs in several conditions:

i. Inside the mucosal cells in *catarrhal inflammation* of the upper respiratory tract.

ii. *Obstruction of ducts* of small salivary gland leads to formation of *mucocele*, a retention cyst filled with mucin. Mucin is also seen in the cytoplasm of cells on the internal side of the cyst and macrophages, which infiltrate its wall ('foamy macrophages').

iii. Obstruction of the gallbladder neck leads to *mucocele of the gallbladder*.

iv. *Cystic fibrosis* of the pancreas (previously called 'mucoviscidosis') is marked by the obstruction of pancreatic ducts by viscous mucin and retention of mucus in acinar cells.

v. *Mucin-secreting tumours* are often marked by the accumulation of mucin in tumour cells which have the appearance of 'signet ring cells'.

IV. **Myxoid change ('degeneration')** Accumulation of mucoid material in the connective tissue is by convention called 'myxoid'. Histochemically, it differs from mucin: mucin is PAS positive, whereas myxoid stroma is PAS negative. Both substances are alcian blue positive.

Myxoid change is seen in the following conditions:
i. Dissecting aneurysm of the aorta
ii. Myxoid degeneration of cardiac valves
iii. Myxoedema of subcutaneous tissue in hypothyroidism.

V. **Fatty change** Most often, it occurs in the liver (hepatic steatosis in obese persons or due to alcohol abuse), but it may be found less often in the kidneys, heart or other parenchyma organs (discussed on page 45).

Q34. What is necrosis? Describe its types and their salient pathologic features.

Definition Necrosis is localised area of tissue death in living organism, followed by degradation of tissue by hydrolytic enzymes liberated from dead cells; it is invariably accompanied by an inflammatory reaction.

Pathologic types There are five types of necrosis: i) coagulative, ii) liquefactive, iii) caseous, iv) fat, and v) fibrinoid necrosis.

I. **Coagulative necrosis** It is the most common form of necrosis.
- Most often caused by ischaemia, and less often by bacterial and chemical agents.
- Most often affected organs: heart, kidney and spleen.

Gross Pale area which becomes yellow, solid. With time, it becomes softer and shrunken.

Microscopy Cells retain their shape (appear like 'tombstones' of healthy cells), but loose nuclear and cytoplasmic details.

i. Cytoplasm become eosinophilic and the nuclei undergo pyknosis, karyorrhexis, karyolysis **(Fig. 3.8)**.

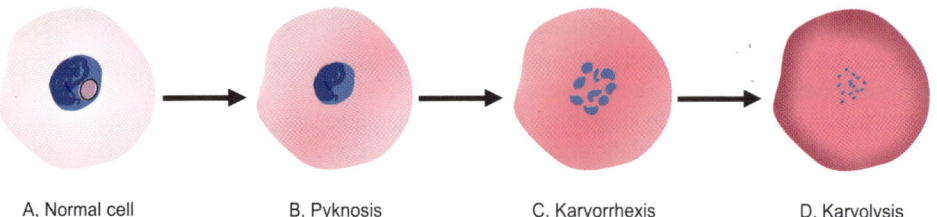

A, Normal cell   B, Pyknosis   C, Karyorrhexis   D, Karyolysis

FIGURE 3.8: Nuclear and cytoplasmic changes in necrosis. A, Normal cell. B, Cytoplasm is more pink and nucleus is shrunken (pyknosis). C, Cytoplasm is more pink and the nucleus is fragmented (karyorrhexis). D, The cytoplasm is intensely pink and nuclear material has disappeared (karyolysis).

ii. Inflammatory reaction (neutrophils) appears 24 hours after onset of necrosis, and finally digest the necrotic tissue **(Fig. 3.9)**.
iii. Acute inflammatory cells are replaced by macrophages and granulation tissue.
iv. If the patient survives, infarct is replaced by fibrous tissue scarring.

II. **Liquefactive necrosis** The necrotic tissue is semiliquid due to the action of hydrolytic enzymes.
- Typically, occurs in the brain.
- *Secondary liquefactive necrosis* occurs in bacterial and fungal abscesses where the liquefaction is caused by purulent inflammatory exudate and lytic enzymes released from neutrophils.

Gross Soft, semiliquid material, well demarcated from the normal brain parenchyma.
Microscopy Necrotic material without preservation of cell outlines.

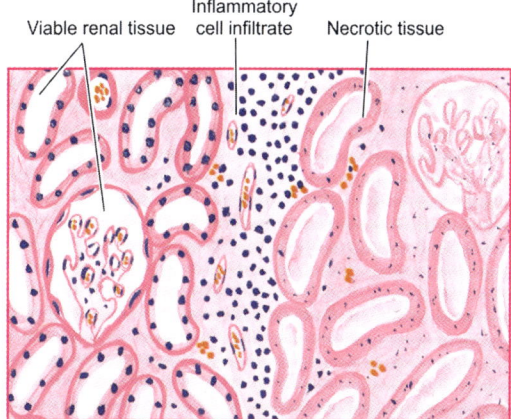

FIGURE 3.9: Coagulative necrosis in infarct kidney. The affected area on right shows cells with intensely eosinophilic cytoplasm of tubular cells but the outlines of tubules are still maintained. The nuclei show granular debris. The interface between viable and non-viable area shows non-specific chronic inflammation and proliferating vessels.

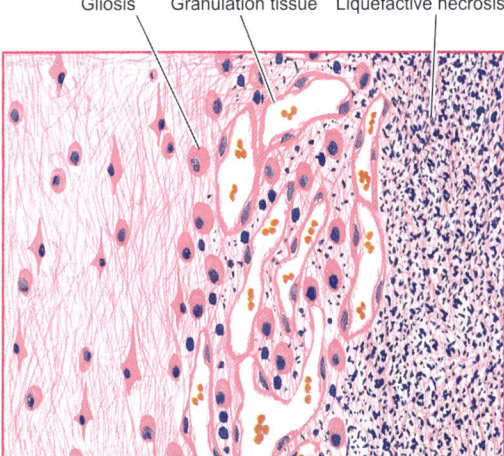

FIGURE 3.10: Liquefactive necrosis brain. The necrosed area on right side of the field contains cell debris, infiltration with microglial cells and some surviving blood vessels while the surrounding zone shows gliosis.

i. On the periphery the necrotic brain tissue, it is separated from normal tissue by gliosis, macrophages and capillaries **(Fig. 3.10)**.
ii. In the brain, it transforms into a pseudocyst filled with fluid.
iii. In an abscess, the semiliquid material is surrounded by a 'capsule', composed of granulation tissue admixed to chronic inflammatory cells.

III. **Caseous necrosis** This descriptive name indicates that the necrotic material resembles cottage cheese.
- It combines features of coagulative and liquefactive necrosis.

Gross It is white or yellow and granular.
Microscopy Typically, it is a feature of tuberculosis, but may also be seen in some fungal granulomas.

i. At the periphery of the necrotic material, there are typically granulomas composed of T-lymphocytes, epithelioid macrophages, and multinucleated giant cells **(Fig. 3.11)**.
ii. It tends to calcify, and ultimately heal by scarring.

IV. **Fat necrosis** It occurs in fat tissue, such as peripancreatic fat tissue or fat tissue of the breast.
- *Enzymatic fat necrosis* of abdominal fat tissue is typically seen in acute pancreatitis. Destruction of pancreatic acinar cells leads to a release of *lipase*, which then acts on fat cells cleaving triglycerides into free fatty acids and glycerol. Free fatty acid may bind calcium and thus form deposits of *calcium soaps*.

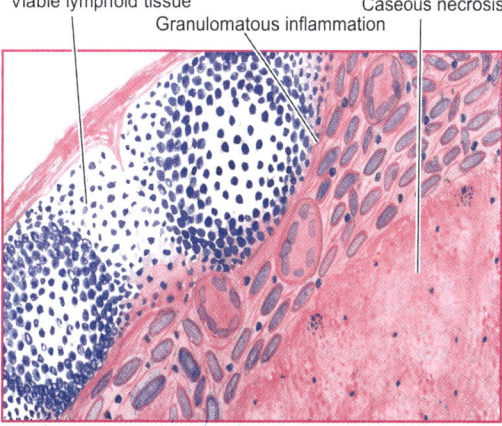

FIGURE 3.11: Caseous necrosis lymph node. There is eosinophilic, amorphous, granular material, while the periphery shows granulomatous inflammation.

- *Traumatic fat necrosis* of the breast may cause rupture of fat cells and a release of triglycerides, which are then cleaved into free fatty acids and glycerol.

Gross Areas of fat necrosis → white speck, much firmer than normal surrounding fat.

Microscopy Adipocytes have lost their nuclei and partially their cell membrane; their cytoplasm appears as cloudy eosinophilic material.

i. Adipocytes are ultimately transformed into finely granular amorphous material.
ii. Calcium salt deposit imparts the necrotic tissue a blue colour in H&E stained section.
iii. Foci of necrosis are usually surrounded by acute inflammatory cells.

V. **Fibrinoid necrosis** It is characterised by a deposition of fibrin-like material in the wall of blood vessels (arteries and arterioles) or glomerular capillaries.

i. It is usually caused by autoimmune mechanisms involving blood vessel injury by immune complexes.
ii. Most often, seen in polyarteritis nodosa and other immune vasculitides.
iii. May be seen in renal vessels and glomeruli in malignant hypertension (rare today!).
iv. It is diagnosed only microscopically—there are no diagnostic macroscopic features.

Q35. Tabulate the salient distinguishing features of coagulative, liquefactive and caseous necrosis.

Contrasting features of three major forms of necrosis—coagulative, liquefactive and caseous, are given in **Table 3.5**.

TABLE 3.5 Contrasting features of three major forms of necrosis.

FEATURE	COAGULATIVE NECROSIS	LIQUEFACTIVE NECROSIS	CASEOUS NECROSIS
1. *Definition and etiology*	Infarction due to lack of blood supply, i.e. hypoxia-ischaemia	Due to hypoxic injury in brain and bacterial or fungal infection elsewhere; dead cells broken down to form a liquid mass or cystic space	Cheese-like necrosis in mycobacterial infection
2. *Common examples*	Infarcts, e.g. heart, spleen, kidney, etc. (but not brain)	➤ Infarct brain from hypoxia ➤ Abscess from microbial infection	➤ Lungs, lymph nodes, intestines ➤ Miliary tuberculosis of any organ
3. *Pathogenesis*	Changes of irreversible cell injury due to interruption in blood supply, i.e. ➤ Intracellular acidosis ➤ Nuclear changes ➤ Membrane damage ➤ Denaturation of proteins and enzymes, but no proteolysis ➤ Phagocytosis of necrotic debris	➤ Liberation of hydrolytic enzymes ➤ Digestion of dead cells from proteolysis (unlike coagulative necrosis) ➤ Central liquefaction, i.e. formation of pus in microbial inflammation, cystic cavity in infarct brain	➤ *Mycobacterium tuberculosis* engulfed by macrophages but not degraded ➤ Host responds to persisting tubercle bacilli by type 4 delayed hypersensitivity reaction ➤ Accumulation of modified macrophages (epithelioid cells) ➤ Central caseous necrosis having high lipid content derived from microbial cell wall
4. *Gross appearance*	Affected part of organ pale, firm, slightly swollen	➤ Soft liquefied centre ➤ Formation of pus in microbial infection	Dry, yellow, cheesy and granular appearance of necrotic area
5. *Microscopic features*	➤ Architecture of tissue retained but cellular details lost ➤ Cells swollen ➤ Cytoplasm more eosinophilic ➤ Necrotic changes in nuclei	➤ Architecture lost ➤ Centre of lesion necrotic, contains debris or creamy yellow pus ➤ Surrounded by gliosis in infarct brain, and granulation tissue in microbial infection	➤ Caseous centre eosinophilic and has granular debris of disintegrated nuclei ➤ Periphery composed of granulomas (epithelioid cells, giant cells, lymphocytes)

Q36. What is gangrene? Discuss salient features of its main types.

Definition Gangrene is a form of necrosis with superimposed putrefaction.
Classification Two main types of gangrene are recognised: dry gangrene and wet gangrene **(Fig. 3.12)**.

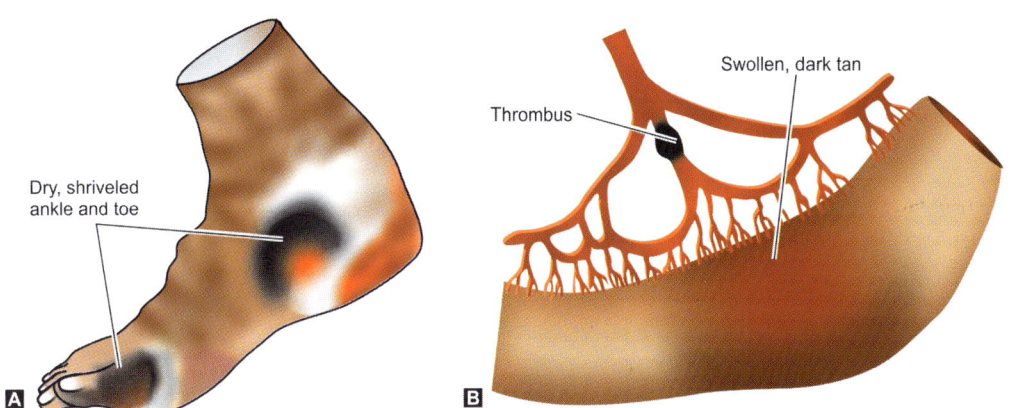

FIGURE 3.12: A, Dry gangrene of the foot. The gangrenous area is dry, shrunken and dark and is separated from the viable tissue by clear line of separation. B, Wet gangrene of the small bowel. The affected part is soft, swollen and dark. Line of demarcation between gangrenous segment and the viable bowel is not clear-cut.

I. **Dry gangrene** is an ischaemic necrosis of the *distal parts of the extremities,* with drying out of the soft tissue and skin ('mummification') and weak bacterial overgrowth.
Etiology Most often, it is caused by severe atherosclerosis and progressive ischaemia.
Less common causes are Buerger disease, ergot poisoning, and trauma.
Pathogenesis Ischaemia affects most often one of the toes, and then progressively extends to other parts of the foot.
- A line of separation is seen between the necrotic and viable tissue.
- Bacteria are present but the severe ischaemia impedes major bacterial overgrowth.

Gross The necrotic tissue is dry, black and appears 'mummified'.
Necrotic tissue may fall off the bones.
Microscopy Coagulation necrosis with smudging of all tissue outlines. The line of separation from toward normal tissue is occupied by granulation tissue.
Amputation of the gangrenous part is the treatment of choice.

II. **Wet gangrene** is ischaemic necrosis of naturally wet tissue, with massive bacterial overgrowth.
Etiology Ischaemia of rapid onset combined with bacterial overgrowth.
Pathogenesis Ischaemia and infection may affect intestines, lungs and other internal organs or the lower extremities and the skin.
- It develops faster and in a shorter period than dry gangrene.
- Ischaemia is related to the occlusion of arteries, but often amplified by venous blockade.
- Stagnant venous blood imparts the tissues a dark blue hue.
- Bacterial overgrowth because the stagnant blood provides a fertile soil.
- It lacks the demarcation line (seen in dry gangrene).
- Bacteria may enter systemic circulation, liberate bacterial toxins that are absorbed into the blood and cause generalised septicaemia with fever, leucocytosis and even septic shock.

Gross The tissue is dark, wet, swollen and has a putrid smell.
Microscopy Ischaemic necrosis of tissue suffused with blood, and liquefaction.
NOTE: *Gas gangrene* is a special form of wet gangrene caused by gas-forming Clostridia.
- Occurs following contamination of an open wound by toxin and gas-producing Clostridia, which cause tissue necrosis, oedema and *gas bubbles*. Such air bubbles cannot be seen under the microscope but can be seen on gross examination and are recognised by crepitation upon palpation.

- Tissues appear dark black and foul smelling.
- Histopathology is the same as in wet gangrene.

Q37. What are the contrasting features of dry and wet gangrene?

Contrasting features of dry and wet gangrene are shown in **Table 3.6**.

TABLE 3.6 Contrasting features of dry and wet gangrene.

FEATURE	DRY GANGRENE	WET GANGRENE
1. *Common etiology*	Arterial occlusion, e.g. atherosclerosis	Commonly venous occlusion, e.g. thrombosis
2. *Common site*	Commonly limbs	More common in bowel
3. *Mechanism*	Ischaemic-hypoxic injury → Coagulative necrosis → Little blood supply → Fewer bacteria	Infarction → Affected part stuffed with blood → Favours profuse overgrowth of bacteria
4. *Gross appearance*	i. Organ dry, shrunken and black ii. Less smell from putrefaction due to very little blood supply iii. Line of demarcation present at the junction between healthy and gangrenous part	i. Part moist, soft, swollen, rotten and dark ii. Marked odour due to profound putrefaction iii. No clear line of demarcation
5. *Microscopy*	i. Coagulative necrosis ii. Inflammatory reaction and limited bacterial growth iii. Line of demarcation at the junction of viable with gangrenous part present	i. Liquefactive necrosis ii. Inflammatory reaction and numerous bacteria iii. No clear line of demarcation at the junction
6. *Systemic manifestations*	Less pronounced	Pronounced (fever, leucocytosis)
7. *Prognosis*	Generally better due to little septicaemia	Generally poor due to profound toxaemia

Q38. Define pathologic calcification. What are its types and general morphologic features?

Definition Pathologic calcification is deposition of calcium salts in tissues other than osteoid or enamel.

Classification Two types of calcification are recognised: i) dystrophic, and ii) metastatic calcification.

I. *Dystrophic calcification* is characterised by deposition of calcium salts into:
- Dead tissues
- Degenerated tissues

II. *Metastatic calcification* is caused by deranged calcium metabolism and hypercalcaemia and it involves deposition of calcium salts in normal tissues.

Microscopy Although etiology and pathogenesis of two forms of pathologic calcification are distinct, their morphologic appearance in routine H&E stained slides is similar.
- Calcium salt deposits appear as basophilic (bluish) irregular clumps.
- They may be intracellular or extracellular or both.
- Calcium can be demonstrated by histochemical stains such as impregnation according to von Kossa (stains calcium salts black) or alizarin red S (which stains them red).

Q39. Discuss salient features of etiology and pathogenesis of dystrophic calcification.

Pathogenesis Dystrophic calcification depends on the following:
i. Very high local concentration of calcium ions.
ii. Ratio of calcium to phosphates that favours the precipitation of calcium phosphate to form hydroxyapatite.
iii. The presence of substances that promote calcification.

These events resemble calcification that occurs physiologically in the bone:
- The initiating event is cell injury and necrosis accompanied by an influx or calcium and the concomitant liberation of calcium ions from intracellular stores.
- Phosphate is liberated locally from phospholipids in damaged cell membrane and organelles.

- The high concentration of Ca and P leads to their deposition and formation of hydroxyapatite crystals.

Etiology It may occur in dead or degenerated tissues:

I. **Calcification in dead tissue** Clinically important examples are:
i. *Caseous necrosis* in lungs and lymph nodes, as well as in other sites of tuberculosis. Healed foci of tuberculosis in the lungs, seen on X-rays, are the most common form of dystrophic calcification encountered in clinical medicine.
ii. *Liquefaction necrosis* of chronic abscess
iii. *Fat necrosis* following pancreatitis or breast trauma
iv. *Gamna-Gandy bodies* in chronic passive congestion of the spleen consisting of haemosiderin encrusted fibrous scars with focal calcification
v. Damaged heart valves
vi. Venous thrombi (phleboliths, especially in the pelvic veins)
vii. Haematomas, especially in the vicinity of bones
viii. Dead parasites and their eggs (e.g. *Schistosoma haematobium* in the wall of the urinary bladder)
ix. Congenital toxoplasmosis of CNS
x. Microcalcifications in the malignant and benign beast lesions seen by mammography

II. **Calcification in degenerated tissue** Clinically important examples are:
i. Old scars
ii. Atheroma and other atherosclerotic lesions of the aorta and major arteries
iii. Mönckeberg sclerosis of arteries
iv. Stroma of some tumours, such as breast cancer, uterine fibroids, thyroid cancer
v. Nodular goitre of thyroid
vi. Psammoma bodies (calcospherites), concentric calcifications in some tumours such as meningioma, papillary serous carcinoma of the ovary, papillary carcinoma of the thyroid
vii. Cysts, such as pillar and epidermal cysts of the skin
viii. Calcinosis cutis, a disease of unknown etiology, marked by deposits of calcium salt in the skin and subcutaneous tissue
ix. Senile degenerative changes, such as calcification in tracheal and laryngeal cartilage, costal cartilage, pineal gland of the brain

Q40. Briefly discuss features of etiology and pathogenesis of metastatic calcification.

Pathogenesis Calcium which is present in blood in very high concentration binds to inorganic phosphorus and these newly formed calcium phosphates are deposited in tissue.
Metastatic calcification occurs selectively; it preferentially affects some tissues:
i. Tissues that are most frequently affected are known to produce acidic fluids (e.g. *stomach*).
ii. Organs involved in the regulation of acid-base balance (e.g. *kidneys and lungs*) are also commonly affected.
iii. For unknown reasons, calcification also occurs in *cornea* in band keratopathy and in internal elastic lamina of the *arteries*.

Etiology It occurs under two groups of conditions: i) excessive mobilisation of calcium from bone, and ii) excessive absorption of calcium from the gut.

I. **Excessive mobilisation of calcium from the bone** Clinically important examples are:
i. Hyperparathyroidism, which may be primary (e.g. parathyroid adenoma) or secondary (e.g. parathyroid hyperplasia secondary to chronic renal failure)
ii. Bone destruction by tumours (e.g. multiple myeloma, metastatic carcinoma from the breast or prostate)
iii. Paraneoplastic syndrome hypercalcaemia (e.g. breast carcinoma)
iv. Prolonged immobilisation and disuse atrophy of skeleton

II. **Excessive absorption of calcium from the gut** Clinically important examples are:
i. Hypervitaminosis D due to intake or some diseases such as sarcoidosis
ii. Milk-alkali syndrome caused by excessive intake of calcium in form of milk, pills of calcium carbonate
iii. Idiopathic hypercalcaemia of infancy (Williams syndrome)
iv. Renal tubular acidosis

Q41. Tabulate the contrasting features of dystrophic and metastatic calcification.

Contrasting features of two main forms of pathologic calcification are outlined in **Table 3.7**.

TABLE 3.7 Contrasting features of dystrophic and metastatic calcification.

FEATURE	DYSTROPHIC CALCIFICATION	METASTATIC CALCIFICATION
1. *Definition*	Deposits of calcium salts in dead and degenerated tissues	Deposits of calcium salts in normal tissues
2. *Calcium metabolism*	Normal	Deranged
3. *Serum calcium level*	Normal	Hypercalcaemia
4. *Reversibility*	Generally irreversible	Reversible upon correction of metabolic disorder
5. *Common causes*	Necrosis (caseous, liquefactive, fat, old infarcts), thrombi, haematomas, dead parasites, old scars, atheromas, Mönckeberg's sclerosis, certain tumours, cysts, calcinosis cutis	Hyperparathyroidism (due to adenoma, hyperplasia, CRF), bony destructive lesions (e.g. myeloma, metastatic carcinoma), prolonged immobilisation, hypervitaminosis D, milk-alkali syndrome, hypercalcaemia of infancy
6. *Pathogenesis*	Increased binding of phosphates with necrotic and degenerative tissue, which in turn binds to calcium forming calcium phosphate precipitates	Increased precipitates of calcium phosphate due to hypercalcaemia at certain sites
7. *Common sites*	i. Tuberculous lymphadenitis ii. Advanced atheromas iii. Medial calcification of uterine arteries in multigravida iv. Gamna-Gandy bodies in CVC spleen v. Psammoma bodies in papillary tumours, meningioma	Along the epithelial lining of intact normal tissues, e.g. i. Basement membrane of tubules in kidney ii. Alveolar lining in lungs iii. Fundic mucosa of stomach iv. Internal elastic lamina of blood vessels v. Band keratopathy in cornea

■ PROGRAMMED CELL DEATH (APOPTOSIS)

Q42. What is apoptosis?

Definition Apoptosis is a form of programmed cells death, i.e. 'coordinated and genetically programmed cell suicide', in which the cells are eliminated by activation of intrinsic enzymes in a variety of physiologic and pathologic conditions.

Q43. How does apoptosis participate in physiologic conditions?

Apoptosis is essential for maintenance of constant cell population and elimination of unwanted cells as follows:

i. *Embryonic development* and formation of tissue and organs, e.g. formation of digits and toes by apoptosis of interdigital cells; lack of apoptosis results in syndactyly.

ii. Physiologic involution and elimination of cell in *hormone-dependent tissues*, e.g. menstrual shedding of the endometrium.

iii. Programmed destruction of *surface epithelial cells* in the intestinal or skin epithelium, followed by regular replacement proliferation from the stem cells.

iv. *Loss of immature B and T cells* in the bone marrow and thymus by clonal deletion.

v. Elimination of *peripheral blood cells* that have reached the end of their life span.

Q44. How does apoptosis participate in pathologic conditions?

Apoptosis is essential for the elimination of abnormal cells, and cell that have been irreparably damaged, as follows:

i. Cells whose DNA has been *irreparably damaged* by radiation or drugs, thermal injury or hypoxia.

ii. Cells under *endoplasmic stress* which have accumulated excessive amounts of misfolded proteins (e.g. Alzheimer and Parkinson disease).

iii. Cells infected with *viruses*, such as Councilman bodies in yellow fever, HIV-infected CD4+ T lymphocytes.

iv. T-cell mediated death in *transplant rejection reactions*.
v. Pathologic atrophy of organs and tissues on *withdrawals of trophic stimuli* as in prostate atrophy after orchiectomy, atrophy of kidney due to obstruction of the urinary flow through the ureters.

Q45. Give some common examples of conditions with abnormal apoptosis.

I. **Conditions with defective apoptosis and increased cell survival:**
i. Gene *TP53* mutations lower the rate of apoptosis and, thus, enable the tumour cells to avoid apoptosis, prolonging their survival.
ii. In autoimmune diseases, defective lymphocytes are not eliminated by apoptosis, and remain in the body where they react against 'self-antigen'.

II. **Conditions with exaggerated apoptosis with higher rate of cell death:**
i. Apoptosis of non-ischaemic cardiac myocytes around the myocardial infarction may augment the initial injury and contribute to mortality in these patients.
ii. In various neurodegenerative disorders (e.g. Alzheimer or Parkinson disease), misfolded proteins and genetic events increase apoptosis of nerve cells.

Q46. What are the typical morphologic features of apoptosis?

The changes in apoptosis can be seen best by light microscopy or electron microscopy (EM) and include the following features; these are schematically shown in **Figure 3.13** in comparison with changes in necrosis:
i. Single cells or small groups of cells are affected.
ii. Apoptotic cells are round or oval shrunken and have intensely eosinophilic cytoplasm. ('mummified cells') that contain cytoplasmic organelles.
iii. Nuclear pyknosis, i.e. small shrunken and hyperchromatic nuclei.
iv. The cell membrane may form blebs or projections best seen by EM.
v. Apoptotic bodies are formed from fragmented cytoplasm.
vi. Apoptotic bodies contain intact organelles and may even contain parts of the segmented nucleus.
vii. There is no acute inflammation mediated by neutrophils.
viii. Apoptotic bodies are phagocytosed by macrophages.

NOTE: Apoptotic cells can be visualised and counted using immunohistochemical stains such as antibody to *active caspase 3* or *annexin V*; and by *fluorochrome-based TUNEL* (terminal nucleotidyl transferase dUTP end-labelling) assay by flow cytometry).

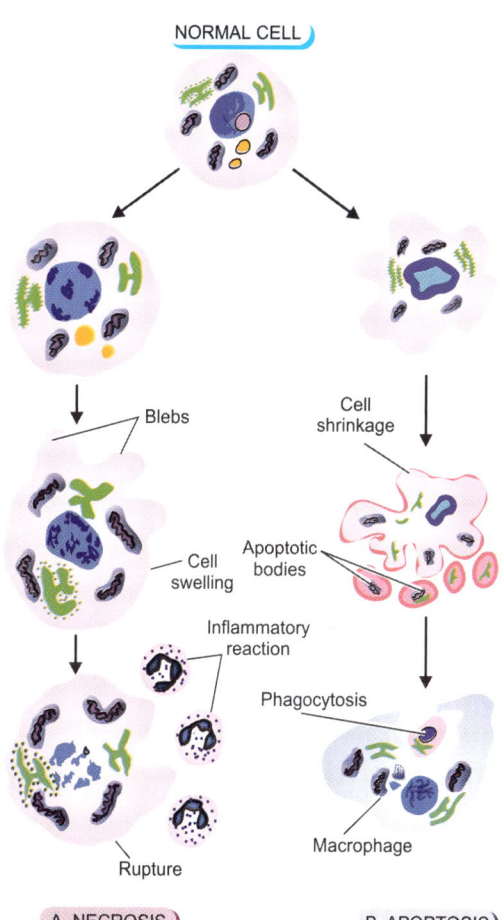

FIGURE 3.13: Necrosis and apoptosis. A, Cell necrosis is identified by homogeneous, eosinophilic cytoplasm and nuclear changes of pyknosis, karyolysis, and karyorrhexis. B, Apoptosis consists of condensation of nuclear chromatin and fragmentation of the cell into membrane-bound apoptotic bodies which are engulfed by macrophages.

Q47. What are the most important sequential biochemical changes during apoptosis?

i. *Activation of proapoptotic regulators and enzyme pathways* leading to proteolysis of cytoskeletal and nuclear proteins.

ii. *Protein-protein cross-linkage* by transaminases leading to the formation of apoptotic bodies.
iii. *DNA condensation and fragmentation* by activated endonucleases which form oligonucleosomes.
iv. *Recognition and removal of dead cells by phagocytosis.* Macrophages recognise the apoptotic cells by their surface expression of phosphatidylserine and thrombospondin.

Q48. What are the molecular mechanisms of apoptosis?

Five phases of apoptosis are recognised as follows **(Fig. 3.14)**:

I. Initiation of apoptosis
i. Withdrawal of normal cell survival signals (e.g. hormones, growth factors, cytokines, etc.)
ii. Agents of cell injury (radiation, hypoxia, toxins, free radicals, etc.)

II. Initiation of death-signaling pathway
Activation of caspases by one of two pathways:
i. *Intrinsic (mitochondrial) pathway*—antiapoptotic proteins (BCL2, BCL-XL, MCL1) in a balance with proapoptotic (BAX, BAK) and sensory proteins (BAD, BIM)
ii. *Extrinsic (cell death receptor) pathway*—Tumour necrosis factor receptor 1 (TNFR1), Fas (CD95) and Fas ligand (FasL) which activate the Fas-associated death domain (FADD). For example, FasL is expressed on cytotoxic CD8+T cells, involved in killing of virus infected and tumor cells.

III. Activation of initiator caspases
i. Forming of the apoptosome and activation of caspase 9 in mitochondrial pathway
ii. Activation of caspase 8 in the FADD pathway

IV. Activation of apoptosis-executing caspases
Two pathways of activation converge from here to *activate executioner caspases* (caspases 3 and 6) which have many DNAases, proteolytic and disruptive functions

V. Removal of dead cells
i. *Phosphatidyleserine molecule* which is normally present on the inside of the cell membrane is now on the surface of apoptotic bodies.
ii. Apoptotic bodies are also coated with *thrombospondin*.

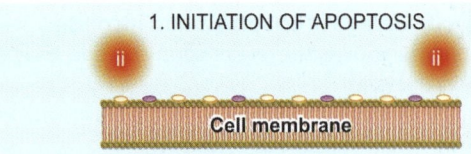

1. INITIATION OF APOPTOSIS

Cell membrane

i) *Withdrawal of normal cell survival signals*
(e.g. absence of certain hormones, growth factors, cytokines)
ii) *Agents of cell injury*
(e.g. heat, radiation, hypoxia, toxins, free radicals)

2. INITIATION OF DEATH-SIGNALLING PATHWAYS

i) *Intrinsic (mitochondrial) pathway*
(Antiapoptotic BCL family: BCL2, BCL-XL, MCL1;
proapoptotic BCL family: BAX, BAK, BAD, BIM, BID, Puma, Noxa)
ii) *Extrinsic (cell death receptor-initiated) pathway*
(TNFR1, Fas or CD95, and its ligand FasL)

3. ACTIVATION OF INITIATOR CASPASES
i) *Mitochondrial pathway*
Binding   Binding
Cytochrome-c → APAF-1 → Apoptosome → Precursor caspase-9
ii) *Death receptor-initiated pathway*
TNF-TNFR1 and Fas-Fas-L → FADD → Caspase-10 ✗→ Caspase-8
(inhibited by a protein FLIP,
FLICE-inhibitory proteins)

4. ACTIVATION OF APOPTOSIS-EXECUTING CASPASES

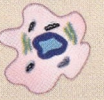 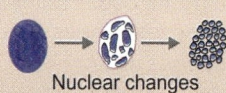

Shrunken cell   Nuclear changes

Both mitochondrial and death receptor-initiated pathways converge
Executioner caspases (3 and 6) → DNAase →
Chromatin clumping, Cytoskeletal damage, Disrupted ER,
Mitochondrial damage, Disturbed cell membrane

5. REMOVAL OF DEAD CELLS (PHAGOCYTOSIS)

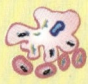

- Phosphatidylserine molecule promotes phagocytosis
- Coating with thrombospondin
- Complement system (C1q)

FIGURE 3.14: Molecular mechanism of apoptosis contrasted with sequence of morphologic changes.

Q49. What is necroptosis?

Definition Necroptosis is a form of programmed cell death that has some features of necrosis.
Pathogenesis and significance It begins with TNFR1 Fas or viruses but does not use caspases. There are many biochemical similarities with necrosis, but the contents of the cell do not leak out.
Necroptosis is involved in the following processes:
i. Formation of normal bony growth plate
ii. Viral defense
iii. Steatohepatitis
iv. Inflammatory disease like Crohn disease, pancreatitis

Q50. What are the salient contrasting features of necrosis and apoptosis?

Main distinguishing features between apoptosis and necrosis are summarised in **Table 3.8**.

TABLE 3.8 Contrasting features of necrosis and apoptosis.

FEATURE	NECROSIS	APOPTOSIS
1. Definition	Cell death along with release of hydrolytic enzymes	Programmed and coordinated cell death
2. Causes	Always pathological, various etiologic agents	May be physiological or pathological process
3. Types	Three major types: coagulative, liquefactive, caseous; others fat and fibrinoid	Classically single type; infrequently atypical types (necroptosis, pyroptosis, ferroptosis)
4. Morphology	i. Inflammatory reaction always present ii. Death of many adjacent cells iii. Cell swelling initially iv. Membrane disruption v. Damaged organelles vi. Nuclear disruption vii. Phagocytosis of cell debris by macrophages viii. Light microscopy only ix. Lysosomal breakdown with liberation of hydrolytic enzymes	i. No inflammatory reaction ii. Death of single cells iii. Cell shrinkage iv. Cytoplasmic blebs on membrane v. Apoptotic bodies vi. Chromatin condensation vii. Phagocytosis of apoptotic bodies by macrophages viii. Light microscopy, IHC for caspase-3 ix. Lysosomes and other organelles intact
5. Molecular changes	i. Initiated by various etiologic agents (ischaemia-hypoxia, toxins, chemicals, microbes, immunologic) ii. Cell death by ATP depletion, membrane damage, free radical injury	i. Initiation by loss of signals of normal cell survival and by action of agents injurious to the cell ii. Triggered by intrinsic (mitochondrial) pathway (pro- and anti-apoptotic members of BCL-2 family), extrinsic (cell death receptor initiated) pathway (TNF-R1, Fas, Fas-L) and finally by activated capases
6. Fate	i. Presence of variable inflammatory reaction ii. Phagocytosis of necrosed tissue present	i. No inflammatory reaction ii. Brisk phagocytosis of apoptotic bodies

Q51. What is pyroptosis?

Definition Pyroptosis is a form of apoptosis which is characterised by a release of fever producing interleukin 1.
Pathogenesis and significance Pyroptosis is triggered by the intracytoplasmic entry of microbial products which activate the *inflammasomes*.
i. Inflammasomes activate caspases.
ii. Caspase 11 generates interleukin 1, causing fever.
iii. Pyroptosis differs from classical apoptosis in several aspects:
- Cell swells rather than shrink or fragment.
- There is damage to the plasma membrane.
- Damaged cells release a fever-producing interleukin 1 in the cells.

Q52. What is ferroptosis?

Definition Ferroptosis is a form of cell death triggered by iron dependent (i.e. by Fenton reaction) accumulation of reactive oxygen radicals.
Iron chelating substances like desferrioxamine prevent cell death.

Q53. Define autophagy. Briefly discuss its major features.

Definition Autophagy is a physiologic process used by the cells to remove damage or effete organelles and maintain normal architecture of the cytoplasm. It is activated in response to stress, nutritional deficiency, lack of trophic hormones and various forms of cell injury, and ageing.

Pathogenesis Autophagosomes are formed from lysosome by passing through four stages (initiation, elongation, maturation into autophagosome), and achievement of the full function at the autophagolysosome stage, during which it is capable of degradation of ingested material **(Fig. 3.15)**.

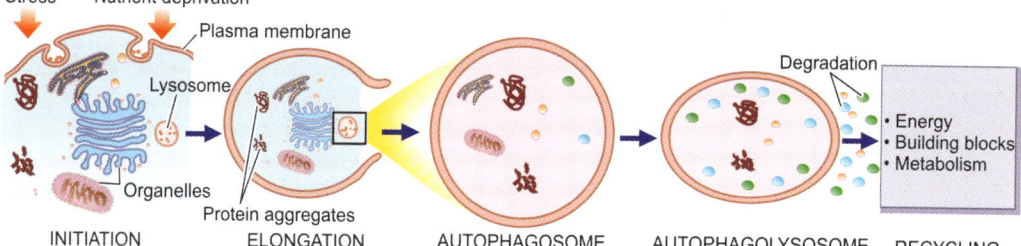

FIGURE 3.15: Mechanism and types of autophagy.

Dysregulated autophagy Autophagy plays an important role in many diseases such as:
i. Cancer: limiting cancer cell growth, reducing mutagenesis and by killing developing cancer cells.
ii. Myopathies (e.g. glycogenosis type II (Pompe disease).
iii. Neuromuscular disorders (e.g. inclusion body myositis).
iv. Neurodegenerative diseases (e.g. accelerated autophagy in Alzheimer disease).
v. Infectious diseases (autophagosomes degrade various pathogens such as mycobacteria, HSV-1, *Shigella*).
vi. Chronic inflammatory diseases such as ulcerative colitis and Crohn disease.

INTRACELLULAR ACCUMULATIONS AND PIGMENTS

Q54. What are the most important intracellular accumulations?

Abnormal intracellular accumulations can be divided into three groups:
 I. Accumulation of normal metabolites (e.g. fats, proteins and carbohydrates)
 II. Accumulation of abnormal substances produced by abnormal metabolism
 III. Abnormal of pigments

Q55. What is fatty liver? Discuss salient features in its etiology, pathogenesis and pathologic changes.

Definition Fatty liver is characterised by excessive accumulation of fat inside the hepatocytes.
- It may be mild and reversible, or severe producing irreversible cell injury and death.
- It may progress to steatohepatitis and cirrhosis, which occurs in a minority of cases.

Etiology Fatty liver can occurs in various conditions that are characterised by i) excess fat in the body, or ii) liver cell damage.
I. *Conditions with excess fat*
i. Obesity
ii. Diabetes mellitus
iii. Congenital hyperlipidaemia
II. *Liver cell damage*
i. Alcoholic liver disease
ii. Starvation

iii. Protein caloric malnutrition
iv. Chronic systemic diseases (e.g. tuberculosis)
v. Acute fatty liver of pregnancy
vi. Hypoxia (e.g. anaemia, cardiac failure)
vii. Hepatotoxins (e.g. carbon tetrachloride, chloroform, ether, aflatoxin, etc.)
viii. Drug-induced liver cell injury
ix. Viral hepatis C
x. Reye syndrome

Pathogenesis Fatty liver, characterised by excessive accumulation of triglycerides (TG), occurs due to a disturbance of one or more of the following six steps in the normal fat metabolism **(Fig. 3.16)**:
i. Increased entry of free fatty acids into the liver
ii. Increased synthesis of fatty acids by the liver
iii. Decreased conversion of fatty acids into ketone bodies resulting in increased esterification of fatty acids to TG
iv. Increased α-glycerophosphate causing increased esterification of fatty acids to TG
v. Decreased synthesis of 'lipid acceptor protein' resulting in decreased formation of lipoprotein from TG
vi. Block in excretion of lipoproteins from the liver into plasma

Pathology Grossly, the liver is enlarged, has rounded edges, and appears heavy, greasy and yellow.

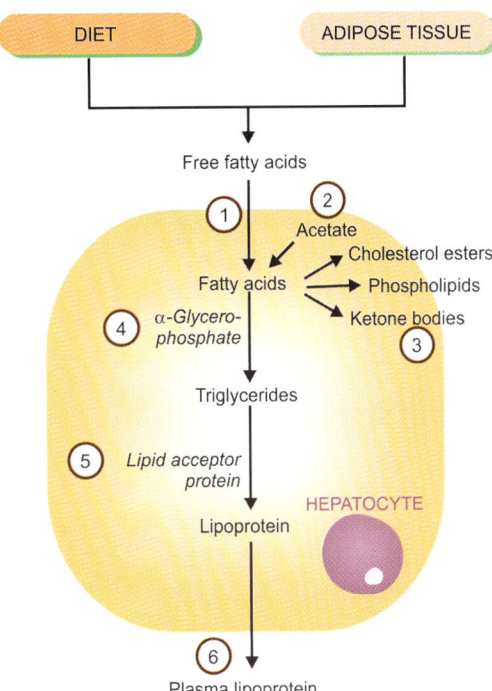

FIGURE 3.16: Lipid metabolism in the pathogenesis of fatty liver. Defects in any of the six numbered steps (corresponding to the description in the text) can produce fatty liver by different etiologic agents.

Microscopy
i. Fat accumulation leads to vacuolisation of liver cell cytoplasm (*microvesicular or macrovesicular steatosis*).
ii. Fat-laden liver cells may rupture, forming fatty cysts, and eliciting formation of lipogranulomas or pericellular fibrosis and inflammation (in transition to *steatohepatitis* and *cirrhosis* in a minority of cases) **(Fig. 3.17)**.
iii. Fat can be demonstrated in frozen sections histochemically with special stains such as Sudan II or IV, Oil Red O; osmic acid stain for fat is the best method for electron microscopic studies.

NOTE:
- Parenchymal fatty change can occur in *other organs* besides the liver (e.g. heart, kidney). It occurs less often, and is of no clinical significance.
- *Stromal fatty infiltration*, i.e. appearance of fat cells in the stroma of parenchymal organs (e.g. heart, or skeletal muscle), is encountered in obese persons, but it is of no clinical significance.

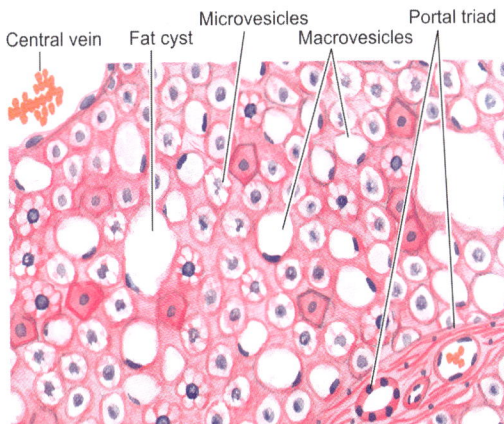

FIGURE 3.17: Fatty liver. Many of the hepatocytes are distended with large fat vacuoles pushing the nuclei to the periphery (macrovesicles), while others show multiple small vacuoles in the cytoplasm (microvesicles).

Q56. What is the significance of intracellular glycogen accumulation?

Glycogen accumulation occurs in several diseases and is usually associated with i) hyperglycaemia or ii) disturbances of intermediary metabolism, as follows:

I. *In diabetes mellitus*, glycogen accumulates in patients with poorly controlled diabetes and long-standing hyperglycaemia. Glycogen accumulates in renal tubules, hepatocytes, cardiac myocytes and the cells of pancreatic islets.

II. *Genetic glycogen storage diseases* lead to the accumulation of glycogen in various organs such as liver, skeletal and cardiac muscle.

Pathology The cells containing large amounts of glycogen have clear cytoplasm. Glycogen can be demonstrated histochemically with Best carmine, or PAS reaction, combined with predigestion of the tissue with amylase (it removes glycogen from the tissue).

Q57. What are pigments in the body and their types?

Pigments are coloured substances, which in the human body can be classifies as a) endogenous, or b) exogeneous **(Table 3.9)**.

Q58. What is melanin? Give a list of the most important melanin-related pathologic changes.

Definition Melanin is brown-black pigment formed from tyrosine through action of tyrosinase. It is normally present in the melanocytes of the skin and hair, choroid of the eye, meninges and adrenal medulla; it is also seen in some mucosal sites such as the oral cavity, oesophagus and anal canal. Melanin can be stained with the Masson-Fontana silver stain and can be demonstrated by the dihydroxy phenyl alanine (DOPA) reaction.

TABLE 3.9 Pigments of the body.

A. ENDOGENOUS PIGMENTS
1. Melanin
2. Melanin-like pigment
    i. Alkaptonuria
    ii. Dubin-Johnson syndrome
3. Haemoprotein-derived pigments
    i. Haemosiderin
    ii. Haematin (Haemazoin)
    iii. Bilirubin
    iv. Porphyrins
4. Lipofuscin (Wear and tear pigment)

B. EXOGENOUS PIGMENTS
1. Inhaled pigments
2. Ingested pigments
3. Injected pigments (Tattooing)

Melanin-related pathologic conditions Pathologic conditions related to melanin can be classified as:
- *Hyperpigmentation*: generalised and focal
- *Hypopigmentation*: generalised and localised

I. **Generalised hyperpigmentation**

i. *Addison disease* causes hyperpigmentation of the skin, especially sun-exposed areas, and oral mucosa.

ii. *Chloasma* is the hyperpigmentation of skin of the face, nipples and genital organs during pregnancy under the influence of oestrogen. Oral contraceptives and exogenous oestrogen can produce the same changes, which are, however, reversible.

II. **Focal hyperpigmentation**

i. *Café-au-lait spots* on the skin in neurofibromatosis type I and Albright syndrome.

ii. *Freckles* are genetically determines small hyperpigmented macules in fair skinned persons similar to café-au-lait spot, but smaller. They contain a normal number of melanocytes which have an increased number of cytoplasmic melanosomes, becoming darker upon exposure to sunshine.

iii. *Lentigo* is a pigmented small skin macule which contains an increased number of melanocytes. It does not become darker upon exposure to sunshine. Some lentigines are composed of malignant melanocytes and these tend to grow by spreading laterally (*'lentigo maligna'*, or *'superficial spreading melanoma'*).

iv. *Naevus* is congenital pigmented skin lesion ('mole') composed of pigmented naevus cells.

v. *Malignant melanoma* is a pigmented malignant tumour composed of malignant melanocytes.

vi. *Peutz-Jeghers syndrome* is characterised by focal peri-oral pigmentation associated with intestinal polyposis.

vii. *Dermatopathic lymphadenitis* is a characterised by the deposition of melanin pigment in macrophages in lymph nodes draining irriated skin lesions.

III. **Generalised hypopigmentation**

Albinism is a genetic deficiency of tyrosinase resulting in a lack of skin and eye pigmentation.
- Affected persons are sensitive to sunlight and develop skin cancer at an increased rate.

- They have blond hair.
- They lack eye pigmentation and suffer from poor vision and severe photophobia.

IV. **Localised hypopigmentation**

i. *Leucoderma* begins as localised hypopigmentation, often with family history and may start following physical trauma, but eventually leads to total loss of pigmentation.

ii. *Vitiligo* is an ongoing loss of pigmentation, often on sunexposed areas. It is mainly triggered by autoimmune conditions.

iii. *Acquired local hypopigmentation* develops as a consequence of various skin diseases, such as leprosy, discoid lupus erythematosus, irradiation of the skin or at the site of wound healing.

NOTE: Melanin must be distinguished from melanin-like pigments, including the following:
- *Ochronosis pigment* in alkaptonuria, a genetic disease related to deficiency of an oxidative enzyme that is essential for the breakdown of homogentisic acid. Homogentisic acid gets deposited in tissues and becomes yellowish-brown when oxidised. Oxidation of homogentisic acid in urine occurs when urine turns its colour to black if the sample is allowed to stand on fresh air.
- *Dubin-Johnson syndrome*, a form of familial conjugated hyperbilirubinaemia, is characterised by the deposition of a melanin-like pigment in liver cells, rendering the liver black on gross examination.

Q59. What are the most important haemoprotein-derived pigments?

I. **Hemosiderin**

i. Brown granular pigment derived from aggregates of transferrin (iron complexed to apoferritin).

ii. It contains ferric iron that can be demonstrated by the Prussian blue reaction (potassium ferrocyanide reacting with ferric iron of haemosiderin forms deep blue ferric-ferrocyanide).

II. **Haematin (haemazoin)**

i. Also known as brown-black pigment of malaria, found in liver cells and tissue macrophages.

ii. Also formed after massive haemolysis due to mismatched blood transfusions.

iii. It contains ferric iron in an acid medium.

iv. Cannot be demonstrated by the Prussian blue reaction.

III. **Bilirubin**

i. Yellow non-iron containing pigment of the bile.

ii. Also present in small amounts in the circulating blood, accounting for its yellow colour of serum.

iii. Excessive hyperbilirubinaemia produces jaundice, which appears as yellow sclerae, skin and many other tissue and fluids. Deposits of bilirubin in the basal ganglia of the brain lead to brain injury (kernicterus).

IV. **Porphyrins**

i. Porphyrins are normal pigments present in haemoglobin, myoglobin and cytochrome.

ii. Clinical porphyria with an excess of porphyrin pigment results from genetic deficiency of the enzyme required for the synthesis of haem.

iii. Porphyrias are associated with excretion of intermediate products in urine: delta aminolevulinic acid, porphobilinogen, uroporphyrin, coproporphyrin, protoporphyrin.

iv. Often precipitated by drugs.

Q60. What is haemosiderosis? Brielfy discuss its classification and salient clinicopathologic features.

Definition Haemosiderosis is excessive accumulation of haemosiderin in the body.

Types (Fig. 3.18)

I. ***Based on pathogenesis and morphologic location***, it may occur in two forms:

i. *Reticuloendothelial (RE) deposition* of haemosiderin occurs in the cells of the liver, spleen and bone marrow. It is caused by repeated blood transfusions and/or parenteral administration of iron.

HAEMOSIDEROSIS	
LOCALISED	GENERALISED (SYSTEMIC)
LOCAL TISSUES (Macrophages, fibroblasts, endothelial and alveolar cells)	PARENCHYMAL DEPOSITS (Liver, pancreas, kidney, heart, skin) RE CELL DEPOSITS (Liver, spleen, bone marrow)
Examples: i. Haemorrhage in tissues ii. Black eye iii. Brown induration lung iv. Infarction	Examples: I. Acquired haemosiderosis (Chronic haemolytic disorders, blood transfusion, parenteral administration of iron) ii. Excessive dietary intake (African iron overload) iii. Haemochromatosis (inborn error of metabolism, autosomal recessive)

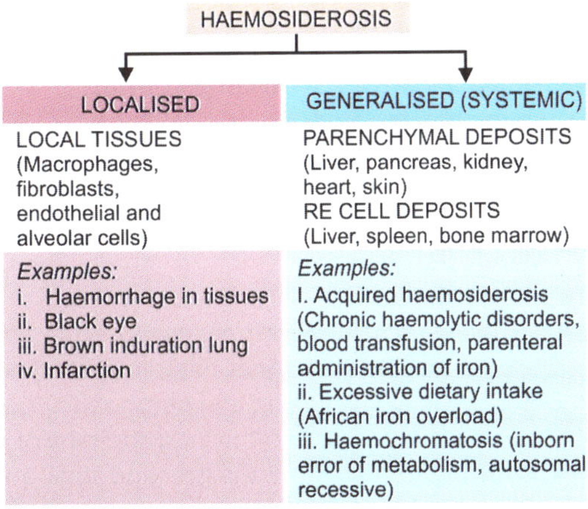

FIGURE 3.18: Consequences of iron overload in the body.

ii. *Parenchymal deposition* of haemosiderin involves the liver, pancreas, kidney, heart. It is caused by genetic haemochromatosis.

II. **Based on etiology and distribution,** there are four types of excessive iron storage:

i. *Localised haemosiderosis* develops following haemorrhage into the tissue. Haemoglobin is taken up from haemolysed RBCs and stored in macrophages. Examples are:
a. Organising haematoma
b. Brown induration of the lungs linked to repeated extravasations of blood in left heart failure and consequent pulmonary hypertension
c. Pigmented villonodular synovitis, a tumour-like proliferation of synovium, with accumulation of haemosiderin inside the joint

ii. *Systemic (generalised) haemosiderosis* is related to systemic iron overload. For example:
a. Chronic haemolytic anaemia with excessive breakdown of RBCs and release of iron from haemoglobin
b. Multiple blood transfusions
c. Sideroblastic anaemia
d. Alcohol-related liver cirrhosis with an overload of iron in Kupffer cells

iii. *African iron overload*, though originally to be related consumption of alcohol brewed in iron utensils, but now known to be related to the mutation of the gene ferroportin, not fully known yet but possibly a *variant of HFE gene*.

iv. *Haemochromatosis,* a hereditary disease characterised by excessive absorption of iron.
- Autosomal recessive mutation of haemochromatosis genes, like *HFE,* which control the synthesis of hepcidin.
- *Hepcidin* regulates absorption of iron in the small intestine and its malfunction leads to excessive absorption of iron from food.

Pathology Deposits of haemosiderin are found in the liver, pancreas, skin and heart.

Clinical features Bronze diabetes with liver and heart disease that includes:
i. Skin hyperpigmentation
ii. Diabetes mellitus
iii. Cirrhosis of the liver
iv. Heart failure

Q61. What is porphyria? Discuss its classification and salient features of main types.

Definition Uncommon genetic disorder of porphyrin metabolism due to the deficiency of one of the several genes involved in the synthesis of haem, with subsequent excessive production of porphyrins.

Classification Porphyrias are broadly of two types: i) erythropoietic porphyria, and ii) hepatic porphyria.

I. **Erythropoietic porphyrias** are due to defective synthesis of haem in red blood cell precursors in the bone marrow. Two subtypes:
i. *Congenital erythropoietic porphyria*—accumulation of uroporphyrin and coproporphyrin.
- Red urine due to excretion of porphyrins
- Skin is photosensitive
- Skin and bones show red-brown discoloration

ii. *Erythropoietic protoporphyria* marked by excessive protoporphyrin but no excess of porphyrin in urine.

II. **Hepatic porphyrias** are more common. They have normal erythroid precursors but a defect in synthesis of haem in the liver. Clinical subtypes are as follows:
i. *Acute intermittent porphyria*, characterised by acute episodes.
- Episodes may be abdominal, neurological or psychotic.
- Delta aminolaevulinic acid and porphobilinogen are excreted in urine.

ii. *Porphyria cutanea tarda* is the *most common* of all porphyrias.
- Porphyrins accumulate in the liver and small amounts are excreted in urine.
- Skin lesions are similar to variegate porphyria.

- Most patients have haemosiderosis and cirrhosis with a potential to develop hepatocellular carcinoma.

iii. *Mixed (variegate) porphyrias* are rare. Its features are:
- Skin photosensitivity.
- Acute episodes with abdominal and neurological manifestations.

Q62. What is lipofuscin? Describe its salient features.

Definition Lipofuscin is the yellowish-brown, lipid rich, intracellular pigment found in atrophic and ageing cells (also known as 'brown pigment of ageing', and 'wear and tear pigment'). It may be seen in:
i. Cardiac myocytes in brown atrophy of the heart
ii. Hepatocytes of ageing persons
iii. Leydig cells in testicular atrophy
iv. Neurons in ageing brains and senile dementia
v. Cells of any tissue in chronic wasting diseases

Pathogenesis
- In ageing or debilitating diseases, the phospholipid end-products of membrane damage, mediated by oxygen free radicals, fail to get eliminated by intracellular lipid peroxidation.
- These, therefore, persist as collections of indigestible material in the *lysosomes*; thus lipofuscin is an example of *residual bodies*.

Pathology
- By *light microscopy*, the pigment is coarse, golden-brown granular and often accumulates in the central part of the cells around the nuclei (**Fig. 3.19**). The pigment can be stained by fat stains but differs from other lipids in being fluorescent and having positive acid-fast staining.
- By electron microscopy, lipofuscin appears as intralysosomal electron-dense granules in perinuclear location.

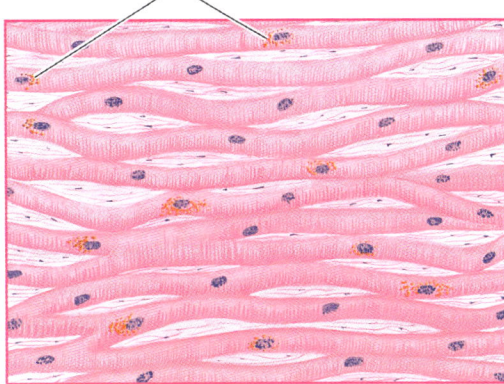

FIGURE 3.19: Brown atrophy of the heart. The lipofuscin pigment granules are seen in the cytoplasm of the myocardial fibres, especially around the nuclei.

Q63. What are the exogenous pigments?

Exogenous pigments can be classified according to their entry into the body as i) inhaled, ii) ingested, and iii) injected pigments

I. **Inhaled pigments** These pigments are inhaled in polluted air and are deposited in the lung macrophages and interstitial tissue spaces. They may cause fibrosis and pneumoconiosis. For example:
i. *Anthracosis*—carbon particles; most prominent in coal miners, and smokers (**Fig. 3.20**).
ii. *Silico-anthracosis*—silica crystals combined with carbon particles, most often in stone masons.

II. **Ingested pigments** Examples are:
i. *Argyria*—silver compounds that cause brownish pigmentation of the skin, bowel, kidneys.
ii. *Lead poisoning*—blue lines on the gums and in the teeth appear in chronic poisoning.
iii. *Melanosis coli*—chronic ingestion of cathartics leads to grossly visible brown discoloration of the

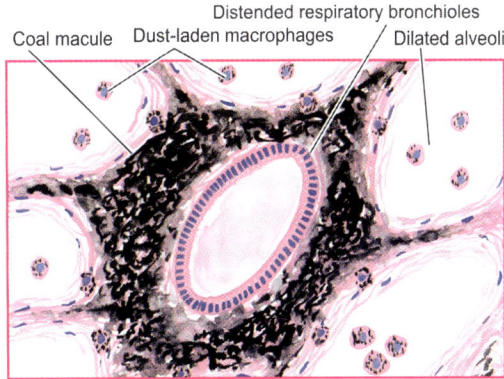

FIGURE 3.20: Anthracosis lung. There is presence of abundant coarse black carbon pigment in the septal walls and around the bronchiole.

colon. There is microscopic accumulation of pigment in macrophages in the lamina propria of the mucosa.

iv. *Carotenaemia*—ingestion of carrots that contain carotene causing yellowish-red discoloration of the skin.

III. **Injected pigments**

i. The best known example is dermal tattoos.

ii. Injected pigments such as India ink, cinnabar or particulate carbon are taken up by macrophages and lie permanently in the dermal connective tissue.

iii. Accidental introduction of pigments into tissue (e.g. during dental procedures or dust particle entry into wounds) has the same consequences.

> **Chapter 3e Supplement: Online Content**
>
> *Digital content of this chapter available with this book is meant for enhanced learning and self-assessment. In addition, it contains 25 Multiple Choice Questions (MCQs), 05 Clinicopathologic Vignettes, and 06 Image-based Questions; these are followed by their answers along with explanatory notes of correct and incorrect answers.*

CHAPTER 4

Inflammation and Repair

■ DEFINITION AND GENERAL FEATURES

Q1. Define inflammation. Briefly comment on its etiology.

Definition Inflammation is local response of living mammalian tissues to injury from any agent. It is a body defense reaction to eliminate or limit the spread of injurious agent, followed by removal of the necrosed cells and tissues.
Etiology Inflammation may be caused by numerous injurious agents, the most important of which are the following:
i. Infectious agents
ii. Necrotic tissues resulting from the action of ischaemia, physical agents (e.g. heat, cold, mechanical force, etc.), chemical agents
iii. Immunologic agents
iv. Inert foreign material such as sutures or thorns
Pathophysiology Infection involves two processes: *inflammatory response* and *repair*.
Classification According to the duration and the defense capacity of the organism, there are two principal forms of inflammation: *acute and chronic inflammation*.

Q2. What are the cardinal signs of inflammation?

The cardinal signs of inflammation, as described by the Roman medical writer Celsus, and expanded by Galen are as follows:
i. *Rubor* (redness)
ii. *Tumor* (swelling)
iii. *Calor* (heat)
iv. *Dolor* (pain)
v. *Functio laesa* (loss of function)

■ ACUTE INFLAMMATORY RESPONSE

Q3. How does inflammation begin?

Inflammation begins through the interaction of i) receptors on the etiologic agent and the host cells, as well as ii) some host proteins in the interstitial tissue and blood.
I. Receptors on etiologic agents and host cells Three sets of receptors play a key role in the initiation of inflammation. They are expressed on: i) infectious agents (e.g. pathogen associated molecular patterns, PAMPs), ii) necrotic cells, and iii) leucocytes.
i. *Receptors for the recognition of microbes* These include several proteins expressed on lymphocytes, macrophages and many other participating cells. The most important of these receptors are toll-like receptors (TLR), NOD-like receptors (NLRs) and RIG-like receptors (RIR).

ii. *Receptors for recognition of necrotic cells* Cytosolic and nuclear molecules released from necrotic leucocytes react with cytosolic receptors such as NLRs, forming inflammasomes, which directly activate caspase-1, triggering the release of proinflammatory cytokines, such as interleukin-1.

iii. *Receptors for the opsonised microbes* Two most important opsonins, the Fc component of immunoglobulins and C3 component of the complement system, are ligands for the receptors on leucocytes, thus stimulating inflammation.

II. **Circulating host proteins** These initiators of inflammation are certain circulating proteins liberated by activation of complement system after microbial infection. These include:
i. mannose-binding lectins, and
ii. collectins.
These act against invading organisms and trigger inflammation.

Q4. What are the key events in acute inflammatory response?

There are two principal components of the acute inflammatory response:
I. **Vascular events** These include:
i. Haemodynamic changes
ii. Altered vascular permeability
II. **Cellular events** These are:
i. Exudation of leucocytes
ii. Phagocytosis

Q5. What is the sequence of haemodynamic changes in acute inflammation?

i. *Transient vasoconstriction* of arterioles, that lasts 3–5 seconds, except in more severe injury when it can last longer, up to 5 minutes.
ii. *Persistent progressive vasodilatation*, involving all compartments of the microcirculation. It is obvious within half an hour and it accounts for the increased blood volume and redness of the involved area.
iii. *Increased local hydrostatic pressure* and transudation of the fluids into the extracellular space.
iv. *Slowing or stasis* of microcirculation and increased viscosity of the blood.
v. *Margination of leucocytes* along the endothelium, followed by their emigration into the perivascular spaces.

Q6. What is the triple response in Lewis 'flare and wheel' experiment?

Lewis experiment included stroking the skin of the forearm with a blunt point object. The response included sequentially the following changes, corresponding to signs of inflammation (redness, heat and swelling) as follows **(Fig. 4.1)**:
i. *Red line* due to the dilatation of the capillaries and venules.
ii. *Flare* of reddish colour surrounding the red line due to the vasodilation of arterioles.
iii. *Wheel* of the surrounding skin due to transudation of fluids to form oedema.

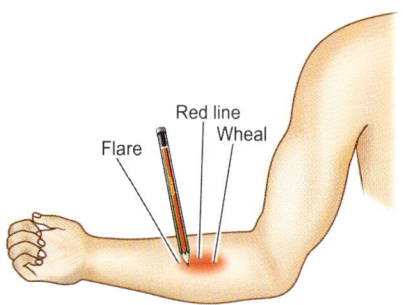 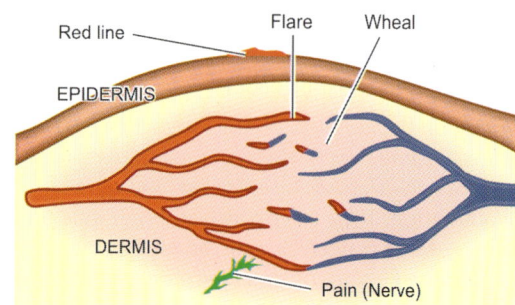

FIGURE 4.1: A, 'Triple response' elicited by firm stroking of skin of forearm with a pencil. B, Diagrammatic view of microscopic features of triple response of the skin.

Q7. What are the mechanisms of oedema formation due to altered vascular permeability?

These are as under **(Fig. 4.2):**

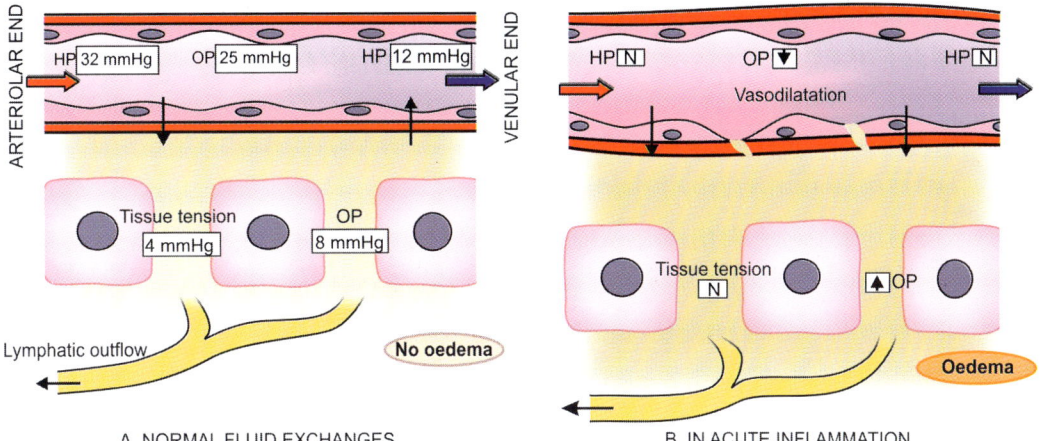

FIGURE 4.2: Fluid interchange between blood and extracellular fluid (ECF).
(HP, hydrostatic pressure; OP, osmotic pressure).

i. Transudation of fluid due to increased intravascular pressure following vasodilation of arterioles and the flooding of the microcirculation with arterial blood.
ii. Increased permeability of blood vessel walls.
iii. Increased colloid osmotic pressure of the interstitial fluid that now contains more albumin.
iv. Decreased intravascular colloid osmotic pressure due to a loss of albumin from circulating blood.

Q8. What are the mechanisms of increased vascular leakiness?

These changes include the following **(Fig. 4.3):**

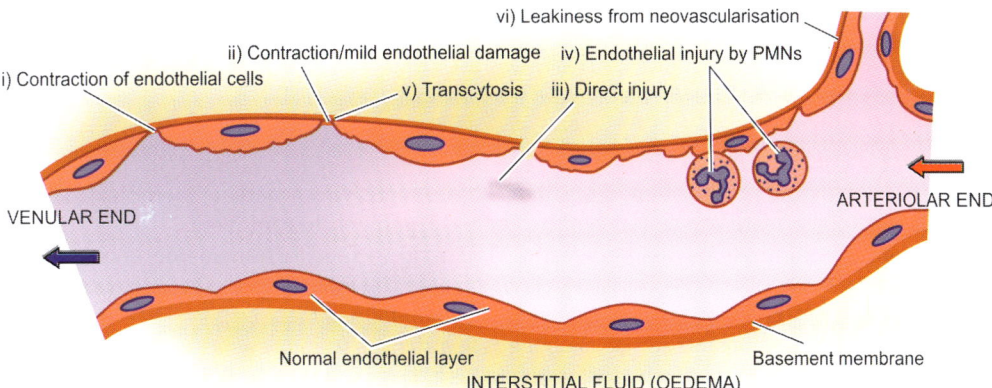

FIGURE 4.3: Schematic illustration of pathogenesis of increased vascular permeability in acute inflammation. The serial numbers in the figure correspond to six numbers described in the text.

i. *Contraction of endothelial cells,* e.g. transient, short (15–30 minutes) response to mild thermal injury. It is mediated by histamine and bradykinin and other mediators of inflammation. It affects venules and it is the most common form of increased vascular leakiness.
ii. *Contraction/mild damage of endothelial cells,* e.g. longer reaction (4–6 hours) sunburn skin injury, mediated by interleukin-1 (IL-1) and tumour necrosis factor-α (TNF-α).
iii. *Direct injury,* e.g. severe bacterial infection or moderate thermal and irradiation injury. It may start immediately or be delayed in onset. It affects all parts of the microcirculation, and lasts hours and days and may be associated with thrombosis.
iv. *Endothelial cell injury by PMNs,* e.g. pulmonary oedema due to the adherence of leucocytes to endothelial cells in lung capillaries. It is a late response affecting venules.

v. *Transcytosis,* e.g. VEGF-induced oedema.
vi. *Leakiness from neovascularisation,* e.g. granulation tissue or oedema in tumours.

Q9. What are the cellular events during the exudation of leucocytes?

The sequential changes are illustrated in **Figure 4.4** and listed as follows:

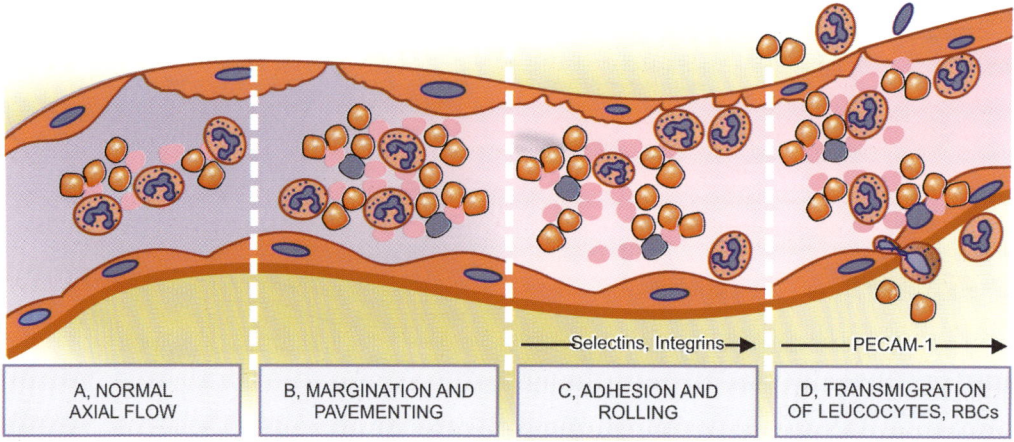

FIGURE 4.4: Sequence of changes in the exudation of leucocytes. A, Normal axial flow of blood with central column of cells and peripheral zone of cell-free plasma. B, Margination and pavementing of neutrophils with narrow plasmatic zone. C, Adhesion of neutrophils to endothelial cells with pseudopods in the intercellular junctions. D, Emigration of neutrophils and diapedesis with damaged basement membrane.

i. **Margination** of PMNs due to the blood flow changes, followed by pavementing of PMNs on the surface of endothelial cells.
ii. **Rolling** of PMNs and their early contact with endothelial cells mediated by selectins. Stronger **adhesion** of PMNs to endothelial cells is mediated by integrins.
iii. **Transmigration** or **diapedesis** is mediated by platelet-endothelial cell adhesion molecule (PECAM-1 or CD31). RBCs may passively follow it and this gives the exudate a haemorrhagic appearance.
iv. **Chemotaxis** and movement of PMNs toward the chemoattractants.

Q10. What are chemoattractants? How are they classified?

Definition Chemoattractants are biologically active compounds, which mediate chemotaxis, i.e. they direct the neutrophils (PMNs) to migrate along a chemical gradients toward them.
Pathogenesis of cell movement Chemoattractants bind to specific transmembrane G-protein coupled receptors (GPCR), which upon activation, increase the influx into the cytoplasm of PMNs, leading to cytoskeletal changes, resulting in directional migration of these cells.
Classification Chemoattractants can be exogenous (e.g. derived from bacteria) or endogenous:
I. *Exogenous chemoattractants* are mostly formylated peptides.
II. *Endogenous chemoattractants* include several groups of substances as given below:
i. Leukotriene B4 formed from arachidonic acid through the lipoxygenase pathway
ii. Activated fragments of the complement system like C5a
iii. Cytokines such as IL-8, MCP-1, MIP
iv. Kallikrein

Q11. Define phagocytosis. How do leucocytes phagocytise microbes?

Definition Phagocytosis is a cellular process during which the cells engulf solid particles. Microbes are phagocytised like any other foreign material by two types of cells:
- Polymorphonuclear leucocytes (PMNs) called microphages
- Circulating monocytes and their descendant in tissue called macrophages

Phagocytosis of microbes is a specialised form of phagocytosis, which occurs in three phases: i) recognition, ii) engulfment, and iii) killing and degradation **(Fig. 4.5)**.

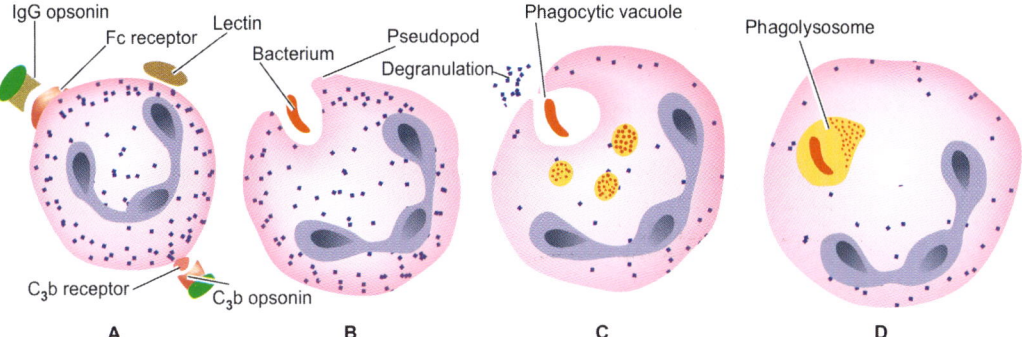

FIGURE 4.5: Stages in phagocytosis of a foreign particle. A, Opsonisation of the particle. B, Pseudopod engulfing the opsonised particle. C, Incorporation within the cell (phagocytic vacuole) and degranulation. D, Phagolysosome formation after fusion of lysosome of the cell.

I. *Recognition* is mediated by mannose receptor and scavenger receptor on the cell membrane of macrophages. It is facilitated by opsonisation with one of the following three *opsonins:*
i. C3b component of complement
ii. Fc part of IgG
iii. Collectins (carbohydrate binding lectin in the plasma which bind to the bacterial wall).
II. *Engulfment* involves formation of a phagocytic invagination of the plasma membrane which becomes a vesicle called phagosome.
Phagosomes fuse with lysosomes forming *phagolysosomes*. Phagolysosome is a membrane-bound vesicle that contains the microbe and is full of lysosomal lytic enzymes.
III. *Killing and degradation* in the phagolysosomes is mediated by the following substances:
i. Reactive oxygen species generation which may be:
- myeloperoxidase (MPO) dependent, or
- myeloperoxidase independent
ii. Nitric oxide (mostly in macrophages and endothelial cells)
iii. Lysosomal enzymes (in PMNs and macrophages)

Q12. Which is the most efficient form of bacterial killing?

Reactive oxygen species (ROS) are the most potent bactericidal substances in the phagolysosomes containing microbes. They include superoxide, hydrogen peroxide and hydroxyl radical, and halide derivatives such as hypochlorous acid.
ROS are generated by two ways:
- MPO dependent, and
- MPO independent pathway.

These include several steps:
i. Both processes begin with an oxygen burst mediated by *NADPH oxidase,* resulting in the production of superoxide anion.
ii. *MPO dependent system* works in PMNs and monocytes. It involves a conversion of superoxide into hydrogen peroxide, which is then converted by MPO into *hypochlorous acid,* in the presence of chloride ion.
iii. *MPO independent system* takes place in mature macrophages which lack the enzyme MPO and, therefore, cannot form halide derivatives like hypochlorous acid. Instead, macrophages form *hydroxyl radical and superoxide* that have a less potent bactericidal activity.

Q13. Which extracellular mechanisms are used for bacterial killing?

i. **Release of granules** from the cytoplasm of PMNs and macrophages floods the tissue with lytic enzymes, which have bactericidal activity. Unfortunately, these lytic enzymes act non-selectively; they not only kill microbes but may also cause tissue damage by proteolysis.
ii. Another mechanism is formation of **neutrophil extracellular traps** (NETs), a fibrillar network composed of nuclear material of dead neutrophils. This fibrillar network may trap microbes and prevent the spread of infection.
iii. **Immune mechanism** also provides a defense against the bacteria.

CHEMICAL MEDIATORS OF INFLAMMATION

Q14. What are the common properties of all chemical mediators of inflammation?

Mediators of inflammation have the following common properties:
i. They belong to two groups: cell derived and plasma derived.
- *Cell derived mediators* are stored in cytoplasmic granules from which they are released when needed.
- *Plasma derived mediators* circulate in an inactive form in blood and require activation. Most of these plasma proteins are synthesised by the liver.

ii. Spectrum of their actions include the following: increased vascular permeability, vasodilation, chemotaxis, fever, pain and tissue damage.
iii. Mediators have a short life span after their release.
iv. All mediators are released in response to certain stimuli.
v. Mediators act on different targets.

Q15. Classify chemical mediators of inflammation.

Two main groups of substances acting as chemical mediators of inflammation—released from the cells and those from the plasma proteins, and members in each group are listed in **Table 4.1**.

TABLE 4.1 Mediators of inflammation.

I. CELL-DERIVED MEDIATORS
1. Vasoactive amines (Histamine, 5-hydroxytryptamine, neuropeptides)
2. Arachidonic acid metabolites (eicosanoids)
i. Metabolites via cyclo-oxygenase pathway (prostaglandins, thromboxane A_2, prostacyclin, resolvins)
ii. Metabolites via lipo-oxygenase pathway (5-HETE, leukotrienes, lipoxins)
3. Cytokines: interleukins (IL-1, IL-6, IL-8, IL-12, IIL-17) TNF -α, TNF-β; IFN-γ; other chemokines
4. Platelet activating factor
5. Free radicals (oxygen intermediates, nitric oxide)
II. PLASMA PROTEIN-DERIVED MEDIATORS (PLASMA PROTEASES) PRODUCTS OF:
1. The kinin system (kallikrein, bradykinin)
2. The clotting system (fibrin, firinopeptides)
3. The fibrinolytic system (plasmin)
4. The complement system (C3a, C3b, C5a, MAC)

Q16. Discuss histamine as a chemical mediator of inflammation briefly.

Storage site Biogenic amine stored in cytoplasmic granules of basophils, mast cells and platelets.
Stimulants for release Agents in acute inflammation, e.g. heat, cold, trauma, irritant chemicals, irradiation, type I hypersensitivity (anaphylactic or allergic) reaction.
Actions Acts on blood vessels and nerves:
i. Vasodilation of arterioles
ii. Increased vascular permeability
iii. Itching
iv. Pain
NOTE: Histamine is similar to another biogenic amine which has similar actions, i.e. *serotonin (5-hydroxytryptamin);* the latter is stored in platelets granules. Serotonin has similar pro-inflammatory activities as histamine, even though serotonin actions are much weaker.

Q17. Which are the mediators of inflammation produced from the arachidonic acid and how are they formed?

Arachidonic acid (eicosanoids) derivatives are the most potent mediators of inflammation. They are fatty acids released from the phospholipids in the cell membrane through the action of phospholipases. The biologically active derivatives are formed through one of the two pathways: cyclo-oxygenase pathway and lipo-oxygenase pathways **(Fig. 4.6)**:
I. **Cyclo-oxygenases** (two enzymes, COX-1 and COX-2) generate the following biologically active compounds:
i. Prostaglandins

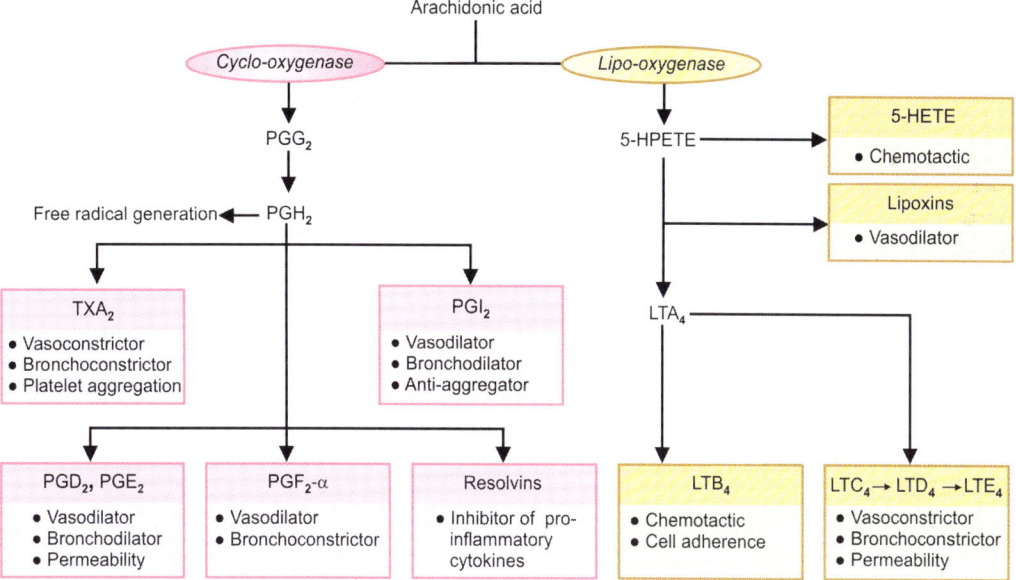

FIGURE 4.6: Arachidonic acid metabolites via cyclooxygenase and lipo-oxygenase pathway and their major actions.

ii. Prostacycline (also known as PGI_2)
iii. Thromboxane
iv. Resolvins

II. **Lipo-oxygenase** (an enzyme most abundant in PMNs) acts on the activated arachidonic acid to form hydroxyperoxy-eicosatetraenoic acid (5-HPETE), which then gives rise to:
i. 5-HETE, a potent chemoattractant of neutrophils
ii. Leukotrienes (chemoattractants, bronchoconstrictors, and vasoconstrictors)
iii. Lipoxins (vasodilators, bronchodilators, counteracting leukotrienes)

Certain key facts on arachidonic acid metabolites:
i. Arachidonic acid derivatives are called **autacoids** because they have predominantly autocrine and paracrine actions.
ii. **Prostaglandins** act on blood vessels, bronchial smooth muscles, or uterine smooth muscle, in synergy or opposing each other's actions (for details see **Fig. 4.6**).
iii. **Thromboxane and prostacyclin** counteract one another: Thromboxane is produced by platelets favouring aggregation of platelets and promoting vasoconstriction. Prostacyclin is produced by endothelial cells, counteracting aggregation of platelets and acting as a vasodilator.
iv. **Resolvins** inhibit production of pro-inflammatory cytokines.
v. The effects of pro-inflammatory prostaglandins can be inhibited by *acetylsalicylic acid* (aspirin), which **inhibits COX-2**.
vi. **Leukotrienes** are synthesised and slowly releases from mast cells as type I hypersensitivity (anaphylactic) reactions, e.g. hay fever or bronchial asthma. Therefore, they are also known as slow reacting substances of anaphylaxis SRS-As.
vii. **Lipoxins** counteract leukotrienes.

Q18. What are cytokines and chemokines? Discuss their classification and their major functions.

Definition Cytokines are polypeptides produced by activated lymphocytes (thus also known as *lymphokines*) or monocytes (*monokines*). Cytokines may act on 'self' cells (autocrine action) or on other cells. The term *chemokine* is used for small cytokines that act as chemoattractants.

Sources Most cytokines are produced by a variety of cells:
i. The most common sources of cytokines are monocytes/macrophages, lymphocytes, dendritic cells, mast cells, neutrophils.
ii. Some connective tissue cells such as fibroblasts, endothelial cells and smooth muscle cells.

iii. Some epithelial cells such as pulmonary alveolar cells.
Targets Many cytokines have multiple target cells, and many act on almost all cells in the body. Selective targets are most often T or B lymphocytes, NK cells and other white blood cells
Classification Several groups of cytokines are recognised, the most important of which are as follows: i) interleukins, ii) tumour necrosis factor family, and iii) interferons **(Table 4.2)**.
I. *Interleukins (IL-1, IL-2, IL-3, etc.)* which have the following main functions:
i. Emigration of neutrophils and macrophages
ii. Expression of adhesion molecules
iii. Regulation of fever, shock
iv. Hepatic production of acute phase reactants
v. Increased production of IFN-γ or other cytokines
vi. Induction of formation of T-cell subsets, like T helper or cytotoxic T cells
vii. Promote CTL activity
viii. Stimulate angiogenesis
II. *Tumour necrosis factors (TNF-α TNF-β)* which is produced by T cells and NK cells and has the following main functions:
i. Fever, shock, anorexia
ii. Hepatic production of acute phase reactants
iii. Increased production of pro-inflammatory cytokines
iv. Expression of endothelial cell adhesion molecules
III. *Interferon (IFN-γ)*:
i. Activation of macrophages and NK killer cells
ii. Stimulation of immunoglobulins by B cells
iii. Differentiation of T helper cells
IV. **Chemokines** (*monocyte chemoattractant protein, MCP-1; macrophage inflammatory protein, MIP1-α; eotaxin; regulated and normal T cell expressed and secreted, RANTES*):
i. Chemoattractant action for specific inflammatory cell types
ii. Release of histamine from basophils

Q19. What is platelet activating factor (PAF)?

Definition PAF is a phospholipid-derived mediator of inflammation, initially identified as a mediator of platelet aggregation and degranulation. It is a multifunctional molecule synthesised by leucocytes, endothelial cells and many other cells. Receptors of PAF are found on numerous cells.
Main functions Binding of PAF to cell receptor may have the following effects:
i. Increase vascular permeability
ii. Vasodilatation or vasoconstriction depending on the concentration of PAF
iii. Bronchoconstriction
iv. Chemotaxis
v. Adhesion of PMNs to endothelium

Q20. What are the main plasma-derived mediators of inflammation?

Mediators circulating in the blood are mostly synthesised by the liver and belong to four interlinked systems:
i. Kinin
ii. Clotting
iii. Fibrinolytic
iv. Complement
Hageman factor (clotting factor XII) plays a key role in interactions of the four systems **(Fig. 4.7)**.

Q21. What are the components of the kinin system and the main functions?

Kinin system is involved in the production of bradykinin from kininogen which is activated by kallikrein. Kallikrein is formed from prekallikrein under the action of prekallikrein activator derived from Factor XII **(Fig. 4.8)**.

TABLE 4.2 Major cytokines in inflammation.

CYTOKINE	CELL SOURCE	CELL TARGET	MAIN ACTIONS
I. INTERLEUKINS			
IL-1	Monocytes/macrophages, B cells, fibroblasts, endothelial cells, some epithelial cells	All cells	➢ Expression of adhesion molecules ➢ Emigration of neutrophils and macrophages ➢ Role in fever and shock ➢ Hepatic production of acute phase reactant
IL-6	Same as for IL-1	T and B cells, epithelial cells, hepatocytes, monocytes/macrophages	➢ Hepatic production of acute phase reactant ➢ Differentiation and growth of T and B cells
IL-8	Monocytes/macrophages, T cells, neutrophils, fibroblasts, endothelial cells, epithelial cells	Neutrophils, basophils, T cells, monocytes/macrophages, endothelial cells	➢ Induces migration of neutrophils, macrophages and T cells ➢ Stimulates release of histamine from basophils ➢ Stimulates angiogenesis
IL-12	Macrophages, dendritic cells, neutrophils	T cells, NK cells	➢ Induces formation of T helper cells and killer cells ➢ Promotes CTL cytolytic activity ➢ Increases production of IFN-γ ➢ Decreases production of IL-17
IL-17	CD4+T cells	Fibroblasts, endothelial cells, epithelial cells	➢ Increases secretion of other cytokines ➢ Migration of neutrophils and monocytes
II. TNF FAMILY			
TNF-α	Monocytes/macrophages, mast cells/basophils, eosinophils, B cells, T cells, NK cells	All cells except RBCs	➢ Hepatic production of acute phase reactant ➢ Systemic features (fever, shock, anorexia) ➢ Expression of endothelial adhesion molecules ➢ Enhanced leucocyte cytotoxicity ➢ Induction of pro-inflammatory cytokines
III. INTERFERON FAMILY			
IFN-γ	T cells, NK cells	All cells	➢ Activation of macrophages and NK cells ➢ Stimulates secretion of Igs by B cells ➢ Differentiation of T helper cells
IV. OTHER CHEMOKINES (BESIDES IL-8)			
MCP-1	Fibroblasts, smooth muscle cells, blood mononuclear cells	Monocytes/macrophages, NK cells, T cells	➢ Chemoattractant for monocytes, T cells and NK cells ➢ Stimulates release of histamine from basophils
MIP-1α	Monocyte—macrophages	Monocyte-macrophages, T cells, NK cells	Chemoattractant for monocytes, dendritic cells, T cells, NK cells
Eotaxin	Alveolar cells, myocardium	Eosinophils, basophils	➢ Chemoattractant for eosinophils and basophils ➢ Induces allergic pulmonary disease
RANTES	Monocytes—macrophages, T cells, fibroblasts and eosinophils	Monocytes-macrophages, T cells, NK cells, dendritic cells, eosinophils	Chemoattractant for monocytes—macrophages, T cells and NK cells
Lymphotactin	NK cells, T cells, mast cells	T cell and NK cells	Chemoattractant specific for lymphocytes
Fractalkine	Endothelial cells	NK cells, T cells, monocytes-macrophages	Dual role for monocytes and T cells: ➢ as cell-surface chemoattractant ➢ as cell adhesion molecule

(IL, interleukin; TNF, tumour necrosis factor; IFN, interferon; MCP, monocyte chemotactic protein; RANTES, regulated and normal T cell expressed and secreted).

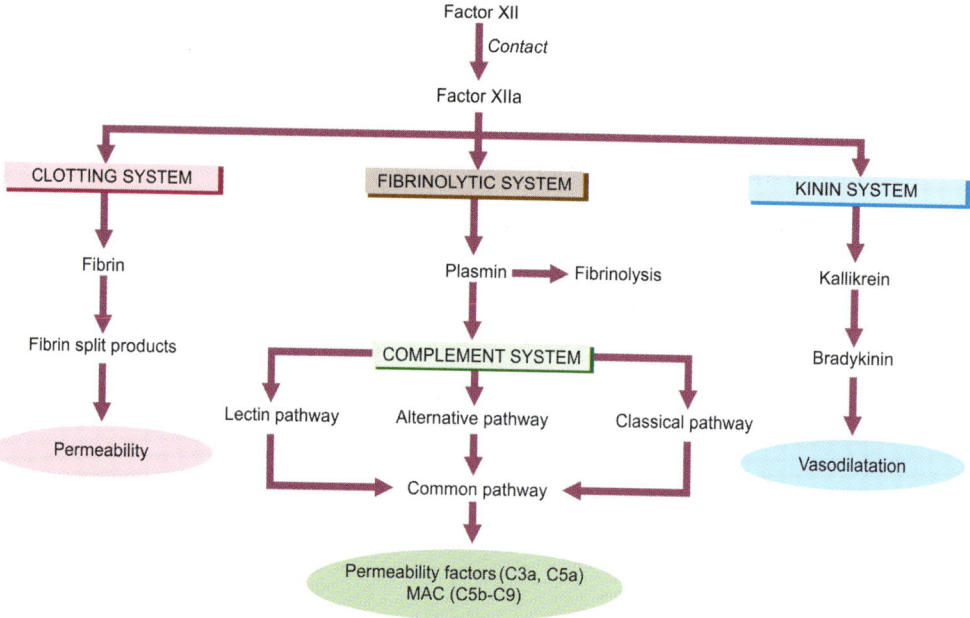

FIGURE 4.7: Inter-relationship among clotting, fibrinolytic, kinin and complement systems.

Bradykinin participates in early stages of inflammation and has the following effects:
i. Smooth muscle contraction
ii. Vasodilatation
iii. Increased vascular permeability
iv. Pain

Q22. What are the main components of the clotting system and their major functions?

Activation of Factor XII through contact of the blood with a hard surface leads to the initiation of the clotting cascade that ends in the formation of fibrin and clot formation **(Fig. 4.9)**.

Plasmin acts on fibrin, splitting it into **fibrinopeptides,** which may act on the inflammatory process as follows:
i. Increased vascular permeability
ii. Chemotaxis for leucocytes
iii. Anticoagulant activity

Q23. What are the main functions of the fibrinolytic system in inflammation?

Plasmin, the most important fibrinolytic protein, is formed from plasminogen. There are several plasminogen activators, including kallikrein, endothelial cells or leucocytes **(Fig. 4.10)**.
Plasmin has the following effects in the inflammatory process:
i. Activation of factor XII to form prekallikrein, ultimately leading to the formation of *bradykinin*.

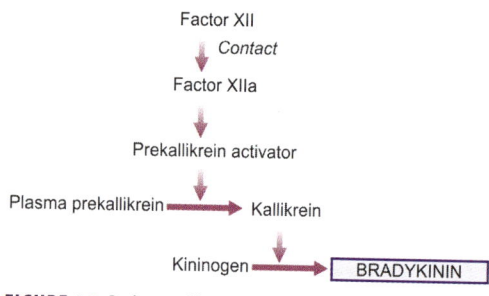

FIGURE 4.8: Pathway of kinin system.

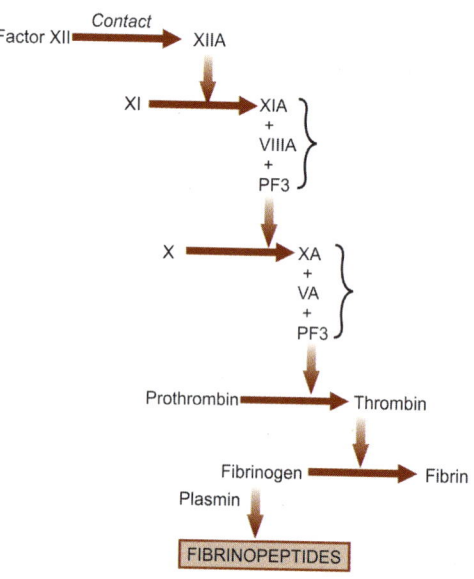

FIGURE 4.9: Pathway of the clotting system.

ii. *Splitting of complement* component C3 to form *C3a*, which leads to increased vascular permeability.
iii. Breakdown of fibrin which gives rise to *fibrinopeptides or fibrin split products*. These compounds increase vascular permeability and are chemotactic for leucocytes.

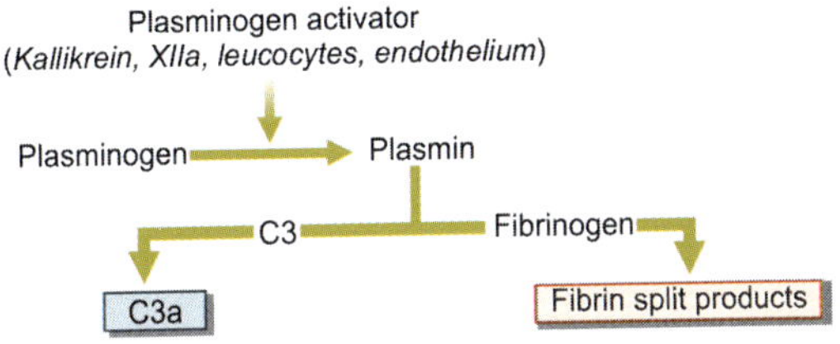

FIGURE 4.10: The activation of fibrinolytic system.

Q24. What is the complement system? Briefly discuss its main features and its pathways of generation.

Definition Complement system comprises some 30 plasma proteins, cell surface proteins and receptors, as well as specific inhibitors.

Main features
i. Complement plasma proteins, which circulate in blood in an inactive form, are labeled numerically from 1 to 9.
ii. Upon activation, complement proteins form *fragments* which are labeled such as 3a, 3b, 5a, etc.
iii. Fragments and activated complement proteins assemble into *intermediate complexes* and also form the final *membrane attack complex (MAC)*, comprising C5b, C6, C7, C8, and C9).
iv. *Activation of the complement pathway* by one of the three pathways **(Fig. 4.11)**:
a. *Classical pathway*, activated by antigen-antibody complexes containing IgG or IgM.
b. *Alternative pathway* which can be activated by a non-immunologic agent such as bacterial toxins or lipopolysaccharides and cobra venom.
c. *Mannose-binding lectin pathway* in which this lectin binds to mannose residues on the microbial surface and activates serine protease.
v. All three pathways converge on the activation of *C3 convertase* which activates more complement proteins that have an important role in inflammation.
vi. Excessive activity of complement components is controlled by specific inhibitors. Clinically, the most important *inhibitors* are as follows:
- *C1 inhibitor*, blocking the first step of the classical pathway. Congenital deficiency of C1 INH causes *hereditary angioedema*.
- *Decay accelerating factor (DAF)* prevents formation of C3 convertase. It is linked to plasma glycophosphatidyl and its deficiency causes *paroxysmal nocturnal haematuria*.
- *CD59* prevents the formation of MAC.

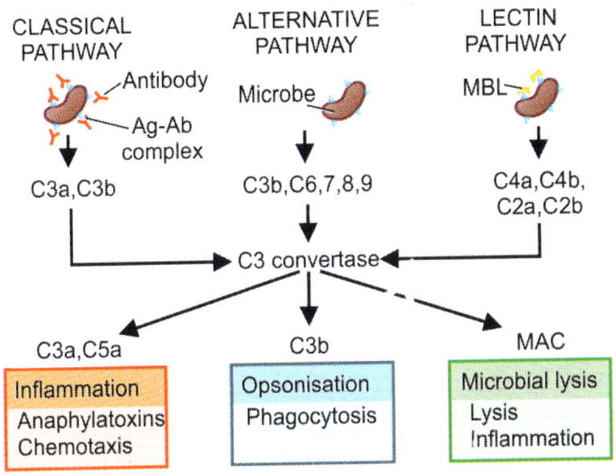

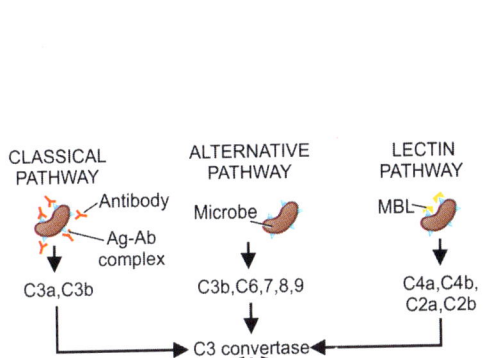

FIGURE 4.11: Activation pathways of complement system and actions of activated products.

Q25. What are the principal functions of complement in the inflammatory process?

Proteins forming the complements have many important functions in the inflammatory process in which they act as:
i. **Anaphylatoxins**, which activate mast cells, stimulate release of histamine and increase vascular permeability.
ii. **Chemoattractants,** which attract leucocytes to the area of inflammation.
iii. **Opsonins,** which coat microbes and facilitate their phagocytosis.
iv. **Membrane attack complex** (MAC), which leads to perforation of the phospholipid cell membrane and lysis of cells (e.g. lysis of RBC in haemolysis) and killing of microbes.

INFLAMMATORY CELLS

Q26. What are the principal inflammatory cells and what are their major functions?

The principal inflammatory cells are: i) polymorphonuclear neutrophils (PMNs), ii) eosinophils, iii) basophils/mast cells, iv) lymphocytes, v) plasma cells, and vi) monocytes/macrophages **(Table 4.3)**. They are all found in the circulating blood except macrophages, mast cells and plasma cells, which are found only in tissues.

I. **Polymorphonuclear leucocytes**

i. Most numerous white blood cells in circulation (40–75% of all leucocytes).
ii. Nucleus is polymorphous, i.e. segmented in up to 5 lobes.
iii. Cytoplasmic granules are classified as primary, secondary, tertiary → rich in lytic enzymes.
iv. Phagocytic activity strong → killing of microbes.
v. Lytic enzymes released from granules → damage tissues and basement membranes.
vi. They are the first inflammatory cells to reach the area of bacterial infections.
vii. In tissues, they live only 2 days.
viii. *Main function:* Most prominent cells in acute inflammation caused by microbes or tissue necrosis.

TABLE 4.3 Morphology and functions of inflammatory cells.

MORPHOLOGY	MAIN FUNCTIONS	FEATURES
A, POLYMORPH	i. Initial phagocytosis of bacteria and foreign body ii. Engulfment of antigen-antibody complexes iii. Basement membrane destruction iv. Acute inflammatory cell	i. Primary granules (MPO, lysozyme, cationic proteins, acid hydrolases, elastase) ii. Secondary granules (lysozyme, alk. phosph, collagenase, lactoferrin) iii. Tertiary granules (gelatinase, cathepsin)
B, EOSINOPHIL	i. Allergic states ii. Parasitic infestations iii. Dermatoses iv. Malignant lymphomas v. Chronic inflammatory cell	i. Contains MPO ii. Granules contain major basic protein, cationic protein iii. Lack lysosomes
C, BASOPHIL/MAST CELL	i. Receptor for IgE molecules ii. Electron-dense granules	i. Histamine ii. Leukotrienes iii. Platelet activating factor
D, LYMPHOCYTE	i. Humoral and cell-mediated immune responses ii. Chronic inflammatory cell iii. Regulates macrophage response	i. B cells: antibody production ii. T cells: delayed hypersensitivity, cytotoxicity
E, PLASMA CELL	i. Derived from B cells ii. Plasma cell dyscrasias iii. Chronic inflammatory cell	i. Antibody synthesis ii. Antibody secretion
F, MONOCYTE/MACROPHAGE	i. Microbial phagocytosis and killing ii. Induce repair by fibrosis iii. Chronic inflammatory cell iv. Regulate lymphocyte response	i. Require activation by: classic (non-immunologic) or alternate (IL-4, IL-13) way ii. Release proteases (collagenase, elastase) iii. Activation of coagulation pathway iv. Prostaglandins, leukotrienes v. Chemoattractant for other leucocytes

(MPO, myeloperoxidase).

II. **Eosinophils**
i. Comprise 1–6% of all leucocytes in blood, but may be found in tissues as well.
ii. Nucleus is usually bilobed.
iii. Cytoplasmic granules are eosinophilic → toxic activity against parasites.
iv. In tissues, live longer than neutrophils.
v. *Main function:* Allergic inflammation and defense against parasites.
III. **Basophils/mast cells**
i. 1% of all leucocytes in blood; mast cells are tissue basophils.
ii. Coarse basophilic granules → contain heparin and histamine.
iii. Surface receptors for IgE.
iv. *Main function:* Binding of antigen in type I hypersensitivity reaction, release of histamine.
IV. **Lymphocytes**
20–45% of all leucocytes in blood but many are in lymph nodes and tissues.
i. Scant cytoplasm, round nucleus (no granules and no nuclear segmentation).
ii. Divided into several classes (B and T lymphocytes, NK cells).
iii. They have long lives.
iv. *Main function:* Immune response and chronic inflammation
V. **Plasma cells**
i. Plasma cells are not seen in blood but only in tissues.
ii. They develop from B lymphocytes.
iii. They have a bluish cytoplasm due to prominent stack of rough endoplasmic reticulum.
iv. Secrete immunoglobulins.
v. They have long lives.
vi. *Main function:* Antibody mediated immune reactions and chronic inflammation.
VI. **Monocytes/macrophages**
i. Monocytes account for 4–8% of leucocytes in blood.
ii. Macrophages are monocyte derived tissue cells.
iii. *Main function:* Phagocytosis and secretion of cytokines, participate in chronic inflammation and repair.

Q27. What are various specialised forms of macrophages found in the tissues?

Specialised forms of macrophages in different locations in tissues are as follows:
i. Kupffer cells in the liver
ii. Alveolar macrophages in lungs
iii. Microglia cells in the CNS
iv. Epithelioid macrophages in granulomas
v. Littoral cells in splenic sinusoids
vi. Osteoclasts in bones
vii. Dendritic cells (Langerhans cells) under mucosal surfaces and in lymph nodes
viii. Hoffbauer cells in the placenta
ix. Mesangial cells in the glomerulus

Q28. What are various types of multinucleated giant cells?

Multinucleated giant cells are formed by:
- either fusion of preexisting cells (e.g. macrophages in granulomas),
- or endoreduplication of the nucleus without a division of cytoplasm (e.g. megakaryocytes in the bone marrow or syncytiotrophoblastic cells in the placenta).

In histopathology, the most important multinucleated giant cells are derived from the fusion of macrophages. These include the following **(Fig. 4.12)**:
i. **Langhans giant cells** in granulomas such as tuberculosis, histoplasmosis or sarcoidosis.
ii. **Foreign body giant cells** that are formed in chronic inflammation elicited by particulate foreign material (e.g. surgical suture material, starch, talc, vegetable material, tattoo, wood particles), or endogenous crystals (e.g. urate crystals in gout, oxalate crystals in the kidneys, and particles (e.g. keratin in ruptured epidermoid cysts).

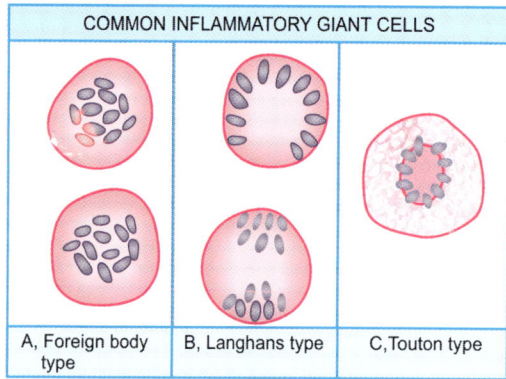

FIGURE 4.12: Inflammatory giant cells. A, Langhans giant cells with uniform nuclei arranged peripherally or clustered at the two poles. B, Foreign body giant cell with uniform nuclei dispersed throughout the cytoplasm. C, Touton giant cell with central circular pattern of nuclei and peripheral vacuolated cytoplasm.

iii. **Touton giant cells** found in lipogranulomas, xanthomas, or fat necrosis. Their cytoplasm is filled with droplets of fat.

NOTE: Giant cells derived from macrophages need to be distinguished from *epidermal cell derived giant cells* (also known as Tzank cells), which are seen in the skin infected with some viruses (e.g. herpes simplex virus, herpes zoster and varicella, cytomegalovirus). Similar cells can be seen is some chronic dermatoses.

ACUTE INFLAMMATION—FACTORS IN RESPONSE, MORPHOLOGIC TYPES, EFFECTS AND OUTCOME

Q29. What are the factors that determine variation in response to acute infection?

There are two sets of factors that determine the type of inflammatory response to microbes: i) factors relating to the infecting organism, and ii) factors involving the host.

I. **Factors involving the organism**

i. *Type of the agent* causing the infection. For example, herpes simplex virus infection of the skin elicits formation of vesicles, whereas leprosy and tuberculosis produce granulomas.

ii. *Virulence* Strains of microbes may vary in their virulence, depending on the amount of toxin that they produce.

iii. *Dose* Large dose of microbes generally causes a more extensive inflammation than a small dose.

iv. *Portal of entry* Some organisms are infectious only if entering the organism through a specific portal. For example, cholera causes infection only by entering through the intestines.

v. *Products of organism* Specific bacterial organisms produce specific enzymes, such as streptococcal streptokinase, or staphylococcal staphylokinase and coagulase.

II. **Factors involving the host**

i. *Systemic diseases* that reduce resistance to infection such as diabetes, chronic alcoholism, etc.

ii. *Immune status* of the host will determine the response to infection. For example, acquired immunodeficiency caused by HIV will facilitate many forms of infection. Leucopenia and congenital neutrophil defects will reduce the capacity of the organism to combat infection.

iii. *Leucopenia and congenital neutrophil defects* Inability of the organism to mobilise leucocytes will markedly reduce prevention of infection.

iv. *Site of infection* For example, skin is more resistant to bacterial infection than mucosa of the respiratory tract.

v. *Local host factors* such as ischaemia, or preexistent injury that has caused necrosis of tissue, will facilitate infection.

Q30. How are inflammatory reactions classified?

Inflammatory lesions are classified based on: i) duration of infection, ii) type of exudate, and iii) anatomic location of infection.

I. **Duration of infection** Infections of short duration (usually a few days) are called *acute,* and those that last longer (many weeks or months) are termed *chronic.* The term *subacute* is used for those in between, i.e. of a few weeks duration.

II. Type of exudates Inflammation may produce the following forms of exudates:
i. *Serous*—exudate is watery and resembles serum, e.g. blister in burns.
ii. *Fibrinous*—the fluid forming the exudate is rich in fibrin, which may form coating of the inner surfaces of the lesion, e.g. rheumatic pericarditis.
iii. *Purulent (or suppurative)*—creamy pus is permeating the affected organ (e.g. purulent appendicitis) or filling a cavity (e.g. abscess).
iv. *Haemorrhagic*—the exudate is red due to extravasation of blood (e.g. haemorrhagic viral pneumonia in influenza).
v. *Catarrhal*—exudate is admixed to mucus secreted by the affected mucosa (e.g. mucus-rich nasal discharge in common cold).
III. Anatomic location of infection Morphology of lesions varies depending on which organs is affected; e.g. solid organ such as liver hepatitis, mucosal surface such as enterocolitis, or serosal surface of an organ such as pericarditis and peritonitis, etc.

Q31. What is pseudomembranous inflammation and what are its main features?

i. Pseudomembranous inflammation involves usually mucosal surfaces of the gastrointestinal and respiratory tract.
ii. It is caused by bacteria that produce a toxin, which kills off the epithelial cells, upon which the exudate of plasma covers the ulceration and forms a fibrin-rich exudate.
iii. These pseudomembranes occur in the throat in diphtheria or pseudomembranous colitis caused by *Clostridioides difficile* in patients who have been treated with broad-spectrum antibiotics.
iv. The 'pseudomembranes' can be wiped off by scraping, consist of necrotic epithelial cells, fibrin-rich inflammatory exudate, admixed in the colon to mucin and even faecal material. If removed mechanically, pseudomembranes expose the underlying ulcerated mucosa which bleeds profusely.

Q32. Define an ulcer. What are its main features?

i. An ulcer is a defect of the mucosa or skin.
ii. Mucosal ulcers include peptic ulcer of the stomach or duodenum, ulcerative colitis, caecal ulcers in amoebic dysentery.
iii. Skin ulcers are seen on legs affected by varicose veins which cause stagnation of blood and ischaemia.
iv. The bottom of a typical peptic ulcer is denuded of mucosa and, instead contains granulation tissue covered with an acute inflammatory exudate composed of neutrophils and necrotic cell debris.
v. Healing of the ulcer includes formation of granulation tissue, which will replace the acute inflammation and then transform into a fibrous scar.

Q33. What is an abscess?

Abscess is a localised suppurative inflammation, leading to accumulation of pus in a cavity formed by the destruction of the infected tissue **(Fig. 4.13)**. The semiliquid content of the abscess cavity is surrounded by a fibrovascular capsule composed of granulation tissue. Removal of pus will allow the abscess to heal by scarring.
Some of the common clinical examples of abscesses are as follows:
- *Boil (furuncle)* is formed from pus accumulating in a hair follicle and extending into the surrounding connective tissue of the skin.
- *Carbuncle* is a more extensive suppurative lesion which most often develops due to confluence of several furuncles.

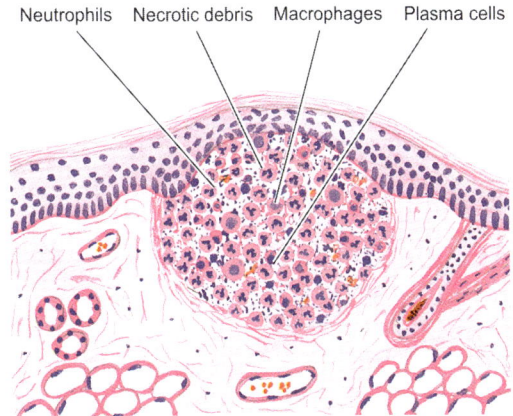

FIGURE 4.13: An abscess in the skin. It contains pus composed of necrotic tissue, debris, fibrin, RBCs and dead and living neutrophils. Some macrophages are seen at the periphery.

Q34. What is bacteraemia and how does it differ from septicaemia and pyaemia?

Bacteraemia is a condition in which bacteria enter the blood but do not multiply significantly. It is typically detected by blood culture and involves pathogens such as *Streptococcus viridans, Escherichia coli,* or *Salmonella typhi*.

Septicaemia means presence of rapidly multiplying, highly pathogenic bacteria in blood, such as pyogenic cocci. Septicaemia is accompanied by systemic effects like toxaemia, purpuric haemorrhage, fever, leucocytosis and even disseminated intravascular coagulation.

Pyaemia is haematogenous dissemination of small septic thromboemboli with formation of small abscesses in various tissues **(Fig. 4.14)**:

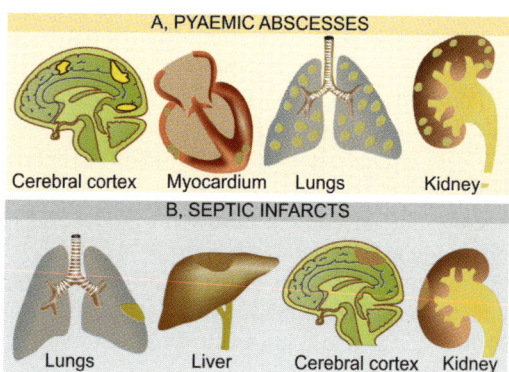

FIGURE 4.14: Sequelae of pyaemia.

Pyaemic abscesses contain a central core of bacteria surrounded by a zone or suppuration and a layer of acute inflammation.

Septic infarcts result from septic thromboemboli occluding large blood vessels and causing visible area of necrosis. Septic infarcts are a common complication of bacterial endocarditis, and atypically seen in the brain, lungs, spleen or kidneys.

Q35. What are the systemic effects of acute inflammation?

Systemic effects of inflammation include the following:

i. **Fever** It is mediated by a release of exogenous pyrogens from the bacteria which induce the production of endogenous pyrogens, prostaglandins, IL-1 and TNF-α. Endogenous pyrogens act on the thermoregulatory centre in the hypothalamus, which acts as a thermostat.

ii. **Leucocytosis** Usually in the range of 15,000 to 20,000 or higher. Leucocytosis is usually neutrophilic in most bacterial infections. Viral infections cause lymphocytosis. Parasitic infections are marked by eosinophilic leukocytosis. Some infections may even cause leucopenia, as seen in typhoid fever.

iii. **Release of acute phase reactants (APRs)** These are produced by the liver in response to infection. The primary stimulus acting on the liver are IL-1 and TNF-α, released from inflammatory cells responding to the infection. APRs cause accelerated erythrocyte sedimentation rate (ESR).

iv. **Lymphadenitis and lymphangitis** Lymph nodes enlarge and show follicular hyperplasia and sinus histiocytosis. The lymphatics draining in and out of these lymph nodes become dilated and are seen as red lines. These changes are a response to mediators released at the site of infection, but also they may represent part of the immune response to infection.

v. **Septic shock** Sepsis leads to a massive release of cytokines. TNF-α is one of the most prominent cytokines released. TNF-α causes profuse systemic vasodilatation, increased vascular permeability, and loss of intravascular fluid with hypotension. Activation of the coagulation system may produce disseminated intravascular coagulation (DIC), bleeding and death.

Q36. What are the acute phase reactants?

Acute phase reactants (APRs) are proteins secreted by the liver, and to smaller extent, by macrophages in response to acute inflammation. They include several groups of proteins as given here:

i. *Cellular protection proteins* (e.g. α1-antitrypsin, plasminogen activator inhibitor).
ii. *Coagulation proteins* (e.g. fibrinogen, plasminogen, factor VIII).
iii. *Transport proteins* (e.g. transferrin, caeruloplasmin, haptoglobin).
iv. *Immune agents* (e.g. amyloid A and P component, C-reactive protein or CRP, which acts as an opsonin).
v. *Stress proteins* (e.g. heat shock protein, ubiquitin).
vi. *Antioxidants* (e.g. ceruloplasmin).

In clinical practice it is customary to measure the serum levels of CRP as a representative of all other APRs. Alternatively, one can measure the erythrocyte sedimentation rate (ESR), which is accelerated in the presence of APRs in blood.

Q37. What are the possible outcomes of acute inflammation?

Possible outcomes of acute inflammation are as follows **(Fig. 4.15)**:
- Resolution
- Healing by fibrous scarring
- Suppuration
- Transition to chronic inflammation

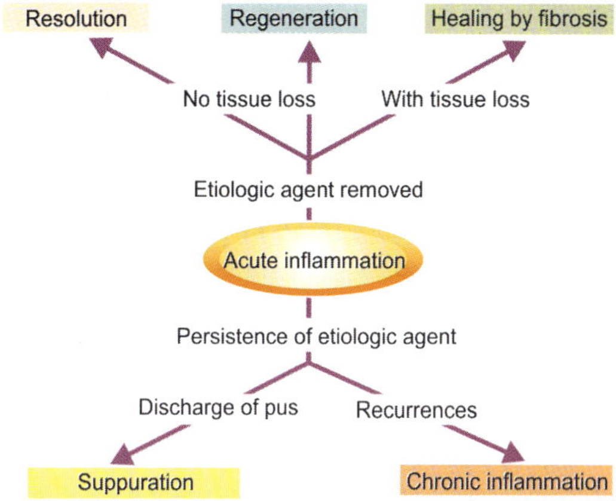

■ CHRONIC INFLAMMATION—TYPES AND GENERAL FEATURES

Q38. What is chronic inflammation? How does it occur?

FIGURE 4.15: Fate of acute inflammation.

Definition Chronic inflammation is a long lasting inflammation with concomitant destruction of tissue and repair.
Mechanism It occurs by one of the following three ways:
i. *Following acute inflammation,* usually because of the persistence of causative agent or extensive destruction of tissues.
ii. *Recurrent attacks of acute inflammation*
iii. *Chronic inflammation which starts as such de novo* This happens with certain pathogens of low virulence, which do not produce an obvious acute phase of inflammation (e.g. *Mycobacterium tuberculosis*) and in infections that are immune-mediated (e.g. autoimmune diseases).

Q39. What are the general common features of most forms of chronic inflammations?

There are certain similarities between various types of chronic inflammation which share the following features:
I. **Mononuclear cell infiltration** Macrophages, lymphocytes and plasma cells accounting for most of the cells; eosinophils and basophils are in a minority.
Macrophages play a key role in chronic inflammation. Their functions include phagocytosis of pathogens, removal of necrotic cells, secretion of cytokines and other mediators of inflammation, and presentation of antigens to lymphocytes. Lymphocytes interact with macrophages and also initiate immune responses. B-lymphocytes differentiate into plasma cells.
II. **Tissue destruction** results primarily due to the action of macrophages which release lytic enzymes and cytokines.
III. **Proliferative changes** include formation of granulation tissue encompassing proliferation of angioblasts, fibroblasts and laying down of interstitial matrix proteins. Cytokines secreted by macrophages play a critical role in these proliferative processes.

Q40. What are the systemic effects of chronic inflammation?

The following systemic effects are seen in most chronic inflammations:
i. **Fever,** usually low grade and persistent.
ii. **Anaemia**, known as the anaemia of chronic disease.
iii. **Leucocytosis**, usually with a relative lymphocytosis.
iv. **Erythrocyte sedimentation rate** (ESR) elevation.
v. **Amyloidosis**, which usually occurs in long-standing chronic suppurative inflammation.

Q41. What are the main forms of chronic inflammation?

Chronic inflammation occurs in two forms: chronic nonspecific inflammation, and chronic granulomatous inflammation.
I. **Chronic nonspecific inflammation** has no specific characteristics. It presents with the usually infiltrates of macrophages, lymphocytes and plasma cells and proliferation of fibroblasts and

angioblasts. In *chronic suppurative inflammation*, there is a combination of chronic inflammation and acute suppuration, characterised by PMN infiltrates and formation of pus.

II. **Chronic granulomatous inflammation** is characterised by the formation of granulomas. Granulomas are composed of T lymphocytes and epithelioid macrophages, which may fuse to form multinucleated giant cells. Granulomas are a typical feature of type IV hypersensitivity reaction and are best studied in the pathogenesis of tuberculosis.

Q42. How are granulomas formed?

The sequence of events leading to the formation of granulomas is presented in **Figure 4.16**.

i. The process starts with an uptake of pathogen or antigenic material into the cytoplasm of macrophages.

ii. Antigen that cannot be digested persists in the macrophages and elicits the reaction of CD4+ T cells which release several important cytokines:

a. IL-1 and IL-2, which stimulate proliferation of additional T cells.

b. Interferon-γ, which activates macrophages and also transform them into epithelioid macrophages, i.e. cells that have abundant cytoplasm and adhere firmly one to another.

c. Tumour necrosis factor-α (TNF-α) promotes proliferation of fibroblasts and activates endothelial cells.

d. Transforming growth factor-β (TGF-β) and platelet derived growth factor (PDGF) activate macrophages and stimulate the growth of fibroblasts.

Q43. What are the typical morphologic features of granulomas?

i. Granuloma is formed of *T-lymphocytes, epithelioid macrophages* and *fibroblasts* that form an external rim around it; epithelioid cells may fuse to form *multinucleated giant cells (see* **Fig. 4.16)**.

ii. Necrosis may be found in the centre of some granulomas, most often those of infectious origin.

iii. Granulomas can be divided into two groups: infectious, and noninfectious.

a. *Infectious granulomas* can be caused by mycobacteria (e.g. tuberculosis, leprosy), bacteria (e.g. actinomycosis), fungi (e.g. cryptococcosis), parasites (e.g. schistosomiasis).

b. *Noninfectious granulomas* as seen in diseases of unknown or presumed immune origin (e.g. sarcoidosis, Crohn disease), diseases caused by inhalation of exogenous material (e.g. silicosis, berylliosis), foreign bodies (e.g. talc, surgical sutures).

Q44. Tabulate the major differences between acute and chronic inflammation.

The differences between acute and chronic inflammation are listed in **Table 4.4**.

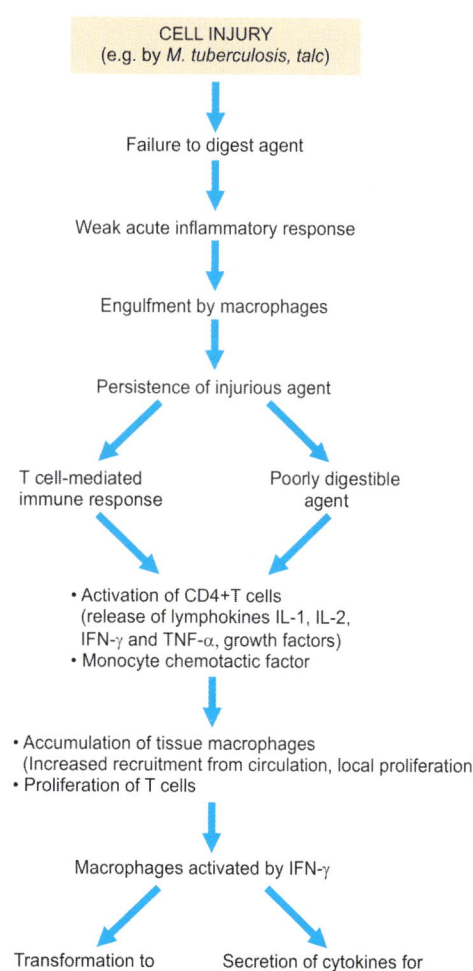

FIGURE 4.16: Mechanism of evolution of a granuloma. (IL, interleukin; IFN, interferon; TNF, tumour necrosis factor, TGF, transforming growth factor; PDGF, Platelet-derived growth factor).

TABLE 4.4 Major differences between acute and chronic inflammation.

FEATURE	ACUTE INFLAMMATION	CHRONIC INFLAMMATION
1. Onset and duration	➤ Within short time ➤ Lasts for short duration	➤ After delay ➤ Lasts longer
2. Cardinal signs	Invariably present	Generally imperceptible
3. Pathogenesis	➤ Vascular events: haemodynamic changes, increased vascular permeability ➤ Cellular events: exudation of leucocytes, phagocytosis ➤ Role of chemical mediators	➤ Following acute inflammation ➤ Recurrent attacks of acute inflammation ➤ Chronic inflammation from beginning ➤ Role of chemical mediators
4. Main inflammatory cells	➤ Neutrophils ➤ Eosinophils ➤ Lymphomononuclear cells (late) ➤ Pus cells	➤ Lymphocytes ➤ Plasma cells ➤ Monocytes/macrophages (epithelioid cells in granulomas) ➤ Giant cells (foreign body, Langhans')
5. Plasma exudation	Present	May or may not be present
6. Systemic effects	➤ Fever: high grade ➤ Leucocytosis (neutrophilic, eosinophilic) ➤ Acute phase reactant proteins ➤ Lymphadenitis-lymphangitis ➤ Septic shock (in severe acute infection)	➤ Fever: mild ➤ Leucocytosis (lymphocytic, monocytic) ➤ Lymphadenitis-lymphangitis ➤ Raised ESR ➤ Anaemia ➤ Amyloidosis (in long-lasting cases)
7. Main morphology	➤ Abscesses (suppuration) ➤ Ulcers ➤ Through blood (bacteraemia, septicaemia, pyaemia)	➤ Chronic non-specific inflammation (infectious, others) ➤ Granulomatous inflammation (tuberculosis, leprosy, sarcoidosis, syphilis, actinomycosis, Crohn's disease, foreign bodies, etc.)
8. Fate	➤ Resolution ➤ Repair (regeneration common, fibrous healing sometimes) ➤ Progression to chronicity	➤ Resolution ➤ Repair: fibrous healing more common; regeneration may accompany fibrosis ➤ Dystrophic calcification
9. Common examples	Pyogenic abscess, cellulitis, bacterial pneumonia, pyaemia	Granulation tissue, granulomatous inflammation (tuberculosis, leprosy, etc.), chronic osteomyelitis

■ COMMON GRANULOMATOUS DISEASES

Q45. What is tuberculosis? Comment on its epidemiology, predisposition and etiologic agent.

Definition Infection caused by *Mycobacterium tuberculosis*, human strain.
Epidemiology Widespread, affecting 25% of the world population.
Ten million new cases are diagnosed yearly, 95% in developing countries of Asia, Africa and South America; India accounts for a quarter of the global burden of tuberculosis.
Predisposing conditions Malnutrition, poverty, crowding, inadequate medical care, immuno-suppressed states (especially HIV), alcoholism and diabetes mellitus.
Etiologic agent *M. tuberculosis* is a bacillus measuring 0.5 -3 µm.
i. It is acid fast and stains with Ziehl-Neelsen stain, which is positive because of the mycolic acids, cross linked fatty acids and other lipids in their cell wall.
ii. It can be cultured in Lowenstein-Jensen medium, but grows slowly (4–8 weeks).
iii. Molecular diagnostic techniques such as PCR are useful for species confirmation.
NOTE: *M. tuberculosis* must be distinguished from **atypical mycobacteria** (non-tuberculous mycobacteria, TBM) that share some properties with it and *Mycobacterium leprae*:
• *Mycobaterium avium intracellulare (MAI)*, and *M. kansasii*, causing pulmonary and lymph node infections. MAI with extrapulmonary spread is especially common in AIDS.
• *M. ulcerans* and *M. marinum* causes skin infections.
• *M. fortiutum* and *M. chelonae* causes abscesses.

Q46. How is tuberculosis transmitted?

The most common forms of transmission are as follows:

i. **Inhalation** Most often, *M. tuberculosis* is transmitted in cough droplets from another infected person.
ii. **Ingestion** This is the usual mode of infection with milk containing *M. bovis*. It can also occur by self-swallowing of *M. tuberculosis* in bronchial contents in a person with active pulmonary tuberculosis.
iii. **Inoculation** Infected material may be the source during autopsy or surgery, which occurs rarely.
iv. **Transplacental route** Infection of the foetus in utero from an infected mother occurs rarely.

Q47. How does tuberculosis spread in the body?

Several ways of spread of *M. tuberculosis* can occur:

I. **Local spread** It occurs in the infected organ and it is mediated by macrophages, which carry live *M. tuberculosis*.

II. **Lymphatic spread** In the lungs, the *primary complex* involves a parenchymal focus and local spread may occur through the lymphatics into the regional lymph nodes, which become infected and enlarged. Such *local lymphadenitis* is seen in lymph node-rich organs such as pharynx or intestines. Regional tuberculous lymphadenitis is typical of *childhood tuberculosis*.

III. **Haematogenous spread** It can occur either through the drainage of the main lymphatic vessels into the vena cava and from there into the systemic circulation, or by the erosion of the local blood vessels in the lungs by a necrotising granuloma. Spread through blood may result in formation of numerous small granulomas typical of *military tuberculosis*, and *systemic dissemination* of tuberculosis in distant organs such as kidneys, bones, brain, etc.

IV. **Spread through natural passages and cavities** Examples of such spread are as follows:

i. Transbronchial spread from one lobe of the lung to another.
ii. Infection of the upper respiratory tract from the lungs through the bronchi and trachea.
iii. Swallowing of the infectious sputum into the gastrointestinal tract, resulting in gastric and intestinal tuberculosis.
iv. Tuberculous pleuritis by the entry of *M. tuberculosis* into the pleural space.
v. Spread of renal tuberculosis through the ureters into the urinary bladder and testis.

Q48. How does immune system of human body respond to *Mycobacterium tuberculosis* infection?

- *M. tuberculosis* elicits **delayed type hypersensitivity (type IV)** and **cell-mediated immunity.**
- Two major participants in this response are **CD4+ and CD8 + T cells and macrophages.**
- Macrophages ingest *M. tuberculosis* and then secrete **cytokines** that activate T cells, which in turn transform the macrophages into epithelioid cells.
- **Granulomas** form and undergo central caseous necrosis **(Fig. 4.17)**.
- This **primary infection** heals; however, upon **secondary infection**, or injection of **tuberculin** extract into the skin, an anamnestic response will occur indicative of **acquired immunity**.

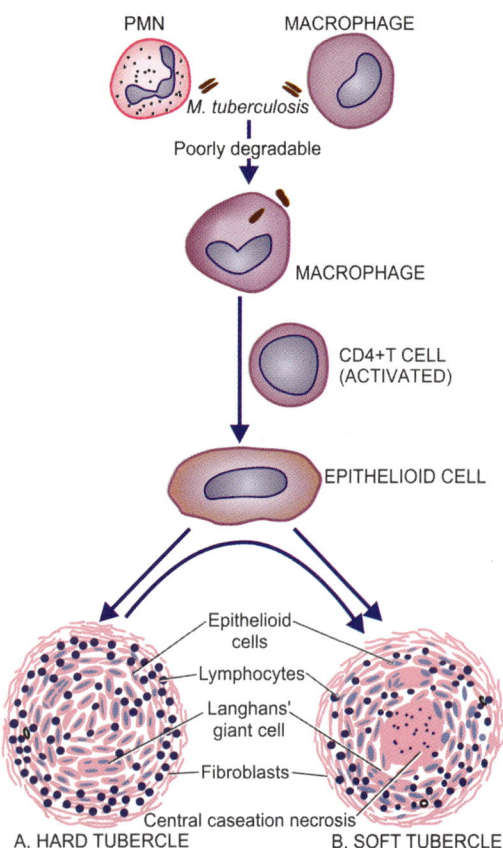

FIGURE 4.17: Schematic evolution of tubercle. In fully formed tuberculous granuloma, the centre is composed of granular caseation necrosis, surrounded by epithelioid cells and Langhans' giant cells and peripheral rim of lymphocytes bounded by fibroblasts.

- Injection of **purified protein derivative (PPD) (Mantoux test)** may be used to determine if a person was infected with *M. tuberculosis*.
- Injection of attenuated bacilli, **Bacille Calmette-Guérin (BCG)**, will induce formation of granulomas in non-immune persons, and induce cell-mediated immunity.
- **BCG vaccination** is used at birth in countries with high prevalence of tuberculosis but is not routinely done in the US. BCG-vaccinated person will have a positive reaction to the Mantoux test.

Q49. What are the two main clinicopathologic forms of tuberculosis? Tabulate their differences.

Two forms of tuberculosis which must be distinguished from each other are: primary and secondary tuberculosis. Their salient contrasting features are given in **Table 4.5**.

TABLE 4.5 Differences between primary and secondary tuberculosis.

FEATURE	PRIMARY TUBERCULOSIS	SECONDARY TUBERCULOSIS
1. Age and evolution	Mostly children who are not previously sensitised to tubercle bacilli	Children and adults, either due to reactivation of primary focus or by reinfection
2. Organs	Almost exclusive in lungs	Lungs, lymph nodes, other organs (genitourinary tract, bones, meninges, brain, eye, liver, spleen, intestines, skin, etc.
3. Distribution	Lower part of upper lobe and upper part of lower lobe	Apex of lungs where oxygen tension is high
4. Lesions	Ghon complex (lung lesion as consolidation, lymphatic vessel and hilar lymph nodes lesions)	Simon focus (lung lesion as tubercles, extensive caseation, miliary lesions, cavitary lesions, fibrocaseous lesions, caseous pneumonia, pleurisy/effusion)
5. Severity	Generally asymptomatic, less severe	Usually symptomatic, more severe
6. Fate	Healing by fibrosis, calcification, may get reactivated in weakened immunity	Consolidation, parenchymal nodules, thickened pleura, amyloidosis, reactivation of healed lesion in impaired immunity and AIDS

Q50. Discuss primary tuberculosis briefly.

Definition Primary tuberculosis occurs in a person who has not been infected previously. It presents in form of the Ghon complex and it is also called childhood tuberculosis.

Ghon complex More commonly, it occurs in the lungs although extrapulmonary primary tuberculosis too may occur.

I. **Pulmonary Ghon complex** has three components **(Fig. 4.18)**:
i. *Pulmonary component* (Ghon focus) comprising tuberculous pneumonia located underneath the pleura in peripheral parts of the lung parenchyma.
ii. *Lymphatic vessels* draining the primary Ghon focus contain bacilli and military tubercles.
iii. *Lymph node component* showing lymph node enlargement due to numerous caseating granulomas.

II. **Extrapulmonary primary tuberculosis** is less common than pulmonary.
i. It usually occurs in the *intestines*.
ii. Like the pulmonary tuberculosis, it has also *three components* (intestinal lesion, lymphangitis and lymph node involvement).
iii. It is called *tabes meseneterica*.
iv. Rupture of mesenteric lymph nodes may result in *tuberculous peritonitis*.

Outcome of primary tuberculosis includes several possibilities **(Fig. 4.19)**:
i. *Healing* of granulomas in all three locations usually involves fibrosis and frequent calcification. The foci thus remain visible by X-rays. They may contain dormant *M. tuberculosis* bacteria.

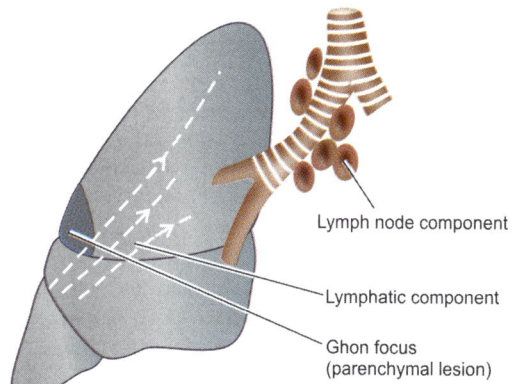

FIGURE 4.18: Primary complex in the lungs is composed of three components: Ghon focus (lower part of upper lobe and upper part of lower lobe), draining lymphatics, and hilar lymph nodes.

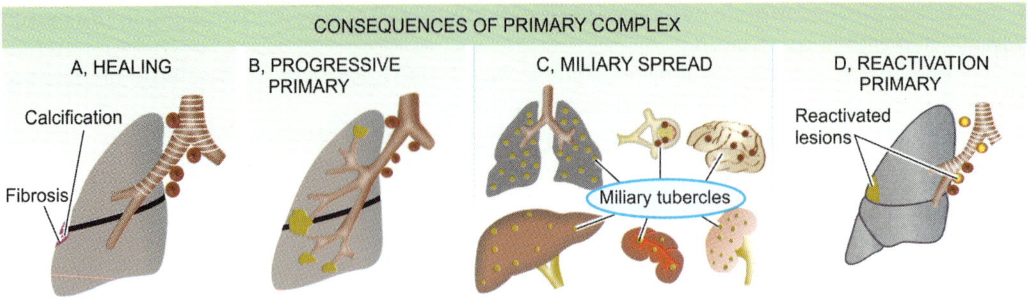

CONSEQUENCES OF PRIMARY COMPLEX

A, HEALING — Calcification, Fibrosis
B, PROGRESSIVE PRIMARY
C, MILIARY SPREAD — Miliary tubercles
D, REACTIVATION PRIMARY — Reactivated lesions

FIGURE 4.19: Possible consequences of primary complex. A, Healing by fibrosis and calcification. B, Progressive primary tuberculosis spreading to the other areas of the same lung or opposite lung. C, Miliary spread to lungs, liver, spleen, kidneys and brain. D, Progressive secondary pulmonary tuberculosis from reactivation of dormant primary complex.

ii. *Progressive primary tuberculosis* occurs less commonly. It occurs when the primary focus in the lungs keeps growing and the infectious material is disseminated through the bronchi to the same and even the opposite lung.

iii. *Primary miliary tuberculosis* with systemic dissemination is a less common outcome, which occurs if the granulomas erode the blood vessel wall and the bacteria enter the bloodstream with subsequent *dissemination* through the entire body.

iv. *Progressive secondary tuberculosis* occurs in immunosuppressed persons and children. It results from *reactivation of dormant bacilli* in the fibrosed or calcified primary lesion.

Q51. What is secondary tuberculosis? Discuss main features of secondary pulmonary tuberculosis.

Definition Secondary tuberculosis is the infection in a person who has been previously infected or sensitised. It is also called post-primary tuberculosis, or reinfection, or chronic tuberculosis.
The source of infection may be endogenous or exogenous **(Fig. 4.20)**:
- **Endogenous infection** stems from the healed primary focus containing dormant bacteria which have been reactivated.
- **Exogenous bacteria** enter the body from outside and represent reinfection.

Pulmonary tuberculosis is the most common form of secondary tuberculosis. Most often, the lesions are in the apical part of the lungs, favouring the growth of mycobacteria which are strict aerobe and thrive best in high oxygen tension in the apex.

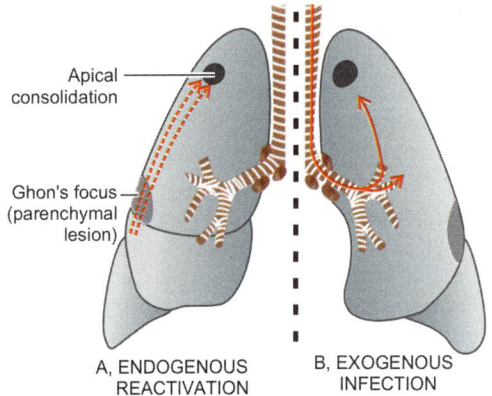

FIGURE 4.20: Progressive secondary tuberculosis. A, Endogenous infection from reactivation of dormant primary complex. B, Exogenous infection from fresh dose of tubercle bacilli.

Outcome of secondary pulmonary tuberculosis may be as under:
I. Fibrocalcific healing
II. Progression to several non-healing forms of tuberculosis which include:
i. fibrocaseous tuberculosis
ii. tuberculous caseous pneumonia
iii. military tuberculosis
iv. tuberculous empyema

Q52. Discuss major features of various possible outcomes of secondary pulmonary tuberculosis.

The possible outcomes of secondary pulmonary tuberculosis are as under:
I. **Fibrocaseous tuberculosis** develops at the site of the original tuberculous pneumonia in the lung parenchyma. Pneumonic area undergoes peripheral fibrous healing and central part undergoes massive caseous necrosis **(Fig. 4.21)**.

- If the necrotic material breaks through into the bronchus and is expectorated, leaving behind a fibrous tissue enclosed cavity, it is called *cavitary or open fibrocaseous tuberculosis*. The external fibrous tissue contains consolidated parts of the lung parenchyma. The inside of the cavity may be traversed by remnants of the bronchi and blood vessels, some of which are patent and functional, and some are thrombosed and occluded.
- If the necrotic tissue remains encased in the fibrous capsule, it remains as a *solid non-cavitary focus*. Solid areas contain numerous confluent granulomas, fibrous tissue and foci of calcification (Fig. 4.22). The overlying pleura may also show fibrosis or tuberculous granulomas.

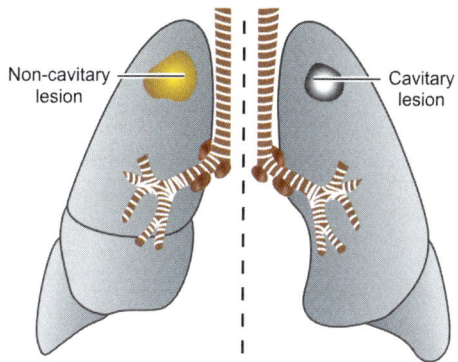

FIGURE 4.21: Fibrocaseous tuberculosis. Chronic fibrocaseous non-cavitary tuberculosis (left) and cavitary/open fibrocaseous tuberculosis (right).

Complications of fibrocaseous tuberculosis include the following pathologic changes:

i. *Aneurysms of arteries* crossing the lumen of the cavity are prone to rupture and bleed with massive haemoptysis.

ii. Formation of *bronchopleural fistula* connecting bronchus on side with the pleural cavity on the other side.

iii. *Tuberculous empyema,* occurring from the rupture of the pulmonary lesion into the pleural cavity and intrapleural discharge of the caseous material and bacteria.

iv. *Fibrosing pleuritis* with obliteration of the pleural cavity.

II. **Tuberculous caseous pneumonia** develops in persons with high degree of hypersensitivity and low resistance. In addition to necrotising granulomas, the lung alveoli of entire lobes are filled with an exudate that contains oedema fluid, neutrophils, macrophages and numerous bacilli (Fig. 4.23).

III. **Miliary tuberculosis** results from a lympho-haematogenous spread of mycobacteria through the lungs. If the spread is through the lymphatics and pulmonary artery branches, military tuberculosis remains restricted to the lungs. If the mycobacteria

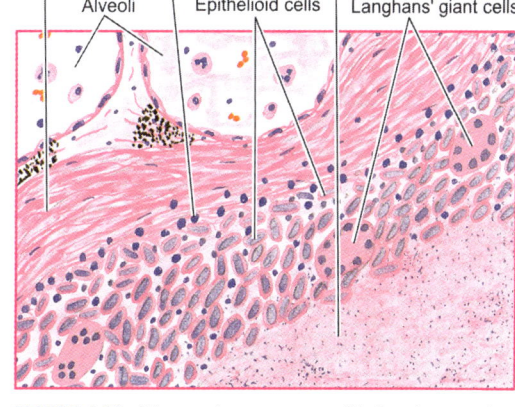

FIGURE 4.22: Microscopic appearance of lesions in secondary fibrocaseous tuberculosis of the lung showing wall of the cavity.

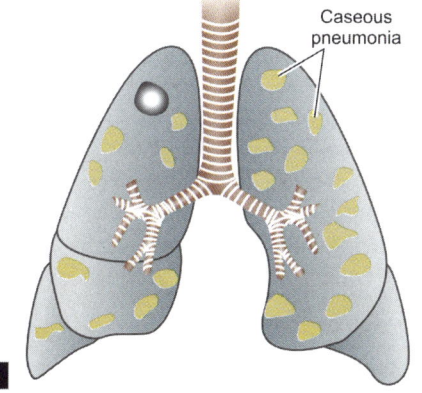

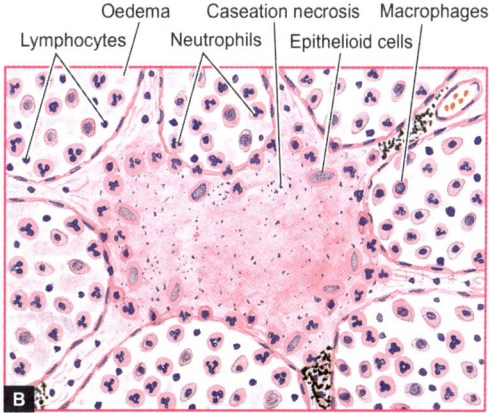

FIGURE 4.23: A, Bilateral tuberculous caseous pneumonia. B, Tuberculous caseous pneumonia showing exudative reaction.

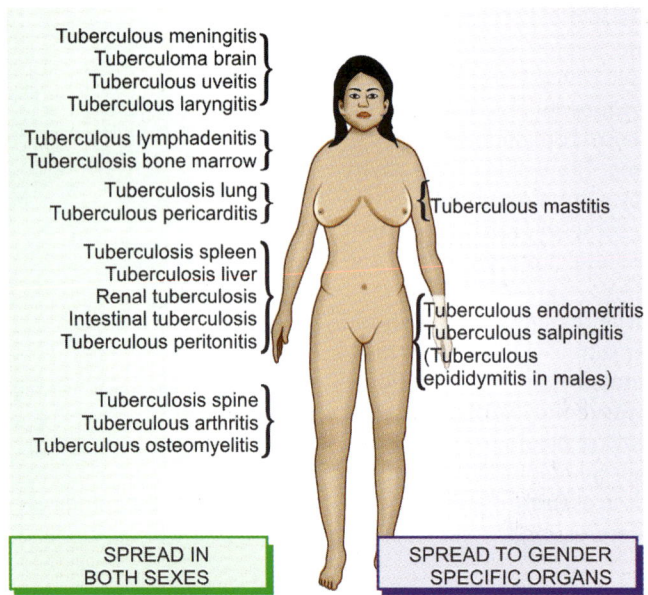

FIGURE 4.24: Miliary spread to different organs by lymphohaematogenous route.

enter into the pulmonary vein, they may reach the systemic circulation and disseminate through the entire body **(Fig. 4.24)**.

On gross examination, the military lesions are millet-sized, 1–2 mm in diameter, and microscopically composed of caseating granulomas **(Fig. 4.25)**.

IV. **Pleurisy and tuberculous empyema** Pleurisy presents as *serous or fibrinous pleuritis,* which tends to progress to *obliterative fibrosing pleuritis.* In *tuberculous empyema,* the cavity is filled with necrotic material discharged into the cavity from a primary pulmonary lesion.

The cause of death in secondary tuberculosis of the lungs is usually pulmonary insufficiency, cor pulmonale, pulmonary haemorrhage, sepsis due to dissemination of mycobacteria or military tuberculosis, and systemic amyloidosis.

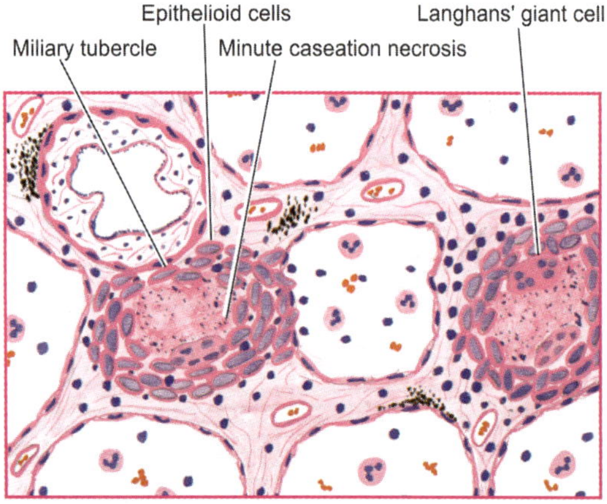

FIGURE 4.25: Microscopy of miliary tubercles in lung having minute areas of central caseation necrosis.

Q53. How is tuberculosis diagnosed clinically?

Tuberculosis may have many clinical presentations. Secondary pulmonary tuberculosis, which still represents the most important clinical form of tuberculosis, presents with the following signs and symptoms:

i. *Symptoms referable to lungs*, such as cough, dyspnoea, haemoptysis, etc. Chest X-rays show typical apical changes and pleural effusion, or military dissemination involving large portion of one or both lungs.

ii. *Systemic features*, such as night sweat, fever, fatigue, loss of appetite, weight-loss, and weakness.

iii. *Bacteriologic findings*, which are essential for diagnosis include: demonstration of AFB in the sputum, or in bacterial culture. Molecular biology tests may be used if other tests are inconclusive.

iv. *Complete haemogram* and laboratory studies, most notably evidence of lymphocytosis and elevated ESR.

v. *Tuberculin skin test.*

vi. *Interferon gamma release assay (IGRA),* measuring the cytokine release in blood may be used as a substitute for the tuberculin test.

vii. *Fine needle aspiration biopsy* of enlarged lymph nodes with cytologic examination of the aspirate, combined with microbiologic studies.

Q54. Enumerate the spectrum of lesions in pulmonary tuberculosis.

Figure 4.26 illustrates the entire spectrum of lesions in the lungs and pleura in pulmonary tuberculosis.

Q55. What is leprosy? Briefly discuss its etiologic agent and modes of transmission.

Definition Leprosy is a chronic, non-fatal infectious disease caused by *Mycobacterium leprae*. It affects mostly cooler parts of the body, such as the skin, mouth, eye, respiratory tract, peripheral nerves, superficial lymph nodes and testes.

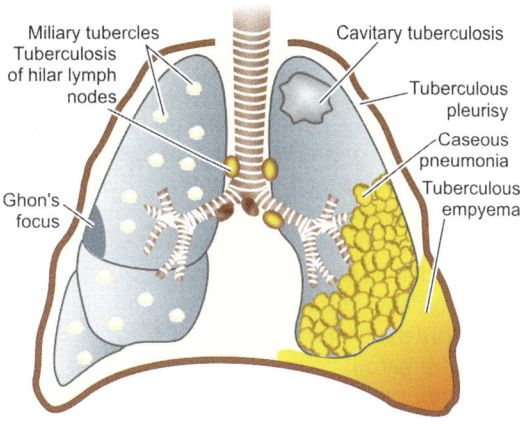

FIGURE 4.26: Spectrum of lesions in the lungs and pleura in various types of pulmonary tuberculosis.

- The early changes are seen in the skin and nerves.
- If bacteraemia develops, many internal organs can be affected.
- Chronic advanced disease may be complicated by amyloidosis and renal disease.

Bacteriology *Mycobacterium leprae* is an acid fast bacterium resembling *M. tuberculosis*. In tissue, it appears as compact masses (*globi*) or arranged in parallel fashion like *cigarettes-in-pack*. *M. leprae* has characteristic *neurotropism* and binds to basal lamina of Schwann cells in nerves.

Sampling → *'split skin scrapings'* from the cut edges of the dermis or *nasal smears*. The following techniques are used for the examination of these samples:

i. *Acid-fast stains* according to Ziehl-Neelsen or Fite-Faraco. AFB stains can be used to assess the density of bacteria (bacillary index), and decide if the disease should be classified as multibacillary or paucibacillary.
ii. *Gomori methenamine silver stain*
iii. *Molecular methods such as PCR*
NOTE: IgM antibodies to *PGL-1 antigen* are found in 95% cases of lepromatous leprosy, but only in 60% cases of tuberculoid leprosy.

Incidence The disease is prevalent in countries with hot and moist climates.
- Affected countries are predominantly in Asia, Africa and Latin America.
- India constitutes about 60% of new cases. The disease is uncommon in Europe and North America.

Mode of transmission Leprosy is a *slow communicable disease* with *long incubation* between first exposure and the appearance of symptoms (2–20 years). It is most often transmitted by *direct contact* as the microbes are shed from damaged skin, nasal secretions, mouth and hair follicles.

Q56. Discuss immunologic aspects of leprosy.

Immunology of leprosy *M. leprae* elicit a *delayed cell mediated immune response*.
i. *Antigens* evoking the immune response are: *M. leprae* specific phenolic glycolipid (PGL-1) and lipoarabinomannan (LAM).
ii. *Genotype* of the host determines the type of immune reaction.
iii. *Two classes of T cells* are activated:
- CD4+ helper T cells which also have cytotoxic effects. In tuberculoid leprosy, CD4+ T cells predominate.
- CD8+ cytotoxic/suppressor T cells. In lepromatous leprosy, CD8+ cells predominate but are inefficient in destroying the bacilli.
iv. *Humoral response* is reflected in a high level of immunoglobins in serum, but these antibodies have no protective effect.

Lepromin test is not used for diagnostic purposes. It is used for *classifying types of leprosy*. It is negative in lepromatous leprosy and it is positive in tuberculoid leprosy, where it can elicit two types of reaction:

- Early positive reaction *(Fernandez reaction)* 24–48 hours induration of skin.
- Late positive reaction *(Mitsuda reaction)* in the form of granulomas, 3–4 weeks after injection.

Q57. Discuss classification of leprosy.

According to the **original Ridley and Jopling classification**, two major forms of leprosy are recognised:
i. *lepromatous type,* representing low resistance, and
ii. *tuberculoid type* representing high resistance.
Using a **modified Ridley and Jopling classification**, five clinicopathologic groups are recognised:
i. TT-tuberculoid polar (high resistance)
ii. BT-borderline tuberculoid
iii. BB-borderline tuberculoid
iv. BL-borderline lepromatous
v. LL-lepromatous polar (low resistance)
In addition, not included in Ridley-Jopling classification, are cases of indeterminate leprosy, pure neural leprosy, and histoid leprosy that resembles a nodule of dermatofibroma and positive for lepra bacilli.

Q58. What are the basic principles of histopathologic examination in classification of lepra lesions?

Histopathologic classification of leprosy is performed on **skin biopsy** samples.
Following **broad guidelines** are followed during the histopathologic examination:
i. Cell type of granuloma
ii. Nerve involvement
iii. Bacterial load
iv. Presence of absence of lymphocytes
v. Relationship of granulomas to epidermis and the adnexa
NOTE: Caution should be used for the following reasons:
- *Multibacillary leprosy* like LL and BL, presents no diagnostic problems on histopathologic examination.
- *Paucibacillary leprosy* like indeterminate and tuberculoid lesions, may be more problematic and are usually interpreted in context of clinical evidence.

Q59. What are the major clinicopathologic features of two polar forms of leprosy?

Polar forms of leprosy are lepromatous and tuberculoid.
I. **Lepromatous leprosy**
Histopathology (Fig. 4.27, A)
i. Characterised by *dermal infiltrates of foamy macrophages* ('lepra cells' or Virchow cells).
ii. Infiltrates are located around nerves, blood vessels or dermal appendages.

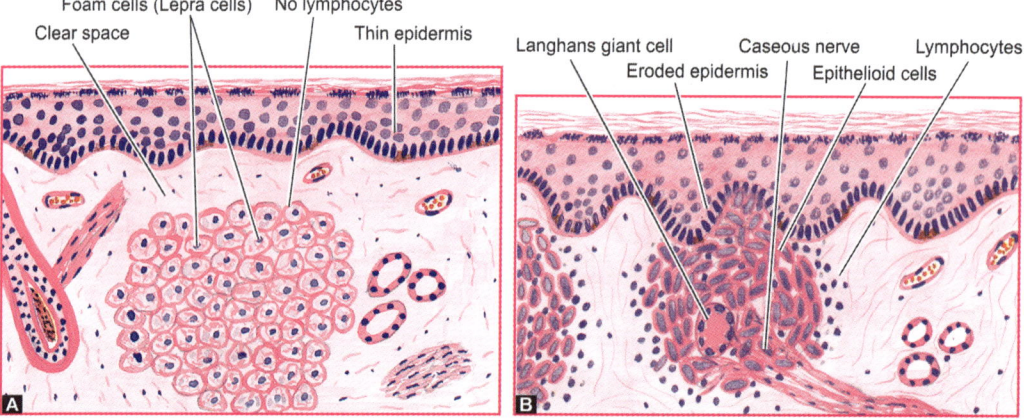

FIGURE 4.27: A, Lepromatous leprosy (LL). There is collection of proliferating foam macrophages (lepra cells) in the dermis, sparse lymphocytes and a clear subepidermal zone. B, Tuberculoid leprosy (TT). Granuloma eroding the basal layer of the epidermis. The granuloma is composed of epithelioid cells with sparse Langhans' giant cells and many lymphocytes.

iii. There are no lymphocytes.
iv. The infiltrate does not encroach upon the thin epidermis, from which it is separated by a clear zone.
v. AFB stains demonstrates numerous bacilli in globules or in form of 'cigarettes-in-pack'.
Clinical features
i. Skin lesions are multiple, symmetrical and slightly hypopigmented.
ii. They include macules, papules, nodules or diffuse infiltrates.
iii. Nodular lesions on the face may coalesce and give a leonine facies.
iv. The lesions are hypoaesthetic or anaesthetic but the sensory disturbance is not as distinct as in tuberculoid leprosy.

II. Tuberculous leprosy
Histopathology (Fig. 4.27, B)
i. Characterised by *hard granulomas in the dermis*.
ii. Granulomas consist of epithelioid cells and giant cells, surrounded at the periphery by a mantle of lymphocytes.
iii. Granulomas erode the basal layer of the epidermis.
iv. There is no clear zone between the granulomas and the epidermis.
v. AFB are few and usually in the nerves.
Clinical features
i. Skin lesions are either solitary, or present as a few asymmetrical lesions.
ii. Lesions present in the form of hypopigmented and erythematous macules.
iii. Sensory impairment is prominent.

Q60. Tabulate the major contrasting features of lepromatous and tuberculoid leprosy.

Table 4.6 summarises the salient differences between lepromatous and tuberculoid leprosy.

TABLE 4.6 Differences between lepromatous and tuberculoid leprosy.

FEATURE	LEPROMATOUS LEPROSY	TUBERCULOID LEPROSY
1. Skin lesions	Symmetrical, multiple, hypopigmented, or erythematous, or maculopapular, or nodular lesions (leonine facies)	Asymmetrical, single or a few lesions, well-defined, hypopigmented and erythematous, macular lesions
2. Nerve involvement	Present but late and sensory disturbance is less severe	Present with distinct sensory disturbance
3. Histopathology	Collection of foamy macrophages or lepra cells in the dermis separated from epidermis by a 'clear zone', lymphocytes absent or a few only	Hard tubercle similar to granulomatous lesion, eroding the basal layer of epidermis; no clear zone, lymphocytes plenty
4. Bacteriology	Lepra cells highly positive for lepra bacilli seen as 'globi' or 'cigarettes-in-pack' appearance (multibacillary type)	Lepra bacilli few, seen in destroyed nerves as granular or beaded forms (paucibacillary type)
5. Complications	Type 2 reactional leprosy (ENL) may occur	Neurologic damage causing sensory loss and paralysis may occur
6. Immunity	Suppressed (low resistance)	Good immune response (high resistance)
7. Lepromin test	Negative	Positive
8. Prognosis	Progressive disease, bad prognosis	Milder disease, better prognosis

Q61. What is syphilis? Discuss its etiologic agent and modes of transmission.

Definition Syphilis is a sexually-transmitted (venereal) disease caused by spirochetes *Treponema pallidum*, characterised by episodes of active disease interrupted by periods of latency.
Etiologic agent *T. pallidum* is a spirochete, 10 μm long, actively moving in fresh preparations
- Live movable spirochetes best seen by dark ground illumination (DGI) microscopy.
- *T. pallidum* can be visualised by antibodies in a fluorescence test and by silver impregnation.
- Molecular biology useful for diagnosis (PCR).
- *T. pallidum* cannot be grown in the laboratory media, but can be propagated in rabbits and chimpanzees.

Epidemiology Global health problem especially in underdeveloped countries.

Modes of transmission It can occur by the following four routes:
i. Sexual transmission, heterosexual or homosexual
ii. Intimate person-to-person contact on lips, tongue or fingers
iii. Transfusion of infected blood
iv. Transplacental maternal to fetal transmission

Q62. Discuss immunologic aspects of syphilis and diagnostic tests based on it.

Immunology Syphilitic infection typically stimulates a local inflammation at the site of entry and the appearance of antibodies in blood.
- Inflammatory infiltrates in the primary lesion contain T and B lymphocytes, plasma cells and macrophages, which, however, provide no significant defense against the spirochetes.
- Spirochetes do not produce toxins and the lesions are due to host immune response and especially small blood vessel vasculitis which causes ischaemia.
- Antibodies produced in response to the infection generate no defense against *T. pallidum*.

Diagnostic tests These tests are classified as i) treponemal, and ii) nontreponemal.
I. *Treponemal tests* measure antibodies to *T. pallidum* antigen. These are:
i. Fluorescent treponemal antibody-absorbed (FTA-ABS) test
ii. Agglutinin assays
II. *Nontreponemal tests* are more often used. They measure IgM and IgG antibodies against cardiolipin-lecithin-cholesterol complex. These are:
i. Reiter protein complement fixation (RPCF) test is the test of choice for rapid diagnosis.
ii. Venereal Disease Research Laboratory (VDRL) test against an antigen in human syphilis tissue that is fixing complement if exposed to reactive serum.

Q63. What are the stages of acquired syphilis? Discuss pathologic lesions recognised in each stage.

Syphilis has three stages: i) primary, ii) secondary, and iii) tertiary **(Fig. 4.28)**.
I. **Primary syphilis** produces lesions on the genitalia or extragenital sites of entry.
Pathology Chancre is the prototypical lesion of primary syphilis, appears 2–4 weeks after the exposure.
i. It begins as a painless papule.
ii. Papule ulcerates and transforms into chancre with indurated margin accompanied by regional lymphadenitis.
iii. Spirochetes can be sampled and seen by DGI microscopy.

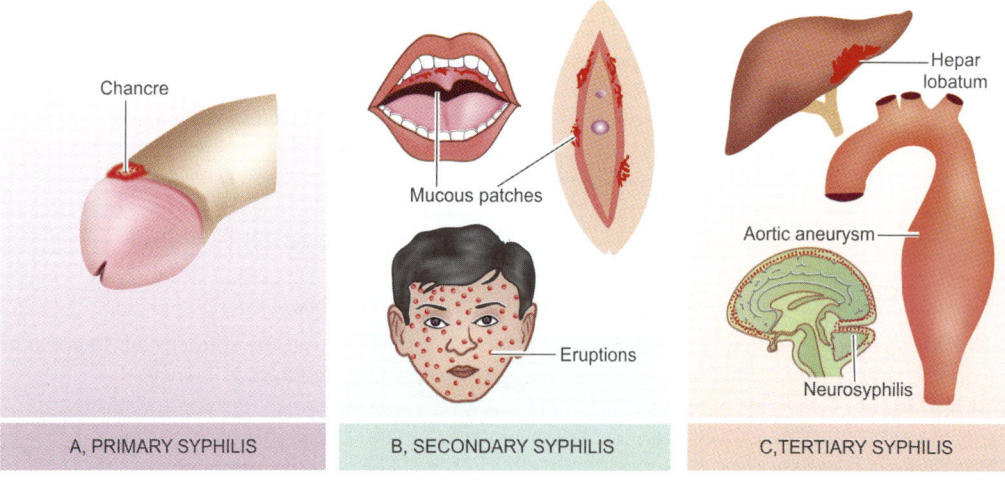

FIGURE 4.28: Organ involvement in various stages of acquired syphilis. A, *Primary syphilis*: Primary lesion is 'chancre' on glans penis. B, *Secondary syphilis:* Mucocutaneous lesions—mucous patches on oral and vaginal mucosa and generalised skin eruptions. C, *Tertiary syphilis:* Localised lesion as gumma of liver with scarring (hepar lobatum); diffuse lesions (right) in aorta (aneurysm, narrowing of mouths of coronary ostia and incompetence of aortic valve ring) and nervous system.

iv. Antibodies appear 1–3 weeks after the appearance of chancre.
v. Chancre heals even without treatment.

II. **Secondary syphilis** develops in inadequately treated or untreated infected person.
Pathology It presents with *mucocutaneous lesions and lymphadenopathy*, 2–3 months after the exposure.
i. Mucocutaneous lesions include patches in the mouth, pharynx and vagina, generalised skin *eruptions* and *condyloma lata* in the anogenital region.
ii. Antibodies are always present in the serum.
iii. Lesions contain numerous spirochetes and are highly contagious.

III. **Tertiary syphilis** develops after a latent period of 2–3 years after the first exposure. The lesions are less contagious and spirochetes are not readily demonstrable.
Pathology Two main types of lesions are seen: i) syphilitic gumma, or ii) diffuse lesions of tertiary syphilis.
i. *Syphilitic gumma* presents as a solitary rubbery nodular lesion in organs like liver, testis, bone or brain.
Microscopically, gumma consists of central necrosis surrounded by macrophages, lymphocytes, plasma cells and giant cells **(Fig. 4.29)**.
ii. *Diffuse lesions of tertiary syphilis* are caused by dissemination of spirochetes throughout the body. Most often, they are seen in the cardiovascular system and central nervous system.
a. *Cardiovascular syphilis* includes *syphilitic aortitis* resulting in aneurysmatic dilatation of thoracic aorta, incompetence of *aortic valves,* and narrowing of the ostia of coronary arteries.
b. *Neurosyphilis* may present as *meningovascular syphilis* involving predominantly the meninges; *tabes dorsalis* involving the spinal cord; or *general paresis* affecting the brain.

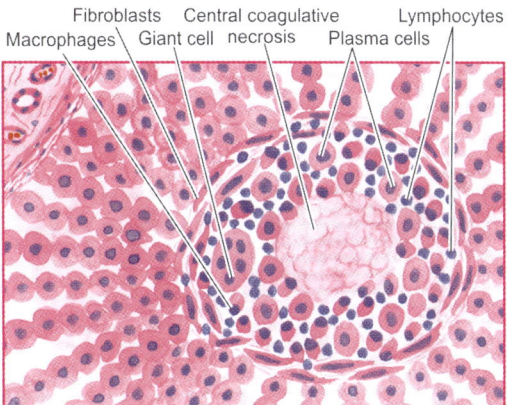

FIGURE 4.29: Typical microscopic appearance in the case of syphilitic gumma of the liver. Central coagulative necrosis is surrounded by palisades of macrophages and plasma cells marginated peripherally by fibroblasts.

Q64. What are the features of congenital syphilis?

The disease affects the foetus *in utero* after the 16th week of pregnancy. The disease is characterised by the following clinicopathologic features:
i. Saddle-shaped nose due to the destruction of bridge of the nose
ii. Characteristic 'Hutchinson teeth' which are small, widely spaced, peg-shaped permanent teeth
iii. Mucocutaneous lesions of secondary syphilis
iv. Bone lesions such as epiphysitis and periostitis
v. Interstitial keratitis with corneal opacities
vi. Diffuse fibrosis of the liver
vii. Interstitial fibrosis of the lungs
viii. Foetal death is common
Microscopy The changes include plasma cell rich chronic perivascular infiltrates. Spirochetes are numerous and can be demonstrated by special stains.

Q65. What is sarcoidosis? Briefly discuss its etiopathogenesis.

Definition Sarcoidosis is a chronic granulomatous systemic disease of unknown origin, most often affecting the lymph nodes, lungs, liver, skin and eyes. However, it can involve many other organs.
Etiopathogenesis Unknown, but three interlinked factors may play a role: i) genetic predisposition, ii) exposure to environmental agents, iii) cellular immune response **(Fig. 4.30)**. Except for the

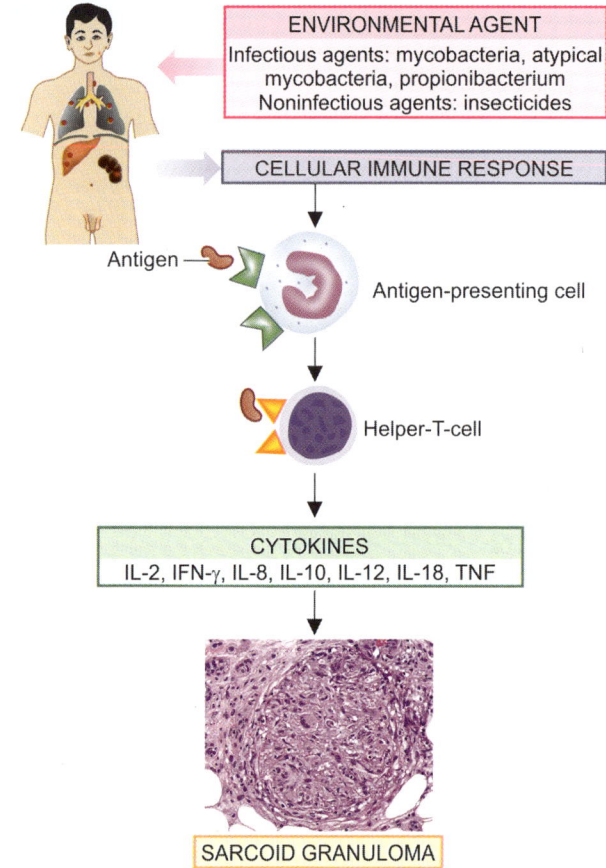

FIGURE 4.30: Schematic events in pathogenesis of lesions in sarcoidosis.

consensus about the importance of *T cell-mediated immune response* and the formation of *granulomas,* all other aspects of sarcoidosis are debatable.

Q66. What are the major clinicopathologic features of sarcoidosis?

Pathology The lungs are most often affected, usually in combination with the involvement of thoracic lymph nodes. Other commonly involved organs are the meninges, the uvea of the eye, lacrimal and salivary glands, skin, liver and spleen **(Fig. 4.31)**.

Microscopy The disease is characterised by the appearance of 'naked' *granulomas* composed almost exclusively of epithelioid cells and scattered multinucleated giant cells. There are

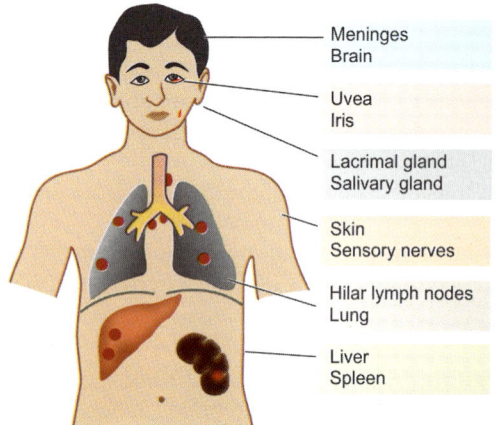

FIGURE 4.31: Common locations of lesions in sarcoidosis. The lesions are predominantly seen throughout lung parenchyma. Other common sites are lymph nodes, skin, liver and eye.

almost no lymphocytes; if lymphocytes are present they are scarce **(Fig. 4.32)**.

Clinical features
i. The disease may be asymptomatic or present with major organ dysfunction.
ii. Lung involvement is found in 90% of all patients causing a variety of symptoms that vary in intensity.
iii. Other organ involvement includes skin lesions and enlargement/dysfunction of parenchymal organs.
iv. Constitutional symptoms are usually non-specific and vary in intensity. These include low grade fever, night sweats, and weight loss.

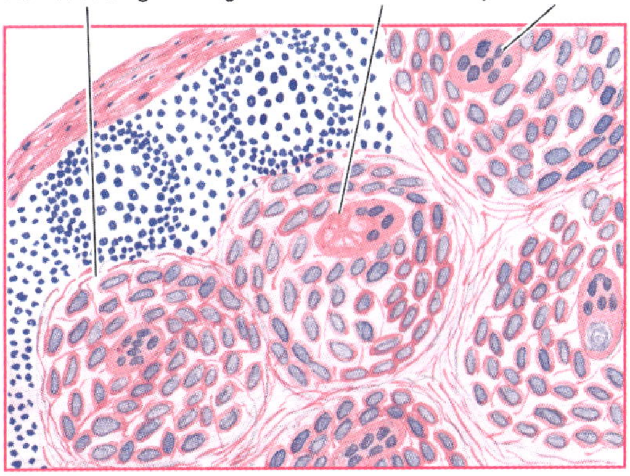

Diagnosis
i. Imaging studies usually show lung changes and lymphadenopathy.
ii. Serum levels of *angiotensin-converting enzyme* are elevated in 60% of acute disease cases and 20% of chronic cases.
iii. Cytologic studies *(bronchoalveolar lavage)* and *biopsy* of lungs, lymph nodes or other internal organs provide support the diagnosis.
Tuberculosis always remains in the differential diagnosis and must be excluded clinically **(Table 4.7)**.

FIGURE 4.32: Peribronchial lymph node involvement in pulmonary sarcoidosis. Characteristically, there are non-caseating epithelioid cell granulomas which have paucity of lymphocytes. A few giant cells with inclusions are also seen in the illustration.

Q67. What are the major differences between tuberculosis and sarcoidosis.

Table 4.7 sums up the salient distinguishing features between tuberculosis and sarcoidosis.

TABLE 4.7 Distinguishing features between tuberculosis and sarcoidosis.

FEATURE	TUBERCULOSIS	SARCOIDOSIS
1. *Definition*	Classic example of caseating granulomatous inflammation caused by Mycobacterium tuberculosis	Multisystem inflammatory disease of unknown etiology characterised by non-caseating granulomas
2. *Location of lesions*	Most commonly lungs; other common location lymph nodes; miliary spread by haematogenous route to various organs	Most commonly lungs; other common locations lymph nodes, skin, liver, eyes
3. *Pathogenesis*	Delayed hypersensitivity (type IV reaction), caseous necrosis due to mycobacterial cell wall or its cytoplasm	In genetically predisposed host (most common HLA-DRB1), exposure to infectious or noninfectious environmental agent, followed by cellular immune response
4. *Clinical features*	Respiratory complaints: productive cough, may be with haemoptysis, low-grade fever, night sweats	Range from asymptomatic to those with organ failure; most common respiratory complaints: dry cough, dyspnoea
5. *Morphology*	i. Typically, granulomatous inflammation with caseation necrosis ii. Lymphocytes present in and around granulomas iii. No inclusions in giant cells iv. AFB staining may be positive	i. Typically, non-caseating granulomas, may have fibrinoid necrosis ii. Naked granulomas, devoid of lymphocytic infiltration iii. May have inclusions in the giant cells iv. AFB staining negative
6. *Diagnosis*	X-ray chest, AFB microscopy, blood profile (raised ESR), tuberculin skin test	X-ray chest, serum ACE levels (>2 times), biopsy or cytology material (BAL or EBUS-NA), elevated serum ACE level
7. *Prognosis and complications*	Better prognosis if good compliance with ATT; main complications haemoptysis, respiratory insufficiency	Treated with immunosuppressive therapy, advanced disease may lead to irreversible fibrosis of lungs

TISSUE REPAIR

Q68. How does tissue injury heal?

Following injury, body attempts to restore its normal structure and function by two processes: regeneration and repair. These two processes are distinguished from each other by the type of tissue replacing the injured tissue, as under:

I. **Regeneration** when the healing involves proliferation of surrounding undamaged specialised cells and resulting in complete restoration of the original tissue.

II. **Repair** when the healing takes place by the formation of granulation tissue and subsequent fibrosis and scarring. Repair includes the participation of connective tissue stem cells, fibroblasts, endothelial cells, macrophages, platelets and the parenchyma cells of the injured organ.

Q69. How are the cells of the body classified according to their capacity for division?

Depending of their capacity to divide, the cells of the body are divided into three groups: i) labile cells, ii) stable cells, and iii) permanent cells **(Fig. 4.33)**.

I. **Labile cells** contribute to multiply throughout life. These include: cells of the epidermis, mucosa of internal organs haematopoietic cells of the bone marrow, and cells of the spleen and lymph nodes.

II. **Stable cells** decrease or lose their ability to proliferate after adolescence but retain the capacity to multiply in response to stimuli throughout adult life. These cells include: those of the liver, kidney and other parenchymal organs and mesenchymal cells like smooth muscle cells, fibroblasts, endothelial cells of the vessels, bone and cartilage.

III. **Permanent cells** are those cells which lose their ability to proliferate around the time of birth. These include: neurons of the central nervous system, skeletal muscle and myocardium.

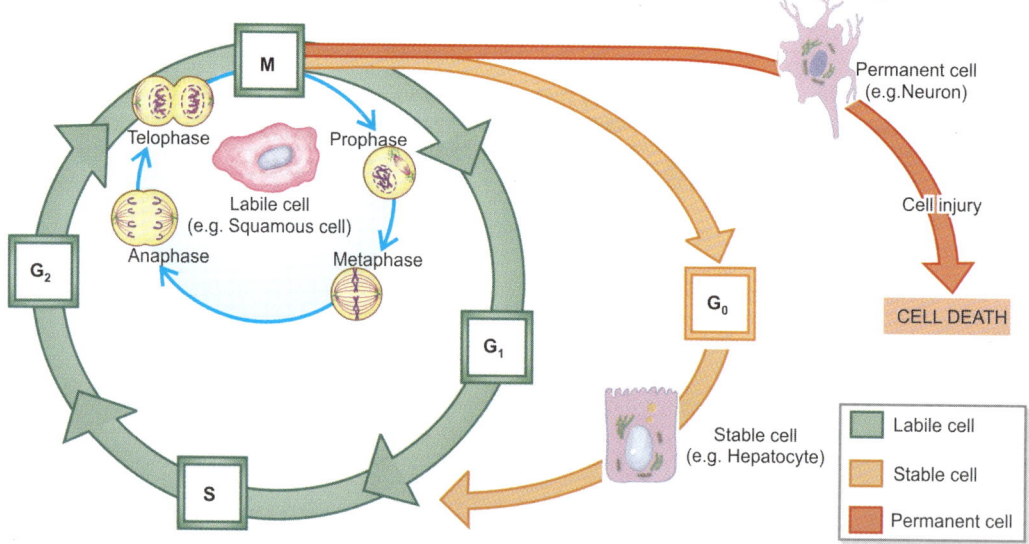

FIGURE 4.33: Parenchymal cells in relation to cell cycle (G_0–Resting phase; G_1, G_2–Gaps; S–Synthesis phase; M–Mitosis phase). The inner circle *shown with green line* represents cell cycle for labile cells; circle *shown with yellow-orange line* represents cell cycle for stable cells; and the circle *shown with red line* represents cell cycle for permanent cells. Compare them with traffic signals—green stands for 'go' applies here to dividing labile cells; yellow-orange signal for 'ready to go' applies here to stable cells which can be stimulated to enter cell cycle; and red signal for 'stop' here means non-dividing permanent cells.

Q70. What is granulation tissue and how is it formed?

Granulation tissue, named after the granular tissue forming the bottom of a wound, forms during repair, most prominently during the proliferative phase of healing **(Fig. 4.34)**.

Healing occurs in four partially overlapping phases: i) bleeding phase, ii) inflammatory phase, iii) proliferative phase, and iv) remodelling phase.

I. **Bleeding phase** occurs due to the rupture of blood vessels and lasts a few hours until clotting takes place.

II. **Inflammatory phase** is an essential phase which involves a vascular and a cellular phase, and is regulated by chemical mediators. Initial infiltration includes *neutrophils* and the entire area is flooded with plasma containing many biologically active proteins. Neutrophils begin the removal of tissue debris and parts of the clotted blood. Neutrophils are replaced by *macrophages,* which continue the demolition and also begin secreting cytokines, which will attract additional cells, and regulate the proliferation of cells already present in the area.

III. **Proliferative phase** begins 1–2 days after injury and reaches its peak 2–3 weeks thereafter. It involves angiogenesis and fibrogenesis:

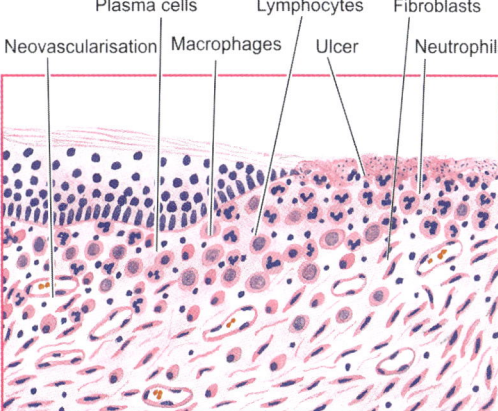

FIGURE 4.34: Active granulation tissue has inflammatory cell infiltrate, newly formed blood vessels, fibroblasts and myofibroblasts in loose extracellular matrix.

i. *Angiogenesis,* i.e. formation of new blood vessels under the influence of vascular endothelial growth factor (VEGF), which has its corresponding receptor only on endothelial cells. Other growth factors also contribute: platelet derived growth factor (PDGF), transforming growth factor-β (TGF-β), basic fibroblast growth factor (b-FGF), and surface integrins.

ii. *Fibrogenesis* begins with the laying down of amorphous extracellular matrix (ECM) which contains various substances including adhesive glycoproteins, basement membrane proteins, elastic fibres, proteoglycans, and fibronectin, a large molecule that tends to bind other molecules together.

The cells involved in the production of the matrix include *myofibroblasts,* which have hybrid features of fibroblasts and smooth muscle cells. The fibrillar matrix first includes collagen type III, which is then removed through the action of collagenase and is replaced by collagen type I.

IV. **Remodelling phase** begins when the proliferation phase is at its peak 2–3 weeks after injury. It involves reduction of blood vessels which are replaced by collagen type I and cross-linking of the collagen fibres. This leads to scar formation (*cicatrisation*).

Q71. Which factors influence tissue repair?

Certain local and some general factors may promote repair or delay it.
I. **Local factors** that delay repair and wound healing are as follows:
i. Infection
ii. Poor blood supply
iii. Foreign bodies
iv. Movement
v. Exposure to ionising radiation
II. **General factors** playing a role in healing are:
i. Age
ii. Nutritional status
iii. Systemic infections
iv. Glucocorticosteroid and non-steroidal anti-inflammatory drug (NSAIDs) administration
v. Uncontrolled diabetes mellitus
vi. Haematologic abnormalities like defects in neutrophil functions, neutropenia and bleeding disorders
vii. Colder temperature

Q72. Which wounds heal by primary intention?

Healing by first intention (primary union) occurs in wounds that have the following characteristics:
i. Clean and uninfected
ii. Surgically excised
iii. Without much loss of cells and tissue
iv. Edges of the wound are approximated by surgical sutures

Q73. What are the phases of wound healing by first intention?

The sequence of events is illustrated in **Figure 4.35** and includes the following phases:
i. Initial haemorrhage
ii. Acute inflammatory response
iii. Epithelial changes and proliferation of the epidermal cells from the edges of the wound
iv. Organisation by an ingrowth of fibroblasts
v. Suture track healing, which occurs in same order as wound healing itself

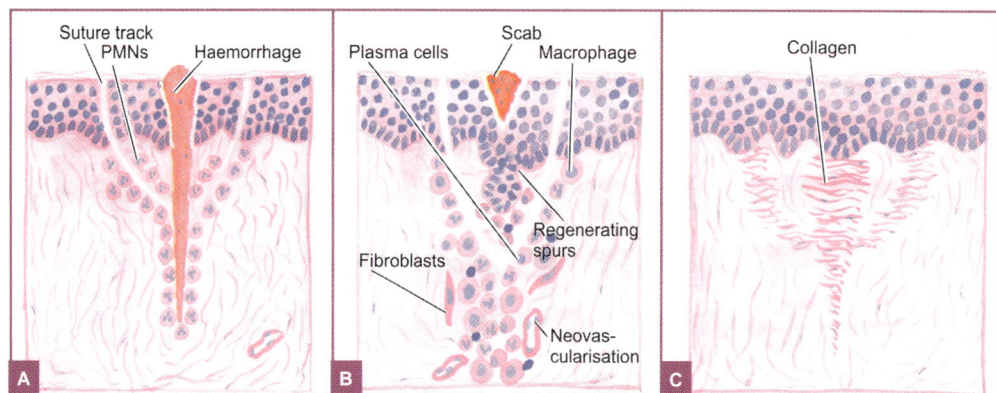

FIGURE 4.35: Primary union of skin wounds. A, The incised wound as well as suture track on either side are filled with blood clot and there is inflammatory response from the margins. B, Spurs of epidermal cells migrate along the incised margin on either side as well as around the suture track. Formation of granulation tissue also begins from below. C, Removal of suture at around 7th day results in scar tissue at the sites of incision and suture track.

Q74. Which wounds heal by secondary intention?

Healing by secondary intention occurs in wounds that have the following characteristics:
i. Open wounds that are infected
ii. Open wounds with extensive tissue loss
iii. Open wounds with gaping edges that could not be approximated or held together

Q75. What are the phases of healing by secondary intention?

The sequence of events is illustrated in **Figure 4.36** and includes the following phases:
i. Initial haemorrhage
ii. Inflammatory response
iii. Epithelial changes at the edges of the wound which occurs after the formation of a scab filling the defect and covering the formation of the granulation tissue

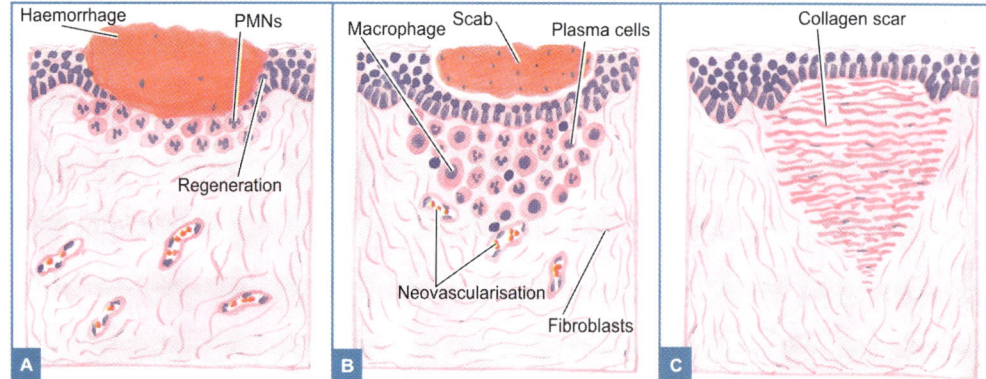

FIGURE 4.36: Secondary union of skin wounds. A, The open wound is filled with blood clot and there is inflammatory response at the junction of viable tissue. B, Epithelial spurs from the margins of wound meet in the middle to cover the gap and separate the underlying viable tissue from necrotic tissue at the surface forming scab. C, After contraction of the wound, a scar smaller than the original wound is left.

iv. Granulation tissue formation
v. Wound contraction through the action of myofibroblasts
vi. Collagenous scar formation

Q76. What are the differences in healing by primary and secondary healing of wounds?

The differences between primary and secondary union of wounds are presented in **Table 4.8**.

TABLE 4.8 Differences between primary and secondary union of wounds.

FEATURE	PRIMARY UNION	SECONDARY UNION
1. Cleanliness of wound	Clean	Unclean
2. Infection	Generally uninfected	May be infected
3. Margins	Surgical clean	Irregular
4. Sutures	Used	Not used
5. Healing	Scanty granulation tissue at the incised gap and along suture tracks	Exuberant granulation tissue to fill the gap
6. Outcome	Neat linear scar	Contracted irregular wound
7. Complications	Infrequent, epidermal inclusion cyst formation	Suppuration, may require debridement

Q77. What are the complications of skin wound healing?

i. Infection
ii. Implantation (epidermal) cyst formation
iii. Pigmentation which may be a consequence of previous bleeding and accumulation of haemosiderin, or retention of pigmented material inside the wound.
iv. Deficient scar formation, usually due to inadequate formation of granulation tissue
v. *Incisional hernia*, which usually occurs after weak healing with dehiscence of the wound and protrusion of the abdominal contents through the gap.
vi. Hypertrophied scar and keloid formation.
a. *Hypertrophied scar* is confined to the site of primary injury. It contains hyalinised collagen fibres that are laid down in parallel.
b. *Keloid* extends beyond the boundaries of the injury and is composed of haphazardly arranged collagen fibres.
vii. Excessive contraction of the wound results in *contracture* or *cicatrisation*. Its clinical examples are:
a. Dupuytren's palmar contracture
b. Plantar contracture
c. Peyronie's disease (contracture of the cavernous tissue of the penis)

Q78. What are the clinical factors that will determine whether bone fracture will heal primary or secondary union?

This depends on the nature of fracture which may be:
I. *Traumatic* (previously normal bone) or *pathological* (in previously diseased bone).
II. *Complete* through entire thickness of the bones or *incomplete* like green stick fracture.
III. *Simple* (closed), *comminuted* (splintering of bone) or *compound* (communicating with skin surface).

Q79. What are the differences between primary and secondary union of fractures?

I. **Primary union of fractures** occurs when the ends of the fracture are approximated surgically. It takes place by the formation of medullary callus without the formation of periosteal callus.
II. **Secondary union of fractures** occurs when plaster casts are applied for immobilisation and it evolves through following three phases **(Fig. 4.37)**:
i. *Procallus formation* which includes four phases:
a. Haematoma
b. Local inflammation
c. Ingrowth of granulation tissue
d. Formation of callus composed of woven bone and cartilage
ii. *Osseous callus formation*
iii. *Remodelling*

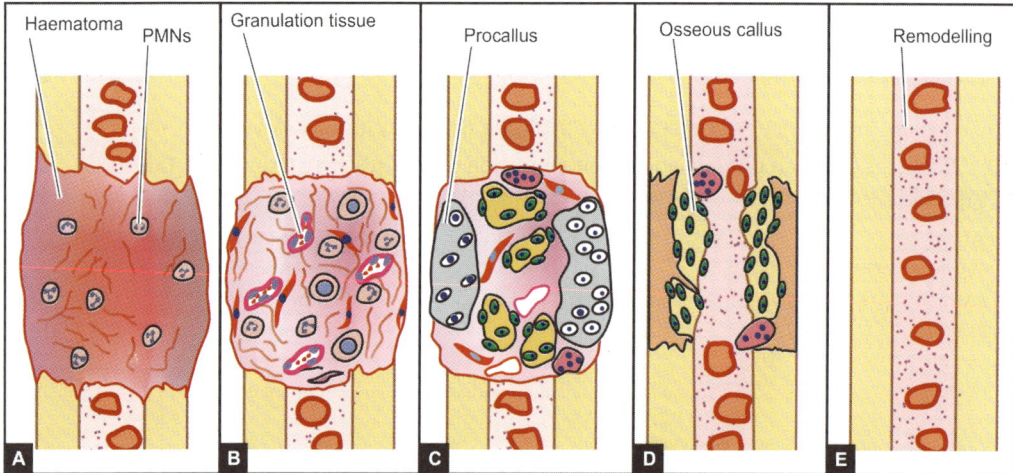

FIGURE 4.37: Fracture healing. A, Haematoma formation and local inflammatory response at the fracture site. B, Ingrowth of granulation tissue with formation of soft tissue callus. C, Formation of procallus composed of woven bone and cartilage with its characteristic fusiform appearance and having three arbitrary components—external, intermediate and internal callus. D, Formation of osseous callus composed of lamellar bone following clearance of woven bone and cartilage. E, Remodelled bone ends; the external callus cleared away. Intermediate callus converted into lamellar bone and internal callus developing bone marrow cavity.

Q80. What are the complications of fracture healing?

The following are the complications of fracture healing:
i. **Fibrous union** when the callus remains composed of fibrous tissue that never becomes ossified. Occasionally a false joint (*pseudoarthrosis*) may develop at the site of incomplete healing, allowing the movement of the adjacent bone parts.
ii. **Non-union** if the soft tissue is interposed between the fractured ends.
iii. **Delayed union** may occur due to the same causes that operate in delayed wound healing, such as infection, inadequate blood supply, poor nutrition, old age.

Q81. How does nervous tissue heal?

I. **Central nervous system** injury cannot be repaired. Brain and spinal cord are composed of permanent nerve cells, which cannot regenerate. Glia cell can proliferate and, therefore, there is gliosis.
II. **Peripheral nerves** show a capacity to regenerate through the proliferation of Schwann cells and sprouting of axons from the main body of the neuron.

Q82. How do muscles heal?

I. **Cardiac muscle** cannot regenerate and the injured or dead cardiac myocytes are replaced by fibrous tissue.
II. **Skeletal muscle cells** can regenerate to some extent, depending on the preservation of the muscle sheath. If the sheath is damaged, no regeneration is possible.
III. **Smooth muscle cells** have a limited capacity for regeneration and large defects cannot be replaced by new smooth muscle cells but are replaced by fibrous tissue.

> ### Chapter 4e Supplement: Online Content
> *Digital content of this chapter available with this book is meant for enhanced learning and self-assessment. In addition, it contains 30 Multiple Choice Questions (MCQs), 05 Clinicopathologic Vignettes, and 03 Image-based Questions; these are followed by their answers along with explanatory notes of correct and incorrect answers.*

CHAPTER 5

Immunopathology Including Amyloidosis

■ NORMAL IMMUNE SYSTEM

Q1. What are the two major types of immunity? List the pathologic conditions caused due to deranged immunity.

Immunity is divided into two types: natural (innate), and specific (adaptive) immunity. Their normal function is to protect the body from microbes and foreign injurious substances. Malfunctions of the immune system causes pathological reactions as under **(Fig. 5.1)**:
i. Immune deficiency disorders
ii. Hypersensitivity reactions
iii. Autoimmune diseases
iv. Amyloidosis

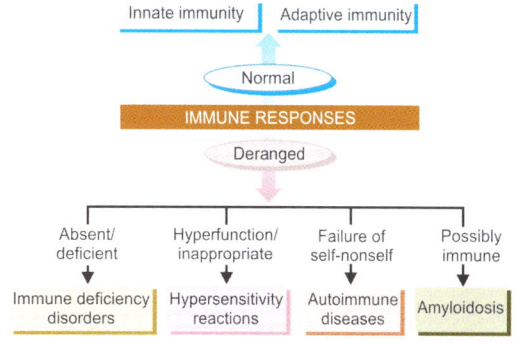

FIGURE 5.1: Normal and deranged immune responses in human beings.

Q2. Define natural (innate) immunity. Enumerate its components and functions.

Definition Innate immune response is inborn and is the first line of defense against pathogens. The basic features of natural immunity are:
i. Lack of antigenic specificity; by nature it is non-specific
ii. Rapid in response-reaction; appears within minutes
iii. No memory; does not confer long-lasting immunity to the host
Components These are distributed throughout the entire body and include:
i. Cells and tissues
ii. Soluble mediators
iii. Recognition receptors
Functions It has many functions but the three most important ones are:
i. Initial inflammatory reactions to various microbes, primarily by neutrophils and macrophages.
ii. Antiviral role played by various cytokines.
iii. Initiation and subsequent direction of adaptive immune response, mostly by antigen presenting cells such as dendritic cells and macrophages.

Q3. What are the tissue and cellular components of the innate immunity and its most important chemical mediators and receptors?

I. **Epithelial barriers** represent the major protective tissue components, including the skin and mucous membranes. Their function is to provide mechanical barrier to microbial invasion.

II. **Cellular defenses** include neutrophils, macrophages, dendritic cells (antigen-presenting tissue cells), natural killer cells, mast cells, innate lymphoid cells which secrete certain cytokines. but do not have T-cell receptors.

III. **Soluble mediators** include kinin-kallikrein system, complement proteins, C-reactive protein, mannose binding lectin, surfactant coating the respiratory passages.

IV. **Pattern-recognition receptors** expressed on cells such as macrophages, dendritic cells, and certain epithelial cells (i.e. cells of innate immune system excluding lymphocytes). Two most important groups of receptors are:

i. *Toll-like receptors* (TLR) on the cell membrane and cytosol and endosomal vesicles for the recognition of microbes expressing their pathogen-associated molecular patterns (PAMPs).

ii. *NOD-like receptors* (NLR; NOD stands for nucleotide oligomerisation domain) NLRs are important for the recognition of microbes and products of host's dead cells and biochemical changes in the metabolism of injured cells.

Q4. What is specific (adaptive) immunity? Briefly discuss its components and functions.

Definition Specific immunity is directed specifically against invading pathogens and foreign substances. It comprises two sets of cells:
i. T cells accounting for the cell-mediated immunity, and
ii. B cells involved in humoral immunity.

Major functions of adaptive immunity are:
i. Recognition of self from non-self antigens, followed by the presentation of non-self antigens to lymphocytes
ii. Specific response to non-self antigen and its elimination
iii. Immunological memory using specific memory cells
iv. Secretion of antibodies

Organs of innate immunity include:
i. Thymus
ii. Bone marrow
iii. Lymph nodes
iv. Spleen
v. Cutaneous lymphoid tissue
vi. Mucosa associated lymphoid tissue (MALT)

Cells involved in the immune system are:
- Lymphoid cells including T and B lymphocytes, NK cells and innate lymphoid cells
- Cells of the mononuclear phagocyte system, including macrophage and dendritic cells

Q5. What are the major contrasting features of innate and specific (adaptive) immunity?

Contrasting features of innate and adaptive immunity are presented in **Table 5.1**.

Q6. What are general features of the lymphoid cells?

i. *Circulation of lymphoid cells through the blood and lymph stream* Lymphocytes circulating from lymphoid organs to other tissue is a continuous process; this also allows lymphoid cells to migrate to the site of pathogen invasion, as part of inflammatory response.

ii. *Maturation and differentiation from lymphoid precursor cells in the bone marrow* B cells mature in secondary lymphoid organs, such as lymph nodes while T cell mature in the thymus.

iii. *Clusters of differentiation (CD)* are molecules, which appear on the surface of differentiated lymphocytes, reflecting their specific functions in the immune system:
- CDs belong to the immunoglobulin superfamily of cell adhesion molecules (CAM).
- They can be recognised with monoclonal antibodies.
- CDs are used clinically in pathology laboratories for cell sorting of lymphocytes and immunohistochemical recognition of various subsets in tissues.

iv. *Naïve lymphocytes* remain as such until they have been exposed to a specific antigen.

TABLE 5.1 Contrasting features of innate and adaptive immunity.

FEATURE	INNATE IMMUNITY	ADAPTIVE IMMUNITY
1. *Definition*	Natural or inborn, first line of defense against pathogen	Specific against invading pathogen
2. *Response time*	Rapid; within minutes to a few hours	Slow; within 4–7 days
3. *Antigenic specificity*	Lacks antigenic specificity	Specific against an invading antigen
4. *Immunologic memory*	Not present	Yes, present
5. *Duration of immunity*	No lasting immunity	Renders immunity (many instances) on next encounter with same pathogen
6. *Key components*	i. Epithelial barriers (skin, mucosa) ii. Cellular defenses (neutrophils, macrophages, dendritic cells, NK cells, mast cells) iii. Soluble mediators (kinins, complements, CRP) iv. Pattern-recognition molecules or receptors (TLRs, NLRs, RLRs, CLRs)	i. Lymphocytes (B, T, subclasses) ii. Antibodies or immunoglobulins iii. Cellular and humoral responses
7. *Major functions*	i. Initial inflammatory reaction ii. Anti-viral role iii. Initiation and direction of subsequent adaptive immune response	i. Recognition of self from non-self antigen ii. Mount a specific response against antigen iii. Develop immunologic memory iv. Secretion of antibodies

v. *Effector lymphocytes* are generated upon contact with antigen which is presented by dendritic cells and macrophages, which perform this function in context of the major histocompatibility complex (MHC) class II.

vi. *Memory cells* are formed as subsets of T and B lymphocytes which give the host long lasting immunity.

Q7. What are the main features of B cells?

i. B cells account for a minority (10–20%) of lymphocytes in blood.
ii. Primary function in antibody-mediated (humoral) immunity.
iii. Antigen recognition is mediated by IgM and IgD in the B-cell receptor (BCR) cell surface complex.
iv. Upon contact with the antigen, B cells will differentiate into plasma cells.
v. Common B cell markers are CD19, CD20, CD21, and CD79a and b. For example, CD21 serves for recognition of products of activated complement, and CD79a and b for signal transduction.

Q8. What are the main features of T cells?

i. T cells account for 70–80% of all lymphocytes in blood.
ii. Primary function is cell-mediated immunity.
iii. Antigen recognition through the cell surface T cell receptor (TCR), which has two chains (α and β), corresponding to α and β regions of the MHC on dendritic cells.
iv. Pan T cell markers are CD3, CD7, CD2.
v. There are three subsets of T cells are: helper T cells (CD4+), suppressor or cytotoxic T cells (CD8+), and regulatory T cells (a subset of CD4+). The ratio of CD4+ to CD8+ cells in circulation is 2:1.

Q9. What are the main features of subsets of T cells?

I. Helper T cells
i. Abbreviated as T_H *cells*, are *CD4+*
ii. They bind to MHC class II of dendritic cells for antigen recognition.
iii. They are activated by cytokines but also produce cytokines.
iv. There are three sets of T helper cells: T_H1, T_H2, T_H17.
v. T_H1 *cells* are activated by IFN-γ, which they also produce, together with IL-12. They participate in delayed hypersensitivity reactions, activation of macrophages and synthesis of IgG.

vi. T_H2 cells are induced by IL-4 and produce several interleukins. They regulate the synthesis of all immunoglobulins and have a role in the defense against parasites.

vii. T_H17 cells which are induced by TGF-β and several interleukins and produce IL-17. These cells release numerous neutrophils and macrophages and combat bacterial and fungal infection.

II. **Suppressor/cytotoxic T cells**

i. Abbreviated as T_s cells, are CD8+
ii. They suppress immune reactions.
iii. They are cytotoxic and destroy cells by direct action (not via cytokines, like CD4 cells!).
iv. Destroy cells infected with viruses, foreign cells, and tumour cells.
v. Bind to MHC class I of dendritic cells for antigen recognition.

III. **Regulatory cells**

i. Abbreviated as *Treg cells*, are CD4+
ii. They comprise a small fraction of CD4+ cells, which express CD25 and FOXP3 (scurfin), which help in their function.
iii. Keep the immune response limited.
iv. Prevent immune reaction against self antigens.

Q10. Tabulate the differences between T and B cells.

The differences between T and B lymphocytes are presented in **Table 5.2**.

TABLE 5.2 Differences between T and B lymphocytes.

FEATURE	T CELLS	B CELLS
1. *Origin*	Stem cells in bone marrow → Maturation in thymus	Stem cells in bone marrow → Maturation in bone marrow and secondary lymphoid organs
2. *Lifespan*	Small T cells: months to years T cell blasts: several days	Small B cells: less than 1 month B cell blasts : several days

3. *Location*
  i. Lymph nodes
  ii. Spleen
  iii. Peyer's patches
	
	Paracortex, deep cortex
	Periarteriolar
	Perifollicular
		
		Germinal centres, superficial cortex
		Germinal centres, red pulp
		Follicular centres

4. *Presence in blood*	70–80%	10–20%

5. *Surface markers*
  i. Ag receptors
  ii. Surface Ig
  iii. Fc receptor
  iv. Complement receptor
  v. CD markers
	
	TCR region
	Absent
	Absent
	Absent
	T_H cells CD4, 3, 7, 2
	T_s cells CD8, 3, 7, 2
		
		BCR region (IgM, IgD)
		Present
		Present
		Present
		CD19, 20, 21, 23

6. *Major functions*	i. Cell-mediated immune reactions ii. Helper T cells: destruction of viruses, tumour cells iii. Suppressor T cells: direct cytotoxicity against viruses, tumour cells iv. T regulatory cells: limit immune response and prevent reaction against self antigens	i. Antibody-mediated humoral reactions ii. Synthesis of specific antibodies (Igs) iii. Precursors of Ig-synthesising plasma cells

Q11. What are the principal features of NK cells?

i. NK (natural killer) cells represent 5–10% of circulating lymphocytes in blood.
ii. They contain granules in their cytoplasm.
iii. They do not have the usual markers of T or B cells, but express CD16 and CD56 and INF-γ.
iv. Their primary function is to kill antibody coated cells (antibody cell-mediated cytotoxicity).
v. Primary targets are virus-infected cells and tumour cells.

Q12. What are innate lymphoid cells?

i. They are a subset of T lymphocytes, that do not express CD3 and lack TCR.

ii. They participate in innate immune reactions.
iii. Produce certain cytokines to kill pathogens, even without priming.

Q13. What are the principal cells of the mononuclear phagocyte system?

The mononuclear phagocyte system includes i) dendritic cells, ii) macrophages in tissues, and c) monocytes in the blood.

I. **Dendritic cells**, so named because of the dendritic processes on their surface.
i. They are located in the skin and mucosae and the germinal centres of lymph nodes.
ii. They have two functions: a) antigen presentation, and b) participating in the secondary antibody response.
iii. Antigen presentation to T and B cell begins by a binding of antigens to dendritic cell surface receptors in the context of MHC class II.
iv. Secondary antibody-mediated response to antigens involves surface receptors for C3b and the Fc component of IgG found on dendritic cells plasma membrane.
v. They are not phagocytic.

II. **Macrophages** have a major role in the immune response, as under:
i. Phagocytosis of microbes → facilitated by the LPS-binding protein which mediates the binding of microbes to the LPS receptor, CD14, on the cell surface of macrophages.
ii. Phagocytosis of microbes and cells that have been opsonised by IgG or C3b (for which macrophages have receptors).
iii. Processing and presentation of antigens to T cell after the antigens have been solubilised in the cytoplasm of macrophages.
iv. Participation in the type IV hypersensitivity reaction in cooperation with T lymphocytes.

Q14. What are cytokines? Discuss their classification and major functions.

Definition Cytokines are biologically active substances, chemically classifies as peptides, proteins, and glycoproteins.

Functions Cytokines stimulate cells in three ways: a) autocrine, b) paracrine, and c) endocrine way. Their major actions include the following:
i. *Regulation of cell growth* This typically involves Janus family of kinases (JAK). JAK-promoting mitogen pathway and transmission of the signals to the nuclear DNA through signal transducer and activator of transcription (STAT) family of transcription factors.
ii. *Stimulation and regulation of inflammation* (page 57).
iii. *Activation of the immune system*.
NOTE: Cytokine storm resulting from an excessive release of cytokines may be fatal.

Classification Based on structural similarity, cytokines are grouped in the following three main categories (also see **Table 4.2**):
i. *Haematopoietic family of cytokines*: colony stimulating factors (G-CSF, GM-CSF), erythropoietin, thrombocytopoietin, several interleukins (e.g. IL-2 and IL-3).
ii. *IL-1α, IL-1β, tumour necrosis factor (TNF, cachectin), platelet-derived growth factor (PDGF), transforming growth factor-β (TGF-β) family*.
iii. *Chemokine family of cytokines* which regulates movement of cells through G-protein derived receptor. This group includes some interleukins (IL-8), monocyte chemokine protein (MCP), neutrophil activating protein (NAP), etc.

■ MAJOR HISTOCOMPATIBILITY COMPLEX AND TRANSPLANTATION

Q15. What is the major histocompatibility complex? Briefly discuss features of its classes.

Definition Major histocompatibility complex (MHC) is a region of chromosome 6 (6.p21.3) containing multiple expressed genes, the products of which are critical for immunologic specificity, histocompatibility, and susceptibility to autoimmune diseases. It is also known as human leucocyte antigen (HLA) region.

A key feature of HLA is its high polymorphism. Thus, there are numerous alleles of MHC genes that must be considered during transplantation of organs.

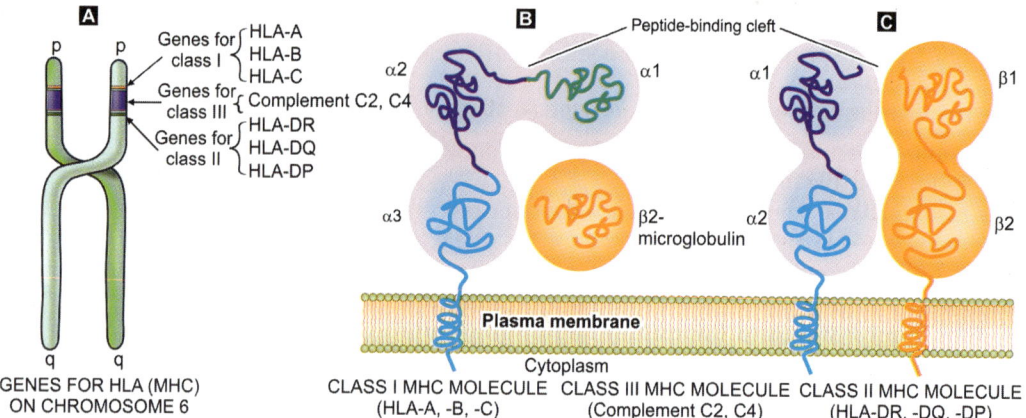

FIGURE 5.2: A, HLA genes and loci on short arm of chromosome 6. B, MHC class I molecules and interaction with CD8+ cells. Upper part of figure B shows configuration of T cell receptor region (TCR) of CD8+ while lower part shows domain structure of MHC class I peptide chains (α1, α2, α3, and β2 microglobulin chain). C, MHC class II chains and biding site for CD4+ cells. Upper part shows TCR of CD4+ cell and lower part shows domain structure of class II molecules (α1, α2, β1 and β2 peptide chains).

Classes of MHC genes MHC genes are divided into three classes **(Fig. 5.2)**:
Class I MHC genes which have 3 loci (HLA-A, HLA-B, HLA-C). T suppressor cells have receptors for this class of MHC proteins, which play a major role in graft rejection, killing of virus infected cells and tumour cells.
Class II MHC genes have a single locus HLA-D, with three subregions HLA-DR, HLA-DQ, HLA-DP. These genes are expressed in on antigen presenting cells, activated B cells and T helper cells. They play a major role in graft-versus-host reaction and immune reaction involving T helper cells.
Class III MHC genes code for some complement components and cytokine TNF but are not used in antigen identification.

Q16. Tabulate contrasting features of MHC class I and class II MHC.

The comparative features of class I and class II MHC are presented in **Table 5.3**.

TABLE 5.3 Comparative features of MHC class I and class II gene molecules.

FEATURE	CLASS I	CLASS II
1. Composition	α1, α2, α3, and β2 microglobulin chains	α1, α2, β1 and β2 peptide chains
2. Location	All nucleated cells, platelets	Antigen presenting cells (macrophages, dendritic cells)
3. Gene coding regions	HLA-A, HLA-B, HLA-C	HLA-DR, HLA-DQ, HLA-DP
4. Recognition of TCR region	CD8+ T cells	CD4+ T cells
5. Functions	i. Graft rejection ii. Lysis of virus-infected cells iii. Destruction of tumour cells	i. GVH reaction ii. T helper cell mediated immune functions
6. Disease associations	Behcet disease, psoriasis vulgaris, spondyloarthritis (HLA-B27 disease)	Coeliac disease, pemphigus vulgaris type I diabetes mellitus, juvenile and rheumatoid arthritis

Q17. What are the main functions of the major histocompatibility complex?

The MHC plays a major role in i) organ transplantation, ii) regulation of the immune system, and iii) determining the susceptibility to diseases.
I. Organ transplantation Donor and the recipient must be matched as closely as possible with regards to their class I and II MHC to prevent alloreactivity, i.e. the anti-graft T cell response. Even so, problems may arise because of the *minor histocompatibility non-MHC loci*.
Both, cell-mediated and humoral antibody response, are involved in graft rejection.

II. Regulation of the immune system Class I MHC regulates the function of T cytotoxic/suppressor cells, whereas class II MHC regulate the function of T helper cells, and, thus, indirectly also affect the function of B cells.

III. Susceptibility to diseases Many diseases are associated with the expression of HLA antigen and especially are linked to certain class II MHC types. A few examples are:
i. *Autoimmune disease,* e.g. rheumatoid arthritis, SLE, coeliac disease, Sjögren syndrome, etc.
ii. *Spondyloarthropathies,* e.g. ankylosing spondylitis, Reiter syndrome.
iii. *Endocrinopathies,* e.g. type I diabetes mellitus.
iv. *Neuro-muscular diseases,* e.g. myasthenia gravis.

Q18. What are the most important types of tissue and organ transplants?

According to the genetic relationship between donor and recipient, transplantation of tissues/organs may be classified into four groups:
i. **Autograft** in which the donor and the recipient is the same individual.
ii. **Isograft** is a graft between the donor and the recipient of the same genotype, e.g. identical twins.
iii. **Allograft** is that in which the donor is of the same species but of different genotype. The best survival is seen when the donor and recipient are HLA-identical.
iv. **Xenograft** is that in which the donor is of a different species from that of the recipient.

Q19. How are organ donor classified?

There are two types of donors:
I. **Living donor** These grafts usually include one of the paired organs (e.g. kidney), or part of a major organ (e.g. part of lobe of liver, lobe of a lung, part of intestine).
II. **Deceased or cadaveric donor** Such donors include two groups:
i. *Brain dead individuals* declared to be dead by the treating team of doctors. The organs of such individuals are still viable because the individual was kept on ventilatory support until the family decided on organ donation.
ii. *Circulatory dead donors* whose organs are harvested from their cadavers within a few hours of death.

Q20. What is transplant rejection? Discuss main features of its types.

Definition Transplant rejection is an immunologic reaction that occurs when the graft is rejected by the recipient body due to the genetic disparity between the donor and the recipient. The greater the disparity, the more likely will the transplant rejection occur and more likely it will be intense or difficult to treat.

Pathophysiology Transplant rejection involves both cell mediated and humoral immune responses:
I. **Cellular transplant reaction** may be acute or chronic.
i. *Acute cellular rejection* involves CD8+ cytotoxic cells which may destroy the donor's cells directly, or CD4+ T helper cells which secrete cytokines, and thus indirectly damage the graft by eliciting an inflammatory reaction.
ii. *Chronic graft rejection* involves T cell acting on the cells in the blood vessel wall, with subsequent ischaemia due to narrowing of the arterial lumen.
II. **Humoral immune reaction** is mediated by antibodies against alloantigens. The mechanisms are as under:
i. *Hyperacute rejection* in the presence of preformed circulating anti-donor antibodies due to the pre-sensitisation of the recipient to the donor, e.g. previous blood transfusions, or pregnancies.
ii. *Acute antibody mediated rejection* in recipients who have not been pre-sensitised but began producing antibodies against antigen of class I and II MHC antigens, resulting in a rejection reaction. It may include any of the following:
- Acute and chronic inflammation
- Complement dependent cytotoxicity
- Antibody-dependent cell-mediated cytotoxicity
- Antigen-antibody complexes

iii. *Chronic antibody mediated graft rejection* is related to a systemic production of antibodies, which enter the graft and damage its blood vessels causing ischaemia many years after the transplantation.

Q21. What are the morphologic features of transplant rejection?

For clinical purposes, the transplant rejections are classified as i) hyperacute, ii) acute or iii) chronic.

I. **Hyperacute rejection** occurs within minutes or hours after transplantation. It is mediated by preformed antibodies. Cross-matching of donor's and recipient's lymphocytes has diminished the frequency of hyperacute rejections.

Grossly, the rejection can be recognised by surgeon shortly after vascular anastomosis.
- The organ becomes swollen purple and cyanotic (rather normally pink) with foci of hemorrhage.

Microscopy The rejection has the features of Arthus reaction.
- There is focal necrosis of the arterial wall with deposition of fibrin, accompanied by an accumulation of neutrophils.
- Microcirculation is interrupted by fibrin thrombi and neutrophils.
- There is also necrosis of parenchymal cells and foci of haemorrhage.

II. **Acute rejection** becomes evident a few days, weeks or even month after transplantation.

i. It is based on *cell-mediated reaction.*

Microscopy There are cellular infiltrates with the destruction of parenchymal cells (e.g. tubules in the kidney or bile ducts in the portal tracts of the liver).
- Medium-sized and larger arteries are accompanied by focal infiltrates of lymphocytes in the vessel wall.

ii. *Humoral antibody mediate rejection* is seen usually in hosts who had a poor response to immunosuppression.
- There is small vessel vasculitis with deposition of antibodies and activation of complement (e.g. in peritubular capillaries in the transplanted kidney).

III. **Chronic rejection** follows after repeated bout of acute rejection, or it may slowly develop over many months and years.
- It is a mixed cell-mediated and antibody-mediated process, primarily affecting arteries which become narrowed causing ischaemia.

Q22. What is graft-versus-host disease (GVHD)? Comment on its main features.

Definition GVHD occurs following transplantation of immunocompetent cells into an immunosuppressed host, whereupon the grafted cells attack the host tissues.

Pathogenesis Host tissues are attacked by grafted T lymphocytes. Most often, it follows transplantation of bone marrow haematopoietic/lymphoid cells into patients who have been treated by high dose whole body irradiation for leukaemia or, less often, other malignancies.

Clinicopathologic features There are two forms of GVHD: acute and chronic.

I. *Acute GVHD* develops within days or weeks after bone marrow transplantation. It affects preferentially some organs as follows:

i. *Skin,* most often on the neck and behind the ears, palms and soles, to become generalised later involving the entire body.

ii. *Liver,* typically associated with destruction of small bile ducts in portal tracts, causing jaundice.

iii. *Gastrointestinal tract,* causing diarrhoea.

II. *Chronic GVHD* is the result of repeated attacks of acute GVHD or it may develop insidiously. Typically, it occurs several months after transplantation.
- It produces sclerosis of the dermis and atrophy of epidermis combined with small blood vessel changes, all of which resemble those in *systemic sclerosis.*

IMMUNODEFICIENCY DISEASES

Q23. What are the differences between primary and secondary immunodeficiency?

I. **Primary immunodeficiencies (PIDs)** result from genetic or developmental disorders and usually become clinically evident in early life.

II. **Secondary immunodeficiencies** result from acquired suppression of the immune system. These may occur in children or adults. The most important causes are:

i. Human immunodeficiency virus (HIV) infection → acquired immunodeficiency syndrome (AIDS).

ii. Chemotherapy or radiation therapy of cancer

iii. Haematologic and lymphoid neoplasia (leukaemias and lymphomas)
iv. Severe malnutrition and cachexia
v. Autoimmune disorders, and their treatment
vi. Post-transplant immunosuppressive therapy

Q24. What are the salient general features of primary immunodeficiencies (PIDs)?

i. PIDs are *rare* genetically determined diseases occurring overall at a rate of 5 per 100,000.
ii. Typically, PIDs present with *recurrent infections in infancy and early childhood*. However, some remain asymptomatic (e.g. selective IgA deficiency), or present only in late childhood and adolescence (e.g. common variable immunodeficiency).
iii. Many PIDs have been linked to a *specific gene mutation* (e.g. BTK on X-chromosome in Bruton agammaglobulinaemia), but the cause of many still remains obscure (e.g. selective IgA deficiency, common variable immunodeficiency).
iv. May involve *any part of the immune system:* i) innate immunity, ii) B cell, or iii) T cell system.

Q25. How are PIDs classified?

I. Innate immunity disorders
i. Deficiencies of leucocyte function, such as leucocyte adhesion deficiency, chronic granulomatous disease, or myeloperoxidase deficiency.
ii. Complement system deficiencies; the most common is C2 deficiency.
iii. Deficiency of complement inhibitors; C1 inhibitor is the cause of hereditary angioedema.

II. B-cell disorders
i. Brutton agammaglobulinaemia
ii. Selective (isolated) IgA deficiency
iii. Common variable immunodeficiency

III. T cell disorders
DiGeorge syndrome

IV. Combined B and T disorders
i. Hyper-IgM syndrome
ii. Severe combined immunodeficiency (SCID)
iii. Wiskott-Aldrich syndrome
iv. Ataxia telangiectasia

Q26. Discuss main features of Bruton disease.

Definition PID disorder of B cell maturation → *agammaglobulinaemia in male infants with frequent infections.*

Etiopathogenesis
i. Mutation of gene for BTK (Bruton tyrosine kinase), which is important for light chain rearrangement during B cell maturation.
ii. Defective maturation of B cell precursors (pre-B) into mature B cells
iii. X-linked recessive, affects only male infants → the gene is on X-chromosome

Pathology Lymph nodes depleted of B cell and there are no plasma cells.
Laboratory findings Agammaglobulinaemia or highly reduced γ-globulin in blood.
Clinical aspects Symptoms appear by 6 months (when the maternal immunoglobulins are depleted).
i. Recurrent bacterial, viral and parasitic infections
ii. T cell functions preserved
iii. 25% develop autoimmune diseases

Q27. What is isolated IgA deficiency?

Definition The most common PID (1:700), but usually asymptomatic. So far, not linked to any gene mutation.
Pathogenesis Block of terminal differentiation of IgA-secreting B cells and plasma cells; IgG and IgM normal.

Laboratory finding No IgA in blood, no IgA+ plasma cells. Other immunoglobulins normal or even increased. T cell functions normal.
Clinicopathologic aspects Often asymptomatic.
i. Weakened mucosal defense due to lack of IgA → recurrent sinonasal infections and infectious diarrhoea.
ii. Increased incidence of autoimmune disorders is seen later in life.

Q28. Describe main features of common variable immunodeficiency.

Definition A *heterogeneous group* of disorders characterised usually by *hypogammaglobulinaemia* or selective IgG deficiency, occurring at a rate of 1:50 000.
Etiology Genetic basis unknown in most instances; probably variable causes.
Clinicopathologic aspects
i. Plasma cells missing from tissues.
ii. B cell areas of lymph nodes hyperplastic.
iii. Recurrent sinonasal infection.
iv. Recurrent herpes in 20% cases.
v. Autoimmune diseases and lymphoid neoplasia I later life.

Q29. What is DiGeorge syndrome?

Definition PID with a severe isolated T cell deficiency, reducing the capacity of the immune system to fight infections. Often presents as part of developmental defect.
Etiology del (22q11.2), i.e. a deletion of long arm of chromosome 22 is found in 90% of cases.
Often part of the *CATCH syndrome* (*c*ardiac and *a*ortic arch abnormalities, *T* cell deficiency and thymic aplasia or hypoplasia, *c*left palate, and *h*ypocalcaemia (missing parathyroids).
Pathogenesis Aplasia or hypoplasia of thymus results in faulty T cell development. It is related to defective development of the third and fourth *pharyngeal pouches* (branchial clefts), which is also the primordium of the parathyroids, parts of the mouth and aortic arch.
Clinicopathologic aspects
Recurrent infections with underlying clinical features of the *CATCH syndrome* including hypocalcaemic cramps or seizures.

Q30. Discuss major features of severe combined immunodeficiency (SCID).

Definition SCID is a PID characterised by deficient functions of B cells, T cells and NK cells.
Etiopathogenesis There are two forms of SCIDs:
i. *X-linked SCID* limited to boys is more severe. The gene encoding *γ-chain cytokine receptor*, which leads to reduced formation of precursors of all lymphoid cells.
ii. *Autosomal dominant SCID* due to the mutation of gene encoding *adenosine deaminase (ADA)*, leading to an accumulation of toxic intermediary metabolites which hamper the formation and function of mature lymphocytes.
Clinicopathologic aspects
i. Early onset of oral thrush, skin rash and slow growth.
ii. Recurrent infections associated with high mortality in early life.
NOTE: SCID is the first PID treated successfully by gene therapy.

Q31. What is Wiskott-Aldrich syndrome (WAS)?

Definition WAS is a rare recessive X-linked disease caused by mutation of *WASP gene*, resulting in defective function of T cells, dendritic cells and platelets.
Clinical aspects It affects only boys. It presents with recurrent infections, eczema, and a bleeding tendency due to thrombocytopenia.

Q32. What is ataxia telangiectasia (AT)?

Definition AT is an autosomal recessive disorder caused by mutation of gene coding the *ATM (AT mutated)*, protein resulting in a B cell deficiency and progressive T cell dysfunction.

Pathogenesis ATM protein is a kinase, involved in DNA repair. The mutation results in the following changes:
i. *Cerebellar ataxia* with abnormalities of gait and posture
ii. *Telangiectasia* evident as malformed and dilated vessels
iii. *Immunodeficiency*
- B cell dysfunction resulting in reduced antibody production (typically low IgA and IgG2)
- T cell defects and recurrent infections

Clinicopathologic aspects
i. Increased incidence of malignant tumours
ii. Autoimmune disease occur at an increased rate in later life

Q33. What is acquired immunodeficiency syndrome (AIDS)? Describe its etiologic agent briefly.

Definition AIDS is a disease caused by human immunodeficiency virus (HIV), characterised by severe immunodeficiency, which is complicated by opportunistic infections, neurologic disorders, and an increased incidence of malignant tumours.

Etiology AIDS is caused by human immunodeficiency virus (HIV), a non-transforming virus belonging to the lentivirus group. It includes two distinct but related viruses:
- HIV1 which is most prevalent in the US, Europe and Central Africa, and
- HIV2 which causes AIDS in India and West Africa.

Etiologic agent The HIV-1 is presented in **Figure 5.3**. It shows the following features:
i. Cone-shaped *core*, containing two strands of viral RNA and the enzyme *reverse transcriptase*.
ii. *Capsid*, which contains the major capsid protein *p24*; this is the most abundant protein important for laboratory diagnosis.
iii. *Inner membrane* containing *p17*.
iv. *Outer membrane* (which is host-derived) is a lipid-rich layer, studded externally with *gp120*, and in a transmembranous manner with *gp41*.

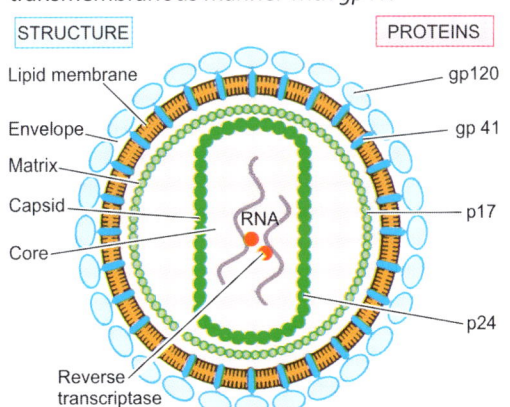

FIGURE 5.3: Schematic representation of structure of HIV. The virion has a cone-shaped *core* that contains major capsid protein *p24*; other components of core are matrix protein p17 on inner membrane, nucleocapsid protein *p7/9*, two strands of viral genomic RNA and three viral enzymes (reverse transcriptase, protease, integrase). Outer *envelope* of virion is studded with two viral glycoproteins at different locations: *gp120* (externally) and *gp41* (transmembranous).

Q34. What are modes of transmission of HIV?

Mode of transmission varies in different populations but in all it includes the following routes:

I. **Sexual transmission** accounts for 75% of cases. In the industrialised world, it affects predominantly homosexual and heterosexual males, whereas in Africa and Asia, heterosexual promiscuity seems to be dominant route.

II. **Transmission via blood and blood products**, accounts for 2% of all cases. It includes three risk groups:
i. Intravenous drug abusers.
ii. Haemophiliacs receiving large amounts of clotting factor concentrates (NOTE: Not any more a risk group since the introduction of genetically modified clotting factors produced commercially).
iii. Transfused persons receiving HIV infected blood, or blood components, like platelets or plasma, pooled from several donors.

III. **Transplacental and perinatal transmission** from infected mother. Virus can be transmitted:
i. Transplacentally from mother to foetus.
ii. From mother to neonate during delivery or the immediate postpartum period by contaminated blood, infected amniotic fluid or breast milk.
IV. **Occupational transmission** including healthcare workers, laboratory personnel and those engaged in disposal of waste.
V. **Transmission by other body fluids such as saliva, tears, sweat, etc.,** which occurs rarely.

Q35. What are the chief events in the pathogenesis of the HIV infection?

I. Events from primary HIV infection to established persistent infection are illustrated in **Figure 5.4**.
II. Destruction of the immune system is shown in **Figure 5.5**.
III. The nervous system is affected in most AIDS patients and microscopic signs of infection are found in 75–90% of all those who were autopsied.
IV. Major abnormalities of the immune system in AIDS are given in **Table 5.4**.

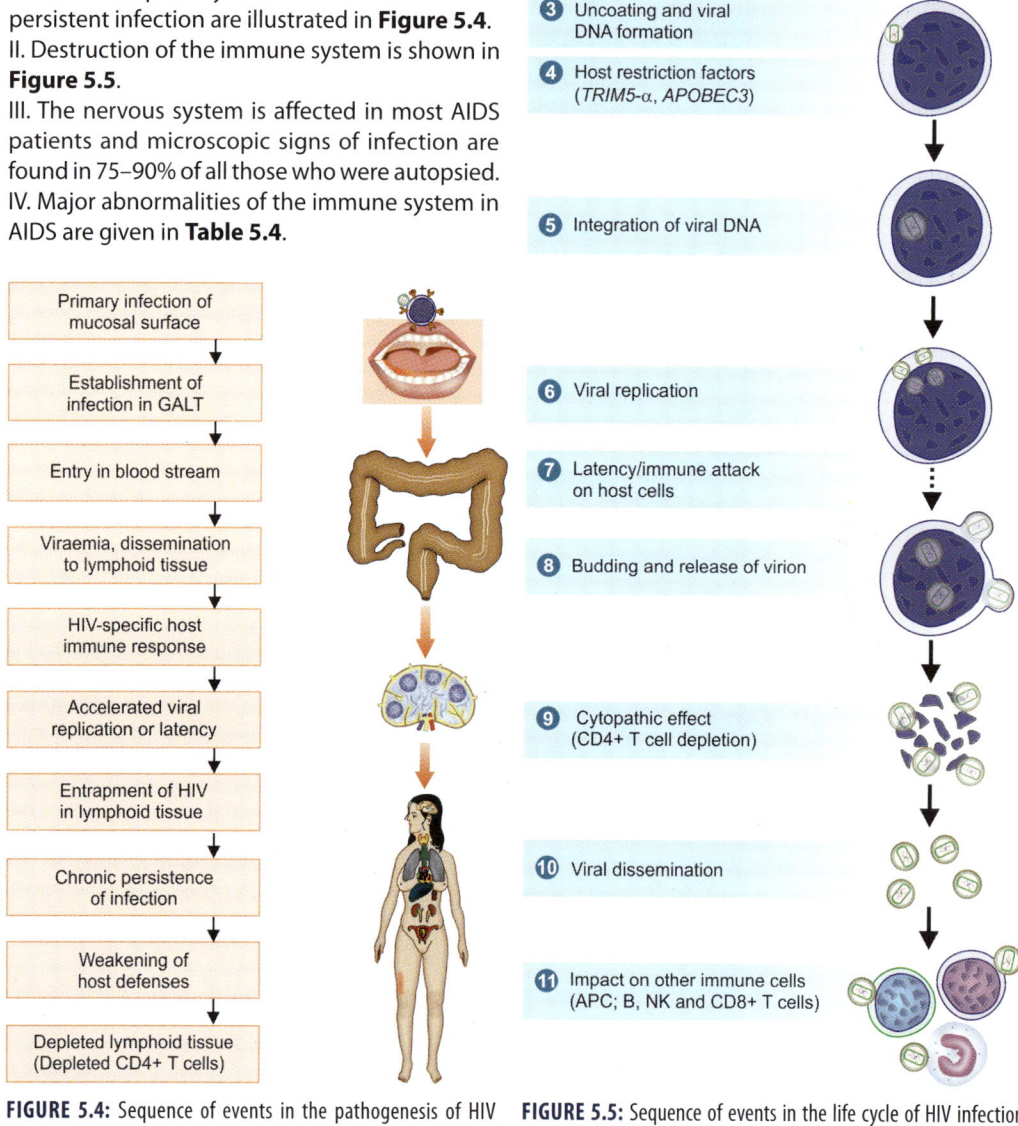

FIGURE 5.4: Sequence of events in the pathogenesis of HIV disease from initial primary infection to persistence of infection with destruction of immune system.

FIGURE 5.5: Sequence of events in the life cycle of HIV infection in the target cell.

TABLE 5.4 Major abnormalities in immune system in AIDS.

1. T CELL ABNORMALITIES

 i. Lymphopenia
 ii. CD4+ T cell depletion
 iii. Selective loss of CD4+ memory T cells
 iv. CD8+ T cell lymphocytosis
 v. Reversal of CD4: CD8 cell ratio
 vi. Decreased production of cytokines (IL-2, IFN-γ) by CD4+ T cells
 vii. Decreased antibody-dependent cellular cytotoxicity (ADCC) by CD8+ T cells

2. B CELL ABNORMALITIES

 i. Not infected, no viral damage
 ii. Polyclonal activation with hypergammaglobulinaemia
 iii. Circulating immune complexes
 iv. Impaired antibody response to newer antigens
 v. Decreased antibody production due to decreased T helper cell function

3. NK CELL ABNORMALITIES

 i. Not infected, no viral damage
 ii. Depressed number, impaired function
 iii. Increased inhibitory NK cell receptors (iNKRs), decreased cytotoxicity

4. MONOCYTE-MACROPHAGE CELL ABNORMALITIES

 i. No destruction
 ii. Decreased chemotaxis
 iii. Decreased phagocytosis
 iv. Decreased HLA class II expression
 v. Decreased antigen presentation

Q36. What are the principal clinical phases of HIV infection leading to AIDS?

I. **Acute HIV syndrome** which includes the following:
i. Viraemia due to replication of the virus.
ii. Seroconversion marked by the appearance of anti-HIV antibodies.
iii. CD4+ cells reduction followed by a return to normal levels.
iv. CD8+ cells rise.
v. Acute self-limited viral illness:
- It occurs in 50–70% of all adults within 3–6 weeks of initial infection.
- It presents with fever, sore throat, myalgia, skin rash and, sometimes with aseptic meningitis. It lasts 2–3 weeks and resolves spontaneously.

II. **Middle chronic phase** which includes competition between HIV and the host immune system.
i. It is of variable duration but may be as long as 10 years.
ii. Viraemia, initially mild but gradually progresses as the host defenses crumble.
iii. CD4+ count slowly drops but is still moderately low.
iv. CD8+ count remains high.
v. Clinically, the patient may be asymptomatic or have only minor constitutional symptoms and generalised lymph node enlargement.

III. **Final crisis phase** is characterised by profound immunosuppression.
i. Viraemia markedly increased.
ii. CD4+ count very low (below 200 per µl).
iii. Opportunistic infections.
iv. Death; average survival of an untreated patient is 2 years after the diagnosis of AIDS.
v. In children, the course of the disease is more rapid than in adults.

Q37. Describe the CDC clinical classification scheme of HIV-AIDS.

According to the CDC, clinical classification of progressive phases of HIV infected adults and adolescents is given in **Table 5.5**.

TABLE 5.5 CDC classification system (2013) for HIV-infected adults and adolescents.

CLINICAL PHASE	EARLY, ACUTE	MIDDLE, CHRONIC	FINAL, CRISIS
Period after infection	3–6 weeks	10–12 years	Any period up to death
CDC clinical category	Category A: Asymptomatic infection Acute HIV syndrome PGL	Category B: Symptomatic disease (neither A nor C) Conditions secondary to impaired CMI	Category C: AIDS- indicator conditions (constitutional disease, neurologic features, neoplasms)
CDC CD4 + T cell stage			
1. >500/µl	A1	B1	C1
2. 200–499/µl	A2	B2	C2
3. <200/µl	A3	B3	C3

(CDC, Centers for Disease Control, US; PGL, persistent generalised lymphadenopathy; CME, cell-mediated immunity).

Q38. What are the pathological and clinical manifestations of HIV-AIDS?

Pathological lesions and clinical manifestations can be explained by four mechanisms:
i. Direct effects of viral infection
ii. Opportunistic infections
iii. Secondary tumours
iv. Treatment effect

Pathological and clinical features and manifestations include the following **(Fig. 5.6)**:

i. **Wasting syndrome**, i.e. involuntary loss of body weight by more than 10% due to multiple factors such as malnutrition, increased metabolic rate, malabsorption of nutrients, anorexia, and the ill effects of opportunistic infections.

ii. **Persistent lymphadenopathy**, which is defined as enlarged lymph nodes >1 cm, at two or more locations, persisting for more than 3 months. It is marked by follicular hyperplasia due to proliferation of CD8+, B cells and dendritic cells. HIV infected CD4+ T cells are seen in the mantle zone. Later in the course of the disease, there is depletion of lymphocytes.

iii. **Gastrointestinal manifestations** are seen in almost all HIV infected persons. These include: oral and oropharyngeal or esophageal candidiasis, mucosal ulcers, watery or haemorrhagic diarrhoea,

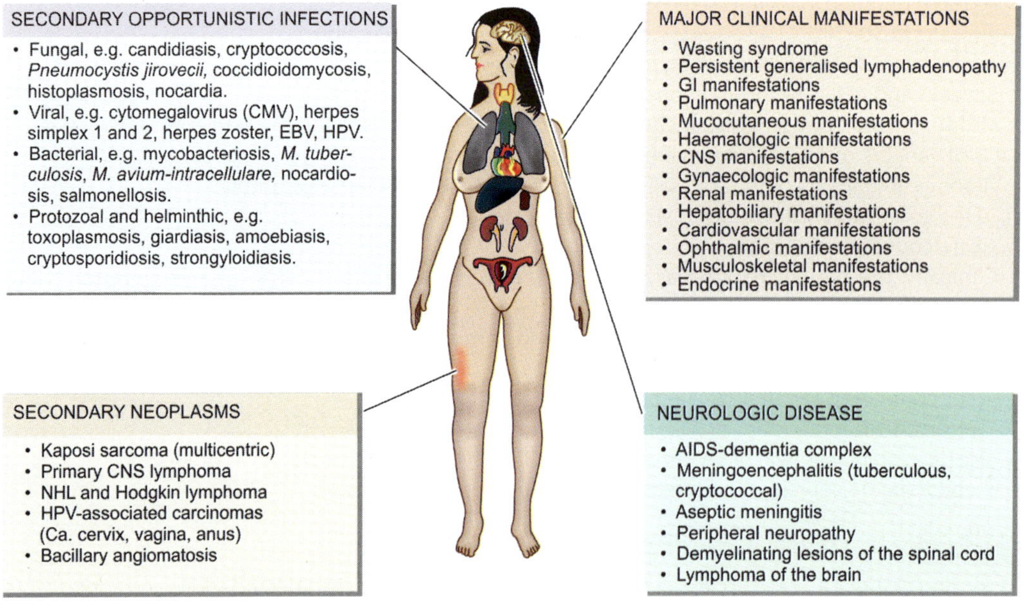

SECONDARY OPPORTUNISTIC INFECTIONS
- Fungal, e.g. candidiasis, cryptococcosis, *Pneumocystis jirovecii*, coccidioidomycosis, histoplasmosis, nocardia.
- Viral, e.g. cytomegalovirus (CMV), herpes simplex 1 and 2, herpes zoster, EBV, HPV.
- Bacterial, e.g. mycobacteriosis, *M. tuberculosis*, *M. avium-intracellulare*, nocardiosis, salmonellosis.
- Protozoal and helminthic, e.g. toxoplasmosis, giardiasis, amoebiasis, cryptosporidiosis, strongyloidiasis.

MAJOR CLINICAL MANIFESTATIONS
- Wasting syndrome
- Persistent generalised lymphadenopathy
- GI manifestations
- Pulmonary manifestations
- Mucocutaneous manifestations
- Haematologic manifestations
- CNS manifestations
- Gynaecologic manifestations
- Renal manifestations
- Hepatobiliary manifestations
- Cardiovascular manifestations
- Ophthalmic manifestations
- Musculoskeletal manifestations
- Endocrine manifestations

SECONDARY NEOPLASMS
- Kaposi sarcoma (multicentric)
- Primary CNS lymphoma
- NHL and Hodgkin lymphoma
- HPV-associated carcinomas (Ca. cervix, vagina, anus)
- Bacillary angiomatosis

NEUROLOGIC DISEASE
- AIDS-dementia complex
- Meningoencephalitis (tuberculous, cryptococcal)
- Aseptic meningitis
- Peripheral neuropathy
- Demyelinating lesions of the spinal cord
- Lymphoma of the brain

FIGURE 5.6: Major pathological lesions and clinical manifestations of HIV/AIDS.

vomiting, anorexia. GI lesions are caused by opportunistic infections caused by *fungi* such as Candida; *bacteria* such as Clostridia, *Shigella, Salmonella*; *protozoa* like *Giardia, Entamoeba histolytica*; *viruses* like CMV.

iv. **Pulmonary manifestations** are found in 50–70% of cases, which all present with some form of pneumonia or adult respiratory distress syndrome. The major pathogens are *Pneumocystis jirovecii, M. tuberculosis*, CMV, *Histoplasma capsulatum* and *Staphylococcus aureus*.

v. **Mucocutaneous manifestations** occur in 50–70% cases. In early stage of HIV infection, patients may present with skin rash. Later on, there are many skin lesions considered to be either infectious (viral, fungal, bacterial), allergic, and, finally neoplastic such as Kaposi sarcoma.

vi. **Central nervous system manifestations** are present in almost all patients and include inflammatory, demyelinating, degenerative conditions and neoplasms (CNS lymphoma).
- *HIV encephalopathy or AIDS-associated dementia complex* is an AIDS-defining condition, presenting with deteriorating neurocognitive symptoms, also known as *HAND (HIV-associated neurocognitive disorder)*.
- CNS infections may be caused by *M. tuberculosis, Cryptococcus, Toxoplasma*.
- Demyelinating disease and peripheral neuropathy are common.

vii. **Other organs** HIV infection spares no organs and, thus there may be lesions in *all major organ systems*.

Q39. How is HIV-AIDS diagnosed in the clinical laboratory?

Three sets of tests are used **(Table 5.6)**:
I. To establish HIV infection
II. To diagnose immunodeficiency
III. Diagnose opportunistic infections and secondary tumours

I. **Tests for establishing HIV infection,** by detecting antibodies to HIV or the virus itself.
i. *Serologic test for antibodies to HIV p24* antigen by enzyme-linked immunosorbent assay (ELISA) which has a sensitivity of 99.5%. It can give false-positive results and, therefore, if positive, it must be repeated. *Nucleic acid testing (NAT) for p24* shortens the testing period ('window') from infection to detection to 12 days.
ii. *HIV Western blot* is used to confirm the repeat positive ELISA test. It is based on the detection of three major HIV genes: *gag, pol, env*.
iii. *Direct detection of HIV* is based on following tests:
a. p24 capture assay
b. HIV RNA detection
c. DNA-PCR by amplification of proviral DNA
d. Culture of HIV from blood monocytes

TABLE 5.6 Tests for diagnosis of HIV/AIDS.

1. Tests for establishing HIV infection
   i. *Antibody tests:*
      a. Serologic testing by ELISA
      b. HIV Western blot
   ii. *Direct detection of HIV*
      a. p24 antigen capture assay
      b. HIV RNA detection methods
      c. DNA-PCR
      d. Culture of HIV in neoplastic T cell lines
2. Tests for defects in immunity
   i. CD4+ T cell count: Fall
   ii. CD8+ cell count: Increased
   iii. Ratio of CD4+ T cell/CD8+ T cell count: Reversed
   iv. Lymphopenia
   v. Hypergammaglobulinaemia
   vi. Increased β-2 microglobulin level
   vii. Platelet count: Thrombocytopenia
3. Tests for detection of opportunistic infection and secondary tumours
   i. FNAC/exfoliative cytology
   ii. Biopsy

II. **Tests for detection of changes in the immune system,** which are used for diagnosis as well as for monitoring of treatment and progression of the disease:
i. *Cell counts of T lymphocytes and total lymphocytes*
a. CD4+ count monitoring for decline
b. CD8+ rise
c. Reversal of CD4+/CD8+ cell ratio
d. Lymphopenia
ii. *β_2-macroglobulin* to monitor rising levels
iii. *Immunoglobulins* to monitor for hypergammaglobulinaemia
iv. *Platelet count* to monitor thrombocytopenia

III. **Detection of opportunistic infections and tumours** is based on standard microbiologic and pathologic techniques, including sampling of tissues by biopsy.

HYPERSENSITIVITY REACTIONS

Q40. What is hypersensitivity and how are various hypersensitivity reactions classified?

Definition Hypersensitivity is an *exaggerated or inappropriate immune response* which is associated with adverse effects on the body. Its salient features are:
- The *immune reaction* may be to endogenous or exogenous antigens.
- *Immunologic tissue injury* accounts for the pathological findings in these immune reactions.
- Many hypersensitivity reactions are *genetically-determined* or associated with certain *HLA types*.

Classification There are four types of hypersensitivity reactions:
Type I: Anaphylactic (or atopic) hypersensitivity
Type II Antibody-mediated cytotoxic hypersensitivity
Type III: Immune complex-mediated hypersensitivity
Type IV: Delayed (cell-mediated) hypersensitivity
- Type I, II, III are grouped under the heading of *immediate reactions,* and are mediated by antibodies produced by *B cells* and their derivative.
- Type IV is considered to be a *delayed reaction* and it is mediated by *T cells*.

Q41. Discuss main features of type I anaphylactic (atopic) hypersensitivity.

Definition Type I hypersensitivity is characterised by a rapid IgE-mediated immune response to an antigen to which the body was previous sensitised.

Key features
i. The reaction appears 15–30 minutes of exposure to antigen.
ii. In some instances, a second late phase reaction develops 2–24 hours later.
iii. The reaction depends on the following:
a. Genetic factors of the host (familial predisposition!)
b. Nature of the environmental pollutants (e.g. some are more potent allergens)
c. Concomitant factors (e.g. concomitant infection)

Q42. What are the sequential events in the pathogenesis of type I hypersensitivity reactions?

The following events occur sequentially during the type I hypersensitivity reaction:
I. **First contact** of the host with the antigen results in the *activation of T_H2 cells*.
i. T_H2 produce *cytokines* which cause *a class switch in B cells*, transforming them into *IgE-secreting plasma cells*.
ii. IgE released from plasma cells *binds* to the Fc receptor on the plasma membrane of *mast cells,* making them thus sensitised to re-exposure to the same antigen.
II. Upon **second exposure**, the antigen will bind to *Fab portion of IgE* antibody, firmly attached by its Fc portion to the mast cells.
Antigen bound to IgE will cause cross-linking of these molecules *triggering mast cell degranulation* and an extracellular release of their contents which include the following:
- Biogenic amines (like histamine)
- Chemotactic factors for PMNs and eosinophils
- Enzymes, such as proteases, hydrolases that damage the tissue.

III. **The second (synthesis) phase** of the immune response follows the initial rapid reaction and degranulation. During this phase, the activated mast cells begin *synthesising de novo and releasing with some delay* into the extracellular spaces various mediators including the following:
- Arachidonic acid derivatives such as leukotrienes, prostaglandins, thromboxane A2
- Platelet activating factor(PAF)
- Cytokines (TNF, IL-1, etc.)

IV. **The effector phase** comprises tissue reaction to various mediators of inflammation, clinically presenting with signs and symptoms, which can be classified clinically as:
- *Local anaphylaxis* (e.g. bronchospasm in asthma).
- *Systemic anaphylaxis* (e.g. anaphylactic shock).

Q43. What are the principal effects of mediators of inflammation released from mast cells?

i. Increased vascular permeability
ii. Smooth muscle contraction
iii. Increased nasal and lacrimal gland secretion
iv. Early vasoconstriction followed by vasodilatation
v. Increased gastric secretion
vi. Increased attraction of eosinophils and neutrophils accompanied by identical increase of these cells in blood.

Q44. Give examples of diseases caused by type I hypersensitivity reactions.

These diseases can be classified as systemic or local:
I. **Systemic anaphylaxis** *Clinical findings* vary from mild to severe:
i. Itching with generalised erythema of the skin
ii. Laryngeal oedema with dyspnoea and choking
iii. Bronchospasm with dyspnoea, coughing and expectoration
iv. Pulmonary oedema with dyspnoea
v. Diarrhoea
vi. Hypotensive shock may result and even death may occur.
Clinical examples of systemic anaphylaxis:
i. Anaphylactic reaction to the repeated injection of horse antiserum
ii. Anaphylactic reaction to various drugs, such as penicillin
iii. Sting by wasp or bee
II. **Local anaphylaxis** is much more common that systemic anaphylaxis.
Clinical examples of local anaphylaxis:
i. Hay fever (seasonal allergic rhinitis) to pollen, which involves nasal passages and conjunctiva of the eye.
ii. Bronchial asthma in response to inhaled antigens such as dust or dander.
iii. Food allergy, to nutrients such as fish, milk, eggs, etc.
iv. Cutaneous anaphylaxis in response to various contact antigens causing urticaria, wheal and flare.

Q45. What is type II antibody-mediated (cytotoxic) hypersensitivity? Briefly discuss its mechanisms.

Definition Type II hypersensitivity is based on an antibody-mediated reaction to antigens on specific cells and tissues with subsequent lysis and destruction of target cells.
Antibodies are mostly of IgG and IgM type which elicit activation of the complement system and the participation of macrophages, platelets, natural killer cells, neutrophils and eosinophils.
Mechanism Following three mechanisms operate and can lead to the destruction of target cells:
i. **Opsonisation** This is mediated by the binding of Fab of IgG to the surface of microbe or cells. The unbound part of IgG, the Fc component, sticks out from the cell surface and interacts with the Fc receptors on PMNs and macrophages, enabling the *phagocytosis* of the opsonised microbe or cell. For example, opsonised blood cells are removed and phagocytised in the spleen.
ii. **Antibody-mediated cellular cytotoxicity** Binding of antibodies to cell surface or basement membrane activates complement which forms chemotactic fragments attracting inflammatory cells, such as PMNs and monocytes/macrophages. *Inflammatory cells release granules* and kill the target cells or damage basement membranes, as in glomerulonephritis.
iii. **Antibody-mediated cellular dysfunction** Binding of antibody does not kill the cell and will only cause change in the function of the target cells. It may *stimulate* the function of target cell as in Graves' disease with hyperthyroidism, or impair the function of the target cell as in myasthenia gravis.

Q46. What are the diseases caused by type II hypersensitivity reactions?

These diseases can be classified as caused by i) cytotoxic antibodies to blood cells, and ii) cytotoxic antibodies to tissue components.
I. **Cytotoxic antibodies to blood cells**
i. Autoimmune haemolytic anaemia
ii. Transfusion reaction due to incompatible or mismatched blood transfusion

iii. Haemolytic disease of the newborn due to materno-foetal blood group incompatibility and antibodies crossing the placenta and haemolysing the foetal RBCs
iv. Immune thrombocytopenic purpura
v. Drug-induced haemolytic anaemia or leucopenia and thrombocytopenia, in which the drugs act as haptens, eliciting an immune reaction leading to destruction of targeted cells.

II. **Antibodies to tissue components** which may kill cells, damage them change their function as given below:
i. Graves disease with antibodies to the TSH receptor on thyroid follicular cells
ii. Myasthenia gravis with antibodies to acetylcholine receptor
iii. Male sterility with antisperm antibodies
iv. Type I diabetes mellitus with antibodies against islet cells
v. Pernicious anaemia with antibodies to intrinsic factor
vi. Hyperacute transplant rejection with antibodies against donor antigens
vii. Goodpasture syndrome with antibodies against components of the glomerular basement membrane
viii. Pemphigus vulgaris with antibodies against epidermal cell adhesion molecule

Q47. Describe main features of type III (or immune complex-mediated) hypersensitivity.

Definition Type III hypersensitivity results from deposition of antigen-antibody complexes on tissues, that is followed by activation of the complement system and an inflammatory reaction which is damaging the target tissue.

Key features
i. The immune complexes may be formed *locally* in tissues, or may be found in the *circulation*, and from it deposited into the tissues.
ii. The immune injury will depend on the site of antibody production.
iii. The antigens can be either *exogenous* (e.g. viruses, or inhalation antigens like moulds, plants or animal material), or *endogenous* (e.g. self antigen from the nucleus, cytoplasm, or extracellular matrix).
iv. The immune reaction is mediated by *IgG and IgM* and includes the participation of *complement* and *inflammatory cells*, such a neutrophils, macrophages and mast cells.

Q48. What are the differences between the tissue injury caused by circulating immune complexes and those formed locally in tissues?

I. **Circulating immune complexes** are formed in the blood due to the binding of antibody to soluble or insoluble antigens in the circulation.
i. Large immune complexes formed in this interaction are readily removed by macrophages, whereas the medium-sized and smaller are deposited in tissues, causing injury.
ii. Preferred sites of immune complex deposition are tissues where the filtration of blood takes place; for instance: kidney (formation of urine), serosal surfaces like pleura or pericardium (where the serous fluid in the body cavities is formed), joints, and small blood vessels in the skin and other tissues.
iii. Immune complex deposits activate complement which in turn stimulates acute inflammation by attracting neutrophils.
iv. The inflammatory reactions are named after the tissue that is affected, such as glomerulonephritis, vasculitis, pericarditis, vasculitis, etc.

II. **Local immune complex** injury occurs in an individual who has abundant preformed antibodies in circulation, and is then injected locally into the skin with the inciting antigen. Antigen reacts with the antibodies and the formed immune complexes elicit local activation of complement, acute inflammation and necrosis of the tissue.

This reaction was experimentally induced some 100 years ago by *Dr Arthus,* after whom it has been named. He originally elicited it by injecting immunised rabbits with the same protein locally into the skin. Upon injection of antigen, it diffused toward the blood vessels and formed the immune complexes with the circulating antibody in the vessel wall, i.e. the site where the diffusing antigen and circulating antibody met.
i. *Polyarteritis nodosa* is a human disease that has the same microscopic features.
ii. *Hypersensitivity vasculitis* of the skin is yet another example.

Q49. What are the most important diseases caused by type III hypersensitivity reactions?

The disease caused by type III hypersensitivity can be systemic (like SLE) or localised to a specific tissue. The most important clinical entities caused by this mechanism are given below:
i. Post-streptococcal or any other post-infectious glomerulonephritis and the intraglomerular deposition of microbe-related antigen-antibody complexes.
ii. Systemic lupus erythematosus caused by an immune response to endogenous antigens, such as nuclear proteins, RNA and DNA.
iii. Farmer's lung with antibodies reacting with actinomycetes-containing hay and forming immune complex deposits in the lungs.
iv. Polyarteritis nodosa with antibodies to hepatitis B antigen-antibody complexed deposited in the blood vessel walls.
v. Drug-induce vasculitis in which the drug reacts as antigen. Serum sickness in response to foreign-protein antigens.
vi. Cutaneous vasculitis to a variety of external antigens.

Q50. Define type IV delayed (cell-mediated) hypersensitivity. Discuss its key features.

Definition Type IV reaction, also known as delayed type hypersensitivity (DTH), is a T cell-mediated, slow and prolonged immune response with tissue injury.

Key features
i. The reaction occurs 24–48 hours after exposure to antigen, and it may last up to 14 days.
ii. It is mediated by *CD4+ T cells and CD8+ T cells,* and also involves macrophages, mast cells and basophils.
iii. The antigen can be exogenous (e.g. mycobacteria, viruses, fungi), or endogenous (e.g. nucleus, collagen, myelin).

Types of DTH DTH can by of two types:
- Classic mediated by CD4+ T cells
- Directly cytolytic due to direct cell toxicity of CD8+ T cells.

I. Classic DTH Reaction to purified protein derivative (PPD) following tuberculosis is the prototype of DTH. It involves the following sequence of events:
i. First injection of PPD (or tuberculous infection) leads to immunisation to tubercular antigen. CD4+ cells recognise the antigen on dendritic cells and differentiate into T_H1 and T_H17 cells.
ii. Upon reinjection of PPD, it is recognised by *T_H1 memory cells* and become activated to produce cytokines (IL-2, IL-12, TNF- α, γ-IFN). Interferon gamma is the most important as it will activate macrophages and transform them into *epithelioid cells.*
iii. After 24–48 hours, the immunised person will respond with a DTH reaction.

II. Direct CD8+ T cell mediated cytolysis occurs after injection of the antigen.
i. Antigen is recognised by CD8+ T cells.
ii. Antigen stimulated CD8+ T cells produce perforins, granzymes and similar toxic proteins.
iii. Perforins drill holes in the plasma membrane of target cells causing cell death by cytolysis.
iv. Granzymes are proteolytic. They enter the cytoplasm of target cells activating caspases, thus inducing apoptosis.

Q51. What are the most important diseases caused by type IV hypersensitivity reactions?

Type IV hypersensitivity reactions present either with granulomas, or in form of chronic inflammation, and are the basis of several important diseases as listed below:
i. Mycobacterial infections, such as tuberculosis or leprosy.
ii. Viral infections, such as encephalitis, chronic hepatitis, myocarditis, etc.
iii. Contact dermatitis following exposure to chemical, metals, plants (e.g. poison ivy).
iv. Transplant rejection and graft-versus-host reaction.
v. Rheumatoid arthritis self antigens, including collagen.
vi. Multiple sclerosis which involves a reaction to myelin related self-antigens.
vii. Inflammatory bowel disease in which the immune system reacts either to bacteria or self antigens.

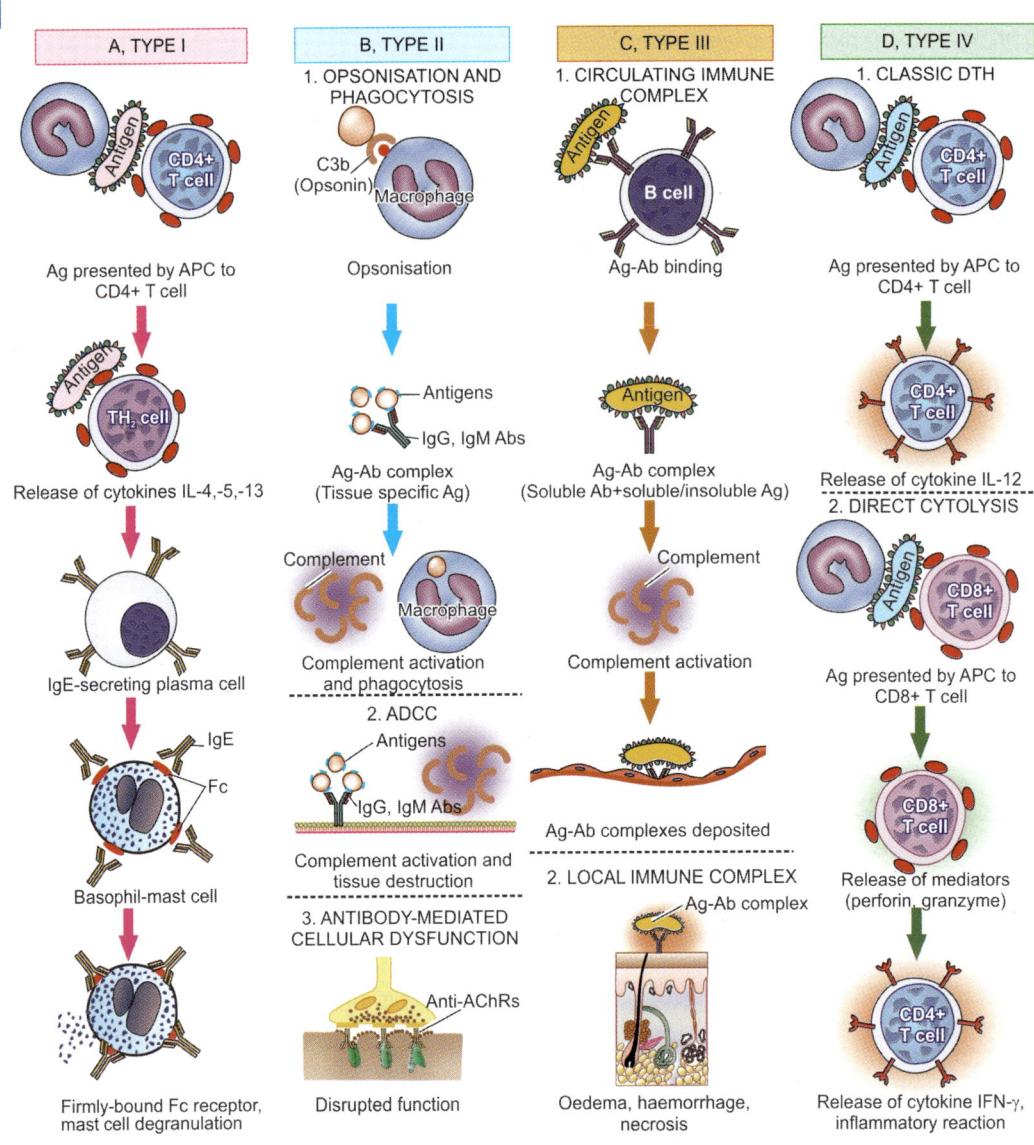

FIGURE 5.7: Schematic representation of pathogenesis of 4 types of immunological tissue injury.

Q52. Tabulate and illustrate the main comparative features of various types of hypersensitivity reactions.

Figure 5.7 illustrates the main features of type I, II, III and IV hypersensitivity reactions. Their comparative features are summarised in **Table 5.7**.

■ AUTOIMMUNE DISEASES

Q53. What are autoimmune diseases?

Definition Autoimmune diseases are immunologically mediated diseases that develop because of the failure of the immune system to distinguish self from non-self and a loss of tolerance to one's own tissue antigens.
- Autoimmunity always results in cell/tissue/organ injury or a loss of specific functions.
- It can be mediated by antibodies to self antigens (autoantibodies) or T cell against-self reactivity, always resulting in tissue injury.

FEATURE	TYPE I	TYPE II	TYPE III	TYPE IV
1. Reaction type	Anaphylactic	Cytotoxic	➤ Serum sickness ➤ Arthus reaction	Delayed type hypersensitivity
2. Definition	Rapidly developing immune response in a previously sensitised person	Reaction of humoral antibodies that attack cell surface antigens and cause cell lysis	Results from deposition of antigen-antibody complexes on tissues	T cell-mediated slow and prolonged response
3. Mediated by	IgE antibodies	IgG or IgM antibodies	IgG, IgM antibodies	T cell-mediated
4. Etiologic factors	Genetic basis, pollutants, viral infections	Exposure to foreign antigens (drug metabolites, microbial products), self antigens	Persistence of low-grade infection, environmental antigens, autoimmune process	Microbial antigens, self antigens
5. Pathogenesis	➤ Formation of IgE antibodies ➤ Release of pro-inflammatory mediators	➤ Opsonisation and phagocytosis ➤ Antibody-dependent cellular cytotoxicity ➤ Antibody-mediated cellular dysfunction	➤ Circulating immune complex-mediated cell injury ➤ Local immune complex injury (Arthus reaction)	➤ Classic DTH mediated by CD4+ T cells ➤ Direct CD8+ T cell mediated lysis
6. Examples	i. Systemic anaphylaxis (administration of antisera and drugs, stings) ii. Local anaphylaxis (hay fever, bronchial asthma, food allergy, cutaneous, angioedema)	i. Cytotoxic antibodies to blood cells (autoimmune haemolytic anaemia, transfusion reactions, erythroblastosis foetalis, ITP, leucopenia, drug-induced) ii. Cytotoxic antibodies to tissue components (Graves' disease, myasthenia gravis, male sterility, type I DM, hyperacute reaction against organ transplant, Goodpasture's syndrome, RHD, pemphigus vulgaris)	i. Immune complex glomerulonephritis ii. SLE iii. Rheumatoid arthritis iv. Farmers lung v. PAN vi. Drug-induced vasculitis vii. Serum sickness viii. Arthus reaction ix. Reactive arthritis	i. Reaction against mycrobacterial antigen (tuberculin reaction, tuberculosis, tuberculoid leprosy) ii. Reaction against virus-infected cells iii. Organ transplant reaction iv. Contact dermatitis v. Rheumatoid arthritis vi. Multiple sclerosis vii. Inflammatory bowel disease

TABLE 5.7 Comparative features of 4 types of hypersensitivity reactions.

Q54. What is immune tolerance? Discuss its mechanisms.

Definition Immune tolerance is an ability of an individual to recognise autoantigens and show selective unresponsiveness to autoantigens; it is the opposite of autoimmunity **(Fig. 5.8)**.

Mechanisms Immune tolerance is based on three general processes: i) sequestration of self antigens, ii) generation and maintenance of self-tolerance, and iii) altered immunoregulatory controls.

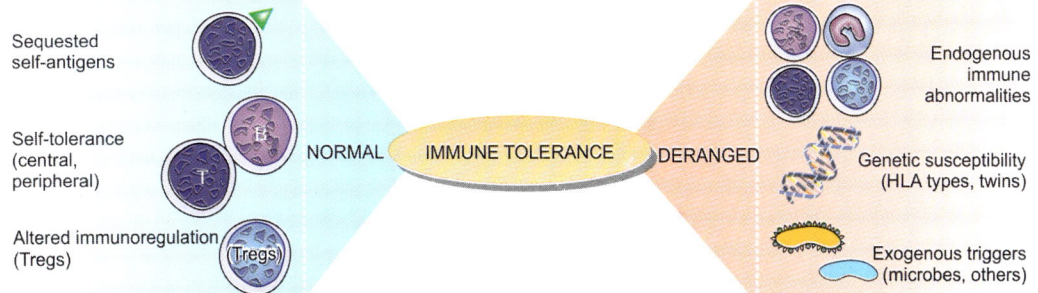

FIG. 5.8: Pathogenesis of autoimmunity as contrasted with normal immune tolerance.

I. **Sequestration self antigens** at so called 'privileged sites' (e.g. anterior eye chamber or brain) where they are 'hidden' from lymphocytes, are protected by immunosuppressive cytokine (e.g. TGF-β).

II. **Generation and maintenance of self-tolerance**

i. Self-tolerance may be achieved by deletion of autoreactive lymphocytes in central organs (thymus and bone marrow), also known as *central tolerance*.

ii. Alternatively, B or T lymphocytes show *clonal anergy* and do not respond to stimuli of self-antigens because of the following events:

a. Lack of a co-stimulatory signal by the antigen presenting cells.
b. Lack of helper cell support.
c. Activation of inhibitory surface receptors.

III. **Altered immunoregulatory controls** due to the downregulation of *Treg function*, i.e. cells that normally prevent T cell attack on self-antigen. This is accomplished by cytokines secreted by CD4+ T helper cells.

Q55. What is the pathogenesis of autoimmunity?

In general terms, autoimmunity results from the interaction of three factors: i) endogenous abnormalities of the immune system, ii) genetic susceptibility, and iii) triggers of exogenous agents.

I. **Endogenous abnormalities of the immune system**

i. *Altered antigen presentation* due to faulty processing of the antigen which leads to presentation of newer or cryptic antigen on these molecules. Presentation of antigens by B cells, or in context of wrong cytokines, may also impair antigen presentation.

ii. *Increased T and B cell stimulation*, which may result in polyclonal B cell activation.

iii. *Defective clearance* of apoptotic material by the immune system, whereupon that material becomes immunogenic.

iv. *Release of sequestered self-antigens* For example in multiple sclerosis, brain antigens which are normally not accessible to immune cells become apparent and immunogenic. Sperm antigens, which are sequestered in seminiferous tubules from immune system, become auto-antigenic after testicular trauma or vasectomy.

II. **Genetic susceptibility** Clinical evidence indicates that the genetic factors have a role in autoimmunity.

i. Certain *type II MHC alleles (mostly HLA-27 and DRB1)*, predispose to certain diseases, such as ankylosing spondylitis, type I diabetes mellitus, rheumatoid arthritis, SLE, multiple sclerosis.

ii. *Identical twins* have a far higher incidence of autoimmune diseases than non-identical twins.

iii. *Inherited deficiency of early complement proteins* (C1q, C2 and C4) is associated with higher incidence of SLE.

III. **Exogenous agents** Bacterial and viral infections have been implicated in triggering autoimmune diseases.

The best explored is the *theory of molecular mimicry* between microbial antigens and human tissue antigens. Accordingly, antibodies to certain microbial antigens could act with similar antigen on the host tissues. For example, antibodies to streptococcal M protein will cause rheumatic fever by reacting with structurally similar antigens on the human heart valves, joints and brain.

Q56. How are the autoimmune diseases classified?

Depending upon whether autoantibodies target a single organ or the disorder is systemic, the autoimmune diseases can be classified as under **(Table 5.8)**:

I. *Organs specific (localised)*
II. *Non-organs specific (systemic)*

These can be subclassified as B cell (antibody and immune complex) or T cell-mediated.

Q57. What is systemic lupus erythematosus? Briefly discuss its pathogenesis.

Definition Systemic lupus erythematosus (SLE) is a systemic autoimmune disease, predominantly based on type III hypersensitivity and to a lesser degree on type II hypersensitivity reactions.

- *Most pathologic tissue changes* are related to deposition of immune complexes and antibody activity against numerous autoantigens, accompanied by complement activation and inflammation in almost all organs of the body.
- *Haematologic findings* are mostly due to type II antibody related cytotoxicity.
- *Serologically,* it is characterised by the appearance of diagnostic antinuclear antibodies.
- In addition to the systemic form of SLE, there is a localised *discoid form, DLE,* affecting the skin of the face.

Etiopathogenesis Complex and not fully understood but we know that certain factors play an important role as under:

i. *Sex predominance and hormones* Females are affected more often than males (9:1). Before puberty and after menopause, this difference between females and males disappears. Oestrogens exacerbate symptoms.

ii. *Genetic predisposition* Evidenced by a high occurrence of SLE in:
a. Identical twins (25%).
b. Persons with genetic complement deficiencies.
c. Certain class II HLA types.

iii. *Exogenous precipitating factors* These include:
a. UV light.
b. Drugs like procainamide and hydralazine.
c. Infectious agents like EBV.

TABLE 5.8 Classification of autoimmune diseases.

ORGAN NON-SPECIFIC (SYSTEMIC)
1. Systemic lupus erythematosus
2. Rheumatoid arthritis
3. Scleroderma (systemic sclerosis)
4. Inflammatory myopathies (polymyositis, dermatomyositis, inclusion body myositis)
5. Polyarteritis nodosa (PAN)
6. Sjögren syndrome
7. IgG4-related disease

ORGAN SPECIFIC (LOCALISED)
1. *ENDOCRINE GLANDS*
   i. Hashimoto (autoimmune) thyroiditis
   ii. Graves disease
   iii. Type 1 diabetes mellitus
   iv. Autoimmune Addison's disease
   v. Autoimmune polyglandular syndrome
2. *ALIMENTARY TRACT*
   i Autoimmune atrophic gastritis in pernicious anaemia
   ii. Inflammatory bowel disease
3. *BLOOD CELLS*
   i. Autoimmune haemolytic anaemia
   ii. Autoimmune thrombocytopenia
   iii. Pernicious anaemia
   iv. Antiphospholipid syndrome
4. *OTHERS*
   i. Myasthenia gravis
   ii. Multiple sclerosis
   iii. Gullian-Barré syndrome
   iv. Immune-mediated infertility
   v. Goodpasture syndrome
   vi. Autoimmune hepatitis
   vii. Autoimmune skin diseases (e.g. pemphigus, psoriasis, dermatitis herpetiformis, vitiligo, autoimmune alopecia)

Q58. What are the most important antibodies in systemic lupus erythematosus?

SLE is characterised by polyclonal activation of B cells and hypergammaglobulinaemia.
The most important **diagnostic autoantibodies** are as follows:

i. **Antinuclear antibodies (ANA)**—present in almost all patients, and used for screening.

ii. **Antibodies to double-stranded DNA (anti-dDNA)**—highly specific for SLE and found in 70% cases

iii. **Anti-Smith antibody (anti-Sm)**—directed at the Sm part of the ribonucleoproteins, highly specific for SLE, but found only in 25% cases.

iv. **Other antibodies** There are also several antibodies that are frequently found in SLE patients, and especially in patients with certain organ involvement, but are not diagnostic of SLE. These antibodies include the following:

a. *Anti-ribonucleoprotein antibody (anti-RPN)* It is seen in 40% of SLE, but is more common in Sjögren syndrome.

b. *Anti-Ro or anti Sjögren syndrome antibody (anti-SS-A or B)* Found in 30% of SLE cases, but is more specific for the sicca syndrome.

c. *Anti-histone antibody (AHA)* against DNA associated histones in the nucleus, seen particularly in drug-induced SLE.

d. *Antiphospholipid antibody (APLA)* or lupus anticoagulant is a test for the thrombotic complications of SLE and the antiphospholipid syndrome.

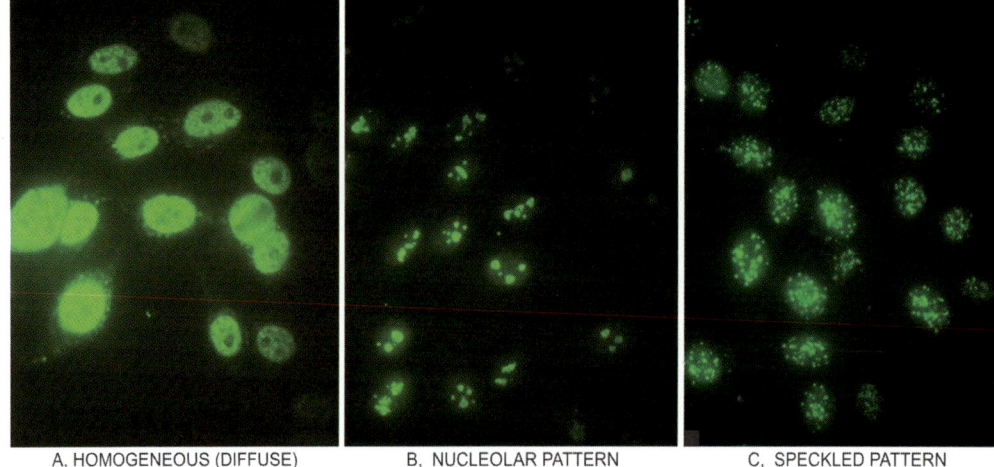

A, HOMOGENEOUS (DIFFUSE) NUCLEAR PATTERN   B, NUCLEOLAR PATTERN   C, SPECKLED PATTERN

FIGURE 5.9: Patterns of autoantibodies in blood in SLE in immunofluorescence microscopy.

e. *Anti-ribosomal P antibody* against proteins in ribosome, especially prominent in CNS SLE.
f. *Anti-neuronal antibody* is seen in 60% of patients with CNS SLE.
NOTE: Using the immunofluorescence test on normal cell smears, these antibodies can be recognised by their patterns of reactivity **(Fig. 5.9)**:
- Diffuse, reflecting the antibodies to chromatin, histones, and ds-DNA
- Peripheral or rim due to antibodies to ds-DNA
- Nucleolar reflecting the anti-RNA antibodies
- Speckled reflecting the antibodies to non-DNA antigens such as Sm

Q59. What are the most important clinicopathologic changes in SLE?

Almost all organs in the body can be affected. The patients usually have some **constitutional signs** of systemic disease, such as low grade fever, malaise, anorexia, weight loss, fatigue.
The most important organ-centered changes are as under:
I. **Cutaneous changes**
i. Butterfly rash on the face (over the nose and cheeks)
ii. Photosensitivity
iii. Skin lesions due to deposits of immune complexes along the dermal-epidermal junction with degeneration of the epidermal basal layer
II. **Renal changes**
i. Immune complex-mediated glomerulonephritis
ii. It is clinicopathologically classified I-VI
iii. Often combined with tubulo-interstitial nephritis.
III. **Cardiovascular changes**
i. Libman-Sacks endocarditis with sterile deposits of immune complex on both sides of valves, most prominently on the mitral valve.
ii. Vasculitis involving small blood vessels of various organs, most often in dermis.
IV. **Joint changes** Acute or chronic arthritis involving various small and large joints.
V. **Serous membranes** Clinically, these inflammatory lesions present as pericarditis, pleuritis, peritonitis.
VI. **Less common lesions** are inflammatory lesion in the eyes, CNS, skeletal and cardiac muscle, lungs, liver.
VII. **Haematologic changes** due to antibody-mediated cytotoxicity and inflammation are:
i. Anaemia
ii. Thrombocytopenia
iii. Leucopenia
iv. Hypergammaglobulinaemia

v. Elevated erythrocyte sedimentation rate
vi. Low complement levels reflecting the activity of the disease

Q60. What are the most common causes of death in patients with systemic lupus erythematosus?
i. Lupus nephritis related end-stage renal failure (35%)
ii. Cardiovascular complications, including hypertension (30%)
iii. Infections including those due to immunosuppression therapy (20%)
iv. Malignancy, such as lymphoma and HPV-related genital cancers (5%)

Q61. What is scleroderma (systemic sclerosis)? Briefly discuss its pathogenesis.
Definition Scleroderma, also known as systemic sclerosis (SS), is a systemic disease associated with signs of cellular and humoral autoimmunity, and characterised by microvascular changes associated with excessive fibrosis of the connective tissue, affecting the skin and numerous internal organs.
Classification Two major forms are known: systemic scleroderma and CREST syndrome.
Etiopathogenesis Unknown, but presumably of autoimmune nature.
i. *Sex* Affects predominantly middle-aged women (F:M= 4:1)
ii. *Racial difference* More common in African and some Native American Indian populations.
iii. *Autoantibodies* such as anti-DNA topoisomerase (previously known as anti-Scl-70) present in blood.
iv. *CD4+ T_H2 cells* increased in affected skin of extremities.
v. T_H2 cells produce *cytokines (IL-13 and TGF-β)* which activate inflammatory cells and fibroblasts, and may affect endothelial cells, which secrete PDGF and TGF-β. These cytokines favour perivascular fibrosis.
vi. *Endothelial cell injury* of arteries of the digits results in a decrease of vasodilator substances (NO and PGI_2) and more vasoconstrictor substances (endothelin) leading to progressive chronic ischaemia.

Q62. What are the clinicopathological features of systemic sclerosis?
I. **Skin** is the most commonly affected organ.
i. First changes are seen on fingers and hands that become oedematous in early stages of the disease.
ii. Raynaud phenomenon, characterised by vascular spasm in response to cold, is the most common complaint.
iii. Chronic thickening of the skin of the fingers and hand ensues leading to 'claw-like' flexion deformities (sclerodactyly) of the fingers. These changes are related to the abundance of sclerotic collagen fibres homogeneously filling the dermis.
iv. Small blood vessels have thick hyalinised walls and narrow lumina contributing to ischaemia, which leads to atrophy of the epidermis.
v. Facial skin appears tightened producing a radial furrowing around the mouth. Additional atrophy of the lips gives mouth a 'pursed-lip' appearance. The face becomes 'mask-like'.
vi. Telangiectatic small blood vessels are common.
vii. Dystrophic calcifications of the subcutaneous tissue.
II. **Kidneys** are involved in most patients, ultimately leading to renal insufficiency.
i. Principal lesions are seen in arterioles which show narrowing due to concentric proliferation of smooth muscle cells ('onion skinning') and even fibrinoid necrosis, similar to malignant hypertension.
ii. Medium-sized arteries and even interlobar arteries also, show luminal narrowing due to concentric proliferation of fibroblasts and smooth muscle cells in their walls.
iii. Vascular changes cause ischaemia with glomerular sclerosis and tubular atrophy and loss, reducing the function of the kidneys and contributing to arterial hypertension.
III. **Gastrointestinal changes** are found in 90% cases and are characterised by extensive fibrosis of the wall of the tubular GI organs.
i. Oesophagus shows fibrosis with a loss of peristalsis, dysphagia and G-E reflux.
ii. Intestinal fibrosis leads to malabsorption syndrome, cramps and bloating, and formation of colonic diverticula.
IV. **Pulmonary interstitial fibrosis** causes progressive ischaemia, often accompanied by pulmonary hypertension. Respiratory failure is the most common cause of death in SS patients.
Outcome 10 year survival is approximately 80% with modern thearpy.

Q63. What is CREST syndrome?

CREST syndrome is a form of scleroderma that includes the following five features:
i. Calcinosis
ii. Raynaud phenomenon
iii. Oesophageal hypomotility (E in CREST syndrome from 'Esophageal hypomotility' in American spelling)
iv. Sclerodactyly
v. Telangiectasia

Q64. Which serologic tests are positive in systemic sclerosis and CREST syndrome?

i. Anti-nuclear antibody test (ANA) is positive in 70–90% of all patients with systemic sclerosis.
ii. Anti-DNA topoisomerase antibody test is positive in 30–70% patients with systemic sclerosis and 10–20% with CREST syndrome.
iii. Anticentromere antibodies are present in 20–30% of CREST patients.

Q65. What are noninfectious inflammatory myopathies? Comment on their salient features.

Definition Group of immunologically mediated muscle diseases usually with an involvement of other internal organs. The group includes polymyositis and dermatomyositis. A rare form of muscle disease, inclusion body myositis, needs to be taken into differential diagnosis in older adults.
Etiopathogenesis Unknown, but presumably of immune origin, as suggested by the following findings:
i. Association with other autoimmune diseases is common.
ii. Presence of autoantibodies against nuclear and cytoplasmic antigens found in 20% of cases.
iii. B cell infiltrates in dermatomyositis; T cell infiltrates in polymyositis and inclusion body myositis.
iv. Some non-immune factors (like viral infections) may be involved in triggering the inflammation.
Clinical features Common features are:
i. Weakness of proximal muscles of the extremities and girdle/shoulder muscles of the trunk.
ii. Increased creatine kinase and myoglobin and aldolase in blood.
iii. Muscle biopsy confirms the diagnosis.

Q66. Discuss major features of polymyositis.

Definition Polymyositis is an autoimmune myositis associated with an increased expression of class-I MHC molecules on myofibres.
Epidemiology Predominantly affects adult women, 40–60 years of age (F:M = 2:1).
- African American women most often affected.
- May be paraneoplastic; increased incidence of neoplasms, such as lung and bladder cancer, lymphoma, noted in up to 20% of cases.

Pathology Proximal muscle injury by T cells (can be proven by muscle biopsy for diagnostic purposes!).
i. Predominantly endomysial infiltration of CD8+ T cells and macrophages.
ii. Myofibre necrosis and regeneration.
iii. Muscle atrophy is a not prominent (in contrast to dermatomyositis!).
Clinical features Muscle disease with signs of the systemic nature of the disease.
i. *Symmetric proximal muscle weakness* of extremities and shoulder girdle, with or without pain.
ii. Electromyography (EMG) shows signs of muscle dysfunction and injury.
iii. Constitutional signs including low grade fever, weakness, fatigue weight loss.
iv. Internal organs may be affected—dysphagia due to the involvement of oesophagus, and dyspnoea due to pulmonary disease.
v. Good response to treatment with corticosteroid and immunosuppressive agents; survival 80%.
Antibodies ANA and anti-transfer RNA synthetase (Jo-1) positive in 30% cases.

Q67. Discuss salient features of dermatomyositis.

Definition Dermatomyositis is a rare autoimmune disease involving the muscles and the skin.
Epidemiology It may occur in childhood or adulthood (F:M = 2:1).
- It is quite rare; 3 per one million in children and 10 per million in adults.
- Still in children, it is the most common form of inflammatory myopathy.

- In children, it is a well-defined clinicopathologic entity.
- In adults, it may also be paraneoplastic and one should search for the underlying neoplasia!

Pathogenesis CD4+ T cells infiltrate the muscle targeting the capillaries.
i. Antibodies and complement contribute to microvascular injury.
ii. Vascular injury causes ischaemic perifascicular atrophy of muscle fibres, that is seen in peripheral parts of the muscle fascicles.

Clinical features Proximal and shoulder/girdle *muscle weakness*, with or without pain, similar to polymyositis.
i. Skin changes are most prominent in children and typically include *purple-red discoloration of eyelids* ('heliotrope rash' or 'racoon eyes').
ii. Gottron red papules are found on knuckles in children and adults.

Outcome Most children recover completely. Adults who have cancer have bad prognosis related to neoplasia.

Q68. Tabulate the contrasting features of inflammatory myopathies.

Inflammatory myopathies include three conditions (polymyositis, dermatomyositis and inclusion body myositis) having overlapping clinical feature of progressive skeletal muscle weakness but distinctive age at presentation and some other features. These are presented in **Table 5.9**.

TABLE 5.9 Contrasting feature of inflammatory myopathies.

FEATURE	POLYMYOSITIS	DERMATOMYOSITIS	INCLUSION BODY MYOSITIS
1. Age at onset	>18 years	Children and young adults	>50 years
2. Familial association	Absent	Absent	Present
3. Extramuscular manifestations	Present	Present	Present
4. Association with other autoimmune diseases	Yes, frequent (SLE, RA, SS)	Yes, infrequent (scleroderma, mixed connective tissue disease)	Yes, 20% cases (SLE, RA, SS)
5. Preceded with exposure to exogenous agents	➢ Infections (viruses, bacteria) ➢ Drugs	➢ Cancers ➢ Drugs rarely	➢ Infections (viruses)

Q69. Discuss salient features of Sjögren syndrome.

Definition Sjögren syndrome is an autoimmune disease caused by immunologic destruction of lacrimal and salivary glands, clinically presenting with dry mouth and eye (*sicca syndrome*).
It may occur in an *isolated form,* or in *association with other autoimmune diseases (60%),* most often rheumatoid arthritis.

Pathogenesis Salivary and lacrimal glands destruction involves *CD4+ T helper cells and antibodies.*
- The initial injury may be a viral infection, but in most instances it remains unrecognised.
- The disease is associated with some class II HLA genes.

Clinicopathologic features It affects most often women in the 50–60 age group.
i. *Immunologic infiltrates* in the glands consist of T helper cells, B cells and some plasma cells.
ii. Initially the glands are enlarged but with time they become smaller.
iii. As the infiltrates destroy the glands, acini atrophy or disappear and are replaced by fibrosis, lymphoid and fat tissue.
iv. Lack of saliva leads to *xerostomia* (dry mouth), complicated by infections, cracks and fissures or shallow ulcerations, accompanied by difficulty in eating and swallowing. Upper and respiratory infections can ensue.
v. Lack of tears causes *xerophthalmia,* blurred vision, itching, and ulceration.

Complications Lymphoma, pathologically mostly classified as marginal zone B-cell lymphoma, develops in salivary glands of 5% of patients, which is 40 times more common than in other people.

Serology All findings must be interpreted in context since none of them is pathognomonic.
i. ANA positive in up to 80% cases.
ii. Rheumatoid factor in 75%.
iii. Anti-ribonucleoprotein antibodies SS-A (Ro), and SS-B (La) are found in over 90% of cases (not entirely diagnostic since it is positive also in some SLE cases).

Q70. What is IgG4 related disease?

Definition A localised or multiorgan disease characterised by infiltrates of IgG4 lymphocytes and plasma cells accompanied by fibrosis.

Clinicopathologic features It can affect any organ in the body.

i. Infiltrates of IgG4+ cells and fibrosis destroy the organs causing clinical symptoms of organ hypofunction.

ii. IgG4 is elevated in serum.

iii. Good response to corticoid treatment.

iv. Clinically, most important forms of IgG4 disease are: chronic pancreatitis, sialadenitis, cholangitis, chronic thyroiditis or lymphadenopathy.

AMYLOIDOSIS

Q71. Define amyloid. What are its key characteristics?

Definition Amyloid is a hyaline extracellular material that by light microscopy appears amorphous and eosinophilic, which upon additional examination with special stains and techniques, has certain well-defined characteristics.

Key characteristics

i. It binds *Congo red*, a special dye that stains all forms of amyloid red.

ii. Upon examination of the Congo red-stained tissue under polarised light, amyloid deposits in tissue sections are *birefringent* and have an *apple green colour*.

iii. Under the electron microscope, i.e. ultrastructurally, amyloid has a *fibrillar structure* and consists of fibres composed of 4–6 fibrils, each measuring 7.5–10 nm in diameter **(Fig. 5.10)**.

iv. These fibrils are wound up on each other and are separated by a clear space which contains regularly placed binding sites for Congo red dye.

v. By X-ray crystallography and infra-red spectroscopy, the fibrils are shown to have *cross-β-pleated sheet configuration* producing a 100 nm periodicity. Hence, amyloid is also called *β-fibrillosis*.

vi. *Chemical analysis* of amyloid shows the heterogeneity of fibrillar proteins in various forms of amyloidosis. Two major chemical forms of amyloid are:
- AL (amyloid light chain), and

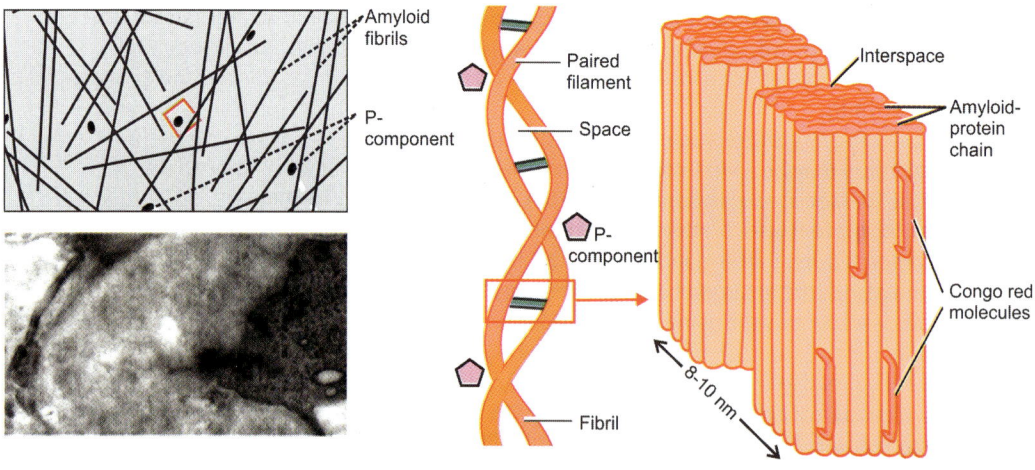

A, EM STRUCTURE B, STRUCTURE OF FIBRIL AND P-COMPONENT C, β-PLEATED STRUCTURE

FIGURE 5.10: Diagrammatic representation of the ultrastructure of amyloid. A, Electron microscopy shows major part consisting of amyloid fibrils (95%) randomly oriented, while the minor part is essentially P-component (5%). B, Each fibril is further composed of double helix of two pleated sheets in the form of *twin filaments* separated by a clear space. P-component has a pentagonal or doughnut profile. C, X-ray crystallography and infra-red spectroscopy shows fibrils having *cross-β-pleated* sheet configuration which produces periodicity that gives the characteristic staining properties of amyloid with Congo red and birefringence under polarising microscopy.

- AA (amyloid associate protein).

Besides, over 20 other chemical forms of amyloid are found in various clinical forms of amyloidosis.

Q72. Discuss main features of AL fibril protein.

i. AL fibril protein is derived from immunoglobulin light chain.
ii. It may include either the entire light chain, or its amino-terminal segment and part of C region.
iii. AL fibril is more often derived from lambda than kappa chain, but in any single case, there is amino acid sequence homology.
iv. Rarely, heavy chain of immunoglobulin may be associated with AL fibril protein.

Q73. What are the major features of AA fibril protein?

i. AA fibril protein is composed of protein derived from a larger serum precursor protein, called SAA (serum amyloid associated protein), which circulates in blood associated with HDL3 (high density lipoprotein 3).
ii. Unlike AL, the deposits of AA do not have sequence homology.
iii. SAA is an acute phase reactant synthesised by the liver in response to chronic inflammation and traumatic events, which raise its levels in serum.

Q74. Besides AL and AL proteins, what are the other important amyloid fibril proteins?

I. **Transthyretin (TTR)** ATTR is derived from TTR, a serum protein synthesised by the liver.
i. TTR functions as serum *trans*porter of *thy*roxine and *retin*ol (trans-thy-retin).
ii. Single amino acid substitution mutation in the structure of TTR results in a variant form, which is responsible for ATTR.
iii. There are some 60 types of such mutations described.
iv. ATTR is the most common form of heredofamilial amyloidosis seen in *familial amyloid polyneuropathies*.
v. Deposits of ATTR without any mutations are found in *senile cardiac amyloidosis*.

II. **Aβ$_2$-microglobulin (Aβ$_2$M)** This protein forms amyloid in long-term haemodialysis patients.
i. β$_2$M, the precursor of amyloid, is a small protein, forming the normal component of the major histocompatibility complex.
ii. It has a β-pleated structure, and since it is not filtered from serum during prolonged haemodialysis, it may be deposited in tissue as amyloid.
iii. Although it is a form of systemic amyloidosis, the deposits are predominantly seen in bones and joints.

III. **Amyloid β-peptide** is deposited in the brain in *Alzheimer disease*.
i. Aβ is derived from amyloid beta precursor protein (AβPP).
ii. AβPP is a cell surface protein having a single transmembrane domain that functions as a receptor, partially extending into the extracellular region.
iii. AβPP has three cleavage sites for secretases α, β, and γ.
iv. Partial proteolysis of AβPP by β-scretase and γ-secretase generates the soluble fragment Aβ, the amyloidogenic protein in Alzheimer disease **(Fig. 5.11)**.

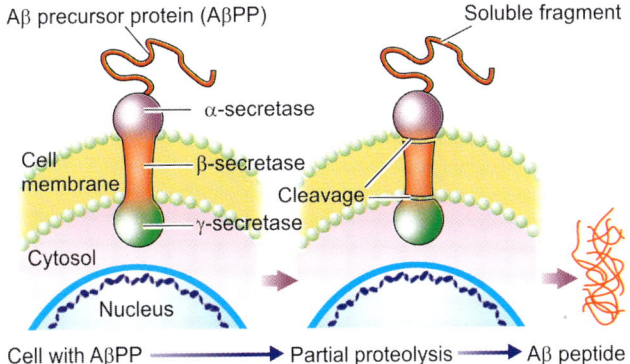

FIGURE 5.11: Mechanism of amyloid deposits in Alzheimer disease.

IV. **Endocrine amyloid from hormone precursor proteins** Amyloid can be formed from several precursor molecules.
i. The precursor molecules include: pro-calcitonin (ACal), islet amyloid polypeptide (AIAPP, amylin), pro-insulin (AIns), prolactin (APro), etc.
ii. Tumours of endocrine cells may contain deposits of endocrine amyloid. For example, medullary carcinoma of thyroid has stromal deposits of ACal, islet cell tumour of pancreas have AIAPP.
iii. Type 2 diabetes may present with deposits in the islets of Langerhans of pro-insulin derived AIns.
V. **Amyloid of prion protein (APrP)** It is derived from precursor prion protein which is a plasma membrane glycoprotein.
i. Prions are proteinaceous infectious particles lacking RNA or DNA.
ii. Amyloid in prionosis occurs due to abnormally folded isoforms of the PrP.

Q75. What are the non-fibrillar components of amyloid?

Non-fibrillar components of amyloid comprise approximately 5% of the amyloid material. Two most important components are as follows:
I. **Amyloid P (AP) component** It is synthesised in the liver and found in all types of amyloid.
- It is derived from circulating serum amyloid P-component, a glycoprotein derived from normal serum $α_1$-glycoprotein, an acute phase reactant.
II. **Apolipoprotein E (apo E)** It is a regulator of lipoprotein metabolism and it is found in all forms of amyloid.
- One allele, *apoE4*, has been found to increase the risk of APP deposition in the brain in Alzheimer disease, but not in other forms of amyloid.

Q76. Describe salient features of pathogenesis of amyloidosis.

Amyloidosis is a term used to denote several diseases related to excessive deposits of amyloid in tissue. It develops under the following conditions **(Fig. 5.12)**:

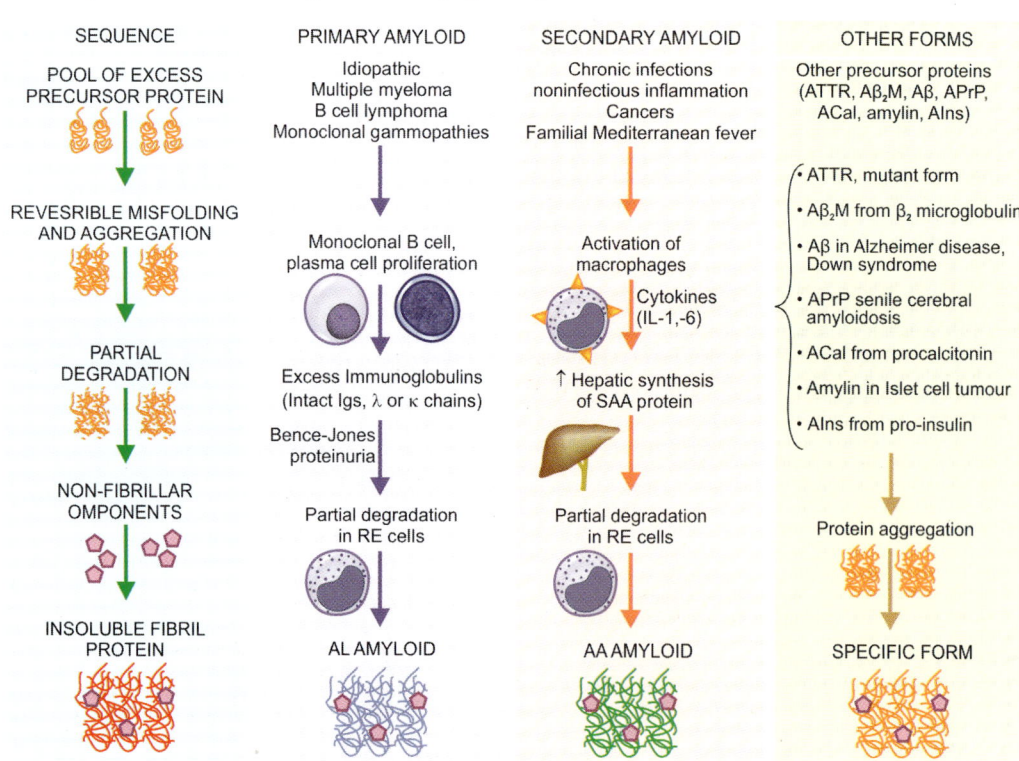

FIGURE 5.12: Pathogenesis of major forms of amyloid deposition.
(AL, amyloid light chain; AA, amyloid-associated protein; GAG, glycosaminoglycan; AP, amyloid P component; RE cells, reticuloendothelial cells). The sequence on left shows general schematic representation common to most forms of amyloidogenesis.

i. *Pool of excess precursor protein*—such as AL in multiple myeloma or AA in chronic infection.
ii. *Reversible misfolding and aggregation*—because of reduced elimination by proteolysis, as in mutant proteins like ATTR due to a single amino acid substitution in the mutant protein.
iii. *Non-fibrillar protein integration into the fibrils*—making them resistant to proteolysis and removal by macrophages.

Q77. Describe classification of amyloidosis.

Historically, classification of amyloidosis used to include two categories:
I. **Primary** (caused by plasma cell dyscrasias, such as multiple myeloma)
II. **Secondary** caused by chronic disease.
These two terms are still retained and are included in other forms of amyloidosis in a extended **clinicopathologic classification** which is based on the following data **(Table 5.10)**:
• *Clinical association* of amyloidosis with certain underlying diseases (e.g. AL amyloidosis and multiple myeloma).
• *Anatomic distribution* of amyloid deposits (*systemic versus localised*) and *organ involvement* (e.g. cardiac amyloidosis, polyneuropathic amyloidosis, etc.).
• *Chemical composition* of amyloid, i.e. the nature of precursor molecule (e.g. AL from light chain, AA from SAA).

TABLE 5.10 Classification of amyloidosis.

CATEGORY	ASSOCIATED DISEASE	BIOCHEMICAL TYPE	ORGANS COMMONLY INVOLVED
A. SYSTEMIC (GENERALISED) AMYLOIDOSIS			
1. *Primary*	Plasma cell dyscrasias	AL type	Heart, bowel, skin, nerves, kidney
2. *Secondary (Reactive)*	Chronic infections, chronic inflammation, cancers	AA type	Liver, spleen, kidneys, adrenals
3. *Haemodialysis-associated*	Chronic renal failure	Ab_2M	Synovium, joints, tendon sheaths
4. *Heredofamilial*	—	ATTR	Peripheral and autonomic nerves, heart
i. *Hereditary polyneuropathies*	—	AA type	
ii. *Familial Mediterranean fever*	—	AApoAI, AGel	Liver, spleen, kidneys, adrenals
iii. *Rare hereditary forms*		ALys, AFib, ACys	Systemic amyloidosis
B. LOCALISED AMYLOIDOSIS			
1. *Senile cardiac*	Age >70 years	ATTR	Heart
2. *Cerebral*	Alzheimer, transmissible encephalopathy, prionosis	$A\beta$, APrP	Cerebral vessels, plaques, neurofibrillary tangles
3. *Endocrine*	Medullary carcinoma Type 2 diabetes mellitus	Procalcitonin Proinsulin	Thyroid Islets of Langerhans
4. *Tumour-forming*	Lungs, larynx, skin, urinary bladder, tongue, eye	AL	Corresponding anatomic location

Q78. What are the features of primary systemic (AL) amyloidosis?

Primary amyloidosis is a systemic disease, characterised by *AL deposits*, most often derived from immunoglobulin lambda light chains.
i. In 30% of cases, AL is related to *plasma cell/B cell dyscrasias* such as multiple myeloma or B cell lymphoma.
ii. The remaining 70% of patients do not have undetectable malignancy and are *idiopathic*.
iii. Some of these patients have an increased number of plasma cells in bone marrow or show subtle *functional abnormalities of plasma cells* detectable by the techniques of molecular biology.
iv. Deposits of AL can be found in *most organs,* but occur most often in some of them; most prominently involved are the kidneys, intestines, hear and peripheral nerves.
v. The urine contains excreted light chains, known under the name of *Bence-Jones protein*.
vi. *Lambda chains* are 2-times more common precursors of AL than kappa chains.

Q79. Describe the main features of secondary/reactive amyloidosis.

i. Secondary/reactive amyloidosis is a systemic or generalised amyloidosis characterised by deposition of *AA amyloid*.

ii. It is usually a complication of *chronic infections* (e.g. pulmonary tuberculosis, chronic osteomyelitis, leprosy), *autoimmune diseases,* or *neoplasia* (e.g. renal cell carcinoma, Hodgkin disease). *Familial Mediterranean fever*, an autosomal recessive disease, affecting people who live in the Mediterranean region (e.g. Jews, Arabs, Turks, Armenians) is also associated with AA amyloidosis.

iii. Deposits of AA are usually found in *abdominal organs* such as the kidney, liver, spleen, adrenals.

iv. It can occur at any age and affects even children.

v. Treatment should be directed at the underlying chronic disease that has caused AL overproduction.

Q80. Tabulate the contrasting features of primary and secondary amyloidosis.

The contrasting features of primary and secondary amyloidosis are presented in **Table 5.11**.

TABLE 5.11 Contrasting features of primary and secondary amyloidosis.

FEATURE	PRIMARY AMYLOID	SECONDARY AMYLOID
1. *Biochemical composition*	AL (Light chain proteins); lambda chains twice more common than kappa; sequence homology of chains	AA (Amyloid associated proteins); derived from larger precursor protein SAA; no sequence homology of polypeptide chain
2. *Associated diseases*	Plasma cell dyscrasias, e.g. multiple myeloma, B cell lymphomas, others	Chronic inflammation, e.g. infections (TB, leprosy, osteomyelitis, bronchiectasis), autoimmune diseases (rheumatoid arthritis, IBD), cancers (RCC, Hodgkin disease), FMF
3. *Pathogenesis*	Stimulus → Monoclonal B cell proliferation → Excess of Igs and light chains → Partial degradation → Insoluble AL fibril	Stimulus → Chronic inflammation → Activation of macrophages → Cytokines (IL-1, IL-6) → Partial degradation → AEF → Insoluble AA fibril
4. *Incidence*	More common in US and other developed countries	Most common in developing countries
5. *Age*	>40 years	Any age including children
6. *Course and prognosis*	Rapidly progressive, dismal outcome	Better, improves on treating underlying cause
7. *Organ distribution*	Kidney, heart, bowel, nerves	Kidney, liver, spleen, adrenals
8. *Stains to distinguish*	Congophilia persists after permanganate treatment of tissue section; specific immunostains anti-λ, anti-κ	Congophilia disappears after permanganate treatment of section; specific immunostain anti-AA

Q81. What are the general pathologic features of amyloidosis? Briefly comment on its management and prognosis.

I. Location of deposits
In general terms, the amyloid deposits are formed in the following locations:

i. At the sites of plasma filtration (e.g. renal glomeruli)

ii. Wall of arteries and arterioles

iii. The perivascular interface between the capillaries and the parenchymal cells (e.g. the Disse space between hepatic sinusoids and liver cells)

II. Diagnosis
i. Biopsies of the affected organ, e.g. kidney or nerve biopsy.

ii. If systemic amyloidosis is suspected, it is possible to make the diagnosis on biopsy/fine needle aspiration of subcutaneous fat tissue, or rectal biopsy.

iii. Tissue obtained by biopsy is sectioned in the laboratory and the slides are stained with Congo red, followed by examination under polarising microscopy.

iv. Immunohistochemical stains can also be employed against specific amyloid antigen, e.g. anti-kappa and anti-lambda light chains, anti-AA, or anti-AP immunostain, etc.

v. Alternatively, the tissue can be submitted for electron microcopy and special molecular biology testing.

vi. In AL amyloidosis, such a diagnostic biopsy is typically followed up by *additional studies* such as serum electrophoresis and bone marrow biopsy to determine the source of AL and the nature of the underlying disease.

III. **Treatment and prognosis**
i. The treatment of amyloidosis is directed at the underlying disease.
ii. The prognosis for patients with systemic amyloidosis is generally poor with the overall survival around 2 years after diagnosis.

Q82. What are the staining characteristics of amyloid?

Various stains and techniques employed to distinguish and confirm amyloid deposits in tissue sections are given in **Table 5.12**.

TABLE 5.12 Staining characteristics of amyloid.

STAIN	APPEARANCE
1. H & E	Pink, hyaline, homogeneous
2. Methyl violet/Crystal violet	Metachromasia: rose-pink
3. Congo red	Light microscopy: pink-red Polarising light: red-green birefringence
4. Thioflavin-T/ Thioflavin-S	Ultraviolet light: fluorescence
5. Immunohistochemistry (antibody against fibril protein)	Immunoreactivity: Positive

Q83. Discuss briefly clinicopathologic features of amyloidosis of kidneys.

Amyloidosis of the kidneys is most common and most serious because it causes major renal dysfunction.
Clinical and gross features
i. The deposits in the kidneys are found in most cases of secondary amyloidosis and in about one-third cases of primary amyloidosis.
ii. Amyloidosis of the kidney accounts for about 20% of deaths from amyloidosis.
iii. Even small quantities of amyloid deposits in the glomeruli can cause proteinuria and nephrotic syndrome.
iv. *Grossly*, the kidneys may be normal-sized, enlarged or terminally contracted due to ischaemic effect of narrowing of vascular lumina. Cut surface is pale, waxy and translucent.

Microscopy
Amyloid deposition occurs primarily in the glomeruli, though it may involve peritubular interstitial tissue and the walls of arterioles as well **(Fig. 5.13)**:
i. *Glomeruli* Amyloid deposition occurs primarily in the glomeruli. The deposits initially appear on the basement membrane of the glomerular capillaries, but later extend to produce luminal narrowing and distortion of the glomerular capillary tuft. This results in abnormal increase in permeability of the glomerular capillaries to macromolecules with consequent proteinuria and nephrotic syndrome.
ii. *Tubules* The amyloid deposits begin close to the tubular epithelial basement membrane. Subsequently, the deposits may extend and produce degenerative changes in the tubular epithelial cells and amyloid casts in the tubular lumina.

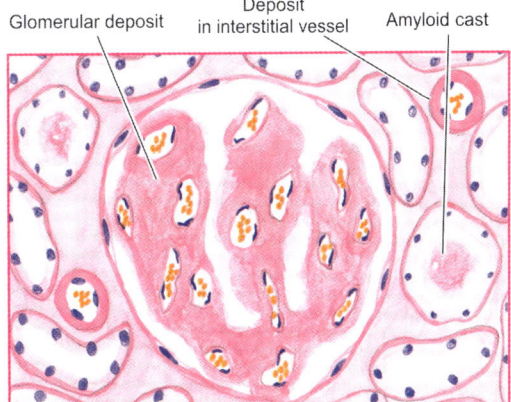

FIGURE 5.13: Amyloidosis of kidney. The amyloid deposits are seen mainly in the glomerular capillary tuft. The deposits are also present in peritubular connective tissue producing atrophic tubules and amyloid casts in the tubular lumina, and in the arterial wall producing luminal narrowing.

iii. *Interstitial vessels* Vascular involvement affects chiefly the walls of small arterioles and venules, producing narrowing of their lumina and consequent ischaemic effects.
iv. *Congo red staining* It imparts red pink colour and polarising microscopy shows apple-green birefringence which confirms the presence of amyloid.

Q84. What are the salient pathologic features of amyloidosis of spleen?

Amyloid deposition in the spleen may have one of the following two patterns **(Fig. 5.14)**:

I. **Sago spleen**
Grossly, splenic enlargement is not marked. Its cut surface shows characteristic translucent pale and waxy nodules resembling sago grains and hence the name.
Microscopically, the amyloid deposits begin in the walls of the arterioles of the white pulp and may subsequently extend out and replace the follicles.

II. **Lardaceous spleen**
Grossly, there is generally moderate to marked splenomegaly (weight up to 1 kg). Cut surface of the spleen shows map-like areas of amyloid (lardaceous-lard-like; *lard* means fat of pigs).
Microscopically, the deposits involve the red pulp in the walls of splenic sinuses and the small arteries and in the connective tissue.
• Confirmation is by observing congophilia in Congo red staining and demonstration of apple-green birefringence under polarising microscopy in the corresponding positive areas.

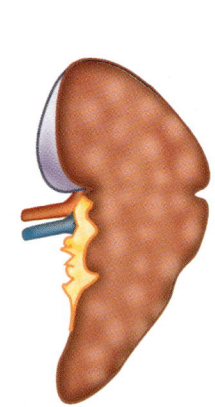
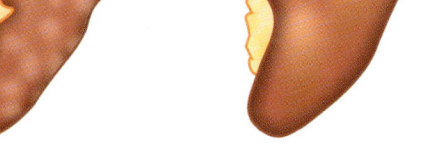

A, SAGO SPLEEN   B, LARDACEOUS SPLEEN
FIGURE 5.14: Gross patterns of amyloidosis of the spleen.

Q85. Briefly discuss pathologic features of amyloidosis of liver.

Clinical and gross features
i. In about half the cases of systemic amyloidosis, liver is involved by amyloidosis.
ii. The liver is often enlarged, pale, waxy and firm.

Microscopy
i. The amyloid initially appears in the space of Disse.
ii. Later, as the deposits increase, they compress the cords of hepatocytes. Eventually, the liver cells are shrunken and atrophic and replaced by amyloid **(Fig. 5.15)**. However, hepatic function remains normal even at an advanced stage of the disease.
iii. To a lesser extent, portal tracts and Kupffer cells are involved in amyloidosis.

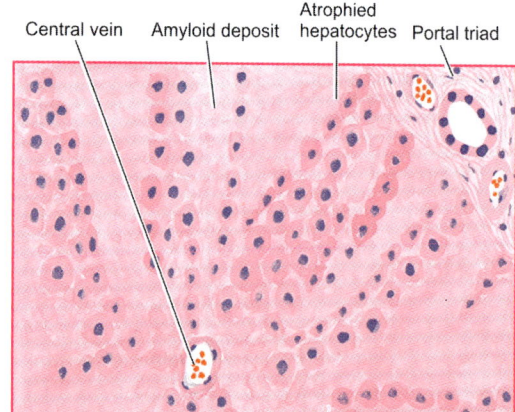

FIGURE 5.15: Amyloidosis of the liver. The deposition is extensive in the space of Disse causing compression and pressure atrophy of hepatocytes.

Chapter 5e Supplement: Online Content

Digital content of this chapter available with this book is meant for enhanced learning and self-assessment. In addition, it contains 26 Multiple Choice Questions (MCQs), 09 Clinicopathologic Vignettes, and 02 Image-based Questions; these are followed by their answers along with explanatory notes of correct and incorrect answers.

Derangements of Homeostasis and Haemodynamic Disorders

■ HOMEOSTASIS

Q1. What are the body water compartments?

Water comprises 60% of the body weight (BW) of a normal male and 50% of the body weight of an adult female. It is distributed into two main compartments: intracellular and extracellular fluid compartment **(Fig. 6.1)**:

I. **Intracellular compartment** comprises about 33% of BW. The bulk of it is contained in the skeletal muscles. The main cations of this fluid are potassium and magnesium, and the main anions are phosphates and proteins.

II. **Extracellular fluid** (ECF) constitutes the remaining 27% of BW. The predominant cations of ECF is sodium and principal anions are chrloride and bicarbonate. ECF has four subcompartments:

i. *Interstitial fluid* including lymph fluid (12% of BW), forming the major proportion of the ECF.

ii. *Intravascular fluid or blood plasma* (5% of BW), totaling about 3 litres, or 3/5 of the total blood volume, which is 5 litres.

iii. *Mesenchymal tissues* such as bone, cartilage and dense connective tissue (9% of BW).

iv. *Transcellular fluid* (1% of BW), found in the secretions formed by various excretory organs such as salivary glands, pancreas, gastrointestinal tract, kidneys and skin.

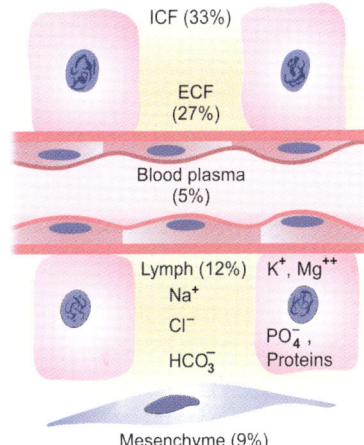

FIGURE 6.1: Body fluid compartments. (ICF, intracellular fluid compartment; ECF, extracellular fluid compartment).

Absorption of water occurs in the intestines. The average intake is 2800 ml per day.
Elimination of water occurs via:
i. Kidneys (urine, 1500 ml per day)
ii. Skin (insensible perspiration and sweat, 800 per day)
iii. Lungs in exhaled air (400 ml per day)
iv. Minor losses such as faeces (100 ml per day) and lacrimal, nasal, oral, sexual and mammary (milk) secretion.

Q2. What is the effective osmotic pressure between the extracellular fluid and plasma?

- **Osmotic pressure** is exerted by the chemical constituents of the body fluids, mostly electrolytes and proteins. The pressure exerted by electrolytes is called *crystalloid pressure,* and the pressure mediated by proteins is called *colloid osmotic pressure* or *oncotic pressure.*

- **Effective oncotic pressure** is the difference between the higher oncotic pressure of the plasma and the lower oncotic pressure of the interstitial fluid. Since the plasma contains more proteins than the intertitial fluid, oncotic pressure of the plasma tends to draw fluid into the vessels.

Q3. What is effective hydrostatic pressure?

i. **Hydrostatic pressure** is the pressure exerted by the capillary blood or the interstitial fluid. *Capillary hydrostatic pressure* has a gradient, which is the highest at the arteriolar end (32 mmHg), and lowest at the venularend of the capillaries (12 mmHg). *Hydrostatic pressure of the interstitial fluid (tissue tension),* is much lower (4 mmHg) and the same on both ends of the capillary bed.

ii. **Effective hydrostatic pressure** is the difference between the higher pressure in the capillaries and the lower tissue tension. It drives the the fluid through the wall of capillries into the intestitial space.

iii. The normal **fluid exchange** between the capillaries and the interstitial space depends on the hydrostatic and oncotic pressure in these two compartments:
- *At the arteriolar side* of the capillaries the difference between the hydrostatic pressure (32 mmHg) and plasma oncotic pressure (25 mmHg) is 7 mm, which is the *outward-driving force* directing the fluid into the interstitial space.
- *At the venular end* of the capillaries the difference between the hydrostatic pressure (12 mmHg) and the plasma oncotic pressure (25 mmHg) reulsts in 13 mmHg *inward-driving force* so that the fluid and solutes could reenter into the venous circulation.
- Tissue fluid remaining after exchanges across the vessel wall escapes into the lymphatics and ultimately reenters the venous circulation.

■ DERANGEMENTS OF BODY WATER

Q4. What is oedema? What are its types?

Definition Oedema is abnormal and excessive accumulation of free fluid in interstitial tissue spaces and in serous cavities.

In practical terms, the term *oedema* (swelling) is used for the accumulation of fluid in the interstitial spaces. Accumulation of free fluid in serous cavities is called *effusion*.

Types
- Oedema may be *localised* or *generalised* (also knowns as *anasarca or dropsy*).
- Depending on fluid composition, oedema fluid can be classified as *transudate* (as in cardiac or renal oedema) or *exudate* (as in inflammatory oedema).

Q5. What are the differences betweeen transualte and exudate?

The differences between transudate and exudate are presented in **Table 6.1**.

TABLE 6.1 Differences between transudate and exudate.		
FEATURE	TRANSUDATE	EXUDATE
1. *Definition*	Filtrate of blood plasma without changes in endothelial permeability	Oedema of inflamed tissue associated with increased vascular permeability
2. *Character*	Non-inflammatory oedema	Inflammatory oedema
3. *Protein content*	Low (less than 1 g/dL); mainly albumin, low fibrinogen; hence no tendency to coagulate	High (2.5–3.5 g/dL), readily coagulates due to high content of fibrinogen and other coagulation factors
4. *Cells*	Few cells, mainly mesothelial cells and cellular debris	Many cells, inflammatory as well as parenchymal
5. *Examples*	Oedema in congestive cardiac failure	Purulent exudate such as pus

Q6. How does oedema develop?

Oedema develops due to mechanisms which interfere with the normal fluid exchange and balance between the plasma, interstitial fluid and lymph flow.

The following mechanisms may lead to oedema formation **(Fig. 6.2)**:
i. decreased plasma oncotic pressure

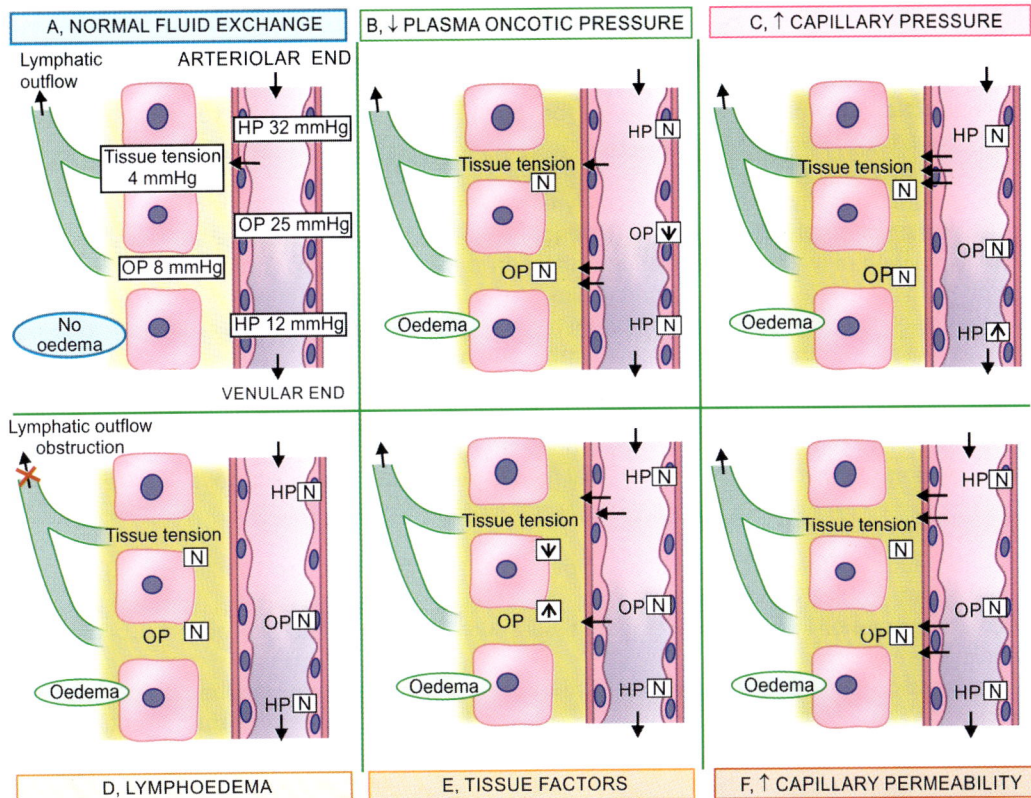

FIGURE 6.2: Diagrammatic representation of pathogenesis of oedema. A, Normal pressure gradients and fluid exchanges between plasma, interstitial space and lymphatics. B, Mechanism of oedema by decreased plasma oncotic pressure and hypoproteinaemia. C, Mechanism of oedema by increased hydrostatic pressure in the capillary. D, Mechanism of lymphoedema. E, Mechanism by tissue factors (increased oncotic pressure of interstitial fluid and lowered tissue tension). F, Mechanism of oedema by increased capillary permeability.
(OP, oncotic pressure; HP, hydrostatic pressure).

ii. increased capillary hydrostatic pressure
iii. obstruction of lymph flow
iv. tissue factors (increased oncotic pressure or decreased hydrostatic pressure)
v. increased capillary permeability
vi. sodium and water retention

I. Decreased plasma oncotic pressure occurs due to *hypoproteinaemia*, i.e. decreased concentration of plasma proteins below 5 g/dL. Since the albumin contributes four times more to the total plasma oncotic pressure than globulins, *hypoalbuminaemia* of less than 2.5 g/dL is the most common of oncotic oedema. At such a low concentration of albumin, plasma cannot prevent the fluid from leaking out of the capillaries.

Clinical examples of oncotic oedema include various causes of hypoalbuminaemia such as:
i. Cirrhosis leading to the formation of ascites due to reduced hepatic synthesis of albumin.
ii. Nephrotic syndrome leading to generalised oedema due to increased renal loss of albumin.
iii. Protein-losing enteropathy resulting in hypoproteinaemia and generalised oedema.

II. Increased capillary hydrostatic pressure at venular end of the capillaries, exceeding the inward effects of oncotic pressure, will increase filtration of fluid from capillaries into the interstitial space.

Clinical examples of hydrostatic oedema include conditions interfering with venous drainage of blood from tissue such as:
i. *Cardiac oedema* of lower extremities in right heart failure.
ii. *Postural oedema* involving feet and ankles due to increased backward leg vein pressure. Typically it is encountered in professions requiring prolonged standing.

iii. *Thrombosis related oedema* due to thrombotic occlusion of leg veins, which results in passive venous congestion and oedema.

iv. *Ascites* due to increased portal vein pressure due to obstruction of the blood flow by the fibrotic liver.

III. **Obstruction of lymph flow** leads to the formation of lymphoedema. It is typically localised and most frequently involves the arms or legs.

Clinical examples are:

i. Arm oedema following removal of axillary lymph nodes for treatment of breast cancer.

ii. Obstruction of lymphatics by malignant tumour.

iii. Inflammation of lymphatics in filariasis (infection with *Wuchereria bancrofti*) resulting in chronic lymphedema of legs (elephantiasis) or scrotum.

iv. External compression of the main abdominal or thoracic duct by tumours, or effusion in serous cavities resulting in thoracic or abdominal lymphoedema.

v. Rupture of the lymphatic channel may cause a formation of chyle rich effusion (chylous ascites or chylothorax).

IV. **Tissue factors** may cause oedema due to increased oncotic pressure of interstitial fluid or increased tissue tension. Oncotic pressure of interstitial fluid is caused by proteins accumulating in interstitial spaces.

Clinical examples are:

i. Accumulation of proteins due to increased permeability of capillaries (as in inflammation).

ii. Inadequate removal of proteins by lymph.

iii. Low tissue tension in some subcutaneous tissues such as eyelids (periorbital oedema), or male and female external genitalia.

V. **Increased capillary permeability** due to injury of endothelial cells by histamine, ischaemia, venom or toxins. The gaps that form in injured capillaries allow the entry of proteins into the interstitial spaces, increasing the oncotic pressure of this fluid and reducing the oncotic pressure of plasma.

Clinical examples are:

i. Generalised oedema in anaphylactic shock, systemic infection, anoxia or adverse drug reaction.

ii. Localised inflammatory oedema due to infection, insect bite, allergic reaction, irritant chemicals or drugs.

iii. Angioneurotic oedema most often involving lips and larynx, pharynx and even lungs. It is most often caused by a genetic defect of a complement system inhibitor (C1IN).

VI. **Sodium and water retention** occurs due to renal problems. *The basic physiologic facts* to understand this important clinical problem are as follows:

i. Some *80% of sodium* filtered through the glomeruli is *reabsorbed* in the proximal tubules.

ii. *Tubular reabsorption* of sodium is controlled by an intrinsic renal and an extrinsic extrarenal mechanism:

- *Intrinsic renal mechanism* (e.g. in response to hypotension) activates the arterial *baroreceptors* to send central vasomotor center to increase *sympathetic outflow*. It will reduce glomerular filtration rate and decrease excretion of sodium.
- *Extrarenal mechanism* involving the release of *renin-angiotnesin-aldosterone system*, increasing the reabsorption of sodium in renal tubules and causing high blood pressure. *Antidiuretic hormone (ADH)* is released from the hypothalamus in response to high concentration of sodium in plasma and hypovolaemia. The resulting retention of sodium is followed by retention of water. ADH will produce antidiuresis and production of highly concentrated urine **(Fig. 6.3)**.

Clinical examples are:

i. Oedema of cardiac disease

ii. Oedema of renal disease

iii. Oedema of chronic liver disease (cirrhosis)

Q7. What is the pathogenesis of renal oedema?

Three important causes of renal oedema are i) nephrotic syndrome, ii) nephritic syndrome, and iii) acute tubular injury.

i. **Nephrotic syndrome** is characterised by severe proteinuria and causing decreased oncotic pressure and generalised oedema. Decreased plasma volume activates the renin-angiotensin-aldosterone system resulting in sodium and water retention.

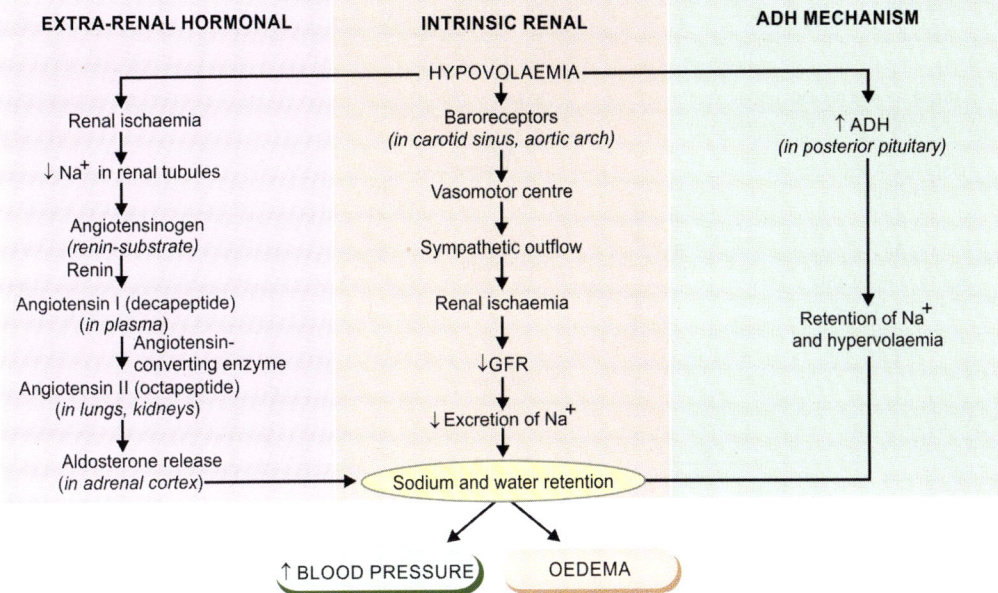

FIGURE 6.3: Mechanisms involved in oedema by sodium and water retention.
(ADH, anti-diuretic hormone; GFR, glomerular filtration rate).

ii. **Nephritic syndrome** is caused by acute glomerulonephritis, which leads to a retention of sodium and water. Nephritic oedema is usually mild in comparison with generalised oedema of nephrotic syndrome, and is limited to loose connective tissue such as around the eyes and face in general, as well as on ankles and genitalia. It is not affected by gravity as cardiac oedema.

iii. **Acute tubular injury** following shock or ingestion of toxic chemicals results in oliguria and retention of water and minerals. It is typically of sudden onset and generalised.

Q8. What are the differences between oedema due to nephrotic and nephritic syndrome?

The differences between nephrotic and nephritis oedema are presented in **Table 6.2**.

TABLE 6.2 Differences between nephrotic and nephritic oedema.

FEATURE	NEPHROTIC OEDEMA	NEPHRITIC OEDEMA
1. Cause	Nephrotic syndrome	Glomerulonephritis (acute, rapidly progressive)
2. Proteinuria	Heavy	Moderate
3. Protein content	High (>1 g/dL)	Low (<0.5 g/dL)
4. Main mechanism	↓ Plasma oncotic pressure (hypoproteinaemia)	Na^+ and water retention
5. Degree of oedema	Severe, generalised	Mild
6. Distribution	Subcutaneous tissues as well as visceral organs	Loose tissues mainly (face, eyes, ankles, genitalia)

Q9. What is the pathogenesis of cardiac oedema?

Cardiac oedema develops due *congestive heart failure* as follows:

i. **Left ventricular failure** is characterised by *reduced cardiac output* that causes *hypovolaemia* which stimulates the renin-angiotensin-aldosterone system as well as the ADH secretion. The net results of these two processes is sodium and water retention and generalised oedema. Hypoxia from hypoperfusion of the vasculature may contribute to an increased permeability of capillaries (*forward pressure hypothesis*), but this hypothesis is not fully documented.

ii. **Right heart failure** results in *elevated central venous pressure*, that is transmitted backward to the venous end-capillaries, raising the capillary pressure, that leads to transudation of fluid into the interstitial spaces (*back pressure hypothesis*) **(Fig. 6.4)**.

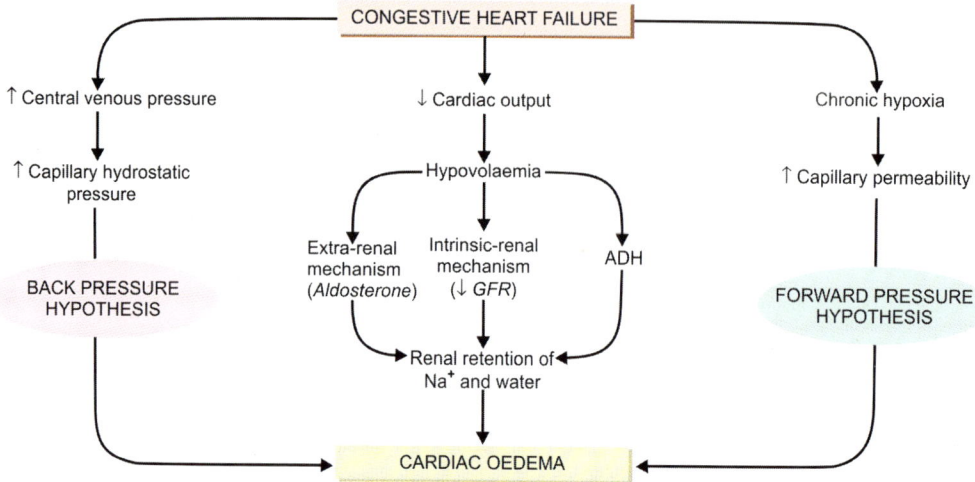

FIGURE 6.4: Mechanisms involved in the pathogenesis of cardiac oedema. (ADH, anti-diuretic hormone; GFR, glomerular filtration rate).

NOTE:
- Cardiac oedema is influenced by gravity (*dependent oedema*), and thus more pronounced in lower extremities of *ambulatory patients*.
- In *bed-ridden patients*, it is most pronounced on the sacrum and the back.
- In both instances, it also accumulates in *serous cavities* of the abdomen and thorax.

Q10. What are differences between cardiac and renal oedema?

The differences between cardiac and renal oedema are shown in **Table 6.3**.

TABLE 6.3 Differences between cardiac and renal oedema.

FEATURE	CARDIAC OEDEMA	RENAL OEDEMA
1. *Main causes*	i. Congestive heart failure ii. Right heart failure	i. Nephrotic syndrome ii. Acute nephritic syndrome iii. Acute tubular injury
2. *Proteinuria*	Absent	Present, amount varies
3. *Serum albumin*	Normal	Decreased
4. *Main mechanism*	↓ Cardiac output	i. Hypoalbuminaemia ii. ↓ plasma oncotic pressure iii. Na⁺ and water retention
5. *Distribution of oedema*	Dependent oedema i. Sacral area in bed-ridden ii. Lower limbs in ambulatory	i. Nephrotic: Severe, generalised ii. Nephritic: Loose tissues mainly (face, eyes, ankles, genitalia)

Q11. What is the pathogenesis of pulmonary oedema? Briefly comment on its pathologic features.

Pulmonary oedema is characterised by an accumulation of fluid in the interstitial spaces and inside the alveoli. It may be caused by: i) elevation of pulmonary vascular hydrostatic pressure, or ii) increased vascular permeability.

I. **Elevation of pulmonary vascular hydrostatic pressure (haemodynamic oedema)** is a consequence of heart failure and resulting back pressure into the pulmonary circulation. When the hydrostatic pressure exceeds the oncotic pressure of the blood, fluid begins seeping out into the loose interstitial spaces around the bronchi and blood vessels of the lung **(Fig. 6.5)**.
- This *interstitial oedema* fluid drains through the lymphatics.
- When the influx of fluid exceeds the capacity of the lymphatics to drain it, a spill-over into the alveolar spaces occurs (alveolar *oedema*).

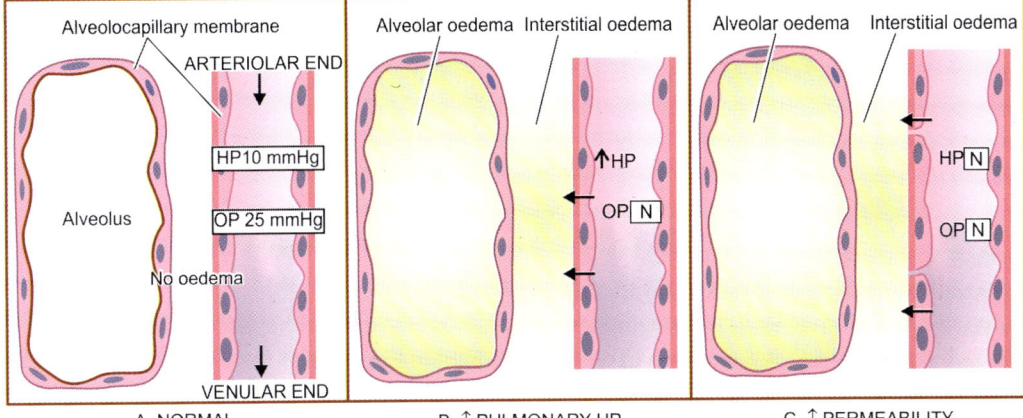

FIGURE 6.5: Mechanisms involved in the pathogenesis of pulmonary oedema. A, Normal fluid exchange at the alveolocapillary membrane (capillary endothelium and alveolar epithelium). B, Pulmonary oedema via elevated pulmonary hydrostatic pressure. C, Pulmonary oedema via increased vascular permeability.
(OP, oncotic pressure; HP, hydrostatic pressure).

- Furthermore, prolonged interstitial oedema will also damage the alveolar lining, facilitating further accumulation of fluid in alveoli.

II. **Increased vascular permeability (irritant oedema)** occurs due to a damage of the *alveolar-capillary unit*, the basic functional unit of each alveolus. The injury may begin from inside the alveoli, like following inhalation of toxic fumes or accumulation of bacteria in the alveolar lumen in early stages of pneumonia. Alternatively, the injury could damage the endothelial cells of alveolar capillaries, as in toxaemia or bacteraemia and shock. In both instances, oedema develops due to increased permeability of alveolar capillaries.

High altitude oedema develops in mountain climbers who reach rapidly altitude over 2,500 metres without proper gradual acclimatisation. High altitude hypoxia damages the alveolar-capillary units causing defects in the capillary wall, increased permeability of the alveolar capillaries with oedema and small intra-alveolar haemorrhages. If acclimatisation is allowed to take place during gradual ascent to higher altitude, the pulmonary arterial pressure and heart output will gradually rise and the pulonary ventilation will increase, preventing the adverse effect of high altitude.

Pathology Irrespective of the initial pathogenesis, lung oedema has the same morphologic features.

X-ray examination of patients suffering from pulmonary oedema will reveal so called *Kerley lines*, corresponding to thickened alveolar septa and dilated lymphatics.

Gross If the patient dies, gross examination at autopsy shows oedematous lungs that are heavy, moist, and less crepitant on palpation than normal lungs, because they contain more fluid and less air.

Microscopy The alveolar septa are widened by the fluid, which also fills the alveolar spaces **(Fig. 6.6)**. Superimposed bacterial pneumonia is a common complication.

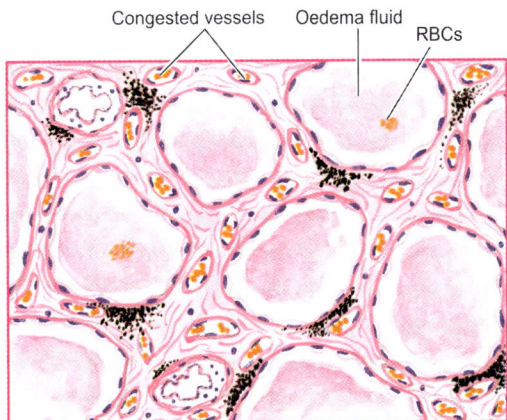

FIGURE 6.6: Pulmonary oedema. The alveolar capillaries are congested. The alveolar spaces as well as interstitium contain eosinophilic, granular, homogeneous and pink proteinaceous oedema fluid along with some RBCs and inflammatory cells.

Q12. Write briefly on cerebral, hepatic and nutritional oedema. How is myxoedema different from other forms of oedema?

I. **Cerebral oedema** is the most life-threatening form of localised oedema. Skull bones prevent unlimited expansion of the oedematous brain. The swelling of the brain due to the accumulation of fluid will compress the vital centres in the medulla oblongata and cause death.
Pathology Grossly, at autopsy the brain is moist. Its gyri are widened compressing the sulci which appear narrowed. The size of lateral ventricles is reduced.
Microscopy Oedema fluid separates the cellular components of the brain one from another, and dilates the perivascular (Virchow-Robin) spaces.

II. **Hepatic oedema** is characterised by formation of ascites and accumulation of fluid in lower extremities. The main reasons for oedema formation is loss of some vital hepatic functions:
i. Hypoalbuminaemia due to reduced synthesis of proteins in the diseased liver
ii. Hyperaldosteronism due to inadequate inactivation of aldosterone in the liver
iii. Secondary stimulation of the renin-angiotensin mechanisms promoting sodium and water retention.
NOTE: Formation of ascites in cirrhosis has several causes including hypoalbuminaemia, increased hydrostatic pressure in the portal system, and the reduced excretion of water through the kidney due to the effects of aldosterone.

III. **Nutritional oedema** may occur due to a deficiency of proteins (kwashiorkor, prolonged starvation, famine, fasting), or vitamins (beri-beri due to B_1 deficiency). Metabolic abnormalities in these conditions also cause sodium-water retention, contributing to oedema formation.

IV. **Myxoedema** in hypothyroidism is a form of non-pitting oedema of the facial skin and other parts of the body, as well as internal organs. It is caused by a deposition of glycosaminoglycans in the interstitium. That can be demonstrated microscopically.

Q13. What is dehydration? Enumerate various factors causing dehydration.

Definition Dehydration is a state of water deprivation or loss with sodium retention leading to hypernatraemia.
Clinically, it presents with intensive thirst, oliguria, mental confusion and fever. There are no particular pathological changes.
Biochemical and haematological changes include haemoconcentration with increased PCV and haemoglobin concentration. In later stages, there is rise in serum urea and sodium concentration. Ultimately there is complete renal shutdown and a state of shock may develop.
Etiopathogenesis may be considered under five headings as follows:
i. *GI excretion* (e.g. vomiting, diarrhoea, cholera)
ii. *Renal excretion* (e.g. acute renal tubular necrosis in the diuretic phase, extensive use of diuretics, endocrine disorders marked by polyuria such as diabetes mellitus, diabetes insipidus, Addison disease)
iii. *Loss of blood or plasma* (e.g. severe burns, during childbirth)
iv. *Loss through skin* (e.g. excessive perspiration, hyperthermia)
v. *Accumulation of fluids in body cavities* (e.g. ascites, accumulation of fluid in dilated intestines).

Q14. What is overhydration? Comment on its etiology and pathogenesis.

Definition Overhydration is an increase of extracellular fluid volume due to pure water excess or water intoxication.
Clinically, it presents with severe weight gain.
Laboratory findings include reduced PCV and reduced plasma electrolyte and protein concentration.
Etiopathogenesis Overhydration is generally a medically induced condition that may occur under the following circumstances:
i. Excessive unmonitored intravascular infusion of normal saline (0.9% of NaCl) or Ringer lactate
ii. Renal retention of sodium and water
iii. Congestive heart failure
iv. Acute glomerulonephritis
v. Chronic renal failure
vi. Cirrhosis
vii. Cushing syndrome

DISTURBANCES OF ELECTROLYTES AND pH OF BLOOD

Q15. How are the acid-base balance and pH of the blood maintained?

- The acid-base balance and the normal pH of the blood, which is 7.4, are maintained by the buffering systems of the blood (especially the bicarbonate buffering system), and the excretion of carbonic acid and metabolic acids formed in the body.
- The pH of the blood depends on the serum concentration of bicarbonate and partial pressure of CO_2 that determines the concentration of carbonic acid. Acidosis is marked by a pH of less than 7.4 and alkalosis by a pH higher than 7.4.
- Alterations in the blood bicarbonate levels are *metabolic acidosis and alkalosis*.
- Alterations in the blood pCO_2 (which depends on the ventilatory function of the lungs) are *respiratory acidosis and alkalosis*.

Q16. What are the most important causes of metabolic acidosis?

Metabolic acidosis is characterised by excess of H^+ ions and a fall of pH below 7.4. The most important causes are:
i. Lactic acidosis in shock or strenuous overexertion
ii. Diabetic ketoacidosis in uncontrolled diabetes mellitus
iii. Starvation
iv. Chronic renal failure
v. Drugs such as ammonium chloride or acetazolamide

Clinical and laboratory features
- High levels of H^+ ion in metabolic acidosis stimulate deep and rapid breathing (*Kussmaul respiration or air hunger*).
- There is a fall in bicarbonate levels.

Q17. What are the most common causes of metabolic alkalosis?

Metabolic alkalosis is characterised by a rise of serum bicarbonates and a loss of H^+ ions. Its main causes are:
i. Severe and prolonged vomiting
ii. Administrations of alkaline salts such as sodium bicarbonate
iii. Hypokalaemia as in Cushing syndrome or due to increased secretion of aldosterone

Clinical and laboratory features
- Clinically, it is characterised by depression of respiration, depressed renal function and uraemia.
- Bicarbonate levels are elevated in blood and in urine.

Q18. What are the most important causes of respiratory acidosis?

Respiratory acidosis is characterised by by raised pCO_2 due to its retention related to pulmonary hypoventilation. It can occur in the following circumstances:
i. Air-obstruction due to pulmonary diseases such a chronic bronchitis and emphysema or asthma
ii. Restricted thoracic respiratory movements due to pleural effusion, large ascites, pregnancy, kyphoscoliosis
iii. Impaired neuromuscular function affecting the respiration such as poliomyelitis or apoplexy.

Clinical and laboratory features
- Clinically, there is peripheral vasodilatation and increased intracranial pressure.
- In severe cases of CO_2 retention (CO_2 *narcosis*), the patients show signs of confusion, drowsiness, and even coma.
- The arterial level of pCO_2 is raised.

Q19. What are the most important causes of respiratory alkalosis?

Respiratory alkalosis is characterised by a lowered pCO_2 consequent to hyperventilation and excess removal of CO_2. It can occur in the following circumstances:
i. Hysterical overbreathing
ii. Working at high temperature

iii. At high altitude
iv. Meningitis, encephalitis
v. Drug overdose, e.g. salicylate poisoning

Clinical and laboratory features
- peripheral vasoconstriction
- pallor of the skin
- light headedness
- tetany in severe cases

■ HAEMODYNAMIC DERANGEMENTS

Q20. What is the difference between active and passive hyperaemia?

Hyperaemia is a localised increase in the volume of blood within dilated blood vessels of an organ or tissue. With regards to its pathogenesis, hyperaemia is classified as active or passive **(Fig. 6.7)**.

I. **Active hyperaemia** (also known simply as *hyperaemia*) occurs due to dilatation of arteries or arterioles and increased inflow of blood. The hyperaemic area is red and warm.
Examples:
i. Inflammation
ii. High grade fever
iii. Blushing, i.e. redness of the face in response to emotions
iv. Menopausal flush
v. Muscular excercise

II. **Passive hyperaemia**, also known as *venous congestion*, results from impaired venous drainage causing decreased outflow of blood. It may be localised or systemic. Both local and systemic may be acute or chronic (chronic venous congestion or CVC):

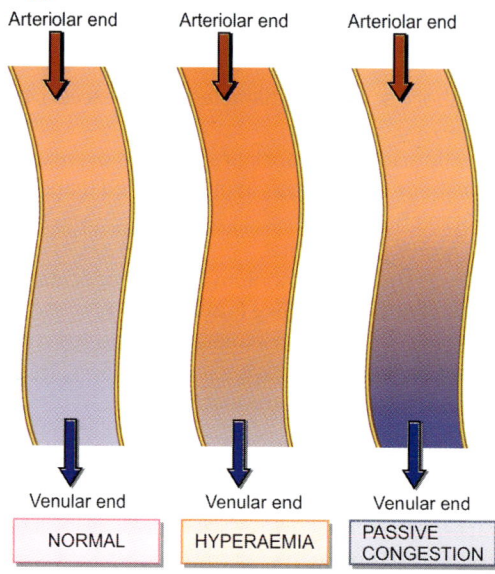

FIGURE 6.7: Schematic representation of abnormal accumulation of blood in the arteriovenous capillary bed causing hyperaemia and passive congestion.

i. *Local venous congestion* occurs when the outflow from an organ or part of the body is obstructed.
Examples:
a. Portal venous obstruction in cirrhosis leading to CVC of the intestines and spleen
b. Venous thrombosis of the leg causing CVC of the leg
c. Tight bandages applied to a leg or arm can cause acute or chronic congestion of the extremities.
ii. *Systemic venous congestion* occurs due to heart failure **(Fig. 6.8)**.
Examples:
a. Left-sided heart failure leads to congestion of lungs
b. Right-sided heart failure leads to congestion of liver, spleen, intestines, other abdominal organs, and lower extremities

Q21. What is the sequence in development of pathologic changes in chronic venous congestion (CVC)?

CVC is characterised by chronic stagnation (*stasis*) of blood in the venous system of various organs. The sequence of events includes the following steps:
i. *Initial enlargement* of a particular organ is related to the *reduced outflow of venous blood*, which accumulates in the veins, venules and capillaries. As the CVC persists, the organ may actually regain its previous normal size and just become firmer due to fibrosis.
ii. *The back-pressure* from venous and capillary part of the circulation leads to *transudation* of plasma and oedema of the perivascular tissue.

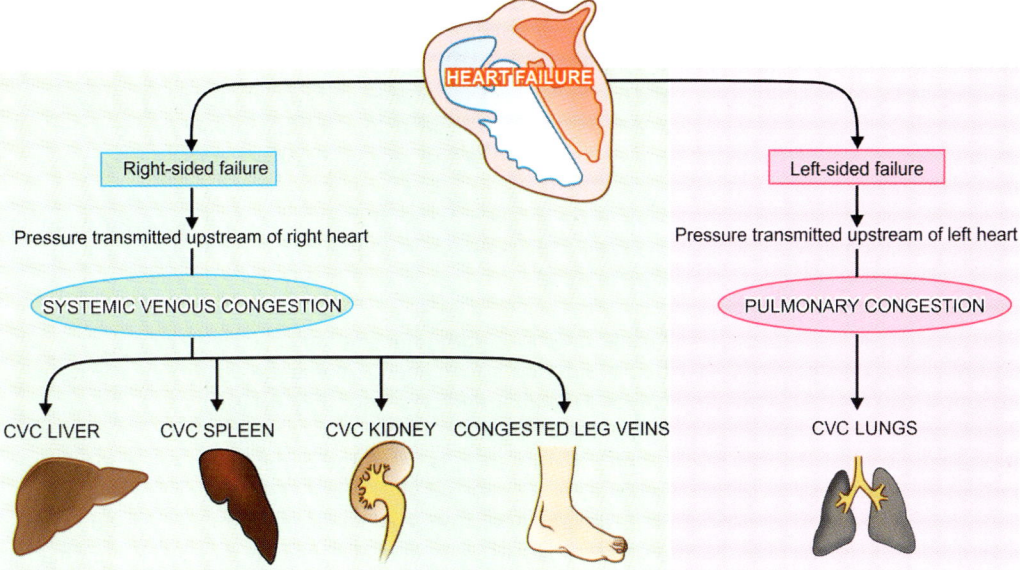

FIGURE 6.8: Schematic representation of mechanisms involved in chronic venous congestion (CVC) of different organs.

iii. *Chronic oedema* impedes the delivery of oxygen and nutrients.
iv. *Hypoxia and mechanical compression* by the stagnant blood will cause *necrosis or atrophy* of parenchymal cells.
v. *Perivascular fibrosis* will start replacing the lost parenchymal cells.
vi. *Fibrosis* will become more prominent with time, further impeding the delivery of oxygen and nutrients.
vii. *Damage* of the capillary walls allows *extravasation* of red blood cells into the perivascular tissue.
viii. Extravasated red blood cells *haemolyse*. The released haemoglobin transforms into an iron-rich pigment (*haemosiderin*) which accounts for the *brownish discoloration* of fibrous tissue.

Q22. What are the principal gross and microscopic pathologic features of chronic venous congestion (CVC) of major organs?

CVC affects most prominently: i) lungs, ii) the liver, and iii) the spleen.

I. **Lungs** CVC of lungs is a common autopsy finding in persons suffering from congestive heart failure.
Gross On cross section of the lungs, the parenchyma appears brown and fibrotic, i.e. a set of changes known as *brown induration of lungs*.
Microscopy Congestion of dilated capillaries and veins is focally accompanied with intra-alveolar haemorrhage:
i. Interstitial fibrosis surrounds the alveoli impeding the respiration **(Fig. 6.9)**. Macrophages containing haemosiderin granules can be seen in the alveoli where they are removing the fragmented RBCs.
ii. Haemosiderin-laden macrophages can be expectorated in sputum and are called *heart failure cells*.

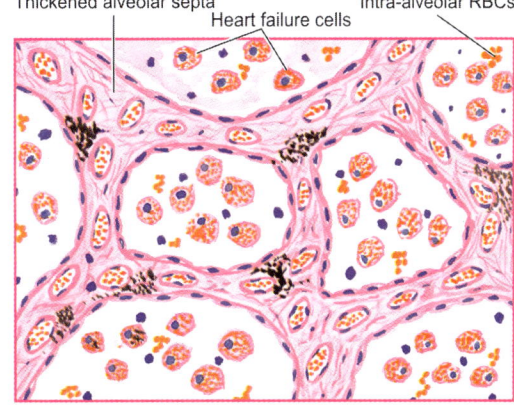

FIGURE 6.9: CVC lung. The alveolar septa are widened and thickened due to congestion, oedema and mild fibrosis. The alveolar lumina contain heart failure cells (alveolar macrophages containing haemosiderin pigment).

iii. Haemosiderin-laden macrophages also move into the fibrotic interstitium.

iv. When these macrophages die, they release haemosiderin granules into the interstitial space, imparting the fibrous tissue its brown colour.

Clinically, CVC of the lungs affects the gas exchange in the lungs and contributes to dyspnoea.

II. **Liver** CVC of liver is usually caused by right-sided heart failure and back-pressure from the right ventricle into the right atrium, inferior vena cava and hepatic vein all the way to the centrilobular zone of liver lobules.

Gross Liver is enlarged and its capsule is tense. On cross section at autopsy, it has a 'nut-meg like appearance', comprising congested central darker zones surrounded by a lighter zone composed of fat-laden and normal hepatocytes **(Fig. 6.10, A)**.

Microscopy

i. Centrilobular vein (terminal venule) and the surrounding sinusoids are filled with blood.

ii. Centrally located hepatocytes and sinusoids undergo ischaemic/compression atrophy and necrosis, accompanied by an accumulation of blood (*haemorrhagic necrosis*) **(Fig. 6.10, B)**.

iii. Lost hepatocytes may be replaced by fibrous tissue.

iv. In long-lasting CVC, the centrilobular fibrous strands can interconnect with those in adjacent lobules, thus producing *cardiac cirrhosis*.

Clinically, CVC of the liver is associated with a *right subcostal pain* resulting from the distention of the hepatic capsule by the retained blood. This is because the capsule is the only part of the liver that has sensory nerve endings.

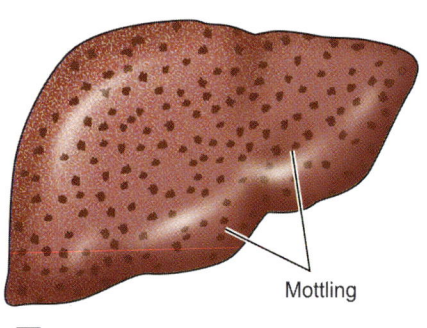
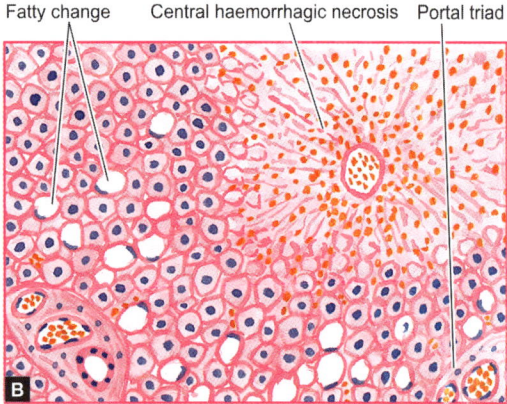

FIGURE 6.10: A, Nutmeg liver. The cut surface shows mottled appearance—alternate pattern of dark congestion and pale fatty change. B, CVC liver. The centrilobular zone shows marked degeneration and necrosis of hepatocytes accompanied by haemorrhage while the peripheral zone shows mild fatty change of liver cells.

III. **Spleen** CVC related changes may be a a consequence of i) right-sided heart failure or, ii) cirrhosis related portal hypertension.

Gross In cardiac failure, the spleen is moderately enlarged (250 g, versus 150 g of a normal spleen). In patients with cirrhosis, the spleen is much more enlarged and may weigh 800–1000 g *(congestive splenomegaly)*.

i. On cross section, enlarged spleen is initially dark bluish-red and soft.

ii. Long-lasting congestive splenomegaly becomes permeated by fibrous tissue.

iii. Splenomegaly appears dark brown on cross section; its colour stemming from the accumulation of haemosiderin.

iv. Fibrous scars may be seen focally, especially underneath the splenic capsule.

v. The capsule may become focally or diffusely fibrotic and thickened.

Microscopy

i. Sinusoids of the red pulp are dilated and filled with blood.

ii. Stagnant RBC are prone to haemolysis. Haemosiderin from haemolysed RBC is taken up by macrophages.

iii. Haemosiderin released from dead macrophages enters into the interstitial spaces.

iv. Interstitium becomes fibrotic, focally coalescing even into larger fibrous scars **(Fig. 6.11)**.
Clinically Congestive splenomegaly is the most common cause of *hypersplenism*, a syndrome characterised by anaemia, leukopenia, and thrombocytopenia.

Q23. What is haemorrhage and how is it classified?

Definition Haemorrhage is the scientific term for bleeding, i.e. escape of blood from blood vessels or the heart.
Classification Clinicopathologic classification takes into account several parameters:
i. **Based on duration:** Haemorrhage of sudden onset and short duration is called *acute*, and the longer lasting haemorrhage is called *chronic*.
Clinical consequences depend on the amount of blood loss and duration:
a. The loss up to 20% has little clinical effects.
b. Acute loss of 33% of blood may be lethal.
c. Loss of 50% of blood over some time may be tolerated.

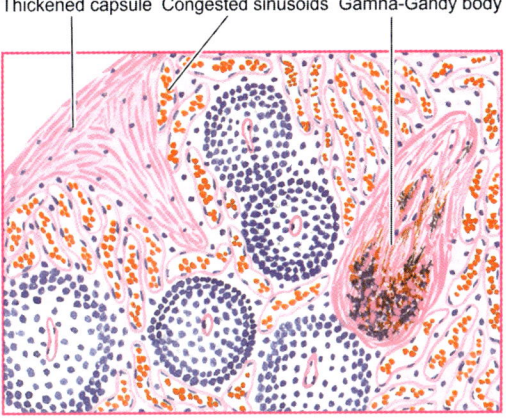

FIGURE 6.11: CVC spleen. The sinuses are dilated and congested. There is increased fibrosis in the red pulp, capsule and the trabeculae. Gamna-Gandy body is also seen.

ii. **Based on location:** Haemorrhage can be *external* (outside of the body), or *internal* such as into a serous cavity (e.g. haemothorax, haematoperitoneum, haematopericaridum), or into the lumen of hollow viscera (e.g. gastrointestinal bleeding, haematometra or bleeding into the uterine cavity), haematocephalus (bleeding into the lateral ventricles of the brain).
iii. **According to the anatomic site of origin:** Haemorrhages can be classified as *cardiac, aortic, arterial, capillary or venous*.
a. Bleeding into the tissues results in a swelling called *haematoma*. The process allowing the microscopic escape of blood from small blood vessels is called *diapedesis*.
b. Haemorrhages into the *skin and mucous membranes* are classified according to their size and extent:
- *Petechiae*—small pinhead hemorrhages (1 mm in size).
- *Purpuras*—haemorrhages measuring up to 1 cm.
- *Ecchymoses*—haemorrhages larger than 1 cm.

NOTE: In clinical practice the term *purpura* also denotes several diseases characterised by a bleeding tendency (e.g. *thrombotic thrombocytopenic purpura*).

Q24. What are the most important causes of haemorrhage?

Haemorrhage may result from an injury or rupture of the vessel wall or due to a bleeding diathesis caused by the disturbances of the coagulation system. The most important causes are listed below:
i. Trauma
ii. Infection (e.g. syphilis, Rickettsioses like Rocky Mountain spotted fever)
iii. Inflammation of the vessel wall (e.g. hypersensitivity vasculitis, polyarteritis nodosa)
iv. Chronic vascular diseases (e.g. atherosclerosis, aneurysm)
v. Inflammation of the tissue eroding the vessel wall (e.g. bleeding peptic ulcer)
vi. Neoplasms invading or eroding the vessel wall
vii. Increased intravascular pressure (e.g. cerebral haemorrhage from ruptured blood vessels in hypertension)
viii. Coagulation problems
ix. Idiopathic bleeding, the cause of which cannot be determined

Q25. What is shock and what are its major types?

Definition Shock is a life-threatening clinical syndrome of cardiovascular collapse characterised by:
- an acute reduction of effective circulating blood volume (hypotension), and

- an inadequate perfusion of cells and tissue (hypoperfusion).

If uncompensated, these changes may lead to impaired cellular metabolism, production and release of damage-associated molecular patterns (DAMPs or danger signals) and death. In other words, it is a circulatory imbalance between oxygen supply and oxygen requirements.

Classification There are three major forms of shock, and a few other variants: i) hypovolaemic, ii) cardiogenic, and iii) septic shock, and iv) variants such as traumatic, neurogenic and hypoadrenal shock.

i. **Hypovolaemic shock** results from:
a. *inadequate blood volume*, such as major haemorrhage, or
b. from the *loss of plasma volume* due to dehydration, diarrhoea, burns or acute pancreatitis with ascites.

ii. **Cardiogenic shock** results from a sudden reduction of cardiac output, without actual loss of blood volume (*normovolaemia*).

iii. **Septic (toxaemic) shock** develops in severe bacterial infections or septicaemia. It may be endotoxic (in Gram-negative septicaemia) or exotoxic (Gram-positive septicaemia).

iv. **Traumatic shock** is caused by severe trauma, resulting initially in hypovolaemia due to blood loss. However, even after the blood loss has been compensated, these patients continue to lose plasma into interstitial spaces and remain in shock.

v. **Neurogenic shock** results from a failure of sympathetic innervation of blood vessels, which tend to dilate and thus cannot be filled adequately by the existing volume of blood.

Q26. Briefly discuss the pathogenesis of shock.

All forms of shock are based on three fundamental derangements **(Fig. 6.12)**: i) reduced effective blood volume, ii) impaired tissue oxygenation, and iii) release of inflammatory mediators.

i. **Reduced effective blood volume** It may be caused by a loss of blood or plasma, or inadequate filling of peripheral blood vessels due to reduced cardiac output.

ii. **Impaired tissue oxygenation** Peripheral hypoxia is related to reduced cardiac output, which is even more aggravated by reduced venous return to the heart causing reduced diastolic filling.

iii. **Release of inflammatory mediators** The release of cytokine is triggered by cell injury caused by hypoxia, activation of the macrophages and other parts of the natural immune system. In septic shock, cytokine release is stimulated further by bacterial endotoxins or exotoxins. The most important cytokines in shock are tumour necrosis factor (TNF) and interleukin 1 (IL-1).

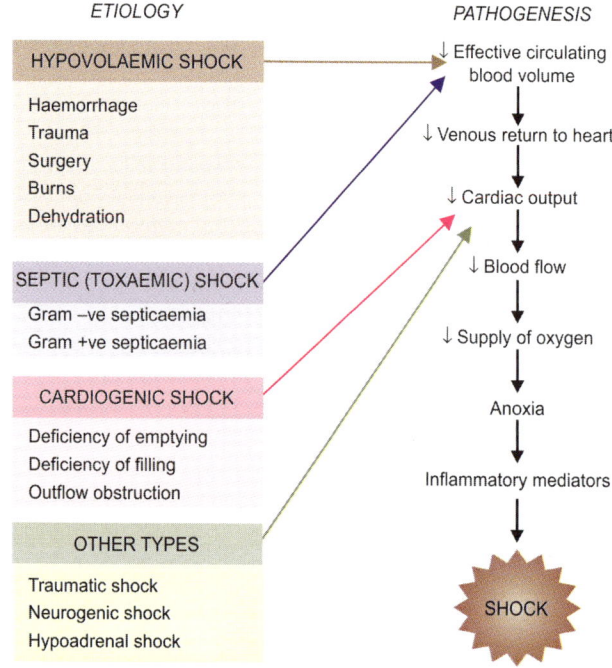

FIGURE 6.12: Pathogenesis of circulatory shock.

Q27. What are the clinical types (or stages) and symptoms of hypovolaemic shock?

The severity of hypovolaemic shock depends on the degree of blood loss:
- <1000 ml: Compensated
- 1000–1500 ml: Mild

- 1500–2000 ml: Moderate
- >2000 ml: Severe

Major clinical features of shock include:
i. Tachycardia
ii. Hypotension
iii. Oliguria progressing to anuria
iv. Mental state changes, from agitation to confusion and lethargy.

Q28. What is the pathogenesis of septic shock?

Septic shock results from bacterial infections, two-third of which are caused by Gram-negative organisms. Polymicrobial infections are common. Fungal infections are less common, and usually found in immunosuppressed persons.

The sequence of events in septic shock is outline below **(Fig. 6.13)**:

i. **PAMPs** (pathogen-associated molecular patterns), including bacterial peptides and lipopolysaccharides, are released from pathogens and react with TLRs (toll-like receptors) and NODs (nucleotide oligomerisation domains) on macrophages and PMNs.

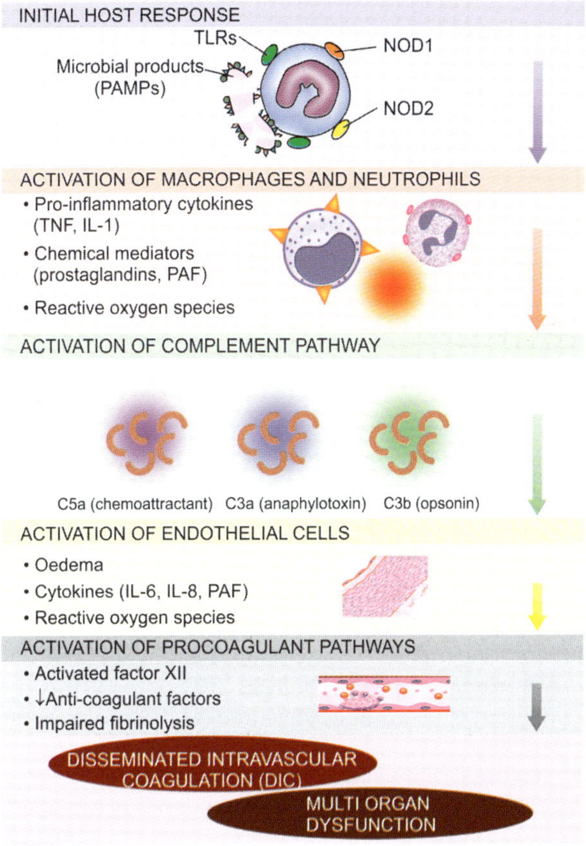

ii. **Activation of macrophages and PMNs** leads to a release of pro-inflammatory cytokines, such as TNF and IL-1, chemical mediators, such as prostaglandins, and reactive oxygen species (ROS).

iii. **Activation of the complement pathway**, forming chemoattractants, anaphylatoxins and opsonin, that stimulate endothelial cells.

iv. **Activation of endothelial cells**, which contribute to dilatation of vessels, increased permeability of capillaries and the formation of oedema. Endothelial cells also produce additional cytokines and ROS, and change their synthetic/secretory activity leading to pooling of venous blood in peripheral circulation.

v. **Activation of the procoagulant pathway** is combined with reduced fibrinolysis, leading to disseminated intravascular coagulation (DIC) and reduced return of blood into the right heart.

INITIAL HOST RESPONSE
- TLRs
- Microbial products (PAMPs)
- NOD1
- NOD2

ACTIVATION OF MACROPHAGES AND NEUTROPHILS
- Pro-inflammatory cytokines (TNF, IL-1)
- Chemical mediators (prostaglandins, PAF)
- Reactive oxygen species

ACTIVATION OF COMPLEMENT PATHWAY
C5a (chemoattractant)   C3a (anaphylotoxin)   C3b (opsonin)

ACTIVATION OF ENDOTHELIAL CELLS
- Oedema
- Cytokines (IL-6, IL-8, PAF)
- Reactive oxygen species

ACTIVATION OF PROCOAGULANT PATHWAYS
- Activated factor XII
- ↓Anti-coagulant factors
- Impaired fibrinolysis

DISSEMINATED INTRAVASCULAR COAGULATION (DIC)

MULTI ORGAN DYSFUNCTION

FIGURE 6.13: Major pathways in pathogenesis of septic shock.

Q29. What is the pathogenesis of three main stages of shock? How are these stages recognised clinically?

Although the various features of shock are interconnected into a continuous sequence of events, for practical purposes, one can recognise three stages: i) compensated shock, ii) progressive decompensated shock, and iii) irreversible decompensated shock **(Fig. 6.14)**:

I. **Compensated shock**, also known as initial, reversible, or non-progressive shock, is characterised by an attempt of the body to maintain adequate cerebral and coronary blood and oxygen supply by redistributing the blood flow through the body. This is achieved through the following mechanisms:

i. *Vasoconstriction,* which is widespread but most prominent in the skin and viscera.
a. It involves the reaction of baroreceptors, chemoreceptors.
b. It is mediated by a release of catecholamines (from adrenal medulla), renin (from ischaemic kidneys) and angiotensin-II.

Clinically, vasoconstriction causes peripheral resistance and hypertension, as well as tachycardia. It accounts for the pale, cold skin in this stage of shock.

STAGE	PATHOGENESIS	EFFECTS
COMPENSATED (INITIAL) SHOCK	i) Widespread vasoconstriction ii) Fluid conservation by kidney iii) Stimulation of adrenal medulla	• Tachycardia • Cool clammy skin
PROGRESSIVE DECOMPENSATED SHOCK	i) Pulmonary hypoperfusion ii) Tissue ischaemia	• ↓ Cardiac output • Mental confusion • ↓ Urinary output • Tachypnoea
IRREVERSIBLE DECOMPENSATED SHOCK	i) Progressive vasodilatation ii) ↑ Vascular permeability iii) Myocardial depressant factor (MDF) iv) Pulmonary hypoperfusion v) Anoxic damage vi) Hypercoagulability	• Brain: Hypoxic encephalopathy • Heart: Focal myocardial necrosis • Lungs: ARDS • Kidney: ATN • Adrenals: Necrosis • GI: Haemorrhagic gastroenteropathy • Liver: Necrosis • Blood: DIC

FIGURE 6.14: Mechanisms and effects of three stages of shock.
(ARDs, acute respiratory distress syndrome; ATN, acute tubular necrosis; DIC, disseminated intravascular coagulation).

NOTE: In septic shock vasoconstriction is preceded by vasodilation, which is then counteracted by a release of thromboxane A_2, a potent vasoconstrictor.

ii. *Fluid conservation* by the kidneys. It is mediated by the following factors, some of which have been listed above as mediating vasoconstriction:

a. Renin-angiotensin-aldosterone system
b. ADH mediated reduced diuresis
c. Reduced glomerular filtration rate due to arteriolar constriction in the kidneys
d. Shifting of fluid from the interstitial space into the capillaries due to peripheral hypotension

II. **Progressive decompensated shock** develops in patients who most often have some other preexistent aggravating clinical condition (e.g. cardiovascular or pulmonary problems). Its two main features are as under:

i. *Pulmonary hypoperfusion* leading to acute respiratory distress syndrome (ARDS) with dyspnoea and tachypnea.
ii. *Tissue ischaemia* which leads to a shift from oxidative phosphorylation to anaerobic glycolysis. Consequent *lactic acidosis* makes the vasomotor response ineffective, leading to vasodilatation and *peripheral pooling of blood*.

Clinically, this stage of shock is characterised by a worsening of renal function and mental confusion.

III. **Irreversible decompensated shock** develops when the compensatory mechanisms fail to reverse shock and the treatment becomes ineffectual. Widespread cell injury leads to the following changes:

i. *Progressive vasodilatation* due to paralysis of arteriolar sphincters and pressure induced dilation of capillaries and venules, reducing even further the effective circulating blood volume.
ii. *Increased vascular permeability* due to hypoxia-induced endothelial cell injury and the effects of pressure of stagnant blood on the endothelial lining of capillaries and venules.
iii. *Myocardial depressant factor* released in the hypoperfused heart.
iv. *Worsening pulmonary hypoperfusion* with formation of chronic pulmonary oedema and alveolar hyaline membranes.
v. *Anoxic damage of cells in vital organs* (cardiac myocytes, neurons of the brain, proximal tubules of kidneys). These cells are especially sensitive to hypoxia because they generate ATP exclusively through aerobic phosphorylations and cannot compensate the deficiency by anaerobic glycolysis.
vi. *Hypercoagulability of blood* due to the activation of the coagulation pathway, platelet aggregation and a release of procoagulants from them and hypoxic endothelial cells.

Clinically, there is progressive multisystem organ failure dominated by worsening of the heart function, renal failure due to acute tubular necrosis, and coma.

Q30. What are the pathologic changes in severe shock?

All major organs are affected and show either macroscopic of microscopic pathologic changes or both, as follows **(Fig. 6.15)**:

i. **Hypoxic encephalopathy** If the systolic blood pressure falls below 50 mmHg and if hypoxia or anoxia persist for 12–24 hours, the brain will show microscopic signs of inadequate oxygen supply. Neurons, and especially the Purkinje cells in the cerebellum, are most prominently affected. These cells have pink eosinophilic cytoplasm and pyknotic nuclei. The border zone between the supply zone of anterior and middle cerebral artery is most affected.

ii. **Heart ischaemia** is usually zonal and related to hypoperfusion of the myocardium. It is most prominent in the subendocardial zone, which is the least perfused layer of the ventricular wall. It includes necrosis of cardiac myocytes, contraction band necrosis, and foci of microscopic haemorrhage.

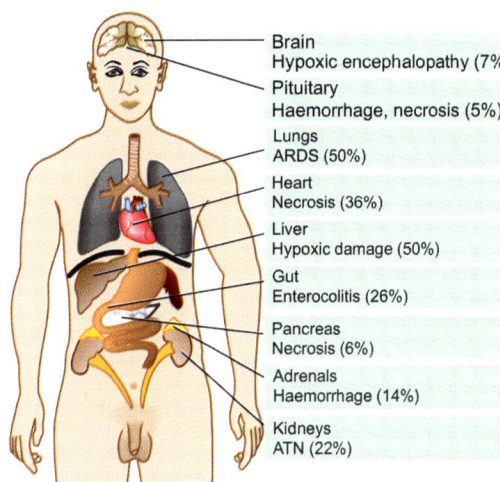

FIGURE 6.15: Morphologic features of shock.

iii. **Shock lung** characterised by congestion, oedema, alveolar hyaline membranes and platelet microthrombi in microvasculature.
iv. **Shock kidney** which is primarily characterised by acute tubular necrosis.
v. **Haemorrhagic gastroenteropathy** marked by focal surface mucosal ulceration of the stomach and intestines with intraluminal bleeding. Acute gastric or duodenal ulcer seen in patients with severe burns is called *Curling ulcer*.
vi. **Focal microscopic areas of necrosis,** with or without concommittant haemorrhage, may be seen in many organs, including adrenals, pancreas and centrilobular necrosis of the liver.
vii. **Reduced immune capacity** makes the surviving patients prone to overwhelming infections and sepsis.

Q31. What are the key clinical features of decompensated shock?

Decompensated shock is characterised by multiple organ failure. It is clinically recognised by the following features:
i. Hypotension
ii. Subnormal temperature
iii. Feeble and irregular pulse
iv. Shallow and sighing respiration

OBSTRUCTIVE CIRCULATORY DISTURBANCES

Q32. What is thrombosis? Write briefly on thrombogenesis.

Definition Thrombosis is a coagulation disorder characterised by the formation of one or more thrombi, i.e. solid intravascular masses composed of clotted blood components.

Thrombogenesis (thrombus formation) is a physiologic process used by the body to prevent excessive bleeding from a ruptured or damaged blood vessel.
i. Thrombus formation depends on the interaction of coagulation factors and platelets in the blood and the damaged vessel wall. It begins with the formation of a *haemostatic plug,* which is lysed once the bleeding has been stopped.
ii. *Thrombosis as pathologic process* is characterised by excessive thrombus formation at a site of vascular injury, or formation of thrombi without obvious vascular injury, or the persistence of thrombus after its useful haemostatic functions have ceased.
iii. *Prevention of thrombus formation* is mediated by intact endothelium which has the two *antithrombotic functions:*
a. Protection of the flowing blood from thrombogenic influence of subendothelial tissue.
b. Production of *anti-thrombogenic factors* which include the following:

- Heparin-like substance, which accelerates the action of antithrombin III and inactivates other clotting factors.
- Thrombomodulin which converts thrombin into activator of protein C, an anticoagulant.
- Inhibitors of platelet aggregation such as ADP and PGI_2 (prostacyclin).
- Tissue plasminogen activator which accelerates fibrinolytic activity.

NOTE: Normal endothelial cells also produce a few *prothrombotic factors*, but their function is outweighed by the predominant antithrombogenic factors. These factors, which can be produced in much higher amounts upon endothelial cell injury, include the following:

i. Thromboplastin or tissue factor (coagulation factor III)
ii. von Willebrand factor which promotes firm adherence of platelets to the subendothelium
iii. Platelet activating factor, an activator and aggregator of platelets
iv. Inhibitor of plasminogen activator, a suppressor of fibrinolysis.

Q33. What are the components of the Virchow triad that predispose to thrombus formation?

Some 150 years ago, the great German pathologist, Virchow, described a triad of factors that promote thrombus formation: endothelial injury, hypercoagulability of blood, and altered blood flow. These three elements were later expanded and thus, we will present them as follows: i) endothelial injury, ii) platelet activation, iii) coagulation system activation, iv) alteration of blood flow, v) and hypercoagulability of the blood.

I. **Endothelial injury** exposes to blood the subendothelial extracellular matrix components of the extracellular matrix (ECM) such as collagens, fibronectin, laminin, elastin, glycosaminoglycans. These substances are thrombogenic and play an important role in haemostasis and in initiating thrombus formation **(Fig. 6.16)**. At the same time, there is a brief vasoconstriction reducing the amount of blood inflow to reduce the blood loss.

II. **Platelet activation** plays a key role in haemostasis as well as in thrombosis. The role of platelets includes the following events:

i. *Platelet adhesion*, which occurs following the binding of the glycoprotein Ib (GpIb) receptor on the surface of platelets exposed ECM (*primary aggregation*). The binding is enforced by von Willebrand factor released from damaged endothelial cells.

ii. *Platelet release reaction*, in which two types of platelet granules are released:
- *Dense bodies*, which contain adenosine diphosphate (ADP), ionic calcium, histamine, serotonin, and epinephrine. Released ADP further activates platelets, calcium is essential for the coagulation pathways, and other substances act on the vessel wall, causing vasoconstriction (serotonin and epinephrine) or increasing permeability (histamine).
- *Alpha granules*, which contain fibrinogen, fibronectin, PDGF, and thrombospondin contributing to the coagulation process.

iii. *Platelet aggregation* which follows the release of ADP that promotes the adhesion of additional platelets (*secondary aggregation*), and leads to the formation of *temporary haemostatic plug*. The formation of the *stable haemostatic plug* occurs only after the addition of fibrin, thrombin and thromboxane A_2.

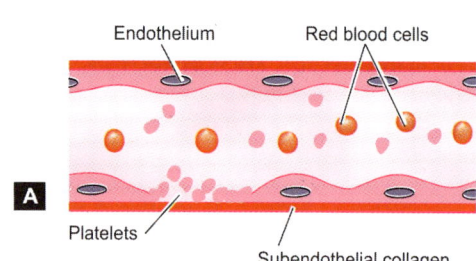
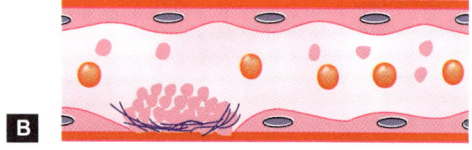
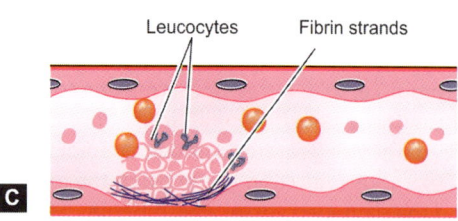

FIGURE 6.16: Role of endothelial injury and platelet activation in thrombosis. A, Endothelial injury exposes subendothelial matrix to circulating blood. B, This triggers three platelet steps involving platelet activation: adhesion, release and aggregation. Platelet release is associated with release of granules (alpha granules and dense bodies). C, Concurrent activation of coagulation cascade generates fibrin strands and thrombin, forming a tight meshwork called thrombus.

III. **Coagulation system activation** results in formation of fibrin from fibrinogen, which can occur through the intrinsic and the extrinsic pathway, leading to the common pathway of the coagulation system **(Fig. 6.17)**.

i. *Intrinsic pathway* involves activation of factor XII, upon contact with abnormal surface (e.g. exposed ECM). Activated factor XII leads to a sequential interaction of factors XI, IX, VIII and finally factor X along with calcium (factor IV) and platelet factor 3 (PF_3).

ii. *Extrinsic pathway* is activated by tissue factor (thromboplastin) released from damaged tissue. It reacts with factor VII and calcium to activate factor X.

iii. *Common pathway* begins with action of factor X at the convergence of the intrinsic and extrinsic pathways. Factor X forms a complex with factor V and PF_3 in the presence of calcium. This complex activates prothrombin to thrombin, which in turn converts fibrinogen to fibrin. Excessive formation of fibrin is controlled by the fibrinolytic system, primarily plasmin, which is formed under the influence of plasminogen activators acting on plasminogen.

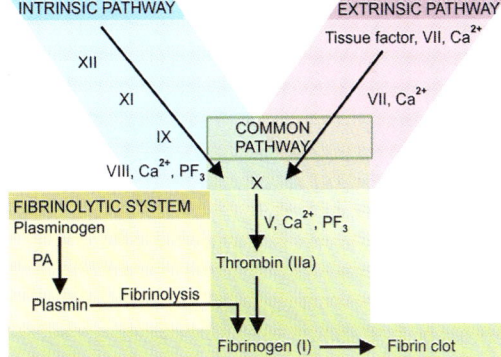

FIGURE 6.17: Schematic representation of pathways of coagulation mechanism and fibrinolytic system.
(PA, plasminogen activator)

IV. **Blood flow alterations** leading to transformation of the axial blood flow into a turbulent stream or promoting slowdown of the blood flow (stasis) **(Fig. 6.18)**.

i. *Turbulence* occurs in the heart chambers and arteries, promoting formation of thrombi in that part of circulation.

ii. *Stasis* promotes the formation of venous thrombi.

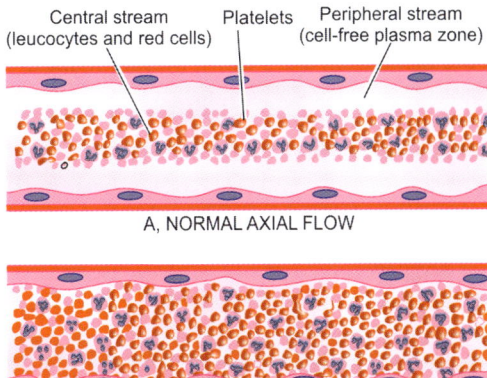

FIGURE 6.18: Alterations in flow of blood.

V. **Hypercoagulability of the blood** (thrombophilia) is a features of several clinical conditions and diseases which can be classified in two groups as follows:

i. *Inherited (genetic)* conditions and diseases such as:
- Deficiencies or excessive amounts of certain coagulation factors or their regulators (e.g. protein C and protein S deficiency, mutation of factor V Leiden)
- Defects of fibrinolysis (e.g. plasminogen disorders)
- Disorders of metabolism (e.g. homocysteinuria, dysfibrogenaemia).

ii. *Acquired (secondary)* conditions and diseases such as:
- Cardiovascular diseases (e.g. myocardial infarction, atherosclerotic aneurysm)
- Hypercoagulable blood diseases (e.g. polycythemia, myeloproliferative disorders, thrombotic thrombocytopenic purpura)
- Paraneoplastic thrombophilia with several forms of cancer
- Shock which often includes DIC
- Late pregnancy
- Certain drugs (e.g. oral contraceptives, corticosteroids).

Q34. Based on location of thrombi, what are the most common diseases predisposing to their formation?

According to their location, thrombi can be classified as i) cardiac, ii) arterial, and iii) venous. The most important clinical conditions and disease in these three groups are given below as follows:

I. **Cardiac thrombi** can occur in the atria and atrial appendages, on the surface of cardiac valves or mural endocardium. They are usually *non-occlusive*, but rarely, if big and pedunculated, may act as a *ball-valve* occluding the mitral orifice. Frequently, they may give rise to pulmonary or systemic arterial *emboli* which produce infarcts.

Examples are as follows:
i. Atrial thrombi in atrial fibrillation
ii. Valvular thrombi in non-bacterial thrombotic endocarditis, or rheumatic fever, or bacterial endocarditis
iii. Mural ventricular thrombi overlying a transmural myocardial infarction or a ventricular aneurysm

II. **Arterial thrombi,** like the cardiac thrombi, are formed in rapidly-flowing blood, usually following an endothelial injury. They may propagate in reverse direction of the blood flow. They may be mural and non-occlusive (as in aorta) or occlusive (as in coronary, cerebral and leg arteries) causing infarcts.

Examples are as follows:
i. Aortic thrombi overlying ulcerated atherosclerosis or in an aortic aneurysm
ii. Coronary thrombus overlying a ruptured atheroma of major coronary arteries
iii. Thrombi in leg arteries affected by atherosclerosis of Buerger disease
iv. Cerebral artery thrombi covering areas of atherosclerosis

III. **Venous thrombi** form in slow-moving venous blood and stasis after some surgical intervention, prolonged bed-confinement, or child-birth. They are often layered due to formation of the lighter stained lines of Zahn (composed of fibrin and platelets) alternating with layers of darker red blood cells. They may grow in the direction of the blood flow and become occlusive, preventing venous return of the blood from areas which they normally drain (e.g. venous infarcts of the intestinal loops). They may fragment to give rise to venous emboli (e.g. pulmonary emboli originating from deep leg veins).

Examples are as follows:
i. Deep vein thrombi of lower extremities, or thrombi in varicose veins
ii. Popliteal, femoral and iliac vein thrombi s in postpartum or postoperative period
iii. Hepatic and portal vein thrombi in cirrhosis and portal hypertension

Q35. What are the major differences between arterial and venous thrombi?

The differences between arterial and venous thrombi are given in **Table 6.4**.

TABLE 6.4 Distinguishing features of arterial and venous thrombi.

FEATURE	ARTERIAL THROMBI	VENOUS THROMBI
1. Sites	➤ Formed in rapidly-flowing blood of arteries and heart ➤ Common in aorta, coronary, cerebral, iliac, femoral, renal and mesenteric arteries	➤ Formed in slow-moving blood in veins ➤ Common in superficial varicose veins, deep leg veins, popliteal, femoral and iliac veins
2. Pathogenesis	Formed following endothelial cell injury, e.g. in atherosclerosis	Formed following venous stasis, e.g. in abdominal operations, child-birth
3. Occlusion	Usually mural, not occluding the lumen completely	Usually occlusive, take the cast of the vessel in which formed
4. Progression	May propagate in reverse direction to the blood flow	Propagates along the direction of blood flow
5. Gross appearance	Grey-white, friable with lines of Zahn on surface	Red-blue with fibrin strands and lines of Zahn, throughout the entire thrombus
6. Microscopy	Distinct lines of Zahn composed of platelets, fibrin with entangled red and white blood cells **(Fig. 6.19)**	Lines of Zahn with more abundant red cells
7. Effects	Ischaemia leading to infarcts of organs, e.g. in the heart, brain, etc.	Thromboembolism, oedema, skin ulcers, poor wound healing

Q36. What is the fate of thrombi?

Following are the four possible outcomes of thrombosis **(Fig. 6.20)**:

i. **Resolution** mediated by the fibrinolytic action of plasmin. It is most effective in small vessels, whereas larger thrombi are not lysed so easily. Thrombolytic substances such as streptokinase may facilitate the removal of thrombi.

ii. **Organisation** occurs in thrombi that are not lysed. The thrombus is invaded by PMNs and macrophages which digest fibrin and also secrete angiogenic cytokines which stimulate the ingrowth of *vascularised granulation tissue* into the thrombus. Ultimately, the granulation tissue transforms into fibrotic tissue which is on the luminal side covered by endothelial cells ingrown over it from lateral sides. Thus, the organised thrombus becomes part of the vessel wall. Fibrous scars formed from granulation tissue may become calcified, giving rise to *phleboliths* (i.e. veinous 'stone-like' calcifications).

Alternatively, the small blood vessels in the granulation tissue may fuse into larger vessels, allowing the blood to flow across a previously occlusive thrombus. This process is called *recanalisation* of the thrombus.

iii. **Propagation** leading to a growth of the thrombus. In the veins, thrombi usually grow in the direction of the blood flow, whereas the arterial thrombi grow in the reverse direction of the blood flow. Propagation converts a non-occlusive into an occlusive thrombus.

iv. **Thromboembolism**, i.e. removal of the thrombi or their fragmented parts by the blood stream. In their final destination, arterial thromboemboli may occlude a blood vessel and cause infarcts. If they end up occluding in the main pulmonary artery or its major branches, thromboemboli stemming from the leg veins may even cause sudden death.

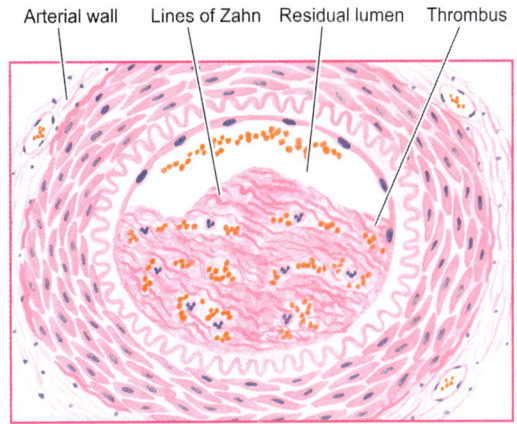

FIGURE 6.19: Thrombus in an artery. The thrombus is adherent to the arterial wall and is seen occluding most of the lumen. It shows lines of Zahn composed of granular-looking platelets and fibrin meshwork with entangled red cells and leucocytes.

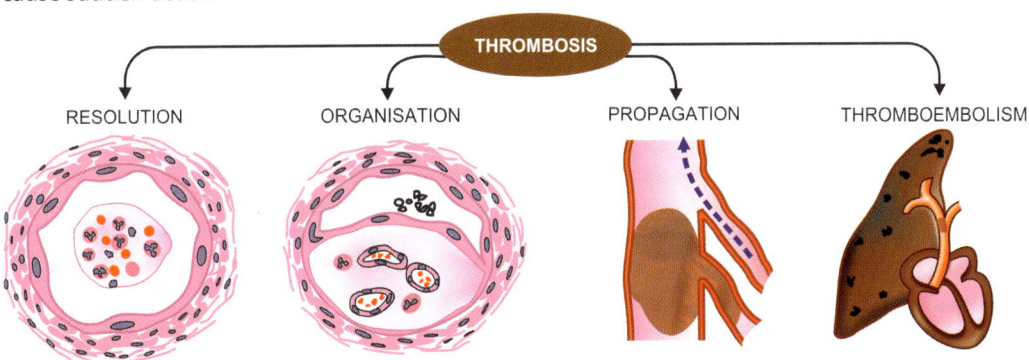

FIGURE 6.20: Fate of thrombus.

Q37. What are the possible clinical features of leg vein thrombosis?

Leg vein thrombosis, also known as *phlebothrombosis* may have the following consequences:
i. Oedema of lower extremities or their parts corresponding the area drained by the thrombosed vein.
ii. Poor wound or skin ulcer healing due to poor venous blood drainage.
iii. Painful white leg (*phlegmasia alba dolens*) due to ileofemoral venous thrombosis in postpartum period.
iv. Thrombophlebitis, i.e. painful inflammation of a thrombosed vein.
v. Pulmonary thromboemboli resulting in pulmonary infarcts or death.
NOTE: Thrombosis of leg veins, following thrombosis of veins in other parts of the body (*thrombophlebitis migrans*) is a paraneoplastic syndrome, most often encountered in patients with pancreatic or gastric cancer).

Q38. What is embolism? How are emboli classified?

Definition Embolism is the process of partial or complete occlusion of some parts of the cardiovascular system by any mass carried in the circulation.
Classification of emboli can be made i) depending on the material in the emboli, ii) presence of microbes, iii) source of emboli, and iv) direction of blood flow.

I. **Material in the emboli**
i. *Solid*, e.g. detached thrombi, atheromatous material, tumour cell clumps, tissue fragments, parasite, bacterial clumps, foreign bodies
ii. *Liquid*, e.g. fat globules, amniotic fluid
iii. *Gaseous*, e.g. air and various gases

II. **Presence of microbes**
i. *Bland,* if sterile
ii. *Infected*, if containing microbes

III. **Source of emboli**
i. *Cardiac*, e.g. mural thrombi or valvular vegetations in endocarditis
ii. *Arterial,* e.g. thrombi from the aorta
iii. *Venous*, e.g. leg vein thrombi giving rise to pulmonary emboli
iv. *Lymphatic*, e.g. cancer cells entering into the lymphatics that drain a neoplasm

IV. **Direction of blood flow**
Paradoxical embolus is carried from the venous to arterial circulation and vice versa, usually though an abnormal communication between the venous and arterial system.

Best examples are paradoxical thromboemboli which begin in leg veins and are carried by venous blood to the heart, where they cross into the arterial circulation through a patent foramen ovale, or septal defects involving the atrium or ventricle. These paradoxical emboli may cause infarcts, most notably in the brain.

Q39. What are important types of emboli?

The important types of embolism are given in **Table 6.5**.

Q40. What are the major sources of thrmboemboli?

A detached thrombus or part of thrombus constitutes the most common type of embolism. These may arise in the arterial or venous circulation as shown in **Figure 6.21**.

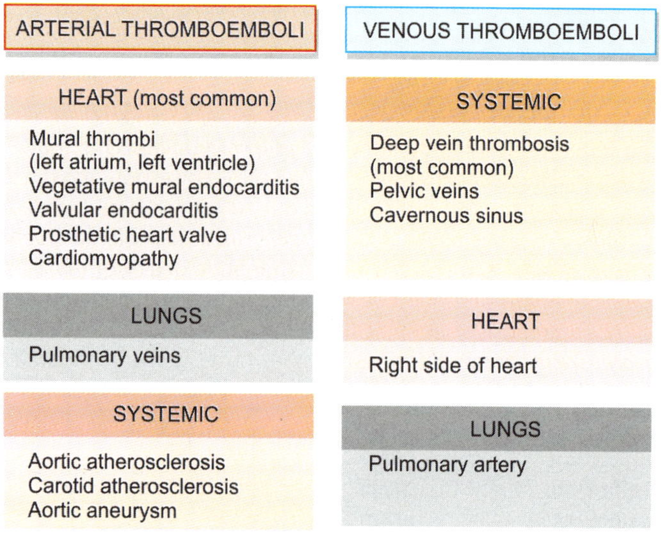

Q41. What are the key features of pulmonary thromboembolism?

Definition Pulmonary thromboembolism is the most common fatal form of venous thromboembolism in which there is occlusion of pulmonary arterial tree by themboemboli.
Key features
i. Most of them (95%) originate in the large lower leg veins.
ii. Risk factors include venous stasis and hypercoagulable states.

TABLE 6.5 Important types of embolism.

TYPE	COMMON ORIGIN
1. Pulmonary embolism	Veins of lower legs
2. Systemic embolism	Left ventricle (arterial)
3. Fat embolism	Trauma to bones/soft tissues
4. Air embolism	Venous: head and neck operations, obstetrical trauma Arterial: cardiothoracic Surgery, angiography
5. Decompression sickness	Descent: divers Ascent: unpressurised flight
6. Amniotic fluid embolism	Components of amniotic fluid
7. Atheroembolism	Atheromatous plaques
8. Tumour embolism	Tumour fragments

ARTERIAL THROMBOEMBOLI	VENOUS THROMBOEMBOLI
HEART (most common)	**SYSTEMIC**
Mural thrombi (left atrium, left ventricle) Vegetative mural endocarditis Valvular endocarditis Prosthetic heart valve Cardiomyopathy	Deep vein thrombosis (most common) Pelvic veins Cavernous sinus
LUNGS	**HEART**
Pulmonary veins	Right side of heart
SYSTEMIC	**LUNGS**
Aortic atherosclerosis Carotid atherosclerosis Aortic aneurysm	Pulmonary artery

FIGURE 6.21: Sources of arterial and venous emboli.

iii. Thromboemboli may occur in several forms:
a. *Saddle embolus*, i.e. large thromboemboli that are impacted at the bifurcation of the pulmonary artery, often causing sudden death due to obstruction of the blood outflow from the right ventricle.
b. *Multiple emboli*, formed from fragmented large thrombi, which occlude smaller branches of the pulmonary artery. This is the most common form of pulmonary embolism.
c. *Paradoxical embolism* entering the arterial circulation through the patent foramen ovale or septal defect.

Q42. What are the possible clinicopathologic consequences of pulmonary embolism?

Clinicopathologic consequences of pulmonary thromboembolism are as follows **(Fig. 6.22)**:
I. **Sudden death**
II. **Acute cor pulmonale**, i.e. acute right-sided heart failure due to the obstruction of pulmonary artery branches by multiple small emboli.
III. **Pulmonary infarction**, which is usually due to the obstruction of a smaller branch of pulmonary artery providing the blood supply to a subpleural portion of the lungs.
Pathology and clinical features of lung Infarcts have following peculiar features:
i. Pulmonary infarcts are *subpleural* and cause *pleuritic pain* and haemoptysis.
ii. *Triangular in shape* (the base being on the pleural surface and the tip pointing toward the hilum).
iii. Infarcts are *red* because of dual circulation of the lungs, which receive blood from pulmonary artery and bronchial arteries. Obstruction of the pulmonary artery flow will be compensated by the inflow arterial blood from bronchial artery branches. This arterial blood flooding the infarct will salvage the affected lung parenchyma from ischaemia.
iv. *Resolution* of most small thromboemboli is common (75%) and involves the fibrinolytic system.
v. *Complete lysis of thromboemboli* assures that there are no residual clinical consequences.
IV. **Pulmonary hypertension with pulmonary arteriosclerosis and chronic cor pulmonale** are usually a consequence of *repeated showers of small emboli* which are organised rather than lysed. Narrowing of pulmonary artery branches provides chronic resistance to blood flow, increasing the work load on the right-sided part of the heart (*chronic cor pulmonale*).

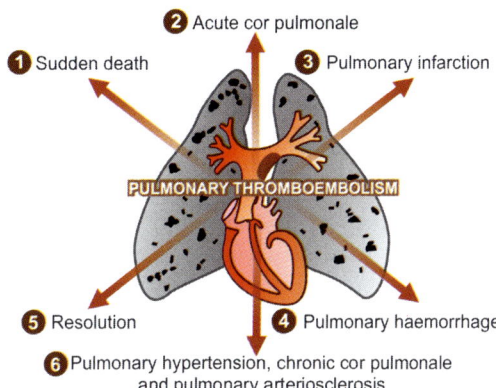

FIGURE 6.22: Major consequences of pulmonary embolism.

Q43. Discuss fat embolism briefly.

Definition Fat embolism is obstruction of arterioles and capillaries by fat globules.
Etiology Trauma is the most common cause of fat embolism leading to lung injury.
i. *Fracture of long bones* will allow the entry of fatty bone marrow contents into gaping veins and thus reach the lungs through the venous blood. Trauma of fat tissue may have similar consequence.
ii. *Non-traumatic hyperlipidaemia* as in patients with diabetes mellitus, hereditary hyperlipidaemia, fatty liver, acute pancreatitis, extensive burns.
Pathogenesis of lung injury Two possible mechanisms of lung injury are as follows:
i. *Mechanical obstruction* of small pulmonary vessels by fat globules, with changes that resemble those to microthromboembolism.
ii. *Biochemical injury of endothelial cells:*
a. Fat globules entering into circulation release triglycerides which break down into glycerin and fatty acid.
b. Fatty acids damage pulmonary endothelial cells.
c. Injured endothelial cells release cytokines.
d. Cytokines induce chemically mediated acute inflammation.
e. Platelets form microthrombi, with consequent pulmonary oedema and ARDS.

Clinicopathologic features Major changes are seen in the lungs and the brain. Petechiae may be seen in the skin and all internal organs.

i. **Lungs** show pulmonary oedema, foci of haemorrhage and ARDS-like changes, such as hyaline membranes. Fat globules can be demonstrated only in frozen sections by special stains (Oil red O). *Clinically*, there is dyspnoea and signs of ARDS.

ii. **Brain** shows oedema and numerous petechial haemorrhages in the meninges and in the white and gray matter of the brain.

Microscopically, there are signs of oedema, small haemorrhages and ischemic brain injury.

Clinically, there are signs of confusion, vertigo and deteriorating consciousness progressing to coma.

Q44. Discuss salient features of air embolism.

Definition Air embolism is a haemodynamic derangement that occurs when air is introduced into venous or arterial circulation.

Etiopathogenesis Air embolism may be venous or arterial and their causes are listed as follows:

I. **Causes of venous embolism** Trauma or medical interventions are the most common cause. For example:

i. Operations on the head and neck with accidental opening of the large neck veins. This event may allow the air to be drawn into the venous circulation.

ii. Obstetrical operations and trauma, childbirth, caesarean section or abortion allowing the entry of air into opened-up uterine venous sinuses and endometrial veins.

iii. Accidental injection of air during intravenous injection or infusion.

iv. Angiography through the entry into the venous system.

Clinical consequences of the entry of air into the venous circulation depends on the amount of air, rapidity of the entry, position of the patient and the general condition of the person affected.

i. Small amounts of air are innocuous.

ii. Larger amounts of air may interfere with circulation and cause ischaemic changes in the major organs.

iii. Death may result from the accumulation of air in the right ventricle and pulmonary artery.

II. **Causes of arterial embolism** Thoracic surgery or chest trauma are the most important causes.

i. Trauma or surgery resulting in rupture of the lungs with or without pneumothorax may cause the entry of large amounts of air into the pulmonary veins or right atrium.

ii. Arteriography may be complicated by an entry of air into circulation.

iii. Paradoxical air embolism through a patent foramen ovale or septal defects.

Clinical effects Arterial air embolism produces typical changes as follows:

i. Marble skin due to the blockage of cutaneous vessels.

ii. Air bubbles seen by ophthalmoscopy in the retinal vessels.

iii. Pallor of parts of the tongue due to the occlusion of a branch or lingual artery.

iv. Coronary or cerebral artery occlusion, with possible lethal outcome. It occurs with smaller amounts of air entering the circulation than in venous air embolism.

Q45. What is decompression sickness? Discuss its main features.

Definition Decompression sickness is a form of gas embolism that occurs suddenly, either from high atmospheric pressure to normal level, or from normal pressure to low atmospheric pressure. It is also known as air embolism, divers' palsy, or caisson disease.

Pathogenesis It affects divers and workers in caissons (diving bells) who descend to high pressure underwater spaces where large amounts of air (mainly nitrogen) are under pressure dissolved in blood and body fluids. Upon rapid ascent, the gases come out of fluids and fat tissue as bubbles, which may coalesce and form larger air emboli. The same can occur during air ascent in an unpressurised aeroplane cabin, when a person enters from normal to a low pressured atmosphere.

The *effects* of decompression depend on the following:

i. Depth or altitude reached

ii. Duration of exposure to altered pressure

iii. Rate of ascent or descent

iv. General condition of the affected person

Clinicopathologic features The changes are more pronounced in *sudden ascent* and decompression from high pressure to normal pressure (e.g. diver returning to surface) than from *sudden descent* from low pressure at high altitude to normal pressure. The changes are more serious in obese persons as nitrogen gas is more soluble in fat than in normal body fluids.

The changes may be acute or chronic:

i. **Acute changes** occur due to the air bubbles obstructing the small blood vessels around the joints, in the lungs, and the brain. The affected persons complain of the following:
a. Severe joint pain forcing persons to double up ('the bends')
b. Respiratory distress ('the chokes')
c. Cerebral changes such as signs of confusion, vertigo and even coma

ii. **Chronic changes** result from focal ischaemic necrosis affecting several organs:
a. *Bones:* avascular necrosis
b. *Skin:* itching, patchy erythema, cyanosis and oedema
c. *Lungs:* oedema and focal haemorrhage, atelectasis
d. *Brain:* focal ischaemia with paresthesia and paraplegia

Q46. Discuss the key features of amniotic fluid embolism.

Definition Amniotic fluid embolism results from the entry of amniotic fluid and various materials normally found in it into the maternal venous circulation during the delivery.

Pathogenesis Amniotic fluid contains epithelial squames, vernix caseosa, lanugo hair, bile from meconium and mucus.

i. All these substances could mechanically block the microcirculation.
ii. These substance also induce *disseminated intravascular coagulation (DIC)*.
iii. DIC results in consumption of platelets and coagulation factors *(thrombocytopenia and afibrinogenemia)*.
iv. *Circulatory shock* that ensues may be lethal.

Clinicopathologic features The symptoms develop rapidly and are progressive. Amniotic fluid embolism is one of the most lethal, unpredictable and unpreventable complication of pregnancy. The findings include the following:

i. Acute respiratory distress syndrome with the pathologic signs of ARDS
ii. Deep cyanosis
iii. Tachycardia and hypotension
iv. Uncontrollable bleeding due to thrombocytopenia and afibrinogenaemia
v. Convulsions and coma

Q47. What is atheroembolism? Discuss its clinical and pathologic features briefly.

Definition Atheroembolism results from the entry of atheromas, which contains cholesterol crystals, hyaline debris and calcified tissue remnants into the arterial circulation.

Clinicopathologic features The aortic atheromas may rupture spontaneously, or are eroded by vascular instrumentation and catheterisation.

i. *Massive discharge of atheromatous material* into the arterial circulation may lead to a blockage of arteries supplying the blood to the brain, kidneys, intestines or extremities, causing massive necrosis of infarcted organs and organ failure or death.

ii. *Minor atheromatous emboli* may cause focal infarcts of the kidney with reactive hypertension, or intestinal haemorrhage, or brain function disturbances.

Q48. Define infarction. What are its main causes? Discuss mechanism of infarction.

Definition Infarction is a localised necrosis caused by ischaemia. Most infarcts show signs of coagulation necrosis, except the brain which shows features of liquefactive necrosis.

Etiology and pathogenesis

i. Most often, infarcts are caused by interruption of arterial blood due to a complete obstruction of the lumen of an artery.
ii. Less commonly, infarcts occur due to venous obstruction causing stagnant hypoxia.

iii. **Non-occlusive infarcts** develop due to hypotension and inadequate filling of the arteries due to circulatory insufficiency.

All forms of ischaemia may produce infarcts:

I. **Heart failure** due to conduction block, fibrillation, infarction, etc. may cause ischaemic infarction of the brain and death, typically ensuing if the heart-standstill lasts 8 minutes or more. Heart failure results in a *hypotensive non-occlusive infarction* of the brain, which at autopsy shows no signs of necrosis.

II. **Arterial occlusion** by thrombi or emboli, atherosclerosis, prolonged vasospasm, or outside pressure due to ligature, tight plaster and bandages or torsion. Common locations of infarcts following arterial embolism are shown in **Figure 6.23**.

III. **Venous occlusion** by thrombi, outside pressure such as in intestinal volvulus, intussusception or strangulated hernia.

IV. **Obstruction of the microcirculation** by microthrombi, macroglobulinaemia, precipitated cryoglobulins, air bubbles in decompression sickness, hyperviscosity of the blood in polycythemia vera, etc.

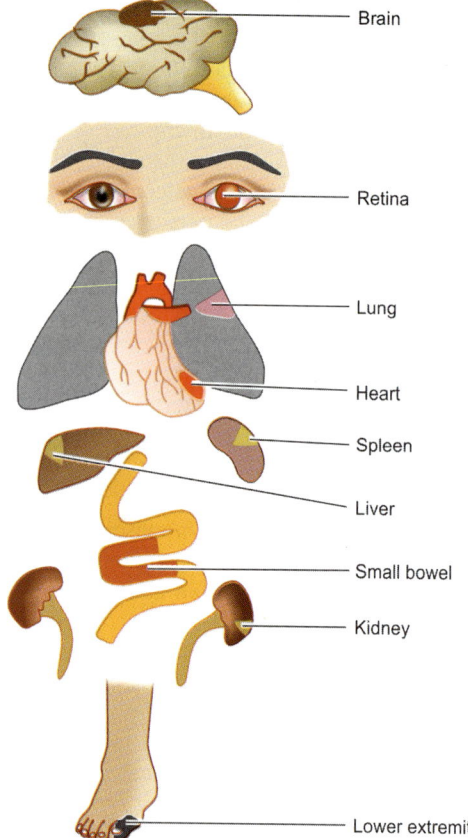

FIGURE 6.23: Common locations of systemic infarcts following arterial embolism.

Q49. What are the factors determining the severity of ischaemic injury?

i. **Anatomy of the blood supply** There are several patterns of arterial supply, that vary from one organ to another. For example,

a. Occlusion of an artery that provides a single artery supply (e.g. central artery of retina) invariably results in an infarction.

b. Occlusion of an artery that is part of a rich anastomotic system, like the intestinal arteries, can be readily compensated by the blood from the anastomotic vessels.

c. Liver that has double supply of blood—from hepatic artery and portal vein, is relatively resistant to ischaemia caused by the occlusion of the vessels of one system.

ii. **General and cardiovascular status of the affected person** Blood loss, anaemia, severe and chronic diseases may make an older person more prone to adverse effects of ischaemia than a healthy young man.

iii. **Type of tissue affected** The following tissues are more vulnerable to ischemia:

a. Brain (neurons)
b. Heart (cardiac myocytes)
c. Kidney (cells of the proximal convoluted tubules)

iv. **Rapidity and degree of vascular occlusion** Occlusion that has a rapid onset and is complete has more adverse effects than a slowly developing and incomplete occlusion.

Q50. What is the difference between pale and red infarcts?

According to their colour, there are two types of infarcts: pale and red.

i. **Pale or anaemic infarcts** are caused by arterial occlusion and are seen in compact organs such as kidney, heart and spleen.

ii. **Red or haemorrhagic infarcts** are seen in soft loose tissues, which have a dual blood supply or supply by anastomosing arteries. These infarcts are typically seen in the lungs following pulmonary embolism, or in the intestines due to arterial or venous occlusion.

Q51. What are the key features of infarcts of commonly affected organs?

The features of infarcts of commonly affected organs are presented in **Table 6.6**.

TABLE 6.6 Infarcts of commonly affected organs.

LOCATION	COMMON CAUSE	GROSS APPEARANCE	OUTCOME
1. *Myocardial infarct*	Coronary arteries	Pale	Frequently lethal
2. *Pulmonary infarct*	Pulmonary artery	Haemorrhagic	Less commonly fatal
3. *Cerebral infarct*	Cerebral arteries	Haemorrhagic or pale	Fatal if massive
4. *Intestinal infarct*	Mesenteric arteries	Haemorrhagic	Frequently lethal
5. *Renal infarct*	Thromboemboli	Pale	Not lethal unless massive and bilateral
6. *Splenic Infarct*	Splenic artery	Pale	Not lethal
7. *Infarct liver*	Hepatic artery	Pale	Not lethal
8. *Lower extremity infarct*	Arteries of lower limb	Pale	Not lethal

> **Chapter 6e Supplement: Online Content**
>
> *Digital content of this chapter available with this book is meant for enhanced learning and self-assessment. In addition, it contains 25 Multiple Choice Questions (MCQs), 05 Clinicopathologic Vignettes, and 04 Image-based Questions; these are followed by their answers along with explanatory notes of correct and incorrect answers.*

CHAPTER 7

Neoplasia

■ NOMENCLATURE AND CLASSIFICATION

Q1. What are neoplasms?

Definition A neoplasm or tumour is a mass of tissue which results from abnormal, excessive, uncoordinated, autonomous, and purposeless proliferation of cells that continues even after removal of stimulus, which has caused it.

Composition of tumours All solid tumours have two basic components:
- *Parenchyma*, comprising proliferating tumour cells, which determine the nature and evolution of the tumour.
- *Supportive stroma* composed of fibrovascular tissue, that provides the framework supporting the growth of tumor cells.

Q2. How are tumours named? Give some common exmaples.

Tumours are named on the basis of cells recognised microscopically as their predominant parenchymal component. That basic name or its essential rudiment are expanded by a suffix or qualifier indicating whether the tumour is benign or malignant.

I. **Benign mesenchymal tumours** are named after the predominant cell expanded by a suffix—**oma** (e.g. fibroma, a tumour composed of fibroblasts).

II. **Epithelial glandular tumours** are called according to their cell type, or site of origin, or key microscopic feature, expanded by the term **adenoma** (e.g. hepatocellular adenoma, gastric adenoma, tubular adenoma of the colon).

III. **Benign epithelial tumours** originating from the skin and mucosae are called **papillomas** (wart-like protruding tumours, e.g. squamous cell papilloma).

IV. **Malignant epithelial tumours** are called **carcinomas** (e.g. squamous cell carcinoma).

V. **Malignant mesenchymal tumours are called sarcoma** (e.g. fibrosarcoma).

VI. Malignant tumours, which are undifferentiated and cannot be classified as carcinoma or sarcoma, are called **undifferentiated malignant tumours.**

VII. **Exceptions** to the general naming principle listed above are worth remembering because they may be encountered in clinical practice. For example,
- *Lymphoma,* a term that sounds like a designation for a benign tumour, is used for all malignant tumours of lymphoid tissue.
- *Seminoma* for the malignant tumour of the testis.
- The correct name for malignant liver cell tumour is *hepatocellular carcinoma*, but still the shorter and more ambiguous term, *hepatoma,* is used quite often.
- To avoid confusion, it is customary to add a qualifier before the name of the tumour, and thus instead of *melanoma,* the proper term is *malignant melanoma*.

VIII. **Special terms for certain tumours** used in clinical practice are as follows:
i. ***Mixed tumour*** of salivary glands (also known as *pleomorphic adenoma*) is a benign tumour composed of an epithelial and mesenchymal component.
ii. ***Carcinosarcoma*** of the uterus is a tumour that has a carcinomatous and a sarcomatous component.
iii. ***Teratoma*** is a benign tumour composed of a mixture of mature, well-differentiated tissues derived from all three germ layers—ectoderm, mesoderm and endoderm.
iv. ***Blastomas (embryomas)*** are composed of embryonic or partially differentiated cells forming the blastema of an organ during foetal organogenesis. Examples of these tumours, which occur during infancy and childhood are: neuroblastoma, nephroblastoma, retinoblastomas, etc.
v. ***Hamartoma*** is a benign tumour composed of abnormally grouped mature cells or tissues indigenous to the organ in which they arise. For example, a naevus of the skin is composed of groups of melanocytes. Hamartoma of the lungs is a mass composed of bronchial epithelium, cartilage and smooth muscle cells.
vi. ***Choristoma*** is a benign lesion composed of heterotopic tissue extraneous to the organ in which it was found (e.g. ectopic pancreas in the stomach, or splenunculi in the pancreas).

Q3. How are tumours classified?

Tumors are classified based on their histogenesis (i.e. cell of origin) and on their anticipated behaviour. A brief list of common examples of tumours is given in **Table 7.1**.

TABLE 7.1 Classification of tumours based on histogenesis.

TISSUE OF ORIGIN	BENIGN	MALIGNANT
I. TUMOURS OF ONE PARENCHYMAL CELL TYPE		
A. Epithelial Tumours		
1. *Squamous epithelium*	Squamous cell papilloma	Squamous cell carcinoma
2. *Transitional epithelium*	Transitional cell papilloma	Transitional cell carcinoma
3. *Urothelium*	Papilloma	Urothelial carcinoma
4. *Glandular epithelium*	Adenoma	Adenocarcinoma
5. *Mesothelium*	Benign mesothelioma	Malignant mesothelioma
6. *Basal cell layer skin*	—	Basal cell carcinoma
7. *Melanocytes*	Naevus	Malignant melanoma (melanocarcinoma)
8. *Hepatocytes*	Liver cell adenoma	Hepatoma (hepatocellular carcinoma)
9. *Placenta (Chorionic epithelium)*	Hydatidiform mole	Choriocarcinoma
B. Non-epithelial (Mesenchymal) Tumours		
1. *Adipose tissue*	Lipoma	Liposarcoma
2. *Adult fibrous tissue*	Fibroma	Fibrosarcoma
3. *Embryonic fibrous tissue*	Myxoma	Myxosarcoma
4. *Cartilage*	Chondroma	Chondrosarcoma
5. *Bone*	Osteoma	Osteosarcoma
6. *Synovium*	Benign synovioma	Synovial sarcoma
7. *Smooth muscle*	Leiomyoma	Leiomyosarcoma
8. *Skeletal muscle*	Rhabdomyoma	Rhabdomyosarcoma
9. *Blood vessels*	Haemangioma	Angiosarcoma
10. *Lymph vessels*	Lymphangioma	Lymphangiosarcoma
11. *Glomus*	Glomus tumour	—
12. *Meninges*	Meningioma	Invasive meningioma
13. *Haematopoietic cells*	—	Leukaemias
14. *Lymphoid tissue*	Pseudolymphoma	Malignant lymphoma
15. *Nerve sheath*	Neurilemmoma, neurofibroma	Neurogenic sarcoma (malignant peripheral nerve sheath tumour)
16. *Nerve cells*	Ganglioneuroma	Neuroblastoma
II. MIXED TUMOURS		
Salivary glands	Pleomorphic adenoma (mixed salivary tumour)	Malignant mixed salivary tumour
III. TUMOURS OF MORE THAN ONE GERM CELL LAYER		
Totipotent cells	Mature teratoma	Immature teratoma, malignant teratoma

CHARACTERISTICS OF TUMOURS

Q4. What are the differences between the benign and malignant tumours?

Benign tumours differ from malignant tumours with regards to their i) clinical and gross features, ii) microscopic features, iii) growth rate, iv) local invasion, v) metastasis (distant spread) and, vi) prognosis **(Table 7.2)**.

TABLE 7.2 Contrasting features of benign and malignant tumours.

FEATURE	BENIGN	MALIGNANT
I. CLINICAL AND GROSS FEATURES		
1. *Boundaries*	Encapsulated or well-circumscribed	Poorly-circumscribed and irregular
2. *Surrounding tissue*	Often compressed	Usually invaded
3. *Size*	Usually small	Often larger
4. *Secondary changes*	Occur less often	Occur more often
II. MICROSCOPIC FEATURES		
1. *Pattern*	Usually resembles the tissue of origin closely	Often poor resemblance to tissue of origin
2. *Basal polarity*	Retained	Often lost
3. *Pleomorphism*	Usually not present	Often present
4. *Nucleo-cytoplasmic ratio*	Normal	Increased
5. *Anisonucleosis*	Absent	Generally present
6. *Hyperchromatism*	Absent	Often present
7. *Mitoses*	May be present but are always typical mitoses	Mitotic figures increased and are generally atypical and abnormal
8. *Tumour giant cells*	May be present but without nuclear atypia	Present with nuclear atypia
9. *Chromosomal abnormalities*	Infrequent	Invariably present
10. *Function*	Usually well maintained	May be retained, lost or become abnormal
III. GROWTH RATE	Usually slow	Usually rapid
IV. LOCAL INVASION	Often compresses the surrounding tissues without invading or infiltrating them	Usually infiltrates and invades the adjacent tissues
V. METASTASIS	Absent	Frequently present
VI. PROGNOSIS	Local complications	Death by local and metastatic complications

Q5. Define the terms differentiation and anaplasia.

Differentiation is the extent of morphological and functional resemblance of parenchymal tumour cells to corresponding normal cells in the organ from which the tumour arose.
• The tumour is called *well-differentiated* if its cells resemble the corresponding normal cells.
• *Undifferentiated or dedifferentiated tumour* is composed of cells, which bear little structural and functional resemblance to equivalent normal cells.

Anaplasia is lack of differentiation. It may be graded as mild, moderate or severe, which is usually a features of undifferentiated tumours.

Q6. What are the morphologic characteristics of anaplasia?

The microscopic features of anaplasia are as follows **(Fig. 7.1)**:

i. **Loss of cellular polarity** Epithelial cells lying on a basement membrane are usually polarised and have a basal and an apical (luminal) pole; the nucleus is typically in a basal location. Cells that have lost polarity do not have a basal and an apical pole; instead their nucleus may be located in any part of the cytoplasm.

ii. **Pleomorphism** The shape and size of tumour cells are variable in contrast to the normal cells, that are uniform. Pleomorphism of nuclei is called anisonucleosis. Extreme anisonucleosis combined with an increased size of tumour cells results in the formation of *multinucleated tumour cells*.

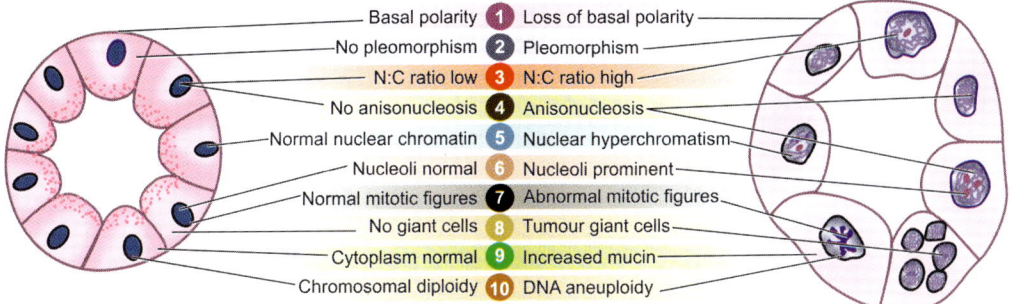

A, NORMAL MORPHOLOGY   B, CYTOMORPHOLOGY IN CANCER

FIGURE 7.1: Diagrammatic representation of cytomorphologic features of malignant cells. Characteristics of cancer cells (B) are contrasted with the normal appearance of epithelial cells in an acinus (A).

iii. **Nucleo-cytoplasmic (N:C) ratio** In normal cells, the cytoplasm is up to 5-times more voluminous than the nucleus. Neoplastic cells have enlarged nuclei and the N:C ratio will thus change from normal 1:5 to 1:3 and even 1:1.

iv. **Hyperchromatism** Chromatin of the nuclei is composed of nucleic acids and proteins clumped together. Tumour cell nuclei contain more DNA which accounts for the dark blue staining of nuclear chromatin with haematoxylin (hyperchromatism). Irregular clumping of chromatin contributes to hyperchromatism of tumour cell nuclei, which is more prominent in malignant than in benign tumours.

v. **Chromosomal abnormalities** Hyperchromatism correlates with the ploidy of tumour cells which is often increased above the normal diploid number (46) of chromosomes (*hyperdiploidy*). Some tumors show *hypodiploidy* due to a loss of chromosomes, whereas many others remain *diploid*. Overall, *aneuploidy* (a chromosome number that is different from normal diploid) is a common feature of malignant tumours. Many tumors contain *abnormal chromosomes* formed by deletion or translocation of parts of their chromatids.

vi. **Nucleolar enlargement** Nucleoli may be prominent, reflecting intense turnover and synthesis of RNA in growing tumour cells.

vii. **Mitotic figures** Mitoses are recognised as parts of the mitotic spindle. They are usually more numerous in malignant than benign tumours, or in normal tissues. Instead of normal mitoses which are bipolar, malignant tumours contain *abnormal mitoses*, which may be tripolar, quadripolar or multipolar.

Q7. What are the factors which determine the tumour growth rate?

Definition Tumour growth rate is objectively measured by additional gain in size or weight it has achieved over a defined period of time compared to the initial observed tumour size and weight.

Factors in tumour growth Rate of tumour growth is, in principle, higher in malignant than in benign tumours; it depends on the following:

i. *Mitotic rate* (or, doubling time, i.e. the time over which the tumour has doubled its size).

ii. *Growth fraction* (i.e. number of cells remaining in proliferating pool).

iii. *Rate of cell loss*, which includes cell shedding, cell death due to apoptosis, or necrosis caused by insufficient supply of oxygen and nutrients.

iv. *Degree of differentiation*, which is inversely proportional to tumour growth rate. The degree of differentiation will also determine tumour's response to growth factors.

Q8. What are the unique features of cancer phenotype that set these cells apart from normal cells?

In contrast to normal cells which respond to physiologic control mechanisms and signals from adjacent cells, cancer cells **escape normal control mechanism** as evidenced by the following:

i. Uncontrolled rapid growth due an escape from growth control signals.

ii. Immortality due to an escape from signals for apoptosis.

iii. Excessive growth due to an imbalance between cell proliferation and cell death.

iv. Loss of function due to a loss of differentiation and functional maturity.

v. Genetic instability with a tendency to develop new mutations.
vi. Parasitic relationship with the rest of the body, in which the tumour cells appropriate common resources for self-nourishment and growth at the expense of all other cells.
vii. Mobility and the ability to travel to distant sites which they colonise during metastasis.

Q9. What are the components of tumour stroma and what are their functions?

Stroma of solid tumours consists of fibrous tissue, blood vessels and peripheral nerves. It also may contain migratory inflammatory cells.

I. **Fibrous stroma** composed predominantly of collagen, forms the scaffold for the growth of tumour cells. Prominent fibrous stroma is called *desmoplasia*. Desmoplastic carcinomas are firm on palpation and gritty on sectioning, and are called *scirrhous carcinomas* (e.g. invasive ductal breast carcinoma).

II. **Tumour angiogenesis** refers to the formation of new blood vessels providing blood, oxygen, and nutrients to tumour cells.
i. Angiogenesis begins with formation of capillaries which sprout on adjacent preexisting blood vessels.
ii. Vascular sprouts elongate to reach the tumour. They fuse with other sprouts to form larger blood vessels, and also grow into the tumour mass to form the vascular part of the neoplastic stroma.
iii. Neoangiogenesis is stimulated by cytokines (growth factors) produced by tumour cells.
iv. These growth factors include vascular endothelium growth factor (VEGF) and basic fibroblast growth factor (bFGF).
NOTE: Neovascularisation of tumour nodules begins from their periphery and, thus, the central part receives the least amount of blood. By the time the blood reaches the central part of the tumour, it is also depleted of oxygen and nutrients. These local circulatory factors account for the common ischaemic necrosis in the centre of tumour nodule. Central necrosis is most evident in metastatic nodules.

III. **Inflammatory cells** may be present inside the tumours and in adjacent normal tissue around the tumours. In some cases, this inflammatory reaction is part of the cell-mediated immune response, as seen in seminoma of the testis, or the Epstein-Barr virus related undifferentiated carcinoma of the nasopharynx (older term 'lymphoepithelial carcinoma').

Q10. How do tumours grow and metastasise?

Key facts:
i. Benign tumours grow by *expansion* compressing the surrounding tissue or pushing it aside.
ii. Malignant tumours grow by *invading or infiltrating or destroying the surrounding tissue*.
iii. Once the tumour cells *penetrate into the lymphatics and blood vessels* or enter into the serous cavities, they metastasise.
iv. *Invasiveness, the capacity to metastasise,* and *anaplasia* are unique features of malignant tumours that distinguish them from benign tumours.
Caveat: The only malignant tumours that do not metastasise are malignant central nervous tumours, basal cell carcinoma of the skin and dermatofibrosarcoma protuberans.

Q11. Define metastasis. What are the main routes of cancer spread?

Definition Metastasis is process during which malignant tumour cells invade into lymphatics or blood vessels or serous cavities and spread to distant sites, where they form a new (secondary) tumour mass that is discontinuous from the primary tumour.
Routes of metastasis include the following three main pathways:
i. Lymphatic spread
ii. Haematogenous spread
iii. Spread along body cavities and natural passages

Q12. Discuss main features of lymphatic spread of tumours.

Lymphatic spread is the preferred route of metastasis for many carcinomas, whereas sarcomas tend to metastasise haematogenously. Lymphatic metastases occur in *several steps* including the following:
i. Entry into the lymphatic spaces

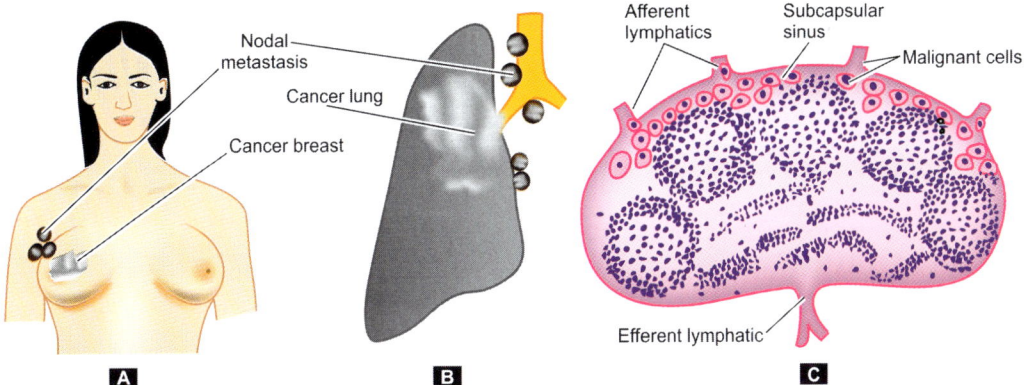

FIGURE 7.2: Regional nodal metastasis. A, Axillary nodes involved by carcinoma breast. B, Hilar and para-tracheal lymph nodes involved by bronchogenic carcinoma. C, Lymphatic spread begins by lodgement of tumour cells in subcapsular sinus via afferent lymphatics entering at the convex surface of the lymph node.

ii. Draining of tumour cells—carrying lymph into regional lymph nodes **(Fig. 7.2)**
iii. Regional lymph node reaction *(lymphadenitis)*
iv. Growth of tumour cells in the lymph node
v. Outflow of tumour cells in effluent lymph through the lymphatics leading to the major lymph vessels
vi. Discharge of tumour cells from the abdominal and thoracic lymph duct into superior vena cava

Q13. What are the key features of haematogenous spread of tumours?

Haematogenous spread is, in general terms, the preferred route of metastasis for sarcomas.
- *Carcinomas of some major organs,* however, metastasise through lymphatics as well haematogenously. These include: carcinomas of liver, kidney, lungs, breast, thyroid, prostate, and ovary.
- *Preferred site for haematogenous metastases* are the blood-rich major organs such as: lungs, liver, bones, brain, adrenals, which also seem to provide the 'good soil for their growth' (if one were to use the 'seed-soil theory of metastasis') **(Fig. 7.3)**.

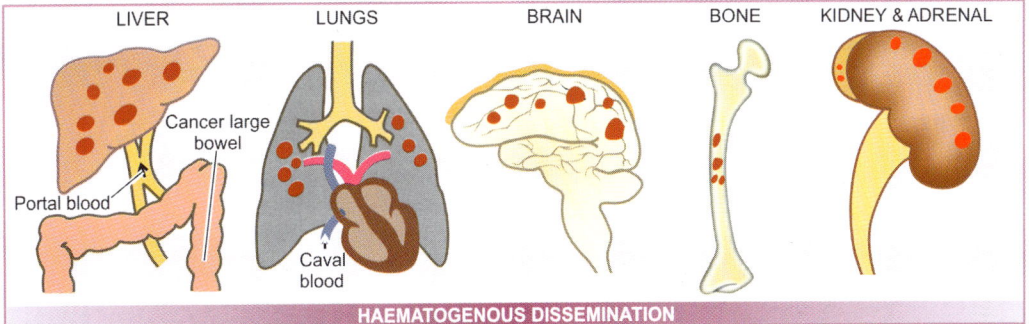

FIGURE 7.3: Appearance of haematogenous metastases at common sites.

Key facts about haematogenous metastases
i. Large systemic veins linked to the right atrium drain the blood from the extremities, head and neck and pelvis, and therefore, the lungs are a frequent site of haematogenous metastases.
ii. Portal veins drain the blood from intestines and pancreas to the liver, which is a common site for metastases from these anatomic sites.
iii. Pulmonary veins are an easy way of dissemination of lung cancer through the arterial blood. The same is true for secondary lung cancers that have arrived to the lungs through the pulmonary artery.
iv. Malignant tumours enter arteries less often than capillaries and veins because arteries have thick walls.
v. Retrograde spread occurs in any venous system that is blocked. Important counter-flow metastases occur in vertebral veins invaded by thyroid and prostate cancer.

Q14. Briefly discuss main features of spread of tumours along natural passages and body cavities.

Spread along body cavities and natural passages occurs when cancer cells enter these spaces. These include following routes and sites:

I. Transcoelomic spread occurs most often in the peritoneal cavity but it can occur in the pleural and pericardial cavity as well.

Clinical examples:
i. *Ovarian cancer* spreading all over the peritoneal cavity without deeper invasion into underlying organs.
ii. *Gastric carcinoma* seeding both ovaries (Krukenberg tumour).
iii. *Pseudomyxoma peritonei* due to peritoneal spread of a mucus-secreting gastrointestinal carcinoma.
iv. *Carcinoma of bronchus* or carcinoma of *breast* invading into and then seeding the pleural cavity.

II. Spread along epithelium-lined surfaces
i. Through fallopian tubes from the uterus to the ovaries and vice versa.
ii. Through the bronchus to the alveoli.
iii. Through the ureters from the kidneys to the bladder.

III. Spread via cerebrospinal fluid
i. Medulloblastoma of the cerebellum or ependymoma of the cerebrum may spread to the spinal cord through the cerebrospinal fluid.
ii. Glioblastoma may spread outside of the cranium through the surgeon-inserted plastic shunts giving cells access to the thoracic cavity.

IV. Implantation
i. This may occur during surgery by inadvertent transfer from one site to another via surgical instruments, needles or sutures.
ii. Inadvertent transplantation of organ that contains cancer from one person to another.
iii. Direct contact from one surface to another (e.g. one lip to another).

Q15. What is the sequence of events in the invasion-metastasis cascade?

Formation of metastases is a complex event involving several steps known as invasion-metastasis cascade, as illustrated in **Figure 7.4** and outlined below under 7 sequential headings:

I. Selective proliferation of aggressive clones within the primary tumour
i. Clonal selection favours the survival and growth of tumour cells that are more invasive and more prone to metastasis.
ii. Clonal selection in heterogeneous tumour populations is, in part, based on their genetic characteristics.
iii. Activation of certain metastatic oncogenes contributes to rapid growth of these cells.
iv. Tumour microenvironment plays an important role in this selection, providing growth advantage to the metastatic clones and facilitating neoangiogenesis.
v. Metastatic clones evade immune control and survive the attacks by immune cells.

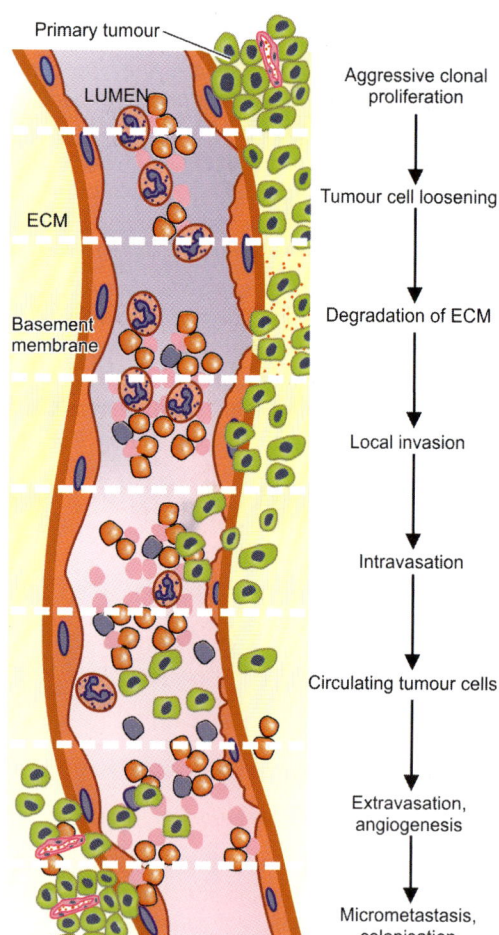

FIGURE 7.4: Invasion-metastasis cascade. Development of clinically detectable metastasis occurs through a series of complex events in cell biology. The figure shows sequential progression: 1) primary tumour, 2) local invasion, 3) intravasation, 4) survival in circulation, 5) arrest at distant organ site, 6) extravasation, 7) initial survival in foreign microenvironment and micrometastasis, 8) metastatic colonisation, and clinically detectable metastasis.

II. Tumour cell dissociation
i. Genes encoding cell-adhesion molecules (CAM) and integrins are downregulated, resulting in reduced cell cohesion.
ii. Genes favouring cell mobility promote emigration of cells from the tumour mass.
iii. Genes favouring epithelial mesenchymal transition (EMT) are upregulated favouring invasiveness of metastatic clones and promoting discohesive tumour growth.

III. Degradation of extracellular matrix (ECM) and basement membranes
i. ECM degradation is based on the action of matrix metalloproteinases (MMPs).
ii. Reduced activity of tissue inhibitor metalloproteinases (TIMP) favours ECM lysis.
iii. ECM changes promote invasive growth of tumour cells, but also stimulate neoangiogenesis and survival of selected tumour cell clones.
iv. Loss of receptors for basement membrane molecules such a laminin and fibronectin contributes to the loss of basal polarity, enhancing cell mobility and invasiveness.
v. Enzymatic degradation of basement membranes removes their barrier function and also generates biologically active fragments that promote cell migration.

IV. Intravasation
i. During this phase of the invasion-metastasis cascade, the tumour cells enter into capillaries, venules or lymphatics.
ii. Tumour entry into intravascular space is propelled by autocrine motility factor (AMF), a tumour cell derived cytokine favouring cell mobility.
iii. Chemotactic action of ECM-derived degradation products direct the migration of cells to the vessels and promote the passage of cells through the vessel wall.

V. Circulating tumour cells in blood and lymph
i. In order to survive in circulation, the cells need to adapt and develop new survival skills, basically alter their metabolism to achieve new homeostasis with the liquid environment.
ii. Most of the tumour cells in circulation will perish due to mechanical, oxidative and chemical stress, the action of cytokines, and natural immunity.
iii. Very few (less than 0.1%) tumour cells survive to the next phase.

VI. Extravasation and organ predilection
i. Circulating tumour cells form small clumps which may occlude the microcirculation and start forming metastatic nodules in that site. However, other factors probably play a role.
ii. Clinical evidence indicates that tumour cells from certain types preferentially extravasate in specific organs, suggesting that the adhesion at those sites is mediated by affinity receptors.
iii. Cytokines and tumour cell surface receptors probably play an important role in this process such as is the case with CD44, a surface molecule on lymphoid malignant cells.
iv. Sinusoids in the liver and the bone marrow have large pores that also probably facilitate extravasation.

VII. Micrometastasis and dormancy and colonisation
These poorly understood processes indicate that the clinical detection of metastases is preceded by some clinically less obvious processes as under:

i. *Micrometastases* This term denotes preclinical events comprising several attempts of the tumour to establish a second site, prior to the successful occurrence of grafting and growth.
ii. *Tumour cell dormancy* At the metastatic site, tumour cells may remain dormant (in translation 'asleep'), i.e. at a stand-still without any clinical evidence of growth. After an unpredictable time, they 'wake up' and begin forming the metastatic nodule. The entire process of tumour cell dormancy is poorly understood.
iii. *Colonisation* Cells forming the initial metastatic nodule may detach and seed the organ, forming new colonies. Alternatively, they may spread through the body and colonise other organs.

EPIDEMIOLOGY OF CANCER

Q16. What is the incidence of tumours?

Definition Cancer incidence is the number of new tumours or tumour deaths registered over a set period of time (typically a year) in a given population or country. Five most common primary cancers in the world are listed in **Table 7.3**.

Variation in incidence The incidence of various cancers varies from one country to another but, in general, the incidence of most common cancers is different in developing and developed countries.
- **In developed countries,** the incidence is highest for cancers of lung, breast, prostate and large intestine.
- **In developing countries,** the incidence is highest for cancers of liver, cervix, oral cavity and large intestine.
- **Etiology of cancers** influences their incidence. One-third of cancers are attributed to following *modifiable risk factors* requiring public health education:
i. Smoking
ii. Diet modification (low fat and high fiber diet)
iii. Physical activity
iv. Energy balance by caloric restriction to avoid obesity
v. Avoidance of excessive sun-exposure.
- **Declining incidence** of some cancers by early detection due to effective periodic screening programmes has been recorded in many developed countries. These cancers include the following:
i. Cancer of the cervix (by Pap screening)
ii. Breast cancer (by screening mammography)
iii. Colorectal cancer (by surveillance colonoscopy)
iv. Prostate (screening by serum prostate specific antigen, PSA)
v. Liver (screening by serum alpha foetoprotein, AFP)

TABLE 7.3 Five most common primary cancers in the world.

MEN	WOMEN	CHILDREN (UNDER 20)
Prostate (oral cavity in India)	Breast (cervix in India)	Acute leukaemia
Lung	Lung	Brain tumours
Colorectal	Colorectal	Lymphoma
Urinary bladder	Endometrial	Bone sarcomas
Melanoma	Thyroid	Soft tissue sarcomas

Q17. What are the most important tumour predisposing factors, in general?

The predisposing factors can be grouped as follows: i) constitutional factors, ii) familial and genetic factors, iii) racial and geographic factors, iv) environmental and cultural factors.

I. Constitutional factors
i. *Age* is one of the most important constitutional factors.
a. Most cancer occur more often in the elderly.
b. Some tumours typically occur during infancy and childhood (neuroblastoma, retinoblastoma, certain forms of leukaemia, etc.).
c. Some tumours have a peak incidence in middle-aged men (e.g. testicular germ cell tumours).
ii. *Gender* is an important constitutional factor.
a. Most malignant tumous are more common in men than women.
b. Important exception to this generalisation are the tumours of the breast, thyroid, gallbladder and hypopharynx, which are more common in women.

II. Familial and genetic factors
Heredity plays a role in the development of cancer.
- Overall the risk of developing cancer in relatives of a known cancer patient are three-times higher than in control subjects.
- Some common cancers show increased familial incidence, such as cancer of colon, breast, ovary, brain and melanoma.
- Cancers of proven genetic origin, however, comprise only 5% of all cancers.
- The incidence is much higher for some well-documented forms of familial (hereditary) tumours.

A few clinical examples are:
i. *Retinoblastoma*: About 40% are familial and show autosomal dominant inheritance, due to the deletion of *Rb* gene on chromosome 13.
ii. *Adenomatous polyposis coli*: Inherited as an autosomal dominant trait, it presents with multiple adenomatous polyps, which invariably (100%) undergo malignant transformation by adulthood.
iii. *Multiple endocrine neoplasia*, MEN-1 and MEN-2.
iv. *Neurofibromatosis type I.*
v. *Carcinoma of the breast* in women who carry the breast susceptibility genes BRCA-1 and BRCA-2.

vi. *Congenital chromosomal syndromes* such as Down syndrome, which is associated with a risk for developing acute myeloid leukaemia.
vii. *DNA-chromosomal instability syndromes* having defects in DNA repair mechanisms, such as xeroderma pigmentosum patients who are at risk for skin cancer.
viii. *Li-Fraumeni syndrome* characterised by familial cancers in multiple sites due to the inheritance of a mutant *TP53* gene.
III. **Racial and geographic factors** which are partly genetic and, in part, reflect the influence of environment, social habits and geography of the habitat. For example:
i. The incidence of gastric cancer is five-times higher in Japan than in the USA, while the incidence of breast cancer is much lower.
ii. India is a country with a high incidence of oral and upper aerodigestive cancer.
iii. South-East Asians have a high incidence of nasopharyngeal cancer and certain forms of lymphoma.
iv. South America has a high incidence of carcinoma of penis in men and cervical cancer in women.
IV. **Environmental and cultural factors** include socially acceptable practices, dietary habits, recreational drinks, and industrial contamination. Some *examples* are as follows:
i. Cigarette smoking is implicated in the pathogenesis of several cancers including carcinoma of the lungs, oral cavity and pharynx, oesophagus, stomach, pancreas, urinary bladder and uterine cervix.
ii. Alcohol abuse predisposes to cancer of oropharynx, oesophagus, liver.
iii. Betel-nut cancer of the oral cavity and tongue is common in parts of India.
iv. Industrial chemicals such as arsenic, asbestos, benzene, vinyl chloride, nickel contribute to the risk of several cancers.

Q18. What are the most important lesions and diseases predisposing to cancer?

Conditions predisposing to cancer are considered under following headings: i) precursor lesions, ii) certain benign tumours, iii) non-neoplastic chronic conditions, and iv) immunodeficiencies.
I. **Precursor lesions** include several forms of metaplasia, dysplasia and preinvasive forms of intraepithelial neoplasia.
i. Cervical intraepithelial neoplasia (CIN, also known as high-grade squamous dysplasia)
ii. Squamous metaplasia and dysplasia of bronchi in smokers
iii. Actinic (solar) keratosis of sun-exposed skin
iv. Oral leukoplakia
v. Barrett esophagus
vi. Atypical ductal hyperplasia of the breast
II. **Some benign tumours** are known to progress to invasive cancer.
i. Adenomas of the large intestine in adenomatous polyposis coli (APC)
ii. Neurofibroma in neurofibromatosis type I, that may progress to sarcoma
III. **Chronic conditions** associated with an increased incidence of malignant tumours in the affected organ as listed below:
i. Chronic ulcerative colitis → colonic adenocarcinoma
ii. Cirrhosis of the liver → hepatocellular carcinoma
iii. *H. pylori* related chronic gastritis → gastric adenocarcinoma or lymphoma
iv. Chronic bronchitis is smokers → bronchial carcinoma
v. Pulmonary asbestosis → pleural mesothelioma and bronchial carcinoma
vi. Chronic osteomyelitis with sinuses draining to skin surface → squamous cell skin carcinoma
vii. Chronic cystitis caused by *Schistosoma haematobium* infection → squamous cell bladder carcinoma
IV. **Immunodeficiencies** Both congenital and acquired immunodeficiencies are risk factors for neoplasia:
i. Congenital (primary) immunodeficiencies → lymphoma
ii. AIDS → lymphoma, Kaposi sarcoma, certain forms of carcinoma (e.g. cervical carcinoma)

Q19. Which hormones promote the growth or contribute to the formation of malignant tumours?

Hormones stimulate the proliferation of cells in hormone-sensitive tissues and contribute to the formation of tumours in the following organs: breast, uterus (endometrium, myometrium), vagina, ovary, prostate, testis, thyroid and liver.

Important **clinical examples** are listed below:

i. *Breast carcinomas* which express oestrogen receptors respond to treatment with anti-oestrogens like tamoxifen and surgical removal of ovaries.

ii. *Prostate carcinomas* are usually initially androgen-dependent and their growth is retarded by castration and anti-androgen therapy.

iii. Oestrogen-producing ovarian *granulosa cell tumour* is known to induce endometrial adenocarcinoma.

■ MOLECULAR BASIS OF CANCER

Q20. What are the most important theories of carcinogenesis?

Modern theories of cancer have concentrated on changes involving the nuclear genetic material and the control mechanisms that fail to eliminate cells that carry altered genes. None of the theories provide definitive answers about key issues of human cancer; thus, it is best to consider them as complementary to one another.

I. **Monoclonal theory** There is strong evidence that most human cancers can be traced to a single transformation or mutation resulting in a clone of neoplastic cells. Supporting data include:

i. The cells of multiple myeloma which all produce the same immunoglobulin or one of its chains.

ii. Inactivation of maternal or paternal X-chromosome shows that in multiple leiomyomas of myometrium, each tumour is monoclonal, i.e. composed of cells that show either paternal or maternal inactivation.

II. **Tissue organisation theory** According to this, neoplasia develops due to disorganisation of tissue and a loss of control of growth of mutated cells, which are normally under the control through cell-to-cell contact and tissue organisation.

III. **Somatic mutation theory and multistep theory of cancer progression** There is general consensus that mutations play a crucial role in the pathogenesis of cancer. The initial mutation may occur at random, or linked to exposure to carcinogenic chemicals, viruses, radiation and other adverse factors. There is overwhelming evidence that carcinogenesis is a multistep process, during which the cells acquire stem cell-like properties and a cancer cell phenotype. It remains to be determined how many mutations occur in addition to an initiator mutation which is followed by driver mutations in a multi-hit process. The role of so called loss-of-function mutations is also debated.

IV. **Epigenetic theory** postulates that the genetic changes are amplified or controlled by epigenetic events such as DNA methylation and histone modification.

Q21. What are the basic concepts of molecular carcinogenesis?

Molecular carcinogenesis is best understood by postulating that cancer results from changes in one or more basic regulatory gene families (**Fig. 7.5**):

i. Proto-oncogenes, i.e. growth promoting genes

ii. Tumour-suppressor genes, i.e. growth inhibitory genes (anti-oncogenes)

iii. Apoptosis regulatory genes which control programmed cell death

iv. DNA repair genes which regulate the repair of DNA damage that has occurred during mitosis

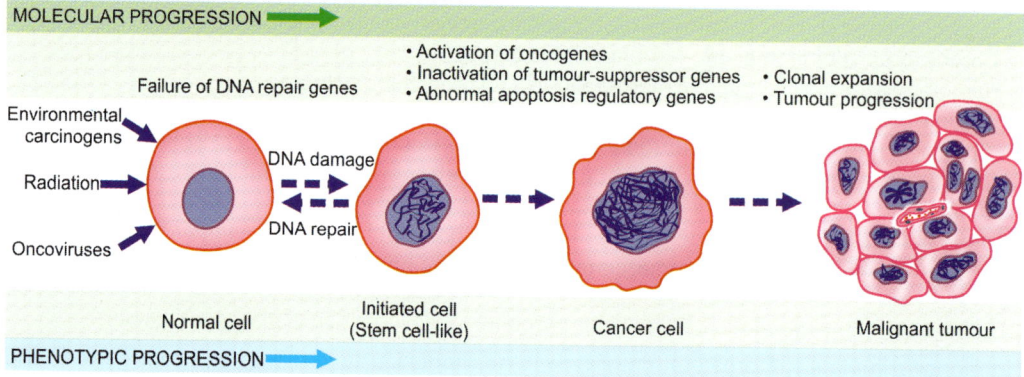

FIGURE 7.5: Schematic illustration to show basic concept of carcinogenesis at molecular level.

I. **Activation of oncogenes**, which are formed through the mutation of proto-oncogenes. Oncogenes promote cell proliferation in a dominant manner; the mutation of a single copy of gene will, thus, transform a normal cell into a cancer cell.
Transformation of proto-oncogene into oncogenes can occur through three mechanisms:
i. *Point mutation*, i.e. alteration of a single DNA base (e.g. *RAS* oncogene).
ii. *Chromosomal translocation*, in which portion of one chromosome carrying proto-oncogene is translocated to another chromosome; e.g.
- *c-ABL* protooncogene on chromosome 9 translocated to the BCR of chromosome 22 in chronic myelogenous leukaemia, thus forming the Philadelphia chromosome.
- *C-Myc* proto-oncogene from its site on chromosome 8 translocated to a portion of chromosome 14 in Burkitt lymphoma.
iii. *Gene amplification* increasing the number of copies of DNA sequence in proto-oncogene, leading to gene overexpression (e.g. *N-Myc* in neuroblastoma).
II. **Inactivation of tumour suppressor genes** permitting the proliferation of transformed cells. Tumour suppressor genes are active in a recessive form, i.e. loss of both alleles is required for neoplastic transformation.
III. **Abnormal apoptosis regulatory genes** may act as oncogenes or tumour suppressor cells, i.e. in a dominant or recessive manner.
IV. **Failure of DNA repair genes** essential for the repair of the altered DNA. Inadequate repair of damaged DNA allows mutations to persist.

Q22. What are the clinicopathologic hallmarks of cancer? Tabulate them in a list.

Definition Cancer hallmarks are acquired characteristics which transform phenotypically normal cells into malignant cells and promote progression of malignant cells while damaging the host tissue.
The main hallmarks of cancer are presented in **Figure 7.6** and listed in **Table 7.4**.

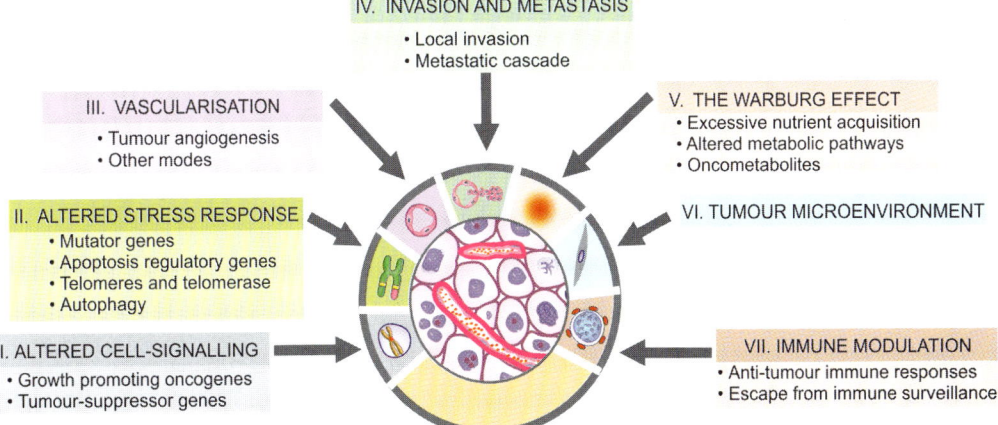

FIGURE 7.6: Schematic representation of revised hallmarks of cancer in terms of molecular carcinogenesis.

Q23. Define oncogenes. What are their main groups?

Definition Mutated form of normal proto-oncogenes in cancer is called oncogenes. In general, overactivity of oncogenes enhances cell proliferation and promotes development of human cancer. Thus, they have a main role in promoting cell proliferation and cell signaling.
Types of oncogenes According to their primary functions, oncogenes can be divided into following five groups:
I. Growth factors
II. Growth factor receptors
III. Cytoplasmic signal transduction proteins
IV. Nuclear transcription factors

TABLE 7.4 Molecular hallmarks of cancer.

I. Growth and proliferation permissive components: Altered growth-signalling
1. Self-sufficiency in growth signals: Growth-promoting oncogenes
2. Refractoriness to growth-inhibitory signals: Tumour-suppressor genes

II. Favouring overall cell survival: Altered stress response
1. DNA damage and repair system: Mutator genes
2. Escaping cell death by apoptosis: Apoptosis regulatory genes
3. Evading cell senescence: Telomere and telomerase
4. Recycling intracellular components: Autophagy

III. Sustained perfusion of cancer: Vascularisation
1. Tumour angiogenesis
2. Other modes of vascularisation

IV. Cancer dissemination: Invasion and metastasis
1. Invasion, intravasation and circulating tumour cells
2. Extravasation, organ predilection, micrometastasis, dormancy and colonisation

V. Growth-promoting metabolic changes: The Warburg effect
1. Excessive nutrient acquisition
2. Altered metabolic pathways
3. Oncometabolites in tumorigenesis

VI. Dynamic tumour microenvironment: The stromal cells
1. Angiogenic vascular cells
2. Cancer-associated fibroblastic cells
3. Infiltrating immune cells

VII. Evasion of host immunity: Immune modulation
1. Tumour antigens
2. Anti-tumour immune responses
3. Escape from immune surveillance

V. Cell cycle regulatory proteins

A list of common examples of each group is given in **Table 7.5**.

Q24. What are the most important oncogenes that encode for growth factors? Give examples of associated tumours in each.

i. *SIS (PDGF-β)*, encoding the platelet derived growth factor beta (PDGF-β). It is overexpressed in gliomas and sarcomas.
ii. *RAS (TGF-α)*, encoding transforming growth factor alpha (TGF-α). It is overexpressed in gliomas and carcinomas.
iii. *HST-1*, encoding fibroblast growth factor (FGF). It is overexpressed in osteosarcoma, breast cancer and gastric adenocarcinoma.

Q25. What are the most important oncogenes that encode for growth factor receptors?

i. *ERB B2* (*HER-2neu, EGFR*), encoding epidermal growth factor receptor. This proto-oncogene is amplified in carcinoma of the breast and ovary.
ii. *c-KIT*, encoding the c-KIT receptor. This proto-oncogene is point mutated in gastrointestinal stromal tumours (GIST).
iii. *RET*, encoding RET (standing for *r*earranged during *t*ransfection) receptor. This proto-oncogene is point mutated in MEN-2A and 2B, and familial medullary carcinoma of thyroid.
iv. *ALKR*, encoding ALK receptor. This proto-oncogene is translocated or point mutated in lymphomas and some lung adenocarcinomas.

Q26. What are the most important oncogenes that encode for cytoplasmic signal transduction proteins?

i. *RAS*, encoding GTP bound (G) proteins. This proto-oncogene is point mutated in 30% of all human malignant tumours, including carcinoma of lung, colon and pancreas.
ii. *ABL-BCR*, encoding non-receptor tyrosine kinase. This proto-oncogene is translocated or point mutated in chronic myeloid leukaemia.

TABLE 7.5 Important oncogenes, their mechanism of activation and associated human tumours.

TYPE/ONCOGENE	PROTO-ONCOGENE	MUTATION	ASSOCIATED HUMAN TUMOURS
1. GROWTH FACTORS			
i. PDGF-β chain	SIS (PDGF-β)	Overexpression	Gliomas, sarcoma
ii. TGF-α	RAS (TGF-α)	Overexpression	Gliomas, carcinomas
iii. FGF	HST-1	Overexpression	Osteosarcoma
	FGF-3	Amplification	Breast cancer, stomach cancer
iv. c-MET	HGF	Overexpression	Follicular carcinoma thyroid, hepatocellular carcinoma
2. GROWTH FACTOR RECEPTORS			
i. EGF receptors	ERB B1(HER-1, EGFR)	Mutation	Adenocarcinoma lung
	ERB B2 (HER-2/neu, EGFR)	Amplification	Carcinoma breast, ovary
ii. c-KIT receptor (steel factor)	c-KIT	Point mutation	GIST
iii. RET receptor	RET	Point mutation	MEN type 2A and type 2B, familial medullary carcinoma thyroid
iv. FMS-like tyrosine kinase receptor	FLT-3 gene	Point mutation	Acute myeloid leukaemia
v. PDGF receptor	PDGFR-B	Overexpression, translocation	Gliomas, leukaemias
vi. ALK receptor	ALKR	Translocation, Point mutation	Adenocarcinoma lung, lymphomas Neuroblastoma
3. CYTOPLASMIC SIGNAL TRANSDUCTION PROTEINS			
i. GTP-bound (G) proteins	RAS (several types)	Point mutation	Common in 1/3rd human tumours, Carcinoma lung, colon, pancreas
ii. Non-receptor tyrosine kinase	ABL-BCR	Translocation, point mutation	CML Acute leukaemias
iii. JAK/STAT signal transduction	JAK2	Translocation	Myeloproliferative disorders, ALL
4. NUCLEAR TRANSCRIPTION FACTORS			
i. C-Myc	Myc	Translocation	Burkitt lymphoma
ii. N-Myc	Myc	Amplification	Neuroblastoma, small cell carcinoma lung
iii. L-Myc	Myc	Amplification	Small cell carcinoma lung
5. CELL CYCLE REGULATORY PROTEINS			
i. Cyclins	Cyclin D	Translocation	Carcinoma breast, myeloma, mantle cell lymphoma
	Cyclin E	Overexpression	Carcinoma breast
ii. CDKs	CDK4	Amplification	Glioblastoma, melanoma, sarcomas

iii. *JAK2*, encoding JAK/STAT signal transduction protein. This proto-oncogene is translocated in acute lymphoblastic leukaemia and myeloproliferative disorders.

Q27. What are most important oncogenes that encode for nuclear transcription factors?

Myc, encoding *C-Myc, N-Myc*, or *L-Myc* proteins. This proto-oncogene is translocated in Burkitt lymphoma (*C-Myc*) or amplified in neuroblastoma and small cell carcinoma of lung (*N-Myc* and *L-Myc*).

Q28. What are most important oncogenes that encode for cell cycle regulatory proteins?

i. *Cyclin D and E*, encoding cyclins. Proto-oncogene cyclin D is translocated or overexpressed in mantle cell lymphoma and multiple myeloma. Proto-oncogene E is overexpressed in breast carcinoma.
ii. *CDK4* encoding cyclin-dependent kinases (CDKs). It is amplified in glioblastoma, melanoma and sarcomas.

Q29. What are tumour suppressor genes? Give their important examples.

Definition Normal tumour suppression genes inhibit cell proliferation. Its mutated form results in removal of brakes for cell growth. Typically, it involves loss of inhibition of G1 → S phase transition.

The loss of this control function may result from point mutations, loss of function mutations, or loss of gene due to chromosomal deletions.

Examples of tumour suppressor genes Most important tumour suppressor genes and related tumours due to mutated forms are listed in **Table 7.6**.

TABLE 7.6 Important tumour-suppressor genes and associated human tumours.		
GENE	MUTATION	ASSOCIATED HUMAN TUMOURS
1. *RB*	Loss of inhibition at G1-S phase transition	Retinoblastoma, osteosarcoma
2. *p53 (TP53)*	➢ Loss of block in mitotic activity ➢ Loss of promoting apoptosis	Most human cancers, common in carcinoma lung, head and neck, colon, breast
3. *TGF-β and its receptor*	➢ Loss of inhibition in cell proliferation by activating CDKIs ➢ Loss of suppression in growth-promoting genes	Carcinoma pancreas, colon, stomach
4. *APC and β-catenin proteins*	Loss of Inhibition in mitosis by WNT pathway and by failure of degrading β-catenin	Carcinoma colon
5. *Others*		
i. BRCA 1 and 2	Loss of repair of damaged DNA	Carcinoma breast, ovary
ii. VHL	Prevents ubiquitination and degradation of HIF-1α and promotes angiogenesis	Renal cell carcinoma
iii. WT 1 and 2	Transcription factor	Wilms' tumour
iv. NF 1 and 2	NF1 (neurofibromin 1a GTPase, NF2 (merlin protein), a cytoskeletal protein	Neurofibromatosis type 1 and 2
v. PTEN	Inhibits P13K/AKT signalling	Breast cancer, other epithelial cancers
vi. PTCH1	Inhibits Hedgehog signalling	Naevoid basal cell carcinoma
vii. CDKN2A	Inhibitor of *p16/INK4* and *CDK4/cyclin D*	Bladder carcinoma, carcinoma cervix

Retinoblastoma *(RB)* is the prototype and best known tumour suppressor gene. It acts as recessive genes and tumours develop only if both alleles are mutated or lost, as seen in retinoblastoma. As shown in **Figure 7.7**, retinoblastoma may be sporadic or inherited:

- For the formation of sporadic retinoblastoma, two somatic mutations must be acquired.
- In hereditary retinoblastoma, there is a germline familial mutation/loss of one allele, and the tumours develop only following second somatic mutation/loss in the cells of the retina.
- Children with hereditary mutated RB gene are at an increased risk of developing other forms of cancers, most notably *osteosarcoma* of long bones.

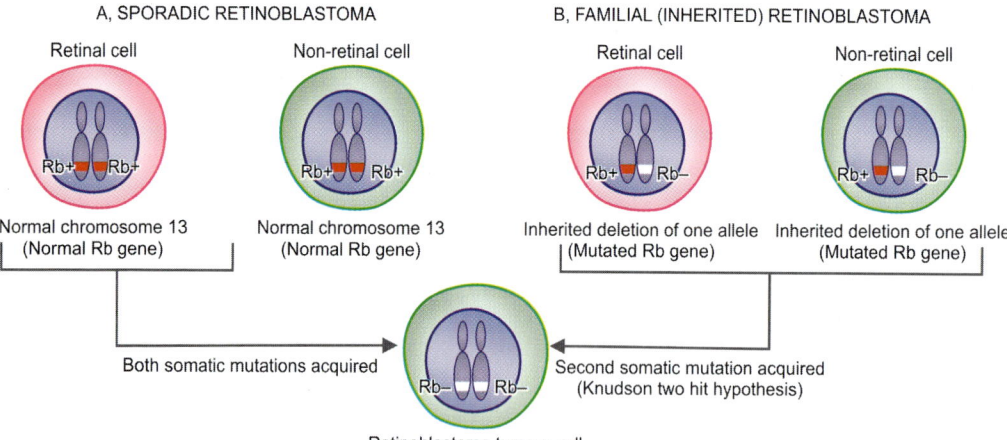

FIGURE 7.7: Schematic representation of role of *Rb* gene in sporadic and familial retinoblastoma. A, In sporadic form, at birth there is no abnormality of either of two alleles of *Rb* gene of retinal and non-retinal cells. Here, two mutations occur after birth involving both alleles of *Rb* gene. B, In familial/inherited retinoblastoma, both retinal as well as non-retinal cells have one germline mutation at birth from one of the parents in one allele that encodes *Rb* protein gene. Second mutational event in these cases in the other allele occurs early during life to form homozygous mutation (two hit hypothesis of Hudson).

Q30. Tabulate the key differences between oncogenes and tumour-suppressor genes.

The comparison of oncogenes and tumour suppressor genes is presented in **Table 7.7**.

TABLE 7.7 Oncogenes versus tumour-suppressor genes (antioncogenes).

FEATURE	ONCOGENES	TUMOUR-SUPPRESSOR GENES
1. *Derived from*	Mutated form of normal proto-oncogenes	Mutated form of normal growth-suppressor genes
2. *Inheritance*	Dominant; mutation of a single copy may transform cell	Recessive; mutation of both alleles (homozygous) required for transformation
3. *Common mutations*	Point mutation, translocation, amplification, overexpression	Deletion, point mutation, loss of function
4. *Major action*	➢ Allows cell proliferation by increased growth promotion pathways ➢ Active action by gene products (oncoproteins)	➢ Allows cell proliferation by removal of brakes in cell proliferation ➢ Passive action, i.e. by loss of normal function
5. *Level of action in cell*	At different levels (cell surface, cytoplasm, mutations)	At different levels (cell surface, cytoplasm, nucleus)

Q31. How does altered stress response favour tumour cell survival and growth?

Cancer cells subvert the stress response in favour of their own survival and growth. This is achieved by:
i. Avoiding DNA repair
ii. Escaping cell death by apoptosis
iii. Avoiding cell senescence
iv. Recycling intracellular component by autophagy

Q32. What are the most important inherited neoplastic diseases characterised by defective or ineffective DNA repair?

Hereditary defective or inefficient DNA repair is linked to mutator genes found in the following diseases:
i. Hereditary non-polyposis colon cancer (HNPCC or Lynch syndrome)
ii. Ataxia telangiectasia (ATM gene): multiple cancers
iii. Xeroderma pigmentosum: skin cancer developing upon exposure to UV rays of sunlight
iv. Bloom syndrome: increased incidence of leukaemia and other neoplasms upon exposure to ionising radiation
v. Hereditary breast cancer: due to mutation of *BRCA1* or *BRCA2*.
NOTE: Overexpression of DNA repair genes may also be accompanied by an increased incidence of certain forms of cancer.

Q33. How does escaping of cell death by apoptosis cause cancer?

By avoiding apoptosis, tumour cells become immortal and persist in the host for long time. This may occur due to several mechanisms, as given below:
i. Reduced cell surface *death receptor CD95/FasL* in hepatocellular carcinoma and certain lymphomas.
ii. Reduced activity of *proapoptotic factors such as BAX* due to a loss of of p53 in Li-Fraumeni syndrome.
iii. Loss of *apoptosis inhibitory factor BCL2* in B-cell lymphoma, resulting in longer survival of malignant cells.

Q34. How does evading cell senescence promote the development of malignancy?

- Cancer cells avoid senescence by upregulating the activity of **telomerase**, an enzyme which is essential for maintaining the normal length of the telomeres in chromosomes of stem cells and dividing cells.
- In contrast to normal senescent cells which lose telomeres after 60–70 mitoses and become mitotically inactive, cancer cells retain telomerase activity and, thus, remain capable of mitosis, avoiding senescence **(Fig. 7.8)**.

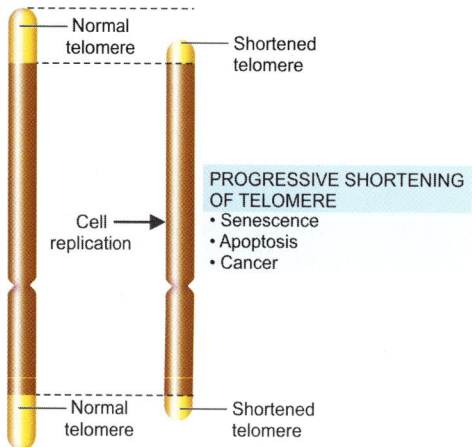

FIGURE 7.8: Telomeres are DNA components located on the tips of chromosomes in cells which are damaged during cell replication which are normally resynthesised by the RNA enzyme, telomerase, but are progressively shortened in senescence due to failure of telomerase for replacement synthesis. In cancer, there is upregulation of telomerase and thus cancer cells escape ageing.

- This process is accelerated by a loss of activity of suppressor genes *p53* or *INK4a/p16*, which normally control senescence.

Q35. How does autophagy promote the development of malignancy?
- Autophagy is upregulated in malignant cells, which is not surprising since it is upregulated in many forms of cell stress.
- Increased autophagy helps cancer cells survive in adverse conditions, such as nutrient deficiency and hypoxia.
- The role of autophagy in cancer is context-dependent and not fully understood.

Q36. What is the role of tumor angiogenesis?
i. Angiogenesis, i.e. formation of blood vessels from the sprouts on pre-existing vessels, plays an important role in tumour growth and metastasis.
ii. It is promoted by cytokines like vascular endothelial growth factor (VEGF) and basic fibroblast growth factor (bFGF) produced by tumour cells. Hypoxia and HIF stimulate VEGF signaling pathway.
iii. Acidic tumour microenvironment (TME) also promotes angiogenesis.
iv. Anti-angiogenesis factors are thrombospondin and several statins (e.g. angiostatin, endostatin, vasculostatin).
v. Mutated p53 removes anti-angiogenesis of thrombospondin.

Q37. What are the most important metabolic changes promoting tumour growth?
The basic metabolic changes in tumours are as follows:
i. *Higher acquisition of essential nutrients* (oxygen, glucose and glutamate).
ii. *Altered metabolic pathways*, including ATP generation, cell signaling, gene expression and nucleotide synthesis.
iii. *Oncometabolite formation* promoting tumour growth.
- Cancer cells *overutilise glucose* (Warburg effect or aerobic glycolysis) and have high activity of *glucose transporter protein (GLUT)*.
- There are several causes for increased activity of GLUT. The known factors that contribute to increased activity of GLUT include high level of *HIF*, mutations of *BRAF* and *K-RAS* and *MYC* oncogenes.

NOTE: *Positron emission tomography (PET)* using the injection of ^{18}F-fluorodeoxyglucose to radiologically localise tumours, is based on these facts.

Q38. Illustrate schematically activation-inactivation of cancer-associated genes in cell cycle.
The molecular properties of cancer cells in are shown schematically in **Figure 7.9**.

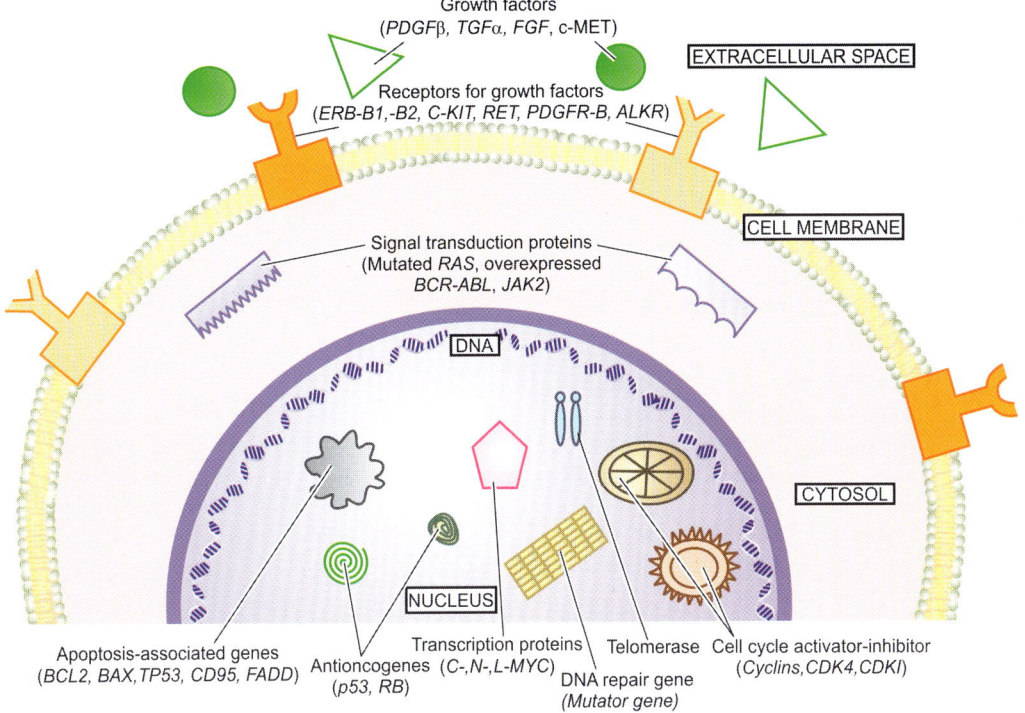

FIGURE 7.9: Schematic representation of activation-inactivation of cancer-associated genes in cell cycle.

Q39. What is the evidence that the immune system may provide a defense against tumours?

The following clinical facts support experimental animal data that the immune system plays a role in the defence against tumours:

i. Certain tumours are *infiltrated densely with lymphocytes* (e.g. seminoma of the testis, medullary carcinoma of the breast).
ii. *Spontaneous regression* of certain primary tumours (e.g. melanoma infiltrated with lymphocytes).
iii. Higher incidence of tumours in *immunodeficient hosts* (e.g. lymphoma in primary immunodeficiencies and AIDS).
iv. *Immunotherapy* is providing more and more encouraging results.

Q40. What are tumour antigens? Briefly discuss its various types.

Definition Tumour antigens are proteins produced by tumour cells that can elicit an immune response or can be recognised as such by immunologic methods in the laboratory.

Types of tumour antigens Following groups of tumour antigens are recognised:

I. *Oncoproteins from mutated oncogenes* They usually appear on the surface of tumor cells. Examples: Proteins encoded by *RAS* or *BCR/ABL*.

II. *Protein products of tumour suppressor genes* Examples: Proteins encoded by mutated *p53* and gene for β-catenin.

III. *Overexpressed normal proteins* Examples: Tyrosinase which is present in small amounts in normal melanocytes is overexpressed in malignant melanoma cells. HER2/neu in breast carcinoma cells.

IV. *Abnormally expressed cellular protein* Examples: Protein MAGE is found in male germ cell line, but may be abnormally expressed in melanoma and carcinomas of major organs.

V. *Viral oncoproteins* Examples: HPV products in carcinoma of the cervix, EBNA protein produced by Epstein-Barr virus in Burkitt lymphoma.

VI. *Cell-specific antigens retained in the tumor cells* Examples: CD3 on T cell lymphoma, and CD20 on B cell lymphoma; PSA in prostate carcinoma cells.

VII. *Oncofoetal antigens* Examples: Antigens expressed on foetal cells, reappearing on tumour cells, such as α-foetoprotein (AFP) in hepatocellular carcinoma, carcinoembryonic antigen (CEA) in colon carcinoma cells.

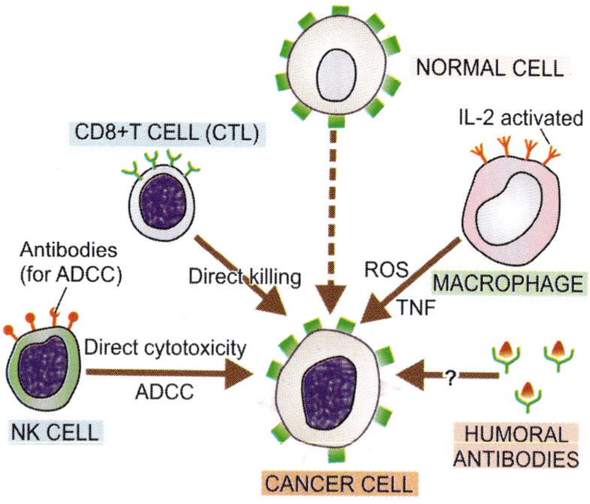

Q41. Which cells participate in the anti-tumour immune response?

Tumours elicit a cell-mediated and an antibody-mediated immune response, but the antibody-mediated immunity is mostly ineffective. The following immune reactions have been documented **(Fig. 7.10)**:

Specifically-sensitised cytotoxic CD8+ T lymphocytes which kill tumour cells in direct contact.

FIGURE 7.10: Schematic illustration of immune responses in cancer. For details see the text.
(CTL, cytotoxic T-lymphocyte; NK cell, natural killer cell; ADCC, antibody dependent cellular cytotoxicity).

Examples: Virus induced cancers such as EBV induced Burkitt lymphoma, or HPV induced carcinoma of the cervix.

Natural killer (NK) cells activated by IL-2 kill tumour cells directly without sensitisation, or by antibody-mediated cellular cytotoxicity (ADCC).

Macrophages activated by interferon-γ secreted by T-cells or NK cells kill tumour cells by reactive oxygen species or TNF.

NOTE: Cancer cells most often evade immune destruction by immunoediting and a variety of intricate escape mechanisms.

■ CARCINOGENS AND CARCINOGENESIS

Q42. Define carcinogens. What are their main types?

Definition Carcinogens are agents that can induce tumour formation, i.e. initiate carcinogenesis.
Classification Carcinogens are classified into following main groups:
I. Chemical carcinogens
II. Physical carcinogens
III. Biological carcinogens

Q43. What are the broad general features of chemical carcinogens?

i. Chemical carcinogens are of two kinds:
• Direct-acting carcinogens (alkylating and acylating agents)
• Indirect-acting carcinogens, which require metabolic conversion to become ultimate carcinogens (e.g. polycyclic aromatic hydrocarbons, aromatic amines, azo dies, naturally occurring biological carcinogens, etc.).
ii. Direct carcinogens are relatively weak carcinogens, and of lesser significance for humans.
iii. Most clinically important carcinogens are indirect-acting.
iv. Carcinogenicity of chemicals is tested by injecting them into experimental animals.
v. An accepted substitute for animal test is the Ames test. It is based on exposing bacteria to chemicals and observing if they are mutagenic.

Q44. What are the most important chemical carcinogens?

The most important examples in direct-acting and indirect-acting groups of human chemical carcinogens and tumours related to each group are given in **Table 7.8**.

TABLE 7.8 Important chemical carcinogens.	
CARCINOGEN	TUMOUR
I. DIRECT-ACTING CARCINOGENS	
i. Alkylating agents	
a. Anti-cancer drugs (e.g. cyclophosphamide, chlorambucil, busulfan, melphalan, nitrosourea, etc.)	➤ Lymphomas
b. β-propiolactone	➤ AML
c. Epoxides	➤ Bladder cancer
ii. Acylating agents	
a. Acetyl imidazole	
b. Dimethyl carbamyl chloride	
II. INDIRECT-ACTING CARCINOGENS (PROCARCINOGENS)	
i. Polycyclic, aromatic hydrocarbons (in tobacco, smoke, fossil fuel, soot, tar, minerals oil, smoked animal foods, industrial and atmospheric pollutants)	➤ Lung cancer
a. Anthracenes (benza-, dibenza-, dimethyl benza-)	➤ Skin cancer
b. Benzapyrene	➤ Cancer of upper aerodigestive tract
c. Methylcholanthrene	
ii. Aromatic amines and azo-dyes	
a. β-naphthylamine	➤ Bladder cancer
b. Benzidine	➤ Hepatocellular carcinoma
c. Azo-dyes (e.g. butter yellow, scarlet red, etc.)	
iii. Naturally-occurring products	
a. Aflatoxin Bl	
b. Actinomycin D	➤ Hepatocellular carcinoma
c. Mitomycin C	
d. Safrole	
e. Betel nuts	
iv. Miscellaneous	➤ Gastric carcinoma
a. Nitrosamines and nitrosamides	➤ Angiosarcoma of liver
b. Vinyl chloride monomer	➤ Bronchogenic carcinoma, mesothelioma
c. Asbestos	
d. Arsenical compounds	➤ Cancer of skin, lung
e. Metals (e.g. nickel, lead, cobalt, chromium, etc.)	➤ Lung cancer
f. Insecticides, fungicides (e.g. aldrin, dieldrin, chlordane, etc.)	➤ Cancer in experimental animals
g. Saccharin and cyclomates	

Q45. What are the three stages of chemical carcinogenesis?

Chemical carcinogenesis evolves through following three stages **(Fig. 7.11)**:
I. **Initiation**, during which the carcinogen interacts with DNA causing mutagenesis. After mutated cells divide, the DNA are transmitted to the progeny and are permanently fixated.
II. **Promotion** during which another chemical called promoter, enhances the effects of the initiating carcinogen and stimulates the clonal proliferation and expansion of the initiated cell population.
III. **Progression** during which the cells assume a cancer phenotype and acquire additional mutations.

Q46. What are the differences between initiator and promoter chemical carcinogens?

These features are summarised in **Table 7.9**.

Q47. What are the most important physical carcinogens? Briefly discuss their key features.

Physical carcinogens can be classified as:
- Radiation (ultraviolet, UV, and ionising radiation); and
- non-radiation physical agents.

I. **Ultraviolet radiation** has the most prominent effects on the skin.
Key facts:
i. Prolonged exposure to UV light has been associated with an increased incidence of basal cell carcinoma, squamous cell carcinoma and melanoma.

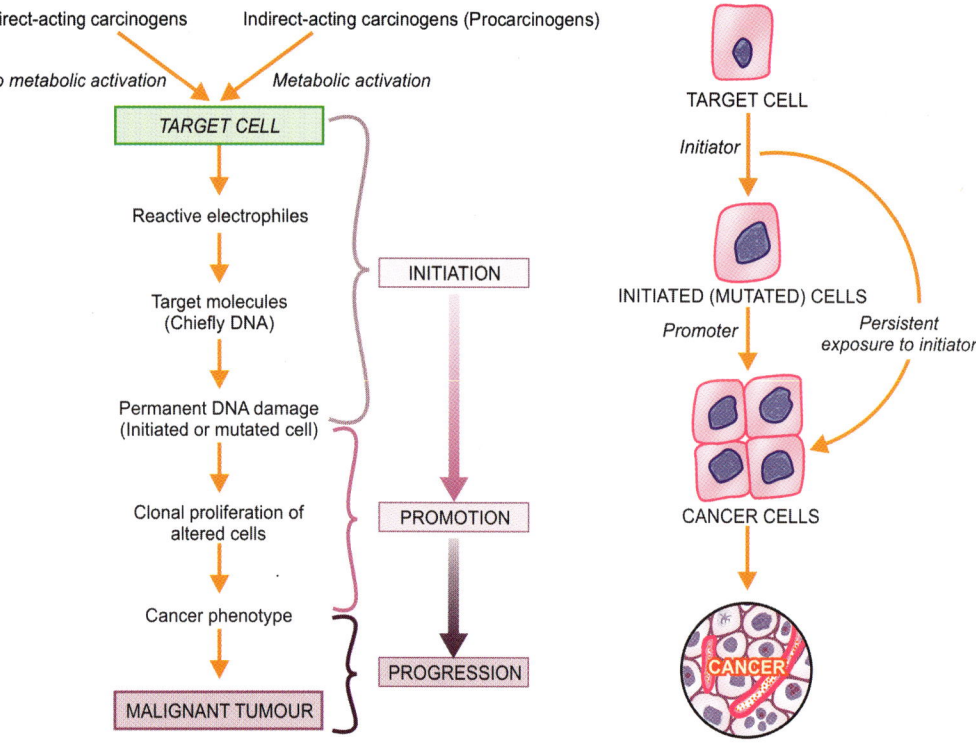

FIGURE 7.11: Sequential stages in chemical carcinogenesis (*left*) in evolution of cancer (*right*).

ii. Highest risk has been recorded in persons with genetic defects in DNA repair, as in xeroderma pigmentosum.
iii. Fair-skinned persons, especially genetic albinos, are at increased risk.
iv. Geographic differences have been noted, with the highest incidence of skin cancer recorded in white populations of in countries like Australia, that are close to the equator.
v. Highest incidence of sun exposure-related skin cancer has been recorded in professions requiring extended outdoor work, like farmers.
II. **Ionising radiation** like X-rays, α-, β- and γ-rays, isotopes, protons, neutrons may induce cancer in experimental animals and humans.
Key facts:
i. Ionising radiation damages *cellular DNA directly*, causing mutations.
ii. Radiation also generates *reactive oxygen species* (ROS) by radio-ionisation of cellular water, with secondary DNA damage from the ROS.

TABLE 7.9 Contrasting features of initiator and promoter carcinogens.

FEATURE	INITIATOR CARCINOGENS	PROMOTER CARCINOGENS
1. *Mechanism*	Induction of mutation	Not mutagenic
2. *Dose*	Single, for a short time	Repeated dose exposure, for a long time
3. *Response*	Sudden response	Slow response
4. *Change*	Permanent, irreversible	Change may be reversible
5. *Sequence*	Applied first, then followed by promoter	Applied after prior exposure to initiator
6. *Effectivity*	Effective alone if exposed in large dose	Not effective alone
7. *Molecular changes*	Most common mutation of *RAS* oncogene, *p53* tumour-suppressor gene	Clonal expansion of mutated cells
8. *Examples*	Most of the chemical carcinogens, radiation	Hormones, phorbol esters

iii. The most common forms of malignancy are various forms of leukaemias (except chronic lymphocytic leukaemia), papillary carcinoma of the thyroid, squamous cell carcinoma of the skin.
iv. Less common, but still related to radiation, are carcinoma of breast, uterus, lungs, salivary gland tumours and multiple myeloma.
v. *Epidemiology* provides strong supportive data about the carcinogenic potential of ionising radiation. Higher incidence of malignant tumours was recorded in several populations such as:
a. Early researchers of radioactivity and in inadequately protected physicians using radioisotopes and X-rays.
b. American workers in watch industry using luminous radium to paint watch dial numbers.
c. Miners working in uranium mines.
d. Japanese atom bomb survivors in Hiroshima and Nagasaki.
e. Persons exposed to radioactive fumes following nuclear power plant melt-down in Chernobyl, Ukraine.
f. Persons treated with therapeutic irradiation for non-neoplastic conditions, such as ankylosing spondylitis or childhood enlargement of the thymus.
III. **Non-radiation physical carcinogens** The data on non-radiation physical carcinogenesis are mostly epidemiologic and based on the association between a certain causative agent and tumours, as given below:
i. *Stones* in the gallbladder and urinary bladder are associated with higher incidence of cancer.
ii. Healed dermal *scars* following burns are associated with higher incidence of skin cancer.
iii. *Occupational exposure* in certain professions. Best known examples are:
a. Asbestos exposure associated with higher incidence of mesothelioma and lung cancer.
b. Workers in hardwood cutting industry at increased risk for carcinoma of nasal sinuses.

Q48. What are the most important agents of biological carcinogenesis?

Epidemiologic data indicate that certain biological agents are carcinogenic in humans, as listed below:
I. **Viruses** that cause cancer include papilloma viruses, such as HPV (carcinoma of cervix), herpesviruses such as EBV (nasopharyngeal carcinoma) and HHV8 (Kaposi sarcoma).
II. **Bacteria**, such as *Helicobacter pylori*, implicated in the pathogenesis of gastric carcinoma and lymphoma.
III. **Fungi**, such as *Aspergillus flavus* producing the potent hepatocarcinogen aflatoxin B1.
IV. **Parasites,** such as *Schistosoma haematobium*, linked to carcinoma of the urinary bladder.

Q49. How do oncogenic viruses cause human cancer?

Oncogenic viruses are classified as **DNA** and **RNA viruses**. RNA virus cause a higher mutation rate than DNA viruses. Each virus has its own mechanism of action but, in general, they promote proliferation pathways and inhibit the action of tumour suppression genes.
I. **DNA virus** infection is recognised by the appearance of T (transformation) antigen on the cell surface **(Fig. 7.12)**.
• Permissive cells alow the replication of DNA virions, resulting in cell death and a release of virion.
• DNA viruses infecting the non-permissive cells are integrated into their own genome and, thus, become transformed into neoplastic cells which transmit the virus to their progeny.
II. **RNA virus (retrovirus)** contains two identical strands of RNA and the enzyme reverse transcriptase, which will transcribe the genetic message into a single strand of matching viral DNA in the host cell's nucleus **(Fig. 7.13)**.
• The single strand DNA is copied resulting in double-stranded viral DNA or provirus, which is then integrated into the host's DNA, resulting in neoplastic transformation.
• Cells allowing replication of integrated retrovirus are called permissive, and those that do not allow the replication as nonpermissive.

Q50. How are human oncogenic DNA viruses classified?

The most important oncogenic DNA viruses belong to five groups:
I. Papova viruses (HPVs)
II. Herpes viruses (e.g. Epstein-Barr or EB virus, human herpes virus 8 or HHV8)

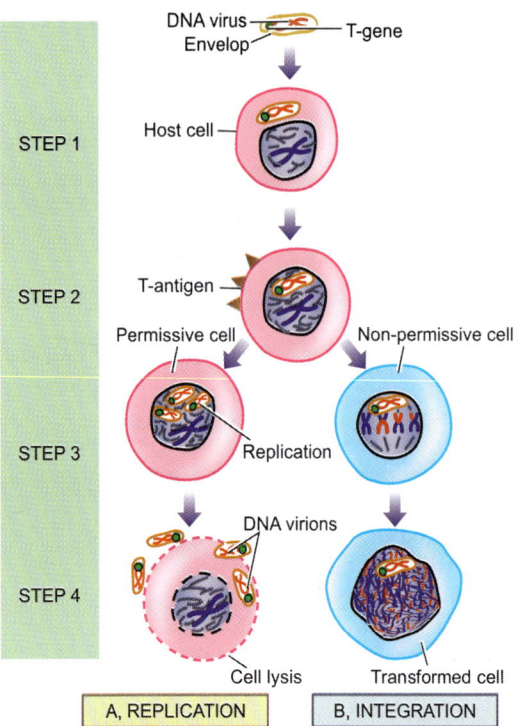

FIGURE 7.12: Replication and integration of DNA virus in the host cell. A, Replication: *Step 1.* The DNA virus invades the host cell. *Step 2.* Viral DNA is incorporated into the host nucleus and T-antigen is expressed immediately after infection. *Step 3.* Replication of viral DNA occurs and other components of virion are formed. The new virions are assembled in the cell nucleus. *Step 4.* The new virions are released, accompanied by host cell lysis. B, Integration: *Steps 1 and 2* are similar as in replication. *Step 3.* Integration of viral genome into the host cell genome occurs which requires essential presence of functional T-antigen. *Step 4.* A 'transformed (neoplastic) cell' is formed.

III. Adenoviruses
IV. Poxviruses (e.g. papilloma pox virus causing benign squamous cell papilloma and molluscum contagiosum)
V. Hepadna viruses (HBV).
All of them induce tumours in humans, except adenoviruses **(Fig. 7.14)**.

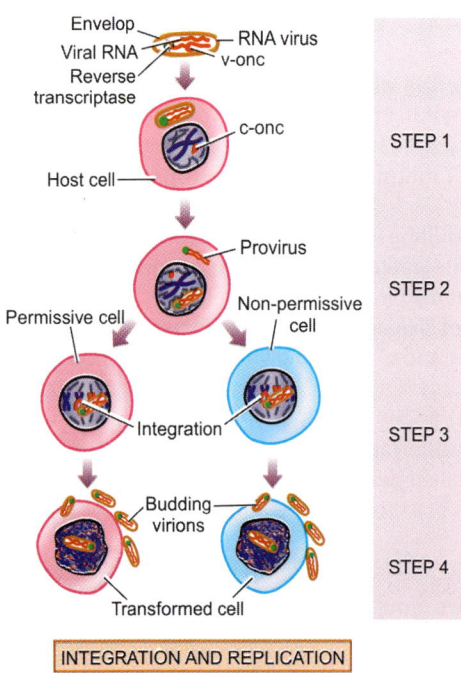

FIGURE 7.13: Integration and replication of RNA virus (retrovirus) in the host cell. *Step 1.* The RNA virus invades the host cell. The viral envelope fuses with the plasma membrane of the host cell; viral RNA genome as well as reverse transcriptase are released into the cytosol. *Step 2.* Reverse transcriptase acts as template to synthesise single strand of matching viral DNA which is then copied to form complementary DNA resulting in double-stranded viral DNA (provirus). *Step 3.* The provirus is integrated into the host cell genome producing 'transformed host cell.' *Step 4.* Integration of the provirus brings about replication of viral components which are then assembled and released by budding.

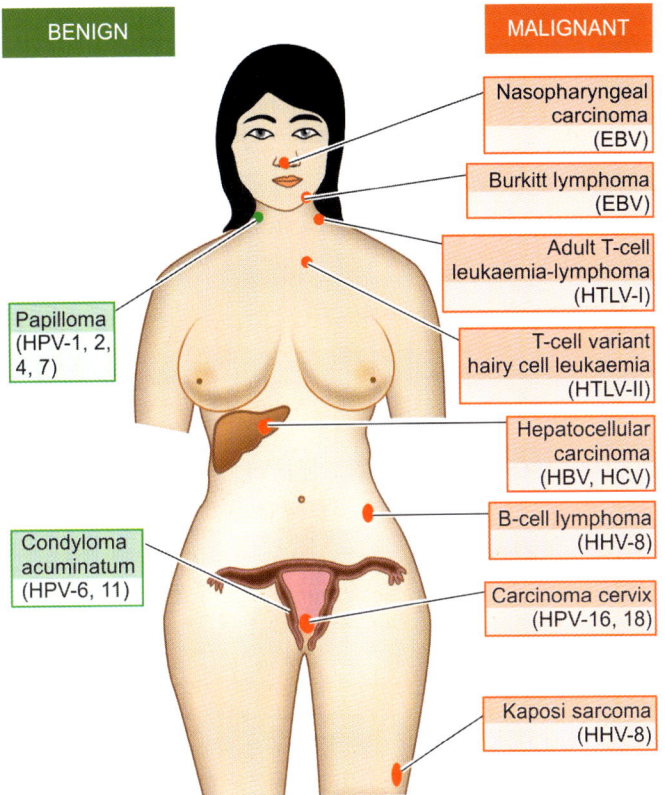

FIGURE 7.14: Viruses (in brackets) in human tumours.

Q51. How do papova viruses cause tumours? Give examples of some common human tumours caused by HPVs.

Human papilloma viruses (HPVs) are the most important groups of papova viruses.
- HPVs infect and proliferate in various squamous cell epithelia.
- HPVs produce either benign wart-like lesions, or preinvasive and invasive carcinomas.

Pathogenesis HPV infection leads to *genomic instability* with a loss of E2 viral repressor, and overexpression of E6 and E7, two components that account for malignant transformation of infected cells **(Fig. 7.15)**.
- **E6** degrades p53, *blocking apoptosis*. It also stimulates telomerase reverse transcriptase (TERT), preventing the age-related *shortening of telomeres* and thus contributing to immortalisation of cells.
- **E7** binds to RB protein *removing the brake on the progression of cell cycle*.

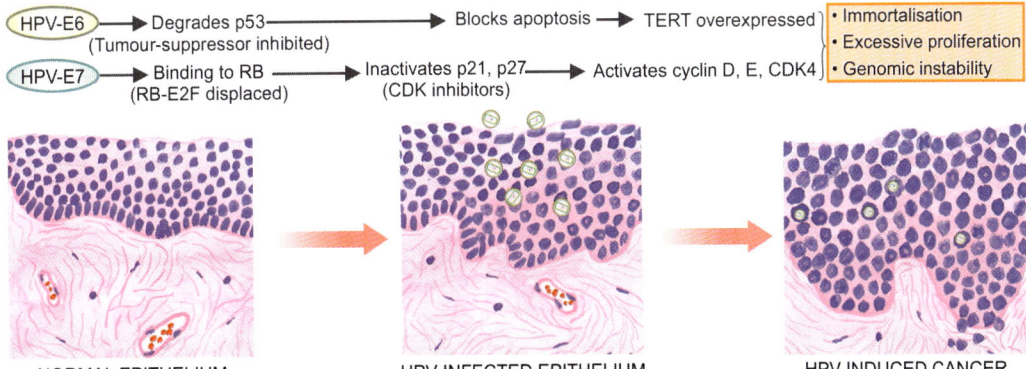

FIGURE 7.15: Oncogenesis by high-risk HPVs. Major oncogenic activities are mediated by genes that encode for E6 and E7 oncoproteins.

Examples More than 100 types are described. From the clinical point of view, they are classified as: *low risk or high risk types*. Examples are:
i. *Warts* (low risk HPV types 1, 2, 4, 7).
ii. Genital warts (*condylomata acuminata*) (low risk HPV types 6 and 11).
iii. *Juvenile papillomas of the larynx* (mostly HPV types 6 and 11 transmitted from the mother during birth, but other types may be found as well)
iv. *Squamous cells carcinoma and precursor* high-grade intraepithelial lesions (dysplasia) of the cervix, vulva, vagina, anus, perianal region, penis and oral cavity (high-risk HPV types 16, 18, 31, 33, 45 found in over 75% of HPV related cancers).

Q52. How does Epstein-Barr virus (EBV) cause tumours?

Pathogenesis
i. EBV infection is almost world-wide. Its oncogenesis, thus, probably depends on some additional factors, such as immunosuppression, or activation of *MYC* gene.
ii. EBV has strong *tropism for B lymphocytes* and is the cause of *infectious mononucleosis*.
iii. Like other herpesviruses, EBV infection persists for life. Infected cells express *latent membrane protein (LMP-1)*, which has a crucial role in the formation of malignant tumours **(Fig. 7.16)**.
iv. LMP-1 *stimulates the proliferation of B cells* acting like a CD40 receptor, and activates *BCL2* thus *preventing apoptosis*.
v. *Immunosuppressed* persons cannot mount an immune response to LMP-1, and, therefore, EBV related malignancies are more common in AIDS. Malaria-related immunosuppression probably plays a role in *African endemic Burkitt lymphoma*.
vi. In immunocompetent persons, LMP-1 is under immune control. Burkitt lymphoma develops only after a 'second hit', i.e. after a translocation t (8;14) of the growth promoting *MYC gene* takes place.
vii. Persistent active EBV infection is associated with the appearance of another viral protein (*EBNA, i.e. EB nuclear antigen*) which activates cyclin D and other oncogenes promoting cell proliferation.

Examples EBV is implicated in the pathogenesis of following human tumours and tumour-like conditions:
i. Anaplastic nasopharyngeal carcinoma, most prominently among the Chinese in South-East Asia, and Eskimos
ii. Burkitt lymphoma (African endemic form and the sporadic form in AIDS)
iii. Primary CNS lymphoma in AIDS
iv. Post-transplant lymphoproliferative disease
v. Hodgkin lymphoma

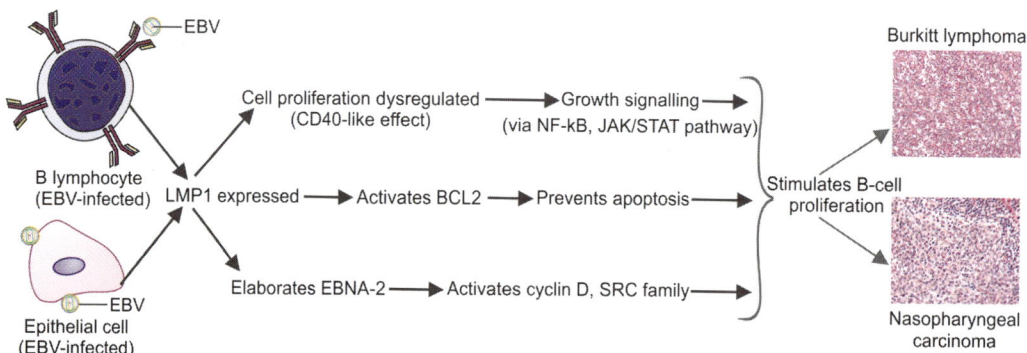

FIGURE 7.16: EBV-induced oncogenesis.

Q53. What is the so called Kaposi sarcoma-associated herpes virus (KSHV)? Briefly discuss its pathogenesis and examples of tumours.

Definition KSHV is the other name for human herpes virus 8 (HHV-8), the cause of Kaposi sarcoma.
Pathogenesis
• Viral DNA is found in 100% of all Kaposi sarcomas, both sporadic and the AIDS-associated form (the more aggressive, multicentric form of tumour).

- Infected cells express several virus related antigens, like *v-interferon regulatory factor* (v-IRF) and *latency-associated nuclear antigen* (LANA), which play a role in promoting tumour cell growth.
Examples HSV-8 is lymphotropic and is also implicated in the pathogenesis of pleural effusion lymphoma and multicentric Casteman's disease, besides Kaposi sarcoma.

Q54. Which hepatitis viruses cause liver cell carcinoma?

Hepatitis B virus (a DNA virus) and **HCV** (an RNA virus) have been implicated in the pathogenesis of 70–80% of all hepatocellular carcinomas.
Pathogenesis The mechanism of cancerogenesis is not understood.
- HBV and HCV induce antibody production and a cell-mediated immune response in the liver that may contribute to the formation of tumours, but the details are not known.
- Neither HBV nor HCV encode for any specific viral oncoprotein.
- Immunisation against HBV has reduced the incidence of hepatocellular carcinoma in Japan. There is no immunisation against HCV.

Q55. Which RNA oncogenic viruses induce malignant neoplasms in humans?

RNA viruses are classified into three groups:
I. Acute transforming viruses
II. Slow transforming viruses
III. Human T-cell lymphotropic viruses (HTLV)
First two groups are animal RNA virsues while only the viruses of the HTLV group cause cancer in humans.
Pathogenesis
HTLV-1 is the cause of adult T-cell leukaemia-lymphoma (ATLL).
- HTLV-1 has tropism for CD4+ T lymphocytes.
- The latent period for the HTLV-1 infection is long (20–30 years).
- Infection with HTLV-1 is endemic in Japan and West Indies.
- Immunosuppression plays a role in its pathogenesis, but the details are not known.
HTLV-2 is the cause of T-cell variant of hairy cell lymphoma, a very rare disease.

Q56. Tabulate the contrasting features of DNA and RNA oncogenic viruses.

Salient contrasting features of DNA and RNA oncogenic viruses are given in **Table 7.10**.

TABLE 7.10 Salient contrasting features of DNA and RNA oncogenic viruses.

FEATURE	DNA ONCOGENIC VIRUSES	RNA ONCOGENIC VIRUSES
1. *Genomic composition*	Double stranded, Deoxyribo Nucleic Acid	Single stranded, Ribo Nucleic Acid
2. *Reverse transcriptase*	Absent	Present, also called retroviruses
3. *Mechanism of transformation*	DNA integrates into genome of host cell nucleus	RNA transcription into DNA that integrates into host cell genome
4. *Mutation rate*	Low	High
5. *Main protein antigen*	T antigen	*SRC* protein
6. *Location of protein*	Mainly nuclear, sometimes on plasma membrane	Plasma membrane
7. *Molecular oncogenesis*	➢ Encodes oncoproteins ➢ Inactivates cell growth regulating proteins p53 and pRB	➢ Overproduction of pro-growth oncoproteins ➢ Integration of cell promoter sequence and viral enhancers ➢ Encode protein *TAX* that transactivates cellular genes
8. *Main virus types and associated tumours*	HPV types 16,18,31: Cervical cancer EBV: Burkitt lymphoma EBV: Anaplastic nasopharyngeal carcinoma KSHV (HHV-8): Kaposi sarcoma HBV: Hepatocellular carcinoma HHV-8: Pleural effusion lymphoma	HTLV-1: Adult T-cell leukaemia-lymphoma HTLV-2: T-cell hairy cell leukaemia HCV: Hepatocellular carcinoma

CLINICAL ASPECTS OF NEOPLASIA

Q57. What are the local effects of neoplasms?

Neoplasms act on the host and the effects can be local or systemic (generalised). Local effects include the following:
i. Compression
ii. Mechanical obstruction
iii. Tissue destruction
iv. Infarction, ulceration, haemorrhage

Q58. What are the systemic manifestations of tumours?

Among the many systemic manifestations of tumours, the following four groups of findings deserve to be outlined as clinically important: i) cachexia, ii) fever, iii) tumour lysis syndrome, and iv) paraneoplastic syndromes.

I. **Cancer cachexia,** i.e. wasting or emaciation (asthenia) caused by malignant tumours and tumour-related anorexia.
Etiopathogenesis Multiple causes, but not fully understood. Contributing factors include the following:
i. Cytokines such as tumour necrosis (TNF) and interleukin-1, and interferon-γ play a role in cachexia.
ii. Tumour necrosis, ulceration, haemorrhage.
iii. Tumour compression or obstruction of oesophagus and other parts of digestive system resulting in reduced calorie intake, malnutrition, or malabsorption.
iv. Hypermetabolism and pyrexia.
v. Pain, anxiety, insomnia.
vi. Infections.

II. **Fever** Its pathogenesis is not understood, although it seems that the tumour cells most likely produce pyrogens. Some tumours cause fever more often than others, e.g. Hodgkin disease, renal cell carcinoma, osteosarcoma.

III. **Tumour lysis syndrome** It is caused by destruction of a large tumour mass, or rapidly proliferating tumours that have outgrown their blood/nutrient supply. Good response to chemotherapy or hormonal treatment is a common cause of tumour lysis syndrome, most often encountered in leukaemia and lymphoma.
Clinical/laboratory findings Hyperuricaemia, hyperkalaemia, hyperphosphataemia, and hypocalcaemia, resulting in acidosis and renal failure.

IV. **Paraneoplastic syndromes** which cannot be explained by direct or distant spread of the tumour, nor the secretion of hormones normally secreted by the organ in which the tumour has arisen. Paraneopalstic syndromes are encountered in 10–15% of patients with advanced cancer.

Q59. How are paraneoplastic syndromes classified?

Paraneoplastic syndromes (PNS) are classified by the organ system that is most affected, such as endocrine, haematologic, vascular, etc. as follows:

I. **Endocrine syndromes** develop due to the secretion of hormones or hormone-like substances by tumours of non-endocrine origin.
i. *Hypercalcaemia* is the most common PNS. This *humoral hypercalcaemia of malignancy* results from the secretion of parathyroid hormone-like polypeptide (PTLP) by tumours like squamous cell carcinoma of the lung, renal carcinoma, and adult T cell leukaemia/lymphoma.
ii. *Cushing syndrome* results from ectopic production of ACTH or ACTH-like substances. Most often, it is related to small cell carcinoma of the lung, but may be also caused by carcinoids and islet cell tumours. Overall, 10–20% of all Cushing syndromes are caused by paraneopalstic ectopic ACTH hyperproduction.
iii. *Ectopic ADH secretion* is found in some patients who have small cell carcinoma of the lung or carcinoids.
iv. *Hypoglycaemia* is related to ectopic production of insulin-like growth factor II (IGF-II) by some sarcomas and hepatocellular carcinoma.

II. **Haematologic syndromes** include increased or decreased production of all or some haematopoietic cell lineages (e.g. pancytosis or pancytopenia, or selective erythrocytosis), as follows:
i. *Erythrocytosis*, i.e. increased RBC count, is related to erythropoietin production by tumours like renal cell carcinoma or hepatocellular carcinoma.
ii. *Leucocytosis* in found in 30% of patients with advanced solid tumours due to the secretion of granulocyte colony stimulation factor (G-CSF). In some patients, there is a leukaemoid reaction.
iii. *Eosinophilia* is seen in lymphomas and leukaemias and is related to the secretion of IL-5.
iv. *DIC* is common in patients with advanced cancer of any kind.
v. *Anaemia* may result as part of bone marrow suppression in advanced cancer. In patients with B cell lymphoma, it may be autoimmune.
III. **Vascular syndromes** related to the hypercoagulability of the blood include:
i. *Deep vein thrombosis*, with or without pulmonary embolism.
ii. *Migratory phlebothrombosis* (Trousseau syndrome) in patients with gastric or pancreatic cancer.
IV. **Bone joint and soft tissue syndromes**
i. *Hypertrophic osteoarthropathy and clubbing* of fingers in patients with lung cancer.
ii. *Oncogenic osteomalacia* in patients with benign soft tissue tumours associated with hypophosphataemia or phosphaturia.
V. **Neuromuscular syndromes**, related to immune mechanisms, typically involve peripheral nerves or the neuromuscular junction.
i. *Peripheral neuropathy* in patients with lung and breast cancer.
ii. *Myasthenia gravis* in patients with thymoma or lung cancer.
VI. **Cutaneous syndromes**, presumably due to immune mechanisms:
i. *Acanthosis nigricans* with hyperpigmented patches of skin in the axillae or groins in patients with gastric, large bowel, and lung cancer.
ii. *Seborrhoeic dermatitis* in patients with colonic cancer.
VII. **Amyloidosis**
i. *Primary* or AL, due to multiple myeloma producing light chains of immunoglobulins.
ii. *Secondary* or AA, due to SAA production by renal cell carcinoma, lymphomas and other solid tumours.

Q60. Define grading of tumours. How are the tumours graded?

Definition Tumours are graded microscopically on the basis of their degree of differentiation and microscopic signs of anaplasia.
Grading systems
I. Tumours are assigned to one of the *descriptive categories*:
- Well-differentiated
- Moderately-differentiated
- Poorly-differentiated

II. Alternatively, these three categories can be numbered and assigned *numerical grades* such as:
- Grade I (well-differentiated)
- Grade II (moderately-differentiated)
- Grade III (poorly-differentiated)

III. In some organs and for some tumours (e.g. neuroendocrine carcinoma of the intestines), it is customary to *grade tumours from I to IV*.
IV. For some organs, such as the urinary bladder, malignant urothelial tumours are assigned *only two grades*: low-grade and high-grade urothelial carcinomas.
V. *Complex grading systems* are used for certain tumours. For example, carcinoma of the prostate is *graded according to Gleason* by using a scale from 1 to 5.
VI. Some tumours are *by definition high grade*, and, thus, need not be graded (e.g. undifferentiated pleomorphic sarcoma of soft tissues or glioblastoma of the brain).
VII. For some tumours (e.g. seminoma of the testis), there are *no clinically useful grading systems*, and, therefore, the pathologists do not grade them.
NOTE: Grading system may be quite subjective. Furthermore, the clinical value of the grading is often dubious for many tumours. On the other hand, some tumours, like carcinoma of the prostate, must

be graded pathologically because such a grade has very high predictive value and must be included in the work-up of each case.

Q61. What are important systems of staging of tumours in clinical medicine?

Definition The extent of spread of cancer in a given case is called staging of cancer.

Staging systems Currently, two common staging systems applied for most of malignant tumours are: TNM staging and AJC staging. However, for soft tissue tumours, staged by Enneking staging system.

I. **TNM staging** TNM staging (T for primary *tumour*, N for regional *nodal* involvement, and M for distant *metastases*) was developed by the UICC (Union Internationale Contre Cancer, Geneva). For each of the three components (T, N and M), numbers are added to indicate the extent of involvement as under:

T0 to T4: In situ lesion to largest and most extensive primary tumour

N0 to N3: No nodal involvement to widespread lymph node involvement

M0 to M2: No metastasis to disseminated haematogenous metastases

II. **AJC staging** American Joint Committee staging divides all cancers into stage 0 to IV, and takes into account all the three components of the preceding system (primary tumour, nodal involvement and distant metastases) in each stage.

III. **Enneking staging** This staging system is accepted by most oncologists and is based on grade and location of tumour as under:
- *According to tumour location*: T1 (intracompartmental) and T2 (extracompartmental)
- *According to tumour grade*: G1 (low grade) and G2 (high grade)

Accordingly, the stages of soft tissue tumours vary from stage I to stage III as under:

Stage I: G1 and T1-T2 tumours, but no metastases.

Stage II: G2 and T1-T2 tumours, but without metastases.

Stage III: G1 or G2, T1 or T2 tumours, but with metastases.

In addition, current clinical staging of tumours rest on more modern non-invasive techniques that include modern imaging techniques, e.g. *computed tomography (CT), magnetic resonance imaging (MRI), positron emission tomography (PET).*

Q62. What are the various methods for tumour diagnosis in clinical medicine?

Diagnostic methods include the following:

i. Histological methods

ii. Cytological methods

iii. Histochemical and cytochemical methods

iv. Immunohistochemistry

v. Electron microscopy

vi. Serologic methods (biochemical assays)

vii. Other modern aids to diagnosis (e.g. flow cytometry, cell proliferation analysis, image analysis, morphometry, DNA microarrays, etc.)

viii. Molecular methods

Q63. How is tissue prepared for histologic examination?

Histologic examination of tissue may be performed on:
- paraffin embedded tissue, or
- freshly frozen tissue sectioned on a cryostat.

I. **For paraffin embedding,** the tissue must be fixed in formalin to neutralise the action of enzymes and thus prevent autolysis.

i. Formalin fixed tissue is firm and practially preserved forever.

ii. Formalin is washed out of the tissue and replaced by paraffin, which allows the technician to prepare a block that can be cut with a microtome in sections that measure a few microns in thickness.

iii. Thin sections cut on a microtome are deparaffinised by solvents.

iv. Sections are then stained with haematoxylin and eosin.

v. Finally, sections are covered with a cover-slip and the slides examined which can be stored for ever.

II. **For frozen sectioning,** fresh tissue is deep-frozen at −20°C to harden.
i. The frozen block is then sectioned in a microtome placed into a deep-freeze box at −20°C.
ii. The frozen sections are mounted on glass slides and stained like the paraffin-embedded sections.
iii. Frozen sections are used for rapid diagnosis *ex tempore* during surgery.
iv. The purpose of intraoperative frozen sections is to make an instant diagnosis for the surgeon, or to determine if the resection margins are free of tumour.
v. Frozen sections are also used for the histochemical demonstration of certain substances (like fat droplets), that would have been lost or dissolved during the processing of the tissue for paraffin embedding.

Q64. How are cytologic methods used for pathologic diagnosis?

There are two approaches for obtaining specimens for cytologic examination: exfoliative cytology, and fine needle aspiration cytology (discussed in detail in Appendix).
I. **Exfoliative cytology** involves scraping or brushing off ('exfoliating') cells from the surface of the skin or mucosa (e.g. mucosa of the mouth, vagina, or cervix). Papanicolau or Pap smear of the uterine cervix is the best known form of exfoliative cytology. Cells can also be obtained by bronchial washings or by centrifuging them from fluids present in serous cavities, cerebrospinal fluid, secretions such as saliva or sputum, urine, etc.
II. **Fine needle aspiration cytology** (FNAC) is based on aspirating cells into a thin needle attached to a syringe that can generate negative pressure allowing sampling of cells from solid tissues. The cells are forced out of the syringe onto a slide, fixed with formalin or alcohol, air-dried and then stained and examined. FNAC may provide rapid diagnosis, with an accuracy between 80 and 95%.

Q65. What is the difference between histochemistry, immunohistochemistry and immunocytochemistry?

The difference is technological as follows:
I. **Histochemistry** is based on applying *biochemical methods* for demonstrating specific chemical components of the tissues, such as fat droplets, glycoproteins, or calcium salts.
Enzyme histochemistry is by use of *enzymatic techniques* to demonstrate the presence of specific enzymes in frozen sections.
II. **Immunohistochemistry** is based on applying *immunological methods* for detecting specific antigens in tissue. For example, immunohistochemistry can be used to identify:
i. Cell surface clusters of differentiation (CD) on subsets of lymphocytes
ii. Specific hormones secreted by endocrine cells
iii. Specific tissue markers (e.g. prostate-specific antigen)
iv. Unique tumour markers
The specificity of immunohistochemistry has been markedly improved by the use of *monoclonal antibodies* produced by the *hybridoma technique*.
Immunoperoxidase technique combined with *antigen retrieval techniques* for demonstrating various antigens in formalin-fixed, paraffin-embedded tissues has contributed to the widespread use of diagnostic immunohistochemistry in clinical pathology. Immunohistochemistry is widely used for the diagnosis of tumours of uncertain origin **(Table 7.11)**.
III. **Immunocytochemistry** is based on applying immunologic methods to cytologic smears. It has been widely used to improve the diagnostic accuracy of cytologic sears. It is also widely used for *flow cytometric examination* of cells in fluids and blood.

Q66. How are tumour markers used for serologic diagnosis of tumours?

Immunologic techniques can be used to detect and measure the concentration of tumour markers in serum. Clinically important serum tumour markers can be classified as under **(Table 7.12)**:
i. Oncofoetal antigen
ii. Enzymes
iii. Hormones
iv. Cancer associated proteins

TABLE 7.11 Common panel of immunohistochemical stains for tumours of uncertain origin.

TUMOUR	IMMUNOSTAIN
1. *Epithelial tumours* (Carcinomas)	i. Pankeratin (fractions: high and low molecular weight keratins, HMW-K, LMW-K) ii. Epithelial membrane antigen (EMA) iii. Carcinoembryonic antigen (CEA) iv. Neuron-specific enolase (NSE)
2. *Mesenchymal tumours* (Sarcomas)	i. Vimentin (general mesenchymal) ii. Desmin (for general myogenic) iii. Muscle specific actin (for general myogenic) iv. Myoglobin (for skeletal myogenic) v. α-1-anti-chymotrypsin (for malignant fibrous histiocytoma) vi. Factor VIII (for vascular tumours) vii. CD34 (endothelial marker)
3. *Special groups*	
a. Melanoma	i. HMB-45 (most specific) ii. Vimentin iii. S-100
b. Lymphoma	i. Leucocyte common antigen (LCA/CD45) ii. Pan-B (Immunoglobulins, CD20) iii. Pan-T (CD3) iv. CD15, CD30 (RS cell marker for Hodgkin's)
c. Neural and neuro-endocrine tumours	i. Neurofilaments (NF) ii. NSE iii. GFAP (for glial tumours) iv. Chromogranin (for neuroendocrine)

Q67. How are molecular biology techniques used in clinical oncology?

Molecular techniques The most important techniques of molecular biology used in clinical medicine are:
i. DNA analysis by Southern blot
ii. RNA analysis by Northern blot

TABLE 7.12 Important tumour markers.

MARKER	CANCER
1. ONCOFOETAL ANTIGENS	
i. *Alpha-foetoprotein (AFP)*	Hepatocellular carcinoma, non-seminomatous germ cell tumours of testis
ii. *Carcinoembryonic antigen (CEA)*	Cancer of bowel, pancreas, breast
2. ENZYMES	
i. *Prostate acid phosphatase (PAP)*	Prostatic carcinoma
ii. *Neuron-specific enolase (NSE)*	Neuroblastoma, oat cell carcinoma lung
iii. *Lactic dehydrogenase (LDH)*	Lymphoma, Ewing sarcoma
3. HORMONES	
i. *Human chorionic gonadotropin (hCG)*	Trophoblastic tumours, non-seminomatous germ cell tumours of testis
ii. *Calcitonin*	Medullary carcinoma thyroid
iii. *Catecholamines and vanillylmandelic acid (VMA)*	Neuroblastoma, pheochromocytoma
iv. *Ectopic hormone production*	Paraneoplastic syndromes
4. CANCER ASSOCIATED PROTEINS	
i. *CA-125*	Ovary
ii. *CA 15-3*	Breast
iii. *CA 19-9*	Colon, pancreas, breast
iv. *CD30*	Hodgkin disease, anaplastic large cell lymphoma (ALCL)
v. *CD25*	Hairy cell leukaemia (HCL), adult T cell leukaemia lymphoma (ATLL)
vi. *Monoclonal immunoglobulins*	Multiple myeloma, other gammopathies
vii. *Prostate specific antigen (PSA)*	Prostate carcinoma

iii. Polymerase chain reaction (PCR) for detecting miniscule amounts of genetic material
Molecular tests These techniques are used for the following investigations:
i. Analysis of molecular cytogenetic abnormalities
ii. Mutational analysis
iii. Antigen receptor gene rearrangement
iv. Study of oncogenes and oncogenic viruses at a molecular level
Applications Molecular methodology is used for three major endeavours in clinical oncology:
i. Detection of minimum residual disease
ii. Genome-wide mutational analysis
iii. Personalised cancer treatment.

> ### Chapter 7e Supplement: Online Content
> *Digital content of this chapter available with this book is meant for enhanced learning and self-assessment. In addition, it contains 34 Multiple Choice Questions (MCQs), 05 Clinicopathologic Vignettes, and 05 Image-based Questions; these are followed by their answers along with explanatory notes of correct and incorrect answers.*

CHAPTER 8

Infectious Diseases

GENERAL ASPECTS

Q1. What are the basic forms of host-microbe relationships?
The basic forms of host-microbe relationship are as follows:
I. Symbiosis → cooperative association between two dissimilar organisms beneficial to both.
II. Commensalism → two dissimilar organisms living together, benefitting one without harming the other.
III. True parasitism → two dissimilar organisms living together, benefitting the parasite but harming the host.
IV. Saprophytism → organisms living on dead tissues.

Q2. What are the main elements in the chain of events leading to transmission of infectious diseases?
Main elements of this process are as follows:
I. **Reservoir of pathogen** It may be i) human beings (e.g. influenza virus), ii) animals (e.g. dogs for rabies virus), iii) insects (e.g. mosquitos for malaria), iv) soil (e.g. enterobiasis).
II. **Route of infection** The infection can occur through the skin or mucosal surfaces of the respiratory, gastrointestinal, or urinary tracts.
III. **Mode of transfection** The infectious organisms can be transmitted by direct contact, by insect bite, body fluids, air carried particles, faecal material.
IV. **Susceptibility of the host** Natural and acquired immunity determine if the host will be infected by a microbial pathogen. Certain people are more susceptible to infections, such as those who are old, debilitated, malnourished or immunosuppressed.

Q3. What are the main routes of infection for various microbes?
The main routes of infection are:
i. Ingestion
ii. Inhalation (respiration)
iii. Inoculation (parenteral route)
iv. Perinatally (vertical transmission)
v. Direct contact with another person (contagious infection)
vi. By contaminated water, food, soil, environment or animals

Q4. What are various host factors favouring microbial infection?
Infection occurs due to inadequate protection, i.e. failure of the following defense mechanisms:
i. Physical barrier → a break in the continuity of the skin or mucous membranes (e.g. wound)
ii. Chemical barrier → lack of tears, saliva or gastric juices
iii. Effective drainage → obstruction of urinary passages, paranasal sinuses, or biliary ducts
iv. Immunity, both natural and acquired → immunosuppression and immunodeficiencies

Q5. How are infectious microbes identified?

Microbes can be seen sometimes in microscopic slides or cell smears but are much easier visualised with special stains **(Table 8.1)**. Final diagnosis is best made by microbiologic culture techniques, sometimes combined with molecular studies.

TABLE 8.1 Methods of identification of microorganisms.

1. BACTERIA
i. Gram stain: Most bacteria
ii. Acid fast stain: Mycobacteria, Nocardia
iii. Giemsa: Campylobacteria
2. FUNGI
i. Silver stain: Most fungi
ii. Periodic acid-Schiff (PAS): Most fungi
iii. Mucicarmine: Cryptococci
3. PARASITES
i. Giemsa: Malaria, Leishmania
ii. Periodic acid-Schiff: Amoebae
iii. Silver stain: Pneumocystis
4. ALL CLASSES INCLUDING VIRUSES
i. Culture
ii. *In situ* hybridisation
iii. DNA analysis
iv. Polymerase chain reaction (PCR)

■ BACTERIAL DISEASES

Q6. What is plague? Discuss its salient features.

Definition Acute bacterial zoonosis, which in the Middle Ages and before that, has caused major epidemics. Today, it is not a significant health problem (global incidence <3,000/year).

Etiopathogenesis *Yersinia pestis*, a gram-negative coccobacillus transmitted by rat-fleas or inhalation from infected persons.

Clinicopathologic aspects Four clinical forms of disease are recognised **(Fig. 8.1)**:

i. *Bubonic form* is the most common, presenting with massive lymphadenopathy.
- Enlarged lymph nodes show areas of necrosis, mononuclear infiltration or granulomas.
- If treated, low mortality (1–15%).

ii. *Septicaemic form* (septic shock without lymphadenopathy), high mortality (40%).

iii. *Typhoidal plague* (with diarrhoea and abdominal organ involvement).

iv. *Pneumonic plague*, the worst form of disease, which is invariably lethal.

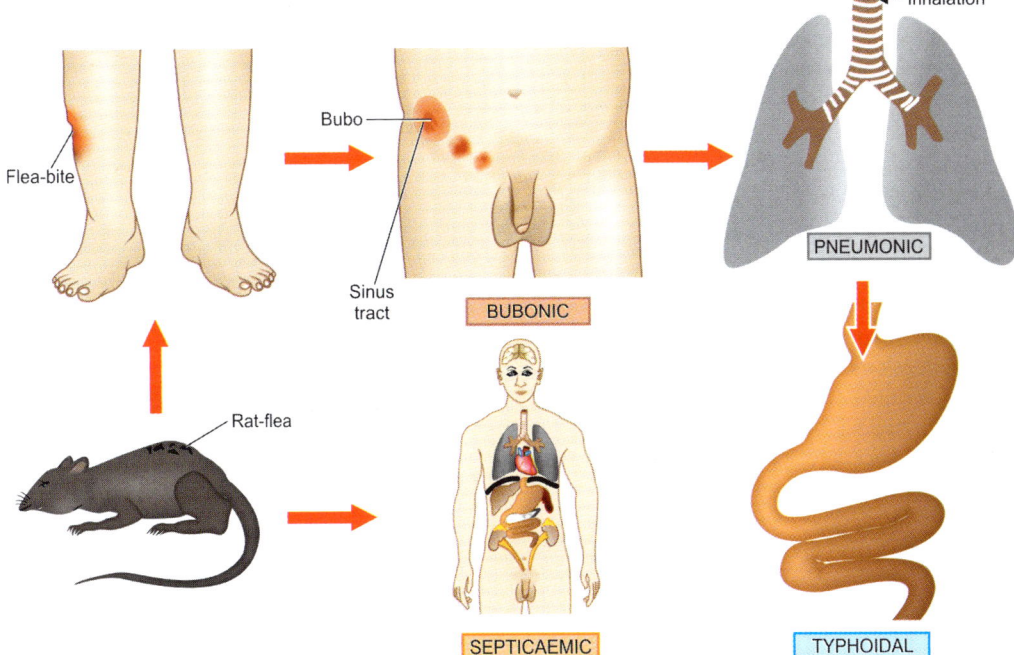

FIGURE 8.1: Forms of plague.

Q7. Discuss main features of anthrax.

Definition Acute bacterial zoonosis, affecting farmers and others who work with infected livestock.

Etiopathogenesis *Bacillus anthracis*, a spore-forming aerobic bacillus. In India, it is endemic in cows and sheep. Infection occurs through contacts with spores in soil or animal products.

Clinicopathologic aspects Clinical findings depend on the portal of entry. Three clinical forms recognised:
i. *Cutaneous form* related to direct contact, is the most common. It presents two ways:
a. Dermal necrosis related to underlying vascular thrombosis.
b. Pimples, which may progress to a necrotic lesion ('malignant pustule').
Lymphadenopathy is seen in both forms.
ii. *Pulmonary infection* ('wool-sorter's disease') presents with necrotising pneumonia, which has high mortality.
iii. *Intestinal anthrax* is rare.

Q8. What is whooping cough? Discuss its key features.

Definition Acute, highly contagious bacterial disease of childhood presenting with respiratory symptoms.

Etiopathogenesis Etiologic agent *Bordetella pertussis* has a strong tropism for the brush border of bronchial epithelium → excessive mucus production causing a cough with a characteristic 'whoop', which may lead to asphyxiation and death. *B. pertussis* secretes endotoxin and exotoxin that damage bronchial mucosa and a lymphocytosis producing factor (histamine-sensitising factor).

Clinicopathologic aspects
i. Necrosis of bronchial epithelium which is covered with mucopurulent exudate.
ii. Lymphocytes infiltrate bronchial mucosa and enlarged local lymph nodes.
iii. Lymphocytosis in blood (90%).
Clinically, the disease begins with a 7–10 days upper respiratory catarrhal phase (most contagious), progressing to the whooping cough stage. It is self-contained. Vaccination is very efficient, but still there are some 20,000 clinical cases per year in the US due to the parental refusal of vaccination.

Q9. What are the most important staphylococcal infections?

Definition Staphylococci are ubiquitous gram-positive cocci found also on the skin, nasal vestibule, stool, etc.

Etiopathogenesis Three species of Staphylococcus are pathogenic to humans: *S aureus, S. epidermidis,* and *S. saprophyticus.*
- Most infections are caused by *S. aureus* unless specified otherwise.
- Staphylococci are among the most common antibiotic-resistant hospital-acquired infections in surgical wounds.

Clinicopathologic aspects Staphylococci may cause infections that may be **(Fig. 8.2)**:
- *Localised* to the skin and specific organs.
- *Systemic disease* with septicaemia or toxaemia.

I. **Skin infections** are quite common and include the following:
i. *Folliculitis* is an infection of hair follicles. It may spread to adjacent follicles (*furuncle*), or deeper parts of the skin (*carbuncle* or *cellulitis*).
ii. *Sty* or *hordeolum* is an eyelid infection involving eyelash follicles and adjacent glands of Zeis and Moll.
iii. *Impetigo* is a childhood superficial purulent infection of the skin. It presents with small pustules which become covered with honey-yellow crusts.

II. **Infection of skin burns and wounds** Infections in these cases are related to contaminations from patient's own nasal secretions or from hospital staff. Infection affects most often the elderly, infants, malnourished and obese patients.

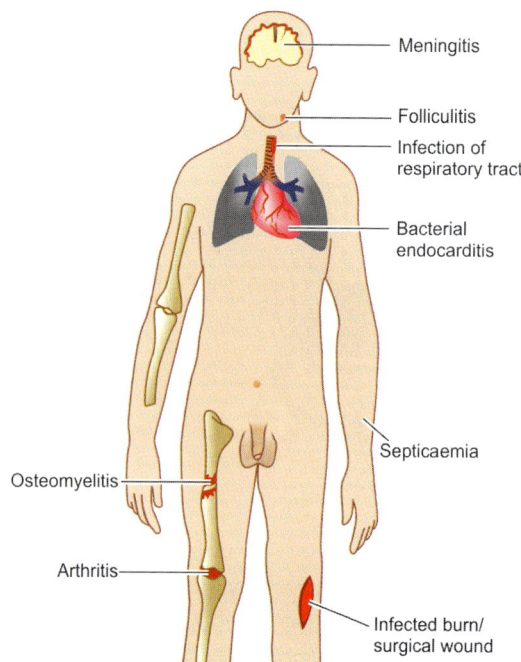

FIGURE 8.2: Suppurative diseases caused by *Staphylococcus aureus*.

III. **Respiratory infections** Upper and lower respiratory tract infections are especially common in children under the age of 2 years. They present as:
i. Acute pharyngitis
ii. Bronchopneumonia
Staphylococcal pneumonia in adults is usually superimposed on some other pre-existing pulmonary infection.
IV. **Arthritis** It is an uncommon infection, affecting mostly the elderly.
V. **Osteomyelitis** It usually affects the long bones of growing boys.
VI. **Endocarditis** It may be caused by *S. aureus* or *S. epidermidis*.
VII. **Meningitis** It most often develops as a complication of CNS surgery.
VIII. **Septicaemia** It occurs in persons with reduced resistance, or from haematogenous dissemination of an internal organ infection.
IX. **Toxic shock syndrome** This serious complication is characterised clinically by fever, hypotension, and exfoliative skin rash. It occurs most often due to staphylococcal toxaemia in menstruating women with retained vaginal tampons that are overgrown by toxin-secreting staphylococci.

Q10. What are the most important streptococcal infections?

Definition Streptococci are gram-positive cocci widely distributed in nature. Type A streptococci are found on the skin and throat of 10–15% persons without any clinical consequences.

Etiopathogenesis and clinicopathologic aspects Specific infections depend on the type of Streptococcus that has caused the infection (Fig. 8.3):
I. **Group A** (β-haemolytic *Streptococcus pyogenes*):
i. Upper-respiratory infection ('strep-throat')
ii. Skin infection (erysipelas)
iii. Rheumatic heart disease
II. **Group B** (*Streptococcus agalactiae*)
i. Newborn infections
ii. Post-streptococcal glomerulonephritis
iii. Rheumatic heart disease
III. **Group C and G** streptococci are responsible for respiratory infections.
IV. **Group D** (*S. faecalis* or Enterococcus)
i. Urinary tract infection
ii. Bacterial endocarditis
iii. Septicaemia
V. **Untypable α-haemolytic** streptococci such as *S. viridans*
Bacterial endocarditis
VI. **Pneumococci** or *Streptococcus pneumoniae*
i. Pneumonia
ii. Meningitis
iii. Septicaemia

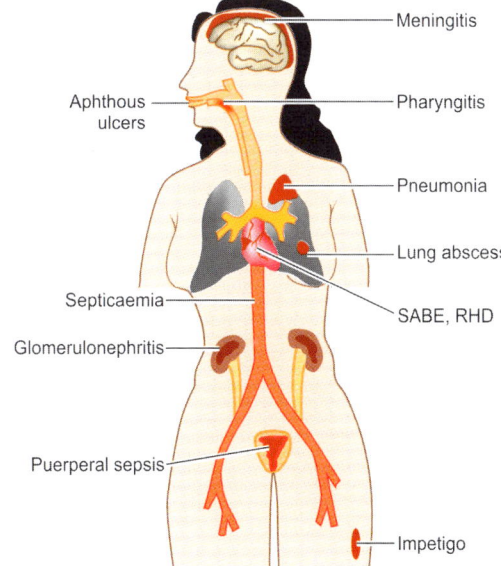

FIGURE 8.3: Diseases caused by streptococci.
(SABE, subacute bacterial endocarditis; RHD, rheumatic heart disease)

Q11. What are the most important clostridial diseases?

Definition Clostridia are gram-positive, spore-forming, anaerobic microbes found in the gastrointestinal tract of herbivorous animals and man.

Etiopathogenesis and clinicopathologic aspects Spores formed under aerobic conditions are passed in faeces and can survive under unfavorable conditions. Plasmids released upon degeneration of clostridia produce toxin which are responsible for the following diseases **(Fig. 8.4)**:
I. **Gas gangrene** caused by *C. perfringens* myotoxin. The disease occurs due to contamination of traumatic or surgical wounds. It is characterised by malodorous muscle necrosis and formation of air bubbles.

II. **Tetanus,** caused by *C. tetani*, which produces a neurotoxin tetanus toxin (tetanospasmin). Tetanus develops following the entry of spores through a penetrating wound. Tetanospasmin causes spasm of skeletal muscles leading to rigidity ('opisthotonos' with backward arching of the body) and respiratory failure due to the spasm of respiratory muscles.

III. **Botulism,** caused by *C. botulinum*, following ingestion of contaminated food. The toxin produced by *C. botulinum* inhibits the release of acetylcholine at cholinergic nerve endings, causing intestinal and respiratory tract paralysis.

IV. **Clostridial food poisoning** It is caused by α-enterotoxin produced by some types of *C. perfringens* ingested in dried meat.

V. **Necrotising enterocolitis** It is caused by β-enterotoxin produced by some *C. perfringens*, ingested in contaminated meat. Mild forms present as gastroenteritis. Severe form was first described in undernourished children overeating contaminated meat in New Guinea and then presenting with painfully distended bellies and bloody diarrhoea; hence the folk name 'pig-bell'.

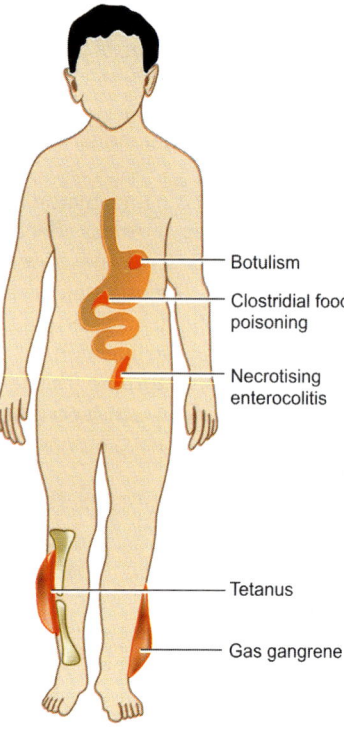

FIGURE 8.4: Diseases caused by clostridia.

Q12. What is Lyme disease? Discuss its salient features.

Definition An endemic multisystemic disease caused by a spirochete, *Borrelia burgdorferi*, transmitted by deer ticks of the *Ixodes* genus.

Clinicopathologic aspects The disease had three stages:
Stage 1 (early localised), presenting with fever and nonspecific symptoms, and a characteristic rash called *erythema migrans*.
Stage 2 (early disseminated infection), presenting with stiffness of neck or meningitis, migratory pain in the muscle and joints, malaise and fatigue.
Stage 3 (late persistent infection), characterised by chronic arthritis, which may be quite disabling. A proportion of treated patients suffer from chronic fatigue for many years.

FUNGAL DISEASES

Q13. What are the main features of fungal diseases?

- There are many species of fungi, but only a few are infective to humans **(Table 8.2)**.
- Some fungi (e.g. *Candida albicans*) are part of the normal flora on human skin and mucocutaneous areas, vagina, and intestines.
- Many fungi become pathogenic upon a loss of balance between the host and fungus, e.g. in immunosuppressed person, long-term antibiotic treatment, diabetes mellitus, pregnancy, etc.

Q14. What is a mycetoma?

Definition Mycetoma is a chronic suppurative infection of subcutaneous tissues that may extend into deeper soft tissues and bone, and is typically accompanied by the formation of pus draining sinuses.

Etiopathogenesis Generic term mycetoma includes two lesions:
- ***Actinomycetoma*** caused by actinomycetic bacteria (Actinomyces or Nocardia).

TABLE 8.2 Diseases caused by fungi.

DISEASE	ETIOLOGIC AGENT
1. Pneumocystis pneumonia	*Pneumocystis jirovecii*
2. Mycetoma	*Madurella mycetomatis*
3. Aspergillosis	*Aspergillus fumigatus, A. flavus, A. niger*
4. Blastomycosis	*Blastomyces dermatitidis*
5. Candidiasis	*Candida albicans*
6. Coccidioidomycosis	*Coccidioides immitis*
7. Cryptococcosis	*Cryptococcus neoformans*
8. Histoplasmosis	*Histoplasma capsulatum*
9. Rhinosporidiosis	*Rhinosporidium seeberi*
10. Superficial mycosis	*Microsporum, Trichophyton, Epidermophyton*

*Conditions discussed in this chapter.

- ***Eumycetoma*** caused by fungi *Madurella mycetomatis* or *Madurella grisea*. Eumycetoma is common in tropical parts of Africa, Southern Asia and South America.

Pathology Madura infection most often involves the foot, causing massive swelling ('madura foot').

Pus containing black grains pours through the draining sinuses that are formed from the mass. *Histologically,* there is purulent inflammation containing brown granules. Granulomas are seen at the border toward normal tissues.

Q15. What are the most important clinicopathologic features of candidiasis?

- *Candida albicans* produces superficial infections of the skin and mucosal membrane.
- Only rarely, it may cause fungaemia with *systemic candidiasis* and infection of internal organs, such as candida endocarditis.

Oral thrush It presents with creamy white pseudomembranes covering the tongue, buccal mucosa or soft palate. It is most often seen in infants and children.

Genital candidiasis In women, most often it presents in form of vaginitis. It is clinically characterised by thick, yellow, curdy discharge and pruritus. Vaginal mucosa is covered with white pseudomembranes. It may extent to the vulva and perineum. In men, it presents as balanoposthitis. In both women and men, genital candidiasis is most often found in diabetes mellitus.

Cutaneous candidiasis It presents most often as dermatitis involving the intertriginous areas or nail plate (paronychia).

Systemic candidiasis It is a rare condition, most often found in persons with impaired immune system. Candida may also be introduced by iatrogenic means such as via intravenous infusions, peritoneal dialysis or urinary catheterisation.

Q16. Which fungi cause cutaneous superficial mycoses?

- The most important dermatophytes are *Microsporum, Trichophyton* and *Epidermophyton*.
- Dermatophytes spread by direct contact, by fomites or infected tissue.
- The diagnosis is made by microscopic examination of the scrapings after addition of sodium or potassium hydroxide solution or by culturing fungi in special media.

Examples of fungal skin diseases are given below:
i. *Tinea capitis* → areas of patchy alopecia.
ii. *Tinea barbae* → acute folliculitis of the beard.
iii. *Tinea corporis* → dermatitis with erythematous papules that have raised margins and depressed center ('ringworm').

■ VIRAL DISEASES

Q17. What are viral haemorrhagic fevers? How are they classified?

Definition Viral haemorrhagic fevers are a group of viral infections presenting clinically with widespread haemorrhages, shock and sometimes, death.

Classification Viral haemorrhagic fevers are classified according to the mode of infection and thus belong to four groups:
i. Mosquito-borne (e.g. yellow fever, dengue fever, Rift Valley fever)
ii. Tick-borne (e.g. Crimean haemorrhagic fever, Kyanasur Forest disease)
iii. Zoonotic (e.g. Korean haemorrhagic fever, Lassa fever)
iv. Marburg virus and Ebola virus disease by unknown route

Q18. What is yellow fever?

Definition Yellow fever is an acute viral disease transmitted by the mosquito *Aedes aegipti*.
- Infections are limited to parts of Africa and South America.
- In endemic countries, the monkeys carry the virus and are the source of human infections.

Clinicopathologic aspects The disease affects the liver and kidneys.
i. Liver shows midzonal necrosis with Councilman bodies and microvesicular steatosis.

ii. Kidneys show proximal tubular necrosis.
iii. Clinically, it presents with jaundice, fever, myalgia, headaches, renal failure and bleeding disorders.
iv. Mortality is 5%, resulting from liver or kidney failure.

Q19. Discuss main features of dengue fever.

Definition Dengue fever is an acute viral disease transmitted by mosquitos *Aedes aegypti*.
- Infections occur in South East Asia, South America and Pacific Island, and North India in post-monsoon rain period.
- Most often affected are children under the age of 15 years.

Etiopathogenesis There are four dengue viruses which all produce the same disease.
- Dengue virus invades lymphocytes, monocytes and endothelial cells.
- Disseminated intravascular coagulation results from endothelial injury.

Clinicopathologic aspects
i. Dengue occurs in two forms:
- *Dengue fever*, a self-limited febrile disease, affecting muscles and joints, thus presenting with severe myalgia ('break bone fever').
- *Dengue haemorrhagic fever* characterised by DIC, widespread haemorrhages, hypovolaemic shock, and neurologic disturbances.

ii. *Laboratory findings* support the diagnosis of DIC and include evidence of thrombocytopenia, consumption coagulopathy, haemoconcentration.
iii. *Definitive diagnosis* of dengue infection is made by finding antiviral antibodies, or by demonstrating virus with monoclonal antibodies and molecular techniques.
iv. *Autopsy findings* include multifocal haemorrhages most prominently in the brain, liver, kidney and muscles.

Q20. What are coronaviruses? Enumerate the disease entities associated with them and their salient clinicopathologic features.

Definition Coronaviruses (CoV) form a large family of single-stranded RNA viruses enclosed in a protein envelope that has external spikes visible by electron microscopy as a crown or corona. Coronaviruses circulate among animals including birds, cats, bats and camels which are their natural habitats. From these animals, the viruses may spread to humans directly or using an intermediary hosts such as palm civets, raccoon dogs and pangolins.

Clinicopathologic aspects Six strains of coronaviruses have proven to be infectious to humans. The following clinicopathologic entities have been linked so far to coronavirus infections:

I. **Common cold** Estimates are that world-wide approximately 30% of all 'common colds' are caused by coronaviruses.

II. **Severe Acute Respiratory Syndrome (SARS)** In 2003, it was caused by SARS-CoV which spread to humans from bats in Guangdong, China. From China, the virus spread to many other countries.
- Clinically, this infection affects the respiratory system, often causing SARS.
- The case fatality rate is 9.5%.

III. **Middle Eastern Respiratory Syndrome (MERS)** Epidemic of MERS appeared in Saudi Arabia in 2012. Almost all cases have been traced to the Arabian Peninsula. It was caused by MERS-CoV transmitted to humans from camels, followed by limited episodes of person-to-person transmission.
- Symptoms of MERS-CoV are initially nonspecific, but soon most patients develop atypical pneumonia and severe acute respiratory distress.
- Up to 80% of patients with MERS require mechanical ventilation, and many of them have prominent GI symptoms and acute kidney failure.
- Case fatality rate is 30%.

IV. **Coronavirus disease 2019 (COVID-19)** The initial cases of this disease were identified in Wuhan, Hubei Province, China in December 2019, and the causative virus was identified soon thereafter (SARS-CoV2). Since then, it has spread throughout the entire world. Millions of people have been infected, and at the time of writing this topic the pandemic is still raging in many countries.

Q21. What are the clinical features of influenza virus infections?

Definition Influenza virus causes respiratory infections which may affect large populations and present as seasonal epidemics.
Etiopathogenesis Influenza virus is a single-stranded RNA coronavirus.
- Three distinct viral types are known (A, B, C).
- Influenza viruses infect humans, but also some home animals such as pigs, horses and birds.
- Type A accounts for most serious and severe outbreaks.

Clinicopathologic aspects Clinical manifestations vary from mild to severe and include the following:
i. Mild upper respiratory symptoms resembling common cold.
ii. Flu-like systemic febrile disease with myalgia and respiratory symptoms.
iii. Severe systemic disease dominated by pneumonia and even mortality.

Two subtypes of A virus have affected humans in a major way: i) avian influenza virus A/H5N1, and ii) swine influenza virus A/H1N1.

I. *Avian influenza virus A/H5N1/SARS-CoV1,* commonly called 'bird flu'.
- Transmitted to humans from infected birds.
- There is no person-to-person transmission.
- Humans have no immune protection against avian flu viruses.
- Vaccination could provide protection, but it is far from ideal (70% conversion rate).

i. *Clinically*, it presents with typical flu symptoms (e.g. sore throat, cough, dyspnoea, fever, muscle aches).
ii. This mild disease may progress to pneumonia and *severe acute respiratory syndrome* (SARS), leading to respiratory insufficiency.
iii. *Autopsy* of those who have died shows signs of acute respiratory distress syndrome (ARDS) with hyaline membranes, pulmonary oedema, and alveolar haemorrhages.
iv. The *diagnosis* is confirmed by documenting A/H5N1 infection with reverse transcriptase PCR.

II. *Swine influenza virus A/H1N1,* commonly called 'swine flu'.
i. Transmitted from infected pigs and subsequent person-to-person transmission.
ii. Clinically, it presents with usual flu-like symptoms.
iii. Additional gastrointestinal symptoms such as vomiting and diarrhoea are found in one third of patients.
iv. Usual vaccines against flu viruses do not protect against A/H1N1 and thus the only protection is by enforcing personal hygiene and washing hands.

Q22. What is coronavirus disease 2019 (COVID-19)? Briefly discuss its features.

Definition COVID-19 is a pandemic disease caused by severe acute respiratory syndrome coronavirus 2 (SARS-CoV-2), initially called novel coronavirus.
- Approximately 80% of infected patients experience mild-to-moderate disease, 14% of patients have a severe course requiring intensive care, and approximately 6% require mechanical ventilation.
- Approximately, 30% of infected persons have no apparent clinical symptoms.

Mode of transmission Human-to-human transmission via respiratory droplets. The initial human infection has been tentatively linked to mutated viruses, which jumped to humans from bats or some intermediary host such as pangolins. However, the exact source of SARS-CoV-2 that initiated the COVID-19 pandemic has not been identified so far.

Pathogenesis Most, if not all, human infections begin with the entry of SARS-CoV-2 into the human body through the lungs.
i. The proteins in the viral capsule have a high affinity for the *angiotensin-converting enzyme 2 (ACE2) receptor* which is expressed on the cell membrane of human type II pneumocytes. Virions attached to the pneumocytes release their RNA into infected cells, where it is replicated and translated into new viral proteins. A release of viral RNA from infected pneumocytes results in viraemia and a spread of the virus to other organs.
ii. Severe infection often provokes a *cytokine release syndrome (CRS)*, also known and 'cytokine storm' or *systemic hyperinflammatory syndrome*. It is marked by elevation serum interleukins (IL-2, IL-7, IL-6) and a number cytokines which can be measured in blood.
iii. In the course of the viral infection and after the cessation of the infection, most patients develop anti-viral antibodies that may cause *immune antibody-mediated complications* such as vasculitis.

iv. *Children and young persons* usually are less affected than the elderly. However, children and some younger persons and under the age of 18 years may develop a Kawasaki disease-like syndrome, known as *multi-inflammatory syndrome in children (MIS-C)*.

Diagnosis A nasopharyngeal swab is taken from the examined person and analysed to detect the viral RNA. Several molecular biology testing methods have been developed to this end.

i. The most widely used technique is *real-time reverse transcription polymerase chain reaction (rRT-PCR)*.
ii. *Laboratory findings* supporting the diagnosis of COVID-19 include the following serologic sign of CRS: C-reactive protein (CRP), lactate dehydrogenase (LDH), D-dimer, and ferritin.

Clinicopathologic aspects Symptoms usually appear 2–14 days after exposure, but in some people the infection is entirely asymptomatic. The median incubation period is 4 to 5 days. Risk factors for severe disease are older age and comorbidities such as hypertension, diabetes, coronary artery disease, chronic pulmonary disease, cancer and immunosuppression.

i. *The most common clinical symptoms* are fever with chills, sore throat, dry cough, dyspnoea and shortness of breath, myalgia, and loss of taste or smell.
ii. *Pathologic findings* are most prominent in the lungs, but may be also found in other major organs such as heart and blood vessels, kidneys, liver, gastrointestinal tract, skin and skeletal muscles.
iii. *Pulmonary symptoms* are related to interstitial viral pneumonia and prominent injury of the endothelial and alveolar cells forming the alveolar-capillary pulmonary units. These changes may heal on their own, or in more severe cases they may progress to acute respiratory distress syndrome (ARDS). Pathologic examination of lungs at autopsy usually shows evidence of alveolar cell injury accompanied by hyaline membrane formations, protein-rich pulmonary oedema and focal intra-alveolar hemorrhage. Bacterial superinfections are common.
iv. Pathologic changes affecting *endothelial cells of capillaries and venules* are seen not only in lungs but also in many other organs, most notably the heart, kidneys, and the gastrointestinal tract. Endothelial injury is often accompanied by *microthrombi* and consequent signs of ischaemic necrosis of adjacent parenchymal cells.
v. Even though there is no definitive evidence of viral infection of the *brain*, severely affected patients often show signs of abnormal mentation, including somnolence, confusion and incoherence. These findings are often ascribed to CRS.

Prognosis Clinical findings predictive of a severe course and poor outcome include:
- Respiratory rate >24 breaths per minute, heart rate >125 beats per minute, and oxygen saturation <90% on room air.
- Case fatality rate is estimated to be 1.4%.

Q23. What are the clinical features of varicella zoster virus infection?

Definition Varicella zoster is a DNA herpes virus which can cause of chickenpox (varicella) in non-immune persons and herpes zoster (shingles) in those who had chickenpox in the past.

Clinicopathologic aspects Two clinical presentations: i) varicella (chickenpox), and ii) herpes zoster.
i. **Varicella** presents as an acute inflammation of the nasopharynx.
a. Viraemia that follows is associated with an appearance of a maculopapular rash over the face and upper trunk, progressing to a vesicular exanthem.
b. Vesicles rupture and transform into scabs.
c. In a small number of infected persons, there is evidence of internal organ infection (e.g. encephalitis, pneumonia, hepatitis, etc.)
ii. **Herpes zoster** is a recurrent, painful, vesicular eruption in persons who have had chickenpox in childhood.
a. Exanthem results from reactivation of varicella zoster virus, residing in dorsal root spinal ganglia or cranial nerve ganglia following previous episode of chickenpox.
b. The virus spreads to sensory nerves and presents as vesicular exanthem limited to specific sensory dermatomes.

Q24. What are the clinical features of herpes simplex infection?

Definition Herpes viruses infections are caused by two DNA viruses: HSV-1 and HSV-2.

HSV-1 causes grouped vesicles of the skin, lips and mucosal surfaces of the respiratory and gastrointestinal tract.
i. Infection is spread by close person-to-person contact.
ii. Virus remains dormant in cranial nerve ganglia, most often trigeminal nerve ganglion.
iii. Virus can be reactivated and descends through the sensory nerves to the sensory area innervated by the corresponding cranial nerve.
iv. Reactivation of the virus follows stress, fever or respiratory infection.
v. Clinical symptoms are more severe in neonates and immunodeficient persons.
vi. Severe forms of HSV-1 infection include encephalitis, keratoconjunctivitis, hepatitis.
vii. HSV-I forms intranuclear inclusions which can be identified microscopically in H&E slides, or by immunohistochemistry.
HSV-2 causes genital herpes presenting with vesicles on the cervix, vagina, vulva.
i. The virus behaves like HSV-1 and remains dormant in the sacral spinal ganglia.
ii. Transmission is by sexual contact.
iii. Reactivation may occur during menstrual bleeding period or sexual intercourse.

Q25. What is rabies?

Definition Rabies is a form of viral encephalitis caused by *Rabies lyssavirus*, a single-stranded neurotropic rhabdovirus, transmitted to humans in saliva of carnivores, such a dogs, foxes, wolves, bats.
Clinicopathologic aspects Following the bite by the infected animal, the virus from the animal's saliva travels centripetally through the sensory nerves to the spinal cord and then to brainstem.
i. Clinical symptoms appear 10 days to 3 months later and include most notably a difficulty of swallowing due to the spasm of the throat muscles ('hydrophobia').
ii. Other symptoms of viral encephalopathy include irritability, seizure and delirium, invariably ending in death.
iii. Negri bodies are the diagnostic eosinophilic intracytoplasmic inclusions seen during microscopic examination of the brain sections.

Q26. What is poliomyelitis?

Definition Poliomyelitis is caused by poliovirus, an enterovirus which enters the body by the faeco-oral route. Most patients remain asymptomatic, but some of them may develop meningoencephalitis with paralysis of muscles.
Clinicopathologic aspects Polio virus has a propensity to invade epithelial cells of the nasopharynx and gastrointestinal tract.
i. From epithelial cells, the virus is transmitted to local lymphocytes and then may enter the blood.
ii. Viraemia is found in 5% infected persons, but most of them remain asymptomatic and recover without consequences.
iii. Meningoencephalitis develops in some infected and some of these develop paralytic polio (less than 1% of all infected).
iv. Paralytic polio is a consequence of motor neuron destruction in the anterior horn of the spinal cord or cerebral motor centers.
v. Clinically, it may be classified as spinal, bulbar or combined bulbospinal paralytic polio.
vi. Immunisation with inactivated oral polio vaccine has almost eradicated polio globally.
vii. *Histopathologic examination* of the spinal cord shows a loss of neurons in motor areas of CNS (e.g. anterior horns of spinal cord, cerebral bulbus), associated with loss of axons in peripheral nerves and denervation atrophy of skeletal muscles.

■ PARASITIC DISEASES

Q27. What is amoebiasis? Discuss its salient features.

Definition Amoebiasis is a chronic infection with *Entamoeba histolytica*, a protozoon most prevalent in tropical and subtropical countries with poor sanitation.

Clinicopathologic aspects The parasite occurs in two forms:

i. *trophozoite*, the active adult form is seen in the tissues and diarrhoeal stools, and

ii. *cystic form*, the infective stage found in faeces, contaminated water or food.

Trophozoites are formed from cysts and colonise the large intestine. They are excreted in faeces but do not survive, and those that survive and are ingested, are killed by gastric hydrochloric acid.

The most important pathologic changes are as under **(Fig. 8.5)**:

I. **Amoebic colitis** Trophozoites colonising the large intestine cause necrosis of the mucosa with subsequent formation of ulcers.

Ulcers are described as 'flask-shaped' due to their undermining margins.

Microscopically, the bottom of the ulcer is formed of granulation tissue, which is covered by an exudate containing PMNs, macrophages and trophozoites.

In some instances, the wall of the large intestine may show thickening resembling carcinoma and is called '*amoeboma*'.

II. **Amoebic liver abscess** It results from the entry of trophozoites into the radicles of portal vein. The abscess contains a yellowish-grey, paste-like, amorphous material composed of necrotic tissue and inflammatory exudate. Trophozoites can be identified at the interface between the necrotic and viable tissue.

III. **Abscesses in other sites** These may result from:
- The rupture of colon or liver abscesses with the dissemination of trophozoites in the peritoneal cavity (e.g. periappendiceal abscess, or subdiaphragmatic abscess).
- Entry of trophozoites into the systemic circulation may lead to formation of pulmonary abscesses, or brain abscesses, which are, however, rare.

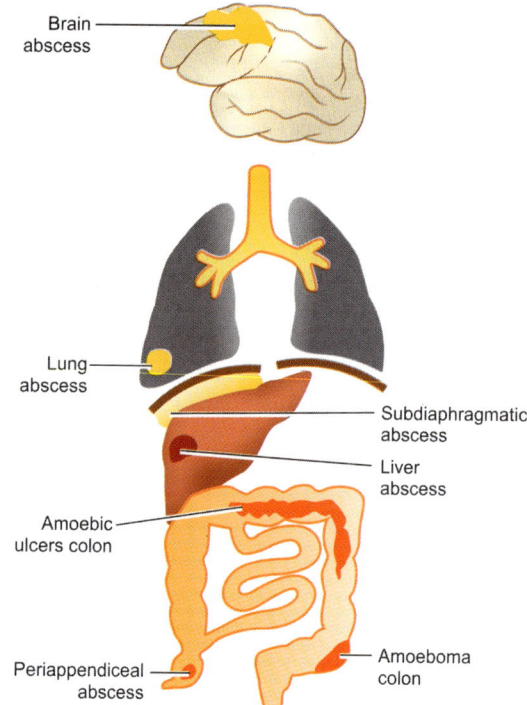

FIGURE 8.5: Lesions of amoebiasis.

Q28. What is malaria? Discuss its main features.

Definition Malaria is a chronic protozoal infection, that is endemic in tropical Africa, parts of Central and South America, India and South-East Asia.

Etiopathogenesis Malaria is caused by four species of plasmodia: *Plasmodium vivax, P. falciparum, P. ovale, P. malariae*. The life cycle of plasmodia is outlined in **Figure 8.6**.

P. falciparum differs from other plasmodia in following respects:

i. It does not have exo-erythrocytic stage.

ii. Erythrocytes of any age are parasitised, while other plasmodia parasitise only juvenile red blood cells.

iii. One red cell may contain more than one parasite.

iv. The parasitised red cells are sticky causing obstruction of small blood vessel thrombi, a feature that is responsible for the high virulence of *P. falciparum*.

Clinicopathologic aspects Parasitisation of RBCs accounts for the major pathologic changes including the following:

i. Malarial pigment liberated from destroyed RBCs accumulated in fixed macrophages, resulting in hepatosplenomegaly.

ii. Congestive heart failure is seen in long lasting disease.

iii. In falciparum malaria, there is massive absorption haemoglobin by renal tubules (*blackwater fever* or *haemoglobinuric nephrosis*).

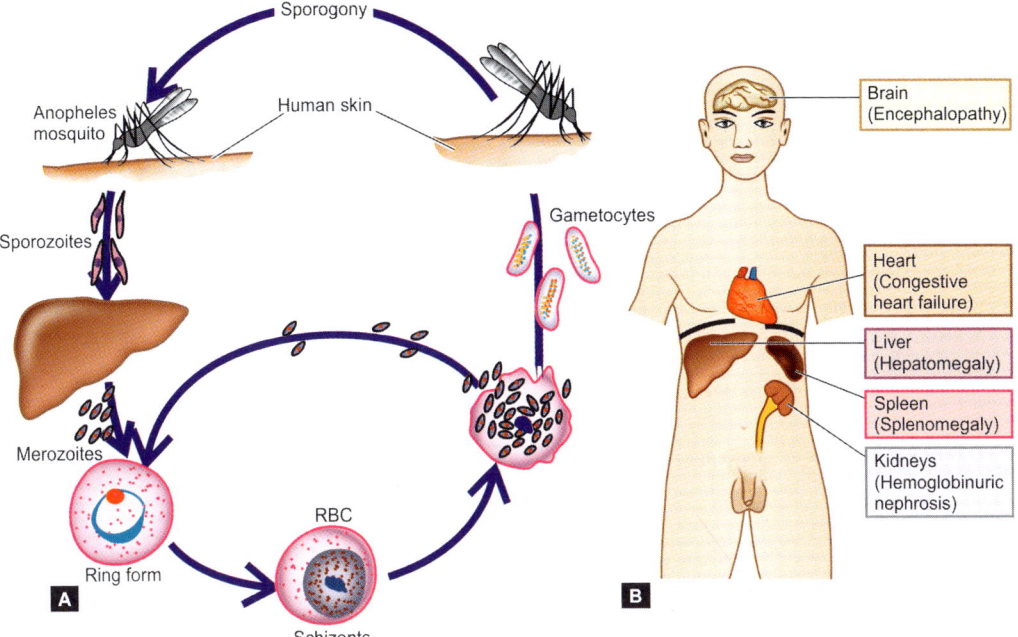

FIGURE 8.6: Life cycle of malaria (A) and major pathological changes in organs (B).

iv. In falciparum malaria, the RBCs are sticky and obstruct capillaries of internal organs and brain causing ischaemia accompanied by microhaemorrhages and microinfarcts.
v. At autopsy, cerebral malaria is characterised by congestion and petechial haemorrhages in the white matter.
vi. The diagnosis is made by demonstrating malarial parasites in RBCs in blood smears.
vii. Malaria parasites must be distinguished from *Babesia microti* or *B. divergens*.

Q29. What is babesiosis? Discuss its key features.

Definition Babesiosis is a deer tick-born infectious disease cause by protozoa of the genus *Babesia*, most often *B. microti*. Ticks transmitting babesiosis belong to the genus *Ixodes* (the same as Lyme disease, page 184).
Clinicopathologic aspects The infection may be asymptomatic or produce nonspecific constitutional symptoms like fever, malaise, fatigue, etc. In some instances it may produce high grade fever.
The diagnosis is made by identifying Babesia trophozoites in blood smears. Extracellular trophozoites can be seen in high grade parasitaemia.

Q30. Briefly discuss main features of filariasis.

Definition Filariasis is a helminthic infection with round worms, such as *Wucheria bancrofti* or *Brugia malayi* belonging to the genus *Filaroidea*. The infection is transmitted by black flies and mosquitoes.
Clinicopathologic aspects Wucheria and Brugia cause lymphatic filariasis.
i. Most infected patients remain asymptomatic.
ii. In acute form, there is lymphangitis, lymphadenitis, epididymo-orchitis, urticaria, eosinophilia and microfilariaemia.
iii. In chronic form, there is lymphoedema, hydrocele and elephantiasis.
iv. The diagnosis is made by identifying microfilaria in blood films.

Q31. What is cysticercosis? Discuss its main features.

Definition Cysticercosis is an infection by the larval stage of *Taenia solium*, the pork tapeworm.

Etiopathogenesis The adult tapeworms reside in the human intestines.
i. Eggs are passed in human faeces and thus passed to pigs, and on to vegetables.
ii. Human infection occurs after eating undercooked pork meat, or by ingesting infected vegetables, or rarely by autoinfection.
iii. Eggs develop into larvae in the host and spread through the host's blood to any site in the body forming cystic larvae called *Cysticercus cellulosae*.

Clinicopathologic aspects Cysticercus cysts may be found in different tissues and organs.
i. Cysts, which measure up to 1 cm in diameter, and are often multiple, produce symptoms most often in the brain, muscles and skin.
ii. The worm may remain viable in the cyst for long time without inducing inflammation.
iii. Once the worm dies, a granulomatous reaction and infiltrates of eosinophils develop around the cyst, which ultimately scars and calcifies.

Q32. What is the TORCH complex?

Definition TORCH is an acronym for the complex of clinicopathologic findings related to intrauterine foetal or perinatal infections caused by *t*oxoplasma, *r*ubella, *c*ytomegalovirus and *h*erpes virus. (Note that 'O' in TORCH stands for 'others', mostly viruses, such as mumps virus, coxsackievirus B, or hepatitis virus B).

Clinicopathologic aspects TORCH complex is diagnosed in 1–5% of neonates. The clinical features of infections caused by TORCH pathogens are indistinguishable one from another. Hence, the affected infant must be tested for all potential causes using serologic or molecular techniques. The most common finding include the following **(Fig. 8.7)**:
i. Microcephaly with neurologic symptoms
ii. Microphthalmia
iii. Sensorineural deafness
iv. Pneumonitis
v. Congenital heart disease
vi. Hepatomegaly with jaundice
vii. Splenomegaly with thrombocytopenia
viii. Skin petechiae and purpura

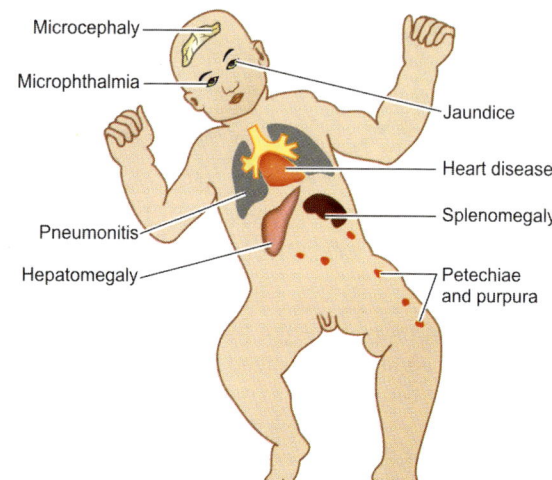

FIGURE 8.7: Lesions produced by TORCH complex infection in foetus *in utero*.

TORCH infection leaves irreparable consequence which cannot be treated. It is thus important to try to prevent these infections by immunisation (e.g. against rubella), or avoidance of exposure to toxoplasma during pregnancy (e.g. in cat faeces or raw meat), or to herpes virus during delivery.

Q33. What are the key features of biological agents used as potential bio-weapons?

Potential bioweapons have the following common features:
i. Cause high morbidity and mortality
ii. Effective in low dose, generally spread by aerosol
iii. Rapid spread from person-to-person
iv. Lack of availability of effective vaccine
v. Feasibility of its production

Q34. How are potential biologic threats classified according to the US Centers for Disease Control (US-CDC)?

Potential biological threats are classified by US-CDC into three categories (A, B, and C)
Category A agents pose greatest risk to life and security because they can be quickly disseminated and cause maximum mortality. This category includes the following disease pathogens:

i. Anthrax (*Bacillus anthracis*)
ii. Botulism (*Clostridium botulinum* toxin)
iii. Plague (*Yersinia pestis*)
iv. Smallpox (*Variola major*)
v. Tularaemia (*Francisella tularensis*)
vi. Viral haemorrhagic fevers

Category B agents fall into the moderate category in terms of their spread, morbidity and mortality and include the following examples:
i. Brucellosis
ii. Agents causing food poisoning (e.g. *Clostridium perfringens, Salmonella* species)
iii. Cholera-contaminated water supplies (*Vibrio cholerae*)

Category C agents which includes some emerging pathogens, mainly viruses, for which humans lack immunity. The examples are:
i. Hanta virus
ii. Respiratory coronaviruses such as influenza A/H5N1 (SARS-CoV1 agent for bird flu), novel coronavirus (SARS-CoV2 agent for covid19) causing severe acute respiratory syndrome (SARS).

> **Chapter 8e Supplement: Online Content**
>
> *Digital content of this chapter available with this book is meant for enhanced learning and self-assessment. In addition, it contains 23 Multiple Choice Questions (MCQs), 06 Clinicopathologic Vignettes, and 03 Image-based Questions; these are followed by their answers along with explanatory notes of correct and incorrect answers.*

CHAPTER 9

Environmental and Nutritional Diseases

ENVIRONMENTAL DISEASES

Q1. What are the most important environmental factors that cause diseases?
The most important environmental aspects of pathology are listed as under:
I. **Environmental pollution**
i. Air pollution
ii. Environmental chemicals
iii. Tobacco smoking
II. **Chemical and drug injury**
i. Therapeutic (iatrogenic) drug injury
ii. Non-therapeutic toxic agents (e.g. alcohol, drug abuse, carbon monoxide)
III. **Physical agents**
i. Thermal and electrical injury
ii. Injury by ionizing radiation

Q2. Discuss air pollution briefly.
Definition Air pollution refers to contamination of the aerial part of our natural environment with substances that could adversely affect human health.
Pollutants Any agent—chemical, physical or microbial, that alters the composition of the environment, is called *pollutant*. Pollutants can be classified as:
- *Visible* (e.g. dust and other particulate material).
- *Invisible* which includes common gases (e.g. carbon dioxide).

With regards to their distribution, pollutants may be found as contaminants of our *common (shared) environment*, such as the earth atmosphere, or they may be found in the *personal environment*, such as a room filled with tobacco smoke.

Q3. What are the main air pollutants?
Air pollutants may be primary or secondary:
- Air pollution results from release of huge amounts of gases generated by various human activities; such pollutants are called **primary pollutants**. The most important primary pollutants are carbon dioxide, sulphur oxide, nitrogen oxide, and dust and various atmospheric particulate matters. The most important source of pollutant gases are fossil fuels used in factories, cars and dwellings for cooking and heating or cooling.
- **Secondary pollutants** are generated in the atmosphere, e.g. free oxygen radicals formed from primary oxides exposed to sunshine. Depletion of the ozone layer by atmospheric pollutants favours the formation of free oxygen radicals, thus contributing to the formation of secondary pollutants.

Q4. What determines the adverse effects of air pollutants?

The adverse effects depend on the following:
i. Duration of exposure.
ii. Total dose of exposure.
iii. Chemical composition of the pollutant.
iv. Particle size; small particles (in the range of 1–5 µm) more likely to get impacted in the lungs than larger particles which are cleared by mucus and ciliary activity of cells of the upper respiratory tract and bronchi.

Q5. Which environmental chemicals have adverse health effects?

i. *Agricultural chemicals* such as pesticides, herbicides, organic fertilisers:
a. Acute poisoning by organophosphate insecticides, which inhibit acetyl cholinesterase and are neurotoxic.
b. Chronic exposure, possibly causing cancer, chronic degenerative diseases, etc.
ii. *Volatile organic solvents and vapours* such as methanol, chloroform, kerosene, petrol, etc.
iii. *Metals* such as mercury, arsenic, nickel.
iv. *Aromatic hydrocarbons* containing polychlorinated biphenyl are common contaminants in herbicides, preservatives and antibacterial substances.
v. *Cyanide* released during combustion of plastic or silk. It is also found in cassava and the seeds of apricots and wild cherries.
vi. *Environmental dust*.

Q6. How does tobacco smoking affect human health?

i. **Tobacco smoking** is the most prevalent and preventable cause of human disease and death. The most important components of tobacco smoke, listed according to the mechanism of their action are listed in **Table 9.1**.

ii. **Other forms of tobacco exposure** are associated with similar adverse effects as seen in India, as below:
- Smoking *bidis* or chewing *pan masala*, *zarda* and *gutka* are more common than smoking but have the same adverse effects.
- Smoking *chutta* in the state of Andhra Pradesh is associated with higher incidence of squamous cell carcinoma of the hard palate.
- Holding a bolus of *paan* admixed to tobacco in the mouth for long time, as practiced by individuals in the states of Uttar Pradesh and Bihar, is associated with an increased incidence of cancer of the mouth and upper aerodigestive system.

TABLE 9.1 Major constituents of tobacco smoke with adverse effects.

ADVERSE EFFECT	CONSTITUENTS
1. *Carcinogenesis*	➢ Tar ➢ Polycyclic aromatic hydrocarbons ➢ Nitrosamines
2. *Tumour promoters*	➢ Nicotine ➢ Phenol
3. *Irritation and toxicity to respiratory mucosa*	➢ Formaldehyde ➢ Nitrogen oxide
4. *Reduced oxygen transport*	➢ Carbon monoxide

Q7. What are the most important tobacco-related diseases?

The risk of developing certain diseases or dying from those diseases is much higher in smokers than non-smokers living under the same circumstances. The estimated risk rates for the most important tobacco-related diseases are presented in **Figure 9.1** and listed in descending order of frequency as follows:
i. Lung cancer (12–23 times)
ii. Chronic obstructive lung disease (10–13 times)
iii. Cancers of upper aerodigestive tract (lip, oral cavity, oesophagus, nasopharynx, larynx) (6–14 times)
iv. Aortic aneurysm (6–7 times)
v. Cancers of internal organs (stomach, pancreas, kidney, urinary bladder, cervix) (2–3 times)
vi. Coronary heart disease and cerebrovascular accidents (2–3 times)
vii. Buerger disease (5–6 times)

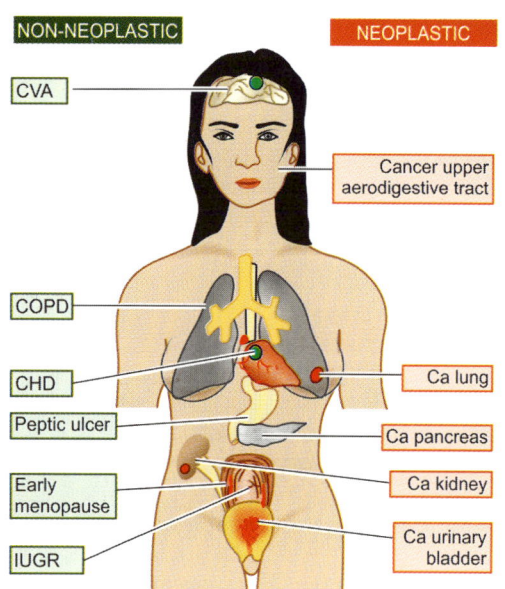

FIGURE 9.1: Major adverse effects of tobacco smoking. *Right side* shows smoking-related neoplastic diseases while *left side* indicates non-neoplastic diseases associated with smoking, numbered serially in order of frequency of occurrence.

viii. Peptic ulcer (70% higher in smokers than in non-smokers)
ix. Early menopause in women smokers
x. Smoking during pregnancy affects the foetus with the following consequences: lower birth weight higher perinatal mortality, and subsequent intellectual impairment.

Q8. What determines the adverse effects of therapeutic (iatrogenic) drug injury?

The adverse effects of drugs depend on the following:
i. Overdose
ii. Genetic predisposition
iii. Exaggerated pharmacologic response
iv. Interaction with other drugs
v. Unknown factors

Q9. What are the main adverse effects of alcohol?

Alcohol is absorbed in the stomach and small intestine. 2–10% of absorbed alcohol is excreted in urine, sweat or breath. As depicted in **Figure 9.2,** alcohol is metabolised in the liver through:
- the alcohol dehydrogenase and aldehyde dehydrogenase system (80%),
- microsomal ethanol oxidizing system (MEOS) (10%), and
- only in small amounts through the catalase in peroxisomes.

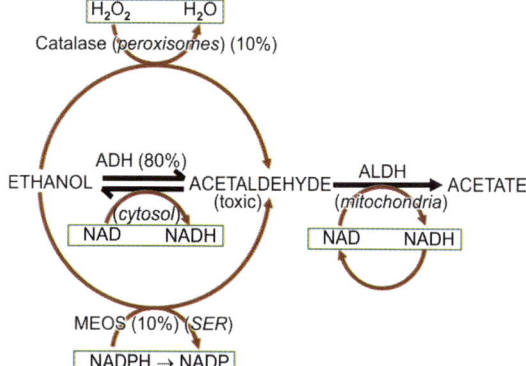

FIGURE 9.2: Metabolism of ethanol in the liver. Thickness and intensity of colour of arrow on left side of figure corresponds to extent of metabolic pathway followed.
(MEOS, microsomal ethanol oxidizing system; ADH, alcohol dehydrogenase; ALDH, aldehyde dehydrogenase; NAD, nicotinamide adenine dinucleotide; NADH, reduced NAD; NADP, nicotinamide adenine dinucleotide phosphate; NADPH, reduced NADP).

The adverse effects are classified as acute and chronic:

I. **Acute adverse effects** are mostly related to the central nervous system and to a lesser extent to irritation of stomach (acute gastritis and ulceration with vomiting and nausea), and liver (fatty change). The effects of alcohol depend on the amount consumed, as reflected by blood levels of alcohol:

i. *Blood level of 100 mg/dL* (the upper limit of sobriety in most western countries) causes behavioural changes, cortical dysfunction and mild motor ataxia.

ii. *Blood level of 100–200 mg/dL* causes depression of cortical centres, lack of coordination, impaired judgement and drowsiness.

iii. *Blood level of about 300 mg/dL* causes stupor and coma.

iv. *Blood level above 400 mg/dL* may cause anaesthesia, depression of vital medullary centres, and death from respiratory arrest.

II. **Chronic alcoholism** affects many organs, reflecting the direct toxic effects of alcohol and its main metabolite *acetaldehyde*. The following are the most important clinicopathologic changes **(Fig. 9.3)**:

i. **Liver** Steatosis, which may be reversible but may also progress to steatohepatitis and then to cirrhosis.

ii. **Pancreas** Acute and chronic pancreatitis.

iii. **Gastrointestinal tract** Gastritis, peptic ulcer and oesophageal varices due to cirrhosis and portal hypertension. Higher incidence of cancer of the mouth, oesophagus and upper aerodigestive system.

iv. **Central nervous system** Peripheral neuropathy, Wernicke-Korsakoff syndrome, cerebellar atrophy, and degeneration with amblyopia.

v. **Cardiovascular system** Alcoholic cardiomyopathy.

vi. **Endocrine system** Testicular atrophy, gynaecomastia, and reduced libido due to low levels of testosterone in blood.

vii. **Blood** Haematopoietic dysfunction with secondary megaloblastic anaemia.

viii. **Immune system** Decreased resistance to infections.

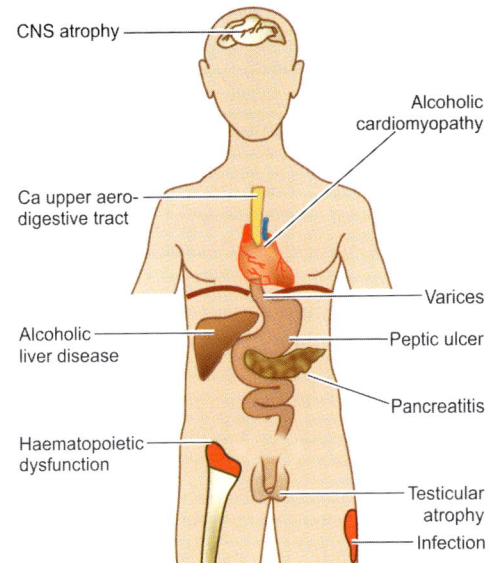

FIGURE 9.3: Complications of chronic alcoholism.

Q10. What are the clinicopathologic features of lead poisoning?

Etiopathogenesis Lead poisoning may be due to *accidental or industrial exposure.*

In children, it is most often accidental, related to chewing lead-containing furniture items, toys and pencils, or eating lead paint flakes from walls.

In adults, it is most often due to occupational exposure (spray painting, production or recycling of car batteries, lead mining or melting). Accidental exposure stems from contaminated water pipes, inhalation of house paint or sniffing lead-containing petrol.

Clinicopathologic aspects Lead enters the body through the GI system and lungs. Lead accumulates in two types of tissues **(Fig. 9.4)**:

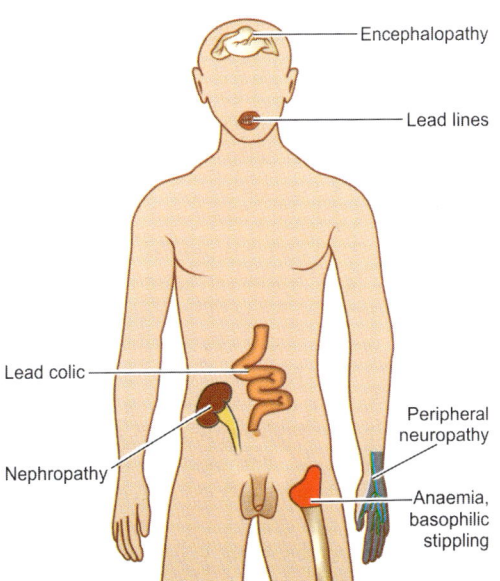

FIGURE 9.4: Complications of lead poisoning.

I. **90%** of lead accumulates in tissues where it causes **no significant harm** (e.g. bone, teeth and gingiva, hair, and nails).
i. On physical examination, one can see dark blue *'lead lines'* on the gingiva.
ii. *Linear bone densities* in the metaphyses of growing bones of children and adolescents are seen by X-rays.
iii. Lead that has accumulated in hair and nails can be demonstrated by chemical analysis. These tests are used to document lead exposure.
II. **10%** of lead accumulates in **internal organs** where it is toxic. These organs include brain, gastrointestinal tract, kidneys and bone marrow.
i. *Central nervous system* Developing brain is most sensitive to lead poisoning.
a. *In children*, lead poisoning presents with headaches, irritability and drowsiness.
- Long-term exposure may retard child's intellectual development.
- Pathologic findings of *lead encephalopathy*, are however, nonspecific.
b. *In adults*, there is *demyelinating peripheral neuropathy* affecting most prominently the radial and peroneal nerve and causing wrist-drop or foot-drop.
ii. *Haematopoietic system* Lead toxicity presents as *microcytic hypochromic anaemia*. It develops due to the inhibition of two enzymes: *delta-aminolaevulinic acid dehydrogenase*, an enzyme that is important for the synthesis of haem; and *ferroketolase*, required for the incorporation of the ferrous iron into the porphyrin ring. Peripheral blood smears show prominent *basophilic stripling of red blood cells*.
iii. *Kidneys* Lead is nephrotoxic and the cumulative renal sings of lead toxicity are known as *lead nephropathy*.
Microscopic changes include formation of lead intranuclear inclusion bodies in proximal tubules associated with functional disorders, such as aminoaciduria.
iv. *Gastrointestinal tract* Lead poisoning affects the intestines. It may cause *colics* and signs of acute abdomen.

Q11. What are the clinicopathologic features of carbon monoxide poisoning?

Definition Carbon monoxide (CO) poisoning, which may be acute or chronic, results from binding of CO to haemoglobin with consequent formation of carboxy-haemoglobin, which interferes with the transport of oxygen.
Etiopathogenesis Carbon monoxide is found in automobile exhaust fumes, fumes generated by burning of fossil fuels in home and industry, and tobacco smoke.
i. CO has a high affinity for haemoglobin (200-times higher than oxygen!).
ii. Carboxy-haemoglobin formed from CO + haemoglobin prevents the binding of oxygen to haemoglobin and the release of oxygen from haemoglobin.
iii. The diagnosis is made by measuring the level of carboxy-haemoglobin in blood.
Pathology Acute CO poisoning may be lethal within minutes.
- At autopsy, there is brain oedema and focal cerebral haemorrhages.
- Chronic lead poisoning presents with nonspecific cerebral changes.
- Clinical findings are also nonspecific and include headache, fatigue, irritability and insomnia.

Q12. What are the clinicopathologic features of drug abuse?

Definition Drug abuse is defined as intake of certain drugs for the purpose of 'mood alteration', 'euphoria', or 'kick', leading to habit-forming dependence and eventually to addiction.
Etiopathogenesis Some of the commonly abused drugs include marijuana, opium derivatives, CNS stimulants or depressants, psychedelic drugs.
Clinicopathologic aspects Drug abuse is associated with a large number of medical and social problems.
i. Many illicit drugs cause behavioural and psychiatric aberrations.
ii. There is an increased incidence of suicides and criminal acts.
iii. Drug overdose is a common cause of death.
iv. Sharing of needles is associated with transmission of viral diseases such as hepatitis C and B, human immunodeficiency virus.
v. *Common infections* in drug addicts are as follows:
a. Cellulitis at the site of infection, complicated by formation of subcutaneous abscess, ulcers and venous thrombosis

b. Thrombophlebitis
c. Bacterial endocarditis
d. Talc granulomas in the lungs
e. Viral infections such as AIDS or viral hepatitis
f. Focal glomerulonephritis

Q13. What are the clinicopathologic features of thermal and electrical injury?

Definition Hypothermia denotes a fall of body temperature below 35°C. Hyperthermia is body temperature above 41°C.
Types and effects Both hypothermia and hyperthermia may be localised or systemic.
i. *Localised hypothermia* → frostbite
ii. Systemic hypothermia → death due to freezing in snow
iii. *Localised hyperthermia* → burns
iv. Systemic hyperthermia → fever
v. *Electrical injury* → local burn at the site of entry, due to electric energy.
NOTE: Electric injury may damage the conduction system of the heart and cause *ventricular fibrillation*.

Q14. What are the clinicopathologic features of radiation injury?

Ionising radiation, the most important cause of radiation injury can produce three types of cell injury:
- cell killing,
- genetic damage causing mutations that are transmitted to next generation, and
- malignant transformation of cells.

These changes are mostly mediated by the radiolysis of the cellular water with subsequent formation of hydroxyl radicals.
Tissue injury results most often from radiation-induced endothelial cell injury and subsequent ischaemic necrosis due to the reduced blood flow. Fibrosis is a common pathologic finding.
Clinicopathologic aspects of ionising radiation-induced are in different organs and tissues:
i. Skin: Radiation dermatitis, cancer.
ii. Lungs: Interstitial pulmonary fibrosis.
iii. Heart: Myocardial fibrosis. Constrictive pericarditis.
iv. Kidney: Radiation nephritis.
v. Gastrointestinal tract: Strictures of oesophagus and intestines.
vi. Gonads: Testicular atrophy and destruction of ovaries.
vii. Haematopoietic tissue: Pancytopenia due to bone marrow depression and fibrosis.
viii. Eyes: Cataracts.

■ NUTRITIONAL DISEASES

Q15. What is the difference between primary and secondary nutritional deficiency?

Primary nutritional deficiency is due to either a lack of a decreased amount of essential nutrients in diet.
Secondary nutritional deficiency results from interference with one or more factors that regulate food intake, metabolism and utilisation as given below:
i. *Interference with ingestion* Intake of nutrients may be interrupted by a variety of gastrointestinal diseases such as stenosis of the oesophagus, malabsorption syndrome, anorexia and psychiatric disorders, food allergy, etc.
ii. *Interference with absorption* Absorption of nutrients may be impeded by achlorhydria in chronic atrophic gastritis, chronic pancreatitis, biliary obstruction, lymphoma of the small intestine, etc.
iii. *Interference with utilisation* Nutrient utilisation is defective in chronic liver disease, malignancy, hypothyroidism.
iv. *Increased excretion and loss* Examples in this category are lactation, diarrhoea, polyuria, perspiration.
v. *Increased nutritional demand* Examples of increased demand is encountered during pregnancy, lactation, fever, hyperthyroidism.

Q16. What is obesity and how does it affect the health?

Definition Obesity is an excess of adipose tissue that imparts health risk; a body weight of 20% excess over ideal weight for age, sex and height is considered a health risk.

Obesity is gauged by calculating the *body mass index (BMI)* which is expressed as body weight in kg/height in m². Obesity is defined as BMI over 30 for men and women alike. Overweight is defined as BMI between 24 and 30.

Etiopathogenesis Obesity is usually multifactorial, including factors of nature and nurture.

i. *Overeating,* i.e. excessive calorie intake.

ii. *Sedentary lifestyle* and a lack of physical activity.

iii. *Genetic predisposition* Obesity runs in families, and has high coincidence among identical twins. Obesity genes are discovered such as *OB* gene and its protein product leptin (energy regulatory hormone) and *DB* gene for leptin receptor.

iv. *Carbohydrates and fat-rich diet* rather than diet based on proteins.

v. *Secondary obesity* due to medical conditions such as hypothyroidism, Cushing syndrome, hypothalamic disorders, etc.

vi. *Hormones and cytokines produced by adipocytes* probably play a significant role in obesity but the details are not fully known. Examples of such molecules are:

a. Leptin, an energy regulatory hormone
b. Insulin sensitivity regulating agents (adiponectin, resistin, and RPB4)
c. Tumour necrosis factor alpha (TNF-α)
d. Interleukin-6

Pathology Obesity is characterised by an excessive accumulation of *lipids* in adipocytes and some parenchymal internal organs.

i. Adipocytes storing fat are found in the subcutaneous tissue, retroperitoneum, omentum, and in a more limited form, in internal organs such as skeletal muscle, heart, kidney, pancreas, liver, to mention just the most important anatomic sites.

ii. Adipocytes enlarge and multiply; accordingly, there is both hypertrophy and hyperplasia.

iii. Fatty liver is common in obese persons.

Q17. What are the major clinicopathologic consequences of obesity?

Obesity has many clinicopathologic consequences; the most important ones are shown in **Figure 9.5** and listed as under:

i. **Hyperinsulinaemia** in response to insulin resistance and tissue insensitivity.

ii. **Type 2 diabetes mellitus,** which is aggravated by obesity and becomes more manageable after weight loss.

iii. **Hypertension,** which may be reduced by weight loss.

iv. **Hyperlipoproteinaemia**, especially with a concentration of very low density lipoproteins.

v. **Atherosclerosis,** which together with hypertension, contributes to an increased incidence of myocardial infarcts and stroke.

vi. **Nonalcoholic fatty liver disease** (NAFLD), which may progress to steatohepatitis and cirrhosis.

vii. **Cholelithiasis**, which is 6-times more common in obese people than non-obese persons of the same age.

viii. **Hypoventilation syndrome** (Pickwickian syndrome), which is marked by shallow breathing, carbon dioxide retention and hypersomnolence, generalised hypoxia and secondary polycythaemia.

ix. **Osteoarthritis** due to accelerated wear and tear of articular cartilage as a result of large body weight.

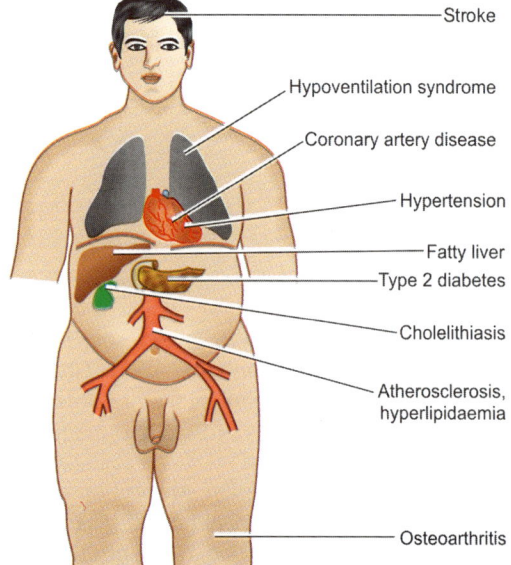

FIGURE 9.5: Major clinicopathologic sequelae of obesity.

x. **Cancer**, which is more common in obese than in non-obese persons. These epidemiologic association data pertain to carcinoma of colon, breast, prostate and endometrium.

Q18. What is starvation? Discuss its etiopathogenesis and pathophysiology.

Definition Starvation is a state of overall deprivation of nutrients. It results in body wasting, reduction of the muscle mass, atrophy of internal organs, and lax atrophic skin.

Etiopathogenesis Starvation has several possible causes:
i. Deliberate fasting, such as political hunger strike, religious fast, etc.
ii. Famine conditions due to poverty, disasters, political events, etc.
iii. Secondary undernutrition due to chronic wasting diseases such as cancer, tuberculosis, cirrhosis, etc.

Pathophysiology Adaptive changes involve the metabolism of glucose, proteins and lipids.
i. *Glucose stores* are enough just for one day and must be maintained. Insulin-dependent tissues like skeletal muscles stop taking up glucose, whereas insulin-independent tissues like brain and blood cells continue utilising glucose. Liver will release glucose into the blood to maintain the normal concentration.
ii. *Proteins* are released from stores that contain reserves for 3 months. Amino acids formed from released proteins are taken up by the liver for neo-glucogenesis and adequate supply of glucose to the brain. Degradation of proteins results in negative nitrogen balance and excretion on nitrogen compounds in urine.
iii. *Fat breakdown* into triglycerides and fatty acids starts after one week to preserve proteins. Ketone bodies produced by the liver become the major source of energy for the brain and many other organs, reducing the need for glucose.

Q19. What is the difference between kwashiorkor and marasmus?

Kwashiorkor and marasmus are two distinct forms of protein-energy malnutrition (PEM):
- *Kwashiorkor* is protein deficiency in the presence of sufficient calorie intake.
- *Marasmus* is starvation of infants under the age of 1 year due to an overall lack of calories.

The clinical findings are most pronounced in infants and small children; contrasting features of the two are illustrated in **Figure 9.6** and summarised in **Table 9.2**.

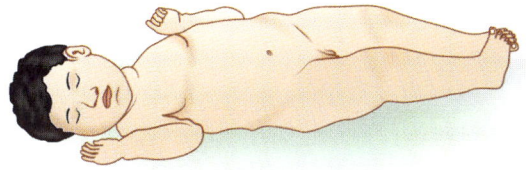 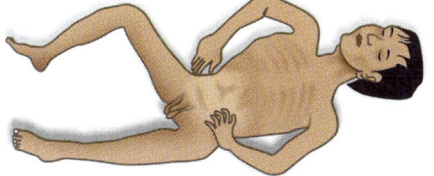

A, KWASHIORKOR B, MARASMUS

FIGURE 9.6: Two forms of PEM.

TABLE 9.2 Contrasting features of kwashiorkor and marasmus.

FEATURE	KWASHIORKOR	MARASMUS
Definition	Protein deficiency with sufficient calorie intake	Starvation in infants with overall lack of calories
Clinical features	➤ Occurs in children between 6 months and 3 years of age ➤ Growth failure ➤ Wasting of muscles but preserved adipose tissues ➤ Oedema, localised or generalised, present ➤ Enlarged fatty liver ➤ Serum proteins low ➤ Anaemia present ➤ 'Flag sign'—alternate bands of light (depigmented) and dark (pigmented) hair	➤ Common in infants under 1 year of age ➤ Growth failure ➤ Wasting of all tissues including muscles and adipose tissues ➤ Oedema absent ➤ No hepatic enlargement ➤ Serum proteins low ➤ Anaemia present ➤ Monkey-like face, protuberant abdomen, thin limbs
Morphology	➤ Enlarged fatty liver ➤ Atrophy of different tissues and organs but subcutaneous fat preserved	➤ No fatty liver ➤ Atrophy of different tissues and organs including subcutaneous fat

Q20. What are the clinicopathologic conditions caused by deficiency of minerals?

Deficiencies of several minerals result in distinct clinicopathologic changes as under:
i. **Iron:** Microcytic hypochromic anaemia.
ii. **Calcium**: Reduced bone mass, osteoporosis.
iii. **Phosphorus:** Rickets, osteomalacia.
iv. **Copper:** Muscle weakness, neurologic defects, anaemia, growth retardation.
v. **Iodine**: Goitre, hypothyroidism, cretinism.
vi. **Zinc:** Growth retardation, infertility, alopecia.
vii. **Fluoride:** Dental caries.

Q21. Define vitamins. How they are classified? List the various vitamin deficiencies.

Definition Vitamins are organic compounds which cannot be synthesised within the body and are essential for normal maintenance of normal cell structure and function.
Classification Vitamins are divided into two groups: fat-soluble and water-soluble **(Table 9.3)**.
I. *Fat-soluble vitamins* include four vitamins: A, D, E and K.
- They are absorbed in the intestine in the presence of bile salts and pancreatic enzymes.
- Deficiency of these vitamins is usually related to conditioning factors (*secondary deficiency*).
- Hypervitaminoses due to excess of vitamin A and D are clinically recognised.

II. *Water-soluble vitamins* include vitamin C and members of the vitamin B group; plus the newly added vitamins, namely choline, biotin, and flavonoids.
- Since they are water soluble, they are lost much easier than fat-soluble vitamins during cooking and processing of food.

TABLE 9.3 Vitamin deficiencies.

VITAMINS	DEFICIENCY DISORDERS
I. FAT-SOLUBLE VITAMINS	
Vitamin A (Retinol)	➢ Ocular lesions (night blindness, xerophthalmia, keratomalacia, Bitot's spots, blindness) ➢ Cutaneous lesions (xeroderma) ➢ Other lesions (squamous metaplasia of respiratory epithelium, urothelium and pancreatic ductal epithelium, subsequent anaplasia; retarded bone growth)
Vitamin D (Calcitriol)	➢ Rickets in growing children ➢ Osteomalacia in adults ➢ Hypocalcaemic tetany
Vitamin E (α-Tocopherol)	➢ Degeneration of neurons, retinal pigments, axons of peripheral nerves; denervation of muscles ➢ Reduced red cell lifespan ➢ Sterility in male and female animals
Vitamin K	➢ Hypoprothrombinaemia (in haemorrhagic disease of newborn, biliary obstruction, malabsorption, anticoagulant therapy, antibiotic therapy, diffuse liver disease)
II. WATER-SOLUBLE VITAMINS	
Vitamin C (Ascorbic acid)	Scurvy (haemorrhagic diathesis, skeletal lesions, delayed wound healing, anaemia, lesions in teeth and gums)
Vitamin B Complex i. *Thiamine (Vitamin B_1)*	Beriberi ('dry' or peripheral neuritis, 'wet' or cardiac manifestations, 'cerebral' or Wernicke-Korsakoff's syndrome)
ii. *Riboflavin (Vitamin B_2)*	Ariboflavinosis (ocular lesions, cheilosis, glossitis, dermatitis)
iii. *Niacin/Nicotinic acid (Vitamin B_3)*	Pellagra (dermatitis, diarrhoea, dementia)
iv. *Pyridoxine (Vitamin B_6)*	Vague lesions (convulsions in infants, dermatitis, cheilosis, glossitis, sideroblastic anaemia)
v. *Folate/Folic acid*	Megaloblastic anaemia
vi. *Cyanocobalamin (Vitamin B_{12})*	Megaloblastic anaemia Pernicious anaemia
vii. *Biotin*	Mental and neurological symptoms
Choline	Fatty liver, muscle damage
Flavonoids	Preventive of neurodegenerative disease, osteoporosis, diabetes

Etiology of deficiency Deficiency may be primary or secondary:
I. *Primary vitamin deficiency* is caused by generalised malnutrition of dietary origin. It occurs more often in underdeveloped countries than in North America and Europe. Usually, it includes the deficiency of several vitamins.
II. *Secondary vitamin deficiency* is related to conditioned nutritional deficiency linked to specific diseases that affect the intake, absorption, digestion or utilisation of nutrients. It usually presents as a deficiency of a single vitamin. Chronic alcoholism is a common denominator in many vitamin deficiencies.

Q22. What are the clinicopathologic features of vitamin A deficiency?

Physiology Vitamin A has several metabolic functions, the most important of which are as under:
- *Maintenance of normal vision* in reduced light by mediating the synthesis of rhodopsin and iodopsins in retinal cells of the eye.
- *Maintenance of structure and function of specialised epithelia*, most notably mucus-secreting cells, respiratory epithelium and urothelium.

Etiopathogenesis
- Nutritional vitamin A deficiency is a component of *general malnutrition* that is common in underdeveloped countries of South-East Asia, Africa and Central and South America.
- In developed countries, it is a *conditioned deficiency* and usually a part of malabsorption syndromes.

Clinicopathologic aspects Vitamin A deficiency-related changes are seen in the eyes, on the skin and in some internal organs **(Fig. 9.7)**:

i. **Eye lesions** include *night blindness*, *xerophthalmia* (dry eyes due to the replacement of mucus-secreting cells by squamous cells in adnexal glands), *ulceration of cornea* with infection, *keratomalacia* with softening of the cornea. *Bitot spots* are triangular keratinised opacities on the cornea that form in some cases. Ultimately, all these changes may progress and cause *blindness*.

ii. **Cutaneous lesions** include papular form of xeroderma due to follicular hyperkeratosis and keratotic plugging of the sebaceous glands at the neck of hair follicles.

iii. **Squamous metaplasia of specialised epithelia**
a. Squamous metaplasia of the respiratory epithelium predisposes to bacterial infections.
b. Squamous metaplasia of the pancreatic duct can cause obstruction and chronic pancreatitis.
c. Squamous metaplasia of the urothelium will predispose to formation of urinary stones and pyelonephritis.

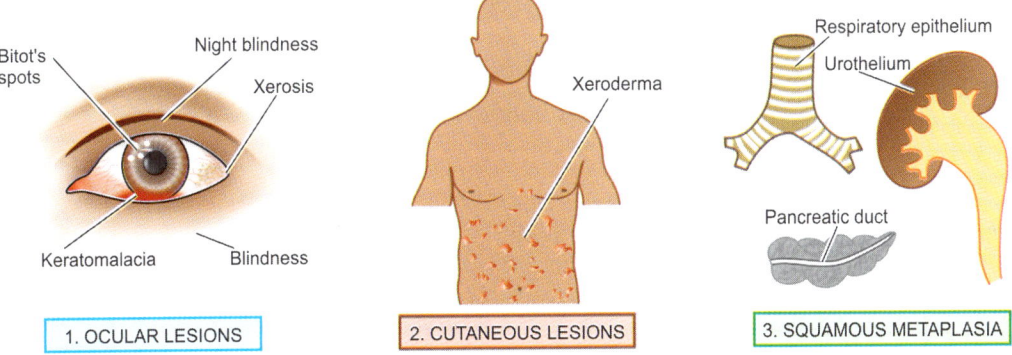

FIGURE 9.7: Lesions resulting from vitamin A deficiency.

Q23. What are the clinicopathologic features of vitamin D deficiency?

Physiology The most important function of vitamin D is the maintenance of normal plasma levels of calcium and phosphorus. It also participates in the mineralisation of bones.
Maintenance of calcium/phosphate levels in blood is accomplished by following mechanisms:
i. Stimulating intestinal absorption of calcium and phosphorus.
ii. Mobilising calcium and phosphorus from bone in hypocalcaemia in collaboration with parathyroid hormone. It is to be noted that this effect is contrary to the effects of the vitamin D on growing bones in normocalcaemia, when this vitamin promotes deposition of calcium into the osteoid facilitating ossification.

iii. Stimulating parathyroid-dependent reabsorption of calcium from the primary filtrate in renal tubules back into the blood stream.

Etiopathogenesis Vitamin D deficiency may develop due to inadequate endogenous synthesis and metabolism or due to dietary deficiency:

i. *Defective endogenous synthesis* Approximately 70% of vitamin D is normally synthesised in the skin under the influence of sunlight. Lack of sun exposure may reduce endogenous vitamin D production.

ii. *Insufficient intake of vitamin D in food* Vitamin D is found in deep sea fish, fish oil, egg, butter, milk and some plants. Restricted or unusual dietary habits in the elderly may cause nutritional vitamin D deficiency.

iii. *Inadequate absorption of vitamin D in the intestine* This occurs in fat malabsorption syndromes due to intestinal, biliary or pancreatic insufficiency.

iv. *Defective conversion of vitamin D into its active form (1,25 dihydroxy vitamin D)* This two step conversion takes place in the liver and the kidneys. It may be blocked in chronic liver and kidney diseases.

Clinicopathologic aspects Vitamin D deficiency presents clinically as:
- rickets in growing children, and
- osteomalacia in adults.

I. **Rickets** It results from defective mineralisation of osteoid. The pathogenesis of rickets is best understood by contrasting the pathologic and physiologic changes **(Table 9.4)**.

TABLE 9.4 Pathogenesis of rickets in comparison with normal bone growth.

NORMAL BONE GROWTH	RICKETS
I. ENDOCHONDRAL OSSIFICATION (occurring in long tubular bones)	
i. Proliferation of cartilage cells at the epiphyses followed by provisional mineralisation	i. Proliferation of cartilage cells at the epiphyses followed by inadequate provisional mineralisation
ii. Cartilage resorption and replacement by osteoid matrix	ii. Persistence and overgrowth of epiphyseal cartilage; deposition of osteoid matrix on inadequately mineralised cartilage resulting in enlarged and expanded costochondral junctions
iii. Mineralisation to form bone	iii. Deformed bones due to lack of structural rigidity
iv. Normal vascularisation of bone	iv. Irregular overgrowth of small blood vessels in disorganised and weak bone
II. INTRAMEMBRANOUS OSSIFICATION (occurring in flat bones)	
Mesenchymal cells differentiate into osteoblasts which develop osteoid matrix and subsequent mineralisation	Mesenchymal cells differentiate into osteoblasts with laying down of osteoid matrix which fails to get mineralised resulting in soft and weak flat bones

The most important pathologic changes are presented in **Figure 9.8** and described as follows:

i. *Craniotabes* (square box-like skull resulting from excess of non-calcified osteoid of fronto-occipital cranial bones)

ii. *Thoracic cage changes* such as *pigeon chest deformity* involving the sternum, *Harrison sulcus* due to inspiratory curve of the lower costal thoracic margin, and rachitic rosary involving the costo-chondral junctions of the ribs.

iii. *Deformities of the extremities* including bow legs, knocked knees enlargement of the lower epiphyses of radius.

iv. *Lumbar lordosis*.

II. **Osteomalacia** is the adult counterpart of rickets. Microscopic examination reveals broad seams of non-calcified osteoid rimming the narrow central calcified bone spicules. Clinical findings include:

i. Fractures following trivial trauma
ii. Incomplete greenstick fractures
iii. Pseudofractures (Looser zones)
iv. Vague bone pain
v. Muscle weakness

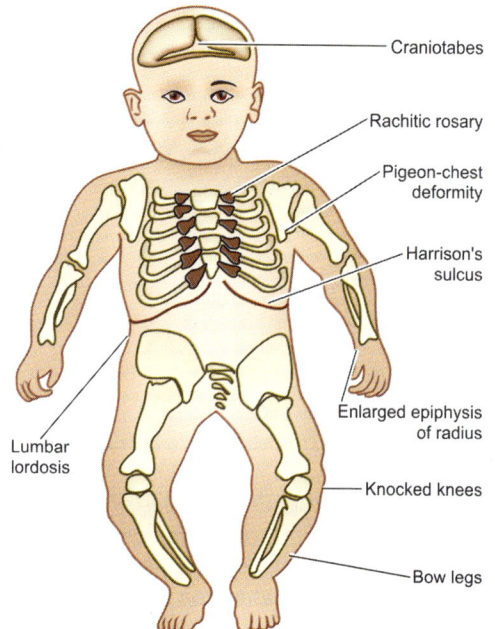

FIGURE 9.8: Clinicopathologic lesions in rickets.

Q24. What are the clinicopathologic features of vitamin D hypervitaminosis?

Vitamin D administered in large amounts will cause hypercalcaemia and hyperphosphataemia due to increased absorption of Ca and P in the intestines, and increased bone resorption.

Hypercalcaemia and **hyperphosphataemia** have the following consequences:
i. Massive excretion of calcium and phosphorus in urine.
ii. Formation of urinary calculi.
iii. Widespread metastatic calcification in the kidneys, heart, arteries, lungs and stomach.
iv. Osteoporosis and loss of calcified bone spicules due to the mobilization of Ca and P from the bone.

Q25. What are the clinicopathologic features of vitamin K deficiency?

Vitamin K is essential for the *synthesis of vitamin K-dependent coagulation factors*: prothrombin (factor II), and factors VII, IX, and X. Hypovitaminosis K leads to *uncontrolled bleeding*.
Physiology Vitamin K is ingested in food and synthesised endogenously.
- Exogenous vitamin K is found in green leafy vegetables as phylloquinone (K_1).
- Vitamin K is fat soluble and its absorption in the small intestine requires bile and pancreatic enzymes.
- Endogenous vitamin K is produced by normal intestinal bacterial flora as menaquinone (K_2).
- Plasma concentration of prothrombin is a reliable indicator of vitamin K stores. If levels of prothrombin are lower than 70% of normal, vitamin K should be administered.

Etiopathogenesis and clinicopathologic aspects Vitamin K deficiency is usually conditioned by other factors and most often can occur under following conditions:
i. *Haemorrhagic disease of the newborn* All newborns are vitamin K deficient because their intestine is not yet colonised by bacteria that can synthesise vitamin K_2, and maternal milk does not provide enough exogenous vitamin K_1. Vitamin K is, therefore, administered to neonates routinely to prevent the haemorrhages.
ii. *Biliary obstruction* Lack of bile impedes absorption of fat-soluble vitamin K_1.
iii. *Malabsorption syndrome* Chronic intestinal diseases such as coeliac sprue and chronic pancreatitis affect adversely absorption of fats and fat-soluble vitamins like K_1.
iv. *Drugs* Administration of warfarin type anticoagulants inhibits biosynthesis of vitamin K in the liver. Broad spectrum antibiotics can alter the intestinal flora and eliminated the vitamin K_2 producing bacteria.
v. *Cirrhosis* Liver microsomal carboxylation of vitamin K does not take place in diseased liver and administering vitamin K has no effect.

Q26. What are the clinicopathologic features of vitamin C deficiency?

Vitamin C (ascorbic acid) is found in citrus fruits, fresh vegetables such as tomatoes and peppers.
Physiology Vitamin C has several functions acting as a coenzyme in reducing and antioxidant substance. Of all functions, the most important is its key role in the *production and maintenance of extracellular matrix* as under:
- Hydroxylation of proline to hydroxyproline, and essential component of collagen type I. Without vitamin C, collagen does not acquire tensile strength.
- Synthesis of ground substance components such as chondroitin sulfate, osteoid, dentin, and intercellular cement of blood vessels.

Clinicopathologic aspects Deficiency of vitamin C causes *scurvy* **(Fig. 9.9)**. Clinical symptoms are most often pronounced in very young and very old person, as under:
i. **Haemorrhagic diathesis** It is caused by the weakness of blood vessels related to defective intercellular cement.

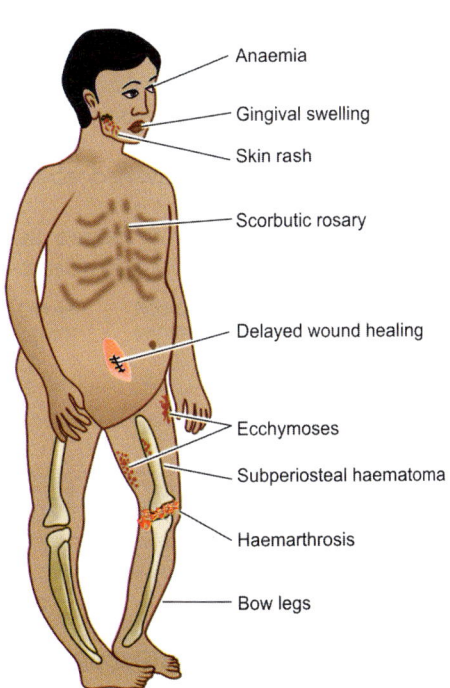

FIGURE 9.9: Clinicopathologic lesions in scurvy.

a. Haemorrhages are seen most often as perifollicular dermal petechiae, which are often accompanied by skin rash.
b. Gums are swollen and bleeding.
c. Skeleton is also often affected; there are haemorrhages into the joints (haemarthrosis), muscles, and long bones (subperiosteal haematomas).

ii. **Skeletal lesions** Weakness and deformities of bones are related to defective production of osteoid.
a. In normal growing bones, osteoid is laid down in the growth plate to replace the provisionally calcified cartilage cells.
b. Vitamin C deficiency impedes formation of osteoid and the calcified cartilage cells are not resorbed, remaining in the growth plate and causing deformity of the bones.
c. These remaining cartilage cells are most prominent at the costochondral zone of the ribs, where they form nodules (*scorbutic rosary*).
d. Abnormal osteogenesis weakens the bones resulting in deformities such as *bow legs*.

iii. **Delayed wound healing** It is related to abnormal production of collagen and extracellular ground substance. Reduced resistance to infections also contributes to delayed wound healing.

iv. **Abnormal dentition** It is related to abnormal dentin production and the weak support of the softened peridental bone tissue. Gingival swelling and haemorrhages also adversely affect tooth growth.

v. **Anaemia** Vitamin C participates in the metabolism of iron and folic acid. Vitamin C deficiency results in normocytic normochromic anemia, which sometimes may be even megaloblastic due to folate deficiency.

Q27. What are the clinicopathologic features of thiamine (vitamin B_1) deficiency?

Thiamine is widely distributed in vegetable and animal derived foods, such as leguminous vegetables, roots, green vegetables and meat. Thus primary nutritional deficiency is uncommon.

Thiamine is not present in sugar, polished rice and white flour. Strong teas and coffee may act as antithiamines.

Physiology Thiamine is a water-soluble vitamin involved in carbohydrate metabolism, synthesis of fat from carbohydrates, and synthesis of ATP. Deficiency of thiamine results in defective utilisation of carbohydrates, accumulation of pyruvic acid, and reduced production of energy-rich ATP.

Etiopathogenesis Thiamine deficiency may be *primary* in parts of Asia where polished rice is consumed. *Secondary* conditioned deficiency in Western world is seen in chronic alcoholics, neglected elderly persons in poor nutritional condition, or food faddists.

Clinicopathologic aspects Thiamine deficiency affects the *central nervous system* and the *heart*. The clinical disease is called *beriberi*, which presents in two forms:
- *Dry beriberi* presenting with neurologic and psychiatric symptoms, or peripheral neuropathy.
- *Wet beriberi* presenting with cardiac failure.

i. **Dry beriberi affecting the brain** Macroscopic changes are found in the mammillary bodies and parts of the brain around the third ventricle.
a. The affected areas are atrophic due to loss of neurons, accompanied by focal perivascular haemorrhages.
b. Clinically, these brain lesions are recognised as *Wernike-Korsakoff syndrome*:
- Wernike syndrome is characterised by progressive dementia, ataxia and ophthalmoplegia.
- Korsakoff syndrome includes additional psychotic features.

ii. **Dry beriberi affecting peripheral nerves** It is characterised pathologically by degeneration of myelin sheaths and fragmentation of axons. It is a sensory-motor neuropathy marked by sensory loss, paraesthesia and muscular weakness.

iii. **Wet beriberi with heart failure** It is characterised by heart failure and generalised oedema. At autopsy, the heart is flabby, enlarged and shows four chamber dilatation **(Fig. 9.10)**.

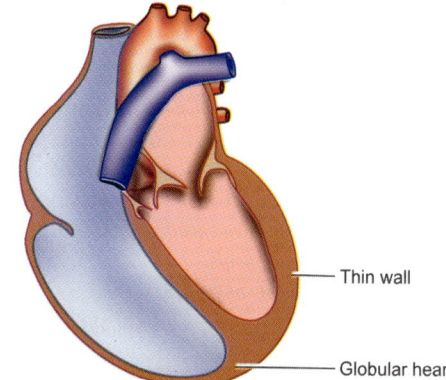

FIGURE 9.10: Wet (Cardiac) beriberi. Flabby, thin-walled, enlarged and globular appearance of the heart due to four-chamber dilatation.

Q28. What are the clinicopathologic features of riboflavin (vitamin B_2) deficiency?

Riboflavin is widely distributed and is found in many foods of plant and animal provenance, such as green vegetables and meats, eggs, milk. Thus, primary nutritional deficiency is uncommon.

Physiology Riboflavin is a coenzyme for cytochrome oxidase and thus important for cellular respiration.

Etiopathogenesis Riboflavin deficiency is uncommon, and usually found in debilitated or neglected persons and chronic alcoholics.

Clinicopathologic aspects Riboflavin deficiency present with oro-facial and eye lesions including the following:

i. *Cheilitis and angular stomatitis*, characterised by fissures and cracks at the angles of the mouth.
ii. *Glossitis* with atrophy of the surface epithelium of the tongue which appears magenta red ('bold tongue').
iii. *Ocular lesions* including vascularisation of normally avascular cornea, progressing to interstitial keratoconjunctivitis and corneal ulceration.
iv. *Skin changes* with scaly dermatitis in the nasolabial folds, scrotum and vulva.

Q29. What are the clinicopathologic features of niacin (vitamin B_3) deficiency?

Niacin is widely distributed in animal and vegetable derived foods. Furthermore, it can be synthesised endogenously from tryptophan. Thus, primary nutritional deficiency is uncommon.

Physiology Niacin includes two compounds: nicotinic acid and its active derivative nicotinamide. Nicotinamide forms coenzymes nicotinamide adenosine dinucleotide (NAD) and its phosphate (NADP), important for the function of dehydrogenases involved in the metabolism of carbohydrates, fats, and proteins.

Etiopathogenesis Niacin deficiency was quite common in previous times but is rare today. It may be still encountered in parts of world relying on maize as the primary food. In Western world, it is seen in chronic alcoholics and debilitated persons, and in malabsorption syndrome.

Clinicopathologic aspects Niacin deficiency presents clinically as pellagra, which is characterised by involvement of skin, gastrointestinal tract and CNS (colloquially known as *3 Ds*):

i. **Dermatitis** It typically presents with erythematous and scaling lesions involving sun-exposed skin of the face feet, and hands ('hand and glove dermatitis'). *Microscopically*, there is chronic dermal vascularisation and lymphocytic inflammation with hyperkeratosis of the overlying epidermis. In chronic stages, there is induration of the skin due to dermal fibrosis. Similar changes can be seen in the mouth with fissuring of the tongue, and the oesophagus.
ii. **Diarrhoea** It is typically watery and relentless, and accompanied by vomiting and nausea. It is caused by mucosal atrophy of the gastrointestinal tract, most prominently involving the colon.
iii. **Dementia** It is characterised by borderline psychotic ideation and motor and sensory defects related to demyelination of ascending and descending spinal cord tracts.

Q30. What are the clinicopathologic features of pyridoxine (vitamin B_6) deficiency?

Pyridoxine is widely distributed in animal and vegetable foods and, therefore, primary nutritional deficiency is uncommon.

Physiology Pyridoxine exists in three closely related naturally occurring compounds (pyridoxine, pyridoxal and pyridoxamine). All three can be converted into the biologically active coenzyme, pyridoxal 5-phosphate, which is important for the function of many enzymes in the intermediary metabolism of lipids, amino acids and proteins, and in synthesis of steroids, neurotransmitters and haemoglobin.

Etiopathogenesis Deficiency of pyridoxine due to inadequate diet is uncommon.

i. Pyridoxine deficiency may be combined with deficiency of other B vitamins in patients with protein energy undernutrition, malabsorption syndrome or chronic alcoholism.
ii. In pregnant and lactating women, and in hyperthyroidism, relative deficiency may appear due to increased demand.
iii. In patients with chronic diseases treated with drugs that interfere with pyridoxine metabolism (e.g. isoniazid treatment of tuberculosis).

Clinicopathologic aspects Pyridoxine deficiency presents with a variety of symptoms, none of which are diagnostic of this vitamin deficiency. The clinical findings are as follows:

i. Skin and oral lesions (dermatitis, cheilitis, glossitis) that resemble those of other B vitamin deficiencies.
ii. Peripheral sensory (stocking-glove) neuropathy.
iii. Central nervous system disorders presenting as confusion, depression and seizures.
iv. Hypochromic microcytic anaemia.
v. In infants and young children born to mothers who have received pyridoxine during pregnancy, it may present with seizures. These seizures do not respond to the usual anti-convulsive therapy, but will respond to injections of pyridoxine.

NOTE: Pyridoxine injected in megadoses for carpal tunnel or premenstrual syndrome may have serious consequences. The most prominent are signs of nerve and spinal cord injury. Injected pyridoxine may cause peripheral sensory neuropathy, presenting in a stocking-glove distribution, associated with sensory ataxia, loss of sense of position and vibration. Infants born to mothers treated with pyridoxine during pregnancy show signs of dependency and could have seizures.

Chapter 9e Supplement: Online Content

Digital content of this chapter available with this book is meant for enhanced learning and self-assessment. In addition, it contains 20 Multiple Choice Questions (MCQs), 05 Clinicopathologic Vignettes, and 02 Image-based Questions; these are followed by their answers along with explanatory notes of correct and incorrect answers.

CHAPTER 10

Genetic and Paediatric Diseases

GENETIC DISEASES

Q1. What are teratogens?

Definition Teratogens are substances (chemicals, drugs, toxins), physical and biologic agents known to induce developmental disorders and birth defects.
Teratology is the study of developmental anomalies (*malformations*), their etiology, pathogenesis, and pathology.

Q2. What are the possible outcomes of the action of teratogens on embryo or foetus in utero?

Action of teratogens could have four possible outcomes:
i. Intrauterine death
ii. Intrauterine growth retardation
iii. Functional defects
iv. Malformations

The effects of teratogens depend on the following factors:
i. *Variable individual susceptibility* to teratogens that is based on genetic features of the exposed individual.
ii. *Developmental stage* at which the exposure to teratogens occurred. Exposure during early stages of embryonic development often results in intrauterine death. Malformations are most often induced during critical stages of embryonic/foetal development, usually involving organogenesis.
iii. *Dose of teratogen and duration of exposure* High dose and prolonged exposure are more dangerous than lower dose and shorter exposure.
iv. *Specificity of developmental defect for specific teratogen* For example, thalidomide, a well-known iatrogenic teratogen, affects the development of extremities resulting in *phocomelia* (limb reduction anomaly of extremities resembling the flippers of a seal).

Q3. Based on pathogenesis, how are the developmental anomalies classified?

The development of organs or parts of the body could be affected by teratogens resulting in the following pathologic conditions:
i. **Agenesis** means complete absence of an organ. EXAMPLE: Unilateral or bilateral agenesis of kidney.
ii. **Aplasia** is the absence of development of an organ with the persistence of its rudiment or anlage. EXAMPLE: Aplasia of one lung, which is replaced by a rudimentary main bronchus.
iii. **Hypoplasia** is incomplete development of an organ not reaching its normal adult size. EXAMPLE: Microphthalmia (small underdeveloped eye).
iv. **Atresia** refers to incomplete formation of lumen in hollow viscus. EXAMPLE: Atresia of oesophagus.
v. **Developmental dysplasia** is defective development of cells and tissues resulting in abnormal structures. EXAMPLE: Renal cystic dysplasia in which renal convoluted tubules transform into cysts and renal stroma forms nodules containing cartilage.

vi. **Dysraphic anomalies** are defects resulting from fusion of its embryonic parts. EXAMPLE: Spina bifida from incomplete posterior closure (midline fusion) of the embryonic neural tube.

vii. **Ectopia or heterotopia** is abnormal location of tissues or parts of an organ outside its normal location. EXAMPLE: Ectopic pancreas in the wall of the stomach.

Q4. What are the most important developmental defects?

Examples of clinically important developmental defects are as under:

i. **Anencephaly-spina bifida complex** This group includes several dysraphic anomalies of the central nervous system. Anomalies may involve the spinal cord and vertebral bones (*spina bifida*) or the cerebrum and the bones of the calvaria (*anencephaly*) and may be associated with the protrusion of meninges (*meningocele*).

ii. **Foetal alcohol syndrome** (recently renamed as *foetal alcohol spectrum disorders* or *FASDs*) is related to drinking of large quantities of alcohol during the first trimester of pregnancy. Alcohol abuse can cause miscarriage due to the death of the embryo, foetal growth retardation, dysmorphic facial features and mental retardation that becomes manifest in infancy and childhood.

iii. **Foetal hydantoin syndrome** Infants born to mothers treated for epilepsy with hydantoin have an increased incidence of congenital heart diseases and have distinct facial features.

iv. **TORCH complex** It results from infection with TORCH group of organisms (*Toxoplasma, Other, Rubella, Cytomegalovirus,* and *Herpes* simplex) (Page 192).

v. **Congenital syphilis** It is characterised by Hutchinson triad: interstitial keratitis, sensorineural deafness, and deformed Hutchinson teeth, with saddle nose deformity.

Q5. What are chromosomes? What are their key features?

Definition Chromosomes are thread-like structures formed of nucleic acids bound to proteins.

Methods of study *Cytogenetics* is the study of chromosomes.

In order to study chromosomes, it is necessary to harvest lymphocytes from peripheral blood, stimulate them to start dividing, and then use colchicine to block them in mitosis.

Chromosome segments are best visualised by the Giemsa stain which demonstrates the dark and light bands of each chromosome. These bands are constant for each chromosome and are given numerical designations enabling scientist to map the location of each gene on the chromosome.

Key facts:

• Chromosomes carry genetic information in the form of *genes*, which are transmitted to the daughter cells during cell division.

• Chromosomes are formed from chromatin of interphase cells at the beginning of mitosis or meiosis.

• Chromosomes are seen only during cell division and are not seen in interphase nuclei.

• Human cells contain 23 pairs of chromosomes, i.e. have 46 chromosomes, which is the normal euploid (*diploid*) number of chromosomes in all somatic cells. Germ cells are *haploid,* i.e. they contain only one set of 23 chromosomes.

• The diploid number of chromosomes includes two *sex chromosomes*, XX for females and XY for males. In females, one X chromosome is inactivated and appears as condensed chromatin or as *Barr body* (drumstick) in neutrophils.

Q6. How are the chromosomes classified?

Depending on the location of the centromere, chromosomes are divided into three groups **(Fig. 10.1)**:

i. *Metacentric chromosomes*, which have a centrally located centromere dividing the chromosome into two equal parts.

ii. *Submetacentric chromosomes*, which are divided by the centromere into a short arm (p) and long arm (q).

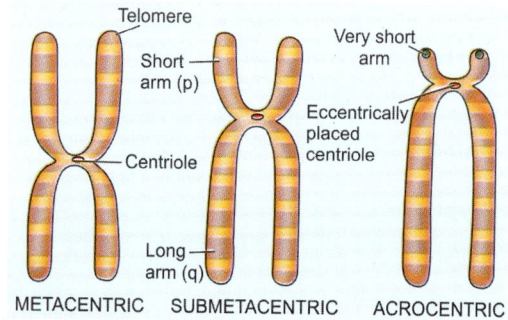

FIGURE 10.1: Classification of chromosomes based on size and location of centromere.

iii. *Acrocentric chromosomes* which are divided by an eccentrically located centromere into a very short arm and a long arm.

Chromosomal abnormalities can be classified as *numerical or structural*.

Q7. What are numerical abnormalities of chromosomes? Briefly discuss their etiopathogenesis.

Definition Numerical chromosomal abnormalities of somatic cells include all chromosome counts that do not equal to 46, i.e. are above or below the normal diploid number of chromosomes.

Classification The most important numerical abnormalities are polyploidy and aneuploidy:

i. **Polyploidy** is the term for chromosome counts that are multiples of the normal haploid number.

Types Polyploid embryos die early in utero and are aborted spontaneously.

Surviving embryos may be malformed and mostly die soon after birth.

Two polyploidies are encountered clinically in the perinatal period:

a. *Triploidy* (3N or 3 x 23 = 69 chromosomes)
b. *Tetraploidy* (4N or 4 x 23 = 96 chromosomes)

ii. **Aneuploidy** is the term for chromosome counts that are not exact multiples of the double haploid number.

Types Aneuploidy results from a deletion of one or more chromosomes, or an addition of a chromosome. Several forms of aneuploidy are recognised:

a. *Monosomy* when one of the paired chromosomes is missing. EXAMPLE: Turner syndrome having monosomy of sex chromosomes, i.e. 45,X0.
b. *Trisomy* if there are three instead of 2 of each chromosome. EXAMPLE: Down syndrome having trisomy 21, i.e. 47,XX+21.
c. *Hypodiploidy* (2N − 1 = 45 chromosomes), is marked by monosomy of one chromosome pair. EXAMPLE: Turner syndrome, i.e. 45,X.
d. *Hyperdiploidy* (2N + 1 = 47 chromosomes), is marked by trisomy of one chromosome pair. EXAMPLE: Klinefelter syndrome having trisomy of sex chromosome, i.e. 47,XXY.

Etiopathogenesis The most common mechanism of aneuploidy is *nondisjunction* during meiosis or mitosis:

i. *Nondisjunction during first meiotic division* results in two gametes with both parental chromosomes and two with no chromosomes (nullisomic).
ii. *Nondisjunction during the second meiotic division* results in one gamete with two identical copies of the same chromosome, one nullisomic gamete and two gametes with normal chromosome number.
iii. *Nondisjunction during mitosis* results in mosaicism, meaning that the individual has two or more types of cell lines derived from the same zygote. This type of mosaicism is common in cancers.
iv. *Anaphase lag* is a form of nondisjunction involving a single chromosome. In this process, chromatid in meiosis or mitosis fails to reach the dividing cell and is left out of the nucleus of the daughter cell. The result is one normal cell and the other monosomic for the missing chromosome.

Q8. What are the most important clinical conditions related to numerical chromosomal anomalies?

Three most important numerical chromosomal abnormalities are: i) Down syndrome, ii) Klinefelter syndrome, and iii) Turner syndrome. Their main features are illustrated in **Figure 10.2**:

I. Down syndrome Trisomy 21 is found in about 95% of all Down syndrome cases. Translocation of chromosome 21 is found in 4%, and accounts for the familial hereditary cases of the syndrome.

- Trisomy 21 is a consequence of nondisjunction in meiosis of one parental germ line, almost all (95%) involving the mother.
- Down syndrome is the most common chromosomal anomaly with an incidence of 1:800.
- Risk is related to maternal age and is increased after the age of 35 years.
- It is the commonest form of mental retardation.
- Cases surviving over 40 years almost all develop Alzheimer disease.

Clinicopathologic features Typical phenotypic features (besides mental retardation) include:

i. Short stature due to shortening of the long bones of extremities.
ii. Dysmorphic facial features including low bridged nose, oblique palpebral fissures with prominent epicanthic folds.
iii. Early cataracts develop in 60% patients.

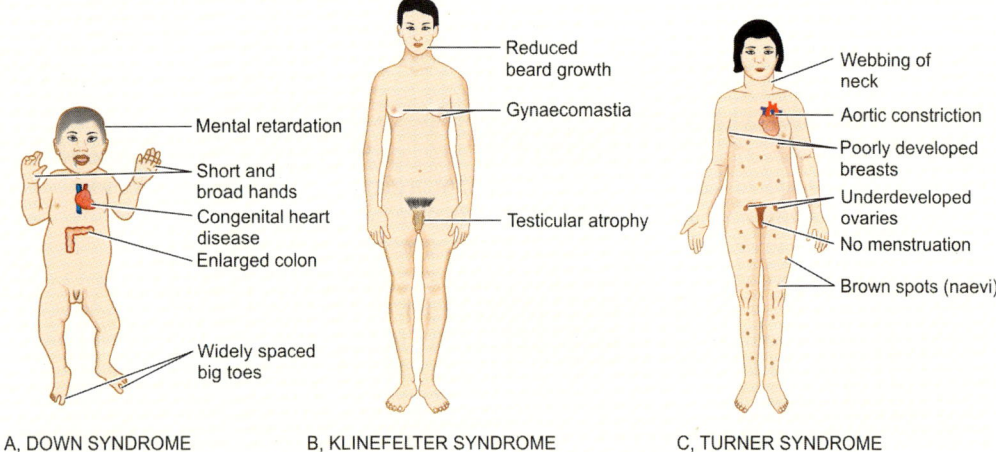

FIGURE 10.2: Clinical features of important forms of numerical chromosomal abnormalities.

iv. Enlarged protruding tongue, which is coarsely furrowed and lacks central grove.
v. Hearing loss in over 70% of patients.
vi. Hand abnormalities showing a horizontal crease (*simian crease*) and clinodactyly of the shortened little finger.
vii. Congenital heart disease found in 40%, mostly septal defects and endocardial cushion defects.
viii. Haematologic and immune system problems favouring recurrent infections, and an increased incidence of acute leukaemia (1–2% develop lymphoblastic or non-lymphoblastic leukaemia).
ix. Colonic agangliosis in 10% cases, presents with megacolon and rectal narrowing

II. Klinefelter syndrome In 80% of all cases, there is trisomy of sex chromosomes (47,XXY).
• The remaining cases are mosaics or have addition X chromosomes (48,XXXY) which usually shows more signs of feminisation.
• The extra chromosome X is due to nondisjunction during *paternal* germ cell meiosis.
• The incidence of Klinefelter syndrome is 1:700.

Clinicopathologic features Phenotypic males usually presenting for treatment of infertility.
i. Infertility is due to azoospermia and atrophic testes.
ii. Physical findings include tall stature with long legs, eunuchoid body proportions.
iii. Female pattern of hair distribution and gynaecomastia.

III. Turner syndrome In 50% of cases, there is monosomy of X chromosome (45,X) due to the loss of one X chromosome during *paternal* germ cell meiosis.
• The remaining cases show *mosaicism* (20%), or *deletion* of the short arm of X chromosome, which may be partial or complete, with *isochromosome* formation of the long arm.
• Most 45,X embryos (>90%) die in utero and are spontaneously aborted.
• The incidence of live born Turner syndrome patients is 1:3000.

Clinicopathologic features Turner syndrome presents with:
i. Short stature, webbed neck, broad chest.
ii. Streak gonad with small underdeveloped uterus.
iii. Primary amenorrhoea (no menstrual bleeding) and infertility.
iv. Increased incidence of aortic and cardiac anomalies, most often bicuspid aortic valve and coarctation of aorta.

Q9. What are the most important structural chromosomal abnormalities?

Chromosomal abnormalities may occur as under:
• During meiosis (*germ line meiotic abnormalities*) that are transmitted to all somatic cell lines in the body, or
• *Somatic cell mitotic abnormalities* limited to a single somatic cell line. Such chromosomal abnormalities are transmitted only to descendants of the parental cell carrying the chromosomal abnormality. Such abnormalities are most often seen in malignant tumours.

Structural abnormalities may be:
- *balanced* (no change in the number of genes), or
- *unbalanced* (with a loss of or gain of genetic material.

The most common structural chromosomal abnormalities are i) translocations, ii) deletions, iii) inversions, iv) ring chromosomes, v) isochromosomes **(Fig. 10.3)**.

I. **Translocations** This abnormality involves the crossing over of chromosome parts to another chromosome.
- Translocation may involve *homologous* (e.g. Chr.1 to Chr.1) or *non-homologous* chromosomes (e.g. Chr. 1 to Chr. 2).
- These translocations can be *reciprocal* (2/3 of all cases) or *Robertsonian* (1/3).

i. *Reciprocal translocation* may be balanced or unbalanced:

a. *Balanced reciprocal translocations* are more common, and the individual is normal.
EXAMPLE: Philadelphia chromosome [t(9;22)] in chronic myeloid leukaemia involves the translocation between long arms (q) of chromosomes 22 and 9.

b. *Unbalanced translocation* is uncommon, and it accounts for repeated abortions and malformed children.

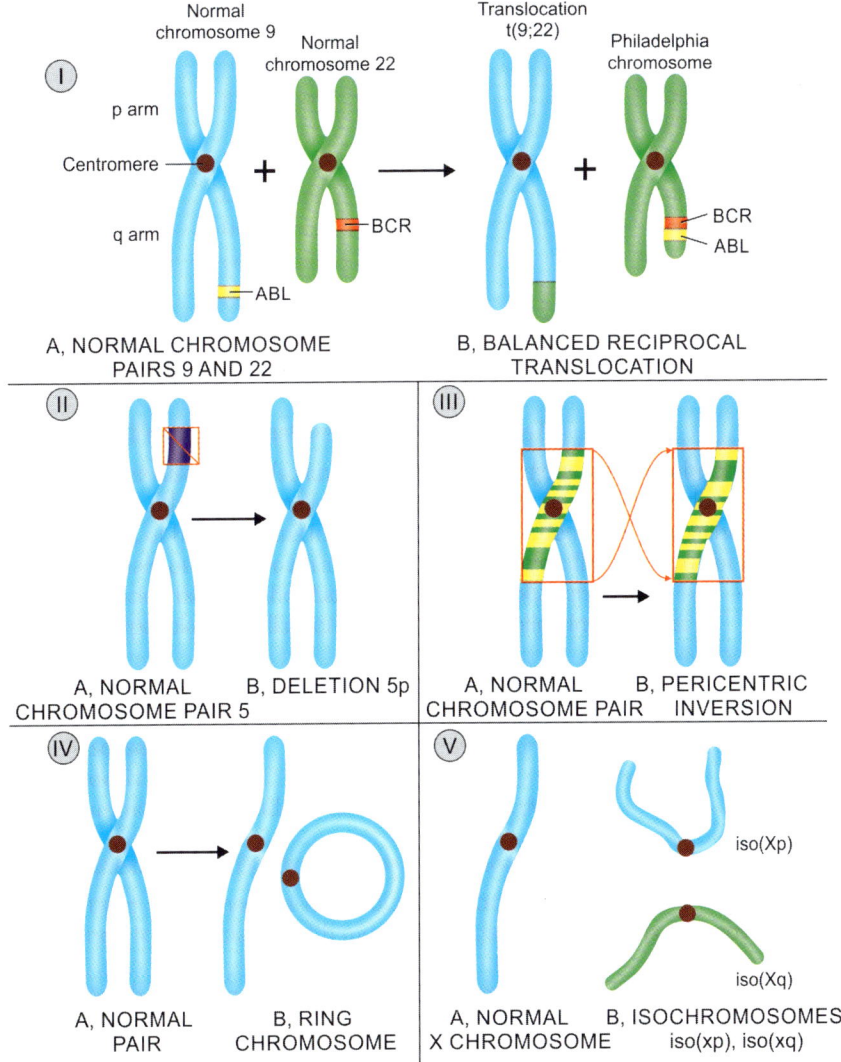

FIGURE 10.3: Common structural abnormalities of human chromosomes.

ii. *Robertsonian translocation* is less common than reciprocal translocation.
a. It involves fusion of the acrocentric chromosomes (with very short arms) at the centromere with a loss of short arms.
b. This translocation results in the formation of one very large and one very small chromosome.
c. Affected persons are phenotypically normal but suffer from infertility and produce often malformed children in the next progeny.
EXAMPLE: Robertsonian translocation of chromosome 21 to chromosomes 22 or 14 in hereditary Down syndrome.

II. **Deletions** Loss of a part of a chromosome which may involve the middle portion or terminal parts of a chromosome.
EXAMPLE: Deletion of the segment of chromosome 13 that contains the *RB* retinoblastoma gene in hereditary retinoblastoma cases.

III. **Inversion** This rearrangement of segments of chromosome that have broken off at two places and were reintegrated into the same chromosome.
Inversion *is not associated* with any clinical abnormality.

IV. **Ring chromosome** Ring chromosome, a rare chromosomal abnormality, is formed by a break at both telomeric ends followed by deletion of the broken fragment and end-to-end fusion of the remaining arms. Any one of the 23 chromosomes may give rise to ring chromosome. Clinical consequences depend on the amount of loss during the break of the chromosome. Most individuals carrying a ring chromosome are growth retarded.
EXAMPLE: Turner syndrome 46,XrX. If significant genetic material is lost this may be lethal resulting in spontaneous abortion.

V. **Isochromosome** This abnormal chromosome is formed due to an abnormal transverse division of the centromere, rather than the normal longitudinal division. It results in a separation of the short from the long arms, each of which can form an isochromosome.
EXAMPLE: The most common isochromosome in live-born infants is Isochromosome of the short arm of X-chromosome due to a loss of the long arm [i(X)(q10)] seen in 15% of Turner syndrome patients.

Q10. Define mutation. What are various types of mutations?

Definition Mutations are permanent changes in the DNA of the cell, that are transmitted to the progeny of dividing cells.
Types Mutations may involve:
i. Substitution of one base in the DNA by another
ii. Insertion of a new base
iii. Deletion of a base
iv. Repeat expansion
Mutations account for most hereditary genetic diseases, and play a role in the pathogenesis of malformations and cancer. The most important functional forms of mutations are as follows:
i. **Point mutation** is the result of substitution of a single nucleotide base by a different base, resulting in a replacement of an amino acid in the encoded protein. EXAMPLE: Sickle cell anaemia, a substitution of glutamic acid by valine in the polypeptide chain.
Missense mutation is a point mutation in which a single nucleotide change results in a codon that codes for a different amino acid. EXAMPLE: Marfan syndrome.
ii. **Stop codon or nonsense mutation** refers to a mutation in which the protein chain is prematurely terminated or truncated. EXAMPLE: Muscular dystrophy and gene for dystrophin.
iii. **Frameshift mutation** occurs when there is insertion or deletion of one or two base pairs in the DNA sequence. EXAMPLE: Cystic fibrosis.
iv. **Trinucleotide repeat mutation** is characterised by amplification of a sequence of three nucleotides. EXAMPLE: Huntington disease.

Q11. What are Mendelian disorders?

Definition Mendelian disorders are a single gene disorders inherited according to the rules of Mendelian genetics as autosomal or sex-linked, dominant or recessive traits.

Patterns of Mendelian inheritance are i) autosomal dominant, ii) autosomal recessive, iii) X-linked autosomal recessive or dominant, as under:

I. *Autosomal dominant* Autosomal dominant genes are expressed in homozygotes (two alleles of the same type) or heterozygotes, i.e. even in the presence of a recessive gene on the other chromosome.
- Patients affected by a mutated autosomal gene transmit it to 50% of next generation descendants.

II. *Autosomal recessive* Autosomal recessive genes are expressed only if both alleles are identical.
- All affected persons are homozygous, i.e. carry the same gene.
- Both parents are asymptomatic carriers of the mutated gene.
- Disease appears in 25% of their offspring, 50% are asymptomatic carriers, and 25% are neither carriers nor affected.

III. *X-linked disorders* These disorders are encoded by genes on the X-chromosome. Most of them are recessive.
- Since males have only one X-chromosome, mutated genes are always expressed in males; females are asymptomatic carriers.
- X-linked dominant diseases are very rare, like vitamin D-resistant rickets transmitted from symptomatic father to his daughters.

NOTE: Y-linked diseases are also very rare and include some forms of male infertility and retinitis pigmentosa.

NOTE: *Multifactorial disorders* are those disorders which result from the combined effects of genetic composition and environmental influences. Some common examples of such disorders are: cleft palate, pyloric stenosis, diabetes mellitus, arterial hypertension and many others.

Q12. Enumerate important clinical forms of Mendelian disorders.

Clinically important Mendelian disorders are listed in **Table 10.1**.

Q13. What are the main types of genetic protein defects?

Genetic protein defects cause diseases that can be divided into the three groups: i) structural protein disorders, ii) receptor proteins disorders, and iii) growth regulatory protein disorder.

I. **Structural protein disorders** These diseases may be caused by genes encoding extracellular matrix or cell membrane proteins. EXAMPLES:

i. *Osteogenesis imperfecta*: Fragility of bones due to a genetic defect in collagen synthesis.

ii. *Ehlers-Danlos syndrome*: Defective collagen synthesis affecting collagen rich tissues, including skin (hyperextensibility), joints (hypermobility), internal organs (lack of tensile strength or colon resulting in diverticulosis or constipation, and large blood vessels resulting in aneurysm formation).

iii. *Marfan syndrome*: Defective synthesis of fibrillin due to the missense mutation in *FBN1* gene. Clinical manifestations include skeletal features (tall and slender stature, long fingers

TABLE 10.1 Important examples of Mendelian disorders (single-gene defects).

I. AUTOSOMAL RECESSIVE INHERITANCE
1. β-thalassaemia
2. Sickle cell anaemia
3. Haemochromatosis
4. Cystic fibrosis of pancreas
5. Albinism
6. Wilson disease
7. Xeroderma pigmentosum
8. Inborn errors of metabolism (Lysosomal storage diseases, glycogenosis, alkaptonuria, phenylketonuria)

II. AUTOSOMAL CODOMINANT INHERITANCE
1. ABO blood group antigens
2. α 1-antitrypsin deficiency
3. HLA antigens

III. AUTOSOMAL DOMINANT INHERITANCE
1. Familial polyposis coli
2. Adult polycystic kidney
3. Hereditary spherocytosis
4. Neurofibromatosis (von Recklinghausen disease)
5. Marfan syndrome
6. von Willebrand disease
7. Hereditary haemorrhagic telangiectasia
8. Acute intermittent porphyria
9. Familial hypercholesterolaemia
10. Osteogenesis imperfecta

IV. SEX-(X-) LINKED RECESSIVE INHERITANCE
1. Haemophilia A
2. G6PD deficiency
3. Diabetes insipidus
4. Chronic granulomatous disease
5. Colour blindness
6. Bruton agammaglobulinaemia
7. Muscular dystrophies

V. SEX-(X-) LINKED DOMINANT INHERITANCE
1. Hypophosphataemic rickets (vitamin D resistant rickets)
2. Incontinentia pigmenti

and toes), and problems related to the eye (subluxation of the lens), and cardiovascular system (mitral valve prolapse, aortic aneurysm, aortic dissection).

iv. *Muscular dystrophy* (Duchenne and Becker dystrophy): Dystrophin defects linking the contractile parts of the muscle with the membrane resulting in muscle weakness and disruption.

v. *Hereditary spherocytosis*: Spectrin or ankyrin defects resulting in increased fragility or RBCs.

II. **Receptor protein defects** These diseases are caused by mutations of genes encoding for receptors.
EXAMPLES:

i. *Familial hypercholesterolaemia*: The mutated gene for LDL receptor defect is inherited as an autosomal dominant trait, resulting in hypercholesterolaemia, high serum lipids, and an accelerated development of atherosclerosis at young age.

ii. *Vitamin D resistant rickets:* The mutated gene encoding for the vitamin D receptor results in an inability to take up vitamin D and rickets that does not respond to vitamin D treatment.

III. **Growth regulatory protein disorders** These diseases are characterised by familial occurrence of tumours.
EXAMPLES:
- Hereditary retinoblastoma (mutation or deletion of RB gene)
- Neurofibromatosis type I (NF1 gene)

Q14. What are glycogenoses? Briefly discuss their pathogenesis and major types.

Definition Glycogenoses (glycogen storage diseases) are a group of at least 10 distinct genetic diseases, each of which is related to a mutation of an enzyme involved in glucose metabolism **(Table 10.2)**. All are rare, with an incidence varying from 1:100 000 to 1: 1 million.

TABLE 10.2 Glycogen storage diseases (inborn errors of metabolism).

DISEASE	ENZYME DEFICIENCY	ACCUMULATING METABOLITE	ORGANS INVOLVED
Type 0	Glycogen synthase	Glycogen	Muscle cramps
Type I (von Gierke disease)	Glucose-6-phosphatase	Glycogen	Liver, kidney
Type II (Pompe disease)	Acid-α-glucosidase (acid maltase)	Glycogen	Heart, skeletal muscle
Type III (Forbes'/Cori disease)	Amyloglucosidase (debrancher)	Limit dextrin	Heart, skeletal muscle
Type IV (Anderson disease)	Amylotransglucosidase (brancher)	Amylopectin	Brain, heart, liver, muscles
Type V (McArdle disease)	Muscle phosphorylase	Glycogen	Skeletal muscle
Type VI (Hers' disease)	Liver phosphorylase	Glycogen	Liver
Type VII	Phosphofructokinase	Glycogen	Muscle
Type VIII/IX	Phosphorylase kinase	Glycogen	Liver

Pathogenesis With one rare exception, all glycogenoses are inherited as autosomal recessive traits. Symptoms are related to adverse effects of:
- *accumulation of glycogen* (e.g. cardiomyopathy in Pompe type II glycogenosis), or
- *a lack of glucose* due to defective release from glycogen (e.g. von Gierke, type I glycogenosis).

Clinicopathologic aspects Depending on the major site of glycogen accumulation, glycogenoses can be divided into three clinical subgroups:

I. **Hepatic forms** The prototype of this form is *type I glycogenosis (von Gierke disease)* due to a deficiency of glucose-6-phosphatase.
Clinically, there is hepatomegaly due to glycogen accumulation, and hypoglycaemia, with retarded growth. Current treatment is quite effective and the patients can live a normal life.

II. **Myopathic forms** The prototype is *type V glycogenosis (McArdle disease),* due to a deficiency of muscle phosphorylase, which hinders the release of glucose-1-phosphate from glycogen, causing accumulation of glycogen in muscles.
Clinically, it presents in adolescence or early adulthood with muscle cramps and fatigue during exercise, and myoglobinuria due myocytolysis in about 50% of all cases.

III. **Other forms** The protype is *type II glycogenosis (Pompe disease),* marked by lysosomal storage in the heart and many other organs. It is related to a deficiency of a lysosomal enzyme, α-glucosidase (acid maltase).
Clinically, heart failure results in death by the age of 2 years.

Q15. What are lysosomal storage diseases? How are these classified broadly?

Definition Lysosomal storage diseases are genetic disorders characterised by deficiencies of lysosomal hydrolases, leading to accumulation of undigested substrates in the lysosomes.
- Lysosomal enlargement occurs at the expense of other cell functions causing cell dysfunction and cell loss.
- Most damaged are the vital organs, most notably the brain.

Classification More than 30 lysosomal storage diseases are known. They are classified according to the metabolites that accumulate in the cells and are divided into two major groups:
I. *Mucopolysaccharidoses* (glycosaminoglycan accumulation) such as Hurler and Hunter syndrome.
II. *Sphingolipidoses* such as Gaucher disease, Tay-Sachs disease, Niemann-Pick disease, Krabbe disease.

Q16. What are mucopolysaccharidoses? Discuss their salient features.

Definition Mucopolysaccharidoses are a group of inherited syndromes characterised by lysosomal accumulation of mucopolysaccharides (glycosaminoglycans or GAGs) numbered consecutively (e.g. MPS I, MPS II etc.), or eponymically as Hurler syndrome, Hunter syndrome, Sanfilippo syndrome, etc.

Etiopathogenesis All mucopolysaccharidoses are related to deficiencies of specific lysosomal enzymes involved in the degradation of mucopolysaccharides/glycosaminoglycans.
- Substances which accumulate in in lysosomes in various MPSs include one of the GAGs: chondroitin sulphate, dermatan sulphate or keratan sulphate.
- All these diseases are inherited as autosomal recessive diseases except MPS II (Hunter syndrome) which has X-linked recessive transmission.

Clinicopathologic aspects These diseases present in early childhood with accumulation of mucopolysaccharides in mononuclear phagocytic cells and fibroblasts in various organs. Typically, the disease affects the brain, skeleton, heart, liver and spleen.

Symptoms and clinical findings of Hurler syndrome (serving as a prototype of other mucopolysaccharidoses) include the following:
i. Progressive mental retardation and neurologic defects
ii. Cranio-facial deformities
iii. Skeletal deformities and joint stiffness, growth retardation
iv. Cardiac valvular defects
v. Hepatosplenomegaly

Q17. What is Gaucher disease? Discuss its key features briefly.

Definition Gaucher disease is a genetic autosomal recessive disorder characterised by lysosomal accumulation of sphingolipid *glucosyl ceramide* in macrophages, and sometimes in nerve cells.
- It is related to a mutation of *GBA* gene encoding for *glucosylceramidase-beta* which breaks down glucosyl ceramide into glucose and ceramide (a lipid).
- It is the most common lysosomal storage disease.
- Carriers of the mutant gene are found in 1 of 100 persons in the US and are ten times more common in Ashkenazi Jews.

Clinicopathologic aspects Clinically, three subtypes of Gaucher disease are identified:
- Most patients (80%) have the classical, type I or *adult form* of Gaucher disease. It is characterised by accumulation of *glucosyl ceramide* in macrophages of the spleen, liver, bone marrow and lymph nodes.
- *Infantile* (type II) form is characterised by progressive CNS involvement and early lethality.
- *Juvenile* (type III) form is a combination of type I and type II.

Grossly, in the adult form there is enlargement of the spleen, liver and lymph nodes as well as microscopic infiltration of the bone marrow.
i. Hypersplenism and bone marrow involvement result in thrombocytopenia and a bleeding tendency, anaemia and leucopenia, with consequent fatigue and reduced resistance to infections.
ii. Patients suffering from type II and III Gaucher disease have additional pathologic changes in the brain and associated neurological symptoms.

Microscopic changes include:
i. Infiltrates of enlarged macrophages known as *Gaucher cells*, most prominently in the spleen, liver and lymph nodes. These cells have enlarged granular and fibrillar cytoplasm that has a crumpled tissue paper appearance. These cells are distinguished from those in *Niemann-Pick disease,* another autosomal recessive disorder, characterised by accumulation of sphingomyelin and cholesterol due to defect in acid sphingomyelinase **(Fig. 10.4)**.
ii. Special stains show that the cytoplasm accumulates lipids and iron pigment (haemosiderin).
iii. Gaucher cells are also seen in the brain of patients with type II and III of Gaucher disease.

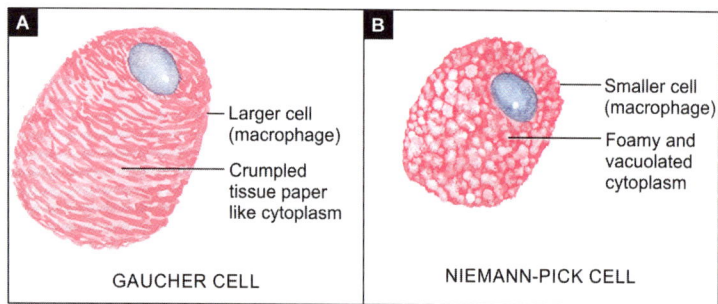

FIGURE 10.4: Diagrammatic view of comparative features of typical Gaucher cell (A) and typical macrophage in Niemann-Pick disease (B).

PAEDIATRIC DISEASES

Q18. What are the four stages of infancy and childhood? Enumerate the main medical problems and diseases encountered in each of these stages.

I. **Neonatal period** (first 4 weeks of life)
Prematurity, low birth weight, birth asphyxia, birth trauma, respiratory distress syndrome, congenital diseases, hydrops.
II. **Infancy** (first year of life)
Congenital anomalies, hydrops, infections of the lung and bowel, sudden infant death syndrome.
III. **Early childhood** (1–4 years of age)
Injuries, certain congenital anomalies, and some tumours.
IV. **Late childhood** (5–14 years of age)
Injuries from accidents, certain congenital anomalies, some malignant tumours.

Q19. What is foetal hydrops? What are its types?

Definition Foetal hydrops is accumulation of oedema fluid in the foetus during intrauterine growth.
Classification Hydrops may be localised or generalised.
There are two types of foetal hydrops: immune and non-immune.
I. *Immune foetal hydrops* EXAMPLE: Erythroblastosis foetalis (haemolytic disease of the newborn) due to materno-foetal blood group incompatibility (Rh or ABO blood group related, with jaundice due to haemolysis of foetal RBCs); kernicterus is bilirubin deposited in cerebral basal ganglia.
II. *Non-immune hydrops*. EXAMPLES:
i. Congenital heart disease
ii. Chromosomal anomalies (e.g. Turner syndrome)
iii. Foetal anaemia (e.g. α-thalassemia, parvovirus infection)

Q20. What are the risk factors for sudden infant death syndrome (SIDS)?

The cause of SIDS is not known but there are some risk factors for it as under:
i. Brain defects
ii. Low birth weight and prematurity
iii. Recent respiratory infection
iv. Sleep posture (sleeping on the stomach or sidewise)

v. Maternal risk factors (e.g. young age, smoking, drug or alcohol abuse, inadequate perinatal care)
vi. Other factors such a history of SIDS in family, exposure to passive smoke

Q21. What is the histogenesis of tumours in infancy and childhood?

I. **Developmental tumours** These tumours develop and grow while the foetus is in utero and can be diagnosed at birth or in early postnatal life.
EXAMPLES: Congenital haemangioma or sacrococcygeal teratoma (the most common solid tumour in newborns).

II. **Embryonic tumours (blastomas)** These tumours develop in abnormally developed organs and organ rests and are composed of undifferentiated or partially differentiated cells.
EXAMPLES: Nephroblastoma, retinoblastoma, hepatoblastoma, neuroblastoma.

Q22. What are the most common benign tumours, tumour-like conditions and malignant tumours in infancy and childhood?

The most common benign tumours and tumour-like conditions are listed in **Table 10.3**.
The most common paediatric malignant tumours are listed in **Table 10.4**.
A few general comments can be made about these malignant tumours as follows:
i. In children under 4 years of age, the most common malignant tumours are blastomas.
ii. In children between 5 and 9 years, haematopoietic malignancies are more common.
iii. In the age group between 10 and 14 years, soft tissue and bone sarcomas predominate.
iv. These malignant tumours are often composed of small round blue cells that have a high N/C ratio. These tumours can be distinguished one from another only by using immunohistochemistry or molecular biology techniques.
v. EXAMPLES: Ewing sarcoma, retinoblastoma, neuroblastoma, Wilms tumour, medulloblastoma, hepatoblastoma, rhabdomyosarcoma, small cell osteosarcoma.

TABLE 10.3 Common paediatric benign tumours and tumour-like lesions.

NOMENCLATURE	MAIN FEATURES
BENIGN TUMOURS	
i. Haemangioma	➤ Most common in infancy ➤ Commonly on skin (e.g. port-wine stain) ➤ May regress spontaneously
ii. Lymphangioma	➤ Cystic and cavernous type common ➤ Located in skin or deeper tissues ➤ Tends to increase in size after birth
iii. Sacrococcygeal teratoma	➤ Often accompanied with other congenital malformations ➤ Majority (75%) are benign; rest are immature or malignant
iv. Fibromatosis	➤ Solitary (which generally behaves as benign) to multifocal (aggressive lesions)
TUMOUR-LIKE LESIONS/BENIGN TUMOURS	
i. Naevocellular naevi	➤ Very common lesion on the skin
ii. Liver cell adenoma	➤ Most common benign tumour of liver
iii. Rhabdomyoma	➤ Rare foetal and cardiac tumour

TABLE 10.4 Common paediatric malignant tumours.

SYSTEM	AGE <4 YEARS	AGE 5–9 YEARS	AGE 10–14 YEARS
1. Haematopoietic	Acute leukaemia	Acute leukaemia Lymphoma	Hodgkin
2. Blastomas	Neuroblastoma Hepatoblastoma Retinoblastoma Nephroblastoma (Wilms' tumour) Pleuropulmonary blastoma	Neuroblastoma Hepatocellular carcinoma	Hepatocellular carcinoma
3. Soft tissues	Rhabdomyosarcoma	Soft tissue sarcoma	Soft tissue sarcoma
4. Bony	—	Ewing's sarcoma/PNET	Osteogenic sarcoma
5. Neural	CNS tumours	CNS tumours	—
6. Others	Teratoma	—	Thyroid cancer

Q23. What are the differences between tumours of infancy and childhood and those in adults?

The main differences are as follows:

i. **Sites** Paediatric tumours most often originate in the haematopoietic and lymphoid system, neural tissue and soft tissues whereas tumours of adults originate in the lungs, prostate, breasts, colon and skin.

ii. **Genetic basis** Many paediatric tumours have underlying genetic abnormalities.

iii. **Regression** Several foetal or neonatal malignancies tend to regress spontaneously or may undergo maturation (e.g. neuroblastoma to ganglioneuroma).

iv. **Histologic features** Many paediatric tumours are composed of uniform primitive small cells, that have an embryonal appearance in contrast to tumours in adults that retain some features of the tissue of their origin or become pleomorphic and anaplastic.

v. **Management** Many of the paediatric malignancies respond well to chemotherapy and could be cured by drugs and radiation therapy.

> **Chapter 10e Supplement: Online Content**
>
> *Digital content of this chapter available with this book is meant for enhanced learning and self-assessment. In addition, it contains 22 Multiple Choice Questions (MCQs), 05 Clinicopathologic Vignettes, and 01 Image-based Questions; these are followed by their answers along with explanatory notes of correct and incorrect answers.*

SECTION II: HAEMATOPOIETIC SYSTEM AND LYMPHORETICULAR TISSUES

CHAPTER 11

Introduction to Haematopoietic System and Disorders of Erythroid Series

■ BONE MARROW AND HAEMATOPOIESIS

Q1. Bone marrows of which bones are involved in haematopoiesis in adult persons?

i. **During adulthood**, haematopoiesis is limited to the bone marrow of the central (axial) skeleton (i.e. bones of the vertebral column, ribs, sternum, sacrum and pelvis), and the proximal ends of the femur, humerus, and tibia (**Fig. 11.1**).

ii. Many other bones contain haematopoietic bone marrow in the **foetus, infants, and young children**. In all those sites, the haematopoietic bone marrow is replaced by fat cells in early infancy and childhood. Note also that foetal haematopoiesis persists in the liver and the spleen during the first two weeks of postnatal life.

iii. In certain pathologic conditions, haematopoiesis can be reactivated in the extra-axial non-haematopoietic bone marrow, the spleen and the liver. In the spleen and liver, this condition is called **extramedullary haematopoiesis**.

Q2. What are the haematopoietic stem cells?

Definition Haematopoietic stem cells (HSC) are the undifferentiated precursors of all blood cells and lymphoid cells.

Key features HSC have the typical features of stem cells that include the following:

i. Small cells with scant cytoplasm resembling lymphocytes.
ii. Self-renewal capacity.
iii. Developmentally pluripotent, i.e. have the capacity to differentiate into all blood and lymphoid cells.

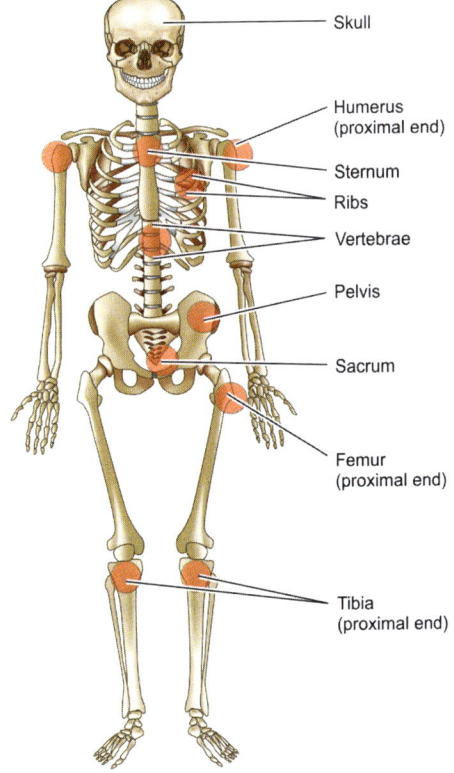

FIGURE 11.1: Sites of haematopoiesis in the bone marrow in the adult.

iv. Cell surface markers typical of their type (e.g. CD34, CD117, CD133, etc.).
v. Cell-cell adhesions molecules that allow them to home in the bone marrow if injected intravenously.

Q3. How do the haematopoietic stem cells (HSC) differentiate?

HSC differentiates into two types of progenitors: i) myeloid stem cell, and ii) common lymphoid progenitor cell **(Fig. 11.2)**:

I. **Myeloid stem cell** is generated through the action of stem cell factor (SCF) and thrombomodulin. This cell is also called *trilineage stem cell* because it can differentiate into the precursors of granulocytic white blood cells on one hand, and to precursors of red blood cells and platelets on the other.

i. **Granulocytic differentiation** occurs through the action of the granulocyte-macrophage colony stimulating factor (GM-CSF), which directs the myeloid stem cell to differentiate into granulocyte-monocyte progenitor.

Granulocyte-monocyte progenitor differentiates into neutrophils, basophils, eosinophils, monocytes and dendritic cells under the influence of specific growth factors (e.g. G-CSF leading to formation of neutrophils) or interleukins (e.g. IL-5 leading to the formation of eosinophils).

ii. **Erythroid differentiation** occurs through the action of erythropoietin.

iii. **Platelet formation** (thrombocytopoiesis) occurs through the action of thrombocytopoeitin.

II. **Common lymphoid progenitor** is formed under the influence of IL-7, which also directs its differentiation into B-cell progenitors and T/NK progenitor cell. Final differentiation into B-cells, T-cells and NK cells occurs under the influence of several interleukins.

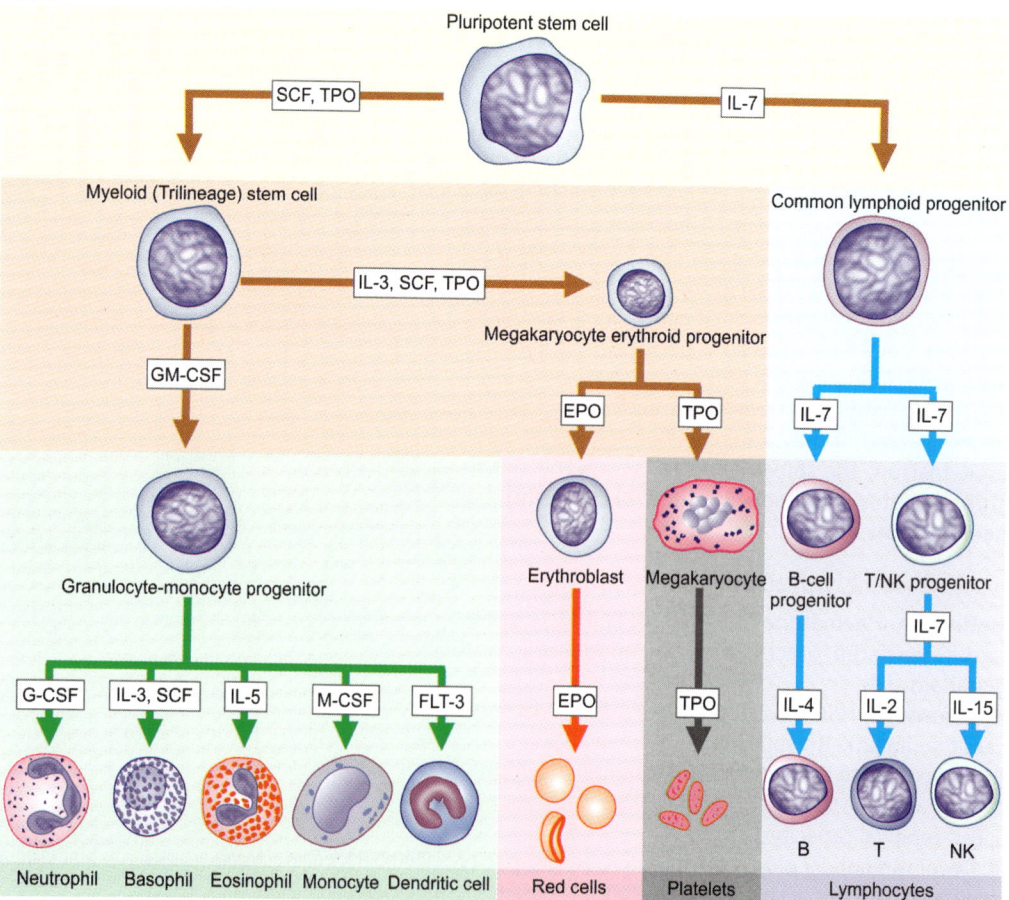

FIGURE 11.2: Schematic representation of differentiation of multipotent stem cells into blood cells.

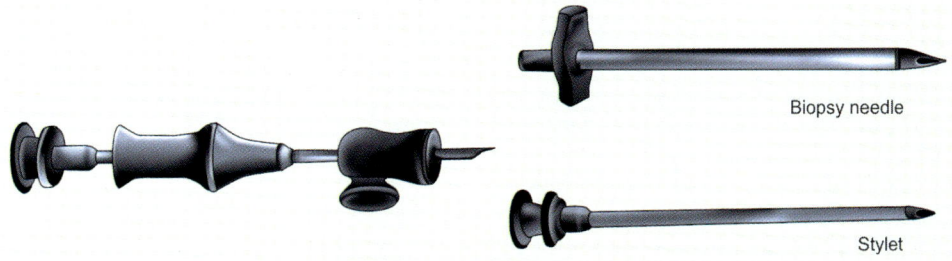

FIGURE 11.3: The Salah bone marrow aspiration needle (A), Jamshidi trephine needle (B).

Q4. What are the differences between bone marrow aspiration and trephine biopsy?

Bone marrow aspiration is performed with a wide bore, short-beveled needle that is ideal for obtaining specimens for cytologic smears **(Fig. 11.3)**.

Major indications include: typing of anaemias and neutropenia, leukaemias, and marrow infiltrations with extracellular matrix (e.g. amyloid) or neoplastic cells.

Trephine biopsy is performed with a longer but thinner needle that will allow preservation of tissues and, thus, allow better assessment of the histologic compartments of the bone from the periosteum to the bone marrow.

Indications are the same as for aspirations. Additionally, trephine biopsy is especially useful in so called 'dry aspirations', myelofibrosis, and aplastic anaemia.

Advantages and disadvantages of bone marrow aspiration and trephine are summed up in the **Table 11.1**.

TABLE 11.1 Comparison of bone marrow aspiration and trephine biopsy.

FEATURE	ASPIRATION	TREPHINE
1. Site	Sternum, posterior iliac crest; tibial head in infants	Posterior iliac crest
2. Instrument	Salah BM aspiration needle	Jamshidi trephine needle
3. Stains	Romanowsky, Perls reaction for iron on smears	Haematoxylin and eosin, reticulin on tissue sections
4. Time	Within 1–2 hours	Within 1–7 days
5. Morphology	Better cellular morphology of aspiration smears but marrow architecture is indistinct	Better marrow architectural pattern but cell morphology is not as distinct since tissue sections are examined and not smears
6. Indications	Anaemias, suspected leukaemias, neutropenia thrombocytopenia, polycythaemia, myeloma, lymphomas, carcinomatosis, lipid storage diseases, granulomatous conditions, parasites, fungi, and unexplained enlargements of liver, spleen or lymph nodes.	Additional indications are: myelosclerosis, aplastic anaemia, in cases with 'dry tap' on aspiration, and for immunohistochemical stains.

Q5. What is a normal myelogram and what is the ratio of myeloid/erythroid cells (M/E)?

Normal bone marrow has a fat cell/haematopoietic cell ratio of 50:50 and a mean M/E ratio of 3:1. Other values of a normal myelogram are given in **Table 11.2**.

Key points:
i. Myeloid cells are the most abundant, but do not exceed 30–45% of all cells.
ii. Erythroid cells account for 10–15% of all cells (one third of the myeloid cell count).
iii. Lymphocytes account for up to 20% cells.
iv. Myeloblast and plasma cells account each for approximately less than 3% of all cells.

TABLE 11.2 Normal adult bone marrow counts (myelogram).

Fat/cell ratio: 50:50
Myeloid/erythroid (M/E) ratio: 2–4:1 (mean 3:1)
Myeloid series: 30–45% (37.5%)
➢ Myeloblasts: 0.1–3.5%
➢ Promyelocytes: 0.5–5%
Erythroid series: 10–15% (mean 12.5%)
Megakaryocytes: 0.5%
Lymphocytes: 5–20%
Plasma cells: ≤3%
Reticulum cells: 0.1–2%

ERYTHROPOIESIS

Q6. What is erythropoietin?

Definition Erythropoietin (EPO) is a glycoprotein hormone regulating erythropoiesis.
Pathophysiology: EPO is synthesised in response to hypoxia.
i. EPO is primarily produced by the kidneys; liver can produce 10% of EPO.
ii. EPO acts on precursors of RBCs in the bone marrow.
iii. It stimulates erythropoiesis and promotes incorporation of haemoglobin into erythrocytes.
iv. There is an increased production of erythropoietin in most types of anaemias, except in anaemia of chronic disease in which EPO blood levels are normal.
v. Depressed levels of EPO are encountered in chronic kidney disease and polycythemia rubra vera.

Q7. What are the stages of erythropoiesis?

Key features
- Erythropoiesis begins with the formation of proerythroblast from the megakaryocytic-erythroid progenitor, and end with the formation of mature red blood cells.
- It takes place in the bone marrow and it is stimulated by erythropoietin.
- All RBC precursors have nuclei up to penultimate stage called reticulocyte, when they lose the nucleus.
- The maturation of RBC precursors is accompanied by a reduction of their size, shrinkage and ultimate loss of the nucleus, and a gradual accumulation of haemoglobin in their cytoplasm.

Maturation stages in erythropoiesis (Fig. 11.4)
i. **Proerythroblast** is a relatively large cell (2–3 times larger than erythrocyte) with a cytoplasm that stains bluish with the routine bone marrow smear stain. The cytoplasm is bluish because it contains abundant RNA needed for the synthesis of proteins. It is a dividing cell that ultimately that gives rise to 16–32 RBCs.
ii. **Erythroblasts** are nucleated intermediary stage cells, which can be classified as early, intermediate, and late, or alternatively named according to the amount of haemoglobin in their cytoplasm as basophilic, polychromatic or orthochromatic. Early and intermediate erythroblasts can divide; late erythroblasts cannot divide.
iii. **Reticulocyte** is the immediate RBC precursor formed from the nucleated orthochromatic erythroblast, which matures by extruding its pyknotic nucleus from its yellow-red cytoplasm.

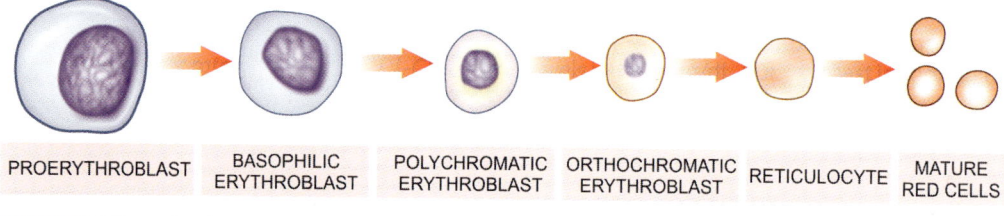

| PROERYTHROBLAST | BASOPHILIC ERYTHROBLAST | POLYCHROMATIC ERYTHROBLAST | ORTHOCHROMATIC ERYTHROBLAST | RETICULOCYTE | MATURE RED CELLS |

FIGURE 11.4: The erythroid series. There is progressive condensation of the nuclear chromatin which is eventually extruded from the cell at the late erythroblast stage. The cytoplasm contains progressively less RNA and more haemoglobin.

Q8. What are reticulocytes? Briefly discuss their normal formation and their alterations in numbers in pathologic conditions.

Definition Reticulocytes are immature RBCs that owe their name to the reticular ribosomal RNA filaments in their cytoplasm, that is demonstrable with vital stains (e.g. methylene blue).
Physiology Cytoplasmic RNA enables them to still synthesise haemoglobin.
- Reticulocyte stays in the bone marrow for 1–2 days from where it enters the circulation. It stays in the circulation for 1–2 days before reaching the spleen for final maturation into RBC.
- Under normal conditions, the blood reticulocyte count is 0.5–2.5 % in adults and 2–6% in infants.

Clinicopathologic aspects Reticulocyte count is increased in conditions marked by rapid red cell regeneration and reduced in bone marrow failure.

EXAMPLES:
- *Increased reticulocyte count:* after recovery from massive haemorrhage, haemolysis and in response to the medical treatment of anaemia.
- *Decreased reticulocyte count:* in aplastic anaemia and chronic anaemia due to RBC production disorders. Low reticulocyte count anaemia successfully treated shows an increased reticulocyte count.

Q9. What are the most important abnormalities of the red blood cell shape?

Normal red blood cells

i. *Shape*: Biconcave discs.

ii. *Size*: 7.2 µm in diameter.

iii. *Life span in circulation*: 120 ± 30 days.

iv. *Biochemistry:* Haemoglobin represents 90% of total dry weight of each RBC. Cell membrane of RBC composed of proteins (band 3 protein, ankyrin, spectrin), lipids (glycolipids, phospholipids and cholesterol), and carbohydrates.

Abnormal shapes of RBCs (Fig. 11.5)

Morphologic abnormalities include changes in the shape of RBCs many of which occur in conditions known under specific names as follows:

i. *Spherocytosis* is characterised by presence of spheroidal biconcave disc-shaped RBCs. Spherocytes are seen in hereditary spherocytosis, autoimmune haemolytic anemia and ABO haemolytic disease of the newborn.

ii. *Schistocytosis* is identified by fragmentation of RBCs. Schistocytes are found in thalassaemia, hereditary elliptocytosis, megaloblastic anaemia, iron deficiency anaemia, microangiopathic haemolytic anaemia and severe burns.

iii. *Irregularly contracted red cells* are found in drug or chemicals or drug-induced haemolytic anaemia and in unstable haemoglobinopathies.

iv. *Leptocytosis* is marked by the presence of unusually thin RBCs. Leptocytes that have a centrally round stained area surrounded by a paler ring and peripheral haemoglobin are called *target cells*. Target cells are found in thalassaemia, chronic liver disease and after splenectomy.

v. *Sickle cells (drepanocytes)* are semilunar-shaped cells seen in sickle cell anaemia.

vi. *Crenated cells* have numerous short projections on their surface. This artefactual change is found in blood that is alkaline, blood that has been allowed to stand overnight, or if the slides on which the smear was made are contaminated with lipid rich substances.

vii. *Acanthocytosis* is marked by coarsely crenated red cells, typically found in chronic liver disease and after splenectomy.

viii. *Burr cells* are cell fragments having one or more spines, found in uraemia and microangiopathic haemolytic anaemia.

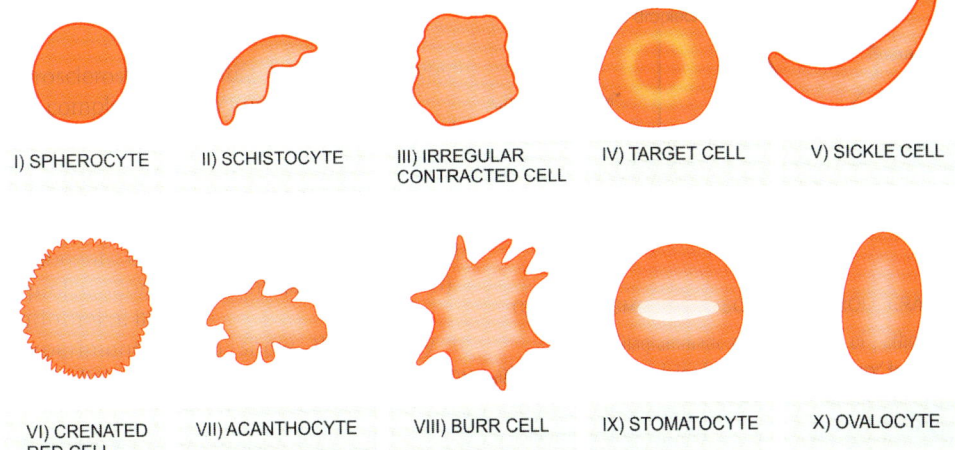

FIGURE 11.5: Common morphologic abnormalities of red cells (The serial numbers in the illustrations correspond to the order in which they are described in the text).

ix. *Stomatocytosis* is marked by the presence of cells that have a central slit-like or mouth-like appearance. They are found in hereditary stomatocytosis or chronic alcoholism.

x. *Ovalocytosis* is marked by the presence of oval or elliptical RBCs, most prominently seen in hereditary ovalocytosis or elliptocytosis. Ovalocytes may be found also in megaloblastic anemia and hypochromic anaemias.

Q10. Which nutritional deficiencies adversely affect red blood cells production?

I. Metals Iron deficiency affects adversely haemoglobin synthesis resulting in microcytic hypochromic anaemia.
- Oligominerals important for erythropoiesis include cobalt and manganese.

II. Vitamins Several vitamins are important for erythropoiesis as under:

i. Vitamin B_{12} and folic acid are essential for the nucleic acid biosynthesis and the deficiency of these vitamins results in megaloblastic anaemia.

ii. Vitamin C facilitates iron turnover in the body and thus has an indirect effect on erythropoiesis.

iii. Vitamin B_6 (pyridoxin), vitamin B_2 (riboflavin) and vitamin E (tocopherol) are also essential for erythropoiesis.

III. Amino acids These nutrients are essential for globin synthesis. Nutritional protein deficiency could adversely affect erythropoiesis.

Q11. What is haemoglobin? Briefly discuss its normal synthesis and degradation.

Definition Haemoglobin is an oxygen transporting protein of red blood cells composed of globin and haem, an iron-porphyrin complex.

Physiology Most of the haemoglobin (65%) is synthesised in nucleated RBC precursors in the bone marrow, whereas 35% is synthesised in reticulocytes in the bone marrow and extramedullary sites (spleen and circulation).

Synthesis Haem is synthesised in the mitochondria which accept the iron from ferritin, a cytosolic protein which in turn has received the iron from transferrin (the plasma transport protein). Iron binds to protoporphyrin to form haem. Four globin chains, synthesised from amino acids on polysomes, combine with 4 haems to form a haemoglobin tetramer, so that each globin has its own haem **(Fig. 11.6)**.

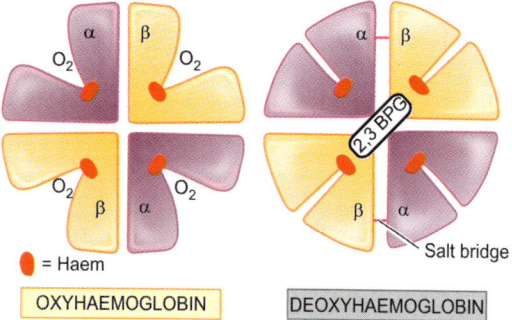

FIGURE 11.6: Normal adult haemoglobin molecule (HbA) consisting of $\alpha_2\beta_2$ globin chains, each with its own haem group in oxy and deoxy state. The haemoglobin tetramer can bind up to four molecules of oxygen in the iron-containing sites of the haem molecules. As oxygen is bound, salt bridges are broken, and 2,3-BPG and CO_2 are expelled.

Degradation Haemoglobin from effete or damaged RBCs is degraded in macrophages of the bone marrow, spleen and the liver. Globin is reutilised whereas the haem component is excreted by the liver in bile as bilirubin, which is partially recirculated and partially excreted in faeces and urine **(Fig. 11.7)**.

Classification All haemoglobins are tetramers composed of two alpha chains and two non-alpha chains, which determine their subclassification. The most important normal haemoglobins are as follows:

- **HbA,** normal adult haemoglobin, composed of 2 alpha and 2 beta chains ($\alpha_2\beta_2$). It accounts for 96–98% of the total haemoglobin in adult RBCs.
- **HbA_2** composed of two alpha and two delta chains ($\alpha_2\delta_2$). It accounts for 1.5–3.5% of total haemoglobin in adults.

- **HbF**, foetal haemoglobin, composed of two alpha and two gamma chains ($\alpha_2\gamma_2$). It accounts for 0.5–0.8% of total haemoglobin in adults.

Q12. What are the normal values and indices for red blood cells?

Normal values
Red blood cell count:
$5.5 \pm 1.0 \times 10^{12}$/L in men
$4.8 \pm 1.0 \times 10^{12}$/L in women
Packed cell volume (PCV) or haematocrit:
0.47 ± 0.07 L/L in men
0.42 ± 0.05 L/L in women
Haemoglobin content:
15.5 ± 2.5 g/dL (13–18 g/dL) in men
14.0 ± 2.5 g/dL (11.5–16.5 g/dL) in women

Red cell indices (absolute values)
Based on these values, one can calculate the normal red blood indices as follows:
Mean corpuscular volume (MCV) = 85 ± 8 fL (77–93 fL)

$$\frac{PCV\,(\%)}{RBC\ count\ (millions)} \times 10$$

Mean corpuscular haemoglobin (MCH) = 29.5 ± 2.5 pg per cell (27–32 pg/cell)

$$\frac{Hb\,(g/dL)}{RBC\ count\ (millions)} \times 10$$

Mean corpuscular haemoglobin concentration (MCHC) = 32.5 ± 2.5 g/dL (30–35 g/dL)

$$\frac{Hb\,(g/dL)}{PCV\,(\%)} \times 10$$

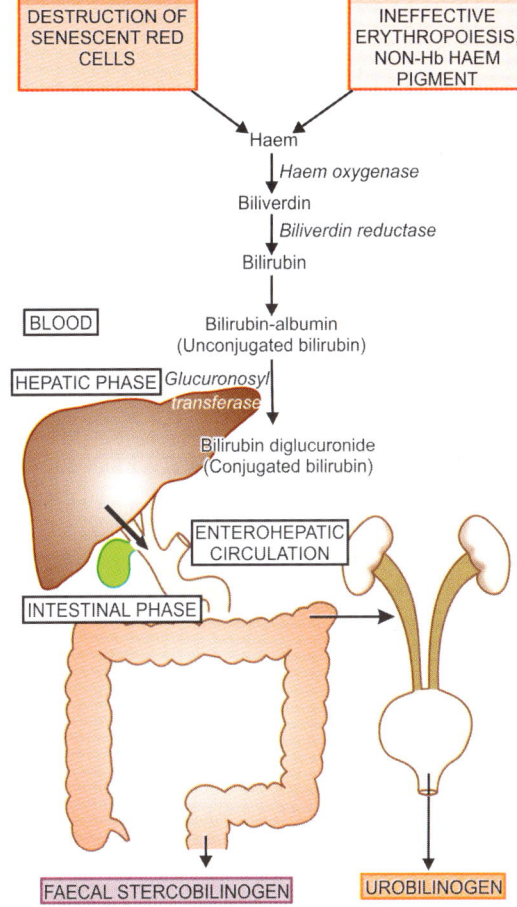

FIGURE 11.7: Normal red cell destruction in the RE system.

GENERAL ASPECTS OF ANAEMIAS

Q13. What is anaemia?

Definition Anaemia is reduced haemoglobin concentration in blood below the lower limit of the normal range for the age and sex of the individual.

Normal range
- At birth: 17 ± 1 g/dL
- Children: 11.5 ± 0.5 g/dL
- Adult men: 16 ± 2 g/dL
- Adult women (menstruating): 13 ± 2 g/dL
- Adult women (post-menopausal): 14 ± 2 g/dL
- Women during pregnancy: 12 ± 2 g/dL

An alternative means of determining whether there is anaemia is by using red cell indices.

Q14. How is grading of anaemias done?

Based on the *haemoglobin value*, severity of anaemia can be classified as mild, moderate, marked/severe or life-threatening **(Table 11.3)**.

Subnormal levels of haemoglobin causes lowered oxygen carrying capacity of the blood. This, in turn, initiates compensatory physiologic adaptations as follows:
i. Increased release of oxygen from haemoglobin
ii. Increased blood flow to the tissues

TABLE 11.3 Grading of anaemia*.		
GRADE	HAEMOGLOBIN VALUE	CLINICAL PRESENTATION
Mild (grade 1)	10 g/dL to lower limit of normal	Compensated <30% loss, no signs and symptoms
Moderate (grade 2)	8 to <10 g/dL	Loss >40%, symptoms and signs present, require treatment
Marked/severe (grade 3)	6.5–8 g/dL	Rapid loss >50%, life-threatening symptoms
Life-threatening (grade 4, 5)	Markedly low	Life threatening to death

*As per National Institutes of Health guidelines, 2011.

iii. Maintenance of the blood volume
iv. Redistribution of blood flow to maintain the cerebral blood supply
Eventually, if anemia persists, tissue hypoxia ensues resulting in impaired function of many organs. Most affected are the organs that have a high demand for oxygen such as the brain, heart and skeletal muscle during exercise.

Q15. What are the main factors that determine the onset of clinical manifestations of anaemia?

Four main factors that determine the haemoglobin level at which symptoms and signs of anaemia will develop are as follows:

i. **The speed of onset of anaemia** Anaemia of rapid onset causes more symptoms and signs than anaemia of slow onset. Furthermore, there is less time for physiologic adaptation.

ii. **The severity of anaemia** Mild anaemia produces no symptoms, but a severe anaemia with haemoglobin values below 6 g/dL may have significant clinical consequences.

iii. **The age of the patient** The elderly patients develop more prominently cardiac and cerebral symptoms due to the presence of cardiovascular disease in old age.

iv. **The haemoglobin dissociation curve** 2,3-Biphosphoglycerate (2,3-BPG) levels in RBC increase in anaemia and hypoxia depressing the affinity of haemoglobin for oxygen, causing a shift of the oxyhaemoglobin dissociation curve to the right.

Q16. What are the main symptoms and clinical signs of anaemia?

I. **Symptoms** of anaemia are usually nonspecific and include the following:
i. Easy fatiguability and lack of energy
ii. Muscle weakness
iii. Headache, inability to concentrate and lethargy
iv. Older patients may have symptoms pertaining to
- Cardiovascular system (e.g. heart failure, angina pectoris, intermittent claudications)
- Nervous system (e.g. confusion, somnolence, visual disturbances)

II. **Clinical signs** of anaemia may relate to many organs as follows:
i. Pallor of the skin, mucosal membranes and conjunctivae.
ii. Cardiovascular system insufficiency (e.g. hyperdynamic circulation with tachycardia and collapsing pulse, dyspnoea on exertion, mid-systolic blood flow murmur, cardiomegaly).
iii. Central nervous system dysfunction (e.g. attacks of fainting, giddiness, headache, drowsiness, tinnitus, tingling sensations in extremities, visual problems).
iv. Reproductive system disorders (e.g. menstrual disorders or amenorrhoea).
v. Gastrointestinal disorders (e.g. anorexia, flatulence, constipation, weight loss).

Q17. What are the peripheral blood smear abnormalities in anaemia?

I. **Anisocytosis** (variation in size and shape of RBCs), which may be due to the presence of RBCs that are larger than normal (*macrocytosis*), or smaller than normal (*microcytosis*). Smears containing both larger and smaller cells are called *dimorphic*.
- **Macrocytes** are typically found in megaloblastic anaemia due to vitamin B_{12} or folic acid deficiency. Other causes are aplastic anaemia, dyserythropoietic anaemias, chronic liver disease, and conditions with increased erythropoiesis.

- *Microcytes* are found in iron deficiency anaemia, thalassaemia and spherocytosis. They also may result from fragmentation of RBCs in haemolytic anaemia.

II. **Poikilocytosis** (increased variation in shape) may be found in many forms of anaemias such as:
i. Iron deficiency anaemia
ii. Megaloblastic anaemia
iii. Thalassaemia
iv. Myelosclerosis
v. Microangiopathic haemolytic anaemia

III. **Hypochromasia** (increased central pallor of RBCs) which may be due to:
i. Low haemoglobin content (e.g. iron deficiency anaemia, chronic disease anaemia)
ii. Thinness of RBCs (e.g. thalassaemia, sideroblastic anaemia)

IV. **Hyperchromasia** (increased haemoglobin concentration) is seen in megaloblastic anaemia, spherocytosis and in neonatal blood.

V. **Compensatory erythropoiesis** can cause several morphological changes visible in blood smears, such as below:
i. **Polychromasia** presenting as RBCs of several shades of red or other colours. Polychromatic RBCs are in most instances reticulocytes, which are larger than normal and appear bluish-grey.
ii. **Erythroblastaemia** is marked by the appearance of red blood cell precursors in peripheral blood.
a. A few nucleated RBC precursors (erythroblasts) may be found in cord blood of the *neonate* but are increased in number in haemolytic disease of the newborn.
b. *In adults,* erythroblastaemia is found in:
- Haemolytic anaemia
- Myelofibrosis and conditions associated with extramedullary haematopoiesis
- Severe form of any other anaemia except aplastic anaemia
- Following splenectomy

iii. **Punctate basophilia** or basophilic stippling, presents as basophilic granularity of RBCs, which does not stain with the Perls' iron stain. It is found in:
- Aplastic anaemia
- Thalassaemia
- Myelodysplasia
- Infections
- Lead poisoning

VI. **Morphologic abnormalities of red blood cells**, such as spherocytosis, sickle cell, etc. (*see* **Fig. 11.5**).

Q18. Which tests are usually performed when investigating the nature of anaemia?

I. **Haemoglobin estimation** is the first and foremost test to be performed when suspecting anaemia.
II. **Peripheral blood smear** is performed routinely on smears stained with one of the Romanovsky dyes (e.g. May-Grünwald-Giemsa stain).
III. **Leucocyte and platelet count** could help distinguish various forms or anaemia from pancytopenia of aplastic anaemia.
IV. **Reticulocyte count** is performed to assess the marrow erythropoietic activity.
V. **Erythrocyte sedimentation rate** is a nonspecific test used for screening. It is elevated in anaemia.
VI. **Bone marrow examination** is performed when the cause of anaemia is not obvious.

Q19. How are anaemias classified?

Two widely used classifications are as under **(Table 11.4)**:
I. **Pathophysiologic classification** is based on identifying the cause and the underlying mechanism of various anaemias, which can be classified as follows:
i. *Anaemia due to blood loss,* which may be acute or chronic.
ii. *Anaemia due to impaired cell formation,* which may include cytoplasmic or nuclear maturation defects, defects in stem cell proliferation, anaemia of chronic disorders, bone marrow infiltration or failure, and congenital anaemias.

iii. *Anaemia due to increased red cell destruction* (haemolytic anaemia), which may be related to extrinsic (extracorpuscular) or intrinsic (intracorpuscular) RBC abnormalities.

II. **Morphologic classification** is based on red cell size, haemoglobin content and red cell indices, and includes three major groups of anaemias:

i. *Microcytic, hypochromic anaemia* MCV, MCH, MCHC are all reduced.
EXAMPLES: Iron deficiency anemia, thalassaemia, anaemia of chronic disorders.

ii. *Normocytic, normochromic anaemia* MCV, MCH, MCHC are all normal.
EXAMPLES: Haemolytic anaemia, major blood loss, bone marrow failure, anaemia of chronic disorders.

iii. *Macrocytic, normochromic anaemia* MCV is raised.
EXAMPLE: Megaloblastic anaemia due to vitamin B_{12} or folic acid deficiency.

TABLE 11.4 Classification of anaemias.

PATHOPHYSIOLOGIC

I. *Anaemia due to increased blood loss*
   a. Acute post-haemorrhagic anaemia
   b. Chronic blood loss
II. *Anaemias due to impaired red cell production*
   A. *Cytoplasmic maturation defects*
      1. Deficient haem synthesis: Iron deficiency anaemia
      2. Deficient globin synthesis: Thalassaemic syndromes
   B. *Nuclear maturation defects*
      Vitamin B_{12} and/or folic acid deficiency: Megaloblastic anaemia
   C. *Defect in stem cell proliferation and differentiation*
      1. Aplastic anaemia
      2. Pure red cell aplasia
   D. *Anaemia of chronic disorders*
   E. *Bone marrow infiltration*
   F. *Congenital anaemia*
III. *Anaemias due to increased red cell destruction (Haemolytic anaemias)* (Details in **Table 11.11**)
   A. *Extrinsic (extracorpuscular) red cell abnormalities*
   B. *Intrinsic (intracorpuscular) red cell abnormalities*

MORPHOLOGIC

I. *Microcytic, hypochromic*
II. *Normocytic, normochromic*
III. *Macrocytic, normochromic*

HYPOCHROMIC ANAEMIAS

Q20. What are hypochromic anaemias?

Definition Hypochromic anaemias are characterised by defective haemoglobin synthesis and reduced MCV, MCH, MCHC.

Pathogenesis The most common cause of hypochromic anaemia is iron deficiency, which most often affects women of child-bearing age. Estimates are that 20% of women of child-bearing age have iron deficiency anaemia.

Classification Hypochromic anaemias are divided into two groups:
- Iron deficiency hypochromic anaemia
- Hypochromic anaemia other than iron deficiency (e.g. sideroblastic anaemia and anaemia of chronic disorders)

Q21. What is iron deficiency anaemia? Briefly discuss its etiology and pathogenesis.

Definition Iron deficiency is a hypochromic microcytic anaemia that develops when the supply of iron is inadequate for the requirements of haemoglobin synthesis.

Etiopathogenesis Iron deficiency anaemia may develop due to the following:

i. *Increased blood loss* In women of reproductive age, the primary cause is blood loss during menstrual bleeding. In post-menopausal women, the cause is uterine or gastrointestinal bleeding. In adult men, the most common cause is GI bleeding.

ii. *Increased requirements* Iron deficiency occurs if the increased requirements are not met adequately by increased intake. Most often, it is found in infants under 2 years of age, growing children, pregnant and lactating women.

iii. *Inadequate dietary intake* This is the most common cause in underdeveloped countries. In the more developed countries, iron deficiency is encountered in poor and neglected elderly persons.

iv. *Decreased intestinal absorption* Iron is absorbed in duodenum and proximal jejunum **(Fig. 11.8)**. Decreased intestinal absorption is an uncommon cause of iron deficiency, usually occurs as part of generalised intestinal malabsorption. It is also found in persons with achlorhydria and gastric resection.

Various conditions and diseases that can be classified under these four pathogenic mechanisms are listed in **Table 11.5**.

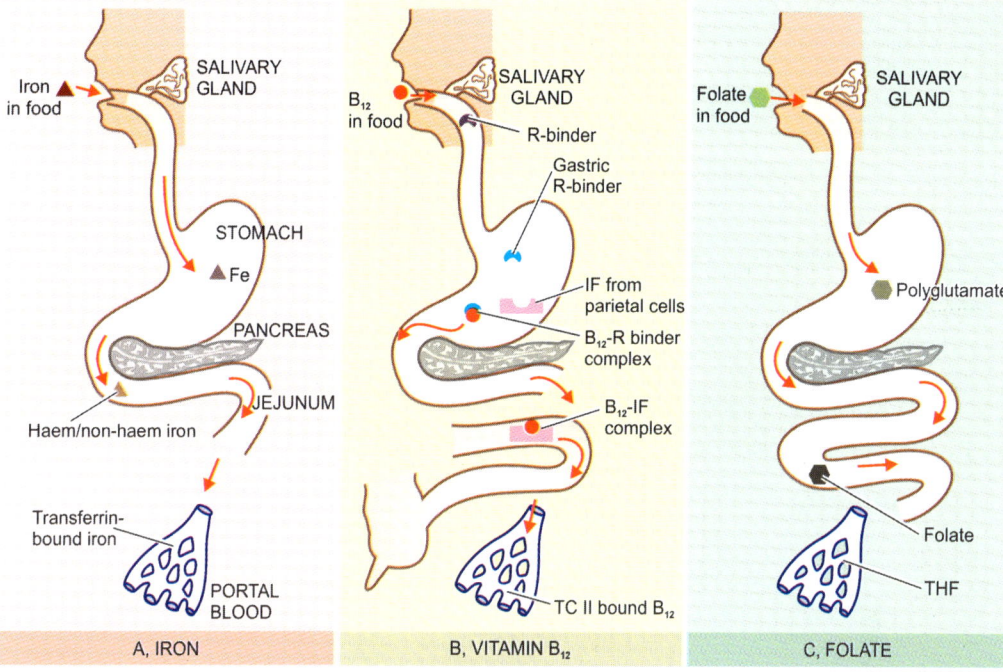

FIGURE 11.8: Contrasting pathways of absorption and transport of iron (A), vitamin B_{12} (B) and folic acid (C). (TC, transcobalamin; THF, tetrahydrofolate; IF, intrinsic factor)

Q22. Comment on various aspects of iron metabolism which are important for understanding iron deficiency anaemia.

Key facts (Fig. 11.9):

i. Iron for the synthesis of haemoglobin is derived from two *sources*: from diet, and from senescent red blood cells taken up by macrophages for recycling.

ii. Normal Western human *diet* contains 10–15 mg of iron, less than 10% of which is absorbed (1–1.5 mg).

iii. Iron is *absorbed* in ferrous form in the duodenum. Haem iron is absorbed better than non-haem iron.

iv. The absorption is limited by the *mucosal block* in the duodenum. It can be raised up to 30% of iron intake in conditions of iron deficiency.

v. Intake of iron corresponds to the *average loss* of iron in faeces, urine and desquamation of cells (1 mg/day). In menstruating women, iron loss is up to 2 mg/day.

vi. Iron absorbed into the intestinal cells is transferred inside the cytoplasm of these cells to *transferrin* by two vehicle proteins (*ferroportin and haphaestin*) which are inversely regulated by *hepcidin*, produced by liver cells.

vii. *Transferrin* is the principal iron transport protein in blood; normally it is one-third saturated.

TABLE 11.5 Etiology of iron deficiency anaemia.

I. INCREASED BLOOD LOSS
1. *Uterine,* e.g. excessive menstruation in reproductive years, repeated miscarriages, at onset of menarche, post-menopausal uterine bleeding
2. *Gastrointestinal,* e.g. peptic ulcer, haemorrhoids hookworm infestation, cancer of stomach and large bowel, oesophageal varices, hiatus hernia, chronic aspirin ingestion, ulcerative colitis, diverticulosis
3. *Renal tract,* e.g. haematuria, haemoglobinuria
4. *Nose,* e.g. repeated epistaxis
5. *Lungs,* e.g. haemoptysis
II. INCREASED REQUIREMENTS
1. Spurts of growth in infancy, childhood and adolescence
2. Prematurity
3. Pregnancy and lactation
III. INADEQUATE DIETARY INTAKE
1. Poor economic status
2. Anorexia, e.g. in pregnancy
3. Elderly individuals due to poor dentition, apathy and financial constraints
IV. DECREASED ABSORPTION
1. Partial or total gastrectomy
2. Achlorhydria
3. Intestinal malabsorption such as in coeliac disease

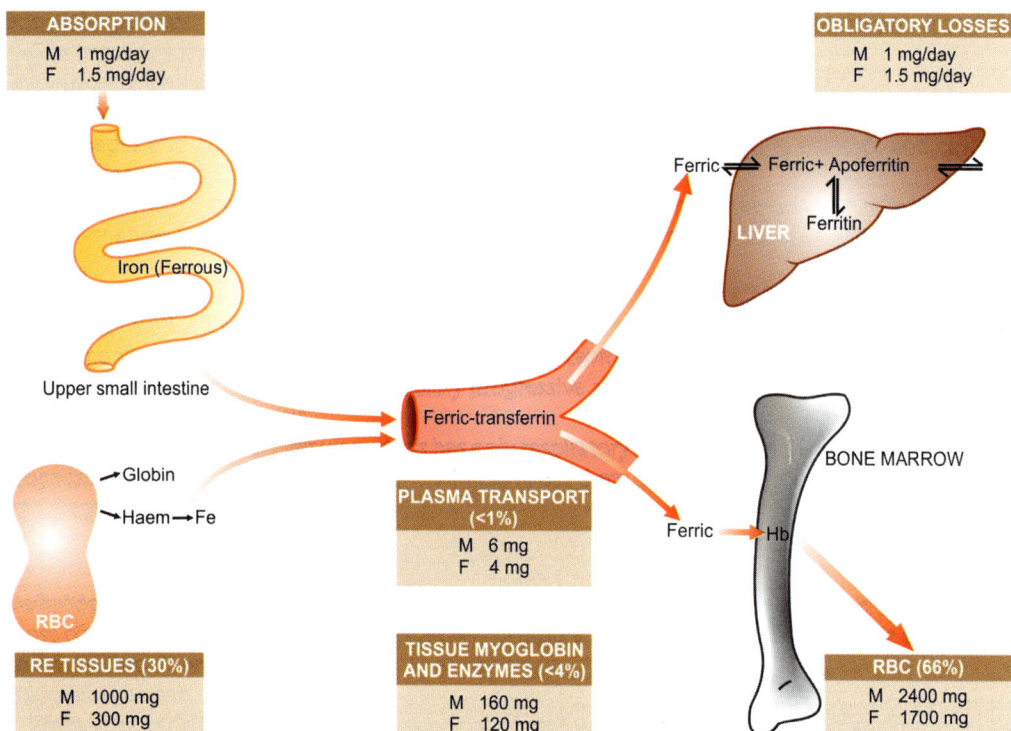

FIGURE 11.9: Daily iron cycle. Iron on absorption from upper small intestine circulates in plasma bound to transferrin and is transported to the bone marrow for utilisation in haemoglobin synthesis. The mature red cells are released into circulation, which on completion of their lifespan of 120 days, die. They are then phagocytosed by RE cells and iron stored as ferritin and haemosiderin. Stored iron is mobilised in response to increased demand and used for haemoglobin synthesis, thus completing the cycle.
(M, males; F, females; RE tissues, reticuloendothelial tissues).

viii. Red cell precursors have the greatest number of *transferrin receptors*, directing the flow of iron into the erythropoiesis.
ix. Excess iron from senescent RBC *phagocytosed* by macrophages is stored in form of *ferritin* in their cytoplasm. From these stores, it can be readily mobilised for erythropoiesis.

Q23. How is iron distributed in the body?

Body iron occurs in two forms (*see* **Fig. 11.9**): i) functional form (70% of total iron), and ii) storage form (30%).
I. **Functional form** of iron is distributed as follows:
i. Haemoglobin (65%)
ii. Myoglobin (3.5%)
iii. Haem and non-haem enzymes such as cytochrome oxidase, succinic dehydrogenase, catalase, peroxidases, etc. (0.5%)
iv. Transferrin bound iron (0.5%)
II. **Storage iron** is stored in form of ferritin and haemosiderin in two kinds of cells:
i. Macrophages of the bone marrow, spleen and liver
ii. Hepatocytes
Iron stores are best evaluated by bone marrow biopsy stained with the Perl Prussian blue reaction.
Pathophysiology of iron deficiency
i. Storage iron depletion is the first step in the sequence of events that leads to iron deficiency anaemia.
ii. The second step is marked by iron deficient erythropoiesis.
iii. The third step is characterised by frank iron deficiency anaemia.
Treatment of iron deficiency anaemia includes:
- Most often, administration of ferrous compounds (e.g. ferrous sulfate).

- Parenteral iron therapy is rarely indicated, and is given only if oral therapy is not tolerated, or if there is a malabsorption syndrome, or if the iron stores need to be replenished fast.

Iron therapy results in *reticulocytosis* within 3–4 days after the onset of treatment, to peak at 10 days.

Q24. What are the laboratory findings in iron deficiency anaemia?

I. **Blood smear and red cell indices** Anaemia is usually mild or moderate and rarely severe.
i. Haemoglobin concentration is low, but usually above 8–10 g/dL.
ii. Red blood cells are microcytic hypochromic and show aniso-poikilocytosis.
iii. Diminished red cell indices (MCV <50 fL, MCH <15 pg/cell, MCHC <20 g/dL).
iv. Leucocytes and platelets normal.
II. **Bone marrow findings** (not essential for diagnosis)
i. Hypercellular bone marrow.
ii. Erythroid hyperplasia, often micronormoblastic.
iii. Iron stores reduced as evidenced by the Prussian blue reaction (Pers iron stain).
iv. Myeloid, megakaryocytic and lymphoid cells are normal.
III. **Relevant biochemical findings** Usually variable, reflecting the severity of anaemia.
i. Reduced serum iron level below 40 µg/dL (normal 40–140 µg/dL).
ii. Serum ferritin level reduced below 30 ng/ml (normal 30–250 ng/ml).
iii. Total iron binding capacity (TIBC) is high (normal 250–450 µg/dL), with low saturation of transferrin- 10% (normal 20–45%).

A summary of laboratory findings is illustrated in **Figure 11.10**.

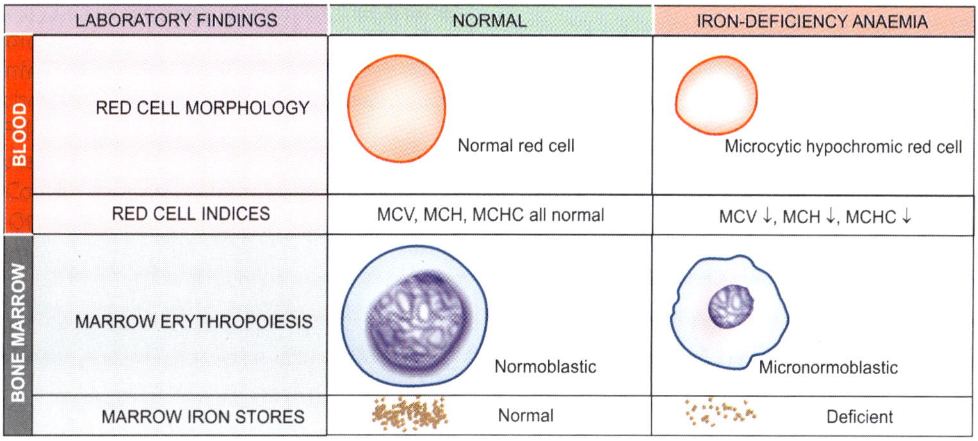

	LABORATORY FINDINGS	NORMAL		IRON-DEFICIENCY ANAEMIA
BLOOD	RED CELL MORPHOLOGY		Normal red cell	Microcytic hypochromic red cell
	RED CELL INDICES	MCV, MCH, MCHC all normal		MCV ↓, MCH ↓, MCHC ↓
BONE MARROW	MARROW ERYTHROPOIESIS		Normoblastic	Micronormoblastic
	MARROW IRON STORES		Normal	Deficient

FIGURE 11.10: Laboratory findings in iron deficiency anaemia.

Q25. What is sideroblastic anaemia? Discuss its salient features.

Definition Sideroblastic anaemia is the term used for a group of hypochromic anaemias characterised by the presence of *ringed sideroblasts* in the bone marrow and *siderocytes* in peripheral blood smears (Fig. 11.11).

Classification Sideroblastic anaemia (SA) may be hereditary or acquired.

I. **Hereditary SA** is due to a rare X-linked disorder due to the mutation of the gene encoding for the enzyme aminolevulinic acid (ALA) synthetase.

II. **Acquired SA** It may be primary or secondary.

i. *Primary acquired SA* Also known as *refractory* or *idiopathic SA,* it occurs spontaneously in middle aged or older men and women. It is associated with chromosomal abnormalities and neutropenia and thrombocytopaenia and is classified as a myelodysplastic disorder. In 10% of cases, it will progress to acute myeloblastic leukaemia.

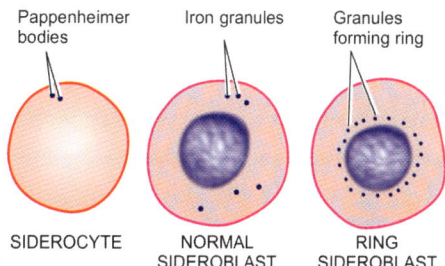

FIGURE 11.11: A siderocyte containing Pappenheimer bodies, a normal sideroblast and a ring sideroblast.

ii. *Secondary acquired SA* It develops after treatment with some drugs (e.g. isoniazid for tuberculosis), chemicals, toxins or haematologic and some systemic diseases.

Clinicopathologic aspects Moderate to severe anaemia.

i. Hypochromic anaemia which may be microcytic or normocytic or dimorphic.

ii. Red cell indices are reduced in hereditary SA but MCV is high in some acquired SA cases.

iii. Bone marrow shows erythroid hyperplasia with macronormoblastic erythropoiesis and ring *sideroblasts*, which contain iron-laden mitochondria around their nuclei. Bone marrow iron stores are elevated.

iv. Serum iron and ferritin levels are raised and TIBC shows almost complete saturation.

v. Iron deposits are seen in many tissues.

Treatment There is no definitive treatment.

- Therapy of primary and hereditary SA usually includes pyridoxine administration, and supportive measures, such as blood transfusion.
- Secondary SA is treated by eliminating the causative agent.

Q26. What is anaemia of chronic disorders? Describe its main features.

Definition Anaemia of chronic disorders is a common form of normochromic normocytic or mildly hypochromic/microcytic anaemia resulting from inefficient iron utilisation in the presence of normal iron stores.

Pathogenesis Anaemia of chronic disorders may be induced by chronic inflammation/infection, chronic renal diseases, or hypometabolic states **(Table 11.6)**.

This anaemia is multifactorial but two factors play a major role: i) defective red cell production, and ii) reduced red blood cell life span **(Fig. 11.12)**.

I. Defective RBC production Iron stores in the bone marrow are normal and even increased because of the action of proinflammatory cytokines (TNF, IL-1, IFN-β and γ) and hepcidin; latter is the principal regulator of iron metabolism. The effects of these mediators include the following:

i. Hyperplasia of macrophages in the bone marrow.

ii. Trapping of iron in macrophages, inhibiting efficient iron transfer to nucleated RBC precursors.

iii. Suppression of erythropoietin production in response to hypoxia.

iv. Blunted response of the erythroid cells in the bone marrow to erythropoietin.

II. Reduced red cell lifespan Most likely, this is due to the activation of macrophages, which phagocytose RBCs at an increased rate.

Clinicopathologic aspects Anaemia is mild to moderate and does not progress below haemoglobin levels of 8 g/dL.

i. Blood smears show usually normocytic normochromic RBCs.

ii. Red cell indices are *usually normal* but the MCHC may be slightly lower than normal.

iii. Bone marrow shows normal maturation and *normal or even increased iron stores*.

iv. *Serum ferritin levels are elevated* in contrast to iron deficiency anaemia, in which it is low.

v. *TIBC is low or normal*, in contrast to iron deficiency anaemia in which TIBC levels are raised.

vi. Serum levels of iron are low in both anaemia of iron deficiency and due to chronic disorders.

TABLE 11.6 Anaemias secondary to chronic systemic disorders.

1. ANAEMIA IN CHRONIC INFECTIONS/INFLAMMATION
   a. *Infections*, e.g. tuberculosis, lung abscess, pneumonia, osteomyelitis, subacute bacterial endocarditis, pyelonephritis.
   b. *Non-infectious inflammations,* e.g. rheumatoid arthritis, SLE, vasculitis, dermatomyositis, scleroderma, sarcoidosis, Crohn disease.
   c. *Disseminated malignancies,* e.g. Hodgkin disease, disseminated carcinomas and sarcomas.
2. ANAEMIA OF RENAL DISEASE, e.g. uraemia, renal failure
3. ANAEMIA OF HYPOMETABOLIC STATE, e.g. endocrinopathies (myxoedema, Addison disease, hyperthyroidism, hypopituitarism, Addison disease), protein malnutrition, scurvy and pregnancy, liver disease.

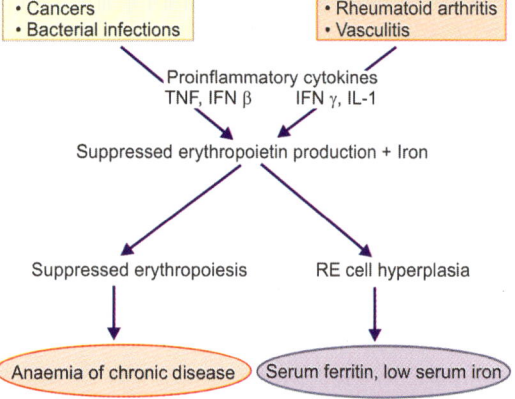

FIGURE 11.12: Pathogenesis of anaemia of chronic disorders through suppression of erythropoiesis by cytokines.
(RE cell, reticuloendothelial cell).

vii. Erythrocyte sedimentation rate is elevated due to the release of acute phase reactants from the liver in response to chronic disease.

Q27. Tabulate the main contrasting features of major forms of hypochromic anaemias.

Comparative features of four most common hypochromic anaemias are presented in **Table 11.7**.

TABLE 11.7 Laboratory diagnosis of hypochromic anaemias.

TEST	IRON DEFICIENCY	CHRONIC DISORDERS	THALASSAEMIA MINOR	SIDEROBLASTIC ANAEMIA
1. MCV, MCH, MCHC	Reduced	Low normal-to-reduced	Very low	Very low (except MCV raised in acquired type)
2. Serum iron	Reduced	Reduced	Normal	Raised
3. TIBC	Raised	Low-to-normal	Normal	Normal
4. Serum ferritin	Reduced	Raised	Normal	Raised (complete saturation)
5. Marrow-iron stores	Absent	Present	High	High
6. Iron in normoblasts	Absent	Absent	Present	Ring sideroblasts
7. Hb electrophoresis	Normal	Normal	Abnormal	Normal

■ MEGALOBLASTIC ANAEMIAS

Q28. What is megaloblastic anaemia? Discuss its etiopathogenesis briefly.

Definition Megaloblastic anaemia is a macrocytic anaemia associated with megaloblastic erythropoiesis in the bone marrow, reflecting impaired DNA synthesis in nucleated RBC precursors due to deficiency of vitamin B_{12} or folic acid.

Etiopathogenesis Vitamin B_{12} is of animal origin while folic acid is from plant and animal origin. Other important differences between these two vitamins are listed in **Table 11.8**.

TABLE 11.8 Salient features of vitamin B_{12} and folate metabolism.

FEATURE	VITAMIN B_{12}	FOLATE
1. Main foods	Animal proteins only	Green vegetables, meats
2. Cooking	Little effect	Easily destroyed
3. Daily requirements	2–4 µg	100–200 µg
4. Daily intake	5–30 µg	100–500 µg
5. Site of absorption	Ileum	Duodenum and jejunum
6. Mechanism of absorption	Intrinsic factor	Conversion to methyl-THF
7. Body stores	2–3 mg (enough for 2–4 years)	10–12 mg (enough for 4 months)

- Metabolic functions of vitamin B_{12} and folates are closely interlinked, and both are critical for the synthesis of DNA **(Fig. 11.13)**.

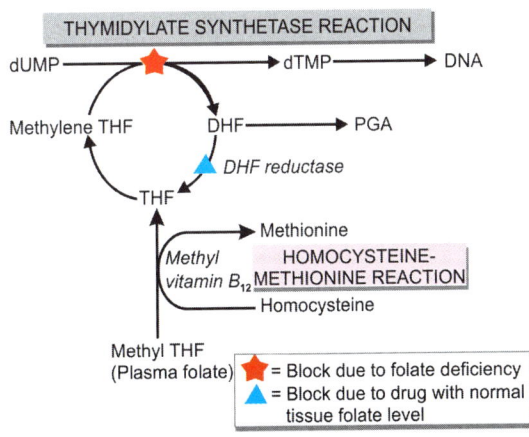

FIGURE 11.13: Biochemical basis of megaloblastic anaemia. (THF, tetrahydrofolate; DHF, dihydrofolate; PGA, pteroyl glutamic acid; dUMP, deoxy uridylate monophosphate; dTMP, deoxy thymidylate monophosphate).

- Vitamin B_{12} is also important for the synthesis of *neuronal lipids,* which accounts for common involvement of the central nervous system in vitamin B_{12} deficiency.

Megaloblastic anaemia may be caused by i) nutritional deficiency of vitamin B_{12} or folic acid, or ii) deficiency of these vitamins caused by other mechanisms, such as abnormal absorption, increased demand, increased loss, metabolic disturbances, drug effects, etc. **(Table 11.9)**.

TABLE 11.9 Etiologic classification of megaloblastic anaemia.

I. VITAMIN B_{12} DEFICIENCY

A. *Inadequate dietary intake,* e.g. strict vegetarians, breast-fed infants.
B. *Malabsorption*
  1. *Gastric causes:* pernicious anaemia, gastrectomy, congenital lack of intrinsic factor.
  2. *Intestinal causes:* tropical sprue, ileal resection, Crohn disease, intestinal blind loop syndrome, fish-tapeworm infestation.

II. FOLATE DEFICIENCY

A. *Inadequate dietary intake,* e.g. in alcoholics, teenagers, infants, old age, poverty.
B. *Malabsorption,* e.g. in tropical sprue, coeliac disease, partial gastrectomy, jejunal resection, Crohn disease.
C. *Excess demand*
  1. *Physiological:* pregnancy, lactation, infancy.
  2. *Pathological:* malignancy, increased haematopoiesis, chronic exfoliative skin disorders, tuberculosis, rheumatoid arthritis.
D. *Excess urinary folate loss,* e.g. in active liver disease, congestive heart failure.

III. OTHER CAUSES

A. *Impaired metabolism,* e.g. inhibitors of dihydrofolate (DHF) reductase such as methotrexate and pyrimethamine; alcohol, congenital enzyme deficiencies.
B. *Unknown etiology,* e.g. in Di Guglielmo syndrome, congenital dyserythropoietic anaemia, refractory megaloblastic anaemia.

Q29. What are the laboratory findings in megaloblastic anaemia?

Laboratory findings Anaemia is variable and may be mild or moderate, and rarely severe. Leucocytes and platelets are affected but to a minor degree. Typical laboratory features include as follows **(Fig. 11.14)**:

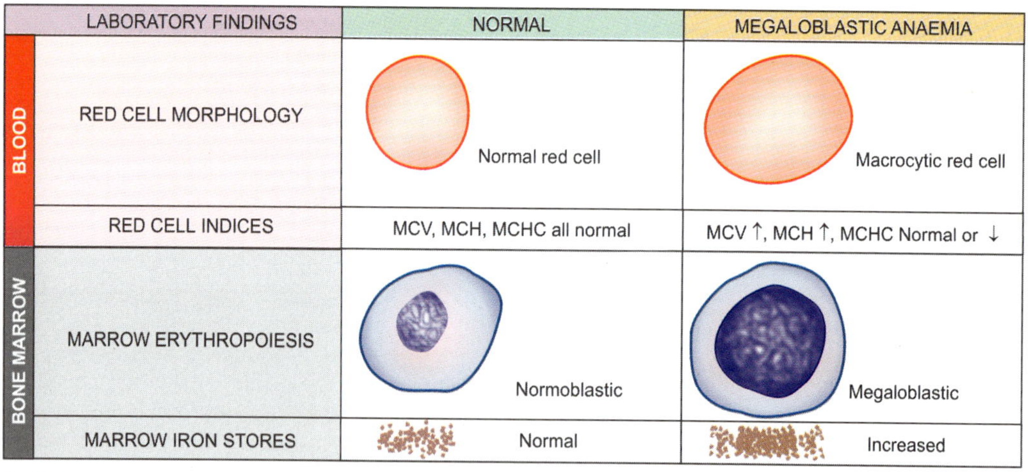

	LABORATORY FINDINGS	NORMAL	MEGALOBLASTIC ANAEMIA
BLOOD	RED CELL MORPHOLOGY	Normal red cell	Macrocytic red cell
BLOOD	RED CELL INDICES	MCV, MCH, MCHC all normal	MCV ↑, MCH ↑, MCHC Normal or ↓
BONE MARROW	MARROW ERYTHROPOIESIS	Normoblastic	Megaloblastic
BONE MARROW	MARROW IRON STORES	Normal	Increased

FIGURE 11.14: General laboratory findings in megaloblastic anaemia.

i. **Haemoglobin** ↓
ii. **RBC indices** MCV ↑ (>120 fL), MCH ↑ (>50 pg/cell), normal or slightly reduced MCHC
iii. **Peripheral blood morphology** RBC macrocytosis, aniso-poikilocytosis, some basophilic stippling
iv. **Leucocytes** Hypersegmented (>5 lobes)
v. **Platelets** Number mildly reduced, bizarre-shaped platelets may be present
vi. **Bone marrow** Nuclear maturation lags cytoplasmic maturation of RBC precursors **(Table 11.10)**
a. Megaloblastic erythropoiesis

TABLE 11.10 Contrasting features of megaloblast and erythroblast.

FEATURE	ERYTHROBLAST	MEGALOBLAST
1. Cell size	Normal	Larger than corresponding stage
2. Nuclear size	Normal	Larger than corresponding stage
3. Nuclear chromatin	Normal for corresponding stage	Lighter, open even in late stage
4. Nuclear maturation	Normal for corresponding stage	Lags behind in late stage
5. Mitosis	Normal	Frequent, abnormal
6. Cytoplasmic maturation	Normal for corresponding stage	Unaffected
7. Colour of cytoplasm	Normal for corresponding stage	Normal for corresponding stage

b. Normal reticulocytes
c. Iron stores ↑
d. Chromosomal abnormalities may be present but are not diagnostic

vii. **Biochemical findings** Unconjugated bilirubin ↑, LDH ↑ due to inefficient erythropoiesis.

viii. **Special tests** Serum vitamin B_{12} or folate tests to distinguish these two forms of vitamin deficiency:

a. *Schilling test:* B_{12} 24 hours urinary excretion following oral administration of radioactive cobalt.
b. *With modifications* it can distinguish dietary B_{12} deficiency from IF deficiency.
c. *Formiminoglutamic (FIGLU) urinary excretion* after histidine injection to test for folate deficiency.

Treatment Most cases of megaloblastic anaemia need therapy with appropriate vitamin:

- Hydroxycobalamin as intramuscular injection and oral folic acid. Severely-anaemic patients in whom a definite deficiency of either vitamin cannot be established with certainty are treated with both vitamins concurrently.
- *Response to treatment:* marrow begins to revert back to normal morphology within a few hours of initiating treatment; becomes normoblastic within 48 hours of start of treatment. Reticulocytosis appears within 4–5 days after therapy is started and peaks at day 7. Haemoglobin should rise by 2–3 g/dL each fortnight.

Q30. What is pernicious anaemia? Discuss its salient features.

Definition Pernicious anaemia (PA) is a megaloblastic anaemia caused by atrophic gastritis-related vitamin B_{12} deficiency, which is secondary to a lack of intrinsic factor (IF).

Etiopathogenesis PA is an *autoimmune disease* characterised by the appearance of autoantibodies to gastric parietal cells or intrinsic factor, which is essential for the absorption of vitamin B_{12}. Autoantibodies belong to three categories:

i. *Blocking or type I antibodies to IF* (55%), preventing the combining of IF to vitamin B_{12}.
ii. *Binding or type II antibodies to IF* (35%), preventing the attachment of IF to ileal mucosa.
iii. *Antibodies to parietal cells,* i.e. cells that secrete IF, in 90% cases.

Facts that support the autoimmune nature of PA include the following:

i. Association with other autoimmune diseases such as Graves disease, Hashimoto thyroiditis, vitiligo, Addison disease.
ii. Familial occurrence of PA and the presence of autoantibodies in the blood of relatives.
iii. Higher incidence of PA in persons of certain HLA haplotypes (HLA-3 and HLA-B8).
iv. Treatment with corticosteroids may improve the symptoms.

Clinicopathologic aspects The average age at presentation is 60 years. It is more common in persons of northern European and African American origin. Clinical findings and symptoms include:

i. Megaloblastic anaemia, sometimes combined with platelet disorders and bleeding tendency.
ii. Glossitis with a beefy red enlarged tongue.
iii. Atrophic gastritis (dyspepsia, anorexia, diarrhoea, weight loss).
iv. Neurologic abnormalities (peripheral neuropathy, subacute combined degeneration of the spinal cord, retrobulbar neuritis).
v. Association with other autoimmune diseases.
vi. Increased incidence of gastric cancer (2–3% develop gastric cancer).

Treatment includes parenteral administration of B_{12} vitamin and supportive measures to combat the complications of anaemia, including the early diagnosis of gastric cancer if it occurs. Neurologic abnormalities are resistant to treatment.

■ HAEMOLYTIC ANAEMIAS AND ANAEMIAS OF BLOOD LOSS

Q31. Define haemolytic anaemias. How are these classified?

Definition Haemolytic anaemias result from increased red cell destruction (haemolysis), which shortens red cell lifespan. Haemolysis is accompanied by compensatory red cell production, which may be increased 6–8 time over the normal (*compensated haemolytic disease*); clinical signs of anaemia develop only after all compensatory measures have been exhausted.

Classification Haemolytic anaemias can be classified as follows:

I. Site of haemolysis

i. *Intravascular haemolysis* (occurring inside the blood vessels and marked by high levels of free haemoglobin in plasma).

ii. *Extravascular haemolysis* (occurring in the fixed macrophages and, thus, not associated with elevated levels of haemoglobin in plasma).

II. Duration of haemolysis

i. Acute anaemia
ii. Chronic anaemia

III. Pathogenesis of haemolysis

i. Acquired haemolytic anaemias caused by extrinsic factors (i.e. *extracorpuscular*)

ii. Hereditary haemolytic anaemias due to intrinsic RBC defects (i.e. *inracorpuscular*)

Pathogenetic classification of haemolytic anaemias is illustrated in **Figure 11.15** and presented in **Table 11.11**.

Clinicopathologic aspects Typically, there is evidence of anaemia and haemolysis.

TABLE 11.11 Classification of haemolytic anaemias.

I. ACQUIRED
A. *Antibody:* Immunohaemolytic anaemias
 1. Autoimmune haemolytic anaemia (AIHA)
  i. Warm antibody AIHA
  ii. Cold antibody AIHA
 2. Drug-induced immunohaemolytic anaemia
 3. Isoimmune haemolytic anaemia (page 267)
B. *Mechanical trauma:* Microangiopathic haemolytic anaemia
C. *Direct toxic effects:* Malaria, bacterial, infection and other agents
D. *Acquired red cell membrane abnormalities:* Paroxysmal nocturnal haemoglobinuria (PNH)
E. *Splenomegaly*

II. HEREDITARY
A. *Abnormalities of red cell membrane*
 1. Hereditary spherocytosis
 2. Hereditary elliptocytosis (hereditary ovalocytosis)
 3. Hereditary stomatocytosis
B. *Disorders of red cell interior*
 1. *Red cell enzyme defects (Enzymopathies)*
  i. Defects in the hexose monophosphate shunt: G6PD deficiency
  ii. Defects in the Embden-Meyerhof (or glycolytic) pathway: pyruvate kinase deficiency
 2. *Disorders of haemoglobin (Haemoglobinopathies)*
  i. Structurally abnormal haemoglobins: sickle syndromes, other haemoglobinopathies
  ii. Reduced globin chain synthesis: thalassaemias

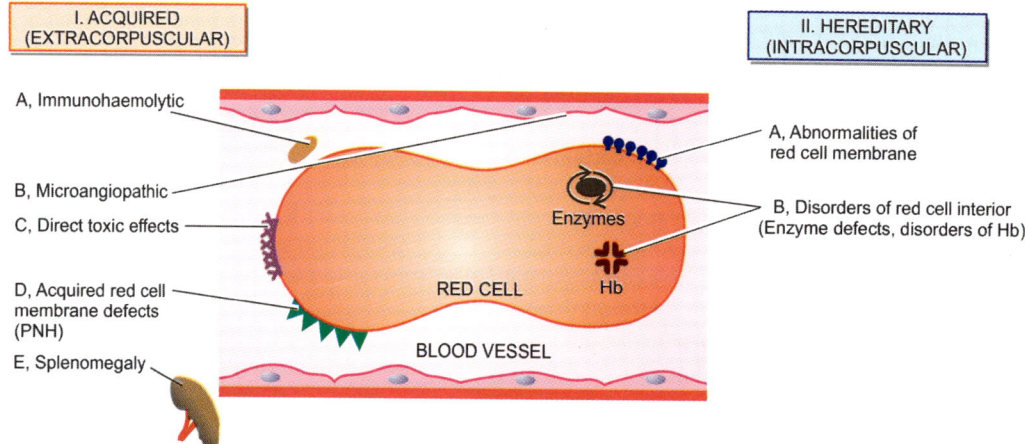

FIGURE 11.15: Diagrammatic representation of classification of haemolytic anaemias based on principal mechanisms of haemolysis.

i. Positive family history in patients with life-long congenital haemolytic anaemia.
ii. Autoimmune phenomena in patients with autoimmune haemolytic anaemia.
iii. History of exposure to infections (e.g. malaria), drugs or some other form of treatment in patients with non-immune extravascular haemolysis.
iv. Pallor of mucus membranes and conjunctiva.
v. Mild fluctuating jaundice due to unconjugated hyperbilirubinaemia.
vi. Urine turns dark on standing due to excess of urobilinogen in urine.
vii. Pigmentary gallstones due to hyperbilirubinaemia.
viii. Splenomegaly in most congenital and acquired haemolytic anaemias.

Q32. List the general tests which should be performed on a patient suspected of having haemolytic anaemia.

The investigations should provide answers to the following three questions:
A. Is there evidence of haemolysis?
B. What is the type of haemolytic mechanism?
C. What is the precise diagnosis?
To find answers to these questions, one must perform laboratory tests which fall in four categories: i) tests of increased red cell breakdown, ii) tests of increased red cell production, iii) tests of damage to red cells, and iv) tests for shortened red cell lifespan.

I. Tests of increased red cell breakdown
i. *Raised levels:*
a. Serum unconjugated (indirect) bilirubin
b. Urine urobilinogen
c. Faecal stercobilirubinogen
d. Plasma lactic dehydrogenase
ii. *Reduced levels:*
Serum haptoglobin, which is bound to haemoglobin released from haemolysed RBCs.
iii. *Negative findings (or normal values):*
Bilirubin in urine, because unconjugated bilirubin does not pass into urine.
NOTE: In patients with intravascular haemolysis there is haemoglobinaemia, haemoglobinuria, methaemoglobinaemia, and haemosiderinaemia. Splenomegaly is found in all forms of haemolytic anaemia.

II. Tests of increased red cell production
i. Reticulocyte count, which rises early and is the most reliable sign of bone marrow erythroid hyperplasia.
ii. Peripheral blood smear showing macrocytosis, polychromasia, and the presence of erythroblasts.
iii. Bone marrow biopsy showing signs of erythroid hyperplasia.
iv. X-ray of bones in chronic haemolytic anaemia shows bone marrow space expansion, especially in tubular bones and skull.

III. Tests of damage to red cells
i. Peripheral blood smears → various abnormal forms (e.g. spherocytes, target cells, etc.) and other morphologic abnormalities **(Table 11.12)**
ii. Osmotic fragility (can be increased or decreased)
iii. Autohaemolysis test, with or without addition of glucose
iv. Coombs' antiglobulin test
v. Estimation of haemoglobins HBA_2 and HBF
vi. Tests for sickling
vii. Screening test for G6PD deficiency and other enzymes (e.g. Heinz bodies test)

IV. Tests for shortened red cell lifespan
i. Best test is ^{51}Cr labeling method.
ii. Normal life span of RBCs is 120 days.
iii. Lifespan is shortened to 20–40 days in moderate haemolysis.
iv. Lifespan is shortened to 5–20 days in severe haemolysis.

TABLE 11.12 Salient red cell morphologic abnormalities in various types of haemolytic anaemias.

FEATURE	ETIOLOGY	TYPE OF HAEMOLYTIC ANAEMIA
1. *Spherocytes*	Loss of spectrin from membrane	Hereditary spherocytosis AIHA
2. *Target cells (Leptocytes)*	Increased ratio of surface area: volume	Thalassaemias Liver disease HbS disease
3. *Schistocytes*	Traumatic damage to red cell membrane	Microangiopathy
4. *Sickle cells*	Polymerisation of HbS	Sickle cell syndromes
5. *Acanthocytes (Spur cells)*	Abnormality in membrane lipids	Severe liver disease
6. *Heinz bodies*	Precipitated Hb, seen by supravital stain	Unstable Hb G6PD deficiency
7. *Howell-Jolly bodies*	Basophilic nuclear remnants	Post-splenectomy

Q33. What are the laboratory and clinical findings that distinguish extravascular and intravascular haemolysis?

Contrasting features of extravascular and intravascular haemolysis are presented in **Table 11.13**.

TABLE 11.13 Contrasting features of extravascular and intravascular haemolysis.

FEATURE	EXTRAVASCULAR HAEMOLYSIS	INTRAVASCULAR HAEMOLYSIS
1. *Frequency*	More common	Less common
2. *Location*	RE system organs (spleen, bone marrow, liver)	In peripheral blood
3. *Iron stores*	Increased	Decreased
4. *Serum ferritin*	Normal to high	Low
5. *Plasma haemoglobin*	Absent	Present
6. *Methaemoglobin*	Absent	Present
7. *Haemoglobinuria*	Absent	Present
8. *Haemosiderinuria*	Absent	Present
9. *Unconjugated hyperbilirubinaemia*	Markedly elevated	Mildly elevated
10. *Serum LDH*	Mildly elevated	Markedly elevated
11. *Serum haptoglobin*	Normal	Decreased
12. *Causes*	i. *Intracorpuscular defects:* haemoglobinopathies, enzymopathies, membrane defects ii. *Extracorpuscular defects:* immune haemolytic (autoimmune, drugs), liver disease	i. Red cell fragmentation (e.g. MAHA, prosthetic valve, TTP/HUS) ii. ABO mismatch transfusion iii. PNH iv. PCH v. Drugs vi. Infections, toxins, snake bite

(LDH, lactic dehydrogenase; MAHA, microangiopathic haemolytic anaemia; TTP/HUS, thrombotic thrombocytopenic purpura/haemolytic uraemic syndrome; PNH, paroxysmal nocturnal haemoglobinuria; PCH, paroxysmal cold hameoglobinuria)

Q34. What are the possible causes of acquired haemolytic anaemias?

Acquired anaemias could be caused by a variety of extrinsic factors as listed earlier in **Table 11.11**; these are as under:
i. Antibodies (e.g. immunohaemolytic anaemias)
ii. Mechanical factors (e.g.microangiopathic haemolytic anaemia or MAHA)
iii. Direct toxic effects of infectious agents or their toxins (e.g. malaria, clostridial infections)
iv. Splenomegaly of any cause
v. Acquired red cell membrane abnormalities (e.g. paroxysmal nocturnal haemoglobinuria or PNH)

Q35. What are immunohaemolytic anaemias and how are they classified?

Definition Immunohaemolytic anaemias are characterised by the production of antibodies against its own RBCs.

Classification There are three types:
I. *Autoimmune haemolytic anaemia (AIHA)*, characterised by the production of antibodies to patient's own RBCs. These are subdivided according to the optimal temperature for the action of their antibodies into:
i. Warm antibody AIHA
ii. Cold antibody AIHA
II. *Drug-induced immunohaemolytic anaemia*
III. *Isoimmune haemolytic anaemia* in which the antibodies are acquired by blood transfusion, pregnancy or haemolytic disease of the newborn

Q36. What is autoimmune haemolytic anaemia? Discuss its types and their main features.

Definition AIHA are characterised by the production of autoantibodies to their own RBCs.

Classification and etiology
- If the antibodies are optimally reactive at 37°C, they are called *warm*.
- If reactive at 4°C, they are called *cold*.

Their causes are presented in **Table 11.14**.

TABLE 11.14 Conditions predisposing to autoimmune haemolytic anaemia (AIHA).

A. WARM ANTIBODY AIHA
1. Idiopathic (primary)
2. Lymphomas-leukaemias, e.g. non-Hodgkin lymphoma, CLL, Hodgkin disease.
3. Collagen vascular diseases, e.g SLE
4. Drugs, e.g. methyldopa, penicillin, quinidine group
5. Post-viral

B. COLD ANTIBODY AIHA
1. Cold agglutinin disease
   a. Acute: *Mycoplasma* infection, infectious mononucleosis
   b. Chronic: Idiopathic, lymphomas
2. PCH (*Mycoplasma* infection, tertiary syphilis)

I. Warm antibody AIHA
Etiopathogenesis AIHA is most often idiopathic and it can occur at any age.
- Approximately 25% of cases are linked to *autoimmune diseases* (e.g. SLE) or lymphoma or drugs.
- Antibodies are usually *IgG which coat the surface of red cells*, facilitating their uptake by fixed macrophages of the spleen and liver, where *extravascular haemolysis* occurs.
- Red blood cells attached to macrophages that are not phagocytosed, loose part of their cytoplasm and transform into *spherocytes*.

Clinicopathologic aspects Chronic anaemia of varying severity with remissions and relapses.
i. Anaemia is normocytic with prominent sphaerocytosis.
ii. Splenomegaly like in most other haemolytic anaemias.
iii. Reticulocytosis to compensate for the red cell loss.
iv. Hyperbilirubinaemia (unconjugated).
v. Positive direct Coombs test for the presence of warm autoantibodies at 37°C on RBCs.
vi. Indirect Coombs test is positive if there are abundant antibodies in the serum.
vii. In severe cases, one may encounter autoimmune thrombocytopenia with venous thrombosis (*Evans syndrome*), or haemoglobinaemia and haemoglobinuria.

Therapy includes removal of the cause of AIHA, corticosteroids. In severe cases, blood transfusion may be indicated.

II. Cold antibody AIHA
Etiopathogenesis This entity includes following two conditions:
i. *Cold agglutinin disease* Caused by viral diseases (e.g. EBV, CMV) or lymphoma.
a. Antibodies are directed to *I antigen* on RBCs.
b. Antibodies of the IgM type bind to RBCs at 4°C causing haemagglutination, which is reversed by heating the blood to 37°C.
c. Antibody binding to RBC will fix C3 complement which mediates haemolysis.
d. Cold antibodies affect juvenile RBCs, and therefore, the reticulocyte count is low.
ii. *Paroxysmal cold haemoglobinuria (PCH)* It is a rare condition seen as a complication of *Mycoplasma pneumoniae* infection and tertiary syphilis.
a. Antibodies directed to *P antigen* on RBCs.
b. Chronic anaemia which is worsened and becomes haemolytic by exposure to cold.
c. Raynaud phenomenon prominent.
d. Cyanosis is precipitated by exposure to cold, affecting the tips pf the nose, ears, fingers and toes.

e. Haemoglobinaemia and haemoglobinuria upon exposure to cold.

Laboratory findings for both types of cold AIHA are similar to warm antibody AIHA, with a few minor differences:
- Reticulocyte count is low in cold agglutinin disease since it affects young RBCs.
- Positive Coombs test detects C3 but IgM is not found.
- Specificity of antibodies to I or P antigen can be demonstrated.

Q37. How does adverse drug reaction cause immunohaemolytic anaemia?

Drugs may cause immunohaemolysis by three different mechanisms:

i. **Induction of warm antibodies** similar to those in warm antibody AIHA (e.g. methyl-DOPA induced antibodies).

ii. **Formation of antigenic complexes** between the drug and the RBCs to which it has attached. These complexes act as 'neoantigens' and elicit an antibody reaction (e.g. penicillin-induced immunohaemolysis).

iii. **Innocent bystander immunohaemolysis** induced by drugs like quinidine, which form antigenic complexes with plasma proteins. Newly formed immune complexes elicit antibody production. Antibodies bind to antigen and activate complement which damages RBCs and platelets.

Q38. What is microangiopathic haemolytic anaemia? Comment on its etiology and pathogenesis.

Definition Microangiopathic anaemia (MAHA) is a form of haemolytic anaemia which is caused by fragmentation of red blood cells as they are passing through abnormal microvasculature.

Etiopathogenesis Damaged RBCs change their shapes and become spiked schistocytes, burr cells (or echinocytes) or helmet cells **(Fig. 11.16)**. Haemolysis may occur due to following factors/conditions:

i. *External impact* Direct external pressure or trauma may cause haemolysis of RBCs as they are passing through the capillaries and venules, especially over bony prominences. Such haemolysis occurs during prolonged marches, long distance running, or karate matches. Heamoglobinemia and haemoglobinuria may be accompanied by myoglobinuria due to muscle injury.

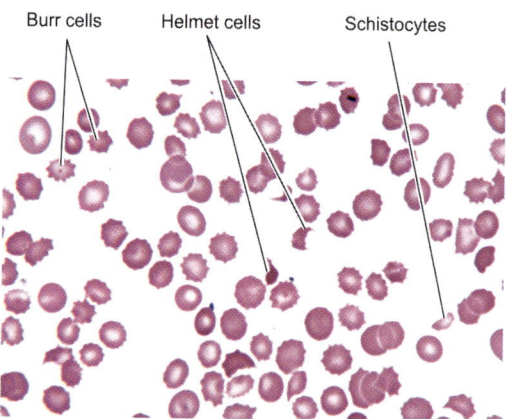

FIGURE 11.16: Microangiopathic haemolytic anaemia (MAHA). Peripheral blood smear shows morphologically abnormal red cells as schistocytes, helmet cells, and burr cells (or echinocytes).

ii. *Fibrin deposition in microvasculature* Fibrin-meshwork may pose a sponge-like barrier to blood cells, which get damaged while trying to pass through the narrow and irregular spaces between the strands of fibrin. Conditions that cause microangiopathic haemolysis include the following:
a. Disseminated intravascular coagulation due to shock or sepsis
b. Dissemination of cancer
c. Transplant rejection
d. Haemolytic uraemic syndrome
e. Thrombotic thrombocytopenic purpura (TTP)
f. Autoimmune disorders with vasculitis
g. Eclampsia

NOTE: Mechanical haemolysis similar to microangiopathic haemolytic anaemia can occur in the heart following installation of prosthetic valves which may cause blood flow turbulence damaging the RBCs.

Q39. What are the most important causes of haemolytic anemia caused by direct toxic effects on the red blood cells?

In general terms, haemolysis could be caused by microbial pathogens directly parasitising the RBCs, pathogens secreting toxin, or by the direct action of chemicals, toxins and physical forces, as under:

i. Malaria
ii. Bartonellosis
iii. *Clostridium welchii* sepsis
iv. Sepsis caused by common bacterial pathogens (e.g. *Streptococcus, Staphylococcus, E. coli,* etc.)
v. Copper (e.g. in patients with Wilson disease)
vi. Haemodialysis-associated haemolysis (due to increased chloramines in the water used for dialysis, or from nitrate contamination)
vii. Lead poisoning (associated with basophilic stippling)
viii. Venomous snake or spider bites
ix. Extensive burns

Q40. What is paroxysmal nocturnal haemoglobinuria? Discuss its key features.

Definition Paroxysmal nocturnal haemoglobinuria (PNH) is a rare acquired condition characterised by an intrinsic red blood cell membrane, rendering these cells unduly sensitive to destructive action of activated complement.

Etiopathogenesis PNH is based on a *somatic mutation* of the X-linked gene *PIG-A* (*phosphatidyl inositol glycan-A*) causing *clonal proliferation* of myeloid progenitor cells and defective haematopoiesis (RBCs, leucocytes, platelets) **(Fig. 11.17)**:

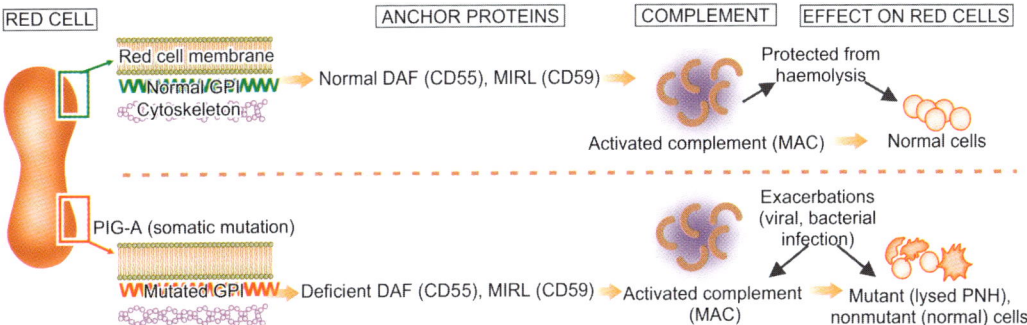

FIGURE 11.17: Pathogenesis of haemolysis in PNH.

- Since the mutation involves somatic cells, the bone marrow and the blood will contain two cell populations: clones of mutant and non-mutant cells.
- The mutations of *PIG-A* leads to a defective synthesis of membrane glycolipid called *glycosyl phosphatidyl inositol* (GPI), which is essential for anchoring of cells.
- GPI defect interferes with the binding of GPI-anchored proteins that *protect the RBC from the attack of activated complement;* these are *decay accelerating factor (DAF or CD55),* and *membrane inhibitor of reactive lysis (MIRL or CD59).*
- Haemolysis of mutant RBCs occurs through the action of membrane attack complex (MAC) formed from activated complement.
- Haemolysis is also exacerbated by infections that may activate complement.

Clinicopathologic aspects
i. Haemolytic anaemia with mild pancytopenia involving WBCs and platelets.
ii. Intermittent attacks of haemolysis are accompanied by nocturnal haemoglobinuria ('brown urine').
iii. Haemosiderinuria is common.
iv. Venous thrombosis due to inappropriate activation of mutant platelets.

Laboratory test Increased sensitivity of red blood cells to complement may be demonstrated by Ham test, which includes haemolysis at acidic pH or sucrose haemolysis test.

Q41. What are the principal forms of hereditary haemolytic anaemia?

Haemolytic anaemias are classified into two groups:
I. **Hereditary abnormalities of red cell membrane**:
i. Hereditary spherocytosis
ii. Hereditary elliptocytosis

iii. Hereditary stomatocytosis

II. **Hereditary disorders of the interior of the red cells:**
i. *Enzymopathies*, such as
a. Hexose monophosphate shunt (e.g. glucose-6-phosphate dehydrogenase)
b. Embden-Meyerhof (glycolytic) pathway (e.g. pyruvate kinase deficiency)
ii. *Haemoglobinopathies*, such as
a. Structurally abnormal haemoglobins, e.g. sickle cell syndrome
b. Reduced globin chain synthesis, e.g. various thalassemias

Q42. What is hereditary spherocytosis? Briefly discuss its main features.

Definition Hereditary spherocytosis is a common type of hereditary haemolytic anaemia in which the red blood cell membrane abnormality leads to spheroidal deformity of RBCs and their increased osmotic fragility. It is the commonest hereditary haemolytic anaemia in persons of northern European descent. In the US, the incidence of clinical cases is 1:5000.

Etiopathogenesis Spherocytosis is caused by mutation of genes encoding proteins which anchor the lipid bilayer of the cell membrane to the cytoskeleton **(Fig. 11.18)**:

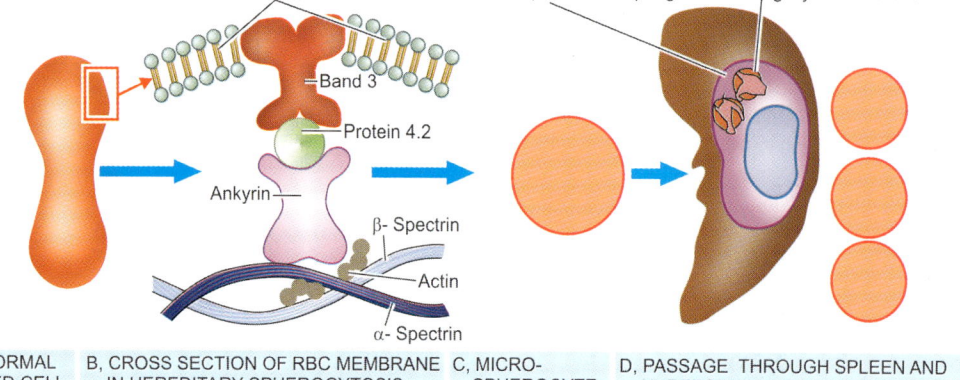

A, NORMAL RED CELL   B, CROSS SECTION OF RBC MEMBRANE IN HEREDITARY SPHEROCYTOSIS   C, MICRO-SPHEROCYTE   D, PASSAGE THROUGH SPLEEN AND HYPERSPHEROIDAL SPHEROCYTES

FIGURE 11.18: Diagrammatic representation of pathogenesis of hereditary spherocytosis. A, Normal red cell with biconcave surface and normal size. B, Red cell membrane as seen in cross section in hereditary spherocytosis. Mutations in membrane proteins—α-spectrin, β-spectrin and ankyrin, result in defect in anchoring of lipid bilayer of the membrane to the underlying cytoskeleton. C, This results in spherical contour and small size so as to contain the given volume of haemoglobin in the deformed red cell. D, During passage through the spleen, these rigid spherical cells lose their cell membrane further. This produces a circulating subpopulation of hyperspheroidal spherocytes while splenic macrophages in large numbers phagocytose defective red cells causing splenomegaly.

- Gene mutations affect the structural stability of the red blood cell membrane leading to cell membrane loss and formation of microspherocytes.
- The most important are the genes encoding ankyrin, spectrin-α and β, protein 4.2 and band 3.
- The disease is most often inherited as an autosomal dominant trait.
- There are also autosomal recessive forms. In approximately 25% of cases, the disease is caused by a new mutation.

Clinicopathologic aspects All patients have anaemia which varies from mild to severe.
i. Haemolysis results in hyperbilirubinaemia and jaundice, which may be the presenting symptom of spherocytosis in early infancy.
ii. Splenomegaly is a constant feature.
iii. Splenectomy may reduce haemolysis and is, therefore, used for the treatment of severe anaemia.
iv. Pigment gallstones are common.
v. Aplastic crisis (10–15% of patients) may occur sometimes after viral infections, especially in children.

Laboratory findings
i. *Microspherocytes* are seen in peripheral blood smears.
ii. *RBC indices:* MCV is normal of slightly decreased, but the *MCHC* is increased.
iii. *Osmotic fragility* is increased as detected by lysis of RBC in solutions at low salt concentration.

iv. *Autohaemolysis* of blood is increased. Blood left overnight in test tubes shows autohaemolysis in the range of 10–15% of all RBCs, in contrast to normal blood, which shows haemolysis of less than 4% RBC. Autohaemolysis is correctable by addition of glucose.
v. *Gel electrophoresis* is used to analyse mutant proteins.
vi. *Coombs test* is negative and important to distinguish hereditary spherocytosis from AIHA, in which it is positive.

Q43. What is hereditary elliptocytosis?

Definition Hereditary elliptocytosis (ovalocytosis) is a hereditary haemolytic anaemia, similar to mild spherocytosis.
The incidence in USA/Europe is 1:5,000 but is much higher in some parts of the world.
Etiopathogenesis Most often, elliptocytosis is caused by mutations of gene encoding for spectrin-α or β, and less often for protein 4.1.
Clinicopathologic aspects Most patients are asymptomatic.
i. Mild haemolytic anaemia with splenomegaly.
ii. In severe haemolytic anaemia, splenectomy may be indicated.
Laboratory findings
i. The peripheral blood smears contain more than 25% elliptocytes, also known as ovalocytes (normal peripheral blood smears contain <15 elliptocytes).
ii. Diagnosis is confirmed by testing RBC for osmotic fragility, and electrophoresis of RBC proteins.
NOTE: Hereditary elliptocytosis must be distinguished from acquired elliptocytosis found in iron deficiency anaemia and myeloproliferative disorders.

Q44. Discuss the main genetic enzymopathies that cause hereditary haemolytic anaemia.

Most important are mutations involving genes which encode enzymes in the *metabolism of glucose* as under:
- Hexose monophosphate shunt (e.g. glucose-6-phosphate dehydrogenase deficiency).
- Embden-Meyerhof (glycolytic) pathway (e.g. pyruvate kinase deficiency).

I. Glucose-6-phosphate (G6PD) deficiency is the most common enzymopathy causing hereditary haemolysis.
- It affects millions of people. Approximately 400 million people are affected world-wide.
- It is most prevalent in Mediterranean countries, Middle East, Africa and India.

Genetics The gene is located on the X-chromosome and thus inherited as X-linked recessive. Symptoms appear only in males, whereas females are asymptomatic carriers. Several genetic variants are recognised.
- Two variants (G6PD A– and G6PD Mediterranean) are the most common in human populations.
- G6PD A– has an occurrence of 10% of Africans and African-Americans while G6PD Mediterranean is prevalent in the Middle East.

Pathogenesis G6PD metabolises glucose-6-phosphate to 6-phosphogluconate involving the *hexose-monophosphate (HMP) shunt*.
Normally, HMP shunt includes NADP reduction to NADPH and glutathione reductase **(Fig. 11.19)**. Reduction of oxidised glutathione provides *reduced glutathione* that protects RBCs from oxidative stress.
In G6PD deficiency, there is reduced capacity to produce reduced glutathione.

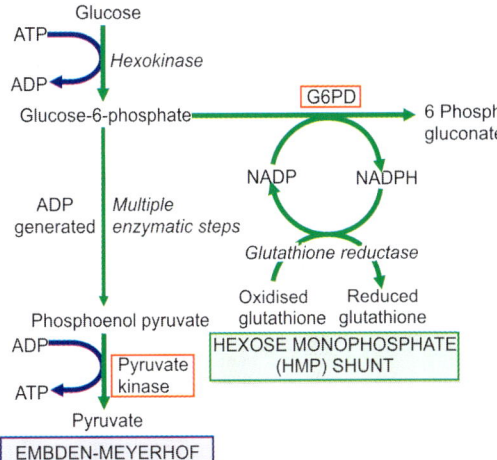

FIGURE 11.19: Abbreviated pathways of anaerobic glycolysis (Embden-Meyerhof) and hexose monophosphate (HMP) shunt in the metabolism of erythrocyte. The two red cell enzyme defects, glucose-6-phosphate dehydrogenase (G6PD) and pyruvate kinase, are shown in bold.

- Reduced levels of reduced glutathione make the affected person susceptible to *oxidative stress* generated by certain drugs (e.g. antimalarials, sulfa drugs, etc.), infections, metabolic acidosis, or foods like fava beans.
- Oxidative stress will cause haemolysis of *older RBCs*, and haemolysis ends when the older cells are eliminated.

Clinicopathologic aspects

i. Anaemia, which is mild to moderate and most of the time affected persons are asymptomatic.
ii. Patients usually have splenomegaly.
iii. *Haemolytic crises* can occur at any age and often begin in early infancy.
iv. Hemolytic crises are precipitated by infection, exposure to oxidants, or certain foods such as fava beans ('favism').
v. *Intravascular haemolysis* is accompanied by a drop of haematocrit (25–30%), hyperbilirubinaemia and jaundice, haemoglobinaemia and haemoglobinuria, low haptoglobin, and reticulosis.
vi. *Heinz bodies* in RBCs (denatured haemoglobin granules) can be seen in peripheral blood smears and even better in smears stained with supravital dies (e.g. crystal violet).
vii. Removal of Heinz bodies in the spleen results in splenomegaly and formation of *'bite cells'* and fragmented RBCs, which are seen in peripheral blood smears.

Laboratory findings The diagnosis is confirmed by screening tests (e.g. methaemoglobin reduction test or MRT), and enzyme testing of RBCs.
Treatment is directed at stoppage of offending drugs and food.

II. **Pyruvate kinase (PK) deficiency** is inherited as an autosomal recessive trait.
- It is rare (1:40,000) showing no predilection for any populations.
- PK deficient persons do not produce ATP in the glycolytic pathway and accordingly their RBCs are more prone to haemolysis.

Clinicopathologic aspects

i. Homozygote individuals present during early childhood with anaemia, splenomegaly and jaundice.
ii. Anaemia is normocytic normochromic and associated with reticulocytosis.
iii. Blood smears contain many bizarre shaped RBCs.
iv. Osmotic fragility of RBC is not increased, unless the blood is preincubated.
v. Autohaemolysis is increased but cannot be corrected by adding glucose (as in spherocytosis!).
vi. The final diagnosis is made by enzyme analysis of RBCs.

Q45. What is sickle cell disease (or sickle syndromes)? What are its main forms.

Sickle cell disease (SCD) or sickle syndromes are caused by the presence of abnormal sickle haemoglobin (HbS) in RBCs. Worldwide, it is the most prevalent haemoglobinopathy. It has the highest prevalence in Africans, especially in Central Africa where falciparum malaria is endemic; patients with HbS are relatively protected from falciparum malaria. In the US, 10% of African-Americans are heterozygous for HbS, and 1:650 are homozygous.

Forms of SCD It occur in three different forms:

I. **Heterozygous state for HbS (sickle cell trait or AS)** In this condition, only one abnormal HbS is inherited.
- The patients have no significant clinical problems except in severe hypoxic states when they may develop sickle cell crisis.
- Haemoglobin electrophoresis studies show HbS accounting for 35–40% of the total haemoglobin.
- Sickling can be elicited under conditions of reduced oxygen tension.

II. **Homozygous state for HbS (sickle cell anaemia or SS)** Clinical signs and symptoms of SS anaemia are present.

III. **Double heterozygote states** in which a combination of HbS occurs with other haemoglobinopathies.
- Most common among these are sickle-β-thalassemia ($b^S b^{thal}$), sickle C disease (SC) and sickle D disease.
- Clinically, these conditions behave like mild sickle cell anaemia. The diagnosis is made by identifying abnormal haemoglobins by haemoglobin electrophoresis.

Q46. What is sickle cell anaemia? Briefly discuss its genetics and pathogenesis.

Definition Sickle cell anaemia is a hereditary autosomal recessive disease involving a point mutation of gene for β-globin. It affects homozygous persons who have inherited the same mutated allele from both parents.

Genetics The basic defect is the single point mutation resulting in the substitution of valine for glutamic acid at 6-residue position of β-globin, producing the abnormal haemoglobin HbS (Hb $\alpha_2\beta_2^s$). The mutation is most common in Central Africa, but is also found in Mediterranean, Middle Eastern and Indian populations **(Fig. 11.20)**.

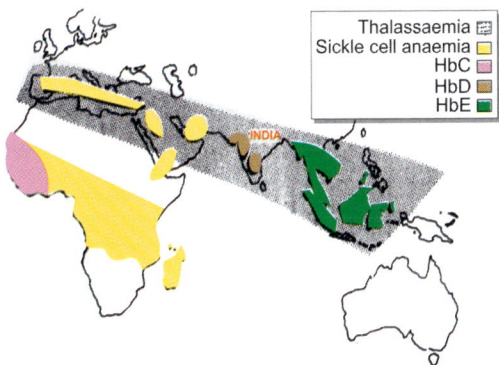

FIGURE 11.20: Geographic distribution of major haemoglobinopathies and thalassaemias. Thalassaemia and HbD are more common haemoglobin disorders in India.

Pathogenesis of sickling (Fig. 11.21)

- During deoxygenation, RBC containing HbS change from biconcave disc shape to an elongated crescent-shaped or sickle-shaped cell.
- This deformity occurs due to the polymerisation of deoxygenated HbS which aggregates to form elongated, rod-like polymers distorting each RBC.
- Sickling is reversible, but if repeated several times it may damage the cell membrane and become irreversible.

Factors which promote sickling include the following:
i. Intracellular concentration of HbS
ii. Total haemoglobin concentration
iii. Extent of deoxygenation
iv. Acidosis and dehydration
v. Increased concentration of 2,3-BPG in red blood cells
vi. Presence of non-HbS haemoglobins, such as HbC
[NOTE: HbF (which may account for 2–20% of total haemoglobin) protects against sickling whereas HbA participates in sickling].

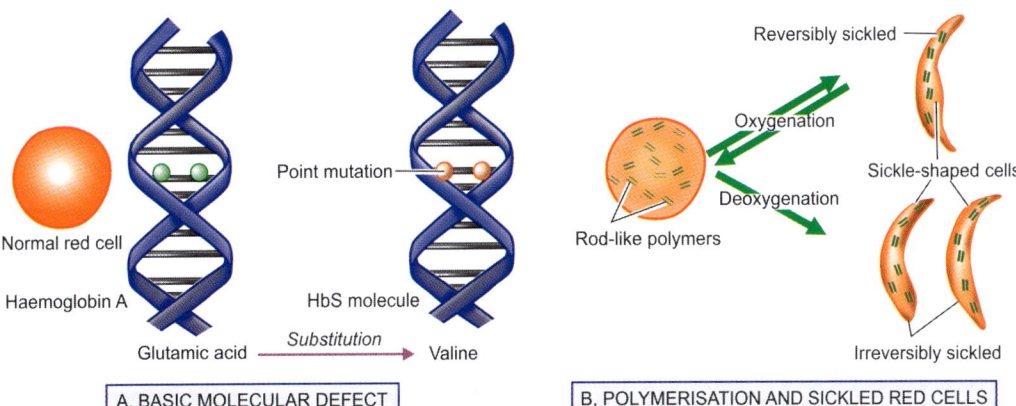

FIGURE 11.21: Pathogenesis of sickle cell anaemia. A, Basic molecular defect. B, Mechanism of polymerisation and consequent sickling of red cells containing HbS. C, Mechanism of sickling on oxygenation-deoxygenation.

Q47. Describe salient clinicopathologic features and laboratory diagnosis of sickle cell disease.

Clinicopathologic aspects Clinical findings can be divide into three groups: i) anaemia, ii) vaso-occlusive phenomena, and iii) constitutional symptoms **(Fig. 11.22)**:

I. *Severe anaemia* Primarily it is extravascular.
i. Iron stores ↑ from haemolysed RBCs and repeat transfusions → hepatic haemosiderosis.
ii. Bilirubin ↑ may lead to pigment gallstone formation.
iii. Anaemia accentuated by aplastic crises when the bone marrow cannot produce enough blood to meet the current needs of the body; most often caused by parvovirus B19 infection.
iv. Splenic sequestration crises with sudden enlargement of the congested spleen, usually in children before autosplenectomy takes place.
v. Cardiomegaly and congestive heart failure due to increased demand for the cardiac output to compensate for hypoxia caused by anaemia.
II. *Vaso-occlusive phenomena* resulting in infarcts, which are classified as micro or macroinfarcts.
i. *Microinfarcts* in the abdomen, chest, back and joints present with painful crises.
ii. *Macroinfarcts* may have numerous clinical consequences such as:
a. *Splenic autosequestration*: Loss of spleen predisposes to infection with encapsulated bacteria (e.g. *Streptococcus pneumoniae*).
b. *Aseptic necrosis of the bone* which may cause severe pain or predispose to osteomyelitis, often caused by *Salmonella typhimurium*.
c. *Pulmonary infarcts* with impaired respiratory function and predisposition to infection. *Acute pulmonary syndrome* presenting as a sudden respiratory crisis may be lethal.
d. *Cerebral infarcts* (strokes and transient ischemic attacks).
e. *Ischaemic retinopathy* (loss of sight).
f. *Skin ulcers* of lower extremities, especially over the ankles.
g. *Priapism* due to thrombosis of corpora cavernosa penis.
III. **Constitutional symptoms** are the result of cumulative effects of the disease, most prominent in children.
i. Affected children are often somnolent, sluggish and less active physically and mentally.
ii. Overall, their growth is impaired, and they have increased susceptibility to infections.

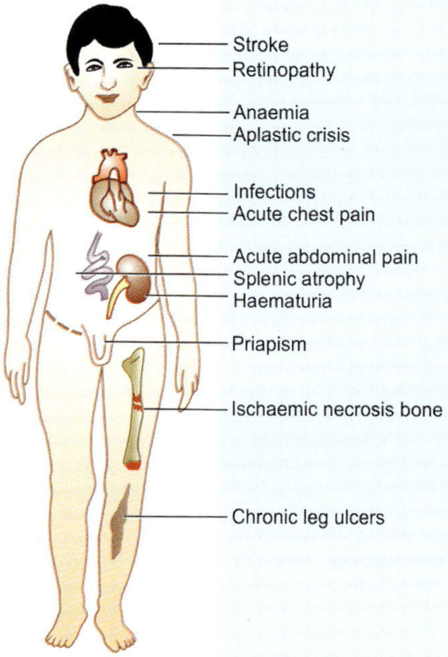

FIGURE 11.22: Major clinical manifestations of sickle cell disease.

Laboratory findings
i. Anaemia, with haemoglobin 6–9 g/dL.
ii. Peripheral blood smears contain sickle cells, target cells and Howell-Jolly bodies (nuclear remnants in the RBC) due to loss of splenic functions.
iii. Sickling can be induced in vitro by adding sodium metabisulphate.
iv. Haemoglobin electrophoresis shows the abnormal HbS, compensatory HbF (2–20%) and no normal HbA.

Q48. Define thalassaemias and their broad classification.

Definition Thalassaemias are a diverse group of hereditary anaemias characterised by *reduced synthesis* of one or more of the globin polypeptide chains. Thus, they represent *quantitative disorders of* globin polypeptide synthesis.

The name of the disease stems from the Greek word *thalassa*, referring to the Mediterranean sea, i.e. the countries surrounding it, where the first cases of thalassaemia were discovered.

Incidence Genetic abnormalities possibly affecting globin polypeptide synthesis that results in thalassaemia are found in 1–2% of the world population but most of the those persons are asymptomatic. Genetic abnormalities are more prevalent in countries around the Mediterranean basin, Middle East, South-East Asia including India and Africa.

Clinical cases of thalassaemia are diagnosed at a rate of 1:100 000 in Europe and America, but are higher in countries with more prevalent genetic.

Classification Thalassaemias are named pathogenetically by the underlying defective synthesis of alpha or beta globin polypeptide chains. Accordingly, they are named as:
- α-thalassaemia having structurally normal α-globin chains but their production is impaired.
- β-thalassaemia in which β-globin chains are structurally normal but their production is decreased.

Q49. What is alpha thalassaemia? Describe its key features.

Definition Alpha thalassaemia is a hereditary haemolytic anaemia that is characterised by deletion of 1,2,3 or 4 alpha globin genes.

Classification The synthesis of all haemoglobins that contain alpha chains (HbA, HbA2, HbF) is interrupted. Depending on how many of the four α globin genes have been deleted, one can recognise four forms of α-thalassaemia, which vary in severity as follows:

i. *Four α-genes deletion: Hydrops foetalis*
a. No HbA, which has been replaced by Hb Bart (tetramer of four gamma chains, γ_4).
b. Peripheral blood smears show profound changes in RBC morphology.
c. The foetus is affected by severe hypoxia and dies in utero or soon after birth.

ii. *Three-genes deletion: HbH disease*
a. Impaired α-chain synthesis, which leads to an increased formation of HbH (tetramer of 4 β-chains).
b. Haemoglobin electrophoresis reveals 2–4% HbH and normal amounts of HbA, HbA_2, HbF.
c. Blood smears show microcytosis, hypochromia, basophilic stippling, target cells and erythroblasts.
d. Clinically, it has an early onset. Anaemia is mild and well compensated.

iii. *Two α-gene deletion: α-thalassemia trait*
a. Present with no clinical signs and symptoms.
b. Haematologic examination reveals microcytic hypochromic anaemia in which iron deficiency and β-thalassaemia minor have been excluded, and the patients belong to one of the ethnic high-risk groups.
c. No signs of haemolytic anaemia, except for minor electrophoretic presence of Hb Bart in neonatal period which usually disappears soon in childhood.
NOTE: HbA_2 is normal or even decreased in contrast to β-thalassaemia trait in which it is increased.

iv. *One α-gene deletion: α-thalassemia asymptomatic carrier*
No signs of haemolytic anaemia

Q50. What is beta-thalassaemia? Comment on its genetics and broad classification.

Definition Beta-thalassaemia is characterised by abnormal synthesis of β-globin chain that may be reduced or completely abolished.
Complete cessation of synthesis of β-chain is marked by the symbol β°, and reduced synthesis as β⁺.

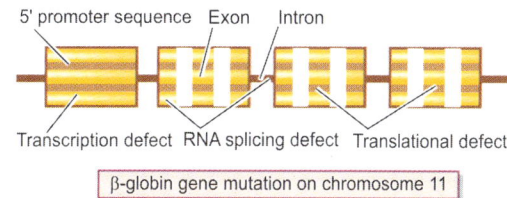

FIGURE 11.23: Schematic representation of sites of β-globin gene mutation in chromosome 11 giving rise to β-thalassaemia.

Genetics Haemoglobin abnormalities are related to β-globin gene mutations on chromosome 11, which may involve three mechanisms, depicted in **Figure 11.23** and as under:

i. *Transcriptional defect* involving the transcriptional promoter resulting in reduced synthesis (β⁺ thalassaemia).
ii. *Translational defect* (stop codon chain termination resulting in β° thalassaemia).
iii. *mRNA slicing defect* which results in intranuclear partial or complete degradation of defective mRNA (resulting in β⁺ or β° thalassaemia)

Classification Depending on the extent of reduction of β-chain synthesis, there are three forms of beta thalassemia:
i. β-thalassemia major
ii. β-thalassemia intermedia
iii. β-thalassemia minor

Q51. Discuss salient clinicopathologic features and laboratory findings in various types of beta-thalassaemia.

I. β-thalassemia major, also known as Mediterranean or Cooley anaemia.
- The most common form congenital hereditary haemolytic anaemia.
- Characterised by complete absence of β-chain (β°), or markedly reduced synthesis of β-chain (β⁺).
- Absence or reduction in the amount of β-chain results in excessive compensatory formation of alternate haemoglobins, HbF ($α_2γ_2$) and HbA$_2$ ($α_2δ_2$).

Clinicopathologic aspects Haemolytic anaemia requiring frequent transfusions with serious consequences in many organ systems **(Fig. 11.24)**:
i. *Early onset of anaemia* in the first 4–6 months, when the switch from γ-chain to β-chain occurs.
ii. *Massive hepatosplenomegaly* due to RBC destruction, extramedullary haematopoiesis, and iron accumulation.
iii. Haemosiderosis due to inefficient haematopoiesis, increased iron absorption and repeated transfusions.
iv. *Deposits of haemosiderin* in the liver, spleen, heart, endocrine pancreas, and pituitary, affecting the function of these organs (respectively fibrosis of liver, splenomegaly, cardiopathy, diabetes mellitus, and reduced pituitary function resulting in slow growth and delayed puberty).
v. *Expansion of bones* due to marked erythroid hyperplasia, most notably involving the skull ('hair on end' appearance of the calvaria of bones on X-rays) and facial bones ('thalassaemia facies' with prominent cheek bones and malocclusion of protruding jaw).

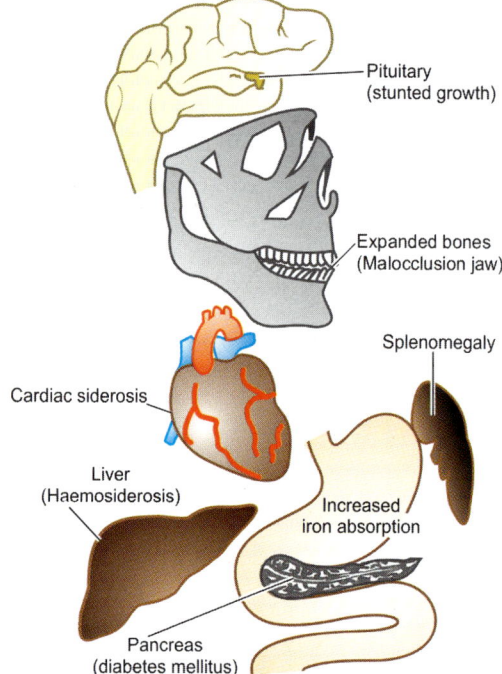

FIGURE 11.24: Major clinical features of β-thalassaemia major.

Prognosis Life expectancy of most patients is markedly reduced. The biggest problem is iron overload from frequent transfusions which damage the heart. Heart failure is the most common cause of death. New treatment modalities are tested, including bone marrow transplantation and gene therapy.

Laboratory findings
i. Microcytic hypochromic anaemia, usually severe, and requiring transfusions to maintain haemoglobin above 8 g/dL **(Fig. 11.25)**.
ii. All red blood cell indices significantly reduced.
iii. Decreased osmotic fragilities of RBCs.
iv. Peripheral blood smears show microcytic hypochromic RBCs, anisopoikilocytosis, basophilic stippling, target cells, tear-drop cells, and normoblasts.
v. Reticulocytosis generally present.

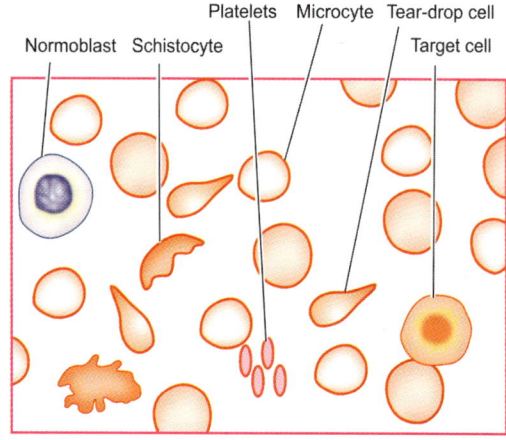

FIGURE 11.25: Peripheral blood smear findings in β-thalassaemia major.

vi. WBCs usually raised with a shift-to-the-left and the presence of nucleated precursor cells.
vii. Platelets normal but may be reduced due to splenomegaly.
viii. Unconjugated bilirubin raised.
ix. *Bone marrow biopsy* shows erythroid hyperplasia with predominance of normoblasts, which often contain siderotic granules. Iron stores in bone marrow macrophages increased.
x. *Haemoglobin electrophoresis*: Increased amounts of HbA2 and HbF, while HbA is reduced or absent.

II. **β-thalassaemia intermedia** is found in genetically heterozygous persons (β°/β or β+/β).
There is moderate anaemia which does not require transfusions.

III. **β-thalassemia minor (trait)** occurs in heterozygotes with moderate suppression of β-chain synthesis and no significant anaemia.
i. Haemoglobin is slightly reduced; up to 15% of normal.
ii. All red blood cell indices are slightly reduced.
iii. Peripheral blood smears show mild anisopoikilocytosis, microcytosis and hypochromasia.
iv. There is decreased osmotic fragility of RBCs.
v. Haemoglobin electrophoresis shows two-fold increased of HbA2 and slight increase of HbF (2–3%).
vi. No treatment is required.

NOTE: If two individuals with thalassaemia minor marry, there is a 25% chance that the offspring will have thalassaemia major. The disease may be diagnosed by antenatal diagnosis.

Q52. Tabulate the salient comparative features of main types of α- and β-thalassaemias.

A classification of various types of thalassaemias along with the clinical syndromes produced and salient laboratory findings are given in **Table 11.15**.

TABLE 11.15 Classification and salient features of types of thalassaemias.

TYPE	HB	HB-ELECTROPHORESIS	GENOTYPE	CLINICAL SYNDROME
α-THALASSAEMIAS				
1. *Hydrops foetalis*	3–10 g/dL	Hb Bart (γ_4) (100%)	Deletion of four α-genes	Fatal in utero or in early infancy
2. *HbH disease*	2–12 g/dL	HbF (10%), HbH (2–4%)	Deletion of three α-genes	Haemolytic anaemia
3. *α-Thalassaemia trait*	10–14 g/dL	Almost normal	Deletion of two α-genes	Microcytic hypochromic blood picture but no anaemia
β-THALASSAEMIAS				
1. *β-Thalassaemia major*	< 5 g/dL	HbA (0–50%), HbF (50–98%)	$\beta^{thal}/\beta^{thal}$	Severe congenital haemolytic anaemia, requires blood transfusions
2. *β-Thalassaemia intermedia*	5–10 g/dL	Variable	Multiple mechanisms	Severe anaemia, but regular blood transfusions not required
3. *β-Thalassaemia minor*	10–12 g/dL	HbA_2 (4–9%), HbF (1–5%)	β^A/β^{thal}	Usually asymptomatic

Q53. What is anaemia due to blood loss? What are its causes and mechanism of anaemia?

Definition Anaemia due to blood loss develops due to acute or chronic bleeding.

Etiopathogenesis

I. **Acute blood loss** may cause hypovolaemic shock, and if massive enough even death.
- If the patient survives, there is acute haemodilution due to a shift of interstitial fluid to the intravascular compartment resulting in a low haematocrit.
- Hypoxia stimulates erythropoietin productions leading to compensatory bone marrow hyperplasia.

Laboratory findings
i. Low hematocrit, normocytic and normochromic anaemia.
ii. Increased reticulocyte count (10–15% after one week).
iii. Bone marrow shows erythroid hyperplasia.

II. **Chronic blood loss** due to prolonged occult bleeding from the gastrointestinal tract, or extensive menstrual bleeding, becomes clinically manifest when the blood loss exceeds the bone marrow production of RBCs and iron stores are depleted.

Laboratory findings
Microcytic hypochromic anaemia with reticulosis consistent with iron deficiency anaemia.

APLASTIC ANAEMIA AND PRIMARY BONE MARROW DISORDERS

Q54. What is aplastic anaemia? Discuss its etiopathogenesis and classification.

Definition Aplastic anaemia is a hypoproliferative anaemia resulting in bone marrow failure and pancytopenia.

Etiopathogenesis Aplastic anaemia results from failure of haematopoietic stem cells which have completely disappeared from the bone marrow, or are present in markedly reduced numbers and fail to differentiate into mature blood cells. In more than 50% of all cases, the cause of this defect is not known.

Classification Aplastic anaemia is classified as primary or secondary **(Table 11.16)**:

TABLE 11.16 Causes of aplastic anaemia.
A. PRIMARY APLASTIC ANAEMIA
1. *Fanconi anaemia (congenital)*
2. *Immune-mediated (acquired)*, e.g. hyperimmunoglobulinanemia, thymoma, GVHD in immunodeficiency
B. SECONDARY APLASTIC ANAEMIA

1. *Drugs*
   i. Dose-related aplasia, e.g. with antimetabolites (methotrexate), mitotic inhibitors (daunorubicin), alkylating agents (busulfan), nitroso urea, anthracyclines.
   ii. Idiosyncratic aplasia, e.g. with chloramphenicol, sulfa drugs, oxyphenbutazone, phenylbutazone, chlorpromazine, gold salts.

2. *Toxic chemicals*, e.g. benzene derivatives, insecticides, arsenicals.
3. *Radiation*
4. *Viral infections*, e.g. hepatitis, EB virus infection (infectious mononucleosis), HIV (AIDS), Parvovirus-B19 (PRCA)
5. *Paroxysmal nocturnal haemoglobinaemia (PNH)*
6. *Idiopathic*

I. **Primary aplastic anaemia** includes cases linked to some hereditary genetic factor, or if no obvious reasons are found. Cases of presumed or suspected immune-mediated injury are also included in this group.

i. **Fanconi anaemia** is caused by mutations of genes encoding for DNA repair enzymes and chromosomal fragility. It presents with multiple congenital deformities and progressive anaemia beginning by the age of 10 years. Aplastic anaemia may progress to myelodysplastic syndrome and acute myelogenous leukaemia, indicating that the haematologic disorders are present due to haematopoietic stem cell defect.

ii. **Presumed immunologic causes** of aplastic anaemia include those that respond to corticosteroid and immunosuppressive drug treatment. This group includes cases associated with hyperimmunoglobulinaemia, thymoma, graft-versus-host reaction in immunodeficiency.

II. **Secondary aplastic anaemia** may be related to a *predictable or unpredictable (idiosyncratic) reaction* to exogenous factors. Predictable reactions are typically dose-related and include bone marrow injury by certain drugs given in high doses, exposure to toxins, radiation, and radioactive substances. Certain viruses are known to induce bone marrow injury. The best known among these are hepatitis virus, EB virus, HIV. Parvovirus B19 infection results in pure red cell aplasia.

Q55. Describe the major clinicopathologic features, laboratory findings and broad outlines of treatment of aplastic anaemia.

Clinicopathologic aspects
i. Pancytopenia.
ii. Anaemia presents as progressive weakness, fatigue.
iii. Leukopenia is marked by reduced resistance and recurrent infection.
iv. Thrombocytopenia with bleeding into skin, gums, from nose, vagina, bowel, etc.
v. *Negative finding*: No enlargement of the spleen, liver, lymph nodes.

Laboratory findings
i. Anaemia is normocytic normochromic, and the reticulocyte number is low (<1%).
ii. Leucopenia with prominent neutropenia (<500/μL).
iii. Thrombocytopenia (<20,000/μL).
iv. Bone marrow biopsy yields a '*dry tap*', largely replaced by fat cells. It is hypocellular (<25%), containing a few haematopoietic cells and a few scattered lymphocytes and plasma cells.

v. Immunohistochemistry shows a markedly reduced number of cells that are positive for CD34, a stem cell marker.

NOTE: Bone marrow must be performed to exclude other possible causes of bone marrow failure and pancytopenia **(Table 11.17)**.

Treatment The most important approaches include the following:

i. *Identification of possible causes* of aplastic anaemia and their elimination/treatment.

ii. *Supportive therapy* with blood transfusions, platelet concentrates and antibiotics to prevent infection (to allow 'recovery of the bone marrow').

iii. *Immunotherapy* and cytotoxic drugs to suppress T cell reaction and corticosteroids to suppress immunoglobulins. Partial response may be expected in 30–50% cases.

iv. *Bone marrow transplantation* to provide new haematopoietic stem cells, if well matched donors are available.

Lethal outcome is high and up to 80% patients may die during the first year.

TABLE 11.17 Causes of pancytopenia.
I. *Aplastic anaemia (Table 11.16)*
II. *Pancytopenia with normal or increased marrow cellularity, e.g.*
1. Myelodysplastic syndromes
2. Hypersplenism
3. Megaloblastic anaemia
III. *Paroxysmal nocturnal haemoglobinuria*
IV. *Bone marrow infiltrations, e.g.*
1. Haematologic malignancies (leukaemias, lymphomas, myeloma)
2. Non-haematologic metastatic malignancies
3. Storage diseases
4. Osteopetrosis
5. Myelofibrosis

Q56. Discuss myelophthisic anaemia briefly.

Definition Myelophthisic anaemia results from the infiltration of the bone marrow by other cells which destroy and replace the haematopoietic cells.

Etiopathogenesis The normal haematopoietic bone marrow may be replaced as under:

i. Haematologic malignancies (e.g. leukaemia, lymphoma, multiple myeloma).

ii. Carcinoma metastatic to the bones (e.g. breast, prostate, stomach, lung and thyroid carcinoma).

iii. Advanced tuberculosis involving bones.

iv. Hereditary lipid storage diseases (e.g. Gaucher disease, Niemann-Pick disease, etc.)

v. Osteopetrosis.

Q57. What is pure red cell aplasia? How is it classified?

Definition Pure red cell aplasia (PRCA) is a rare disease characterised by selective failure in the production of erythroid precursors in the bone marrow and peripheral blood anaemia accompanied by normal granulocyte and platelet counts.

Classification PRCA can be congenital or acquired, acute (transient) or chronic.

i. *Acute and transient (self-limited)*, which is most often caused by parvovirus B19 infection, but also occurs as aplastic crisis of haemolytic anaemia, or transient erythroblastopenia in normal children.

ii. *Acquired PRCA,* most often seen in adult patients with thymoma. Other conditions that could cause PRCA are autoimmune diseases like SLE, and malignancies such as lymphoma, T-lymphocytic leukaemia, and some solid tumours.

iii. *Chronic B19 parvovirus infection,* which occurs most often in children.

iv. *Congenital PRCA (Blackfan-Diamond syndrome)* presenting with anaemia at birth or in early childhood. It is caused by ribosomal RNA processing enzyme encoded by the gene *RPS19*.

Chapter 11e Supplement: Online Content

Digital content of this chapter available with this book is meant for enhanced learning and self-assessment. In addition, it contains 34 Multiple Choice Questions (MCQs), 05 Clinicopathologic Vignettes, and 05 Image-based Questions; these are followed by their answers along with explanatory notes of correct and incorrect answers.

CHAPTER 12

Haemostatic System, Bleeding Disorders and Transfusion Medicine

■ HAEMOSTATIC SYSTEM

Q1. What are the three cardinal components of the haemostatic system?
Haemostatic system has following three key components that halt bleeding by forming a haemostatic plug:
i. Platelets
ii. Coagulation cascade proteins
iii. Blood vessel wall

Q2. How are the megakaryocytes formed and what is their function?
Megakaryocytes are bone marrow cells specialised for the production of platelets.
Key facts (Fig. 12.1):
i. Megakaryocytes are formed from megakaryocyte precursors (megakaryoblasts and promegakaryocytes) in the bone marrow.
ii. The process of maturation involves endoreduplication of the nuclei which ultimately acquire 4–16 lobes and become polyploid containing up to 32-times the normal diploid content of DNA.
iii. Megakaryocytes produce platelets by detachment of their cytoplasmic pseudopods containing granules and other organelles.
iv. One megakaryocyte can produce up to 4,000 platelets and the entire process lasts 10 days.
v. Thrombocytopoiesis is under the control of thrombopoietin, a glycoprotein produced by the liver and kidneys, especially if stimulated by IL-6.

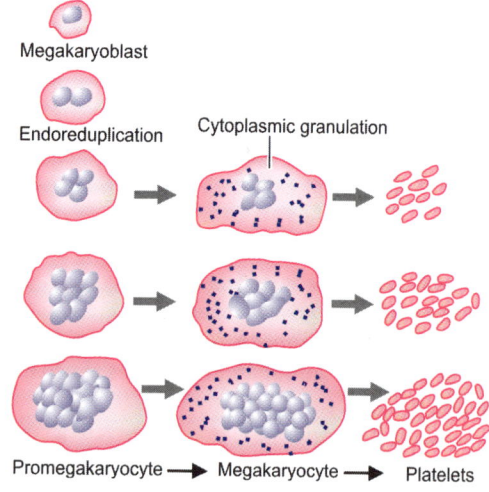

FIGURE 12.1: Thrombopoiesis.

Q3. What are platelets? What is their physiologic role?
Definition Platelets are small, discoid, anuclear blood cells derived from the cytoplasm of megakaryocytes. They participate in haemostasis and inflammation.
Physiology Platelets are found in the bone marrow, spleen, and the circulation.
Key facts:
i. Platelets released from the bone marrow spend the initial 24–36 hours in the spleen before entering the circulation.
ii. About 70% of platelets are in circulation, while the remaining 30% are sequestered in the spleen.

iii. Platelets survive in peripheral blood for 7–10 days.
iv. Normal blood count for platelet is 1,50,000 to 4,00,000/μL.
v. Thrombocytopoiesis is stimulated by stress, epinephrine and exercise.

Q4. What is the mechanism of haemostasis?

Haemostasis occurs through the interactions of vascular endothelial cells, platelets and coagulation cascade proteins, as under:

I. **Endothelial cells** normally secrete antithrombotic factors such as prostacyclin, vasodilators such as nitric oxide, as well as factors that inhibit activation of platelets. In order to stop bleeding, this *antithrombotic activity* of normal blood vessels will change into *prothrombotic activity* marked by secretion of endothelin (a vasoconstrictor), thrombospondin opposing the action of prostacyclin, and activators of platelets.

II. **Platelets participation** in haemostasis includes three phases: i) adhesion, ii) release reaction (activation), and iii) aggregation **(Fig. 12.2)**.

i. **Adhesion** It is mediated by the integrin Ia-IIb on the surface of the platelet surface membrane. The adhesion is stabilised by von Willebrand factor which binds to another platelet receptor, GpIb-IX complex **(Fig. 12.3)**.

ii. **Release reaction** It involves the release of three types of granules: dense granules, α-granules and lysosomal vesicles. These granules contain numerous bioactive substances such as ADP, ATP, calcium, serotonin, platelet factor 4, coagulation factors V and VIII, von Willebrand factor, fibrinogen, fibronectin, thrombospondin, thromboxane A_2, PDGF, etc.

iii. **Aggregation** This process is mediated by fibrin attaching to platelet surface receptors GpIIb-IIIa. Formation of the platelet plug is called *primary haemostasis*.

III. **Coagulation cascade proteins** Coagulation cascade is activated by tissue factor and includes proteins of the extrinsic, intrinsic and common pathway, fibrinolytic system and its inhibitors. It results in the formation of fibrin plug (*secondary haemostasis*).

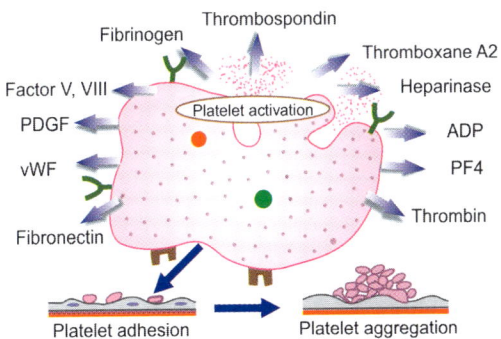

FIGURE 12.2: Main events in primary haemostasis—platelet adhesion, release (activation) and aggregation.

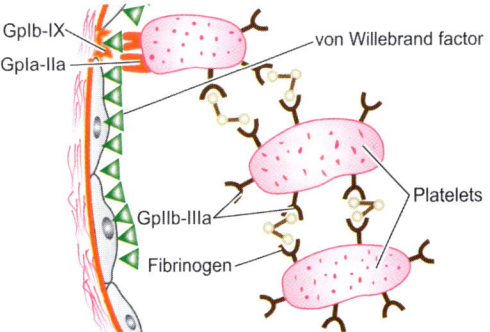

FIGURE 12.3: Molecular mechanisms in platelet adhesion and release reaction.
(Gp, glycoprotein).

Q5. What is the broad scheme of laboratory tests for haemostatic function?

Haemostatic function is tested by evaluating the function of all its components including the following:
i) blood vessels, ii) platelets, iii) plasma coagulation factors, iv) fibrinolytic system, and v) inhibitors of coagulation.

The following course of work up and testing is usually followed:
- *Comprehensive clinical evaluation* to include patient's history, family history, and details of the site, frequency and character of haemostatic disorder.
- *Screening tests* to evaluate abnormalities of various components maintaining the haemostatic balance **(Table 12.1)**.
- *Specific tests* to pinpoint the cause of the bleeding.

TABLE 12.1 Screening tests for haemostasis (coagulation tests).

LABORATORY TEST	FACTOR/FUNCTION MEASURED	ASSOCIATED DISORDERS
1. *Bleeding time*	Platelet function, vascular integrity	i. Qualitative disorders of platelets ii. von Willebrand disease iii. Quantitative disorders of platelets iv. Acquired vascular disorders
2. *Platelet count*	Quantification of platelets	i. Thrombocytopenia ii. Thrombocytosis
3. *Prothrombin time*	Evaluation of extrinsic and common pathway (deficiency of factors I, II, V, VII, X)	i. Oral anticoagulant therapy ii. DIC iii. Liver disease
4. *Partial thromboplastin time*	Evaluation of intrinsic and common pathway (deficiency of factors I, II, V, VIII, IX, X, XI, XII)	i. Parenteral heparin therapy ii. DIC iii. Liver disease
5. *Thrombin time*	Evaluation of common pathway	i. Afibrinogenaemia ii. DIC iii. Parenteral heparin therapy

Q6. What are the tests for evaluating disorders of vascular haemostasis?

Disorders of vascular haemostasis include the following: increased vascular permeability, reduced capillary strength, and failure of vessels to contract after injury.
Two tests are used: i) bleeding time, ii) Hess capillary resistance test (tourniquet test).
I. **Bleeding time** measures the cessation of bleeding following a superficial incision made on the forearm. Normally, the bleeding time is 3–6 minutes, depending on the normal function of capillaries, normal number of platelets and their ability to adhere and form aggregates at the site of incision. The following conditions will prolong the bleeding time:
i. Thrombocytopenia
ii. Functional defects of platelets
iii. Von Willebrand disease
iv. Vascular abnormalities (e.g. Ehlers-Danlos syndrome)
v. Severe deficiency of factors V and XI
II. **Hess capillary resistance test** (tourniquet test) is performed by tying sphygmomanometer cuff to the upper arm and raising the pressure between the systolic and diastolic pressure to 5 minutes. After deflation, one counts the number of petechiae in a 3 cm^2 area.
- The test is positive if there are more than 20 petechiae.
- It is positive in patients with capillary fragility and thrombocytopenia/platelet dysfunction syndromes.

Q7. What are the tests for investigating platelet count, morphology and function?

Haemostatic disorders may be related to abnormalities in platelet number, morphology or function. Tests which are used include screening test and special tests:
I. **Screening tests** include the following:
i. Platelet count in peripheral blood
ii. Peripheral blood smear examination to see morphologic abnormalities of platelets
iii. Bleeding time
II. **Special tests** include the following tests usually performed in reference laboratories:
i. Platelet adhesion tests
ii. Platelet aggregation tests
iii. Granule content of platelets examined by electron microscopy
iv. Platelet coagulant activity measured indirectly by prothrombin consumption index

Q8. What are the tests for investigating blood coagulation?

Coagulation cascade includes intrinsic, extrinsic and common pathway, and the fibrinolytic system **(Fig. 12.4)**. Coagulation tests for components of the coagulation cascade and the fibrinolytic system can be evaluated by screening tests and confirmatory special tests which include the following:

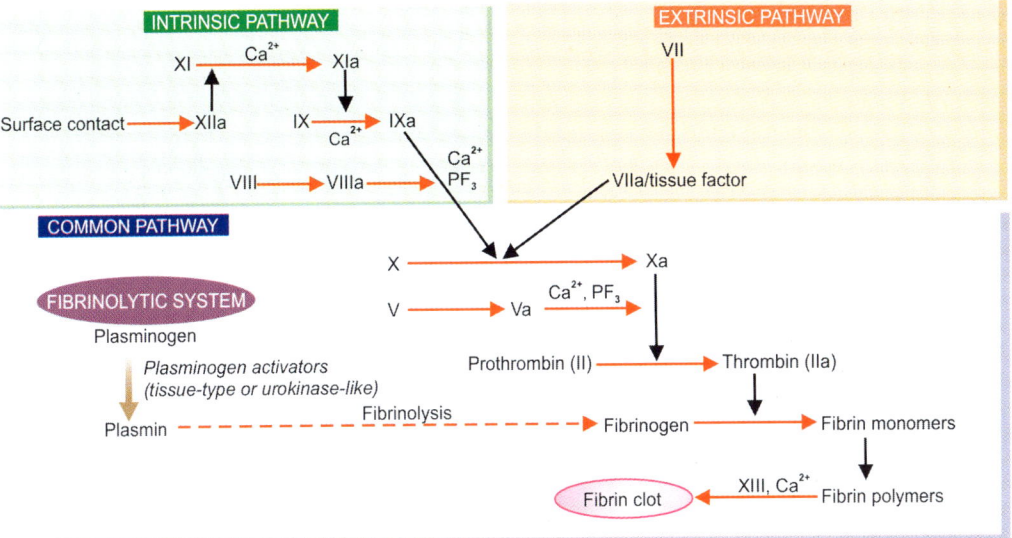

FIGURE 12.4: Pathways of blood coagulation, fibrinolytic system and participation of platelets in activation of the cascade and their role in haemostatic plug formation.

I. **Activated partial thromboplastin time (APTT) or partial thromboplastin time with kaolin (PTTK)** It measures the activity of the factors in *intrinsic pathway* (VII, IX, XI, XII) and *common pathway* (X, V, prothrombin, and fibrinogen). The normal range is 30–40 seconds.
The common causes of a prolonged APTT are as under:
i. Parenteral administration of heparin
ii. Disseminated intravascular coagulation
iii. Liver disease
iv. Circulating anticoagulants

II. **One stage prothrombin time (PT)** It measures the *extrinsic pathway* factor VII and the factors of the *common pathway*. The normal PT is 10–14 seconds. The ratio of PT result of the patient with test results from other laboratories is expressed as *international normalised ratio (INR)*, commonly used to record the PT test results. The normal INR is <1.1. Higher INR means slower, and lower INR means quicker blood clot formation than desired. In patients on blood-thinning drugs (e.g. warfarin), the acceptable INR is 2.0 to 3.0.
The common causes of prolonged PT are as under:
i. Patients of oral anticoagulant drugs (e.g. warfarin)
ii. Liver disease, especially obstructive hyperbilirubinaemia
iii. Vitamin K deficiency
iv. Disseminated intravascular coagulation

III. **Fibrinogen measurement** Screening tests for fibrinogen deficiency are semiquantitative fibrinogen titre and thrombin time (TT). The normal TT is under 20 seconds, while a fibrinogen titre in plasma dilution up to 32 is considered normal.
The common causes of prolonged TT are as under:
i. Hypofibrinogenaemia (as in DIC)
ii. Raised concentration of fibrin degradation products
iii. Presence of heparin

IV. **Coagulation factor assays** Each factor is measured separately by deleting it from the substrate on which the test is performed. The values are compared with the values obtained with standard control plasma and expressed as percentage of normal activity.

V. **Quantitative specific coagulation and fibrinolytic factor and coagulation inhibitor assays**
The concentration of each factor can be measured by direct immunologic and chemical methods. Currently, there are tests for measuring all coagulation and fibrinolytic factors in plasma, as well as inhibitors such as antithrombin III, protein C and S.

BLEEDING DISORDERS

Q9. What are vascular bleeding disorders? What are their causes?

Definition Vascular bleeding disorders (also known as vascular purpuras or non-thrombocytopenia purpuras) are usually mild and characterised by petechiae, purpuras of ecchymoses confined to skin and mucous membranes. They are of unknown etiology and not associated with any abnormal screening tests of haemostasis.

Etiopathogenesis Unknown but presumptively related to lesions of capillary endothelium or subendothelial matrix or extravascular connective tissue that supports the blood vessels, or from abnormally formed new blood vessels. They can be inherited or acquired.

Q10. What are inherited vascular bleeding disorders?

These conditions are rare, each with an incidence of approximately 1:5,000.
EXAMPLES of inherited vascular bleeding disorders are as under:

i. **Hereditary haemorrhagic teleagiectasia (HHT or Osler-Weber-Rendu disease)** is inherited as an autosomal dominant disorder.
a. It is characterised by vascular malformations presenting as telangiectatic (dilated) capillaries of the skin and mucosal surfaces that are prone to spontaneous bleeding.
b. At least four genes have been identified as causing HHT and the symptoms vary depending on the underlying genetic defect.
c. The most commonly involved is the gene for *endoglin*, an endothelial protein important for the formation of blood vessels.
d. Capillary lesions are most prominent on lips, tongue, nose, palms, and soles, but may also involve internal organs.
e. The first symptoms become evident in early childhood presenting with epistaxis or mucosal bleeding from the mouth, stomach or other sites.

ii. **Connective tissue matrix disorders** Bleeding from structurally weak blood vessels occurs in hereditary disease such as Marfan syndrome (gene for fibrillin), Ehlers-Danlos syndrome (gene for some collagens and matrix proteins).

Q11. What are acquired vascular bleeding disorders?

Several acquired conditions are associated with vascular purpuras, as under:

i. **Henoch-Schönlein purpura**, a self-limited type of hypersensitivity vasculitis.
a. Symptoms appear in children and young adults.
b. Clinically, it presents with purpuric rash on extensor surfaces of arms, legs and buttocks.
c. Often associated with internal bleeding such as renal and intestinal bleeding (haematuria, hematochezia) and polyarthritis.
d. Skin biopsy shows leucocytoclastic vasculitis.
e. Circulating immune complexes in blood with deposits of IgA, C3 complement and fibrin in the wall of small blood vessels.

ii. **Haemolytic-uraemic syndrome (HUS)**, a disease of infancy and early childhood.
a. It may have several causes but most often related to infection with *E. coli* (H7:0157) secreting shiga-like verotoxin that damages endothelial cells, especially those in the glomeruli.
b. Clinically, it presents with a bleeding tendency and varying degrees of renal failure.
c. Renal biopsy shows glomerular fibrin thrombi.
d. Central nervous system involvement is a frequently lethal feature of HUS.
e. Haemolysis of RBCs has the typical features of microangiopathic anaemia.
f. Coagulopathy is associated with consumptive thrombocytopenia.

iii. **Simple easy bruising ('Devil's pinches')** This disease of unknown etiology affects women of child-bearing age. It presents with easy bruising.

iv. **Infections** caused by bacteria or viruses may damage endothelium and present with purpura. Septicaemia and overwhelming infection are most often associated with DIC and a bleeding tendency.

v. **Drug-induced hypersensitivity reaction** involving small dermal and mucosal vessels present as a self-limited leucocyctoclastic vasculitis.

vi. **Steroid purpura**, as in Cushing syndrome, due to defective vascular support.
vii. **Senile purpura**, most prominent on the dorsum of the forearm and hand, results from age-related tissue atrophy.
viii. **Scurvy** caused by vitamin C deficiency results from inadequate collagen type I synthesis. It presents with bleeding into gums, skin, mucosae, and muscles.

Q12. What are the platelet disorders that cause bleeding?

Platelet disorders producing bleeding may be related to one of the following three abnormalities:
i. Thrombocytopenia, i.e. reduced number of platelets
ii. Thrombocytosis, i.e. increased number of platelets
iii. Defective platelet function

Q13. What is thrombocytopenia? What are its main causes?

Definition Thrombocytopenia is a reduced number of platelets in peripheral blood below the lower limit of normal (1,50,000/µL).

Clinicopathologic aspects Thrombocytopenia results in a bleeding tendency which may present with spontaneous cutaneous purpura and mucosal haemorrhages, as well as prolonged bleeding after trauma. Clinically, such haemorrhages become evident only after severe depletion of platelets below 20,000/µL.

Etiopathogenesis According to their pathogenesis thrombocytopenias can be classified into five groups as follows:
i. Impaired production
ii. Accelerated platelet destruction
iii. Splenic sequestration
iv. Dilutional loss
v. Inherited

The most important examples of various forms of thrombocytopenia are listed in **Table 12.2**.

TABLE 12.2 Causes of thrombocytopenia.

I. IMPAIRED PLATELET PRODUCTION
1. *Generalised bone marrow failure*, e.g. Aplastic anaemia, leukaemia, myelofibrosis, megaloblastic anaemia, marrow infiltrations (carcinomas, lymphomas, multiple myeloma, storage diseases).
2. *Selective suppression of platelet production*, e.g. Drugs (quinine, quinidine, sulfonamides, PAS, rifampicin, anticancer drugs, thiazide diuretics, heparin, diclofenac, acyclovir), heparin, alcohol intake

II. ACCELERATED PLATELET DESTRUCTION
1. *Immunologic thrombocytopenias*, e.g. ITP (acute and chronic), neonatal and post-transfusion (isoimmune), drug-induced, secondary immune thrombocytopenia (post-infection, SLE, AIDS, CLL, lymphoma).
2. *Increased consumption*, e.g. DIC, TTP, giant haemangiomas, microangiopathic haemolytic anaemia.

III. SPLENIC SEQUESTRATION
Splenomegaly

IV. DILUTIONAL LOSS
Massive transfusion of old stored blood to bleeding patients

V. INHERITED
Macrothrombocytopenia

Q14. Discuss main features of drug-induced thrombocytopenia.

Definition Drug-induced thrombocytopenia is a relatively common form of low platelet count which is preceded by intake of a drug that has presumably caused it. Upon discontinuation of the drug treatment, the platelet count typically returns to normal.

Etiopathogenesis
i. Treatment with most cytotoxic drugs given in high dose or over prolonged periods of time will **predictably** suppress the bone marrow and could thus produce thrombocytopenia.
ii. Many other drugs could cause thrombocytopenia in an **unpredictable manner**.
• These drugs may act by *non-immunologically* suppressing the function of megakaryocytes, or by *immunologically* destroying platelets through the so called 'innocent bystander mechanism'.
• The exact mechanism of such unpredictable thrombocytopenia is often not determined.
• The diagnosis is usually made empirically by eliminating the suspected drug, whereupon the platelet count reverts to normal.

Clinicopathologic aspects This adverse drug reaction presents clinically as a bleeding tendency.
i. The most common sign is acute purpura.
ii. The platelet count is low, usually below 10,000/µL.
iii. The bone marrow contains a normal or slightly increased number of megakaryocytes.

iv. The treatment includes removal of the suspected drug, sometimes combined with corticosteroid treatment, plasmapheresis platelet transfusion.

Q15. What are the salient features of heparin-induced thrombocytopenia?

Definition Heparin-induced thrombocytopenia is the most common unpredictable form of thrombocytopenia, which is distinct from other drug-induced thrombocytopenias because it is not associated with bleeding but thrombosis.

Etiopathogenesis This thrombocytopenia is related to heparin-induced antibodies against platelet factor 4-heparin complex. This antibody activates endothelial cells initiating thrombus formation. Heparin-induced thrombocytopenia occurs in a small number of patients who have been taking heparin for 5–10 days.

Clinicopathologic aspects Clinically it is known as *4T disease* including the following for features:
i. *thrombocytopenia* that has no other cause,
ii. *thrombosis*,
iii. is related to *treatment with heparin*, and
iv. is characterised by *time related* fall of platelet counts (5–10 days after onset of treatment).

Q16. What is immune thrombocytopenic purpura (ITP)? How is it classified? Discuss its main features.

Definition Immune thrombocytopenic purpura (ITP) is a bleeding disorder characterised by immunologic destruction of platelets and a normal or increased number of megakaryocytes in the bone marrow.

Classification ITP occurs in two forms: acute and chronic ITP.

I. **Acute ITP** is a self-limited immune disease, usually affecting children recovering from an acute viral disease (e.g. infectious mononucleosis, viral hepatitis C, CMV or HIV infection), or an upper respiratory illness.
i. Thrombocytopenia is sudden and severe.
ii. Recovery lasts a few weeks to 6 months.
iii. Thrombocytopenia is immune-mediated and involves two mechanisms:
a. Antiviral antibodies may form circulating complexes with virus antigens; such antigen-antibody complexes circulate in blood destroying platelets as innocent bystanders.
b. Alternatively, antibodies to viral antigens cross-react with antigens on platelets and attack platelets destroying them.
iv. Spontaneous recovery in 90% cases.

II. **Chronic ITP** occurs more often in adults and it usually affects women in the 20–40 age group.
i. The disease is insidious and may last several years.
ii. Most often it is idiopathic.
iii. It may occur as a feature of autoimmune diseases such as SLE, autoimmune thyroiditis or even AIDS.
iv. The destruction of platelets is mediated by antibodies to platelet glycoproteins GpIIb-IIIa and GpIb-IX complex.
v. Antibodies are synthesised mostly in the spleen where they coat platelets.
vi. Platelets coated with antibodies are phagocytosed by macrophages in the spleen, leading to splenomegaly.
vii. Some antibodies impair the function of platelets and shorten their survival.

Clinical features include:
i. petechial haemorrhages,
ii. easy bruising,
iii. bleeding from the mucosae such as gums or nose, and
iv. internal bleeding presenting as haematuria, melaena, and menorrhagia in women.

Laboratory findings
i. Low platelet count in the range from 10,000 to 50,000/μL.
ii. Abnormal, enlarged and deformed platelets are seen in peripheral blood smears **(Fig. 12.5)**.
iii. Bone marrow contains an increased number of megakaryocytes which have large non-lobulated single nuclei and have reduced cytoplasmic granularity associated with cytoplasmic vacuolation.

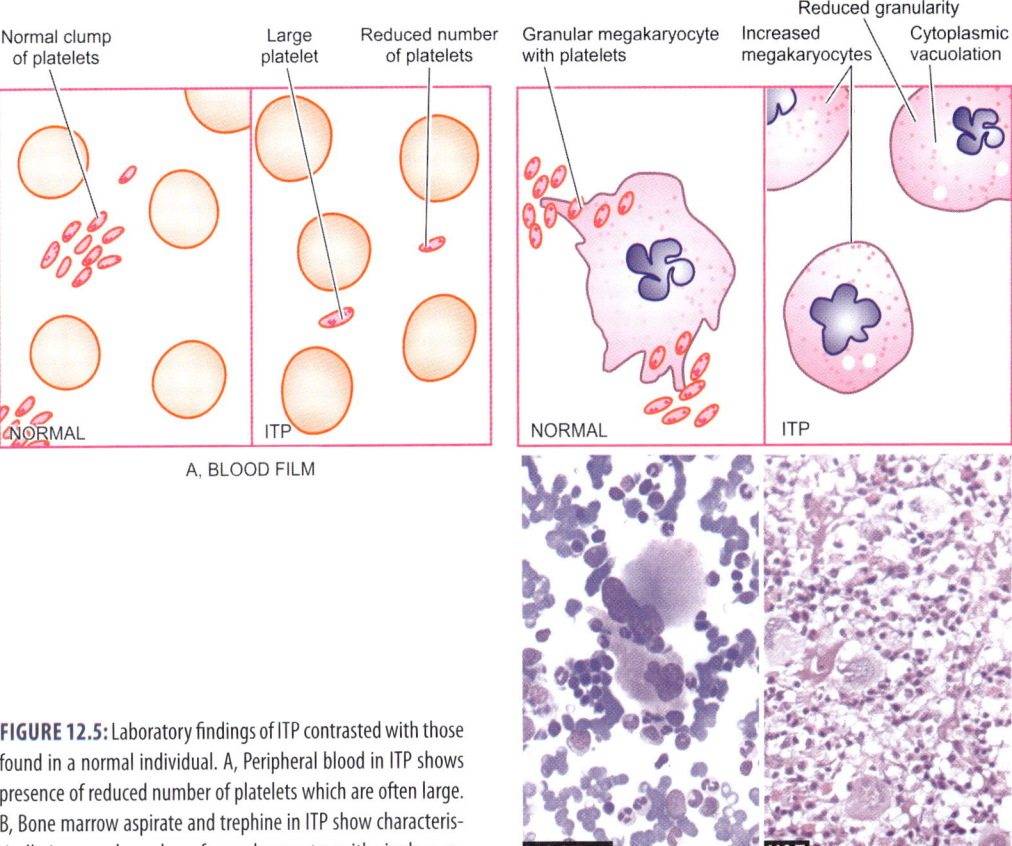

FIGURE 12.5: Laboratory findings of ITP contrasted with those found in a normal individual. A, Peripheral blood in ITP shows presence of reduced number of platelets which are often large. B, Bone marrow aspirate and trephine in ITP show characteristically increased number of megakaryocytes with single non-lobulated nuclei and reduced cytoplasmic granularity.

iv. Special studies show antiplatelet antibodies on the surface of platelets and in serum.
v. Platelet survival studies show reduced platelet lifespan, often less than one hour, in contrast to the normal which is 7–10 days.
Treatment includes immunosuppression and splenectomy to remove the major source of antibodies and the site of platelet destruction.

Q17. Briefly discuss thrombotic thrombocytopenic purpura and haemolytic-uraemic syndrome.

Definition Thrombotic thrombocytopenic purpura (TTP) and haemolytic-uraemic syndrome (HUS) form a group of thrombotic microangiopathies which are characterised by a triad including:
i. thrombocytopenia,
ii. microangiopathic haemolytic anaemia, and
iii. formation of fibrin/platelet microthrombi within the microvasculature.
Pathogenesis Endothelial injury is the primary lesion.
- Endothelial injury may be caused by a variety of factors such as pregnancy, drugs (e.g. mitomycin), high dose chemotherapy, cancer, and various infections. HUS in small children under 5 years of age is most often caused by toxin-producing *E. coli* (O157:7 strain) infection.
- Injured endothelial cells release von Willebrand factor and other procoagulant factors.
- Microthrombi are formed in various parts of the body which account for most of the clinical findings and symptoms.
Clinicopathologic aspects TTP and HUS affect young adults or children.
i. Clinically, these disorders are typically fulminant and often lethal.
ii. Microthrombi are found in all parts of the body in arterioles, capillaries and venules.

iii. Most serious consequences are renal failure (uraemia) and ischaemic central nervous system disturbances. HUS is the most common cause of acute renal failure in small children.
iv. Consumption of coagulation factors leads to thrombocytopenia and hypofibrinogenaemia and a bleeding tendency.
Microangiopathic haemolytic anaemia aggravates the clinical condition.

Laboratory findings
i. Haemolytic anaemia with widespread microthrombi
ii. *Peripheral blood smear* shows anisopoikilocytosis with RBC fragmentation and deformities
iii. Coombs test negative
iv. Thrombocytopenia
v. Leucocytosis, sometime even leukaemoid reaction
vi. *Bone marrow* shows normal or slightly increased number of megakaryocytes and some myeloid hyperplasia
vii. *Biopsy* (e.g. gums or kidney) will show microthrombi

Q18. What are the main disorders of platelet function?

Definition Disorders of platelet function are bleeding disorders caused by platelet membrane or granule dysfunction.
Classification These disorders are classified as hereditary or acquired.
I. **Hereditary platelet disorders** are classified pathogenetically into three groups, each one of which involves a distinct pathophysiological defect as under:
i. *Defective platelet adhesion*, such as seen in Bernard-Soulier disease and von Willebrand disease.
ii. *Defective platelet aggregation*, such as seen in thrombasthenia (Glanzmann disease).
iii. *Defective platelet release reaction*.
EXAMPLES:
i. *Bernard-Soulier syndrome,* also known as giant platelet syndrome, is characterised by defective platelet adhesion to von Willebrand factor.
a. It is inherited as an autosomal recessive trait.
b. The basic defect is a mutation of one of the three genes encoding for components of GpIb, a platelet membrane adhesion molecule that serves as receptor for the von Willebrand factor.
c. GpIb defect prevents the adhesion of platelets to subendothelial collagen after the endothelial defect in an injured blood vessel has been covered with von Willebrand factor (*see* **Fig. 12.3**).
d. It is a very rare disease presenting in childhood with a bleeding tendency.
e. Laboratory studies show thrombocytopenia and giant platelets, which lack GPIb.
ii. *Glanzmann thrombasthenia* is a defect of platelet aggregation.
a. It is related to a defect of platelet glycoprotein GpIIb/IIIa, which serves as a receptor for fibrinogen and von Willebrand factor, thus mediating aggregation of platelets, clot retraction and formation of the fibrin plug.
b. The disease presents with a bleeding tendency in early childhood.
II. **Acquired platelet disorders** Acquired platelet disorders may be caused by the following:
i. *Drugs*, such as aspirin which inhibits cyclooxygenase and synthesis of prostaglandins which are involved in platelet aggregation and release reaction.
ii. *Systemic diseases*, such as chronic liver and kidney disease.
iii. *Haematopoietic malignancies*, such as multiple myeloma and myeloproliferative disorders.

Q19. What are coagulation disorders?

Coagulation disorders present as increased coagulability of blood (thrombophilia) or an increased tendency for bleeding.
• Bleeding disorders caused by a deficiency of plasma coagulation factors could be related to a deficiency of one of the coagulation factors or several coagulation factors.
• Clinically, they present with large ecchymoses, haematomas, bleeding into body cavities such as joints, and internal organs, such as GIT and urinary tract. Thus, they differ in their clinical presentation

from those caused by blood vessel and platelet deficiencies, which are characterised by petechiae and purpura.
Classification Coagulation disorders may be hereditary or acquired.
I. *Hereditary coagulation disorders* are due to quantitative or qualitative defects of a *single* coagulation factor. Three most common disorders in this group are: haemophilia A and B, and von Willebrand disease.
II. *Acquired coagulation disorders* are characterised by deficiencies of multiple coagulation factors. Most common are: vitamin K deficiency, liver disease related coagulopathies, fibrinolytic defects and disseminated intravascular coagulation (DIC).

Q20. Define haemophilia. Discuss its salient features.

Definition Haemophilia is a hereditary bleeding disorder caused by mutations of X-linked genes for plasma coagulation factor VIII (haemophilia A) or factor IX (haemophilia B). Haemophilia A accounts for 80% of all cases.
I. Haemophilia A is caused by a deficiency of coagulation factor VIII or (less commonly) reduced activity of factor VIII which is present in blood in normal concentration.
Genetics The incidence is 1: 4,000–5,000 but shows some geographic variation from one country to another. The highest incidence is in UK and Northern Europe.
- Mutations of the factor VIII gene, a very large gene on the tip of the long arm of X-chromosome, include deletions, inversions, point mutations and insertions.
- Inherited as an X-linked recessive disorder, it affects only males, whereas the women carrying the mutated gene are asymptomatic carriers.
- Haemophilic fathers do not transmit the disorder to their sons, but their daughters are asymptomatic carriers.
- Homozygous symptomatic women, who have inherited a mutated gene from a haemophilic father and a carrier mother, are rare.
- New mutations account for the cases that do not have a history of haemophilia in the family.

Pathogenesis Factor VIII is part of the intrinsic coagulation pathway and its major function is activation of factor X. Bleeding occurs if the plasma levels of factor VIII are reduced.
- In 90% cases, there is a quantitative reduction of factor VIII, whereas 10% have normal or increased levels, but reduced activity.
- Most patients have less than 5% of normal factor VIII plasma levels, much below the 25% that is required for normal coagulation.

Classification Clinical severity of the disease correlates with the degree of reduction of factor VIII in plasma or its activity. According to severity, there are three forms of haemophilia:
i. Severe haemophilia (50% of patients) → less than 1% of normal factor VIII.
ii. Moderate haemophilia (10% of patients) → 2–5% of normal factor VIII.
iii. Mild haemophilia (30–40% of patients) → 5–30% of normal factor VIII, but many with its reduced activity.

Clinicoppathologic aspects Bleeding may involve any organ.
Most often, bleeding involves the large joints (*haemarthroses*) and muscle (*haematomas*), whereas internal organs are involved less often.
Intracranial haemorrhage is rare today, but previously it was the most common cause of death.
Treatment Transfusions of factor VIII concentrates or plasma cryoprecipitates.
NOTE: Modern laboratory testing has reduced the danger of transfusion-transmitted infections such as viral hepatitis C and HIV.
Laboratory findings
i. Reduced activated partial thromboplastin time, and normal prothrombin time.
ii. Specific test for factor VIII shows lowered activity/concentration of factor VIII.
iii. Symptomatic patients have usually less than 25% of factor VIII activity.
iv. Minority of patients with mild haemophilia have normal or elevated concentration of factor VIII, but it has reduced activity.
v. Female carriers have 50% of normal factor VII activity and some have even lower levels due to the selective inactivation ('Lyonisation') of one X-chromosome.

II. **Haemophilia B,** also known as Christmas disease, is based on a hereditary deficiency of factor IX.
i. Approximately 2–4 times less common than haemophilia B, with an incidence of 1:20,000.
ii. The mutated gene is also located on X-chromosome and transmitted as an X-linked trait.
iii. Clinically, it is indistinguishable from haemophilia A.
iv. The treatment includes transfusion of factor IX concentrates.
v. Repeat transfusions may activate the coagulation system and cause thrombosis.

Q21. Define and discuss von Willebrand disease in brief.

Definition von Willebrand disease (vWD) is a hereditary bleeding disorder presenting in several pathogenic forms which are based on *quantitative* or *qualitative defects* of von Willebrand factor (vWF). It is the most common hereditary bleeding disorder affecting 1–2% of the entire world population.
Genetics The mutated gene is located on chromosome 12.
- The vWF gene is transmitted in most instances as an autosomal dominant trait with variable penetrance and expressivity.
- The severe form of vWD is autosomal recessive and found only in homozygotes.
- vWD has an incidence of 1:1,000 affecting equally both men and women.

Pathophysiology vWF is a coagulation protein present in plasma in form of multimers whose molecular weights varies. Only the higher molecular weight multimers are physiologically active.
i. Synthesised by endothelial cells, megakaryocytes and platelets, in contrast for factors VIII and IX which are produced by the liver.
ii. vWF has the following functions in coagulation processes as follows:
a. Mediates the adhesion of platelets to subendothelial collagen.
b. Binds to fibrinogen to facilitate the aggregation of platelets.
c. Serves as the carrier for factor VIII by forming a vWF-factor VIII complex that circulates in plasma. The half-life of complexed factor VIII is 4–5 times longer than in the free form (1–2 hours versus 10 to 12 hours!). Deficiency of vWF will reduce the procoagulant activity of factor VIII.

Clinicopathologic aspects The defects of vWF that cause the bleeding tendency can be quantitative or qualitative.
- vWD may be asymptomatic or present with a mild bleeding diathesis in most instances.
- Clinically, it presents with easy bruising, multifocal mucosal haemorrhages, menorrhagia (in women) and prolonged bleeding from wounds after trauma or surgery.

There are three main forms of vWD, each of which has several distinct subtypes:

Type I vWD accounting for 75% of all cases presents as a quantitative vWF deficiency. It is marked by mild to moderate decrease of vWF (50% activity). Vasopressin analogue, desmopressin (DDAVP), is the treatment of choice because it will release into circulation vWF stored in endothelial cells.

Type II vWD accounting for 20% of all cases, presents with qualitative functional defects of vWF, which cannot normally interact with subendothelial collagen or platelets. Plasma levels of high molecular weight multimers of vWF and factor VIII are low. Abnormal vWF may cause thrombocytopenia. DDAVP is effective in some cases.

Type III vWD is the least common but rather severe form of the disease that occurs only in homozygotes. vWF is absent from plasma and the levels of factor VIII are less than 10% of normal.

Laboratory findings
i. Prolonged bleeding time
ii. Reduced plasma vWF concentration
iii. Reduced factor VIII activity
iv. Normal platelet count and normal concentration of coagulation factors except factor VIII
v. Defective platelet ristocetin aggregation test

Q22. What is disseminated intravascular coagulation? Discuss key features in its etiology, pathogenesis and laboratory findings.

Definition Disseminated intravascular coagulation (DIC) is a syndrome caused by intravascular activation of coagulation with formation of fibrin thrombi in microcirculation and subsequent fibrinolysis. It is also called consumptive coagulopathy or defibrination syndrome occurring as a consequence of some severe systemic disease.

Etiology Numerous conditions and diseases could cause DIC. The most important causes are as under:

i. *Massive tissue injury* It may occur in obstetrical syndromes (e.g. eclampsia, abruptio placentae, amniotic fluid embolism, retained dead foetus), massive trauma, surgery, metastatic cancer, etc.
ii. *Infections*, especially those associated with endotoxaemia, septicaemia, and bacteraemia.
iii. *Widespread endothelial damage* (e.g. severe burns, haemolytic uraemic syndrome, ITP, TTP)
iv. *Shock* of any etiology.
v. *Toxins, poisons or drugs* (e.g. snake bite, mushroom poisoning, intravenous drug abuse)

Pathogenesis The following sequence of event can be seen in most instances as presented in **Figure 12.6**:
i. Activation of coagulation
ii. Thrombotic phase
iii. Consumption phase
iv. Fibrinolysis

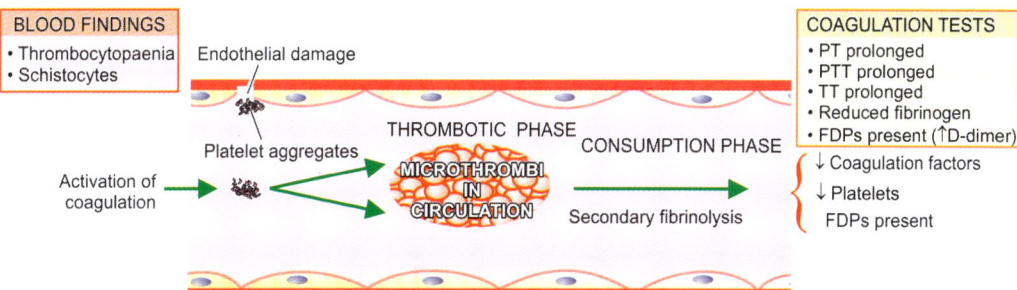

FIGURE 12.6: The pathogenesis of disseminated intravascular coagulation.

Clinicopathologic aspects Pathologic and clinical findings are related to two main components of DIC **(Fig. 12.7)**:
i. Ischaemia caused by thrombotic occlusion of the microcirculation, and
ii. Haemorrhage

Laboratory findings Laboratory findings reflect the consumption of coagulation factors and platelets during intravascular coagulation, damage to endothelial cells and red blood cells, and fibrinolysis.

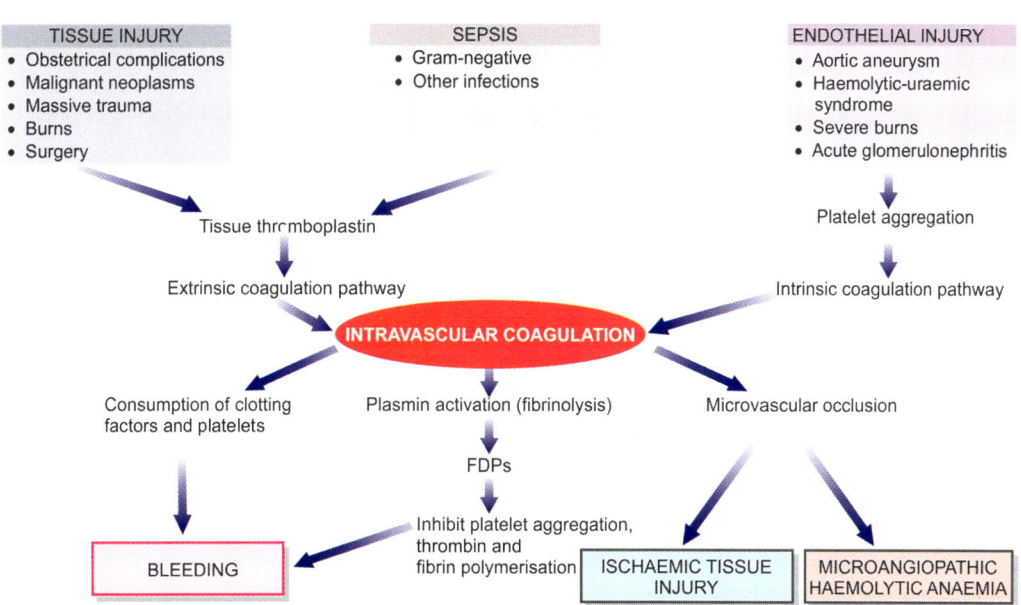

FIGURE 12.7: Pathophysiology of disseminated intravascular coagulation.

i. Thrombocytopenia.
ii. Microangiopathic anaemia, as evidences by haemolysis, and typical changes in the peripheral blood films (e.g. fragmented RBCs, schistocytes).
iii. Prolonged coagulation tests: prothrombin time, activated thromboplastin time, thrombin time.
iv. Reduced concentration of fibrinogen in plasma.
v. Fibrin degradation products (FDPs) are raised in blood and urine due to secondary fibrinolysis.

Q23. Tabulate the important contrasting laboratory findings in important haemostatic disorders.

A summary of important laboratory findings in common conditions causing haemostatic abnormalities are presented in **Table 12.3**.

TABLE 12.3 Major laboratory findings in common haemostatic disorders.

DISORDER	PLATELET COUNT	BT	PT	APTT	TT	FDPS	F-VIII
I. VASCULAR DISORDERS							
Vascular purpuras	N	↑	N	N	N	Absent	N
II. PLATELET DISORDERS							
1. ITP	↓	↑	N	N	N	Absent	N
2. Heparin	↓	↑	N	↑	↑	Absent	N
3. TTP	↓	↑	N	N	N	Absent	N
III. COAGULATION DISORDERS							
1. Haemophilia A	N	N	N	↑	N	Absent	
2. Haemophilia B	N	N	N	↑	N	Absent	
3. von Willebrand	N	↑	N	↑	↑	Absent	
4. Vitamin K deficiency	N	↑	↑	↑	↑	Absent	
5. Liver disease	N	↑	↑	↑	N	Absent	
IV. DIC	↓	↑	↑	↑	↑	Present	

BLOOD TRANSFUSION

Q24. Classify and briefly describe the major blood group systems.

Key Facts:

i. Over 20 blood group systems having approximately 400 blood group antigens are recognised, but only some of them are of clinical significance.
ii. The ABO and Rhesus (Rh) blood group systems are of major clinical significance.
iii. Other minor and clinically less important blood group systems are: Lewis, P, I, MNS, Kell, Duffy and Luther systems.
iv. Individuals who lack the corresponding antigen and have not been previously transfused have *naturally occurring IgM antibodies* in their serum **(Table 12.4)**.
v. *Immune antibodies* to blood group antigens develop in response to blood transfusions and are of the *IgG* type.
vi. *Antigens of the ABO system* are encoded by three allelic genes A, B and O located on chromosome 9.
vii. *Rhesus blood group system* is encoded by allelic genes C or c, D or d, and E or e located on chromosome 1. One set of three genes is inherited from each parent. D antigen is most strongly immunogenic and thus clinically most important. There are no natural antibodies to Rh antigens.

TABLE 12.4 The ABO blood groups.

BLOOD GROUP	ANTIGENS ON RED CELLS	NATURALLY-OCCURRING SERUM ANTIBODIES
A	A antigen	Anti-B
B	B antigen	Anti-A
AB	A and B antigens	None
O	None	Anti-A and anti-B

*Persons with blood group AB Rh-positive are called universal recipients.
**Individuals with blood group O Rh-negative are called universal donors.

Q25. What is a unit of blood? Enumerate infections that can be transmitted by blood transfusion.

Unit of blood bag Blood from a donor is collected as whole blood in a suitable donor bag that contains an anticoagulant. One unit of blood consists of 450 ml of blood in 63 ml of anticoagulant, commonly CPDA in the donor bag (C = citrate, prevents clotting; P = phosphate, source of 2,3 DPG and to maintain pH; D = dextrose, generates ATP by glycolysis; A = adenine, substrate for ATP synthesis).
CPDA preserves the blood for 35 days at 1–6°C.

Infections and tests It must be borne in mind that *several infections may be transmitted by transfusion*. Hence, prior to transfusion of collected blood, it is mandatorily tested for:
i. Hepatitis B (for HBsAg by ELISA)
ii. Hepatitis C (for anti-HCV by ELISA)
iii. HIV (for anti-HIV1,2 by ELISA or spot test)
iv. Syphilis (for treponema antigen by VDRL)
v. Malaria (for malarial antigen by malaria antigen assay)

Q26. How is blood transfusion performed?

Key Facts:
i. Healthy donor selection—typically haemoglobin over 12g/dL, and free of infectious diseases.
ii. Storage of blood in refrigerator at 2–6°C.
iii. Donor testing for ABO-Rh grouping and for infectious organisms (HBV, HBsAg, HCV, HIV, syphilis and malaria).
iv. Blood grouping (ABO and Rh) of recipient.
v. Pre-transfusion compatibility testing of donor and recipient.
vi. Antibody screening of recipient's serum to detect the presence of clinically significant antibodies.
vii. Cross-matching of recipient's serum against donor's red cells to confirm donor-recipient compatibility.
viii. Supervise blood transfusions to observe adverse reactions, if any.

Q27. Describe the steps in the blood compatibility testing (cross-matching).

Before blood transfusion, a cross-match is a pre-requisite so as to avoid untoward reactions of mismatched transfusion. The donor-recipient compatibility is tested by matching recipient's serum and donor red cells.
i. In a small test tube, place a drop of recipient's serum.
ii. Add washed donor red cells suspended in 5% saline.
iii. Mix the two and incubate at 37°C for 30 minutes.
iv. Centrifuge it at 3,000 rpm for one minute.
v. After dislodging the cell palette gently from the centrifuge tube, examine it for presence or absence of agglutination and haemolysis, first grossly and then under the low power of the microscope.

Interpretation
- If there is no agglutination or haemolyis, the donor-recipient blood groups are *matched*.
- In a *mismatch*, there is either haemolysis or agglutination, or both.

Q28. What are the main blood components used for transfusion?

Various components of blood can be prepared from a unit of whole blood collected and thus a single unit of blood can be used for many patients. *Apheresis* refers to a technique in which blood of a donor or a patient is passed through a machine that separates blood into two types of components: *cellular* and *soluble components*.

I. Cellular components
i. *Packed red cells* Red cell concentrate is prepared by centrifuging whole unit of blood at high speed. This way, the unit of blood is separated into two parts: the supernatant *plasma* which is separately collected into another satellite bag, while the parent blood bag is kept in an upright position to allow

sedimentation of red cells (*packed red cells*). In most centres, this process of separation is better done by apheresis machine.
- Packed red cells bag is stored at 2–6°C and can be used for up to 35 days.

ii. **Leucocyte-depleted red cells** Packed red cells contain leucocytes which carry HLA proteins on their surface, and thus have ability to distinguish between *self* and *non-self* (or foreign). Therefore, during transfusion of packed red cells, recipient immune system recognises transfused leucocytes as 'foreign' and the recipient may develop several adverse reactions.
- Leucodepleted red cells can be prepared by filtration procedures and this renders a safer transfusion.

iii. **Platelet concentrates** Platelet concentrates can be prepared from whole blood or by apheresis from healthy donors.
- Platelet concentrate is stored at 20–24°C and its shelf-life of is 3–5 days.

iv. **Granulocyte concentrates** This is prepared from either whole blood or by leucapheresis.
- Separated granulocyte concentrate are also stored at 20–24°C but must be used within 24 hours of collection.

II. **Plasma components**
In earlier times, whole plasma was used for replenishing volume in haemorrhagic shock. Nowadays, separated plasma is used in two forms:

i. **Fresh frozen plasma (FFP)** Plasma separated from whole blood or by apheresis machine is frozen at –70°C and can be used for up to one year.
- FFP contains various coagulation factors and is used after thawing it.

ii. **Cryoprecipitates** These are rich in factor VIII and fibrinogen. Cryoprecipitates are prepared by thawing FFP slowly and then separating the supernatant.
- These can be stored at –30°C and have a shelf-life up to one year.

Q29. What are the main clinical uses of various blood components?

I. **Packed RBCs** are used to increase the oxygen carrying capacity of blood. One pack of RBCs will raise haemoglobin concentration by 1 g/dL.
Its indications are:
i. Symptomatic chronic anaemia, e.g. haemolytic anaemias
ii. Perioperative anaemia
iii. Acute blood loss of >30%
iv. Cardiac failure with anaemia
v. Leukaemias
vi. Aplastic anaemia

II. **Platelet concentrates** are used in bleeding patients with platelet count typically below 10,000/µL. One unit of apheresis platelets raises the platelet count in adults by 30,000–60,000 per µL, while a unit of platelets from whole blood should raise the platelet count by 10,000–12,000 per µL.
Main indications are:
i. Patients of thrombocytopenia
ii. Platelet function defects

III. **Fresh frozen plasma (FFP)** contains plasma proteins including the coagulation factors and anticoagulants, like protein C and S.
Major indications are:
i. Coagulation failure (bleeding disorders) due to deficiency of clotting factors
ii. TTP

IV. **Cryoprecipitates** are the source of insoluble plasma proteins like fibrinogen, factor VIII and vWF. One unit of cryoprecipitate yields about 80 IU of factor VIII.
Indications for cryoprecipitates are:
i. Haemophilia
ii. Hypofibrinogenaemia
iii. von Willebrand disease

V. **Granulocyte concentrates** are transfused as supportive therapy to manage infections in patients who have do not respond to standard medical therapy.

Q30. Define autologous blood transfusion and its principle. What are its procedure types and their indications? Enumerate advantages and disadvantages of this transfusion method.

Definition and principle Autologous blood transfusion means that the blood is collected from the same person (auto = self) who has to be transfused.

It is known that allogenic blood transfusion is a potentially hazardous process. Besides, there is ever shortage of donated blood. Thus, in recent years, autologous blood transfusion has attracted more attention.

Procedures and indications There are three types of autologous blood transfusion procedures and distinct corresponding indications as under:

I. **Preoperative autologous blood donation** This is the banking of blood from the patient before a planned surgery and it is reinfused back during surgery. Its main *indications* are:
i. Patients with rare blood group when difficult to find matched allogenic donor
ii. Patient refusing donor blood transfusion

II. **Intraoperative and postoperative autotransfusion** In this method, blood in the body cavity of a patient, or blood lost during surgery, or lost postoperatively in the drain, is reinfused to the patient after it has been anticoagulated and processed through filtration and washing. Its *indications* are:
i. Patients in which blood loss is more than 20% volume of blood, e.g. due to major accidental haemorrhage, or due to surgery
ii. Patients with risk factors for bleeding tendencies
iii. Those with very low haemoglobin

III. **Acute normovolaemic haemodilution autologous transfusion** This is a perioperative method in which autologous blood is collected before anaesthesia and before start of the main surgery and it is transfused back before the end of surgery when its indications appear. The method includes rapidly withdrawing of a predetermined volume of autologous blood prior to surgery and storing it in operating room. When during surgery, an equivalent volume of intravenous fluids (crystalloids or colloids) have been transfused to the patient that diluted the blood and reduced the haematocrit of patient, at that time autologous blood is transfused back to the patient. Its *indications* are:
i. When there is need for fresh whole blood transfusion that is rich in platelets and clotting factors, e.g. in cardiac bypass surgery
ii. Patients with Rh-negative trait, difficult ABO group typing, or problematic blood cross-matching

Advantages
i. Safer transfusion due to avoidance of autoimmunisation and transmission of infections
ii. Lesser chances of transfusion reactions (e.g. allergic, haemolytic or febrile)
iii. Useful due to shortage of stored blood in blood banks
iv. Useful in rare blood groups or difficult cross-matching

Disadvantages
i. Does not reduce the overall exposure to transfusion process
ii. Does not prevent adverse reaction of wrong blood episode due to error in patient identification or in collection
iii. Increases the chances of unnecessary transfusion due to availability of autologous blood

Q31. What are the principal clinically important complications of blood transfusion?

Minor complications occur in 5–6% of all transfusions but they are of limited clinical significance. Major complications are rare and can be classified as: i) immunologic, and ii) nonimmune complications.

Q32. What are the most important immunologic transfusion reactions?

Immunologic transfusion reactions are mediated by antibodies. The most important are: i) haemolytic transfusion reactions, ii) transfusion-related acute lung injury, and iii) other allergic reactions.

I. **Haemolytic transfusion reactions** may be immediate or delayed, intravascular or extravascular.
i. *Intravascular haemolytic reaction* is due to ABO incompatibility between the donor and the recipient.
a. Reaction involves naturally occurring antibodies which fix complement.
b. The symptoms include restlessness, anxiety, flushing, chest or lumbar pains, tachypnoea, tachycardia and nausea.

c. Haemolytic reaction is often followed by shock and renal failure.
ii. *Extravascular haemolytic reactions* are mediated by immune antibodies to Rh antigens.
a. Acute symptoms are less prominent than in intravascular reactions and include malaise and fever, but no evidence of shock or renal failure.
b. Delayed reactions occurring a week after transfusion (usually in Rh-negative patients sensitised to Rh antigens by previous transfusions or pregnancies).
c. Delayed reactions include extravascular haemolysis of antibody coated RBCs in splenic and hepatic macrophages.
II. **Transfusion-related acute lung injury (TRALI)** is a rare complication that occurs upon transfusion of donor plasma that contains high levels of anti-HLA antibodies reacting with recipient's leucocytes.
i. Leucocytes coated with donor's antibodies aggregate in pulmonary microcirculation.
ii. Upon aggregation, such leucocytes release mediators which increase vascular permeability, resulting in pulmonary oedema and acute respiratory distress syndrome.
III. **Other allergic reactions** include the following:
i. *Febrile reactions* usually directed against leucocytes, platelets or IgA.
ii. *Anaphylactic shock* mediated by pre-existent antibodies to donor's IgA.
iii. *Allergic urticaria*
iv. *Graft-versus-host reaction* mediated by donor's lymphocytes, usually in immunosuppressed recipients.

Q33. What are the most important non-immune transfusion reactions?

The most important non-immune adverse reactions are as follows:
I. **Circulatory overload** It is the most common and most important transfusion complication that may results in death.
i. It presents with pulmonary congestion and acute heart failure.
ii. Symptoms may develop immediately or may be delayed up to 24 hours.
iii. At highest risk are patients who have chronic anaemia, infants and the elderly.
II. **Massive transfusion** It develops when the volume of stored blood transfused to bleeding patients exceeds their normal blood volume. Consequences include dilutional thrombocytopenia and dilution of coagulation factors, predisposing to a bleeding tendency.
III. **Transmission of infections** The most common pathogens transmitted are viruses such as hepatitis viruses B and C, CMV, HIV; protozoa causing malaria and toxoplasmosis; spirochetes causing syphilis; bacteria, causing brucellosis. Blood transfusion-related infections are rare today because of compulsory testing of blood units for most of these pathogens.
IV. **Air embolism** This complication has become very rare since the introduction of plastic transfusion bags with negative pressure. The design of these bags prevents the entry of air into recipient's blood circulation. Debilitated patients are still at risk because they can develop symptoms even after the entry of very small amounts of air (10–40 ml) into circulation.
V. **Thrombophlebitis** Infection may develop at the site of venesection. It is more common if transfusion is performed through saphenous veins rather than the arm veins. Transfusions that last more than 12 hours also increase the risk of thrombophlebitis.
VI. **Transfusion siderosis** Post-transfusion iron overload is a complication of repeated transfusions in patients who have chronic anaemia, such as thalassaemia major. The body cannot eliminate more than 1 mg of iron per day. Since a unit of whole blood (400 ml) contains about 250 mg of iron, it is obvious that iron could easily accumulate following multiple transfusions. Damage of the heart, liver and endocrine glands can be expected after 100 units have been transfused.

Q34. Define haemolytic disease of the newborn. Briefly discuss pathogenesis of its types and their salient features.

Definition Haemolytic disease of the newborn (HDN) results from maternal foetal incompatibility involving the Rh-D or ABO antigens.
It is marked by haemolysis of foetal RBCs caused by antibodies passed across the placenta from the mother that has been previously sensitised to antigens expressed on foetal RBCs.

Pathogenesis of types haemolytic reaction in Rh-D incompatibility is different from that in ABO incompatibility.

I. **HDN due to Rh incompatibility** Since Rh-D is the most antigenic of the three Rh antigens, 95% of Rh incompatibility-related HDH cases are caused by antibodies to Rh-D, whereas reaction to other Rh antigens are rare.

• This form of HDN develops in an Rh positive (Rh-D) foetus in the womb of a Rh negative (Rh-d) mother who was sensitised to Rh-D in a previous pregnancy or by transfusion of Rh positive (Rh-D) blood.

• Immune antibodies to Rh-D produced by the sensitised mother cross the placenta and attack the foetal RBCs causing haemolysis and other symptoms of HDN.

• HDN can be prevented by preventing immunisation of the Rh-negative mother at the end of the pregnancy with an Rh-D foetus. This is accomplished by giving anti-D immunoglobulin within 72 hours after first delivery of an Rh-positive infant.

Clinicopathologic aspects HDN can vary in severity from mild to severe.

i. *Severe intrauterine haemolysis* results in hydrops foetus and intrauterine death.

ii. *Moderate HDN* is characterised by severe haemolytic anaemia, non-conjugated hyperbilirubinaemia and jaundice that are present at birth.

iii. *Mild HDN* presents with neonatal anaemia with or without jaundice.

Laboratory findings Cord blood shows variable degree of anaemia, reticulocytosis, elevated unconjugated hyperbilirubinaemia and positive Coombs test on Rh-D red blood cells.

Maternal blood is Rh negative (Rh-d) with high titre of anti-D IgG.

II. **HDN due to ABO incompatibility** About 20% pregnancies with ABO incompatibility between the mother and foetus develop HDN, which is usually mild.

• Most often, it is encountered in group A or B infants born to blood group O mothers that have in their circulation anti-A or anti-B antibodies of the IgG type.

• In contrast to Rh-related HDN, it can occur in first pregnancy and does not require previous sensitisation.

> **Chapter 12e Supplement: Online Content**
>
> *Digital content of this chapter available with this book is meant for enhanced learning and self-assessment. In addition, it contains 26 Multiple Choice Questions (MCQs), 05 Clinicopathologic Vignettes, and 01 Image-based Questions; these are followed by their answers along with explanatory notes of correct and incorrect answers.*

CHAPTER 13

White Blood Cells—Proliferations and Myeloid Neoplasms

■ WHITE BLOOD CELLS—NORMAL AND REACTIVE PROLIFERATIONS

Q1. Which cells belong to the myeloid series leading to the formation of mature granulocytes?

Key facts:
i. Granulocytes, i.e. polymorphonuclear leucocytes, eosinophils and basophils, originate from myeloid or trilineage stem cells residing in the bone marrow. In addition to granulocytes, the trilineage stem cells differentiate into monocytes, erythroid and megakaryocyte progenitors (see **Fig. 11.3**).
ii. Cells of the myeloid series can be divided into two groups **(Fig. 13.1)**:
- *proliferative or mitotic pool* (myeloblasts, promyelocytes and myelocytes), and
- *mature or post-mitotic pool* (metamyelocytes, band forms and mature granulocytes).

iii. The ratio of myeloid to erythroid cells in the bone marrow is 3:1 on average, but may vary from 2:1 to 15:1. Bone marrow contains approximately 10 to 15 times more granulocytes and their precursors than the circulating blood.

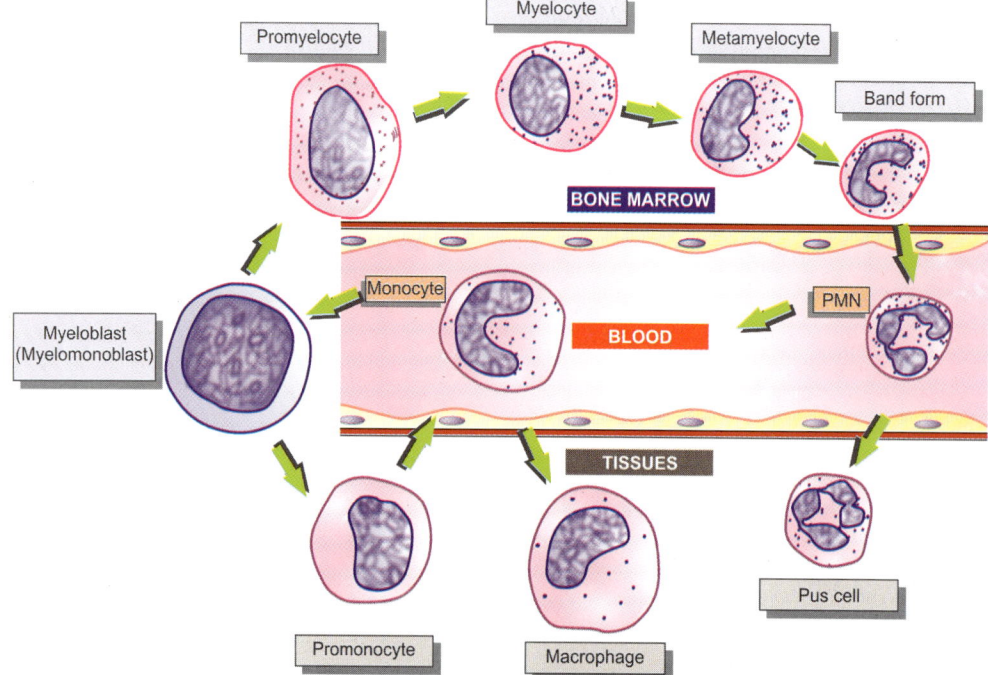

FIGURE 13.1: Granulopoiesis and the cellular compartments of myeloid cells in the bone marrow, blood and tissues.

iv. Following their release from the bone marrow, granulocytes spend about 10 hours in circulation before moving to peripheral tissues. Accordingly, granulocytes can be divided into two groups:
- the *circulating pool,* and
- the *marginating pool.*

v. Granulocytes spend 2–3 days in tissues before they are destroyed or die due to senescence.

vi. Monocytes spend less 20–40 hours in circulation before they enter tissue to differentiate into macrophages. Macrophages have a very long life span.

Q2. In which organs are lymphoid cells formed?

i. The bone marrow and thymus are the *primary organs* of lymphopoiesis. In these organs, lymphoid stem cells undergo spontaneous division independent of antigenic stimulation.

ii. Lymph nodes, spleen and gut-associated lymphoid tissue (GALT) are part of the *secondary or reactive lymphoid tissue.* In these organs, lymphocytes are actively produced in the germinal centres of lymphoid follicles in response to antigenic stimulation.

iii. Functionally, the lymphocytes are divided into T, B and natural killer (NK) cells. B cells mature into plasma cells which secrete immunoglobulin.

iv. Formation of mature lymphocytes occurs through two stages: lymphoblast and prolymphocyte **(Fig. 13.2)**.

v. Differentiation and maturation of lymphocytes occurs in the thymus and secondary lymphoid organs.

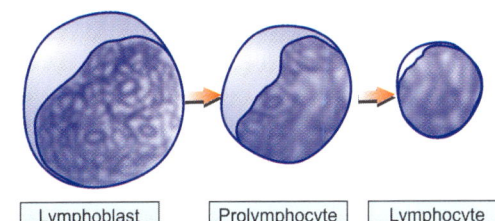

FIGURE 13.2: The formation of lymphoid series of cells.

Q3. How are myeloblasts distinguished morphologically from lymphoblasts?

The distinguishing morphologic features between the myeloblast and lymphoblast are summarised in **Table 13.1**.

TABLE 13.1 Morphologic characteristics of the blast cells in Romanowsky stains.

FEATURE	MYELOBLAST	LYMPHOBLAST
1. Size	10–18 μm	10–18 μm
2. Nucleus	Round or oval	Round or oval
3. Nuclear chromatin	Fine meshwork	Slightly clumped
4. Nuclear membrane	Very fine	Fairly dense
5. Nucleoli	2–5	1–2
6. Cytoplasm	Scanty, blue, agranular, Auer rods may be seen	Scanty, clear blue, agranular

Q4. What are the normal white cell counts?

Normal white cell counts are given in **Table 13.2**.

Key facts:
- Normal white counts are higher in children than in adults, and are even higher in neonates.
- There is a slight diurnal variation in every adult; the highest counts are in the afternoon hours.
- White blood cell counts are elevated in pregnancy, and after delivery they return to normal values.

TABLE 13.2 Normal white blood cell counts in health.

	ABSOLUTE COUNT
TLC	
Adults	4,000–11,000/μL
Infants (Full term, at birth)	10,000–25,000/μL
Infants (1 year)	6,000–16,000/μL
Children (4–7 years)	5,000–15,000/μL
Children (8–12 years)	4,500–13,500/μL
DLC IN ADULTS	
Polymorphs (neutrophils) 40–75%	2,000–7,500/μL
Lymphocytes 20–50%	1,500–4,000/μL
Monocytes 2–10%	200–800/μL
Eosinophils 1–6%	40–400/μL
Basophils <1%	10–100/μL

Q5. Enumerate the principal pathologic variations involving the neutrophils.

The principal pathologic variations from normal include the following:

- *Count*, which involves either neutrophilic leucocytosis or neutropenia
- *Morphology*, which involves cytoplasmic or nuclear changes
- *Function*

Q6. What are the main causes of neutrophil leucocytosis?

Definition Neutrophil leucocytosis (neutrophilia) is, for practical purposes, defined as an increased number of PMNs above 7,500/μL.

Etiology The most common causes of neutrophil leucocytosis are as under:

i. *Acute infections* are the most common cause of neutrophilia. Such infections are most often caused by certain bacilli, but can be caused by viruses, spirohaetes, or parasites as well.

ii. *Other inflammations* in response to tissue damage such as those caused by burns, ischaemia (e.g. myocardial infarction), trauma and surgical interventions, gout, collagen-vascular diseases, hypersensitivity reactions, etc.

iii. *Intoxications and metabolic changes* such as poisoning, drug-reactions, uraemia, diabetic ketoacidosis, eclampsia, etc.

iv. Acute haemorrhage, internal or external.

v. Acute haemolysis.

vi. Disseminated malignancies.

vii. Myeloproliferative disorders (in some cases).

viii. Miscellaneous, e.g. corticosteroid therapy, idiopathic neutrophilia, etc.

Q7. What are the most common causes of neutropenia?

Definition Neutropenia is, for practical purposes, defined as neutrophil count below 2,500/μL.

- Since neutrophils represent the most numerous leucocytes, it is usually associated with absolute leucopenia.
- Typically, neutropenia is associated with an increased incidence of infections.

Etiology Neutropenia may be acute and transient or chronic. The most common causes are:

i. Certain bacterial infections such as typhoid, paratyphoid, brucellosis, influenza, measles, viral hepatitis, malaria, kala-azar, etc.

ii. Overwhelming bacterial infections, especially in patients with reduced resistance, e.g. miliary tuberculosis, septicaemia, etc.

iii. Drugs, chemicals, and physical agents which induce aplasia of bone marrow. These drugs include cytotoxic anticancer drugs, toxins like benzene, or ionising radiation. Neutropenia can be induced by numerous drugs due to individual hypersensitivity of some persons.

iv. Certain haematologic and systemic diseases, e.g. pernicious anemia, aplastic anemia, cirrhosis with splenomegaly, SLE, Gaucher disease.

v. Cachexia and debility.

vi. Anaphylactic shock.

vii. Certain rare hereditary/genetic diseases such as cyclic neutropenia, idiopathic benign neutropenia, primary splenic neutropenia.

Q8. What are the most common variations in morphology of neutrophils?

Pathologic changes may involve granules and other cytoplasmic components or the nucleus of the neutrophils, as under **(Fig. 13.3)**:

I. **Cytoplasmic abnormalities**

i. *Toxic cytoplasmic granules* These dark-staining, heavy granules seen in bacterial infections.

ii. *Vacuoles* Increased cytoplasmic vacuolisation is seen in septicaemia and severe bacterial infections.

iii. *Döhle bodies* These small, round or oval patches, 2–3 μm in diameter are signs of infection.

II. **Nuclear abnormalities**

i. Reduced number of nuclear lobes ('*shift-to-the-left*', i.e. 1–2 lobes from the mean number of 3 lobes per nucleus), seen in severe infection, leucoerythroblastic reactions or leukaemia.

ii. *Hypersegmentation* of nuclei ('*shift-to-the-right*', i.e. more than 5 lobes per nucleus) as seen in megaloblastic anaemia, uraemia, and sometimes in leukaemia.

iii. *Inherited Pelger-Huet anomaly* is presence of bilobed nuclei in most granulocytes.

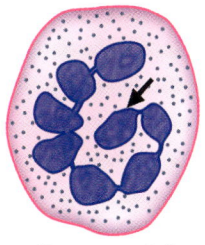 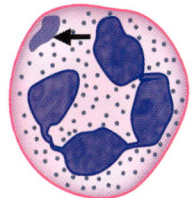 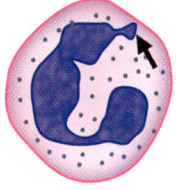 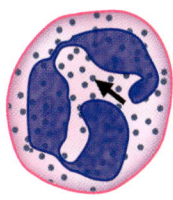 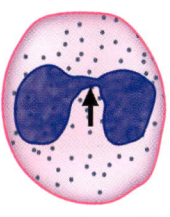

Hypersegmented neutrophil | Döhle body | Female sex chromatin | Toxic granules | Hereditary Pelger-Hüet anomaly

FIGURE 13.3: Common variations in neutrophil morphology.

Q9. What are the most important defective functions of neutrophils?

Neutrophil function abnormalities include the following:
I. **Defective chemotaxis** may be congenital or acquired.
i. *Congenital defects* of chemotaxis such as 'lazy-leucocyte syndrome'.
ii. *Acquired defects* of chemotaxis may be seen after corticosteroid therapy, aspirin ingestion, due to alcoholism or in myeloid leukaemia.
II. **Defective phagocytosis** may be congenital or acquired.
i. It is often related to a lack of opsonisation in hypogammaglobulinaemia or hypocomplimentaemia.
ii. Splenectomy and sickle cell anaemia also cause defective phagocytosis.
III. **Defective killing** is a feature of certain conditions.
i. Some congenital disorders or neoplasia.
ii. Chédiak-Higashi syndrome and chronic granulomatous disease.
iii. Myeloid leukemia.

Q10. What are the common causes of lymphocytosis?

Definition Lymphocytosis is defined as a peripheral blood lymphocyte count of over 4,000/μL. It may be acute or chronic, absolute or relative (due to neutropenia).
Etiology Most often, lymphocytosis is caused by infections and neoplasia.
i. Certain acute bacterial and viral diseases, such as pertussis, infectious mononucleosis, viral hepatitis.
ii. Certain chronic diseases, e.g. brucellosis, tuberculosis, syphilis.
iii. Haematopoietic neoplastic diseases such as lymphocytic leukaemia, lymphoma, heavy chain disease.
iv. Relative lymphocytosis which is encountered in diseases causing neutropenia. Best examples are viral exantemas of childhood, during the convalescence from acute infections, thyrotoxicosis.
NOTE: *Lymphopenia*, the opposite of lymphocytosis (lymphocyte count below 1,500/μL) is an uncommon finding. It is most often seen as a relative lymphopenia in acute infection accompanied by neutrophilia. It can be secondary to treatment with corticosteroids, cytotoxic drugs and irradiation.

Q11. What are the common causes of eosinophilia?

Definition Eosinophilia is defined as an increased number of eosinophils above 400/μL. Eosinopenia is a count below 40/μL.
Etiology The most important causes of eosinophilia are as under:
i. *Allergic and hypersensitivity disorders*, e.g. hay fever, bronchial asthma, drug hypersensitivity, polyarteritis nodosa, rheumatoid arthritis.
ii. *Skin diseases* such as pemphigus, dermatitis herpetiformis, erythema multiforme.
iii. *Parasitic infestations*, e.g. trichinosis, echinococcosis, intestinal parasitoses, *Strongyloides stercoralis* infection causing Löeffler syndrome, *Wucheria bancrofti* causing tropical eosinophilia.
iv. *Haematopoietic disorders*, e.g. chronic myelogenous leukaemia, polycythaemia vera, Hodgkin disease.
v. *Solid malignant tumours* with metastases.
vi. *Diseases of unknown origin*, e.g. sarcoidosis.

vii. *Treatment related*, e.g. post-splenectomy states, post-irradiation.
NOTE: *Eosinopenia* is the oposite of eosinophilia. It is a rare condition, most often caused by corticosteroid treatment or hypercorticism due to ACTH stimulation of adrenals or adrenal cortical tumours.

Q12. What are the causes of basophil leucocytosis?

Definition Basophil leucocytosis of basophilia is defined as a number of basophilic leucocytes in peripheral blood above 100/µL.

Etiology Most common causes are haematopoietic neoplastic disorders, but it can be seen in some other diseases as well, as under:
i. Chronic myeloid leukaemia
ii. Polycythaemia vera
iii. Myelosclerosis
iv. Hodgkin disease
v. Urticaria pigmentosa and mastocytosis
vi. Myxoedema
vii. Ulcerative colitis
viii. Post-splenectomy states

Q13. What is infectious mononucleosis?

Definition Infectious mononucleosis ('glandular fever') is a benign, infectious, self-limiting lymphoproliferative disorder caused by the B lymphotropic Epstein-Barr virus (EBV).

Key features
i. Transmitted by close person-to-person contact (e.g. kissing).
ii. Groups of young people living together (e.g. students, campers, military personel) at highest risk.
iii. Primary infection in childhood usually asymptomatic, whereas 50% of adults have symptoms.
iv. Most adults older than 40 years have antibodies to EBV.
v. EBV plays an important role in the pathogenesis of nasopharyngeal carcinoma, Burkitt and B-cell NH lymphoma **(Fig. 13.4)**.

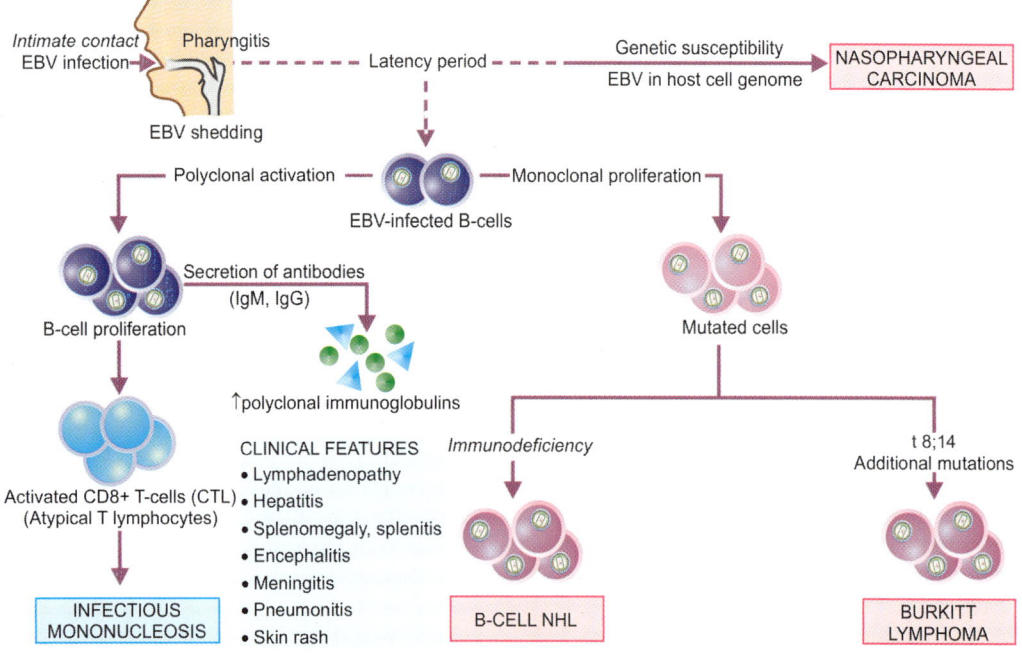

FIGURE 13.4: The role of EBV in the pathogenesis of infectious mononucleosis, nasopharyngeal carcinoma and Burkitt lymphoma.

Q14. How is EBV involved in the pathogenesis of infectious mononucleosis?

The sequence of events is typically as under (*see* **Fig. 13.4**):
i. EBV first enters from saliva during kissing into the epithelial cells of the salivary gland, from where it is transmitted to B lymphocytes, which have receptors for EBV →
ii. Sore throat results from necrosis of infected B cells and salivary gland cells →
iii. Viraemia leads to acute febrile disease and stimulates production of antibodies →
iv. Antibodies peak at 2 weeks post-infection and eliminate virus from blood →
v. Virus persists in B cells as a latent infection →
vi. EBV infected B-cells undergo polyclonal activation and proliferation →
vii. B-cells secrete antibodies, which are first IgM heterophil antibodies used for the diagnosis of IM, followed by IgG antibodies, which persist for life of the infected person →
viii. CD8+ cytotoxic T-cells are activated, proliferate and appear in blood as atypical lymphocytes important for the haematologic diagnosis of IM →
ix. Proliferation of T-cells leads to lymphadenopathy and hepatosplenomegaly →
x. Recovery after 2 months with regression of physical findings.

Q15. What are the clinical features of infectious mononucleosis?

IM has the following phases:
- *Incubation phase* (30–50 days) without clinical symptoms.
- *Prodromal phase* (3–5 days) with nonspecific symptoms such as malaise, myalgia, headache and fatigue.
- *Clinical phase* (1–3 weeks)

Clinical features
i. Fever, sore throat and cervical lymphadenopathy (80–95%)
ii. Splenomegaly (50%)
iii. Less common features (~10%):
a. Hepatomegaly with jaundice
b. Transient erythematous maculopapular rash on trunk and extremities
c. Periorbital oedema

Complications are uncommon and include the following:
i. Neurologic manifestations (in children)
ii. Splenic rupture (in those with splenomegaly)
iii. Autoimmune haemolytic anaemia due to heterophile antibodies
iv. Upper airway obstruction due to lymphadenopathy/tonsillitis
v. Bacterial superinfections

Q16. What are the laboratory tests performed for diagnosis of infectious mononucleosis?

Laboratory tests performed for the diagnosis of IM include i) standard haematologic and laboratory tests, ii) EBV specific serologic test, and iii) molecular biology tests.

I. Standard haematologic and laboratory tests show the following abnormalities:
i. Leucocytosis (10,000–20,000/µL) with absolute lymphocytosis and relative neutropenia.
ii. Atypical lymphocytes (10–12%) seen in peripheral blood smears **(Fig. 13.5)**.
iii. Reversal of CD4+/CD8+ ratio → fall of CD4+, increase of CD8+ cells.
iv. Thrombocytopenia.
v. Abnormal liver function tests (AST, ALT and alkaline phosphatase) are positive in 90% cases.

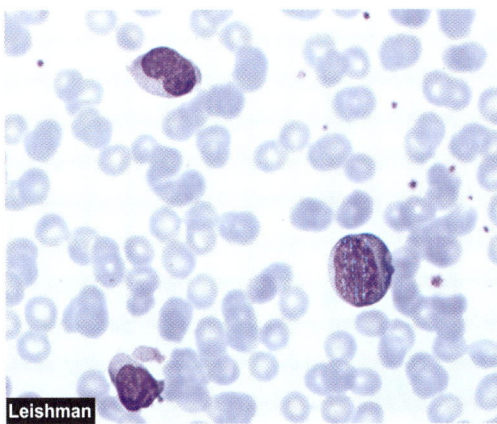

FIGURE 13.5: Peripheral blood film showing atypical lymphocytes in infectious mononucleosis.

II. **Serologic tests for EBV** are important for diagnosis and prognosis, as under:
i. *Test for heterophile antibodies (Paul-Bunnel test)*—In the first week a titre of 40 or more is diagnostic of IM. Currently, this has been replaced by 'monospot test'.
ii. *EBV specific tests* (e.g. antibodies against EBV capsid, antibodies to EBV nuclear antigen)
iii. *EBV tests predicting* possible development of nasopharyngeal carcinoma and African Burkitt lymphoma (e.g. antibodies to early antigen, and IgA antibodies).
III. **Molecular biology tests** for EBV DNA or proteins are performed using PCR.

Q17. Define leukaemoid reactions. What are its types? Describe their salient features.

Definition Leukaemoid reaction is a reactive excessive leucocytosis in the peripheral blood resembling leukaemia in a person who clinically does not have leukaemia, and does not have the usual pathologic features of leukaemia (e.g. splenomegaly, lymphadenopathy, bleeding tendency, lowered resistance to infections).

Types There are two types of leukaemoid reaction: i) myeloid, and ii) lymphoid; the former is much more common than the latter.

I. **Myeloid leukaemoid reaction** involves the granulocyte series.
Etiology It may occur in association with a wide variety of diseases as follows:
i. Infections, e.g. staphylococcal pneumonia, tuberculosis, sepsis.
ii. Intoxications, e.g. mercury poisoning, eclampsia, severe burns.
iii. Malignant diseases, especially those involving the bone marrow such as multiple myeloma, myelofibrosis, bone metastases, or of lymph nodes such as Hodgkin disease.
iv. Severe haemorrhage or haemolysis.
Laboratory findings Typical findings include leucocytosis, with abnormal peripheral blood smears, and negative cytogenetic/molecular biology findings which are important to rule out chronic myeloid leukaemia in questionable cases **(Fig. 13.6)**.
i. Leucocytosis usually moderate and does not exceed 100,000/μL.
ii. Immature myeloid cell precursors in peripheral blood smears include metamyelocytes, myelocytes (5–15%), and fewer than 5% blasts, thus resembling CML.
iii. Anaemia.
iv. Platelet counts are either normal or increased.
v. Leucocyte alkaline phosphatase (LAP) is high (important for excluding CML in doubtful cases!).
II. **Lymphoid leukaemoid reaction** presents with an appearance of numerous small lymphocytes in peripheral blood.
Etiology Infections (some bacterial and viral diseases) and neoplastic diseases (rarely).

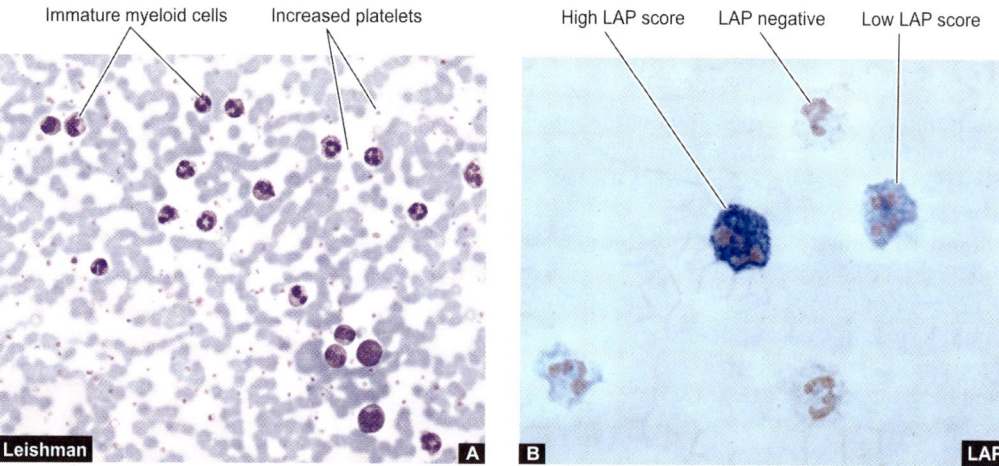

FIGURE 13.6: Leukaemoid reaction. A, Peripheral blood film showing marked neutrophilic leucocytosis accompanied with late precursors of myeloid series. B, Neutrophil (or leucocyte) alkaline phosphatase (NAP or LAP) activity is higher as demonstrated by this cytochemical stain.

Infections causing lymphoid leukaemoid reactions include the same diseases that cause *lymphocytosis*, such as pertussis, infectious mononucleosis, cytomegalovirus infection, and childhood viral diseases (e.g. measles, chickenpox).

Q18. What are the main differentiating features between leukaemoid reactions and chronic myeloid leukaemia?

The contrasting features of leukaemoid reaction and chronic myeloid leukaemia are presented in **Table 13.3**.

TABLE 13.3 Contrasting features of leukaemoid reaction and chronic myeloid leukaemia.		
FEATURE	LEUKAEMOID REACTION	CML
1. TLC	25,000–1,00,000/μL	≥1,00,000/μL
2. DLC	i. Dominant cells PMNs ii. Immature cells predominantly metamyelocytes and myelocytes (5–15%); myeloblasts and promyelocytes ≥5% iii. Basophils normal	i. All maturation stages ii. Immature cells all stages; myeloblasts and promyelocytes ≤10% iii. Basophilia present
3. NAP score	Elevated	Reduced
4. Philadelphia chromosome	Absent	Present
5. ABL-BCR fusion gene	Absent	Present
6. Major etiology	Infections, intoxication, disseminated malignancy, severe haemorrhage	RNA viruses, HTLV oncogenesis, genetic factors, radiations, certain drugs and chemicals
7. Additional haematologic findings	i. Anaemia ii. Normal to raised platelet count iii. Myeloid hyperplasia in bone marrow	i. Anaemia ii. Normal to raised platelet count iii. Myeloid hyperplasia in bone marrow
8. Organ infiltration	Absent	May be present
9. Massive splenomegaly	Absent	Present

■ HAEMATOLYMPHOID MALIGNANCIES—GENERAL ASPECTS

Q19. How are haematolymphoid malignancies broadly classified?

Definition Haematoid malignancies include leukaemias and lymphomas.
- Leukaemias are classified according to their nature as *myeloid or lymphoid*.
- WHO classification has an additional third group of rare malignancies called *histiocytic neoplasms*.
- According to their duration and clinical course, leukaemias are classified as *acute or chronic*.

Classification There are four major types of leukaemia:
i. Acute myeloblastic leukaemia (AML)
ii. Acute lymphoblastic leukaemia (ALL)
iii. Chronic myeloid leukaemia (CML)
iv. Chronic lymphocytic leukaemia (CLL)

Clinicopathologic course
- *Acute myeloblastic leukaemia (AML) and acute lymphoblastic leukaemia (ALL)* have a rapid downhill course. Pathologically, these forms of leukaemias are characterised by the predominance of undifferentiated or earliest leucocyte precursors and blasts in peripheral blood.
- *Chronic myeloid leukaemia (CML) and chronic lymphocytic leukaemia (CLL)* which have a more indolent and prolonged clinical course. These chronic diseases are characterised by an increased number of late precursors of corresponding leucocyte series in peripheral blood.

Age distribution Each leukaemia affects different populations and has a distinct peak age incidence as under:
- Acute lymphoblastic leukaemia is a disease of children and young adults.
- Acute myeloblastic leukaemia occurs in all ages.
- Chronic lymphocytic leukaemia is a disease of older adults.
- Chronic myeloid leukaemia has its peak in middle age persons.

For therapeutic purposes, leukaemias are subclassified into categories based on their *distinct cytogenetic and molecular biologic features.*

Q20. What is the etiology of haematolymphoid neoplasms?

The exact etiology of various haematolymphoid is not known. However, several etiologic factors have been implicated as under:

I. **Hereditary genetic factors** Evidence for the existence of genetic factors stems from studies of identical twins, cancer families, and disease associations.

i. High twin concordance has been shown in leukaemia involving children younger than one year.

ii. Hodgkin disease is 100-times more common in the patient's identical twin than in the general population.

iii. Familial cases of leukaemia are well recognised. There is also a familial predisposition to Hodgkin disease.

iv. Leukaemia is much more common in families affected by some genetic disorders than in the general population.

v. Genetic diseases with an increased incidence of leukaemia include Down, Bloom, Wiskott-Aldrich syndromes, Fanconi anaemia, and ataxia telangiectasia.

II. **Infections**, including primarily some viral diseases, but also some bacterial infections, have been linked to subsequent appearance of leukaemia/lymphoma as under:

i. Human T-cell leukaemia lymphoma virus I (HTLV-I) has been implicated in the etiology of adult T-cell leukaemia-lymphoma.

ii. HTLV II in T-cell variant of hairy cell leukaemia.

iii. Epstein-Barr virus in the etiology of endemic (African) variety of Burkitt lymphoma, post-transplant lymphoma, and Hodgkin disease (mixed cellularity type and nodular sclerosis type).

iv. Human herpes virus 8 (HHV-8) in primary effusion lymphoma.

v. HIV in diffuse large B-cell lymphoma and Burkitt lymphoma.

vi. Hepatitis C virus in lymphoplasmacytic lymphoma.

vii. *Helicobacter pylori* in MALT lymphoma of stomach.

III. **Environmental factors** include ionising radiation, environmental chemical carcinogens and drugs.

i. *Ionising radiation* has been linked to subsequent occurrence of leukaemia/lymphoma in Japanese survivors of the atomic bomb explosion (higher incidence of AML, ALL and CML), inadequately protected professionals exposed to radiation and radioactive materials, and patients receiving radiation therapy.

ii. *Chemicals* found to increase the risk of leukaemia/lymphoma epidemiologically include benzene, tobacco smoke, certain agricultural chemicals and hair dyes.

iii. *Drugs* include chemotherapeutic and alkylating agents. For example, patients treated for Hodgkin disease can develop lymphoma/leukaemia.

IV. **Association with diseases of immunity** Since lymphoid cells are part of the immune system, any disturbance of immunity could promote the development of lymphoma and lymphoid leukaemia.

i. A higher incidence than expected has been found in patients surviving HIV infections, iatrogenic immunosuppression induced by drugs or radiation therapy, as well those born with congenital immunodeficiencies.

ii. A few autoimmune diseases have been associated with an increased incidence of lymphoma. Such diseases include Sjögren disease, coeliac sprue, rheumatoid arthritis, and SLE.

Q21. What is the pathogenesis of haematopoietic neoplasms?

Several pathogenetic pathways have been identified as under:

I. **Genetic damage to single clone of target cells** It is followed by proliferation and expansion of transformed clone. The genetic damage may be related to exposure to chemical carcinogens, or insertion of a carcinogenic virus into the genome of the infected cell.

II. **Chromosomal translocation** Many translocations have been recognised. The first and the best known is the so called Philadelphia chromosome seen in CML, involving reciprocal translocation of parts of the long arm of chromosome 22 to the long arm of chromosome 9, i.e. t(9;22) **(Fig. 13.7)**.

III. **Maturation defect** In acute myeloblstic leukaemia, the most prominent defect is the arrest of maturation of myeloid precursors beyond the myeloblast or promyelocyte stage. In ALL, a similar maturation defect occurs at the level of lymphoblast.

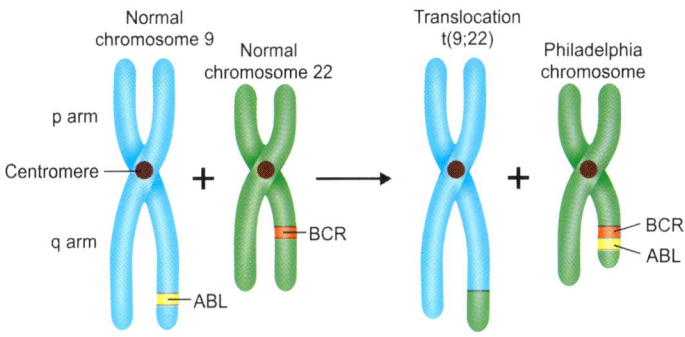

FIGURE 13.7: The Philadelphia (Ph) chromosome. There is reciprocal translocation of the part of the long arms of chromosome 22 to the long arms of chromosome 9 written as t(9;22).

IV. **Myelosuppression** Leukaemic cells may accumulate in the bone marrow, physically replacing the normal haematopoietic cells. Inhibition of haematopoiesis may be mediated by humoral factors, as evidenced by hypocellular marrow in some cases. Following successful treatment, such hypocellular marrow can be repopulated by normal haematopoietic cells originating from residual normal stem cells.

V. **Organ infiltration** Leukaemic cells may exit from blood vessels and infiltrate many organs, in contrast to WBCs in myeloid leukaemoid reaction which do not infiltrate parenchymal organs.

VI. **Cytokines** Some lymphomas are associated with an inflammatory reaction, induced by cytokines secreted by tumour cells. The best example is Hodgkin disease in which the Reed-Sternberg cells secrete IL-5 eliciting an influx of eosinophils, and IL-13 for autocrine stimulation of RS cells, or fibroblast growth factor for fibrogenesis.

MYELOID NEOPLASMS

Q22. How are myeloid neoplasms classified?

Since the myeloid trilineage stem cell differentiates into three series of progenitor cells, that includes granulocyte-monocyte, erythroid and megakaryocytic series, all examples of myeloid neoplasms fall into these three categories of cell-lines **(Fig. 13.8)**. Based on this concept, the myeloid neoplasms can be subdivided into five groups:

I. Myeloproliferative neoplasms (MPN)
II. Myeloid/lymphoid neoplasms with eosinophilia and gene rearrangement

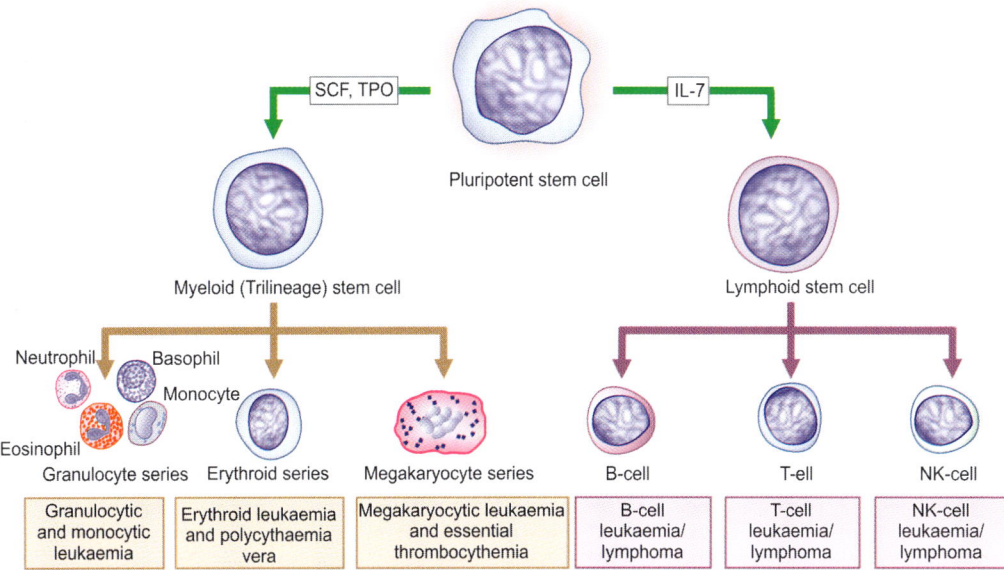

FIGURE 13.8: Maturation stages of myeloid cells in relation to corresponding types of myeloid neoplasms.

III. Myelodysplastic/myeloproliferative neoplasms (MDS/MPN)
IV. Myelodysplastic syndrome
V. Acute myeloid leukaemia
As shown in **Table 13.4**, each of these groups has several subtypes.

Q23. What is chronic myeloid leukaemia? Discuss its genetic basis and main clinicopathologic features.

Definition Chronic myeloid leukaemia (CML) is a clonal malignant disorder characterised by balanced reciprocal translocation between chromosome 9 and 22, forming the Philadelphia chromosome (*see* **Fig. 13.7**).

Genetics The t(9;22) involves fusion of the *BCR* (breakpoint cluster region) gene on chromosome 22q11 with *ABL* (named after Abelson murine leukaemia virus) gene located on chromosome 9q34.
- The fusion product so formed is called '*Ph chromosome t(9;22)(34;q11),BCR-ABL*,' which must be identified for the diagnosis of CML.
- Identification of the diagnostic chromosomal changes is done by FISH (fluorescent in situ hybridisation) or polymerase chain reaction (PCR).
- Activated ABL protein acts as a tyrosine kinase, which activates other kinases to inhibit apoptosis. The ability of ABL protein to bind to DNA is also altered.
- The progression of CML to a blastic phase is not fully understood, but it involves probably some other oncogenes (e.g. *RAS* and *MYC*) and tumour suppressor genes (e.g. *RB* and *TP53*).

Clinicopathologic features
- CML accounts for 20% of all leukemias.
- Peak incidence in 3rd and 4th decades of life.
- Males and females affected equally.
- Insidious onset, but may progress to an accelerated phase, and a blast crisis.
- A distinct variant form, called *juvenile CML* has been identified in children.

Common symptoms and clinical findings reflect a loss of PMN functions, as well as reduced numbers of RBCs and platelets as under:
i. Anaemia with pallor, weakness, fatigue, dyspnoea and tachycardia.
ii. Bleeding tendency with bruising, epistaxis, menorrhagia and formation of haematomas.
iii. Splenomegaly is almost always present, and sometimes painful due to infarcts.
iv. Increased susceptibility to infections (especially in the juvenile form).
v. In juvenile form, there is lymphadenopathy rather than splenomegaly.
vi. The most common cause of death (80%) is disease acceleration or blastic crisis.

Therapy The aim of the therapy is elimination of all malignant clones bearing BCR/ABL fusion protein.
- This is achieved with oral *imatinib* therapy, which inhibits ATP-binding site of the ABL kinase and signal transduction of the BCR-ABL fusion protein. Therapy can induce remission in 97% of cases for ~18 months.
- Additional treatment modalities include allogeneic bone marrow transplantation, interferon-α treatment and chemotherapy or radiation.

Q24. What are the laboratory findings in chronic myeloid leukaemia?

Laboratory finding are based on the study of i) peripheral blood, ii) bone marrow, and iii) biochemical changes in the serum.

I. **Peripheral blood studies** show the following:
i. Anaemia moderate, normocytic normochromic.
ii. Platelet count normal, but may be elevated in 50% of cases.
iii. Leucocytosis of 2,00,000/μL or more at the time of presentation.
iv. Cytochemistry shows reduced score of *neutrophil alkaline phosphatase* (NAP), which helps distinguish CML from leukaemoid reaction. NAP returns to normal with successful therapy.
v. *Peripheral blood smear* shows changes that vary according to the phase of the disease **(Fig. 13.9)**:
a. *Chronic phase* of CML is characterised by the appearance of myeloid cells of intermediate grade (i.e. myelocytes and metamyelocytes), as well as band forms and segmented PMNs. Myeloblasts do not

TABLE 13.4 WHO classification of myeloid neoplasms and acute leukaemias#.

I. Myeloproliferative neoplasms (MPN)
1. Chronic myeloid leukaemia (CML) (*BCR-ABL1*-positive)
2. Chronic neutrophilic leukaemia (CNL)
3. Chronic eosinophilic leukaemia/hypereosinophilic syndrome
4. Polycythaemia vera (PV)
5. Primary myelofibrosis (PMF)
6. Essential thrombocythaemia (ET)
7. Chronic eosinophilic leukaemia, NOS
8. Mastocytosis
9. MPN, unclassifiable

II. Myeloid/lymphoid neoplasms with eosinophilia and gene rearrangement or with *PCM1-JAK2*

III. Myelodysplastic/myeloproliferative neoplasms (MDS/MPN)
1. Chronic myelomonocytic leukaemia (CMML)
2. Atypical CML (*BCR-ABL1* negative)
3. Others

IV. Myelodysplastic syndrome (MDS)
1. MDS with single lineage dysplasia (MDS-SLD)
2. MDS with multi-lineage dysplasia (MDS-MLD)
3. MDS with ring sideroblasts (MDS-RS)
    i. With single lineage dysplasia (MDS-RS-SLD)
    ii. With multi-lineage dysplasia (MDS-RS-MLD)
4. MDS with excess blasts (MDS-EB)
5. MDS with isolated del (5q)
6. MDS-unclassifiable (MDS-U)
7. Refractory cytopenia of childhood
8. Myeloid neoplasms with germ line predisposition

V. Acute myeloid leukaemia (AML) and related neoplasms
1. AML with recurrent genetic abnormalities
    i. AML with t(8;21)(q22;q22); *RUNX1-RUNX1T1*
    ii. AML (M4Eo*) with inv(16)(p13.1;q22) or t(16;16)(p13.1;q22); *CBFB &β-MYH11*
    iii. APML (M3*) with *PML-RARA*
    iv. AML with t(9;11)(p21;q23); *MLLT3-MLL*
    v. AML with t(6;9)(p23;q34); *DEK-NUP214*
    vi. AML with inv(3)(q21q26.2) or t(3;3)(q21;q26.2); *RPN1-EVI1*
    vii. AML (megakaryoblastic) with t(1;22)(p13;q13); *RBM15-MKL1*
    viii. AML with mutated *NPM1*
    ix. AML with mutated *CEBPA*
2. AML with myelodysplasia-related changes
3. Therapy-related myeloid neoplasm
4. AML, not otherwise categorised
    i. AML minimally differentiated (M0*)
    ii. AML without maturation (M1*)
    iii. AML with maturation (M2*)
    iv. Acute myelomonocytic leukaemia (M4*)
    v. Acute monoblastic/monocytic leukaemia (M5a, M5b*)
    vi. Acute erythroid leukaemia (M6*)
    vii. Acute megakaryoblastic leukaemia (M7*)
    viii. Acute basophilic leukaemia
    ix. Acute panmyelosis with myelofibrosis
5. Myeloid sarcoma
6. Myeloid proliferations related to Down syndrome
    i. Transient abnormal myelopoiesis
    ii. Myeloid leukaemia associated with Down syndrome

VI. Blastic plasmacytoid dendritic cell neoplasm

VII. Acute leukaemia of ambiguous lineage

VIII. B-lymphoblastic leukaemia/lymphoma

IX. T-lymphoblastic leukaemia/lymphoma

*Corresponding M type of FAB classification has been shown with asterix wherever applicable.
#Arber et al: The 2016 revision to the WHO classification of myeloid neoplasms and acute leukaemia. Blood. 2016;127:2391-405.

exceed 10%. Basophilia of 10% is a characteristic feature. Increasing basophil count is indicative of impending blastic transformation.

b. *Accelerated phase* of CML is characterised by rising leucocytosis, accompanied by thrombocytosis or thrombocytopenia, and splenomegaly. Bone marrow contains 10–20% blasts, and 20% or more basophils.

c. *Blast crisis* fulfills the criteria for the diagnosis of acute leukaemia. Typically, bone marrow contains more than 20% of blasts, which are most often myeloid, but may also be lymphoid, erythroid or undifferentiated.

II. **Bone marrow studies** show myeloid hypercellularity with predominance of myelocytes. The number of blasts varies from less than 10% in chronic phase to more than 20% in the blast crisis.
Cytogenetic studies show Philadelphia chromosome in 90–95% of cases.

III. **Biochemical studies** of peripheral blood shows elevated serum B_{12} and B_{12} binding capacity. Serum uric acid is elevated.

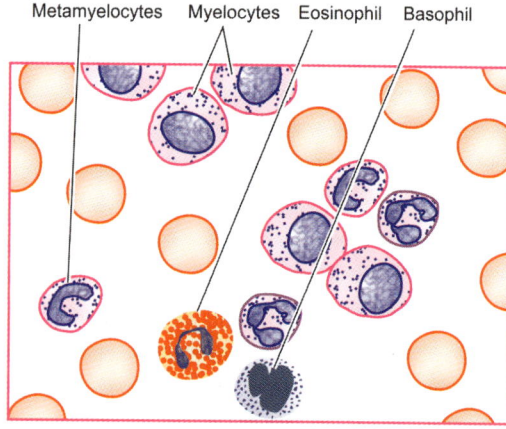

FIGURE 13.9: PBF findings in chronic myeloid leukaemia (CML).

Q25. What is polycythaemia vera? Discuss its salient features.

Definition Polycythaemia vera (PV) is a clonal disorder characterised by increased production of all myeloid elements (RBCs, granulocytes, platelets) resulting in pancytosis in the absence of any recognisable cause.
- It is also called primary or idiopathic polycythemia.
- It is the most common myeloproliferative disorder.

Etiopathogenesis Unknown.
- Tyrosine kinase JAK2 mutation plays a major role in the pathogenesis of PV by removing the autoinhibitory control of kinases.
- One third cases have chromosomal abnormalities, which are, however, inconsistent.

Laboratory findings Erythrocytosis, mild leucocytosis and thrombocytosis.
i. RBC count ↑ >6 million/μL in males and >5.5 million/μL in females.
ii. Haematocrit ↑ >55% in males and >47% in females.
iii. Haemoglobin ↑ >17.5 g/dL in males and >15.5 in females.
iv. Leucocyte count ↑ in the range from 15,000 to 25,000/μL, with basophils↑ and NAP↑.
v. Platelet count ↑, but with defective platelet function.
vi. Bone marrow cellularity ↑ with erythroid hyperplasia and panhyperplasia.
vii. Cytogenetic abnormalities in 30%, but inconsistent.
viii. Erythropoietin levels ↓ in serum and urine.

Clinicopathologic features PV is a disease of late middle age and slightly more common in males. Symptoms result from hyperviscosity of the blood, hypervolaemia, hypermetabolism, and decreased cerebral perfusion, as under:
i. Headaches, tinnitus, vertigo, visual alterations, syncope and even coma.
ii. Increased risk of thrombosis and accelerated atherosclerosis.
iii. Haemorrhagic diathesis due to increased blood volume and platelet dysfunction.
iv. Splenomegaly.
v. Pruritus, especially after a bath.
vi. Hyperuricaemia predisposing to urinary stones.

Therapy
- Phlebotomy (venesection) at regular intervals is the treatment of choice. Survival up to 10–12 years.
- Interferon-α effective in reducing JAK2 expression in patients who have this mutation.
- Chemotherapy may be used to induce myelosuppression.

- Symptomatic therapy includes antithrombotic drugs and uricosuric drugs to prevent secondary gout and urinary stones.

Complications Usually after several years of treatment.
i. About 25% of PV patients develop myelofibrosis.
ii. Some develop leukaemia and lymphoma or multiple myeloma.
iii. Vascular thrombosis is a major cause of death.

Differential diagnosis Secondary polycythaemia is secondary erythrocytosis from various causes; requires to be distinguished from PV. Secondary polycythaemia has:
- Erythropoietin↑.
- Not associated with splenic enlargement, leucocytosis, or platelet abnormalities which are typical of PV.

Etiopathogenesis Possible sources of excessive erythropoietin secretion include the following:
i. High altitude
ii. Cardiovascular disease
iii. Pulmonary disease with alveolar hypoventilation
iv. Heavy smoking
v. Tumour-derived erythropoietin (e.g. renal cell carcinoma, hepatocellular carcinoma, cerebellar haemangioblastoma, massive uterine leiomyoma)
NOTE: *Spurious polycythaemia* may result from plasma loss in burns or dehydration due to vomiting or water deprivation.

Q26. Define essential thrombocythaemia. Discuss its main features.

Definition Essential thrombocythaemia (essential thrombocytosis or primary (essential) thrombocythaemia) is a rare clonal disorder characterised by markedly elevated platelet counts in absence of any recognisable stimulus. Although the elevated platelet count is the dominant feature, other haematopoietic cell-lines may be involved as well.

Etiopathogenesis Unknown.
- Some cases are familial, suggesting a genetic predisposition.
- The basic defect is uncontrollable thrombopoietin stimulation of megakaryocytes and platelet release.

Laboratory findings
i. Thrombocythaemia >4,00,000/μL.
ii. Peripheral blood smears contain large platelets, megakaryocyte fragments and hypogranular forms.
iii. Bone marrow contains an increased number of hyperdiploid magakaryocytes.
iv. Myelofibrosis is focal and variable.

Clinicopathologic features
i. Older persons, affected by spontaneous haemorrhagic and thrombotic events.
ii. Easy bruising after minor trauma.
iii. Spontaneous bleeding.
iv. Transient ischaemic attacks or frank stroke due to platelet aggregation in CNS microvasculature.
v. Acquired von Willebrand disease develops in some patients.

Therapy and prognosis The disease runs a benign course and usually does not require treatment unless the platelet count is above 1 million/μL.

Differential diagnosis Secondary or reactive thrombocytosis that occurs in response to a variety of stimuli. Etiology of secondary thrombocytosis includes: chronic infection, haemorrhage, postoperative states, chronic iron deficiency, malignancy, rheumatoid arthritis and postsplenectomy state.

Q27. What is primary myelofibrosis?

Definition Primary myelofibrosis (PMF, also known as chronic idiopathic myelofibrosis, agnogenic myeloid metaplasia, or myelosclerosis), is a clonal disorder of unknown etiology characterised by proliferation of neoplastic stem cells at multiple sites outsides of bone marrow (i.e. *extramedullary haematopoiesis*, especially in the spleen and liver), associated with fibrosis of the bone marrow.

Etiopathogenesis Unknown.
- The disease evolves though an early *prefibrotic stage* to an overt *fibrotic stage*.
- Fibrosis results from the action of transforming growth factor-β.
- Osteosclerosis is related to the action of osteonectin.
- Marrow angiogenesis is related to the action of endothelial growth factor (VEGF).

Laboratory findings Anaemia, leucocytosis progressing to leucopenia, thrombocytosis progressing to thrombocytopenia.

i. *Peripheral blood smear* shows bizarre red cell shapes, tear drop poikilocytosis nucleated red blood cells, immature leucocytes, basophilia and giant platelet forms.

ii. *Bone marrow aspiration* typically unsuccessful ('dry tap').

iii. *Trephine biopsy* shows initially proliferation of megakaryocytes and atypia without reticulin fibrosis, myeloid hypercellularity and decreased erythropoiesis (*'prefibrotic stage'*).
Later stage of PMF is marked by megakaryocyte proliferation with reticulin fibrosis ('fibrotic stage').

iv. *Extramedullary haematopoiesis* can be documented by liver biopsy or splenic aspiration biopsy.

Clinicopathologic features Symptoms and findings are related to the replacement of haematopoietic bone marrow by fibrous tissue.

i. Anaemia with constitutional symptoms such as fatigue and weakness.

ii. Petechial and other bleeding problems in 20% cases.

iii. Massive splenomegaly causing abdominal discomfort, pain or dyspnoea.

iv. Hepatomegaly in 50% cases.

v. Less common symptoms such as jaundice, lymphadenopathy, bone pain, ascites, hyperuricaemia.

Therapy and prognosis No treatment is required and, in general, it is ineffective. Splenectomy is preformed if there are compression symptoms.

In general, PMF has poorer prognosis than PV or ET.

Q28. What is acute myeloid leukaemia? Briefly describe its main clinicopathologic features.

Definition Acute myeloid leukaemia (AML) is a heterogeneous disease characterised by infiltration of malignant myeloid cells into the blood, bone marrow and other tissues.

AML is the most malignant form of leukaemia, with a median survival of 12–18 months after diagnosis. The median five-year survival is 40%, but it depends on the subtype of leukaemia and varies from 15% to 60%.

Etiopathogenesis Etiology unknown.
- AML develops due to genetic mutation leading to the *inhibition of maturation* of myeloid stem cells and *accumulation* of early myeloid precursors in the bone marrow.
- Mutations are most likely induced by heredity, radiation, chemical carcinogens, anti-cancer drugs, or occur spontaneously.

Classification Two classifications are currently used:
- *WHO classification*, based on clinical, cytogenetic and molecular abnormalities (*see* **Table 13.4**).
- *FAB (French-American-British) classification*, which still serves as the basis for most clinical treatment protocols **(Table 13.5)**.

Clinicopathologic features Symptoms and clinical findings are due to i) bone marrow failure, and ii) organ infiltration by neoplastic cells.

I. **Bone marrow failure** develops due to proliferation of malignant clones which replace the normal blood stem cells. The symptoms and clinical findings result from a deficiency of normal RBCs, leucocytes and platelets and include the following:

i. *Anaemia*, presenting as pallor, fatigue, lethargy and dyspnoea.

ii. *Leucopenia*, i.e. reduced number of normal WBCs, with a predisposition to infections, including those of the mouth, throat, skin, respiratory tract, perianal and other sites.

iii. *Thrombocytopenia* presenting as a bleeding tendency and bleeding from the gums and other mucosae, petechiae, or easy bruising. Major haemorrhages are a common cause of death.

iv. *Fever* that can be attributed to infections, but often occurs even in the absence of infection.

II. **Infiltration of various organs** by neoplastic clones as under:

i. Bone marrow infiltration presenting as *bone pain*.

ii. *Lymphadenopathy* including prominent enlargement of tonsils.

TABLE 13.5 Revised FAB classification of acute myeloblastic leukaemias.

FAB CLASS	OLD NAME	PERCENT CASES	MORPHOLOGY	CYTOCHEMISTRY
M0	Minimally differentiated AML	5	Blasts lack definite cytologic and cytochemical features but have myeloid lineage antigens	Myeloperoxidase –
M1	AML without maturation	20	Myeloblasts predominate; few if any granules or Auer rods	Myeloperoxidase +
M2	AML with maturation	30	Myeloblasts with promyelocytes predominate; Auer rods may be present	Myeloperoxidase +++
M3	Acute promyelocytic leukaemia	10	Hypergranular promyelocytes; often with multiple Auer rods per cell	Myeloperoxidase +++
M4	Acute myelomonocytic leukaemia (Naegeli type)	20	Mature cells of both myeloid and monocytic series in peripheral blood; myeloid cells resemble M2; M4Eo has in addition abnormal eosinophils	Myeloperoxidase ++ Non-specific esterase +
M5	Acute monocytic leukaemia (Schilling type)	10	Two subtypes: M5a shows poorly-differentiated monoblasts, M5b shows differentiated promonocytes and monocytes	Non-specific esterase ++
M6	Acute erythroleukaemia (Di Guglielmo's syndrome)	4	Erythroblasts predominate (>50%); myeloblasts and promyelocytes also increased	Erythroblasts: PAS + Myeloblasts: myeloperoxidase +
M7	Acute megakaryocytic leukaemia	1	Pleomorphic undifferentiated blasts predominate; react with antiplatelet antibodies	Platelet peroxidase +

iii. *Splenomegaly*.
iv. *Hepatomegaly*, which is usually unaccompanied by abnormal liver functions.
v. *Gum infiltration*, most prominently in myelomonocytic (M4) and monocytic (M5) leukaemia.
vi. *Chloroma or granulocytic sarcoma* presenting in form of nodules and tumours of the skin and conjunctiva, that are greenish on cross section due to myeloperoxidase activity in tumour cells.
vii. *Intracranial infiltrates* involving predominantly the meninges. These lead to an elevation of intracranial pressure, headache, nausea, vomiting, blurring of vision and diplopia. (NOTE: Meningeal infiltrates are more common in ALL than in AML).
viii. *Other organ infiltrates* involving kidneys, mediastinum, testes, etc. These infiltrates can be recognised clinically, but usually produce no major symptoms.
Treatment includes the following:
- Symptomatic treatment of anaemia and thrombocytopenia with transfusions.
- Prophylaxis of infection.
- Cytotoxic drug therapy to eradicate the neoplstic cells; it usually includes 3 or more drugs.
- Bone marrow transplantation, especially for young adults in first remission.

Q29. What are the laboratory findings in acute myeloid leukaemia?

Laboratory findings include data obtained by studying: i) peripheral blood, ii) bone marrow (usually combined with cytochemistry and immunophenotyping), and iii) biochemical tests.
I. **Peripheral blood** data show the following:
i. *Anaemia*, which is normochromic, normocytic. It is usually severe and progressive. Reticulocytosis up to 5% is present.
ii. *Thrombocytopenia*, moderate to severe, with platelet counts below 50,000/μL. Spontaneous bleeding occurs when the platelet count drops below 20,000/μL.
iii. *Disseminated intravascular coagulation (DIC)* occurs only in acute promyelocytic leukaemia (M3).
iv. *White blood count* is usually elevated, but may vary from subnormal to extremely high, over 1,00,000/μL. In 25% of patients, the WBC count is lower than normal (1,000–4,000/μL).

v. Most WBC are *blasts* **(Fig. 13.10)**. (NOTE: Myeloblasts may resemble lymphoblasts of ALL, and therefore it helps to *identify them by the company they keep*, i.e. the myeloid cells surrounding them).

vi. In most instances (subtypes M1 to M4, comprising over 80% of cases), leukaemic cells contain myeloperoxidase, a marker of granulocytic differentiation. Non-specific esterase is a marker of monocytic differentiation in in M4 (acute myelomonocytic leukaemia) and M5 (acute monocytic leukaemia).

vii. '*Smear cells*', representing degenerated leucocytes are readily identified.

viii. Characteristic features of malignant cells in various subtypes of AML (M0 to M7) are presented in **Table 13.5**.

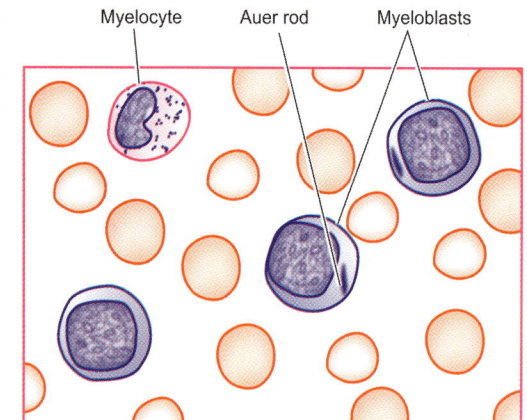

FIGURE 13.10: Peripheral blood findings in a case of acute myeloblastic leukaemia (AML).

ix. The most numerous subtypes of AML are as follows:
a. M2 (AML with maturation), 30%
b. M1 (AML without maturation), 20%
c. M4 (acute myelomonocytic leukaemia), 20%

II. **Bone marrow examination** shows the following:

i. *Hypercellularity* In most case the bone marrow cells are readily sampled.

ii. In some cases there is a '*blood tap*' or '*dry tap*'. This occurs because the malignant clones adhere firmly one to another or are enmeshed in a reticulin network preventing their aspiration.

iii. *Blast cell count* Leukaemic blast cells *exceed 20%* of all bone marrow cells. This is an essential criterion for the diagnosis of AML.

iv. *Erythropoiesis* RBC precursors are reduced in number. Dyserythropoiesis is common and megaloblasts and sideroblasts are readily identified.

v. *Thrombocytogenesis* Megakaryocytes are reduced in number or absent.

vi. *Cytogenetic abnormalities* are found in 75% of cases and are important for treatment and prognosis.

Immunophenotyping is based on CD markers:
- Primary panel (CD13, CD33 and CD117) is used to distinguish AML from ALL.
- Secondary panel of CDs is used for further subtyping of AML.

Cytochemistry is used for confirming the diagnosis and includes the following tests:

i. *Myeloperoxidase*, which is positive in all granule-containing and Auer body-containing cells. It is negative in myeloblasts, which do not contain granules.

ii. *Sudan black*, which is positive in all immature AML cells.

iii. *Periodic acid-Schiff reaction (PAS)*, which is positive in erythroleukaemia (M5) but also (notably!) in immature lymphoid cells.

iv. *Non-specific esterase (NSE)* is positive in monocytic cells (M4 and M5). These cells also show diffuse cytoplasmic staining for acid phosphatase.

III. **Biochemical testing** These test on blood plasma or serum provide additional confirmation of haematopathological diagnosis in some cases and include the following:

i. *Muramidase (lysozyme)*, which leaks into the plasma from monocytic cells in some subtypes of leukaemia (M4 and M5).

ii. *Uric acid* is elevated, as in other neoplastic conditions marked by rapid cell proliferation and breakdown.

Prognostic grouping WHO divides AML into three groups **(Table 13.6)**:
- *Favourable group* (25%) five-year survival 60%: M2, M3 and M4Eo
- *Intermediate group* (50%) five-year survival 40%: M5
- *Poor outcome* (25%) five-year survival 15%: AML-MLD (multilineage dysplasia), dysmegakaryopoiesis, therapy-related AML, and rising basophilia are predictors.

TABLE 13.6 Prognostic stratification of AML as related to mutations in the WHO type and corresponding FAB type*.

PROGNOSIS	5-YEAR SURVIVAL	MUTATIONS AND CYTOGENETICS	FAB TYPE	FREQUENCY
Favourable	~60%	t(8;21); *RUNX1-RUNX1T1*; t(15;17); inv(16) Mutated *NPM1* without *FLT3-ITD* Mutated *CEBPA*	M2, M3 M4Eo	~25%
Intermediate	~40%	Intermediate-I: Mutated *NPM1* and *FLT3-ITD* Intermediate-II: t(9;11); MLLT3-MLL Cytogenetic abnormalities	M5	~50%
Adverse	~15%	Inv(3) or t(3;3);*RPN1-EVI1* t(6;9); *DEK-NUP214* del(5q); abnormal(17p) Complex karyotypes (>3 abnormalities)	AML-MLD, dysmega-karyopoiesis, therapy-related AML, rising basophilia	~25%

*Döhner et al: European leukaemia network recommendations. Blood. 2010;115:453.

Q30. Define myelodysplastic syndromes. How are they classified? Describe their main features.

Definition Myelodysplastic syndromes (MDS) are a group of haematopoietic clonal neoplasms of the bone marrow. They are characterised by ineffective haematopoiesis involving several cell lineages, and presenting with morphologically dysplastic cells, and often peripheral cytopenia. In older literature, they were termed as *preleukaemic syndromes*.

Classification Several classifications have been used up to now resulting finally in the 2016 WHO classification which is used all over the world **(Table 13.7)**.

Important features of this classification are as under:

i. WHO classification divides MDS into several groups, with some subgroups, relying on *three parameters*:
- Degree of dysplasia (involving 1, 2 or 3 lineages)
- Percentage of blasts
- Specific types and extent of cytopenia (involving 1, 2 or 3 lineages)

TABLE 13.7 Laboratory findings in categories of myelodysplastic syndrome (MDS) as per WHO classification (2016).

CATEGORY	DYSPLASTIC LINEAGES (1, 2 OR 3)	CYTOPENIA (1, 2 OR 3)	RINGSIDERO-BLASTS	BM AND PB BLASTS
1. MDS with single lineage dysplasia (MDS-SLD)	1	1 or 2	<15%	BM <5%, PB <1%, no Auer rods
2. MDS with multilineage dysplasia (MDS-MLD)	2 or 3	1–3	<15%	BM <5%, PB <1%, no Auer rods
3. MDS with ring sideroblasts (MDS-RS)				
MDS-RS with single lineage dysplasia (MDS-RS-SLD)	1	1 or 2	≥15%	BM <5%, PB <1%, no Auer rods
MDS-RS with multilineage dysplasia (MDS-RS-MLD)	2 or 3	1–3	≥15%	BM <5%, PB <1%, no Auer rods
MDS with isolated del(5q)	1–3	1–2	None or any	BM <5%, PB <1%, no Auer rods
4. MDS with excess blasts (MDS-EB)				
MDS-EB-1	0–3	1–3	None or any	BM 5%-9% or PB 2%-4%, no Auerrods
MDS-EB-2	0–3	1–3	None or any	BM 10%-19%, or PB 5%-19% , or Auer rods
5. Refractory cytopenia of childhood	1–3	1–3	None	BM <5%, PB <2%

(BM, bone marrow; PB, peripheral blood).
*Adapted from Arber et al: The 2016 revision to the WHO classification of myeloid neoplasms and acute leukaemia. Blood. 2016;127: 2391-405.

The threshold for diagnosing MDS is 10% of dysplastic cells involving any or all of the three cell lineages.

ii. *Cut-off for cytopenia* is defined for all three lineages as follows:
- Haemoglobin <10 g/ml for erythrocytes
- Platelet count of <100,000/μL
- Neutrophil count (absolute) <1,800/μL

iii. *Cytogenetic studies* are performed by conventional karyotyping:
- MDS defining abnormality is isolated del (5q).
- Aneuploidy is found in cases evolving into leukaemia.
- Genetic mutations are common, most often involving genes SE3B1 and TP53.
- Although most cases are sporadic, a category for familial cases and germ line mutations has been formed.

Clinicopathologic features MDS is found in the elderly past 6th decade of life.
Clinical features are nonspecific and the diagnosis is often made upon routine CBC examination. Symptoms and clinical findings include the following:

i. Anaemia
ii. Fever
iii. Weight loss
iv. Neutrophilic dermatoses (Sweet syndrome)
v. Splenomegaly (20%)

Laboratory findings Highly variable as presented in **Table 13.7**.

i. *Peripheral blood* Cytopenia with dysplasia involving 1, 2 or 3 lineages.
a. Anaemia, macrocytic or dimorphic.
b. Leucocyte counts normal but may be elevated.
- Dysplastic PMNs are hyposegmented and hypogranulated.
- Myeloblasts may be seen, correlating with bone marrow findings.
c. Thrombocytopenia with large agranular platelets.

ii. *Bone marrow* Variable cellularity (normal, hypo- or hypercellular)
a. *Erythroid cells*—dyserythropoiesis with abnormally appearing nuclei and ring sideroblasts. Megaloblasts may be seen.
b. *Myeloid series*—myeloid precursors have abnormal nuclei.
- Neutrophils are hypogranular and hyposegmented.
- Myeloblasts may be increased in some forms of MDS (e.g. MDS with excess blasts, MDS-EB-1 and MDS-EB2); these may progress to myeloid leukaemia.
- Blast are by definition below 20% in the bone marrow and peripheral blood, to distinguish these patients from those with AML who have more than 20% blasts.
c. *Megakaryocytes* reduced in number and have abnormal nuclei.

Therapy Not very efficient since MDS usually does not respond to treatment.
- Supportive therapy like in aplastic anaemia.
- Cytopenia may not respond to treatment and is the major cause of complication and death.
- Bone marrow transplantation offers cure sometimes and longer survival.

Prognosis depends on type of MDS.
- MDS with ring sideroblasts and 5q syndrome, may survive for years.
- MDS with excess blasts and severe cytopenia with monosomy-7 survive only a few months.

> **Chapter 13e Supplement: Online Content**
>
> *Digital content of this chapter available with this book is meant for enhanced learning and self-assessment. In addition, it contains 29 Multiple Choice Questions (MCQs), 05 Clinicopathologic Vignettes, and 05 Image-based Questions; these are followed by their answers along with explanatory notes of correct and incorrect answers.*

CHAPTER 14

Lymphoid Cells of Blood and Lymphoreticular Tissues

NORMAL LYMPH NODES AND REACTIVE LYMPHADENITIS

Q1. What are the main anatomic and histologic parts of a lymph node which are important for understanding diseases of this organ?

- Lymph node is composed predominantly of lymphoid tissue which is arranged into several components, comprising the outer part of *cortex*, and the inner part called *medulla* (**Fig. 14.1**).
- The cortex contain several aggregates of lymphoid tissue called *lymphoid follicles* composed of B-cell.
- The central paler zone of the follicle is called *germinal centre*, which is surrounded by a darker zone called the mantle zone.
- The deeper zone of the cortex is called *paracortex* composed of T cells.
- Paracortex separates follicles one from another and also the cortex from the medulla.
- Medulla is composed of cords of plasma cells and some lymphocytes.
- The lymph node has an external capsule, underneath which there is a subcapsular sinus.
- On the convexity of the lymph nodes, these sinuses are connected with afferent lymphatics.
- In the hilum, the sinuses drain into the efferent lymphatics.
- The hilum also contains an artery and a vein.

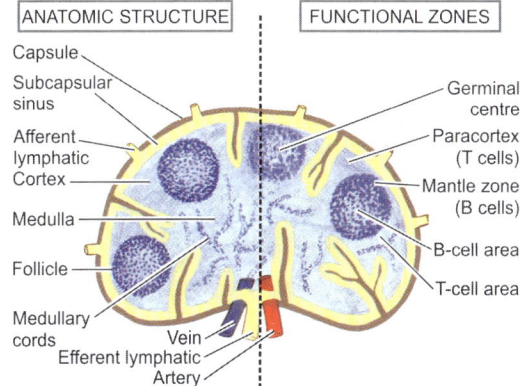

FIGURE 14.1: The anatomic structure and functional zones of a normal lymph node.

Q2. What are the most common causes of lymph node enlargement?

The most common causes of lymph node enlargement are:
i. Infections resulting **lymphadenitis**.
ii. Immune reactions, causing **lymphadenopathy**.
iii. **Other causes** of lymph node enlargement are:
a. Drug reactions
b. Environmental pollutants
c. Necrotic tissue debris draining to the lymph nodes after tissue injury
d. Malignant neoplasms, including lymphomas and metastatic tumour deposits.

Q3. What is acute nonspecific lymphadenitis? Briefly discuss its etiology and pathologic features.

Definition Acute lymphadenitis is an acute infection of the lymph node. Since the causative pathogen is usually not identified bacteriologically, it is called nonspecific.

Etiology Bacterial and viral infections of tissues draining the lymph into the corresponding lymph nodes are the most common cause of acute lymphadenitis. It is usually mild and transient and heals without consequences. Anatomically, these organisms belong to several groups:

i. *Cervical lymphadenitis*—due to the infections of the oral cavity.
ii. *Axillary lymphadenitis*—due to infection of the arm or breast.
iii. *Inguinal lymphadenopathy*—due to the infection of lower extremities or genital organs.
iv. *Mesenteric lymphadenopathy*—due to infections of abdominal organs, e.g. acute enteritis or acute appendicitis.

Pathology *Grossly*, the affected lymph nodes are enlarged and soft. If the infection is massive, the lymph nodes may contain abscesses, which are visible on cross section.

Microscopy
i. Congested sinuses containing neutrophils.
ii. Suppuration with necrosis in severe cases, associated with microabscess formation.
iii. Lymphoid follicles enlarged and contain numerous mitotic figures and macrophages containing phagocytosed material in their cytoplasm.

Q4. Define chronic nonspecific lymphadenitis. Discuss its etiology, types and their clinicopathologic features.

Definition Chronic nonspecific lymphadenitis, also known as lymphoid hyperplasia, is a reaction of draining lymph nodes to a local inflammation, or a response to antigenic stimuli arising in such an inflammation.

Etiology Common causes include:
i. Repeated attacks of acute lymphadenitis
ii. Chronic infection
iii. A reaction to malignant tumours

Types and clinicopathologic features Three microscopic pattern are recognised:

I. **Follicular hyperplasia** is the most common change, especially in children.

Etiology
i. Nonspecific infection or stimulation is the most common cause.
ii. Chronic autoimmune diseases such as rheumatoid arthritis.
iii. Infections with identifiable pathogens including toxoplasmosis, syphilis, or chronic viral infections such as AIDS.
iv. *Diseases of unknown etiology*: For example *angiofollicular lymphoid hyperplasia* (Castleman disease), a well-defined pathologic entity of unknown pathogenesis, probably caused by Epstein-Barr virus.

Microscopy
i. The most prominent change is the enlargement of follicles.
ii. Expansion of germinal centre of follicles due to proliferation of B lymphocytes and increased number of macrophages.
iii. Parafollicular areas are also expanded and contain plasma cells, macrophages, neutrophils and eosinophils.
iv. Lymphatic sinuses lined by enlarged mononuclear cells are expanded and contain inflammatory cells.

II. **Paracortical lymphoid hyperplasia** results from a hyperplastic response of T cells.

Etiology
i. Immune reactions to defined antigens such as drugs or vaccination.
ii. Viral infections (e.g. infectious mononucleosis).
iii. Autoimmune diseases.
iv. *Dermatopathic lymphadenopathy* in areas draining various skin lesions. Melanin, released from damaged melanocytes is seen in macrophages.

v. *Diseases of unknown etiology*: For example, *angioimmunoblastic lymphadenopathy*, a defined pathologic lesion, developing in elderly with hypergammaglobulinaemia.
Microscopy
i. Expansion of paracortical zones impinging upon germinal centres.
ii. Paracortical zones contain numerous stimulated T cells (immunoblasts).
iii. Increased number of macrophages in sinuses.
III. **Sinus histiocytosis**, also known as sinus hyperplasia.
Etiology
i. Most often in lymph nodes draining malignant tumours.
ii. *Diseases of unknown etiology:* as in *sinus histiocytosis with massive lymphadenopathy*. This well-defined clinicopathologic entity of unknown etiology affects adolescents presenting as neck lymphadenopathy, with fever and leucocytosis but has a self-limiting course.
Microscopy
Dilated sinuses are filled with macrophages, which often contain phagocytosed material, such as pigment, bacteria or lipid droplets.

PATHOLOGY OF THE SPLEEN

Q5. What are the main anatomic and histologic and physiologic features of the normal spleen relevant to understanding of its pathology?

Anatomy
- Spleen is the largest lymphoid organ.
- It normally weighs about 150 g in the adults.
- It is located in the left upper abdominal quadrant, covered by the 9th, 10th and 11th rib.
- Externally, the spleen is covered with a layer of peritoneum and a fibrous capsule.

Histology
i. The connective tissue extends from the capsule into the parenchyma of the spleen in form of fibrous trabeculae providing structural support to other splenic cells.
ii. On cross section, the splenic parenchyma comprises two components:
- *Red pulp* composed of venous sinuses and adjacent spaces filled with blood, macrophages and lymphocytes, forming the so called Billroth cords.
- *White pulp* (Malpighian bodies) forming grey-white nodules composed of lymphoid cells.

Physiology The spleen performs the following four functions:
i. *Immune function*.
ii. *Storage and sequestration of blood cells*, including RBCs, leucocytes, and platelets. Spleen is the major organ for the removal of effete or damaged blood cells.
iii. *Regulating of the portal blood flow*.
iv. *Extramedullary haematopoiesis*, as reserve site for the production of blood cells when the bone marrow production fails.

Q6. Define splenomegaly. What are its most common causes?

Definition Splenomegaly is enlargement of the spleen due to increased cellularity or vascularity of splenic parenchyma.

Etiology Spleen is rarely the primary site of disease and thus splenomegaly is usually either part of a systemic multiorgan disease or it is involved secondarily. Splenomegaly may develop through several pathogenetic mechanisms as under:
I. Infections
II. Disorders of immunoregulation
III. Altered splenic blood flow
IV. Haematolymphoid neoplasia
V. Diseases with abnormal erythrocytes
VI. Metabolic storage diseases
VII. Miscellaneous diseases of unknown etiology

A detailed list of diseases and conditions causing splenomegaly is given in **Table 14.1**.

Q7. Describe the clinicopathologic features of splenomegaly.

Clinical features Splenomegaly can be classified as i) mild, ii) moderate, and iii) severe.

I. **Mild splenomegaly** (up to 5 cm in largest diameter) may be caused by:
i. Congestive heart failure
ii. Thalassaemia minor
iii. Certain infections such as typhoid fever, malaria
iv. Autoimmune diseases such as rheumatoid arthritis, SLE

II. **Moderate splenomegaly** (extending up to the umbilicus):
i. Cirrhosis and chronic hepatitis
ii. Infectious mononucleosis
iii. Haemolytic anaemia (e.g. sphaerocytosis)
iv. Lymphoma
v. Splenic abscess
vi. Amyloidosis

III. **Massive splenomegaly** (extending below umbilicus):
i. Chronic myeloid leukaemia
ii. Myelofibrosis
iii. Thalassaemia major
iv. Storage diseases (e.g. Gaucher disease)
v. Chronic malaria
vi. Leishmaniasis
vii. Portal vein obstruction

Pathology *Grossly,* the enlarged spleen is heavy and firm.
i. The capsule is tense and thickened.
ii. On sectioning, the organ is firm.
iii. Trabeculae are prominent and widened.

Microscopy Features of *fibrocongestive splenomegaly* **(Fig. 14.2)**.
i. Sinuses dilated, fibrotic.
ii. Trabeculae prominent and appear thickened.
iii. Foci of haemorrhage which in foci of fibrosis form Gamna-Gandy bodies.

TABLE 14.1 Causes of splenomegaly.

I. INFECTIONS
1. Malaria
2. Leishmaniasis
3. Typhoid
4. Infectious mononucleosis
5. Bacterial septicaemia
6. Bacterial endocarditis
7. Tuberculosis
8. Syphilis
9. Viral hepatitis
10. AIDS

II. DISORDERS OF IMMUNOREGULATION
1. Rheumatoid arthritis
2. SLE
3. Immune haemolytic anaemias
4. Immune thrombocytopenias
5. Immune neutropenias

III. ALTERED SPLENIC BLOOD FLOW
1. Cirrhosis of liver
2. Portal vein obstruction
3. Splenic vein obstruction
4. Congestive heart failure

IV. HAEMATOLYMHPOID MALIGNANCIES
1. Hodgkin disease
2. Non-Hodgkin lymphomas
3. Multiple myeloma
4. Leukaemias
5. Myeloproliferative neoplasms (e.g. CML, polycythaemia vera, primary myelofibrosis)

V. DISEASES WITH ABNORMAL ERYTHROCYTES
1. Thalassaemias
2. Spherocytosis
3. Sickle cell disease
4. Ovalocytosis

VI. STORAGE DISEASES
1. Gaucher disease
2. Niemann-Pick disease

VII. MISCELLANEOUS
1. Amyloidosis
2. Primary and metastatic splenic tumours
3. Idiopathic splenomegaly

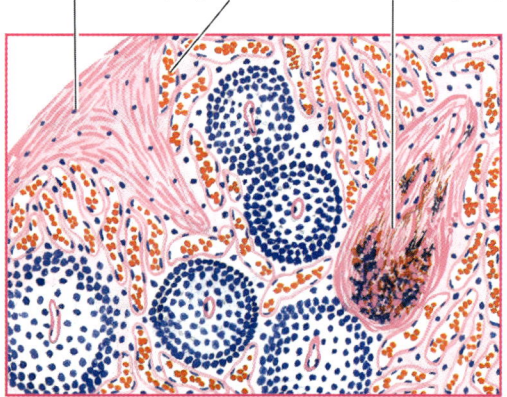

Thickened capsule   Congested sinusoids   Gamna-Gandy body

FIGURE 14.2: CVC spleen. The sinuses are dilated and congested. There is increased fibrosis in the red pulp, capsule and the trabeculae. A Gamna-Gandy body is also seen.

Q8. What is hypersplenism? What are its features?

Definition Hypersplenism denotes conditions which cause excessive removal of erythrocytes, granulocytes or platelets from the circulation. This can be achieved by increased sequestration of cells in the spleen by altered splenic blood flow, or by production of antibodies against some blood cells.

Criteria for the diagnosis of hypersplenism are as follows:
i. Splenomegaly.
ii. Splenic destruction of one or more of the blood cell types causing anaemia, leucopenia, thrombocytopenia, or pancytopenia.
iii. Cellularity of the bone marrow is normal or hyperplastic.
iv. Splenectomy is followed by improvement of cytopenia.

Q9. What are the consequences of splenectomy?

Splenectomy is followed by changes in peripheral blood as follows:
I. **Red blood cells** Abnormal RBC forms appear in circulation because there is no spleen to remove them from circulation.
i. Abnormal RBCs include target cells, RBCs with Howell-Jolly inclusions.
ii. Osmotic fragility test shows increased resistance to haemolysis.
iii. Normoblasts may appear in peripheral blood.
II. **White blood cells** Numbers and morphology changes.
i. Leucocytosis, reaching a peak in 1–2 days after splenectomy.
ii. There is a shift-to-the-left of neutrophils.
iii. Myeloid precursors such as myelocytes may appear in blood.
III. **Platelets** Their number increases 3–4 times over normal within hours after splenectomy.
NOTE: Splenectomy may be used in the treatment of some diseases to reduce splenic sequestration and clearing, as under:
- Hereditary spherocytosis
- Immune haemolytic anaemia
- Thrombocytopenia

Q10. What are the possible causes and consequences of splenic rupture?

Etiology Splenic rupture can be traumatic or nontraumatic (spontaneous).
i. *Blunt trauma* is the most common cause of splenic rupture of laceration.
ii. *Non-traumatic (spontaneous) rupture* involves only enlarged spleen and never affects spleen of normal size. Conditions predisposing to spontaneous rupture are as follows:
a. Acute splenic tumour due to acute infection (enlarging the spleen 2–3 times it normal size). EXAMPLES: Pneumonia, septicaemia, acute endocarditis, infectious mononucleosis.
b. Splenomegaly in chronic diseases. EXAMPLES: Malaria, thalassemia, leukaemia.

Q11. What are the most important splenic neoplasms?

Splenic neoplasms are classified as primary, or secondary.
I. **Primary splenic tumours** are extremely rare.
i. *Benign splenic tumours* are rare: EXAMPLES: Hemangioma and lymphangioma.
ii. *Malignant splenic tumours* include the two types of neoplasms:
- Haematolymphoid tumours originating in the spleen, such as Hodgkin disease, non-Hodgkin lymphoma and leukaemia.
- Angiosarcoma of the spleen.

II. **Secondary splenic tumours** include metastases of solid cancers in other organs or systemic spread lymphoma/leukaemia which may include splenic involvement.
Metastases may reach the spleen through several routes including:
- haematogenous route (e.g. lung and breast cancer),
- by transcoelomic spread (e.g. ovarian cancer), or
- by direct local extension (e.g. pancreatic cancer).

Involvement of the spleen usually occurs in advanced stages of neoplastic dissemination and it is rare in early stages of neoplastic disease.

THYMUS

Q12. Describe in brief normal structure of thymus.

Definition Thymus is a complex lymphoreticular organ located in the anterior mediastinum. It is involved in nurturing and maturation of T-lymphocytes. Thymus also secretes polypeptide hormones, thymopoietin and thymosin-α, which regulate the proliferation and maturation of T-lymphocytes.

Anatomy and histology
- At birth, it is a relatively large organ and continues to grow till puberty, after which it slowly undergoes involution.
- Thymus is a *bilobed* organ subdivided into numerous lobules by fibrous strands extending into the parenchyma from an external fibrous capsule.
- Each lobule has two parts, an *outer cortex* and an *inner medulla*, both of which are composed of epithelial cells and lymphocytes.
- In the medulla, there are Hassall corpuscles composed of keratinised centre, surrounded by concentric layers of epithelial cells.
- Cortical part of the lobules is composed predominantly of immature lymphocytes which move to the medulla to mature.

Q13. What are the most important non-neoplastic pathologic lesions of the thymus?

I. **Developmental lesions** *Thymic agenesis* and *hypoplasia* are the most important developmental lesions. They occur in various forms of congenital immunodeficiency such as DiGeorge syndrome, severe combined immunodeficiency, and reticular dysgenesis.

II. **Acquired thymic atrophy (involution)** occurs mostly in neonates and children due to severe stress.
- Most common causes, especially in underdeveloped countries, are severe infections or malnutrition.
- It may be related to treatment with corticosteroids, cytotoxic drugs and irradiation.

III. **Thymic hyperplasia** is characterised by an appearance of lymphoid follicles in the medulla, which accounts for the alternative designation *thymic follicular hyperplasia*.
- Most often, it is found in persons suffering from myasthenia gravis.
- Other diseases associated with thymic hyperplasia are: Addison disease, Graves disease and systemic autoimmune diseases such as SLE, rheumatoid arthritis and scleroderma.

Q14. What are the most important thymic tumours? Discuss clinicopathologic features of the most common thymic tumour.

- Tumours of the thymus are rare. They may be classified as primary or secondary.
- Primary thymic tumours originating from thymic epithelial cells are called thymomas.
- Non-Hodgkin lymphomas and Hodgkin disease may originate in the thymus, or involve the thymus during systemic dissemination of the disease.
- Hilar lung carcinomas may extend into the thymus.

Thymomas are rare tumours (incidence is 1:750,000) originating from the thymic epithelial cells.

Pathology *Clinically and grossly*, a mass in the antero-superior part of the mediastinum, usually well delimited from adjacent tissues.

Microscopy Thymomas are classified into four subtypes and labeled A, B, AB and C according to the appearance of epithelial tumour cells and the extent of the lymphoid cell infiltration into the adjacent tissue.

i. Most thymomas (65%) are *benign*, but some recur if not completely removed.
ii. In a minority of cases, tumours are obviously malignant and are thus rightfully called *thymic carcinomas*.

Clinical features Most patients are adults.
i. In about half the cases, the tumour is asymptomatic and is discovered accidentally during routine X-rays of the chest.
ii. Symptomatic tumours cause local compression or systemic disorders.

iii. Thymomas are often associated with paraneoplastic syndromes, the most common of which is myasthenia gravis.
iv. Other diseases that may be associated with thymoma are hypogammaglobulinaemia, pure red cell aplasia, peripheral T-cell leukaemia/lymphoma, and several autoimmune diseases.
v. An increased incidence of other malignant tumours has been noted in thymoma patients.

LYMPHOID AND HISTIOCYTIC NEOPLASMS

Q15. What are the broad principles of current classifications of lymphoid neoplasms?

Key features
- Lymphoid neoplasms are grouped together with haematopoietic and histiocytic neoplasms into a unified single category of malignant disorders presenting either as *leukaemia,* or as *lymphoma,* which form solid masses in lymph nodes or infiltrate internal organs and skin.
- The diagnosis of lymphomas can be reliably made only on *lymph node or internal organ biopsy.*
- Initial diagnosis of leukaemia can be made by examining the *peripheral blood,* but it must be confirmed and further elaborated by studies of *bone marrow biopsies.*
- The extent of disease for planning of therapy is done according to the Ann Arbor *staging system* for NHL and Hodgkin lymphoma. Staging is done on the basis of imaging studies including CT and PET and gallium scanning.
- Lymphoid neoplasms may be classified according to *several classifications*, most of which are of historical interest only.
- The latest WHO classification proposed by the international experts (2016), and incorporating the principles of previous REAL classification (*Revised European American classification of Lymphomas*), is currently the most widely used clinicopathologic classification.
- According to *REAL classification,* 80% of all lymphomas are of B-cell origin and 20% of T-cell origin. Leukaemias in 90% cases are of B-cell origin and 10% of T-cell origin. These two groups can be further subdivided clinically into indolent and aggressive forms of lymphoma.
- The WHO (2016) classification is based on clinical and pathologic findings and additional characterisation of neoplastic cells by modern techniques of *immunophenotyping, cytogenetics, and molecular biology.*

According to WHO (2016) classification, lymphoid and histiocytic neoplasms are divided into five major groups as follows **(Table 14.2)**:
I. Precursor lymphoid neoplasms
II. Mature lymphoid, histiocytic and dendritic cells neoplasms
III. Hodgkin lymphomas
IV. Post-transplant lymphoproliferative disorders
V. Histiocytic and dendritic cell neoplasms

Q16. What is the incidence of various forms of lymphoid malignancies?

Five major forms of lymphoid malignancies and their relative frequency is as under:
i. Non-Hodgkin lymphoma = 62% (most common lymphoma)
ii. Hodgkin lymphoma = 8%
iii. Plasma cell disorders = 16%
iv. Chronic lymphocytic leukaemia = 9% (most common lymphoid leukaemia)
v. Acute lymphoblastic leukaemia = 5%

Relative frequency (in descending order) of common NHLs is shown here as follows:
i. Diffuse large B cell lymphoma (*most common NHL*)
ii. Follicular lymphoma (*second most common*)
iii. MALT lymphoma
iv. Small lymphocytic lymphoma
v. Mantle cell lymphoma
vi. Mediastinal large B cell lymphoma
vii. Anaplastic large cell lymphoma
viii. Burkitt lymphoma
ix. Others

TABLE 14.2 Revised WHO classification of lymphoid and histiocytic neoplasms (2016)*.

A. PRECURSOR LYMPHOID NEOPLASMS
  I. *B-lymphoblastic leukaemia/lymphoma, not otherwise specified*
  B-lymphoblastic leukaemia/lymphoma, with recurrent genetic abnormalities (with translocations, hypoploidy, hyperploidy)
  II. *T-lymphoblastic leukaemia/lymphoma*
  III. *NK-lymphoblastic leukaemia/lymphoma*

B. MATURE LYMPHOID, HISTIOCYTIC AND DENDRITIC CELL NEOPLASMS*

I. Mature B-cell neoplasms
1. Chronic lymphocytic leukaemia/small lymphocytic lymphoma (B-CLL/SLL)
2. Monoclonal B-cell lymphocytosis
3. B-cell prolymphocytic leukaemia
4. Splenic marginal zone lymphoma
5. Hairy cell leukaemia and variant
6. Lymphoplasmacytic lymphoma
7. Monoclonal gammopathy of undetermined significance (MGUS)
8. Heavy chain diseases (α,γ,μ)
9. Plasma cell myeloma and plasmacytoma
10. Extranodal marginal zone lymphoma of mucosa-associated lymphoid tissue (MALT lymphoma)
11. Nodal marginal zone lymphoma
12. Follicular lymphoma (and its subtypes)
13. Primary cutaneous follicle centre lymphoma
14. Mantle cell lymphoma
15. Diffuse large B-cell lymphoma (DLBCL) (and its subtypes)
16. T-cell/histiocyte rich large B-cell lymphoma
17. Primary mediastinal (thymic) large B-cell lymphoma
18. Intravascular and ALK-positive large B-cell lymphoma
19. Plasmablastic lymphoma
20. Primary effusion lymphoma
21. Burkitt lymphoma/leukaemia (and its subtypes)
22. High-grade B-cell lymphoma

II. Mature T and NK-cell neoplasms
1. T-cell prolymphocytic leukaemia
2. T-cell large granular lymphocytic leukaemia
3. Aggressive NK-cell leukaemia
4. Systemic EBV-positive T-cell lymphoma of childhood
5. Adult T-cell leukaemia/lymphoma
6. Extranodal NK/T-cell lymphoma, nasal type
7. Enteropathy-associated T-cell lymphoma
8. Hepatosplenic T-cell lymphoma
9. Mycosis fungoides/Sézary syndrome
10. Primary cutaneous T-cell lymphoproliferative disorders
11. Peripheral T-cell lymphoma, NOS
12. Angioimmunoblastic T-cell lymphoma
13. Anaplastic large cell lymphoma (ALCL), ALK-positive and ALK-negative

III. Hodgkin lymphoma (HL)
Nodular lymphocytic predominant HL
Classic HL
1. Nodular sclerosis classical HL
2. Lymphocytic-rich classical HL
3. Mixed cellularity classical HL
4. Lymphocytic depleted classical HL

IV. Post-transplant lymphoproliferative disorders (PTLD)
1. Plasmacytoid PTLD
2. Infectious mononucleosis PTLD
3. Classical Hodgkin lymphoma PTLD

V. Histiocytic and dendritic cell neoplasms
1. Histiocytic sarcoma
2. Langerhans cell histiocytosis
3. Langerhans cell sarcoma
4. Dendritic cell sarcoma, interdigitating and follicular variants

*Swerdlow et al. The 2016 revision of the WHO classification of lymphoid neoplasms. Blood. 2016;127:2375-90.

Q17. Discuss the main features of acute lymphoblastic leukaemia/lymphoma.

Definition Acute lymphoblastic leukaemia/lymphoma (ALL/LBL) is a malignancy of lymphoid precursor cells, i.e. precursors of B, T and NK cells.

Incidence ALL is the most common cancer of children under 6 years of age.

i. ALL is the second most common acute leukaemia in adults, accounting for 25% of all acute leukaemias in adults (AML = 75%).

ii. *The incidence of subtypes varies according to the age group* as follows:
- In children (under 6 years of age) = 75% cases B-ALL, 15% T-ALL, 10% B-LBL.
- In young adults (under 18 years of age) = 90% T-LBL, 10% B-LBL

Clinical features

I. *B-ALL/LBL* presents most often as leukaemia in children or as lymphoma in young adults, that rapidly transforms into leukaemia.

i. Leukaemia includes nodal and extranodal involvement, most often resulting in hepatosplenomegaly.

ii. Other organs may be involved also including CNS, testis and skin.

iii. Cytopenia with infections is common.

II. *T-ALL/LBL* is more aggressive than B-ALL/LBL.

i. T-cell origin accounts for common involvement of thymus followed by pleural effusion.

ii. Bone marrow involvement and leukaemia are common early events, resulting in pancytopenia, infections and bleeding.

iii. Lymphadenopathy, hepatosplenomegaly and CNS infiltrates are common.

Haematologic findings Essential for diagnosis of leukaemia are:

i. *Peripheral blood* shows anaemia, thrombocytopenia and leucocytosis with reduced number of normal myeloid cells. Lymphoblasts (>20%) and small prolymphocytes predominate **(Fig. 14.3)**.

ii. *Bone marrow* contains 20–95% lymphoblasts. Megakaryocytes are reduced in number or absent.

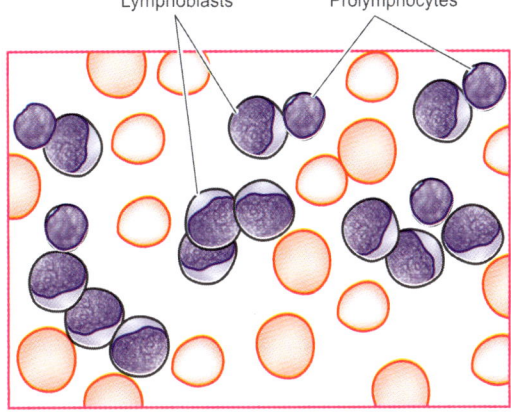

FIGURE 14.3: PBF findings in acute lymphoblastic leukaemia (ALL). The cells are large, with round to convoluted nuclei having high N/C ratio and no cytoplasmic granularity.

Immunophenotyping Terminal deoxynucleotidyl transferase (TdT) is expressed on both B and T-cell precursors.
- B-ALL/LBL has B cell markers (CD19, CD10, CD9a)
- T-ALL/LBL has T cell markers (CD1, CD2, CD3, CD5, CD7)

Cytogenetic prognostic markers have been identified as follows:

B-ALL/LBL
- *Unfavorable prognosis* if containing Philadelphia chromosome with t(9;22), but also t(4;11), t(1;19) and hypodiploidy (<50%).
- *Favorable prognosis* if containing t(12;21) or hyperdiploidy (>50%).

T-ALL/LBL is generally more aggressive than their B cell counterparts.
- *Unfavourable prognosis* with deletion of CDKN2A/B, 6q15 and PTEN.
- *Favourable outcome* with t(10;14), and mutations of NOTCH1, FBXW7 and JAK1.

Clinical features

i. ALL presents with clinical signs of malignant lymphoid cell infiltration of lymph nodes (lymphadenopathy) and involvement of extranodal sites such as mediastinum, liver and spleen (hepatosplenomegaly).

ii. Involvement of testicles, CNS and subcutaneous tissue is common. CNS involvement is usually a prognostically adverse finding.

iii. Bone marrow infiltration is accompanied by signs of bone marrow failure including anaemia, leucopenia and thrombocytopenia. Bleeding disorders and infections are therefore common.

Therapy is based on multi-drug treatment.
i. Overall prognosis is better in children than in adults.
ii. Median survival in adults is only 12–18 months.
iii. Chemotherapy will induce remission in 90% of children.
iv. Bone marrow transplantation after chemotherapy results in complete cure in 50% children.
v. Children suffering from T-ALL/LBL and CNS involvement have a less favourable prognosis. CNS prophylaxis improves prognosis.
vi. Children and adults with limited disease confined to lymph nodes have a better prognosis than those with systemic disease.

Q18. Tabulate the contrasting features of acute myeloblastic (AML) and acute lymphoblastic leukaemia (ALL).

The salient differences between two main forms of acute leukaemia (AML and ALL) are summarised in **Table 14.3**.

TABLE 14.3 Contrasting features of AML and ALL.

FEATURE	AML	ALL
1. Common age	Adults between 15–40 years; comprise 20% of childhood leukaemias	Children under 15 years; comprise 80% of childhood leukaemias
2. Physical findings		
i. Splenomegaly	Less common	Marked
ii. Hepatomegaly	Less common	Prominent
iii. Lymphadenopathy	Less prominent	Prominent
iv. Bony tenderness	Present	Present
v. Gum hypertrophy	Present	Absent
vi. CNS involvement	Infrequent	Common
vii. Bleeding tendencies	Common	Less common
3. Laboratory findings	➢ Low-to-high TLC ➢ Predominance of myeloblasts and promyelocytes in blood and bone marrow ➢ Thrombocytopenia moderate to severe.	➢ Low-to-high TLC ➢ Predominance of lymphoblasts in blood and bone marrow ➢ Thrombocytopenia moderate to severe.
4. Diagnostic criteria	➢ FAB types M0-M7 ➢ WHO criteria = >20% blasts	➢ FAB types L1-L3, WHO types B-ALL/LBL (85%), T-ALL/LBL (15%) ➢ WHO criteria = >20% blasts
5. Cytochemical stains	Myeloperoxidase +, Sudan black +, NSE + in M4 and M5, acid phosphatase (diffuse) + in M4 and M5	PAS +, acid phosphatase (focal) +
6. Specific therapy	Cytosine arabinoside, anthracyclines (daunorubicin, adriamycin) and 6-thioguanine	Vincristine, prednisolone, anthracyclines and L-asparaginase
7. Immunophenotyping	CD13, 33, 41, 42	Both B and T cell ALL TdT +ve Pre B: CD19, 20 Pre T: CD1, 2, 3, 5, 7
8. Common cytogenetic abnormalities	M3: t(15;17) M4: in(16)	B-ALL/B-LBL: t(9;21) T-ALL/LBL: 14q11
9. Response to therapy	Remission rate low, duration of remission shorter	Remission rate high, duration of remission prolonged
10. Median survival	12–18 months	Children without CNS prophylaxis 33 months, with CNS prophylaxis 60 months; adults 12–18 months

Q19. Briefly discuss features of chronic lymphocytic leukaemia/small lymphocytic lymphoma.

Definition Chronic lymphocytic leukaemia/small lymphocytic lymphoma (CLL/SLL) is a clonal disease involving mature B lymphocytes, presenting either as leukaemia or lymphoma.

Incidence CLL is the most common form of leukaemia, whereas SLL accounts for 7% of all NHL. It affects people over 50 years of age, males > females = 2:1.

Clinical features Insidious onset with indolent course and no significant symptomatology.
i. Anaemia
ii. Lymph node enlargement without confluence or tenderness.
iii. Splenomegaly and hepatomegaly common.
iv. Susceptibility to infections and a bleeding tendency may be evident in later stages.
v. Less common findings related to infiltrates of organs such as eyes, CNS, mediastinum, joints.

Haematologic findings
i. Lymphocytosis (50,000 to 200,000/μL). Small, round, mature lymphocytes account for 90% of all cells **(Fig. 14.4)**.
ii. Mild anaemia which may also include Coombs-positive autoimmune haemolytic anaemia found in 20% cases.
iii. Neutropenia but only in late stages of disease.
iv. Platelets normal.

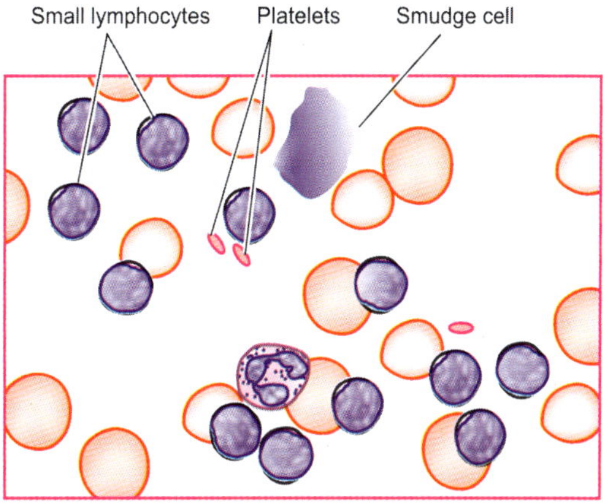

FIGURE 14.4: PBF in chronic lymphocytic leukaemia (CLL). There is large excess of mature and small differentiated lymphocytes and some degenerated forms appearing as bare smudged nuclei.

Lymph node biopsy
i. Architecture effaced due to infiltration of entire lymph node with mature small lymphocytes **(Fig. 14.5, B)**.
ii. Lymphocytes positive for B cell markers (CD5, CD19, CD20, CD23), and monoclonal (kappa or lambda chain positive).
iii. In some patients, the disease may transform into more aggressive lymphoma or macroglobulinaemia.

Treatment Palliative since the disease cannot be eradicated to induce remission.

Prognosis
- Good prognosis of pure CLL presenting with peripheral blood lymphocytosis and no other symptoms. The median asymptomatic survival is approximately 10 years.
- Lymph node involvement, less favourable outcome (~5 years).
- Severe anaemia and thrombocytopenia indicative of bone marrow involvement carries the worst prognosis (<2 years).

Q20. What is follicular lymphoma?

Definition Follicular lymphoma is a slow-growing chronic clonal neoplastic disease of B-lymphocytes expressing BCL2, an antiapoptotic protein.

Clinicopathologic features Follicular lymphoma affects older persons accounting for 22% of all lymphomas.
i. Lymph node architecture is effaced and replaced by small, cleaved or large cleaved lymphocytes, forming follicles with germinal centres and infiltrating the capsule **(Fig. 14.5, C)**.

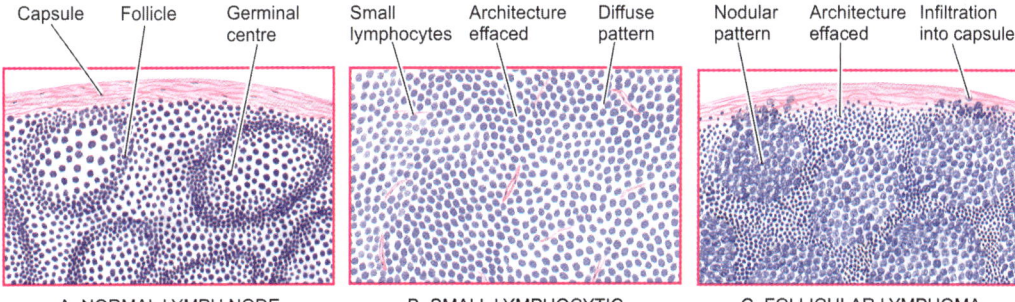

FIGURE 14.5: Prototypes of non-Hodgkin lymphoma—small lymphocytic lymphoma SLL/CLL (B) and follicular lymphoma (C) contrasted with structure of normal lymph node (A).

ii. Extranodal involvement is uncommon.
iii. Approximately 50% of all follicular lymphomas transform into a more aggressive diffuse large B-cell lymphoma.
iv. Median survival is 7–9 years.

Q21. Discuss salient features of diffuse large B-cell lymphoma.

Definition Diffuse large B-cell lymphoma (DLBCL) is a rapidly proliferating clonal B-cell neoplasm infiltrating diffusely lymph nodes and extranodal sites.
- It is the most common form of lymphoma, accounting for 31% of all lymphomas.
- In a significant number of cases, it evolves from preexisting follicular lymphoma.

Clinicopathologic features DLBCL affects older persons and the median age at the time of diagnosis is 60 years.
i. The tumour is composed of large cleaved B cells infiltrating lymph nodes in a diffuse manner.
ii. In about 50% of cases, DLBCL also involves extranodal sites, most often affecting the bone marrow and the gastrointestinal tract.
iii. Primary extranodal presentation may also occur including primary CNS lymphoma.
iv. Immunophenotypically, the neoplastic cells express B-cell markers (CD19, CD20) and BCL-2, and shows kappa or lambda chain monoclonality like follicular lymphoma.
v. *Subtypes* of DLBCL are as follows:
a. Epstein-Barr virus infection related to DLBCL *in immunosuppressed persons*.
b. Human herpes virus type 8 (HHV-8) combined with immunosuppression related to *primary effusion lymphoma*.
c. *Mediastinal large B-cell lymphoma* of young women that spreads to CNS and abdominal viscera.

Q22. Define Burkitt lymphoma. What are its main features?

Definition Burkitt lymphoma is a malignancy of very rapidly dividing B-cell caused by overexpression and dysregulation of translocated *MYC* gene.

Pathogenesis Burkitt lymphoma develops most often after *MYC* gene translocation from its normal location on chromosome 8 to chromosome 14.
- Translocation t(8;14) leads to the juxtaposition of this oncogene to the *IgH* gene, resulting in overproduction of *MYC transcription factor,* a protein which has a transforming capacity.
- A less common translocation of *MYC* gene to chromosomes that carries the genes for kappa or lambda chains results in the same overproduction of MYC protein.
- In most endemic cases and up to 20% of sporadic cases, the lymphoma cells are latently infected with *EBV.*

Classification Three forms of Burkitt lymphoma are recognised:
I. **Endemic Burkitt lymphoma** (also called 'African variant') affects the bone marrow of children and young adults living in malaria-infested equatorial Africa.
i. Almost all patients are latently infected with Epstein-Barr virus.
ii. Clinically the disease presents as a mandibular or maxillary mass.
iii. If not treated, it will spread to the marrow of other bones and internal organs.
II. **Sporadic Burkitt lymphoma** affects children and young adults living outside of malaria-infested tropical countries.
i. Only 20% of patients are latently infected with EBV.
ii. The disease involves most often internal organs, such as the ileocecal region, retroperitoneum and ovaries.
iii. Sporadic Burkitt lymphoma accounts for approximately 30% of childhood lymphomas in children in the US and Europe.
III. **Immunodeficiency-associated Burkitt lymphoma** occurs predominantly in HIV infected persons.
i. It could be one of the manifestations of AIDS.
ii. Rarely it can occur in post-transplant patients taking immunosuppressive drugs.
iii. About 30% of individuals with the immunodeficiency variant are infected with EBV.

Clinicopathologic features Burkitt lymphoma infiltrates are composed of uniform, noncleaved cells of intermediate size.

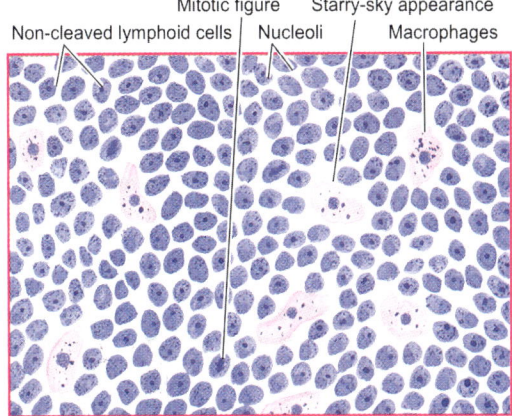

FIGURE 14.6: Burkitt lymphoma. The tumour shows uniform cells having high mitotic rate. Scattered among the tumour cells are benign macrophages surrounded by a clear space giving 'starry sky' appearance.

i. Nuclei contain 2–5 nucleoli and are surrounded by scant cytoplasm that may contain lipid droplets.
ii. Mitoses and apoptotic bodies are numerous.
iii. Scattered among the lymphoma cells are macrophages containing phagocytosed cell fragments. These macrophages are surrounded by a clear space that imports the tumour a *'stary-sky' appearance* (Fig. 14.6).
iv. *Immunohistochemistry* Positive for markers of proliferating germinal centre B cells.
a. B-cell markers: CD20 and surface IgM
b. Germinal centre B cells: CD10 and BCL6.
c. Cell proliferation markers: MIB-1 (Ki-67). It is positive in 95–100% cells, confirming their high mitotic rate.
Therapy Prompt aggressive chemotherapy can cure most of the cases.

Q23. Discuss key features of extranodal marginal zone B-cell lymphoma (MALToma).

Definition Extranodal marginal zone B-cell lymphoma (also known as *MALToma)* is an extranodal type of B-cell lymphoma originating in the mucosa-associated lymphoid tissue (MALT).
Etiopathogenesis MALTomas occur in tissues involved by *chronic inflammation* which stimulates and then maintains the monoclonal proliferation of small B lymphocytes.
- *Gastric MALTomas* are associated with *Helicobacter pylori* infection. About 50% of gastric MALTomas have a translocation t(11,18). Eradication of *H. pylori* infection may lead to regression of MALToma.
- *Salivary glands MALTomas* may develop in context of Sjögren disease or chronic sialadenitis with lymphoepithelial lesions.
- *Thyroid MALToma* may result as a complication of Hashimoto lymphocytic thyroiditis.

Clinicopathologic features MALTomas comprise 8% of all NHL.
i. Median age at diagnosis is 60 years.
ii. The usual site of this lymphoma are stomach, intestines, orbit, lungs, thyroid gland, salivary glands, and CNS.
iii. Lymphoma cells infiltrate the mucosa diffusely, but some epithelial cells may survive forming so called lymphoepithelial lesions.
iv. Lymphoma cells have the features of small B lymphocytes. Mitoses are rare and there is no necrosis/apoptosis.
v. Tumour cells express surface IgM, and CD20, but are negative for CD5.

Prognosis MALTomas have a good prognosis.
- For localised tumours, excision followed by local irradiation may suffice.
- For gastric MALTomas, one must first eradicate *H. pylori* infection.
- In some cases, MALTomas may progress to more aggressive lymphomas which require aggressive chemotherapy.

Q24. What is mantle cell lymphoma? Discuss its key clinicopathologic features.

Definition Mantle cell lymphoma (MCL) is an moderately aggressive but incurable form of B-cell lymphoma, composed of neoplastic cells resembling naive B cells found in the mantle zone that surrounds the germinal centre of the lymphoid follicles.

Pathogenesis Diagnostic *translocation t(11,14)* is found in all patients. This translocation leads to a fusion of *cyclin D_1* gene and *IgH* locus and overexpression of cyclin D_1, which promotes the progression of G_1 phase of the mitotic cycle to the S phase.

Clinicopathologic features MCL comprise 6% of all NHL.

i. Patients are most often older than 50 years of age; males predominate.

ii. Lymph nodes are infiltrated diffusely or in a vague nodular manner by cells that have an irregular nucleus, scant cytoplasm and are slightly larger than normal lymphocytes.

iii. In addition to widespread lymph node enlargement, there is early involvement of the bone marrow, liver, spleen and often the GI tract.

iv. *Immunohistochemistry:* Positive for B-cell markers (surface IgM, CD20 and CD5) and cyclin D_1.

Prognosis The disease is invariably fatal and most patients die 4–6 years after diagnosis.

Q25. Define hairy-cell leukaemia. Discuss its pathogenesis and main features.

Definition Hairy cell leukaemia is a rare form of B cell malignancy characterised by the presence of hairy cells in the blood and bone marrow, liver and spleen.

Pathogenesis *BRAFV600E* mutations found in almost all cases.

Clinicopathologic features The peripheral blood contains hairy cells, which are lymphocytes with surface cytoplasmic projections **(Fig. 14.7)**.

i. Tumour cells express B cell markers and a number of CD markers which confirm the diagnosis by flow-cytometry.

ii. Typically, the cells are also positive for *tartrate resistant acid phosphatase (TRAP)*.

iii. Lymphoid cells infiltrate the bone marrow, with consequent pancytopenia and cause splenomegaly.

iv. Pancytopenia presents with symptoms of anaemia, thrombocytopenia and a susceptibility to infection.

v. Infections with *Mycobacterium avium intracellulare* are common.

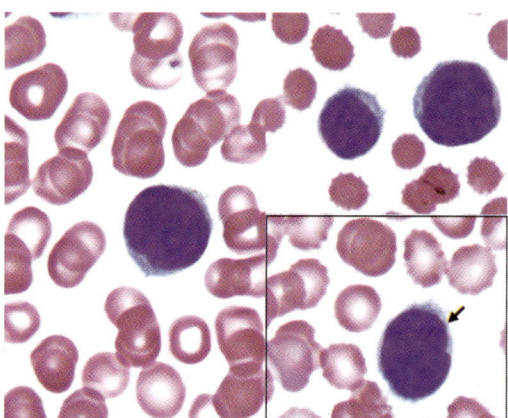

FIGURE 14.7: Hairy cell leukaemia. Peripheral blood shows presence of a leukaemic cells with hairy cytoplasmic projections (arrow).

Prognosis The disease is incurable, and most patients die 4–5 years after diagnosis.

Q26. Discuss briefly the most common mature T and NK cell neoplasms (lymphomas).

Peripheral or mature T-cell lymphomas are much less common than B-cell lymphoma. Mature NK-cell lymphomas are even less common.

Since NK-cells share some features with cytotoxic cells, it is customary to consider all these malignancies together. The most common disease in this category are as follows:

I. **Mycosis fungoides/Sèzary syndrome** is a slowly evolving cutaneous T-cell lymphoma affecting predominantly adult males.

i. It has three stages as under:
- *Premycotic stage* presenting in the form of eczema or dermatitis.
- *Plaque stage* characterised by infiltration of the skin by CD4+ lymphocytes.
- *Tumour stage* with formation of skin nodules.

ii. Dissemination may occur to internal organs, most often lymph nodes, spleen, liver and lungs.

iii. Leukaemic form of the disease is called Sèzary syndrome.

Prognosis Mycosis fungoides has an indolent course, but it does not respond to treatment and most patients die 8–9 years after diagnosis.

II. **Anaplastic large T/NK-cell lymphoma (ALCL)** cells express T-cell markers and are also positive for CD30.
i. A diagnostic translocation t(2;5) can be detected, and the cells may overexpress anaplastic lymphoma kinase (ALK).
ii. ALCL affects young people, with a male predominance.
iii. Clinically, it presents with indolent cutaneous lesions.
iv. Rarely, there is bone marrow and internal organ involvement.

III. **Aggressive T-cell NK-cell lymphomas** form a morphologically heterogeneous group, which however express markers of mature T cells (CD4+ or CD8+ or both).
- They mostly affect young adults.
- Often, there is bone marrow involvement at presentation.

Examples of these disorders are as under:
i. *Angioimmunoblastic lymphoma* (20% of T-cell NHL) presents with profound constitutional symptoms (fever, weight loss, skin rash), generalised lymphadenopathy and hypergammaglobulinaemia.
ii. *Extranodal T/NK cell lymphoma of nasal type* involves preferentially upper airways. Infiltrates of T/NK cells cause destruction of facial bones and nasal sinuses, previously known under the name of *lethal midline granuloma*. Progression of the disease is associated with *haemophagocytic syndrome*, bone marrow involvement and leukaemia.
iii. *Enteropathy type T-cell lymphoma* is an aggressive intestinal form of lymphoma that affects patients with gluten-sensitive enteropathy.
iv. *Hepatosplenic T-cell lymphoma* affects the liver, spleen and bone marrow. Tumour cells do not form nodules, but instead invade through the sinusoids. Hepatosplenomegaly is accompanied by systemic symptoms and a rapid downhill course.

Q27. What is Hodgkin lymphoma? Discuss its classification and key general features.

Definition Hodgkin lymphoma (HL, also known as Hodgkin disease or HD) comprises a group of germinal centre B-cell neoplasms characterised by the presence of diagnostic Reed-Sternberg (RS) cells and unique clinicopathologic features that distinguish them from non-Hodgkin lymphomas (NHL).

Classification There are five subtypes of HL belonging to two main groups **(Table 14.4)**:
I. *Classical HL,* which has four subtypes:
i. lymphocyte-rich HL
ii. nodular sclerosis HL
iii. mixed cellularity HL
iv. lymphocyte depleted HL

TABLE 14.4 Contrasting features of types of Hodgkin's lymphoma (HL) as per the WHO classification 2016.

HISTOLOGIC SUBTYPE	INCIDENCE	MAIN PATHOLOGY	RS CELLS	PROGNOSIS
I. CLASSICAL			HL IHC: CD3-, CD15+, CD20+, CD30+, CD45-, PAX5+, EBV+	
Lymphocyte-rich	5%	Proliferating lymphocytes, a few histiocytes	Few, classic and polyploid type	Excellent
Nodular sclerosis	70%	Lymphoid nodules, collagen bands	Frequent, lacunar type	Very good
Mixed cellularity	22%	Mixed infiltrate	Numerous, classic type	Good
Lymphocyte-depleted (Diffuse fibrotic and reticular variants)	1%	Scanty lymphocytes, atypical histiocytes, fibrosis	Numerous, pleomorphic type	Poor
II. NODULAR LYMPHOCYTE-PREDOMINANT			HL IHC: CD3-, CD15-, CD20+, CD30-, CD45+, PAX5+, EBV-	
	2%	Proliferation of small lymphocytes, nodular pattern of growth	Sparse number of RS cells	Chronic relapsing, may transform into large B cell NHL

II. Nodular lymphocyte predominant HL

Key general features Certain common important facts about various subtypes of HL are as under:

i. **Incidence**

a. Nodular sclerosis is the most common form of HL (70%), followed by mixed cellularity HL (22%).

b. The other forms of HL are less common as indicated by their relative incidence as follows: lymphocyte rich HL (5%), lymphocyte depleted HL (1%), nodular lymphocyte predominant HL (2%).

ii. **Reed-Sternberg cells** The number and morphologic types of Reed-Sternberg cells present in various subtypes of HL varies.

iii. **Age and sex**

a. *Bimodal age distribution*: First large peak is 15–34 years of age, second smaller peak over 50 years of age.

b. *Gender distribution*: All subtypes, except for nodular sclerosis, are more common in males than females.

iv. **Clinical presentation**

a. Painless enlargement of lymph nodes belonging to the same anatomic group.

b. Spread by contiguity from one lymph node group to another.

c. Most often, HL involves lymph nodes above the diaphragm, i.e. cervical, supraclavicular, mediastinal and axillary lymph nodes.

d. Waldeyer ring lymph nodes in the throat and mesenteric lymph nodes are only rarely involved, in contrast to NHL which often involves these sites.

e. Extranodal involvement is rare and usually found only in advanced stages of HL or in chemotherapy-resistant cases.

f. Splenomegaly found in 50% of cases, often accompanied by hepatomegaly. Infiltrates may be diffuse and not visible on gross examination or in form of nodules resembling metastatic carcinoma.

g. Constitutional symptoms ('type B symptoms') are found in 25–40% patients.

v. **Prognosis** Depends on its histologic subtype and the stage of the disease:

a. *Lymphocyte rich HL* tends to show only limited local lymph node involvement, and thus has the *best prognosis*.

b. *Nodular sclerosis HL has very good prognosis*. It is the most common subtype in young people.

c. *Mixed cellularity HL* has good prognosis. Mixed cellularity is the most common subtype in persons older than 50 years. It most often has B symptoms and will most likely disseminate.

d. *Lymphocyte depleted HL* has *worst prognosis*. Furthermore, it is the most common subtype in HIV-infected persons.

e. *Nodular lymphocyte predominant HL* usually presents by involving a localised small group of lymph nodes and thus has an *excellent prognosis*. In 7–10% cases, it may even transform into DLBCL several years after remission.

Q28. What are Reed-Sternberg (RS) cells? Discuss their various morphologic variants.

Definition RS cells are very large B-cells diagnostic of HL. They are often surrounded by atypical Hodgkin cells, which have similar nuclear features as typical RS, but are not bilobed. Atypical Hodgkin cells are most likely precursors of RS cells.

Types of RS Following four types are recognised, each with distinct morphologic features and seen in different histologic subtype of HL **(Fig. 14.8)**:

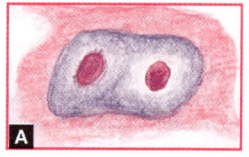
A, Classic RS cell

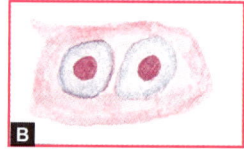
B, Lacunar type RS cell

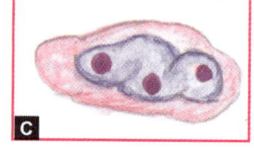
C, Polyploid (popcorn, lymphocytic-histiocytic, i.e. L and H) RS cell

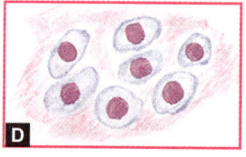
D, Pleomoprhic RS cell

FIGURE 14.8: Morphologic variants of RS cells in different types of Hodgkin lymphoma.

I. **Classic RS cell** measures 15–45 μm in diameter. It has a bilobed nucleus which contains two large nucleoli surrounded by a clear halo, giving it an *owl-eye like appearance*. The cytoplasm is abundant and amphophilic. Classical RS are abundant in mixed-cellularity HL, but may also be found, though less numerous, in lymphocyte-rich HL.

II. **Lacunar type RS cell** has similar nuclear features but is smaller than classical RS. Each cell is surrounded by a clear space or lacuna. This type is characteristically found in nodular sclerosis HL.

III. **Polyploid type RS cell** (also known as *popcorn, or lymphocytic-histiocytic, i.e. L and H cell*) is relatively large and has a lobulated nucleus resembling popcorn. Typically these cells occur in nodular lymphocyte-predominance HL.

IV. **Pleomorphic RS cell** has a pleomorphic highly atypical nucleus. These RS cells are found in lymphocyte-depleted HL.

Immunohistochemical features of RS cells are important for their identification. However, they show some variation from one subtype to another as follows (*see* **Table 14.4**):

- In the majority of HL cases (nodular sclerosis HL, mixed cellularity HL, and lymphocyte depleted HL), RS cells are positive for CD15 and CD30, but negative for CD45 (leucocyte common antigen).
- In lymphocyte-rich HL, RS cells are negative for CD15 and CD30 and T-cell markers, but positive for CD20, a B-cell marker.
- In nodular lymphocyte predominance HL, there are few RS cells; those that are present are negative for CD15 and CD30, and positive for CD45 and EMA.

Q29. What are the principal histopathologic features of the five subtypes of Hodgkin lymphoma?

Key features of histopathology are presented in **Figure 14.9**.

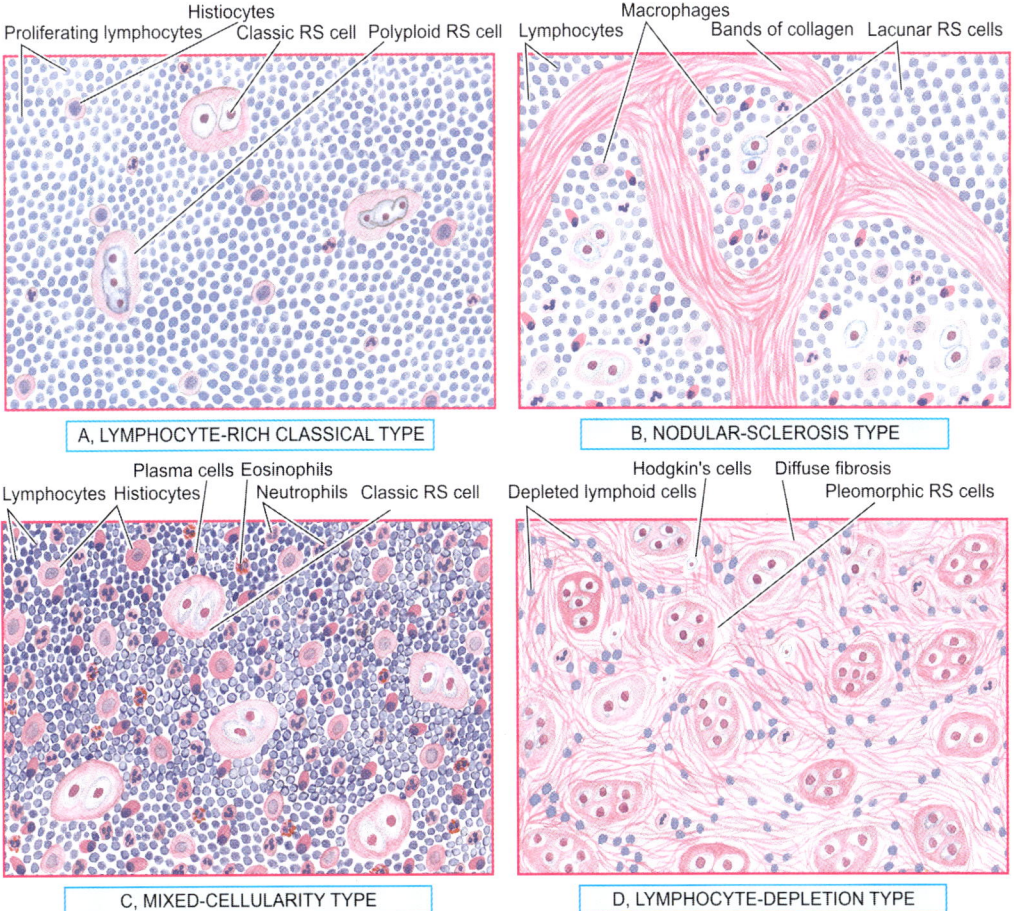

FIGURE 14.9: Microscopic features of four subtypes of classical Hodgkin lymphoma of lymph node.

I. **Lymphocyte-rich HL** The involved lymph node is diffusely infiltrated by small lymphocytes, some histiocytes and sparse RS cells, which are of the *classical or polyploid type*. There are no plasma cells or eosinophils and there is no fibrosis or necrosis.

II. **Nodular sclerosis HL** It is characterised by bands of fibrous tissue, which may replace large parts of the lymph node. The infiltrate comprises of lymphocytes, histiocytes and *prominent lacunar RS cells* and there are scattered areas of necrosis.

III. **Mixed cellularity HL** Typically, a mixed inflammatory infiltrate involves the entire lymph node replacing its normal components. These infiltrates comprise lymphocytes, macrophages, plasma cells, eosinophils, neutrophils. There are numerous *RS cells of the classic type*. Foci of necrosis and fibrosis may be present.

IV. **Lymphocyte depleted HL.** There are two variants:

i. **Diffuse fibrotic variant** presenting as a hypocellular lesion. The entire lymph node is replaced by diffuse fibrosis, which appears like a homogeneous sclerotic material. There are only a few residual lymphocytes, atypical Hodgkin cells (macrophages) and *RS cells of the classical or pleomorphic type*.

ii. **Reticular variant** is more cellular and contains a large number of atypical pleomorphic histiocytes, scant lymphocytes, and pleomorphic RS cells.

V. **Nodular lymphocyte predominant HL** is characterised by a nodular growth pattern, vaguely resembling nodular sclerosis HL. The lymph node is infiltrated with small lymphocytes, a variable number of histiocytes and sparse *polyploid RS cells* with 'popcorn' nuclei; this type of RS cells are also known as 'lympho-histiocytic (L and H) variant of RS cells. On immunohistochemistry, they differ from classical RS: L and H RS cells are positive for CD45 and epithelial membrane antigen (EMA) but negative for CD15 and CD30.

Q30. What are the usual clinical signs, symptoms and laboratory findings in Hodgkin disease?

I. **Lymphadenopathy** presenting as painless, movable and firm lymph node enlargement involving one or more contiguous groups of lymph nodes.

i. Most often, there is palpable cervical and supraclavicular lymph node enlargement.

ii. X-rays show mediastinal lymphadenopathy.

iii. Splenomegaly is found in about 50% cases, sometimes accompanied by hepatomegaly.

II. **Constitutional symptoms** (called type B symptoms, in contrast to type A disease, which does not have constitutional symptoms) include low grade fever, night sweats and weight loss exceeding 10% of normal. Other symptoms include fatigue, malaise, weakness and pruritus. Mixed cellularity subtype most often has these symptoms.

III. **Laboratory findings** include:

i. Normocytic normochromic anaemia.

ii. Low serum iron and TIBC, associated with normal bone marrow irons stores.

iii. Moderate leukaemoid reaction.

iv. Eosinophilia in patients with pruritus.

v. Erythrocyte sedimentation rate is increased.

vi. Bone marrow is normal, except in advances cases with HL involving the bone marrow.

vii. Reduced number of T cells and a reversal of the normal CD4:CD8 ratio, associated with anergy to skin tests.

viii. Normal antibody-mediated immune system.

Q31. How is Hodgkin disease staged clinically?

For planning of treatment and formulating the prognosis of HL, it is important to do the following:
i. Stage the disease
ii. Classify it histopathologically
iii. Determine clinically if there are B symptoms.
Staging is done according to the Ann Arbor system **(Table 14.5)**.
- Patients treated for stage I and II HL have a 100% 5-year survival rate.
- Those with advanced HL survive 5 years in 50% of cases.

TABLE 14.5 Ann Arbor staging classification of Hodgkin disease.

Stage		
Stage I (A or B)	I	Involvement of a single lymph node region.
	I_E	Involvement of a single extra-lymphatic organ or site.
Stage II (A or B)	II	Involvement of two or more lymph node regions on the same side of the diaphragm.
	II_E	(or) with localised contiguous involvement of an extranodal organ or site.
Stage III (A or B)	III	Involvement of lymph node regions on both sides of the diaphragm.
	III_E	(or) with localised contiguous involvement of an extranodal organ or site.
	III_S	(or) with involvement of spleen.
	III_{ES}	(or) both features of III_E and III_S.
Stage IV (A or B)	IV	Multiple or disseminated involvement of one or more extra-lymphatic organs or tissues with or without lymphatic involvement.

(A, asymptomatic; B, presence of constitutional symptoms; E, extranodal involvement; S, splenomegaly).

Q32. What are the salient differences between Hodgkin lymphoma and non-Hodgkin lymphoma?

Since the treatment of Hodgkin disease differs from the treatment of non-Hodgkin lymphoma, it is important to distinguish one from another. Contrasting feature of HL and NHL are presented in **Table 14.6**.

TABLE 14.6 Contrasting features of Hodgkin (HL) and non-Hodgkin lymphoma (NHL).

Feature	HL	NHL
1. Cell derivation	B-cell mostly	90% B / 10% T
2. Nodal involvement	Localised, may spread to contiguous nodes	Disseminated nodal spread
3. Extranodal spread	Uncommon	Common
4. Bone marrow involvement	Uncommon	Common
5. Constitutional symptoms	Common	Uncommon
6. Chromosomal defects	Aneuploidy	Translocations, deletions
7. Spill-over	Never	May spread to blood
8. Overall prognosis	Better (75–85% cure)	Bad (30–40% cure)

Q33. Define plasma cell disorders. What are their principal types?

Definition Plasma cell disorders (also known as *plasma cell dyscrasias*) are abnormal proliferations of B cells that differ from other B-cell malignancies in that they secrete monoclonal immunoglobulins, or light chains (κ or λ), or heavy chains (α, γ or μ) that may be demonstrated in blood and sometimes even in urine (light chain protein known as Bence Jones protein). They account for approximately 15% of all B-cell malignancies. Besides, they lack prominent lymphadenopathy.

Classification Principal plasma cell disorders include the following entities:
i. Multiple myeloma
ii. Localised plasmacytoma
iii. Waldenström macroglobulinaemia (B cell lymphoplasmacytic lymphoma)
iv. Heavy chain disease
v. Primary amyloidosis
vi. Monoclonal gammopathy of undetermined significance (MGUS)

Q34. What is multiple myeloma? Briefly discuss its etiopathogenesis.

Definition Multiple myeloma is a multifocal monoclonal plasma cell malignancy, primarily involving the bones. It is associated with monoclonal gammopathy. It is the most common plasma cell disorder.

Etiopathogenesis The etiology is unknown for most cases.
Epidemiologic evidence of possible causation includes exposure to heavy irradiation, petroleum products, agrichemical toxins used in farming, and chemicals used in wood and leather industry.

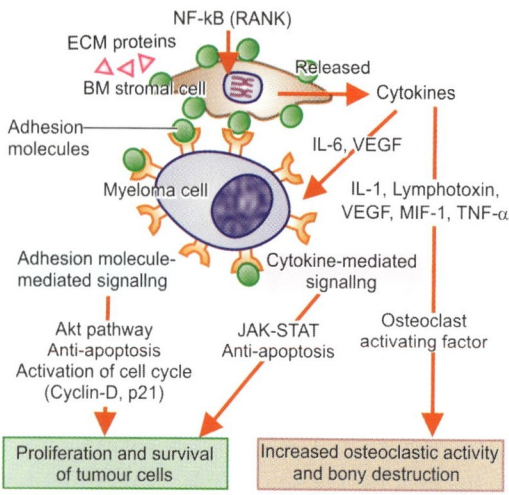

FIGURE 14.10: Schematic diagram showing molecular pathogenesis of multiple myeloma and its major manifestations. (ECM, extracellular matrix; IL, interleukin; EGF, vascular endothelial growth factor; MIF, macrophage inhibitory factor; RANK, receptor activator of nuclear factor-κB; BM, bone marrow; TNF, tumour necrosis factor).

Molecular pathogenesis includes the following **(Fig. 14.10)**:

I. **Genetic changes in the tumour cells** Tumour cells show a constant translocations of immunoglobin heavy chain gene (*IHG*) on chromosome 14q32 to loci that contain *cyclin D_1 and D_3* genes [i.e. t(11,14) q13;q32].

Cyclin D genes dysregulation has the following consequence:

i. Promotes proliferation of myeloma cells.

ii. Has an *anti-apoptotic effect* thus contributing to the longevity and survival of tumour cells.

iii. Stimulates the secretion of *myeloma (M) proteins*.

iv. Stimulates the production of cytokines which have *osteoblast inhibitory functions* and act as *osteoclast activating* factors (OAF). These cytokines act jointly in producing the typical osteolytic lesions in the bones.

II. **Tumour cell-stromal cell interaction** This is crucial for the growth of myeloma cells in the bone marrow and for the pathogenesis of pathologic changes seen in multiple myeloma. Stimulated stromal cells secrete numerous cytokines such as IL-1, IL-6, VEGF, TGF-β and receptor activator of NF-κB ligand (RANKL). These cytokines have multiple functions as follows:

i. Activate cell cycle and stimulate *myeloma cell proliferation*.

ii. Through their *anti-apoptotic activity* assure survival of myeloma cells.

iii. Promote *osteoclastic degradation* of the bone.

iv. Contribute to *drug resistance* of tumour cells.

v. Facilitate the *spread of tumour cells* through the bone marrow.

Q35. What are the typical morphologic findings in multiple myeloma?

Pathologic changes in multiple myeloma can be described under two headings: i) osseous lesions, and ii) extraosseous lesions.

I. **Osseous lesions** are present at the time of diagnosis in 95% of all cases. They are usually multiple and involve predominantly the red bone marrow, i.e. the skull, ribs, vertebrae and pelvis. Other bones may become involved in later stages of the disease **(Fig. 14.11)**.

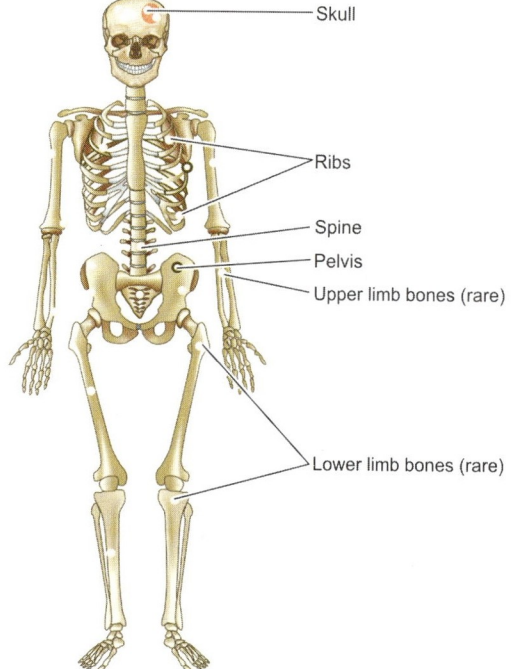

FIGURE 14.11: Major sites of lesions in multiple myeloma.

Gross Visible on X-rays as punched out sharply outlined bone defects.
- On cross section, the tumour tissue is soft, reddish-grey and gelatinous.
- Surrounding areas may show osteoporosis.

Microscopy Myeloma cells constitute more than 10% of the marrow cellularity.
i. Biopsied lesions are composed of myeloma cells that resemble normal plasma cells.
ii. Main features of myeloma cells are **(Fig. 14.12)**:
- Variable in size and shape.
- Cytoplasmic vacuoles may be present and are filled with M protein.
- Some cells are binucleate or show nuclear atypia.

II. **Extraosseous lesions** develop usually in advanced stages of the disease and include the following:

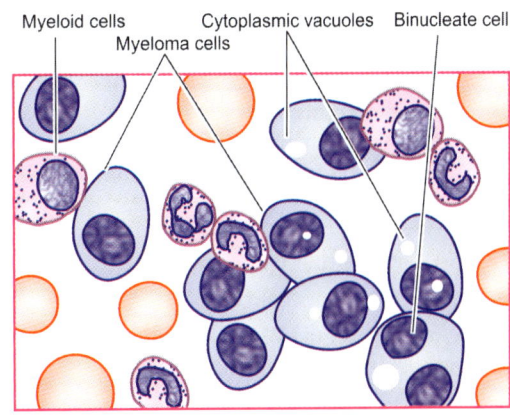

FIGURE 14.12: Bone marrow aspirate in myeloma showing numerous plasma cells, many with abnormal features.

i. **Peripheral blood** shows normocytic normochromic anaemia with prominent rouleaux formation reflecting increased viscosity of the blood. In about 50% of patients, there are occasional myeloma cells in peripheral blood.
ii. **Myeloma kidney** results from the filtration of the light chain proteins (Bence Jones proteins) in the glomeruli and subsequent formation of myeloma casts in the distal convoluted tubules. The casts occlude the tubules and elicit an inflammatory reaction as evidenced by the presence of multinucleated giant cells or neutrophils surrounding the casts.
iii. **Myeloma neuropathy** results from the infiltration of nerve trunk roots by tumour cells, deposits of amyloid or compression by broken bones.
iv. **Systemic amyloidosis** involving multiple sites may be found in 10% of patients.

Q36. What are the major clinical features of multiple myeloma?

Multiple myeloma is a diseases of the elderly (median age at diagnosis is 68 years), with a male predominance.
The clinical findings are related to destruction of bones by myeloma cells and the dysregulated synthesis of immunoglobulins, as follows:
i. **Bone pain** is the most common symptom.
- Usually, it is localised in the back or the ribs.
- It results from proliferation of myeloma cells in the marrow and activation of osteoclasts which destroy the bone.
- Bone fractures are yet another cause of bone pain.

ii. **Susceptibility to infections** due to the suppression of normal immunoglobulin synthesis, granulocyte dysfunction and neutropenia.
- Most common bacterial infections include respiratory and urinary tract infections.

iii. **Renal failure** seen in 25% patients, but laboratory signs of renal disease in 50%. Causes include: hypercalcaemia, amyloid deposits, tubular injury by Bence Jones protein, hyperuricaemia.
iv. **Anaemia** due to infiltration of bone marrow with myeloma cells and inhibition of erythropoiesis.
v. **Hyperviscosity syndrome** due to hyperglobulinaemia presents with headache, fatigue, visual problems and bleeding diathesis.
vi. **Neurologic symptoms** found in a minority of patients, related to hyperviscosity and amyloid deposits.
vii. **POEMS syndrome** (**P**olyneuropathy, **O**rganomegaly, **E**ndocrinopathy, **M**ultiple myeloma, and **S**kin changes) found in 1% of all patients.

Q37. Discuss the salient laboratory findings for diagnosis of multiple myeloma.

Laboratory findings essential for diagnosis
i. Monoclonal gammopathy, which is in 50–60% of cases IgGκ.
ii. Serum M protein > 3g/dL.

iii. Hypercalcaemia due to destruction of bones.
iv. Hyperuricaemia from lysis of tumor cells and renal failure.
v. Increased β-2 microglobulins and other globulins in urine and serum.

Prognosis and treatment
- Without treatment, most patients die within 2–5 years of diagnosis.
- Chemotherapy with proteasome inhibitors and thalidomide may prolong life but it is not curative.

Q38. What are the clinicopathologic criteria for making the diagnosis of multiple myeloma and its variant forms?

I. **Multiple myeloma (MM)**
Original criteria for diagnosis by recognising the *classical triad* as under:
i. Bone marrow showing clonal plasmacytosis >10%, or multiple myeloma diagnosed by biopsy.
ii. Monoclonal protein (M component) in serum or urine electrophoresis.
iii. Related organ or tissue impairment (CRAB = Calcium↑ in serum, Renal insufficiency, Anaemia, Bone lesions)

Revised criteria have been introduced recently as follows:
i. >60% of clonal plasma cells on bone marrow examination.
ii. >100 as the ratio of serum involved/uninvolved free light chain (either kappa or lambda).
iii. >5 mm-sized, more than one focal lesion on MRI.

II. **Variant forms of multiple myeloma and related conditions**
i. ***Smoldering or asymptomatic myeloma*** is diagnosed by the following criteria:
a. Presence of M-component in serum
b. Clonal plasma cells in the bone marrow ≥10%
c. No CRAB (no related organ impairment)
ii. ***Nonsecretory myeloma*** accounts for 1–2% of all cases.
a. >10% myeloma cells in the bone marrow
b. CRAB+
c. No paraproteins in serum or urine (i.e. absence of M band in serum, absence of Bence Jones proteins)
iii. ***Solitary plasmacytoma*** is diagnosed on the basis of the following findings:
a. Plasmacytoma diagnosed pathologically. It may present as a *solitary bone plasmacytoma* or a *solitary extramedullary plasmacytoma*.
b. Clnical/pathologic findings do not meet the classical triad criteria for multiple myeloma.
c. Solitary plasmacytoma differs from classical multiple myeloma as under:
- Patients are usually younger than typical MM cases.
- Most common site of extramedullary solitary plasmacytoma is the lymphoid tissue of nasopharynx or paranasal sinuses.
- Most patients do not have serum M component. It is present in serum of 30% of cases.
- Solitary plasmacytoma of bone is 2 times more common in women than in men.
- *Prognosis:* In 50% cases, may progress to MM in 4–5 years. Extramedullary plasmacytoma will only rarely progress to MM.

Q39. What are paraproteins? Discuss their method of diagnosis and conditions associated with paraproteinaemias.

Definition Paraproteins are abnormal immunoglobulins or their parts circulating in plasma or excreted in urine.

Laboratory findings On serum electrophoresis, the paraproteins usually appear as a single M-band component, most commonly in the region of γ-globulin (**Fig. 14.13**).
i. Monoclonal M band appears as a narrow peak in contrast to the broad band of polyclonal immunoglobulins.
ii. Most frequently paraprotein in multiple myeloma is IgG (50–60%), followed by IgA (20%), and IgD (1%).

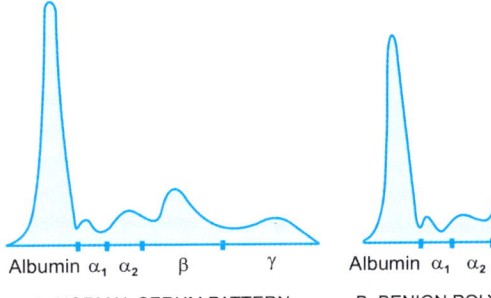
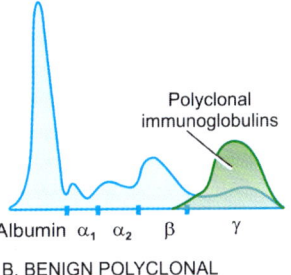
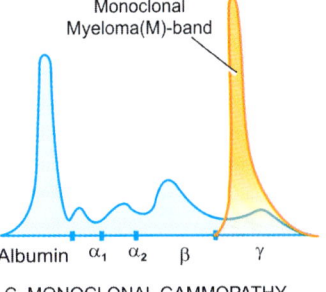

FIGURE 14.13: Serum electrophoresis showing normal serum pattern (A), as contrasted with that in benign polyclonal gammopathy (B) and in monoclonal gammopathy (C), typical of plasma cell myeloma.

iii. In 20% of cases, only immunoglobulin light chains are found in serum and urine.
iv. Two-thirds of myeloma patients have Bence Jones protein in urine.
Etiology The causes of paraproteinemia are as follows:
i. Multiple myeloma
ii. Monoclonal gammopathy of undetermined significance (MGUS) (*most common*)
iii. Waldenström macroglobulinaemia
iv. Benign monoclonal gammopathy
v. B-cell lymphomas
vi. Chronic lymphocytic leukaemia
vii. Light chin disease
viii. Heavy chain disease
ix. Cryoglobulinaemia

Q40. Define monoclonal gammopathy of unknown significance (MGUS). What are its salient features?

Definition MGUS is a laboratory disorder usually discovered in asymptomatic patients by serum electrophoresis.
Epidemiology MGUS has an incidence of 3% individuals over the age of 50 years. It accounts for 50–60% of monoclonal gammopathies and is thus the *most common* monoclonal gammopathy.
Clinicopathologic features
i. Small IgG M-spike seen by electrophoresis in an asymptomatic person.
ii. Serum M protein concentration <3 g/dL.
iii. No Bence Jones protein in serum or urine.
iv. Bone marrow contains <10% plasma cells.
v. Negative findings: scan for skeletal lytic lesions and no CRAB.
vi. Life long risk for progression to MM is 1%.

Q41. What is Waldenström macroglobulinaemia?

Definition Waldenström macroglobulinaemia is an uncommon lymphoplasmacytic lymphoma characterised by the presence of serum IgM paraproteins called macroglobulins as they have high molecular weight.
Genetics Almost all cases of Waldenström macroglobulinaemia have a mutation of *MYD88 gene*, encoding an adaptor protein that supports the survival of cells.
Pathology and laboratory findings
i. The bone marrow is infiltrated with lymphocytes, plasmacytoid lymphocytes and plasma cells, often accompanied by reactive mast cell proliferation.
ii. In contrast to multiple myeloma, there are no visible lytic bone lesions; thus, no hypercalcaemia (unlike multiple myeloma).
iii. Malignant cells infiltrate lymph nodes, spleen and liver causing their enlargement in 50% patients (lymph node enlargement not a feature of multiple myeloma!).

iv. In terminal stages of the disease, malignant cell infiltrates can be found in all organs.
v. Serum protein concentration is elevated due to M component (IgM-macroglobulin).
vi. Bence Jones protein in serum in 80% cases, but no renal failure.
vii. Anaemia results from malignant cells replacing the bone marrow cells. In 10% patients there is autoimmune haemolytic anaemia because IgM may act as cold haemaglutinin.

Clinical features
i. Hyperviscosity syndrome due to IgM is the most common clinical problem presenting with:
a. Constitutional symptoms (e.g. fatigue, weakness, weight loss), which in part can be due to anaemia.
b. CNS ischaemia (sluggish blood flow and minor strokes) resulting in sensory and motor neurologic defects, and confusion or somnolence.
c. Visual problems due to sluggish flow of viscous blood in retinal vessels and haemorhages.
ii. Bleeding tendency due to bindings of IgM to clotting factors and affecting adversely the function of platelets.
iii. Cryoglobulinaemia causing Raynaud syndrome and cold urticaria.
Prognosis Poor response to therapy; average survival 3–5 years.

Q42. Briefly discuss heavy chain diseases.

Definition Heavy chain disease is a rare malignant proliferation of B-cell accompanied by monoclonal excess of one of the heavy chain which may be γ, α or μ.

Clinicopathologic features
I. *Gamma heavy chain disease* is characterised by γ_1 paraprotein in serum and urine.
i. It can develop at any age and presents with fever and generalised lymphadenopathy including the involvement of the Waldeyer ring.
ii. Hepatosplenomegaly is common.
iii. Severe infections are common and lead to rapid downhill course
II. *Alpha heavy chain disease* is the commonest heavy chain disease.
i. It presents with bowel symptoms (diarrhoea, malabsorption, weight loss).
ii. Abdominal lymph nodes are enlarged.
iii. α-heavy chains polymerise rapidly and are difficult to demonstrate by electrophoresis.
iv. Chemotherapy may induce long term remission.
III. *Mu heavy chain disease* is the rarest of all heavy chain disease.
i. Difficult to demonstrate since μ-chains do not appear in urine.
ii. κ-chains, which are also produced in excess, appear in urine.
iii. Malignant lymphocytes contain prominent vacuoles.
iv. Prognosis is like other leukaemia/lymphoma.

Q43. What is Langerhans cell histiocytosis? How is it classified? Briefly discuss their features.

Definition Langerhans cell histiocytosis (LCH) is a term that includes several pathologic entities characterised by proliferation of Langerhans cells (i.e. immature dendritic cells involved in antigen presentation).

Etiopathogenesis Etiology is unknown.
• Mutation of the gene encoding *serine/threonine kinase BRAF* is found in many cases and probably promotes the proliferation of LCH. This kinase is involved in the RAS signaling pathway affected in several other cancers.
• Proliferating cells have the typical *immunohistochemical markers* of Langerhans cells: S100, CD1a, langerin, and MHC class II antigens (HLA-DR).
• *Electron microscopy* shows that they contain *Bierbeck granules* ('tennis racket-like'), known to contain langerin (an adhesion molecule, also known as CD207).

Classification LCH is not a single disease. It includes a spectrum of diseases that vary from clinically benign (eosinophilic granuloma) to potentially disabling (Hand-Schüller-Christian disease) to malignant and incurable diseases (Letterer-Siwe disease).
I. *Eosinophilic granuloma,* a clinically benign condition most often affecting bones; more often solitary (unifocal) (60%) than multifocal.

Clinicopathologic features
i. Affects children or young adults.
ii. *Location* Bones: femur, skull, vertebrae, ribs and pelvis.
iii. Solitary osteolytic lesion seen by X-rays is the most common finding.
iv. Asymptomatic unless it caused a bone fracture.
v. May affect any internal organ.
vi. *Microscopy* Aggregates of macrophages (Langerhans cells) admixed to eosinophils.
vii. Immunohistochemistry supports the diagnosis (CD1a, S100 positive).
viii. *Prognosis* Tends to heal by fibrosis, but if symptomatic it requires surgery.

II. **Hand-Schüller-Christian disease** is a benign disease but it may be potentially disabling.
Clinicopathologic features
i. Affects children under the age of 5 years.
ii. Multifocal bone defects with secondary internal organ derangements.
iii. Microscopically indistinguishable from eosinophilic granuloma.
iv. Diabetes insipidus, because of compression of hypothalamus or posterior pituitary.
v. Exophthalmos, because of retrobulbar lesions.
vi. Hepatic, splenic and lymph node involvement in 50% of children.
vii. *Prognosis* May resolve spontaneously, but some need chemotherapy or radiation treatment.

III. **Letterer-Siwe disease** is an acute disseminated form of LCH affecting infants and children under the age of 2 years that behaves clinically as lymphoma.
Clinicopathologic features
i. Lytic and cystic bone lesions (skull, pelvis, long bones)
ii. Skin lesions
iii. Hepatosplenomegaly
iv. Lymphadenopathy
v. *Prognosis* Treatment is based on chemotherapy

> **Chapter 14e Supplement: Online Content**
> *Digital content of this chapter available with this book is meant for enhanced learning and self-assessment. In addition, it contains 45 Multiple Choice Questions (MCQs), 05 Clinicopathologic Vignettes, and 04 Image-based Questions; these are followed by their answers along with explanatory notes of correct and incorrect answers.*

SECTION III: SYSTEMIC PATHOLOGY

CHAPTER 15

Blood Vessels and Lymphatics

Q1. What are the main components of the vascular and the lymphatic system?
- Vascular and lymphatic systems consist of vessels which transport the blood and lymph.
- The vascular system is linked to the heart which acts as a pump maintaining the circulation of blood from the central to peripheral parts, and vice versa.
- It comprises histologically distinct components including arteries, arterioles, capillaries and veins.
- The lymphatic system consists of lymphatic capillaries, vessels and lymph nodes.

Q2. How are arteries classified?
All arteries have three layers or *tunicae*; these are intima, media and adventitia **(Fig. 15.1)**. On the basis of these histologic features and their calibre, arteries are classified as: large (elastic), medium-sized (muscular), and arterioles:

I. **Large elastic arteries** include the aorta, innominate, common carotid, major pulmonary, and common iliac arteries.
i. These arteries have abundant amounts of elastic tissue, which is most prominently condensed into an *internal elastic lamina*, which separates intima from the media.
ii. *External elastic lamina* and the elastic fibres in the tunica media are less well-defined but can be demonstrated by special stains.
II. **Medium-sized muscular arteries** are smaller than the elastic arteries. Examples of muscular arteries are radial, ulnar, popliteal and renal arteries. They contain less elastic tissue and their media is composed of prominent smooth muscle cells.
III. **Arterioles** measure 20–100 µm in diameter even though they also have three layers. The layers of arteriolar wall are not as distinct as in larger arteries and the elastic laminae are virtually not evident.

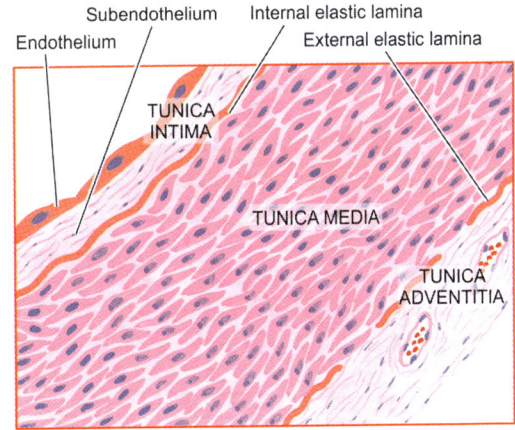

FIGURE 15.1: The structure of a medium-sized muscular artery.

Q3. What are the main histologic features of veins? How do veins differ from lymphatics?
Veins begin at the venous end of capillaries, the terminal part of circulation, still containing arterial blood, which gradually becomes deoxygenated and transforms into the venous blood.

i. Veins have essentially the *same three-layered structure* as the arteries. However, they are much *thinner*, and their layers are not as distinct as those in the arteries.

ii. The media of veins contains less smooth muscle cells and more collagen.

iii. All veins, except the venae cavae and common iliac veins, have *valves*, which prevent any significant retrograde venous flow.

iv. In that respect they resemble *lymphatic vessels* which also have valves.

v. Lymphatic vessels differ from veins in that they do not contain blood; instead they drain lymph from *lymphatic capillary plexuses* in peripheral tissues. Furthermore, in contrast to blood vessels, lymphatics are not directly linked to the heart.

Q4. Define arteriosclerosis. What are its main types?

Definition Arteriolosclerosis is a generic term for degenerative changes resulting in thickening and hardening of arterial wall.

Types The following clinicopathologic entities are included under this term:
i. Senile arteriolosclerosis
ii. Hypertensive arteriolosclerosis
iii. Mönckeberg arteriolosclerosis
iv. Atherosclerosis

Q5. What is senile arteriosclerosis?

i. Senile arteriosclerosis presents with thickening of the intima and media.

ii. It affects non-selectively any or all arteries in the elderly.

iii. Microscopic changes include fibroelastosis of the intima marked by an accumulation of elastic and collagenous fibres and reduplication of the internal elastic lamina.

iv. Hardening of the arterial wall reduces its capacity to expand under pressure during systole leading to age-related blood pressure elevation.

Q6. Discuss salient features of hypertensive arteriolosclerosis and its types.

Definition Hypertensive arteriolosclerosis, as the name implies, affects arterioles and presents in three forms: hyaline, hyperplastic and necrotising arteriolosclerosis **(Fig. 15.2)**. All three forms of arteriolosclerosis are most prominently found in kidneys, but may be seen in other internal organs and brain as well.

I. **Hyaline arteriolosclerosis** is marked by accumulation of hyaline material in the wall of arterioles, with narrowing of the arteriolar lumen.

Etiology It is part of the *ageing*, but also occurs in younger adults who have *hypertension* or *diabetes mellitus*.

Pathogenesis Insudation of plasma proteins and lipids into the arteriolar wall due to increased pressure and altered metabolic conditions (e.g. in diabetes) play a key role.

II. **Hyperplastic arteriolosclerosis** is marked by thickening of arteriolar wall due to an increased number of smooth muscle surrounding concentrically the narrowed lumen (so called 'onion-skin like' changes). Some arterioles show *mucinous degeneration* of their walls, with less prominent cellular proliferation.

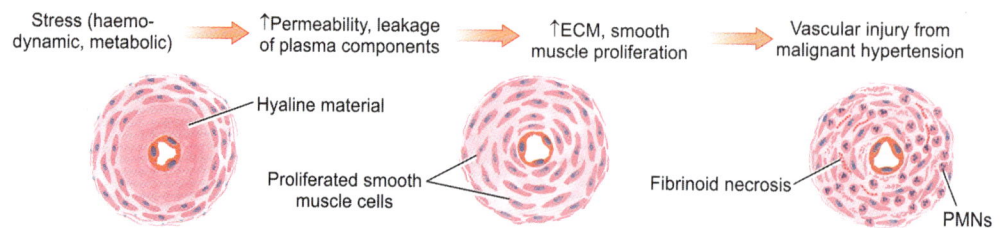

A, HYALINE ARTERIOLOSCLEROSIS   B, HYPERPLASTIC ARTERIOLOSCLEROSIS   C, NECROTISING ARTERIOLITIS

FIGURE 15.2: Schematic illustration to show pathogenesis and morphology of arteriolosclerosis, commonly seen in hypertension. (PMNs, polymorphonuclear leucocytes; ECM, extracellular matrix).

Etiology Hypertension is the major cause and most often it affects the renal arterioles.
Pathogenesis It seems that the smooth muscle cells in the arteriolar wall have a *protective role* preventing arterial pressure induced damage of glomeruli.
- With time, injured arteriolar smooth muscle cells are replaced by collagenous fibrous tissue.
- Fibrous thickening of arterioles is usually combined with intimal fibrosis of larger renal arteries.
- Arteriolar and arterial fibrosis will uncontrollably reduce the blood flow to the kidneys stimulating renin secretion and thus contributing in a vicious cycle to arterial hypertension.

III. **Necrotising arteriolitis** is a feature of *malignant hypertension* affecting primarily the arterioles of the kidney.
i. *Sudden onset* of very high hypertension is a common cause of damage the arteriolar wall.
ii. Arteriolar injury is associated with *fibrinoid necrosis*.
iii. Deposits of fibrin attract neutrophils which infiltrate the vessel wall.

Q7. What is Mönkeberg arteriosclerosis?

Mönkeberg's arteriosclerosis is marked by *dystrophic calcification of the media of muscular arteries*, transforming arteries into pipestem-like rigid tubes.
Calcified arteries can be seen by X-rays (e.g. during mammography or abdominal CT-scan) but are of no clinical significance.

Q8. What is atherosclerosis? Discuss etiologic factors involved in its pathogenesis.

Definition Atherosclerosis is multifactorial disease involving the large and medium-sized arteries, resulting in thickening and hardening of their walls due to intimal fibrofatty plaques progressing to atheromas (derived from Greek words *atheros* meaning porridge, and *sclerosis* meaning scarring).

Etiology Atherosclerosis is a multifactorial disease. Major risk factors are divided into three groups **(Table 15.1)**:

I. *Major risk factors modifiable by life style and/or therapy*:
i. Lipid disorders
ii. Smoking
iii. Life-style factors such as diet, obesity, physical inactivity

II. *Constitutional non-modifiable risk factors*:
i. Age—atherosclerosis is an age-related disease!
ii. Sex—males affected more than female, and develop changes 10 years earlier.
iii. Genetic and familial factors—mostly involving the metabolism of lipids and lipoproteins, e.g. mutations of genes for:
- Lipoprotein-α
- Apolipoprotein-C
- LDL receptor

iv. Racial predisposition—atherosclerosis is less common in Black people than in White people.
III. *Non-traditional emerging risk factors and biomarkers* are of lesser significance and are mostly still under investigation.

TABLE 15.1 Risk factors in atherosclerosis.

I. MAJOR RISK FACTORS MODIFIABLE BY LIFESTYLE AND/OR THERAPY
1. Dyslipidaemia (High LDL, low HDL cholesterol)
2. Hypertension
3. Diabetes mellitus
4. Smoking
5. Lifestyle risk factors (atherogenic diet, obesity, physical inactivity)
II. CONSTITUTIONAL NON-MODIFIABLE RISK FACTORS
1. Age
2. Sex
3. Genetic factors
4. Familial and racial factors
III. NON-TRADITIONAL EMERGING RISK FACTORS
1. Environmental influences
2. Oestrogen hormone
3. Stressful behavioural pattern
4. Hyperhomocysteinaemia
5. Homocystinuria
6. Prothrombotic factors
7. Infectious burden
8. Excessive alcohol consumption
9. Biomarkers for risk assessment

(HDL, high-density lipoproteins; LDL, low-density lipoproteins).

Q9. What are the evidences that lipid disorders (dysplipidaemia) promote the development of atherosclerosis?

Disorders of lipid metabolism (dyslipidaemia) are the most firmly established major risk factors for atherosclerosis. The following data support this assertion as follows:
i. Atheromas and atherosclerotic plaques contain cholesterol and cholesterol esters derived from lipoproteins in the blood.
ii. Atherosclerotic lesions can be experimentally induced in animals by feeding them with a cholesterol-rich diet.
iii. Individuals with hypercholesterolaemia caused by various metabolic diseases such as diabetes mellitus, familial hypercholesterolaemia, myxoedema, etc. are at an increased risk for atherosclerosis.
iv. Treatment of persons with hypercholesterolaemia with cholesterol-reducing drugs lowers the risk of atherosclerosis-related diseases such as ischaemic heart disease or brain infarcts.

Q10. What are lipoproteins? What are their classes?

Definition Lipoproteins are biochemical complexes made up of lipids and proteins (called apoproteins) that circulate in the blood and transport cholesterol, triglycerides and fat-soluble vitamins.

Classification Major plasma lipoprotein fractions are listed in **Table 15.2**. In clinical practice, they are usually measured in conjunction with total serum cholesterol and triglycerides.

TABLE 15.2 Fractions of lipoprotein cholesterol in serum.

CLASSES	SITES OF SYNTHESIS	NORMAL SERUM LEVELS*	ROLE IN ATHEROSCLEROSIS
1. Total cholesterol	Liver, intestine	< 200 mg/dL	Maximum
2. LDL cholesterol	Liver	< 100 mg/dL	Maximum
3. VLDL-C/triglycerides	Intestine, liver	< 150 mg/dL	Less marked
4. HDL cholesterol	Liver, intestine	> 50 mg/dL	Protective
5. Chylomicrons	Liver, intestine, macrophage	—	Indirect

*Easy way to remember optimum desirable cut-off levels of serum lipids in mg/dL: it is a multiple of 50, i.e. <200 for cholesterol, <150 for VLDL (or triglycerides), <100 for LDL, and >50 for HDL.
Lipids can also be measured in plasma (EDTA blood); plasma values are 3% lower than in serum.
(HDL, high-density lipoproteins; LDL, low-density lipoproteins; VLDL, very low-density lipoproteins).

i. *Total cholesterol* Normal levels are 140–199 mg/dL. Levels of 200–240 mg/dL are borderline high. Levels over 260 mg/dL are associated with three time higher risk of atherosclerosis-related diseases.
ii. *Low-density lipoprotein cholesterol (LDL-C)* Optimal levels is <100 mg/dL. LDL is richest in cholesterol and has the maximum association with atherosclerosis.
iii. *Very-low-density lipoprotein cholesterol (VLDL-C)* Optimal level is <150 mg/dL. VLDL carries much of triglycerides and its serum level correlates with the levels of triglycerides.
iv. *High-density lipoproteins cholesterol (HDL-C)* Normal desirable serum level is >50 mg/dL. HDL is protective ('good cholesterol') against atherosclerosis.

Q11. How does hypertension affect the course of atherosclerosis?

Epidemiology Autopsy data show higher incidence of all forms of atherosclerosis in hypertensive persons.
- All major complications of atherosclerosis, such as myocardial infarction, cerebral stroke, aortic aneurysm formation occur at a higher rate in persons with hypertension.
- Incidence of ischaemic heart disease is five times higher in hypertensive persons than in normotensive age-matched controls.
- Medical control of hypertension will usually reduce the incidence of atherosclerosis. However, even treated hypertension is associated with increased incidence of IHD.

Pathogenesis Hypertension contributes to endothelial cell injury, thus initiating the formation of atherosclerotic plaques and atheromas.

Q12. How does smoking promote atherosclerosis?

Epidemiology Epidemiologic population data show that smoking is associated with higher incidence of IHD and sudden cardiac death.
- Geographic difference in the incidence of atherosclerosis correlates with the extent of smoking in various populations.
- Reduced smoking in some has reduced the incidence of IHD.

Pathogenesis Smoking could promote atherosclerosis by several mechanisms:
i. Reducing the serum levels of HDL-C
ii. Promoting blood coagulation
iii. Favouring accumulation of carbon monoxide (CO) in the blood
iv. CO produces carboxyhaemoglobin and eventually causing hypoxia of endothelial cells, thus favouring the formation of atherosclerotic plaques.

Q13. How does diabetes mellitus promote atherosclerosis?

Epidemiology Both type I and type II diabetes mellitus are risk factors for atherosclerosis.
i. The incidence of all forms of atherosclerosis is increased in all persons with diabetes, and especially those with uncontrolled diabetes.
ii. Atherosclerosis in diabetics appears earlier, the lesions are more severe and widespread.
iii. Diabetes is associated with increased incidence of major complications of atherosclerosis:
- Ischemic heart disease (IHD)—risk increased two times
- Cerebral ischaemia—risk increased 2–3 times
- Foot gangrene—risk increased 100 times

Pathogenesis The effects of diabetes on blood vessels are complex and include the following:
i. Endothelial cell injury/dysfunction
ii. Increased aggregation of platelets and increased coagulability of blood
iii. LDL-C levels ↑ in serum
iv. HDL-C levels ↓ in serum
v. Type II diabetes mellitus, frequently characterised by *'diabetic dyslipidaemia'* (high LDL-C, low HDL-C, elevated triglycerides).

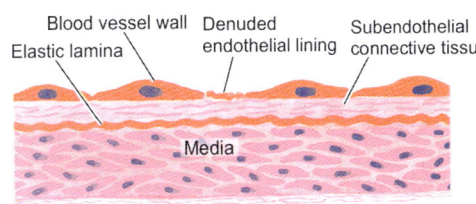

A, ENDOTHELIAL INJURY

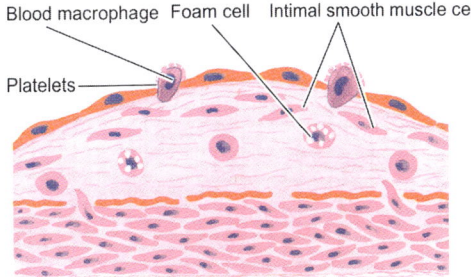

B, PLATELET ADHESION AND MONOCYTE MIGRATION

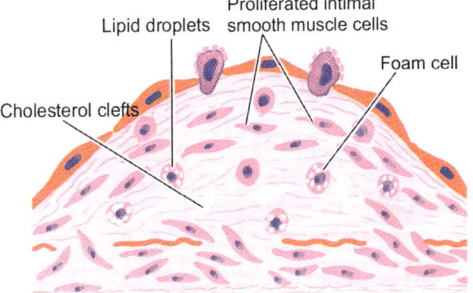

C, INTIMAL SMOOTH MUSCLE CELL PROLIFERATION

FIGURE 15.3: Diagrammatic representation of pathogenesis of atherosclerosis as explained by 'reaction-to-injury' hypothesis. A, Endothelial injury. B, Adhesion of platelets and migration of blood monocytes from blood stream. C, Smooth muscle cell proliferation into the intima and ingrowth of new blood vessels.

Q14. Discuss pathogenesis of atherosclerosis briefly.

Atherosclerosis is a multifactorial disease which is not completely understood.

Historic hypotheses (e.g. insudation hypothesis, encrustation hypothesis, monoclonal theory) have been replaced by **response to injury theory**, which includes the following three key components: endothelial injury, smooth muscle cell proliferation, and inflammation **(Fig. 15.3)**.

I. Endothelial injury
i. Experimental data show that injury to endothelial cells can be induced by many means, but in humans most important factors are *hypertension* and *dyslipidaemia*, leading to the entry of LDL into the vessel wall.

ii. Dysfunctional endothelial cells release *nitric oxide* and *endothelin*.
iii. Endothelial injury is typically followed by *adhesion of platelets* to the inner layer of the arteries.
iv. Aggregated platelets are a source of cytokines, such as *platelet derived growth factor (PDGF)*.

II. **Intimal smooth muscle proliferation and matrix protein secretion**
i. Smooth muscle cells which are normally present in the media are *stimulated by various cytokines* to proliferate and invade the intima.
ii. Inside the intima, smooth muscle cells change their secretory profile and begin *secreting matrix proteins* such as collagen, elastic fibres and proteoglycans.

III. **Inflammation**
i. Plasma LDLs entering into the intima are oxidised whereupon they attract *T-lymphocytes* and *monocytes*, which transform into macrophages.
ii. Oxidised LDLs are taken up by macrophages which transform into *foam cells*.
iii. Oxidised lipids are also cytotoxic for endothelial cells which are killed off, leaving surface defects that are filled with *fibrin, which attracts more platelets*.

Q15. What is the sequence of events in the pathogenesis of atheromas?

The sequence of events is illustrated in **Figure 15.4**.

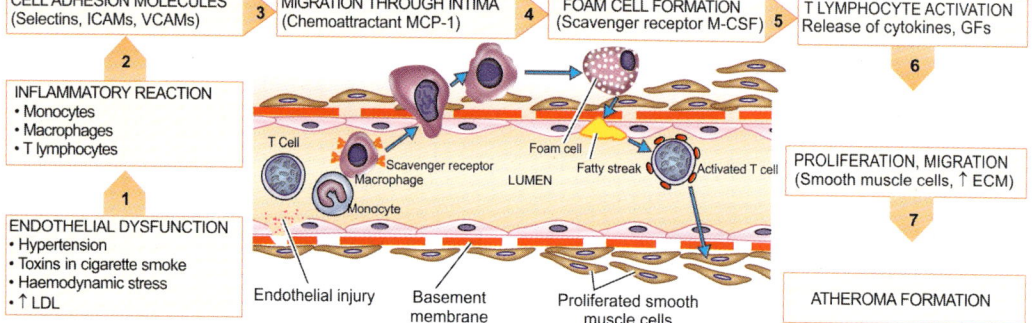

FIGURE 15.4: Pathogenesis of atheromatous plaques by response-to-injury theory. Sequential role of various factors is highlighted: endothelial dysfunction, inflammatory cells (monocytes, T lymphocytes) with release of proinflammatory mediators, modified macrophage foam cells, smooth muscle cell proliferation and ECM production, and evolution of various stages of atheroma (Modified from Kaperonis et al. Inflammation and atherosclerosis. *Eur J Vasc Endovasc Surg* 2006;31:386-93).

(LDL, low-density lipoproteins; ECM, extracellular matrix; VCAM, vascular cell adhesion molecule; ICAM, intercellular adhesion molecule; M-CSF, macrophage colony-stimulating factor; GF, growth factor).

i. Endothelial cell injury is the beginning of the sequence. It can be caused by mechanical factors (e.g. hypertension), chemical injury (e.g. dyslipidaemia, diabetes, smoking) or immunological insult.
ii. Dysfunctional endothelial cells differ from resting endothelial cells in several aspects:
• They secrete cytokines which stimulate inflammation.
• They display cell adhesion molecules for inflammatory cells and platelets which aggregate on the inner vascular surface.
• They are more permeable and allow the entry of LDL into the vessel wall, where these are oxidised.
iii. Endothelial cells and aggregated platelets secrete cytokines which stimulate the proliferation of smooth muscle cells displacing them from media into the intima.
iv. Inflammation mediated by cytokines attracts T-lymphocytes and monocytes, which transform into macrophages.
v. Macrophages produce additional cytokines which amplify the inflammation.
vi. Cytokines of various sources stimulate proliferation of smooth muscle cells and change the secretory functions of smooth muscle cells and fibroblasts.
vii. Oxidised LDLs contribute to the inflammation and are cytotoxic to endothelial cells, producing endothelial defects which are filled with fibrin, which traps more platelets.
viii. Macrophages takeup oxidised lipids transforming themselves into foam cells which account for the earliest changes of atherosclerosis, the *fatty streaks*.

ix. Various cytologic events, combined with inflammation and increased influx of LDL leads to necrosis of vessels wall, accumulation of extracellular lipid and fibrosis typical of fully developed atheroma.

Q16. Describe salient morphologic features of atherosclerosis.

Atherosclerosis begins with early precursor lesions (fatty streaks and dots, gelatinous lesions), which may progress to atheromatous plaques, and ultimately become complicated plaques **(Fig. 15.5)**:

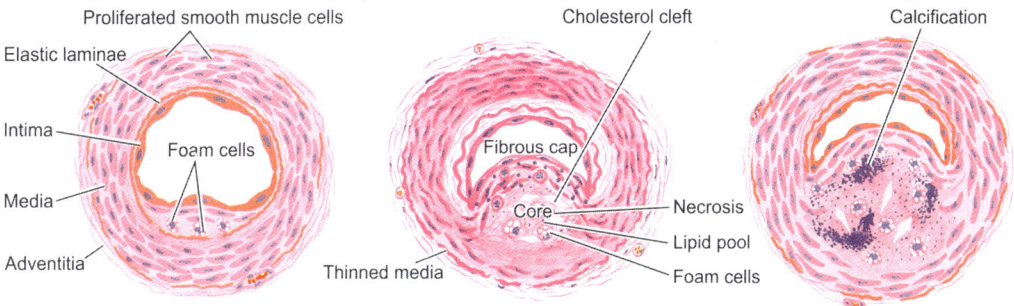

FIGURE 15.5: Schematic evolution of lesions in atherosclerosis.

I. **Early lesions**, such as fatty streaks and dots are flat or slightly elevated yellow intimal lesions, most commonly seen in the aorta.
Microscopy They consist of subintimal aggregates of lipid-laden foamy macrophages or smooth muscle cells. Accumulation of acellular ground substance results in formation of gelatinous lesions **(Fig. 15.5,A)**. All these changes start appearing in the first year of life and are of no clinical significance.
II. **Atheromatous plaques** are fully developed atherosclerotic lesions, also called *atheromas*. Most often, they are found in the aorta and its major branches, especially at their ostia **(Fig. 15.6,A)**. Atheromas protrude into the lumen of the artery and may cause its narrowing as illustrated in the coronary artery **(Fig. 15.5,B)**.
Microscopy Prototypical atheroma has three layers: a fibrous cap, which covers a more cellular area, and a central soft core.

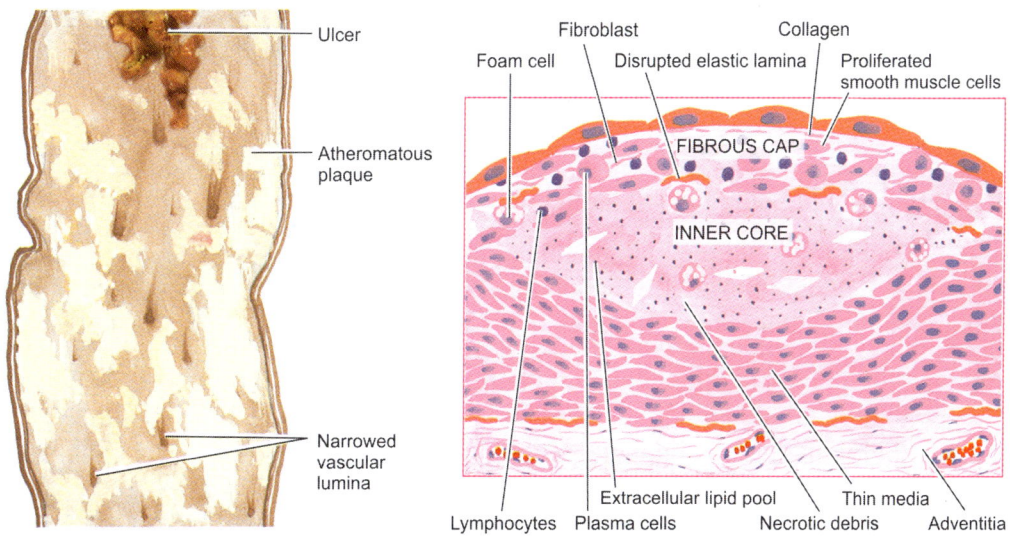

FIGURE 15.6: Structure of a fully-developed atheroma. A, The opened up inner surface of the abdominal aorta shows a variety of atheromatous lesions. While some are raised yellowish lipid-rich lesions elevated above the surface, a few whitish calcified areas and a thrombus overlying an ulcerated area (12 o'clock position). Orifices of some of the branches coming out of the wall are narrowed by the atherosclerotic process. B, Histologic appearance of a fully-developed atheroma in the intimal layer. Schematic image shows layers in the plaque: inner core and outer (luminal) fibrous cap.

i. *Fibrous cap* occupies the space underneath the endothelium and is composed predominantly of collagen, a few smooth muscle cells and fibroblasts. In older lesion, it may be composed of thick, hyalinised collagen.

ii. *Cellular area below the fibrous cap* contains macrophages, foam cell, lymphocytes and a few scattered smooth muscle cells.

iii. *Central soft core* consists of extracellular lipids, cholesterol crystals necrotic debris and fibrin, and scattered foam cells **(Fig. 15.6,B)**.

III. **Complicated plaques** show a variety of secondary changes as under (*see* **Fig. 15.5, C**):

i. *Calcification* contributing firmness to the arterial wall, but also causing fragility and cracking.

ii. *Ulceration* or an endothelial defect caused by the rupture of the fibrous cap of an expanded atheroma. Such rupture is accompanied by a discharge of semiliquid contents of atheroma into the lumen of the artery, and is common cause of thrombosis.

iii. *Thrombosis* may occur at the site of ulceration of atheroma or any other endothelial cell injury. Thrombi may occlude the lumen or medium-sized and smaller arteries. In the aorta, thrombi may fragment and give rise to emboli.

iv. *Haemorrhage* may occur into the lumen of an atheroma, into the wall of a major artery, or into the periarterial soft tissue following arterial rupture.

- Haemorrhage may result from the mechanical effects of atheromas which disrupt the integrity of the blood vessel.
- In the aorta, it may also result from the erosions of vasa vasorum or from rupture of an aneurysm.
- It may be combined with thrombosis.

v. *Aneurysm formation,* i.e. irregular dilatation of the arterial lumen due to pressure-induced thinning and rupture of the arterial wall.

Q17. What are the clinical consequences of atherosclerosis?

The clinical effects of atherosclerosis depend on the size and type of arteries affected, and the nature of the process that has caused the clinical findings. These clinical effects can be caused by the following events:

i. Slow luminal narrowing causing ischaemia and atrophy.
ii. Sudden luminal occlusion causing infarction necrosis.
iii. Propagation of plaque by formation of thrombi and emboli.
iv. Formation of aneurysmal dilatation and eventual rupture.

The most important clinical consequences of atherosclerosis, as they affect the major organ systems, are illustrated in **Figure 15.7** and are listed below:

i. *Heart:* Myocardial infarction, ischaemic heart disease.
ii. *Brain:* Chronic ischemic brain damage, cerebral infarction and stroke.
iii. *Aorta:* Aneurysm formation, thrombosis and embolisation to major organs.
iv. *Small intestine:* Ischaemic bowel disease, infarction.
v. *Lower extremities:* Intermittent claudication, gangrene.

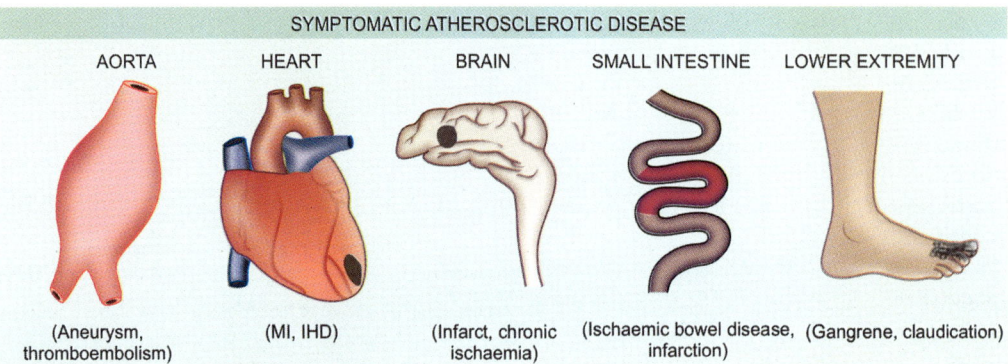

FIGURE 15.7: Major forms of symptomatic atherosclerotic disease.

Q18. Define vasculitis. How is it classified?

Definition Vasculitis is inflammation of blood vessels.
Classification Vasculitis can be classified according to several principles:
I. *Pathophysiologic classification*
i. *Primary vasculitis,* in which the involvement of the vessel is the sole or primary manifestation. For example, polyarteritis nodosa, hypersensitivity vasculitis.
ii. *Secondary vasculitis,* which is part of another disease, or the inflammation of the vessel develops due to the spread of the disease from some other tissue. For example, endarteritis obliterans involving the artery below a gastric peptic ulcer, or in the lungs involved by tuberculosis.

II. **Classification based on the distribution**
i. *Systemic vasculitis* involving the blood vessels of several organ systems or the entire body, such as hypersensitivity arteritis.
ii. *Localised vasculitis* involving only certain organs, such as temporal arteritis.
III. **Anatomic classification** based on the type of blood vessel involved, such as arteritis, aortitis, phlebitis (veins), capillaritis, etc.
IV. **Etiologic classification** is limited to arteries and divides all forms of vasculitis into two groups: infectious arteritis and non-infections arteritis. Various types in each category are listed in **Table 15.3**.

TABLE 15.3 Etiologic classification of vasculitis.

I. INFECTIOUS ARTERITIS
1. Endarteritis obliterans
2. Syphilitic arteritis
3. Non-specific infective arteritis
II. NON-INFECTIOUS ARTERITIS
1. Polyarteritis nodosa (PAN)
2. Hypersensitivity (allergic, leucocytoclastic) vasculitis
3. Wegener granulomatosis
4. Temporal (giant cell) arteritis
5. Takayasu arteritis (pulseless disease)
6. Kawasaki disease
7. Buerger disease (thromboangiitis obliterans)
8. Miscellaneous vasculitis

Q19. What are the typical features of syphilitic arteritis?

Definition Syphilitic arteritis is an infectious disease that involves blood vessels in all three stages of the disease (primary, secondary and tertiary) but is clinically most significant in *tertiary stage of syphilis* when it prominently affects the aorta and cerebral arteries.
Types Based on main sites of location of lesions, two types: syphilitic aortitis and cerebral syphilitic arteritis:
I. **Syphilitic aortitis** is a serious complication of tertiary syphilis predominantly involving the ascending aorta and the aortic arch.
Pathogenesis Treponema pallidum spreads through the lymphatics from infected lymph nodes in the mediastinum, selectively affecting the thoracic part of the aorta. Estimates are that only 10% of persons infected with *Treponema pallidum* develop aortitis.
Pathology The infection produces *endarteritis and periarteritis of aortic vasa vasorum*.
i. *Microscopy* Reveals infiltrates of plasma cells and lymphocytes in and around vasa vasorum **(Fig. 15.8)**.
ii. Obliteration of microvasculature in the wall of the aorta leads to focal ischaemia and subsequent fibrosis of damaged tissue. The puckering of the aortic tissue imparts to the intima a *'tree-bark appearance'*.
iii. The weakening of the aortic wall result in *aneurysmal dilatation* of the ascending aorta and aortic arch. Aneurysms develop in 40% of all cases of syphilitic aortitis. Complications of aortic aneurysms include:
- Rupture

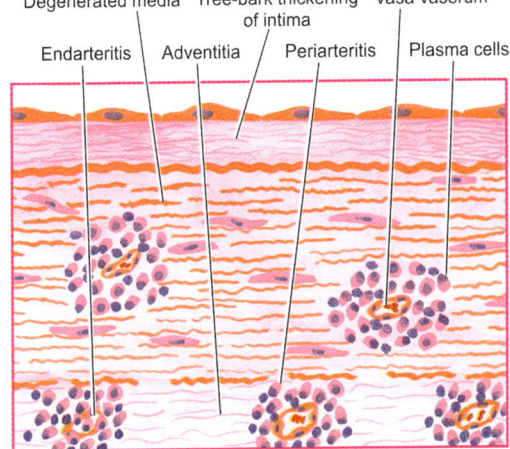

FIGURE 15.8: Syphilitic aortitis. There is endarteritis and periarteritis of the vasa vasorum in the media and adventitia. There is perivascular infiltrate of plasma cells, lymphocytes and macrophages.

- Compression of adjacent structures such as trachea (dyspnoea), oesophagus (dysphagia), recurrent laryngeal nerve (hoarseness), and bones (vertebrae, ribs, sternum).
- Cardiac dysfunction due to dilatation of the aorta that needs to be filled with each heart stroke, dilatation of the aortic valve with aortic insufficiency and compression of coronary arteries.

iv. Infection spreads from the aorta into the aortic valves causing *aortic insufficiency*.

v. Spreading infection may cause *narrowing of the coronary ostia* in 20% cases with myocardial ischaemia presenting as angina pectoris, IHD and even myocardial infarction.

II. **Cerebral syphilitic arteritis** involving small and medium-sized arteries is a feature of tertiary syphilis.

i. Vasculitis is similar to the changes in the aorta and is characterised by infiltrates of plasma cells and lymphocytes.

ii. Obliteration of blood vessels leads to focal ischaemic necrosis of the brain and major mental and neurologic disturbances (*generalised paralysis*).

Q20. Define small vessel vasculitis. Briefly discuss its classification and pathogenesis in general.

Definition Small vessel vasculitis is a group of diseases of unknown etiology, presumably of immune origin, involving arterioles, venules and capillaries.

Classification Following diseases are included as small vessel vasculitis:

i. Wegener granulomatosis (granulomatosis with polyangiitis)
ii. Microscopic polyangiitis
iii. Churg-Strauss syndrome (eosinophilic granulomatosis with polyangiitis)
iv. Henoch-Schönlein purpura (IgA vasculitis)
v. Cryoglobulinaemic vasculitis

Pathogenesis In support of the immune nature of small vessel vasculitis are the serologic data and the findings of autoantibodies, such as ANCA, in some of these patients.

Antineutrophil cytoplasmic antibodies (ANCAs):

- The name 'antineutrophil' is of historical origin since the antibodies were first identified as attacking neutrophils.
- Later, it was shown that these antibodies also react with other cells and with many bacterial polypeptides.
- Neutrophils are still used for their detection by immunofluorescence (IF) microscopy.

Two patterns of IF staining of ANCA are seen (*see* **Fig. 5.9**):

i. *Cytoplasmic (c-ANCA)* which reacts with proteinase-3 (PR-3) in azurophilic cytoplasmic granules in neutrophils, and, therefore, also called PR3-ANCA. This antibody is found in patients with active Wegener granulomatosis (granulomatosis with polyangiitis).

ii. *Perinuclear ANCA (p-ANCA)* which react with myeloperoxidase (MPO) and is, therefore, called MPO-ANCA. It is found in microscopic polyangiitis and Churg-Strauss syndrome, but also can be induced by some drugs, such as propylthiouracil.

Q21. Write briefly on polyarteritis nodosa.

Definition Polyarteritis nodosa (PAN) is a rare autoimmune disease (incidence 4:100,000) involving small and medium-sized arteries and presenting as segmental transmural inflammation with fibrinoid necrosis.

Etiology Unknown in the majority of cases. In 30% of patients it is mediated by antibodies to hepatitis B virus.

Pathogenesis Most often, arteries contain deposits of antibody complexes which activate complement and attract neutrophils. Underlying mechanism is as follows:

i. Circulating antibody reacting with an antigen in the blood vessel will form locally antigen-antibody complexes.

ii. Alternatively, preformed circulating antigen-antibody complexes are deposited in the vessel wall in hepatitis B virus infected persons.

iii. In both scenarios, antibodies activate complement and elicit an acute inflammation.

iv. Inflammation spreads transmurally and is usually accompanied by periarteritis, which accounts for the palpable nodularity of the vessels (hence the name 'nodosa').

v. Inflammation destroys the vessel wall and leads to formation of microaneurysms which often thrombose (another cause of palpable nodularity!).

vi. Inflammation is accompanied by thrombi inside the affected blood vessel that may cause ischaemia.
vii. Healing can lead to endarteritis obliterans occluding the vessel and reducing or interrupting the blood flow.
viii. Acute and chronic and healing stages of vasculitis may be found in the same patient.

Clinical features Symptoms of PAN are protean and vary from one patient to another. Symptoms depend on which organ is affected.
i. Any organ can be affected, but the lungs are typically spared.
ii. The most frequently affected organs are the kidneys and the GI tract.

Prognosis Good response to treatment with corticosteroid and cyclophosphamide induces immunosuppression.

Q22. Describe salient features of hypersensitivity vasculitis.

Definition Hypersensitivity vasculitis is a group of immunologically mediated acute diseases characterised by inflammation of small vessels (arterioles, venules and capillaries). It is also known as *allergic or leucocytoclastic vasculitis,* and *microscopic systemic polyangiitis,* which also indicates that it is not a single entity but rather a group of diseases.

It is the most common form of acute vasculitis.

Etiology
i. Most often, elicited by an immune reaction to drugs, in which case it involves only the skin, or skin and visible mucosae, such as the mouth or genitalia.
ii. Some cases develop as immune response to bacteria, or exogenous allergens.
iii. It may be part of clinicopathologic entities such as serum sickness, Henoch-Schönlein purpura, mixed cryoglobulinaemia.
iv. It may be part of systemic autoimmune diseases such as SLE or rheumatoid arthritis.

Location
i. It most often involves the skin and mucous membranes.
ii. Systemic microscopic polyangiitis involves also internal organs, most often kidneys, lungs, muscles, GI tract and brain.

Clinicopathologic features The findings are variable.
I. **Skin lesions** in early stages show deposits of immunoglobulin in small blood vessels.
i. Immunoglobulin deposits activate complement which attracts neutrophils to infiltrate the vessel wall (hence the alternative name 'leucocytoclastic vasculitis').
ii. The disease presents as 'vascular purpura'.
iii. These skin lesions are palpably indurated and do not blanch upon compression. In chronic form, the small blood vessels are infiltrated and surrounded by lymphocytes and plasma cells.
iv. Treatment with corticosteroids is beneficent.
II. **Henoch-Schönlein purpura** is a childhood disease.
i. The small blood vessels contain deposits of IgA.
ii. Vasculitis is associated with purpura and internal haemorrhage (e.g. GI bleeding or haematuria).
III. **Mixed cryoglobulinaemia** which may be idiopathic or associated with lymphoid malignancies is characterised by deposits of cryoglobulins.
IV. **Systemic microscopic polyangiitis** is usually of unknown etiology.
i. This vasculitis is not associated with immunoglobulin deposits ('pauci-immune').
ii. These patients are positive for MP-ANCA.
iii. They often develop pauci-immune glomerulonephritis, which responds to immunosuppressive treatment.

Q23. What is Wegener granulomatosis?

Definition Wegener granulomatosis (also known as *granulomatosis with polyangiitis*) is a necrotising vasculitis presenting with a triad that includes the following:
i. Necrotising granulomas of the upper and lower respiratory tract.
ii. Necrotising or granulomatous vasculitis affecting small to medium-sized vessels, most prominently in the upper and lower respiratory tract.
iii. Focal or diffuse necrotising crescentic glomerulonephritis.

Etiopathogenesis Unknown, but presumed to be immune mediated because the disease responds well to immunosuppressive treatment and the patients are PR3-ANCA positive.
Pathology Granulomas and polyangiitis (vasculitis) are found in all cases.
i. Granulomas show central fibrinoid necrosis and are infiltrated with neutrophils, lymphocytes, macrophages and multinucleated giant cells. Pulmonary granulomas tend to coalesce and cavitate due to widespread necrosis.
ii. Vasculitis which may be segmental or circumferential shows fibrinoid necrosis with inflammation.
iii. Renal changes vary from mild focal necrosis to diffuse necrotising glomerulonephritis with crescent formation.
Clinical findings
i. Chronic sinusitis, nasal mucosal ulceration with haemorrhage.
ii. Pneumonia with multifocal pulmonary infiltrates and cavities with dyspnoea and haemoptysis.
iii. Renal dysfunction often in form of rapidly progressive renal failure, related to focally necrotising crescentic glomerulonephritis.
iv. *Limited form of Wegener granulomatosis* has only respiratory tract symptoms without renal failure.
Prognosis Immunosuppressive treatment is efficient, but there is high rate of relapses progressing the end stage renal failure.

Q24. Discuss temporal (giant cell) arteritis briefly.

Definition Temporal arteritis is a granulomatous inflammation of medium-sized and large arteries, most often involving cranial arteries, especially temporal arteries, of elderly persons. It is the most common chronic arteritis in the elderly.
Etiopathogenesis Unknown.
- Granulomas and the presence of T lymphocytes in the vessel wall suggest a cell-mediated immune reaction.
- An association with polymyalgia rheumatica has been noted, supporting the immune etiology.

Pathology Non-necrotising granulomas involve the temporal artery and its branches, such as the ophthalmic artery but may also be found in other major arteries and even the aorta.
i. Granulomas are composed of T lymphocytes, macrophages and multinucleated giant cells; they are initially centered on the internal elastic lamina, causing its fragmentation.
ii. Granulomas tend to extend through all the layers of the vessel, causing thickening of the vessel wall.
iii. Intimal proliferation of smooth muscle cells and fibroblasts will markedly narrow the lumen of the artery.
iv. The narrowed lumen may contain a thrombus.
v. Similar changes are seen in the aorta and other arteries.
Clinical manifestations Temporal arteritis is a disease of old age. Its symptoms are related to local ischaemia.
i. Headaches are relentless and predominantly involve the temporal areas.
ii. Visual problems are common and may progress to blindness due to reduced blood flow through the granulomatous vasculitis of the ophthalmic artery.
iii. Thickened arteries can be palpated, and they may appear beaded on palpation.
iv. Surgical biopsy is important for the diagnosis but also may relieve pain.

Q25. What is Takayasu arteritis?

Definition Takayasu arteritis, also known as giant cell aortitis or pulseless disease, is a granulomatous vasculitis affecting chiefly the aortic arch and the major arteries originating from it.
Etiopathogenesis Unknown but presumed to be a disorder of T cell mediated immunity.
Pathology The disease has a predilection for the aortic arch and major arteries originating from it. Other parts of the aorta and the arteries originating from them are less commonly affected.
i. Granulomas are the hallmark of the disease; they are composed of T lymphocytes, macrophages and giant cells.
ii. There are also scattered infiltrates of T lymphocytes.
iii. Reactive fibrosis of intima and media leads to severe narrowing of the lumen of major arteries, resulting in ischaemic changes distal to this progressively obliterative vasculitis.

iv. Thrombosis in affected arteries is common.
v. In 30% of cases, the disease involves other parts of the aorta and its major branches, including the coronary arteries.
vi. In 50% cases, the pulmonary artery and its major branches are also involved.

Clinical manifestations It is most prevalent in Japan but may occur in other geographic regions as well.

i. *Age and sex* Takayasu disease affects predominantly young women; less common in women over the age of 50 years. By clinical convention, the disease in older women is simply called *giant cell arteritis,* rather than Takayasu disease, even though the pathologic changes are the same in both conditions.
ii. The clinical features of Takayasu disease are called *aortic arch syndrome* and include ocular manifestation, arm weakness and a lack of pulse in both arms *'pulseless disease'*).
iii. Advanced lesions cause neurologic deficits, blindness, IHD and myocardial infarction and pulmonary hypertension.
iv. Narrowing of the ostia of renal arteries may cause hypertension and renal insufficiency.

Prognosis The clinical course of the disease is unpredictable: it has a rapid downhill course in some patients, and it stabilises after initial progression in others.

Q26. Discuss Kawasaki disease in brief.

Definition Kawasaki disease, also known as 'mucocutaneous lymph node syndrome' is an acute or subacute febrile illness affecting mainly young children and infants, leading to the formation of aneurysms of coronary and some other arteries.

Etiology Unknown, but considered to be related to some infection and related immune disturbances.

Clinicopathologic features The disease affects children and infants.
i. It begins with fever, conjunctivitis, oral ulceration, skin rash and lymphadenopathy.
ii. Following this acute onset, most children develop necrotising arteritis with fibrinoid necrosis and acute inflammation resembling periarteritis nodosa and resulting in aneurysm formation.
iii. Coronary artery aneurysms are the most common findings at autopsy are most often involved.
iv. Other major arteries such as renal, mesenteric and hepatic arteries, may show aneurysmatic dilatation.

Q27. Discuss salient features of Buerger disease.

Definition Buerger disease is an inflammatory and thrombotic disease involving segments of small and medium-sized arteries and veins of the extremities, and also affecting peripheral nerves.

Etiopathogenesis Unknown, but most likely an interplay of genetic and environmental factors.
i. It affects mostly Asians and people of East European descent.
ii. Consistent association with *heavy cigarette smoking* indicates that tobacco may cause endothelial damage and initiate the disease, leading to thrombosis.
iii. Many patients have *anti-endothelial antibodies,* supporting the view that the endothelial cell injury is the primary event.
iv. *Genetic factors* play a role as evidenced by the fact that many patients have HLA-A9 and HLA-B5 antigens.

Clinicopathologic features
i. The disease begins with *intermittent claudication or Raynaud phenomenon* due to ischaemia caused by thrombotic endarteritis.
ii. Early pathology changes include segmental transmural areas of acute inflammation of arterial wall followed by intraluminal thrombosis **(Fig. 15.9)**.

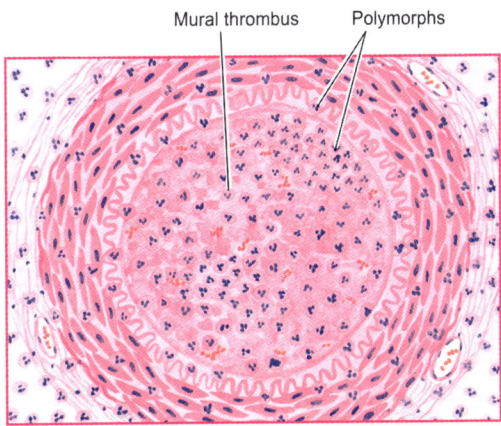

FIGURE 15.9: Buerger disease (Thromboangiitis obliterans). There is acute panarteritis. The lumen is occluded by a thrombus containing microabscesses.

iii. Inflammation is mediated by neutrophils which may even form small sterile abscesses in the wall of the artery or inside the thrombus. In later stages, chronic inflammatory cells replace the neutrophils and even may form granulomas.
iv. Inflammation spread to adjacent nerves and veins causing thrombophlebitis, which can present as palpable nodularity of leg veins.
v. Involvement of the nerves is associated with relentless pain.
vi. Healing of acute inflammation results in fibrosis with organisation of the thrombus and periarterial fibrosis involving the vein and the nerves.
vii. Obliterative endarteritis and venous congestion due to venous thrombi may cause ischaemic leg ulcers or gangrene.
Prognosis In early stages of the disease, cessation of smoking can prevent the progression of the disease, but once the vessel obliteration ensues, the extremities must be amputated.

Q28. What is Raynaud phenomenon?

Definition Raynaud phenomenon is a functional vasospastic condition affecting small arteries and arterioles and resulting in inadequate blood flow to extremities, especially fingers and hands.
Classification Raynaud phenomenon can be primary or secondary:
I. **Primary Raynaud phenomenon** (also known as *Raynaud disease*) is characterised by excessive vasoconstriction of small arteries and arterioles that occurs without any underlying vascular disease.
i. Vasospasms may be precipitated by cold, emotions or occur without any known reasons.
ii. The cause of vasospasms is not known but most likely they result from disautonomia, i.e. dysfunctions of the sympathetic and parasympathetic systems.
iii. It affects 3–5% of the entire population and it is most often seen in young women.
iv. Vasospasms of this kind rarely have significant clinical consequences.
v. In a minority of patients, recurrent vasospasms may impair movements and strength of fingers or cause atrophy of skin and muscles.
NOTE: The diagnosis of primary Raynaud phenomenon should be made only after the major causes of secondary Raynaud disease have been excluded.
II. **Secondary Raynaud phenomenon** is characterised by vasoconstriction related to some identifiable underlying disease such as under:
i. Autoimmune collagen vascular diseases, e.g. scleroderma, SLE
ii. Vasculitis, e.g. Buerger disease, polyarteritis nodosa
iii. Atherosclerosis
iv. Haematologic diseases, e.g. multiple myeloma, Waldenström macroglobulinaemia, polycythaemia.
Clinical features
i. Sudden vasospasm of small arteries and arterioles leads to sudden blanching of the skin.
ii. Pallor is best observed on fingers which become pale and cold, except for their tips and base.
iii. Tips of the fingers appear bluish due to venous congestions over distal phalanges.
iv. Stagnation of arterial blood proximal to the vasospasm accounts for the red color of the base of the fingers and hand.
v. These tricolour changes are transitory and reversible.

Q29. What are aneurysms and how are they classified?

Definition Aneurysms are permanent dilatations of a vessel due to congenital or acquired weakening or destruction of the vessel wall. Most often, they involve large elastic arteries like the aorta and its major branches.
Classification Aneurysms are classified on the basis of composition of the wall, shape, and pathogenesis as under:
I. **Composition of the wall**
i. *True aneurysm* composed of all the layers of a normal vessel wall.
ii. *False aneurysm* whose wall consists of fibrous tissue, most often due to a trauma to the vessel.

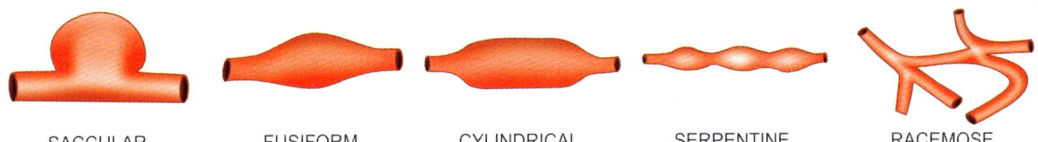

FIGURE 15.10: Common shapes of aneurysms of various types.

II. *Shape*
Aneurysms may have several shapes **(Fig. 15.10)**:
i. *Saccular* in form of a spherical sac-like outpouching.
ii. *Fusiform* in form of a symmetrical spindle shaped dilatation.
iii. *Cylindrical* in form of a cylinder or tube-like dilatation with symmetrical straight sides.
iv. *Serpentine or varicose* in form of a tortuous dilatation along the course of the vessel.
v. *Racemose or cirsoid* comprising a mass of intercommunicating small arteries and veins.

III. *Pathogenesis*
i. *Atherosclerotic* (the most common, typically involving the abdominal aorta).
ii. *Syphilitic*, as a feature of tertiary syphilis.
iii. *Dissecting*, resulting from a haematoma between the layers of the vessel; in the aorta it is also called aortic dissection.
iv. *Mycotic* resulting from weakening of the vessel wall by local purulent bacterial infection, which destroy part of the vessel wall.
v. *Berry aneurysms* are small saccular aneurysms formed at the weak point at the bifurcation of arteries of the circle of Willis.
The most common sites of these various aneurysms are depicted in **Figure 15.11**.

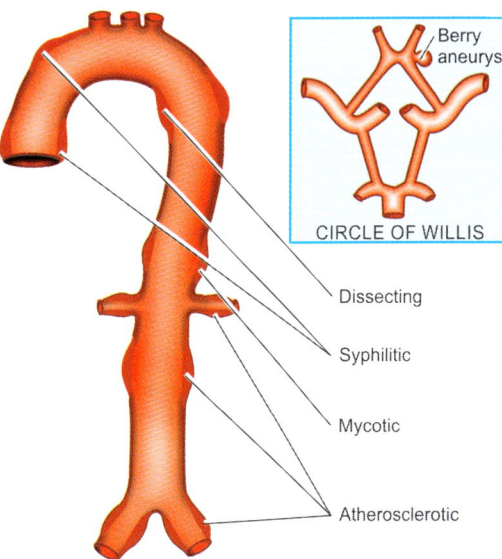

FIGURE 15.11: Sites of major forms of aneurysms.

Q30. Briefly discuss aortic dissection.

Definition Aortic dissection results from accumulation of blood between the layers of the aortic wall forming a slit space transforming into a blood-filled cavity between the separated layers. It is also called dissecting aneurysms of the aorta or dissection aortic haematoma.

Etiopathogenesis Several factors play a role but the most important are mechanical and structural factors in the wall of the aorta, as under:
i. *Hypertension*
a. It is found in 90% of cases.
b. Hypertension damages the media causing cystic medial necrosis.
c. Directs the stream of blood between the separated layers.
ii. *Genetic weakness of the connective* tissue as in Marfan syndrome.
iii. *Old age degeneration of aortic media* (cystic medial necrosis of Erdheim).
iv. *Iatrogenic trauma* during cardiac catheterisation or coronary bypass surgery.
v. *Pregnancy* for unknown reasons (rare).

Pathology Haematoma is the most prominent finding at autopsy **(Fig. 15.12)**.
Gross Haematoma forms most often between the layers of the outer and middle third of the aortic wall. The blood enters the wall of the aorta at the site of an intimal tear. Intramural haematoma extends at a variable length distally into the thoracic and even abdominal aorta.
i. Intimal tear through which the blood enters into the wall of the aorta is located in the ascending aorta in 70% of all cases.

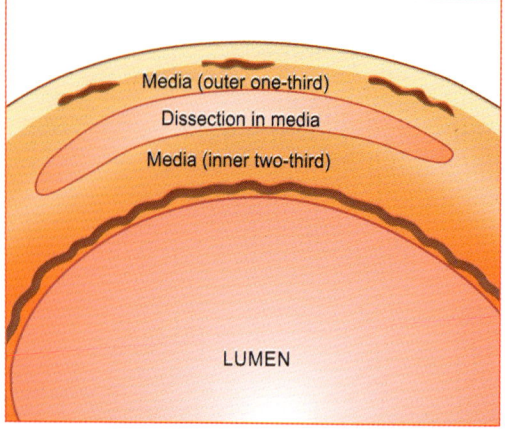

FIGURE 15.12: Aortic dissection (dissecting aneurysm aorta). Schematic drawing showing aortic dissection in cross section, typically separating the intima and inner two-thirds of the media on *luminal* side, from the *outer* one-third of the media and the adventitia.

ii. In 5% cases it is in the arch and in 20% in descending thoracic aorta near the origin of subclavian artery. The site of tear is used for clinical classification of dissections **(Fig. 15.13)**.

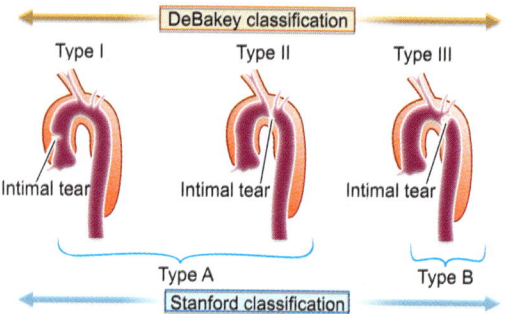

FIGURE 15.13: Two classification schemes of thoracic aortic dissection: Stanford and DeBakey. Stanford type A involving ascending aorta only includes DeBakey's type I (involving ascending aorta and extending into descending aorta as well) and II (limited to ascending aorta only), while Stanford type B is limited to descending aorta corresponds to DeBakey type III.

Microscopy In most cases, features of so called *cystic medial necrosis* are seen as under:
i. Separation of fibromuscular and elastic tissue of the media.
ii. Numerous cystic spaces filled with basophilic ground substance.
iii. Fragmentation of elastic fibres.
iv. Increased fibrosis of the media.

Clinical features and complications
i. Dissection of the aorta is accompanied by *sharp persistent pain in the chest* radiating into the abdomen.
ii. Rupture of the haematoma is accompanied by formation of a *periaortic haematoma*.
iii. Ruptured dissection is lethal in 90% cases. It is accompanied by *massive hypotension*, shock and loss of consciousness.
iv. Haematoma in the ascending aorta may compress the coronaries and cause *myocardial ischaemia* and even myocardial infarction.
v. *Disruption of aortic valves* may cause aortic insufficiency.
vi. Haematoma compressing the branches of the aorta causes *ischaemia in parts of the body*, most prominently evident in the brain.

Q31. What are varicosities?

Definition Varicosities are dilations of veins.
Classification Clinicopathologic terms are applied for varicosities in different parts of the body as under:

i. *Varicose vein* is the term used for varicosities of the leg veins, which may be superficial or deep.
ii. *Oesophageal varices* are a sign of portal hypertension, and are typically seen patients with cirrhosis.
iii. *Haemorrhoids* are submucosal anal varicosities involving the haemorrhoidal plexus.
iv. *Varicocele* involving the testicular veins in the spermatic cord.

Q32. What are varicose veins of lower extremities?

Definition Varicose veins are dilated veins seen most often on lower extremities.
- Varicose veins are found in 10–12% of the general population, clinically appearing most often in the 4th and 5th decade.
- Females are affected more than males, and are especially prone to develop them during pregnancy.

Etiopathogenesis Varicose veins develop due to the interaction of several factors as under:
i. Familial weakness of vein walls and valves is the most common cause.
ii. Increased intraluminal pressure due to prolonged standing posture in various professions (e.g. surgeons, policemen).
iii. Compression of iliac veins, e.g. during pregnancy, pelvic tumours.
iv. Hormonal effects on smooth muscle.
v. Obesity.
vi. Chronic constipation with straining during defaecation.

Pathology Varicose veins of lower extremities most often involve the *saphenous vein* and its tributaries:
i. The veins are tortuous and the venous valves are incompetent for allowing the backflow of the blood.
ii. Stagnant blood causes fibrosis of the venous wall.
iii. There is an increased incidence of venous thrombi.
NOTE: *Phlebothrombosis* of deep veins of extremities or *deep vein thrombosis (DVT)* accounts for 90% of all clinically diagnosed venous thrombi.
iv. Some of the thrombi get organised contributing to fibrous thickening of the venous wall, with foci of calcification.
v. Organising thrombi may be accompanied by inflammation (*thrombophlebitis*).
vi. Some thrombi give rise to emboli and cause pulmonary embolism.

Clinical features Varicose veins cause *venous stasis* in the lower extremities with following consequences:
i. Oedema of the soft tissue and skin.
ii. Capillary bleeding into soft tissue and dermis with accumulation of haemosiderin imparting the skin a brown colour.
iii. Fibrosis of soft tissues and dermis.
iv. Chronic dermatitis.
v. Ischaemic ulceration of the skin (*chronic varicose ulcers*).

Q33. What are the most important clinical variants of phlebothrombosis?

I. **Thrombophlebitis migrans**, also known as *migratory thrombophlebitis* or *Trousseau syndrome*.
i. It is characterised by the appearance of thrombi in large and medium-sized veins that appear and then disappear, to reappear in other sites.
ii. It is a paraneoplastic syndrome originally described in patients with pancreatic and gastric cancer, but also found in other forms of cancer as well.
II. **Phlegmasia alba dolens**, meaning in Latin 'painful white leg' is most often a complication of iliofemoral thrombosis.
i. Typically, it can occur during pregnancy or in patients who had pelvic surgery or cancer.
ii. Pulmonary emboli originating from pelvic venous thrombi are a common complication.
III. **Phlegmasia cerulea dolens**, meaning in Latin 'painful blue leg'.
i. It refers to markedly swollen bluish skin of the leg affected by superficial gangrene.
ii. Similar to white phlegmasia, it is a complication of iliofemoral thrombosis and decreased arterial blood inflow.
IV. **Superior vena caval syndrome** refers to occlusion of the superior vena cava due to thrombosis or external compression of the large veins.
i. It may be caused by lung cancer, mediastinal lymphoma or tuberculosis.
ii. Clinical features include dilated veins of neck and thorax, oedema of the face, neck and upper chest, and visual disturbances.
V. **Inferior vena caval syndrome** refers to obstruction of inferior vena cava.
i. Most often, it is caused by caval venous thrombi representing an extension of thrombi in iliofemoral veins.

ii. External compression and invasion of veins by cancer are other possible causes.
iii. Clinically, it presents with massive oedema of legs, dilatation of leg veins and terminally development of collateral venous channel in the lower abdomen.

Q34. What is lymphangitis? Discuss its etiopathogenesis and clinicopathologic features.

Definition Lymphangitis is an inflammation of the lymphatics that occurs in the course of many bacterial infections, which may be acute or chronic.

Etiopathogenesis
- *Acute lymphangitis* is most often caused by streptococcal or staphylococcal infections but may have other causes as well.
- *Chronic lymphangitis* is a feature of chronic infections such as tuberculosis, syphilis, actinomycosis.

Clinicopathologic features These depend on the duration of infection; i.e. acute or chronic.

I. *Acute lymphangitis*
i. It accompanies local infection of the skin or soft tissue and involves lymphatics draining and infected area.
ii. It is marked by dilatation of inflamed lymphatics which appear as red streaks corresponding to a lymphatic drainage area.
iii. *Microscopy* The lymphatics contain acute inflammatory cells, which may be found around the lymphatics in soft tissue as well.
iv. Typically, it is associated with acute lymphadenitis.
v. It heals spontaneously after the local infection has been cured.

II. *Chronic lymphangitis*
i. It results from recurrent bouts of acute lymphangitis of chronic infections like tuberculosis or syphilis.
ii. Affected lymphatics show persistent fibrosis of their walls and perilymphatic soft tissue and microscopic chronic inflammation.

Q35. What is lymphoedema?

Definition Lymphoedema is a swelling caused by local accumulation of lymph in soft tissues.

Clinicopathologic features Lymphoedema may be primary (idiopathic) or secondary (obstructive), and present in several clinical forms:

I. **Congenital lymphoedema** is primary lymphoedema which occurs in two forms:
i. *Milroy disease* affecting one limb, but sometime also involves the lips and the eyelids. It is inherited as an autosomal dominant trait and often associated with other abnormalities. It results from abnormal development of lymphatics which appear dilated like honeycomb. Recurrent bacterial infections are commonly superimposed on the affected area.
ii. *Simple congenital lymphoedema* occurs at random with no obvious reasons. It involves various parts of the body. The best known example is web-neck oedema in Turner syndrome.

II. **Lymphoedema praecox** is a primary lymphoedema affecting young women. It begins on the foot spread upwards. With time there is induration of the entire limb. Over time, the pitting oedema transforms into a non-pitting form.
Etiology Unknown. Probably it is related to female hormones and genital tract, because it occurs predominantly in women and is aggravation during the menstrual period.

III. **Secondary (obstructive) lymphoedema** is more common than the congenital form.
Etiology Obstruction of the lymphatic drainage can be caused by the following:
i. Lymphatic invasion and obstruction by malignant tumour.
ii. Surgical removal of lymph nodes and lymphatics (e.g. axillary lymph node dissection in breast carcinoma patients).
iii. Postradiation fibrosis of lymphatics.
iv. Parasitic infestation (e.g. filariasis producing elephantiasis of lower extremities).
Clinicopathologic features Obstructive oedema develops only if collateral lymph circulation does not develop to relieve the consequences of obstruction.
i. Lymph accumulates distal to the obstruction. Initially lymph distends the lymphatics, but thereafter it permeates the soft tissues causing more fibrosis and chronic non-pitting oedema.
ii. Fibrosis of interrupted lymphatics is hard to repair and therefore obstructive oedema persists for long time if not for ever.

Complications Dilated lymphatics and distended lymph ducts may rupture and the lymph fluid may enter body cavities (*chylothorax, chylopericardium, chyloperitoneum*) or it appear in urine (*chyluria*).

Q36. How are the vascular tumours classified?

- Vascular tumours can be classified as *benign* or *malignant (sarcomas).*
- Low grade malignant tumours are separated from sarcomas and form the third category named *tumours of intermediate grade*. Haemangioendothelioma is such a tumour of intermediate grade.
- Under the heading of vascular tumours, we currently also include certain *tumour-like malformations* (e.g. arteriovenous malformations) and *reactive proliferations* like bacillary angiomatosis caused by *Bartonella henselae* in immunocompromised persons.

Q37. Briefly discuss the most important benign vascular tumours.

Benign vascular tumours are very common and often quite visible since many of them occur in the skin and mucosal surfaces. The most common tumours in this group are haemangiomas, which are histologically subclassified in several forms. The most important examples are discussed below.

I. **Capillary haemangiomas** are composed of capillaries filled with blood **(Fig.15.14)**.
i. Most often they are small.
ii. They are most often found on the skin and mucosal surfaces of small children.
iii. Many regress spontaneously.

II. **Cavernous haemangiomas** are composed of dilated ('cavernous') vascular spaces lined by flattened endothelial cells and filled with blood **(Fig. 15.15)**.
i. They are usually bigger than capillary haemangiomas.
ii. They may occur both on the skin (especially head and neck) and internal organs.

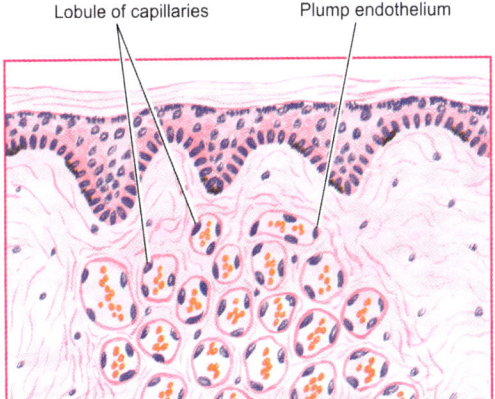

FIGURE 15.14: Capillary haemangioma of the skin. There are capillaries lined by plump endothelial cells and containing blood. The intervening stroma consists of scant connective tissue.

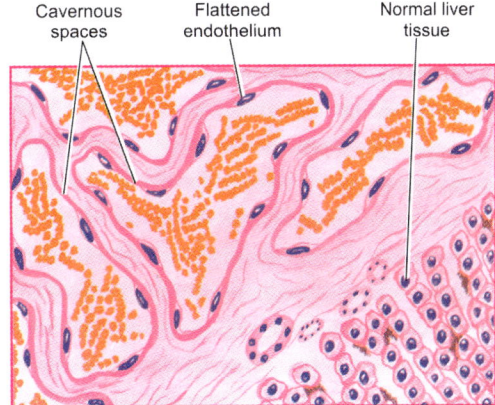

FIGURE 15.15: Cavernous haemangioma of the liver. The vascular spaces are large, dilated, many containing blood, and are lined by flattened endothelial cells. Scanty connective tissue stroma is seen between the cavernous spaces.

III. **Granuloma pyogenicum** presents as a benign nodular exophytic mass on the gingiva, oral mucosa or skin.
i. Typically, these nodules develop following traumatic tissue injury.
ii. *Microscopy* They are composed of capillaries and stroma resembling granulation tissue.
iii. A tumour of the same histologic type occurs on the gingiva of pregnant women and is called *pregnancy tumour* or *granuloma gravidarum*.

IV. **Lymphangioma** is a benign tumour of lymphatic capillaries, corresponding to haemangioma.
i. It can be capillary or cavernous **(Fig. 15.16)**.
ii. Cavernous lymphangioma is most often found in the head and neck region.
iii. In neonates, it may attain a huge size and is then called *cystic hygroma*.

V. **Glomus tumour** is an uncommon benign tumour arising from contractile glomus cells present in the arteriovenous shunts.
i. These tumours are found most often in the dermis of the fingers or toes under a nail.

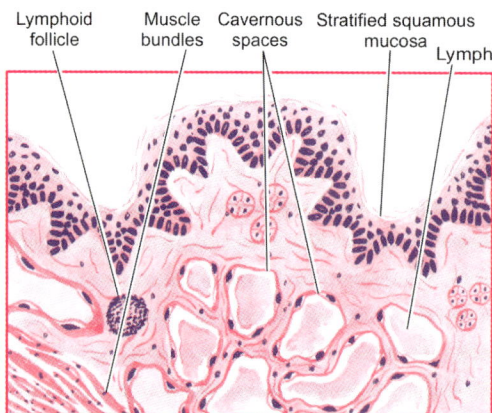

FIGURE 15.16: Cavernous lymphangioma in the soft tissues. Large cystic spaces lined by the flattened endothelial cells and containing lymph are present. Stroma shows scattered collection of lymphocytes.

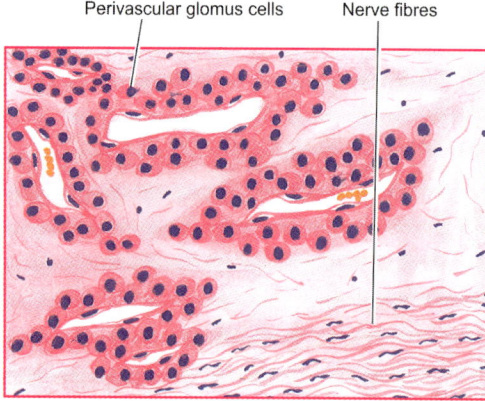

FIGURE 15.17: Glomus tumour. There are blood-filled vascular channels lined by endothelial cells and surrounded by nests and masses of glomus cells.

ii. These lesions are characterised by extreme pain.
iii. *Microscopy* The tumours are composed of small blood vessels surrounded by aggregates, nests and masses of glomus cells **(Fig. 15.17)**. The intervening connective tissue stroma contains some non-myelinated nerve fibres.

Q38. What are the most important malignant vascular tumours?

Two most important malignant vascular tumours are angiosarcoma and Kaposi sarcoma.
I. **Angiosarcoma**
Definition It is a malignant vascular tumour composed of neoplastic endothelial cells forming incomplete vascular spaces.
Etiology The cause of most angiosarcomas is unknown.
i. Some angiosarcomas develop after medical interventions such as angiosarcoma of the breast following therapeutic irradiation, or lymphangiosarcoma following long standing post-mastectomy lymphoedema.
ii. Angiosarcoma of the liver has been recorded in increased numbers in polyvinyl industry workers and farmers exposed to arsenical pesticides.
Clinical and gross Angiosarcomas most often develop in skin and soft tissues, but may occur in any or all internal organs.
i. Tumours of the skin usually begin as circumscribed red nodules. Nodules grow into larger irregularly shaped haemorrhagic masses with invasive margins.
ii. In the internal organs, angiosarcomas are diagnosed as haemorrhagic necrotic masses with indistinct margins.
Microscopy
i. Tumours are composed of plump spindle cells which express immunohistochemical markers of endothelial cells (e.g. CD31).
ii. Tumour cells may be *well differentiated* forming capillary-like spaces or *poorly differentiated* forming solid cords with rudimentary markings of their endothelial nature.
iii. Haematogenous metastases are common and most often found in the lungs.
iv. Overall five-year survival is 30%.
II. **Kaposi sarcoma**
Definition Kaposi sarcoma is a malignant vascular tumour caused by human herpes virus 8 (HSV-8 also known as Kaposi sarcoma-associated herpes virus, KSHV).
Classification Four clinical/epidemiologic forms of Kaposi sarcoma are recognised:
i. *Classic Kaposi sarcoma* affects men over 60 years of age of Eastern European, Mediterranean and Middle Eastern origin.

a. It presents with slow-growing multiple, small, purple plaques and dome-shaped nodules on the skin of the lower extremities.
b. The disease usually remains localised to the extremities and can be treated surgically with excellent results.
c. Spread to internal organs occurs rarely.
ii. *African (endemic) Kaposi sarcoma* is a common disease in equatorial Africa.
a. In addition to skin lesions, lymph node involvement is common, and even visceral lesions could be found.
b. It affects children and young men under the age of 40 years.
c. Clinical course is relatively indolent in adults but in children it could be quite aggressive, involving viscera with a lethal outcome.
iii. *Epidemic (AIDS-associated) Kaposi sarcoma* is seen in AIDS cases, and is actually one of the AIDS defining diseases.
a. Most commonly it affects male homosexuals.
b. The lesions are not limited to the skin of the lower extremities and often involve oral mucosa, other mucosal surfaces, lymph nodes and internal organs.
c. Most of these patients die of opportunistic infections and less than 10% of these patients die of Kaposi sarcoma.
iv. *Transplantation-associated Kaposi sarcoma* is a consequence of immunosuppression induced for transplantation of solid organs.
a. It often involves lymph nodes, mucosal surfaces and internal organs. Skin lesions are less prominent and may not be evident at all.
b. The rapid down-hill course of this form of Kaposi sarcoma may be reversed by reducing the extent of immunosuppression.
Etiopathogenesis Kaposi sarcoma is caused by HSV-8, which can be demonstrated in tumour cells in essentially all cases.
i. Sexual transmission of HSV-8 takes place in AIDS-associated Kaposi sarcoma.
ii. The route of infection is less obvious in other forms of Kaposi sarcoma but could include transdermal or transmucosal virus transmission.
iii. HSV-8 infects endothelial cells stimulating their proliferation and inhibiting apoptosis.
iv. Immunosuppression facilitates the proliferation of infected endothelial cells.
v. HIV interacts with HSV-8 contributing to the proliferation of infected endothelial cells.

Pathology
i. The early skin lesions consist of irregular dilated capillaries surrounded by chronic inflammatory cells and extravasated blood and haemosiderin-laden macrophages.
ii. Subsequently, the lesions are more cellular and consist of spindle cells of endothelial origin surrounded by extravasated red blood cells, which also fill the slit like vascular spaces between the endothelial cells **(Fig. 15.18)**.

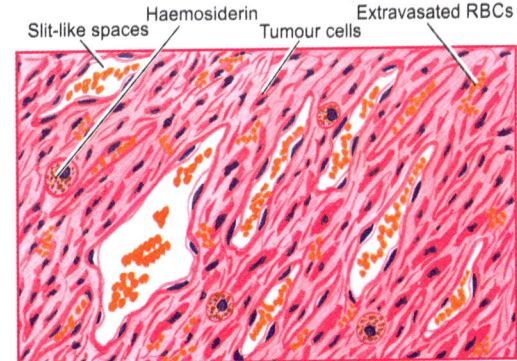

FIGURE 15.18: Kaposi sarcoma in late nodular stage. There are slit-like blood-filled vascular spaces with extravasated RBCs in the intercellular slit-like space. The tumour cells are arranged as bands of plump spindle-shaped cells.

Chapter 15e Supplement: Online Content
Digital content of this chapter available with this book is meant for enhanced learning and self-assessment. In addition, it contains 29 Multiple Choice Questions (MCQs), 05 Clinicopathologic Vignettes, and 07 Image-based Questions; these are followed by their answers along with explanatory notes of correct and incorrect answers.

CHAPTER 16

Heart

Q1. Briefly recall the key aspects of anatomy and histology of heart which are important for learning cardiac diseases.

Chambers Heart has four chambers: a right and a left atrium lying superiorly, and a right and left ventricle lying inferiorly to the atria **(Fig. 16.1)**.
- The atria are separated from each other by a thin fibro-muscular partition called *interatrial septum*.
- Both the ventricles are separated from each other by a thick muscular partition called *interventricular septum*.

Valves They separate atria from ventricles, and ventricles from great vessels.
- Atria are separated from ventricles by the flap-like *atrioventricular valves*, called the tricuspid (3 cusps) and the mitral valve (2 cusps).
- Ventricles are separated from the pulmonary artery and aorta respectively by semilunar tricuspid valves, called *pulmonary and aortic valve*.

Conduction system It regulates the rate of contraction and their rhythm.

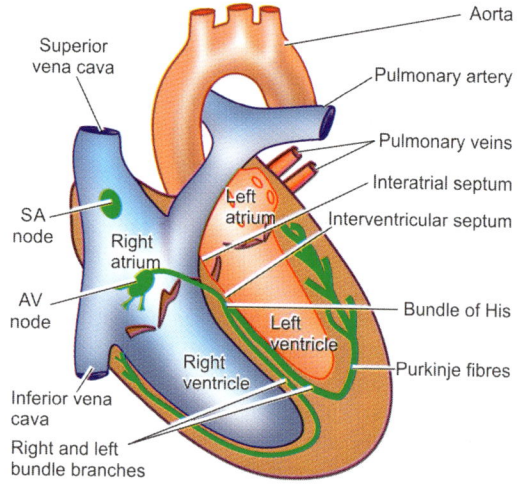

FIGURE 16.1: The normal anatomic structure of the heart. (SA, sinoatrial; AV, atrioventicular).

- The pacemaker of cardiac contractions is *the sinoatrial node*, which is in the right atrium.
- *The atrioventricular node* is located on the top of the interventricular septum, through which it is contiguous with the bundle of His.
- *The bundle of His* extends into left and right bundle branches which arborise in the respected ventricular walls.

Microscopy The heart is composed of three layers:

i. *Endocardium* covers the inside of heart chambers and the valves. It consists of connective tissue which is covered on its inner surface with endothelial cells, similar to those that line the inside of blood vessels.

ii. *Myocardium* is composed of a syncytium of striated muscle cells (cardiac myocytes), terminally differentiated cells that cannot regenerate. The contractile apparatus of cardiac myocytes is arranged into sarcomeres, which represent the structural and functional units of each cell.

iii. *Pericardium* covers the external surface of the heart. It consists of two layers: the inner *visceral pericardium (or epicardium)* and outer fibrous pericardial sac formed by the *parietal pericardium*. The epithelial layer of the pericardium is called mesothelium, like the epithelium of the pleura and peritoneum. Mesothelial cells have a cytoskeleton composed of cytokeratin.

Q2. What are the main coronary arteries?

The arterial blood is supplied to the heart through the coronary arteries which originate from the aorta immediately above the aortic semilunar valves. There are three major coronary trunks, each providing the blood to a defined part of the heart as follows **(Fig. 16.2)**:

I. **The anterior descending branch of the left coronary artery** (also known as left anterior coronary artery, LAD) supplies the apex, anterior surface of the left ventricle, the adjacent third of the anterior wall of the right ventricle, and the anterior two-thirds of the interventricular septum.

II. **The circumflex branch of the left coronary artery** (commonly called left circumflex branch, LCX) supplies the left atrium and a small portion of the lateral left ventricle.

III. **Right coronary artery**, abbreviated RCA, supplies the right atrium, the remainder of the anterior surface of the right ventricle, the adjacent half of the left ventricle, and posterior third of the interventricular septum.

The most common pattern of distribution is based on right coronary artery preponderance.

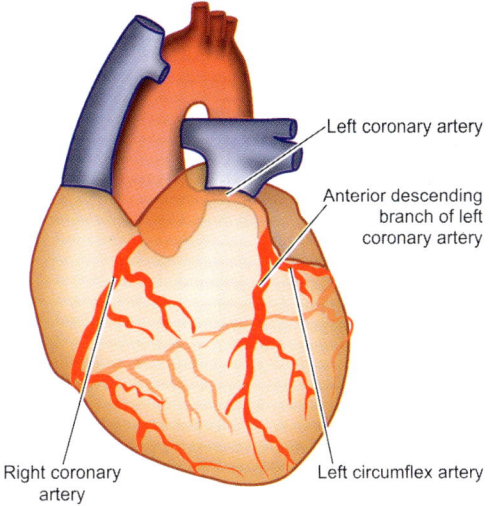

FIGURE 16.2: Distribution of blood supply to the heart.

Q3. Discuss heart failure in brief.

Definition Heart failure is a pathophysiologic state in which the impaired cardiac function is unable to maintain an adequate circulation for the metabolic needs of the organs and tissues of the body.

Etiopathogenesis The causes of heart failure can be grouped under three headings: i) intrinsic pump failure, ii) increased heart workload on the heart, and iii) impaired filling of chambers during diastole.

I. *Intrinsic pump failure* due to weakening of the ventricular muscle is the most cause of heart failure. The common causes include the following:
i. Ischaemic heart disease (IHD)
ii. Myocarditis
iii. Cardiomyopathies
iv. Metabolic disorders (e.g. beriberi)
v. Disorders of rhythm (e.g. atrial fibrillation and flutter)

II. *Increased workload on the heart* with increased myocardial demand, which may be due to increased pressure load or increased volume load.

A. *Increased pressure load*
i. Systemic or pulmonary hypertension
ii. Valvular disease resulting in stenosis of the ostia (e.g. aortic stenosis)
iii. Chronic lung disease

B. *Increased volume load*
i. Valvular insufficiency
ii. Severe anaemia
iii. Thyrotoxicosis
iv. Arteriovenous shunt
v. Hypoxia due to lung disease

III. *Impaired filling of cardiac chambers during diastole*
i. Pericardial tamponade
ii. Constrictive pericarditis
iii. Low diastolic filling due to peripheral venous blood stagnation

Q4. What is the difference between left-sided and right-sided heart failure?

While the heart fails as a whole, but functionally the left and the right heart act as independent units and each fails in its own way, resulting in *upstream* accumulation of excess fluid, i.e. upstream of the left or right ventricle **(Fig. 16.3)**.

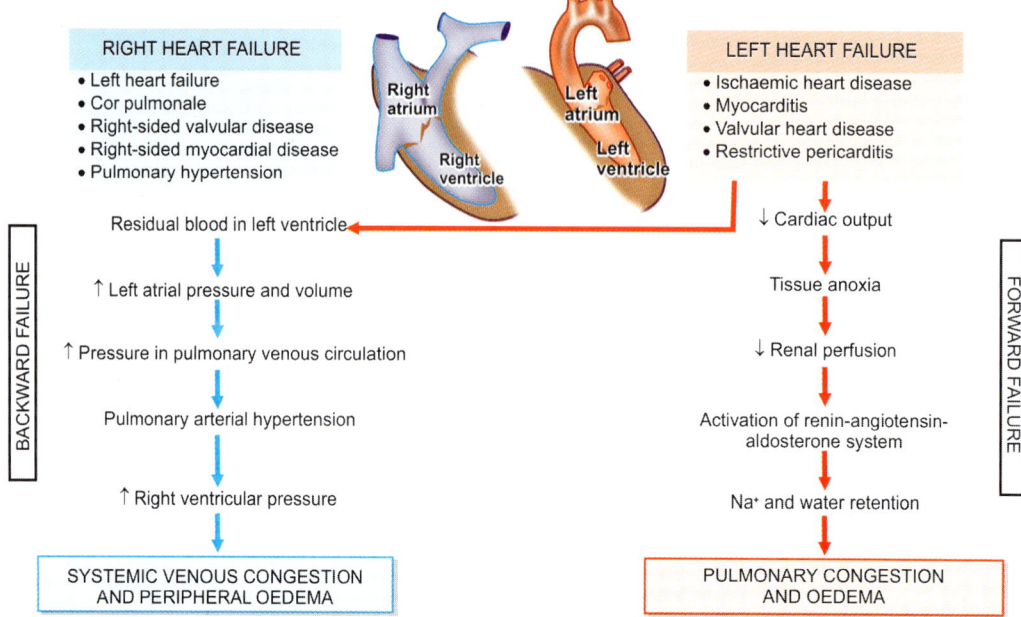

FIGURE 16.3: Schematic evolution of congestive heart failure and its effects.

Etiopathogenesis

A. *Left heart failure* is most often caused by the following:
i. Systemic hypertension (most common)
ii. Mitral and aortic valve disease
iii. Ischaemic heart disease
iv. Myocardial disease (e.g. cardiomyopathy, myocarditis)
v. Restrictive pericarditis
B. *Right heart failure* is most often caused by the following:
i. Left heart failure
ii. Cor pulmonale due to pulmonary hypertension and intrinsic lung disease **(Fig. 16.4)**
iii. Pulmonary and tricuspid valvular disease
iv. Pulmonary hypertension caused by pulmonary thromboembolism
v. Myocardial disease affecting right heart
vi. Congenital heart disease with left-to-right shunt

Clinicopathologic features In order to maintain normal cardiac output, the failing hear will resort to several *compensatory mechanisms* such as *tachycardia, cardiac hypertrophy and dilatation*.
The most visible pathophysiological compensatory mechanisms are hypertrophy and dilatation, which are often combined.

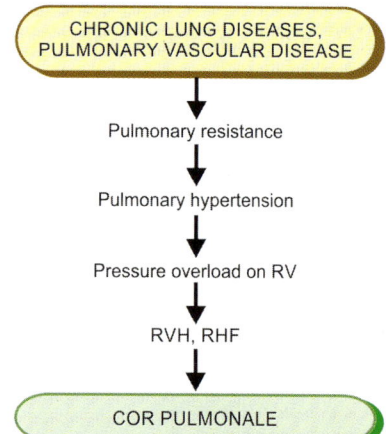

FIGURE 16.4: Pathogenesis of cor pulmonale. (RV, right ventricle; RVH, right ventricular hypertrophy; RHF, right heart failure).

I. **Hypertrophy** may involve *the left ventricle* or *the right ventricle*, depending on the type of heart failure, each of which has *distinct clinicopathological features* **(Fig. 16.5)** as follows:
i. Left ventricular hypertrophy is most prominent in patients with *arterial hypertension*.

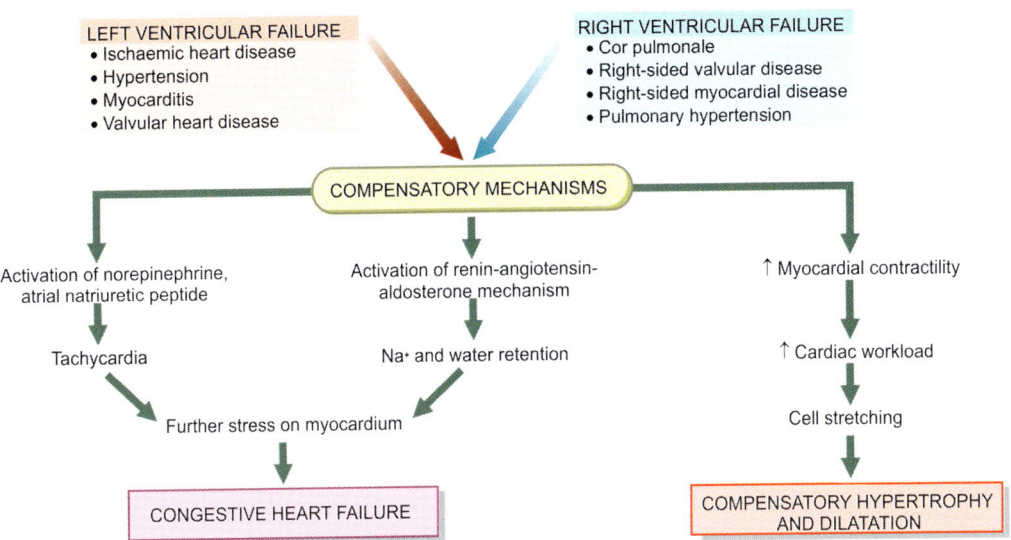

FIGURE 16.5: Schematic pathophysiology of compensatory mechanisms in cardiac failure.

ii. Right ventricular hypertrophy is most often caused by failure of the hypertrophic left ventricle **(Fig. 16.6)**.
iii. *Pulmonary hypertension*, a constant feature of left heart failure, plays a key role in hypertrophy of the right ventricle and the clinical condition called *cor pulmonale*.
iv. Hypertrophic heart muscle may be *relatively hypoxic* (same amount of coronary blood for an increased myocardial mass!) which leads to interstitial myocardial fibrosis.
v. Heart failure results in upstream accumulation of *excess oedema fluid*:
- Left heart failure—pulmonary oedema
- Right heart failure—pedal oedema, ascites and pleural effusion

vi. Heart failure also leads to *venous congestion* in:
- Lungs (in left heart failure); or
- Liver, spleen and abdominal organs (in right heart failure).

II. **Dilatation of single or both ventricles** that occurs with or without coincidental hypertrophy, is seen most often in following conditions:
i. Terminal stages of hypertensive or ischaemic heart failure, when the ventricles dilate and just cannot contract any more.
ii. Valvular insufficiency (mitral and aortic insufficiency causing left ventricular dilatation, and tricuspid or pulmonary insufficiency causing right ventricular dilatation)
iii. Left to right shunt (e.g. in ventricular septal defect)

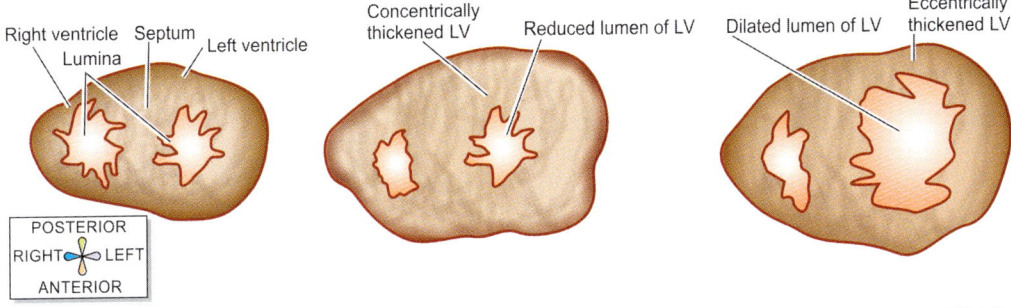

FIGURE 16.6: Schematic diagram showing transverse section through the ventricles with left ventricular hypertrophy (concentric and eccentric). (LV, left ventricle)

iv. High cardiac output conditions (e.g. thyrotoxicosis, or arteriovenous shunt)
v. Myocardial disease (e.g. dilated cardiomyopathy or flabby heart in myocarditis)

Q5. How are congenital heart diseases classified?

Definition Congenital heart disease is the name for a group of diseases related to inborn abnormal development of the heart.

Epidemiology Congenital heart diseases (CHD) are, therefore, the most common and most important heart diseases of infants and children.
- Approximately 1% of all infants are born with some cardiac defect.
- The incidence is higher in premature infants, and even more common in stillborn infants, 30% of which have heart abnormalities.

Etiology Unknown in most instances.
i. These diseases are considered to be of multifactorial origin based on an interaction of genetic and environmental influences.
ii. Some teratogens may play a role such as intrauterine rubella infection and foetal alcohol syndrome.
iii. Chromosomal syndromes (e.g. Down's syndrome and other trisomies) have a high incidence of CHD.

Classification CHD are divided into three groups **(Table 16.1)**: i) malpositions of the heart, which are extremely rare (e.g. extra-thoracic heart), ii) shunts (85%), and iii) obstructions (15%). Ten CHDs listed in the **Table 16.1** account for over 80% of all CHDs.

TABLE 16.1 Classification of congenital heart diseases.

I. MALPOSITIONS OF THE HEART	
II. SHUNTS (CYANOTIC CONGENITAL HEART DISEASE)	
A. *Left-to-right shunts (Acyanotic or late cyanotic group)*	
1. Ventricular septal defect (VSD)	25–30%
2. Atrial septal defect (ASD)	10–15%
3. Patent ductus arteriosus (PDA)	10–20%
B. *Right-to-left shunts (Cyanotic group)*	
1. Tetralogy of Fallot	6–15%
2. Transposition of great arteries	4–10%
3. Persistent truncus arteriosus	2%
4. Tricuspid atresia and stenosis	1%
III. OBSTRUCTIONS (OBSTRUCTIVE CONGENITAL HEART DISEASE)	
1. Coarctation of aorta	5–7%
2. Aortic stenosis and atresia	4–6%
3. Pulmonary stenosis and atresia	5–7%

Q6. What are the congenital heart diseases with left-to-right shunt?

Definition CHD with a left-to-right shunt fall into the group of acyanotic or late cyanotic CHD, and include ventricular septal defect, atrial septal defects, and patent ductus arteriosus.

Pathophysiology The defect allows the flow of blood from the left side (where the blood pressure is higher) to the right side.
i. *Volume overload of the right ventricle* is the main haemodynamic problem.
ii. Inflow of blood into the right heart results in pulmonary hypertension and right atrial/ventricular hypertrophy.
iii. When the pressure on the right side exceeds the pressure on the left side, the shunt will revert into a right-to-left shunt.
iv. Entry of venous blood into the left heart will cause late cyanosis.

Q7. What is ventricular septal defect?

Definition Isolated ventricular septal defect (VSD) is the most common CHD, accounting for more than one-third of all CHD. It is characterised by a defect that may involve the muscular or the membranous part of the interventricular septum, leading to a left-to right shunt **(Fig. 16.7)**.

Clinicopathologic features The shunt most often occurs through a solitary defect of the membranous septum. Defects in the muscular septum are less common, usually smaller and often multiple. Such smaller muscular defects tend to close spontaneously.

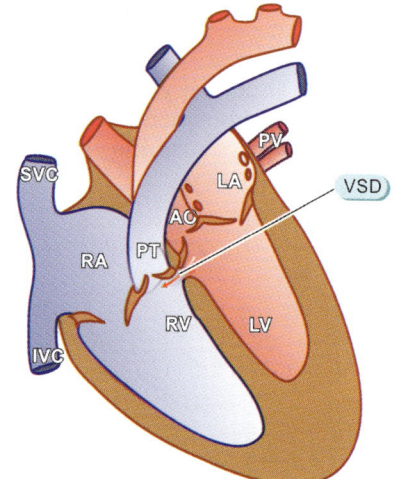

FIGURE 16.7: Ventricular septal defect.
(LA, left atrium; LV, left ventricle; AO, aorta; PV, pulmonary valve; PT, pulmonary trunk; RA, right atrium; RV, right ventricle; SVC, superior vena cava; IVC, inferior vena cava).

i. The large defect allows excess blood to enter into the right ventricle causing pulmonary hypertension and hypertrophy of the left ventricle and atrium.
ii. When the pressure in the right ventricle exceeds the pressure in the left ventricle, the original shunt will revert to a right-to-left shunt.
iii. Entry of venous blood into the arterial circulation will cause late cyanosis.
iv. Surgical treatment ('patching-up') of the defect has excellent results.

Q8. What is atrial septal defect?

Definition Atrial septal defect (ASD) is a congenital heart disease with left-to-right shunting of blood that occurs through a defect in the interatrial septum.

Clinicopathologic features Depending on the location of the defect, there are three types of ASD:
i. *Fossa ovalis* type (*ostium secundum*), the most common type (90%), involving the fossa ovalis **(Fig. 16.8)**.
ii. *Ostium primum*, located lower than the previous defect and lying adjacent to atrioventricular valves. It may be associated with malformations of the atrioventricular valves.
iii. *Sinus venosus type* which is close to the entry of the sinus venosus into the right atrium, just below the superior vena cava.

The left-to-right shunt through these septal defects has the same consequences as the VSD, except for the fact that the symptoms are much less prominent. The treatment is surgical and has excellent results.

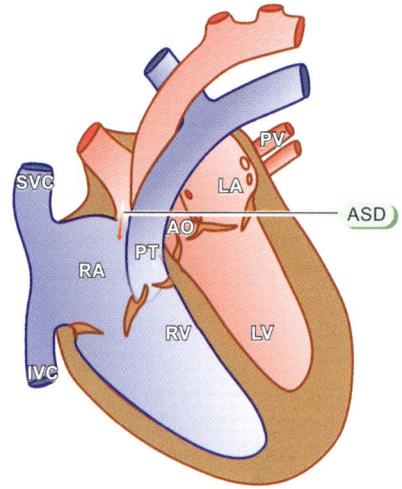

FIGURE 16.8: Atrial septal defect fossa ovalis type, a schematic representation.
(LA, left atrium; LV, left ventricle; PV, pulmonary vein; AO, aorta; PT, pulmonary trunk; RA, right atrium; RV, right ventricle; SVC, superior vena cava; IVC, inferior vena cava).

Q9. What is patent ductus arteriosus?

Definition Patent ductus arteriosus (PDA) is a consequence of incomplete involution/ obliteration of the normal foetal ductus arteriosus, connecting the pulmonary artery with the aorta.

Pathogenesis Normally the ductus arteriosus will close during the first or the second postnatal day. The reasons for it persistence are not known.
- PDA is diagnosed if the ductus does not close 3 month after the birth of the infant.
- It seems that prostaglandin PGE_2 produced locally in the ductus prevents its closure.
- Infusion of indomethacin, an inhibitor of cyclooxygenase, could facilitate the closure of PDA; if it does not, then it must be tied off and resected surgically.

Clinicopathologic features PDA allows the inflow of arterial blood from the aorta into the pulmonary artery **(Fig. 16.9)**. Inflow of blood will cause volume overload and strain the right ventricle.
i. The left ventricle is also under strain because the retrograde flow of blood from the aorta returning into the pulmonary artery requires more contractile cardiac activity.
ii. This blood flow results in an audible systolic-diastolic 'machinery murmur' over the entire left chest.
iii. Surgical treatment is very effective as long as PDA is the only defect. In 10% of cases PDA is combined with other cardiac defects.

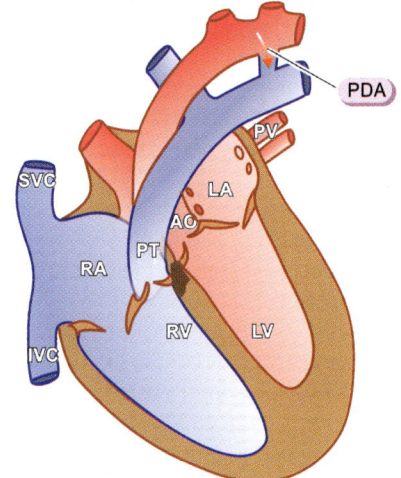

FIGURE 16.9: Patent ductus arteriosus, a schematic representation.
(LA, left atrium; LV, left ventricle; PT, pulmonary trunk; PV, pulmonary vein, AO, aorta; RA, right atrium; RV, right ventricle; SVC, superior vena cava; IVC, inferior vena cava).

Q10. What are the salient features of tetralogy of Fallot?

Definition Tetralogy of Fallot is a complex cardiac malformation including four (Greek, tetra) clinicopathologic components (shunts and obstructions), resulting in a right-to-left shunt and early cyanosis. It is the most common cyanotic CHD.

Clinicopathologic features The four components of the tetralogy of Fallot are as under **(Fig. 16.10)**:
i. Ventricular septal defect (VSD), providing the septal hole for the right to left shunt.
ii. Displacement of the aorta to the right ('dextroposition') so that it overrides the VSD.
iii. Pulmonary stenosis ('obstruction')
iv. Right ventricular hypertrophy
(NOTE: Popular mnemonic is *PROVe*=Pulmonary stenosis, Right ventricular hypertrophy, Overriding of aorta, and Ventricular septal defect.)

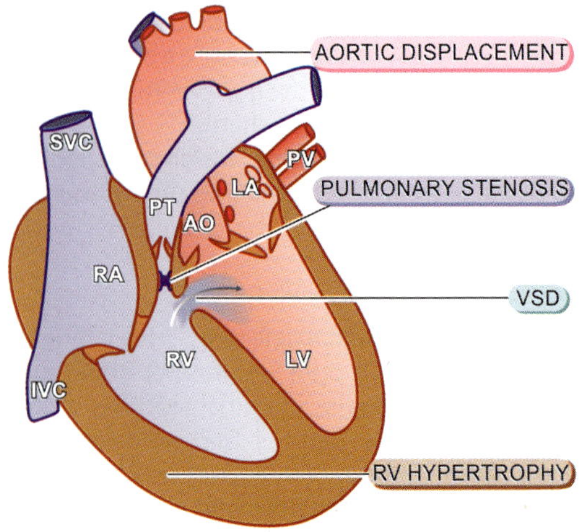

FIGURE 16.10: Tetralogy of Fallot, a schematic representation.
(LA, left atrium; LV, left ventricle; PT, pulmonary trunk; PV, pulmonary vein; AO, aorta; RA, right atrium; RV, right ventricle; SVC, superior vena cava; IVC, inferior vena cava).

The severity of the clinical manifestations depends on the extent of pulmonary stenosis and the size of VSD. Severe pulmonary stenosis aggravates the cyanosis. Large VSD may allow a left-to-right shunt and the disease in such cases could even be acyanotic.

Q11. What is coarctation of the aorta?

Definition Coarctation of the aorta is congenital obstruction of aorta due to the narrowing of its lumen. It is the most common of the three obstructive congenital heart diseases, the other two being *aortic stenosis/atresia* and *pulmonary stenosis/atresia*.

Clinicopathologic features Coarctation of the aorta may present in two forms:
I. **Infantile coarctation**, which includes hypoplasia of the aortic arch and preductal stenosis of it lumen.
i. Venous blood from the pulmonary artery flows through ductus arteriosus accounting for the cyanosis of the lower parts of the body.
ii. The upper part of the body may be oxygenated from the aortic arch proximal to the stenosis.
iii. It is a highly lethal condition; without surgical resection of the affected arch of aorta and its complete replacement, these infants die soon after birth.

II. **Adult type of coarctation** which includes a postductal ridge-like folding of the aortic wall immediately distal to the ductus arteriosus **(Fig. 16.11)**.
i. Due to the narrowing of aorta, the blood for the head and arms flows under high pressure.
ii. In contrast to hypertension in the arms, there is hypotension in the lower parts of the body because the coarctation prevents aortic blood to flow beyond it.
iii. The clinical symptoms are partially ameliorated by a collateral circulation around the coarctation in the aorta linking the subclavian arteries through the intercostal arteries with the distal aorta.

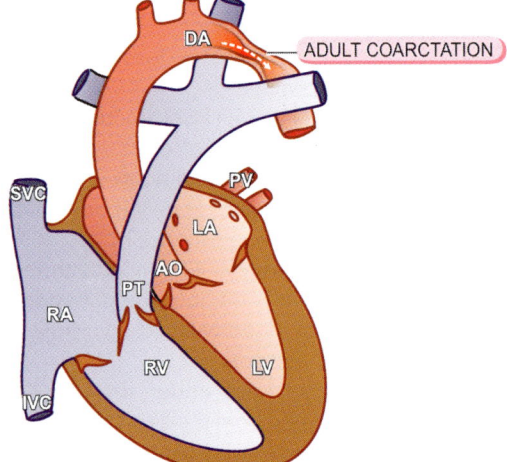

FIGURE 16.11: Postductal or adult type coarctation of the aorta, a schematic representation.
(LA, left atrium; LV, left ventricle; PT, pulmonary trunk; PV, pulmonary vein; AO, aorta; RA, right atrium; RV, right ventricle; SVC, superior vena cava; IVC, inferior vena cava; DA, ductus arteriosus).

iv. The intercostal arteries are dilated and palpable usually causing notching of the compressed ribs.
v. Surgical treatment can markedly improve the clinical condition.

Q12. What is ischaemic heart disease? Discuss its etiopathogenesis briefly.

Definition Ischaemic heart disease (IHD) is a form of acute or chronic cardiac disability arising from the imbalance between the myocardial supply for oxygenated blood and the demand for it. IHD accounts for 30% of world mortality, which is even more prevalent in high-income countries (~40%).

Etiopathogenesis Coronary atherosclerosis is the most common cause accounting for the vast majority of all cases of IHD (90%) (hence the synonym *coronary heart disease*).

I. *Atherosclerosis* with significant narrowing of the lumen (over 75%) involves most often the LAD. In 30% cases, clinically it is a single artery disease, another 30% two-artery disease and remaining 40% three-major artery disease.

II. *Location* The *stenotic lesions* are usually 3–4 cm distal from the ostia, and present in the form of calcific fixed *atheromatous plaques* and *atheromas* eccentrically narrowing the lumen of the artery.

III. *Acute changes* which may aggravate the ischaemia or cause myocardial infarction are as below:
i. Haemorrhage into the plaque or atheroma.
ii. Fissuring and ulceration of fibrous cap or intima overlying the atheroma.
iii. Intraluminal discharge of atheromatous debris.
iv. Thrombosis superimposed on the above changes.

Acute changes may be precipitated by several factors including coronary artery spasm, tachycardia and irregular myocardial contractions, sudden strain and emotional stress.

Q13. What are the non-atherosclerotic causes of ischaemic heart disease?

Non-atherosclerotic causes of IHD are rarely encountered in clinical practice. These are as under:
i. *Vasospasm* which may involve arteries that are altered by atherosclerosis as well as those that appear normal.
ii. *Stenosis of coronary ostia* secondary to aortic diseases such as syphilis or aortic aneurysm and dissection.
iii. *Arteritis* may involve coronary arteries and has been documented in patients suffering from Takayasu, Kawasaki or Buerger disease, polyarteritis nodosa and bacterial infections.
iv. *Embolism of coronary arteries* from mural thrombi in the left atrium or ventricle or ascending aorta, as well from endocardial vegetations in endocarditis.
v. *Trauma of coronary arteries* with subsequent thrombosis.
vi. *Aneurysms of the coronary arteries,* a rare event, may lead to luminal thrombosis.
vii. *External compression of coronaries* by pericardial tumour.

Q14. List the major clinical consequences of myocardial ischaemia.

Clinical consequences of myocardial ischemia depend on the suddenness of onset, duration, degree (completeness), location and the extent of the area affected as under **(Fig. 16.12)**:
i. Asymptomatic state
ii. Angina pectoris (AP)
iii. Myocardial infarction (MI)
iv. Chronic ischaemic heart disease(ischaemic cardiomyopathy)
v. Sudden cardiac death

NOTE: The term *acute coronary syndromes* include a triad of acute myocardial infarction, unstable angina pectoris and sudden cardiac death.

Q15. Define angina pectoris. What are its salient features?

Definition Angina pectoris (AP) is a clinical syndrome of IHD resulting from transient myocardial ischaemia which causes paroxysmal substernal and precordial pain. Anginal pain is aggravated by an increase in demand by increased heart action and is relieved by a decreased heart exertion.

Classification There are three overlapping clinical patterns of AP: i) stable or typical angina, ii) Prinzmetal variant angina, and iii) unstable or crescendo angina.

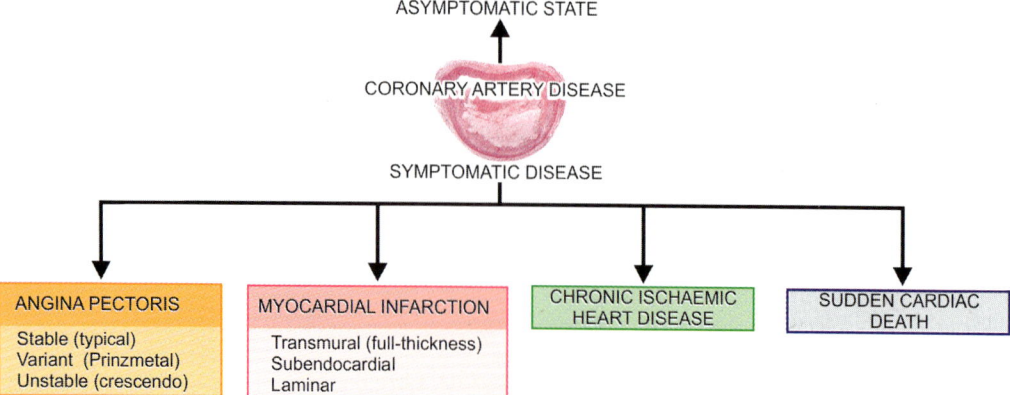

FIGURE 16.12: Spectrum of coronary ischaemic manifestations.

I. **Stable or typical angina** This is the most common patterns.
i. Anginal pain begins following physical exertion or emotional excitement and is relieved by rest.
ii. It is caused by chronic, stable, stenosing coronary atherosclerosis and an inadequate perfusion of the myocardium.
iii. ECG shows temporary depression of ST segment due to poor perfusion of the subendocardial myocardium.
iv. There is no elevation of cardiac enzymes or troponin in blood, and no pathologic evidence of irreversible myocardial injury.

II. **Prinzmetal or variant angina** It is characterised by pain at rest and it has no relationship with physical activity. It is related to coronary vasospasm.
i. Vasospasm is elicited by atherosclerosis or a local release of humoral vasoconstrictors in arteries that show no atherosclerosis.
ii. ECG shows ST elevation due to transmural ischemia.

III. **Unstable or crescendo angina** It is also known as pre-infarctional angina or acute coronary insufficiency.
i. It is characterised by pain that begins at rest, it is more intensive, and lasts longer than in classical angina.
ii. ECG shows non-ST elevation, in contrast to MI which shows ST segment elevation.

Pathology The lesions underlying AP are complex and include the following:
i. Stenosing coronary atherosclerosis.
ii. Stenosis often involves major branches of the main coronary arteries, the occlusion of which is compensated by anastomoses from other coronary arteries.
iii. Complicated atherosclerotic plaques.
iv. Fibrin thrombi which cause narrowing of the lumen but do not occlude the artery.
v. Platelet thrombi overlying plaques.
vi. Vasospasm.

Q16. What is myocardial infarction (MI)? Briefly discuss its etiopathogenesis and pathologic changes.

Definition Focal necrosis of myocardium due to ischaemia is called MI. It may be acute (fresh) or old (healed or organised)
Incidence Acute MI accounts for 10–25% of all deaths; more common in men than women.
Etiopathogenesis Occlusive thrombi are found in 90% cases of acute MI.
Sequence of events of acute MI: Severe atherosclerosis → plaque/atheroma erosion and rupture → aggregation of platelets over the ulcerated intima → activation of coagulation cascade → fibrin thrombus → thrombus enlarges and occludes the lumen of coronary → infarction.
Pathology LAD occlusion in 40–50%, RCA 30–40%, LCX 15–20%. Macroscopic and microscopic changes over time are described in **Table 16.2** and illustrated in **Figure 16.13**.

TIME	GROSS CHANGES	LIGHT MICROSCOPY
First week		
0–6 hours	No change or pale; TTC/ NBT test negative in infracted area	No change; (?) stretching and waviness of fibres
6–12 hours	No change or pale; TTC/ NBT test negative in infracted area	Coagulative necrosis begins; neutrophilic infiltration begins; oedema and haemorrhages present
24 hours	Cyanotic red-purple area of haemorrhage	Coagulative necrosis progresses; marginal neutrophilic infiltrate
48–72 hours	Pale, hyperaemic	Coagulative necrosis complete, neutrophilic infiltrate well developed
3rd -7th day	Hyperaemic border, centre yellow and soft	Neutrophils are necrosed and gradually disappear, beginning of resorption of necrosed fibres by macrophages, onset of fibrovascular response
Second week		
10th day	Red-purple periphery	Most of the necrosed muscle in a small infarct removed; fibrovascular reaction more prominent; pigmented macrophages, eosinophils, lymphocytes, plasma cells present
14th day	—	Necrosed muscle mostly removed; neutrophils disappear; fibrocollagenic tissue at the periphery
Third week	—	Necrosed muscle fibres from larger infarcts removed; more ingrowth of fibrocollagenic tissue
Fourth to sixth week	Thin, grey-white, hard, shrunken fibrous scar	Increased fibrocollagenic tissue, decreased vascularity; fewer pigmented macrophages, lymphocytes and plasma cells

TABLE 16.2 Sequential pathologic changes in myocardial infarction.

(TTC, triphenyl tetrazolium chloride; NBT, nitro blue tetrazolium).

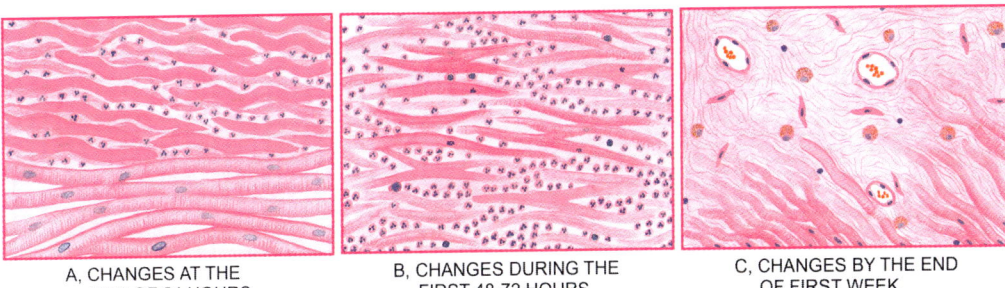

A, CHANGES AT THE END OF 24 HOURS

B, CHANGES DURING THE FIRST 48-72 HOURS

C, CHANGES BY THE END OF FIRST WEEK

FIGURE 16.13: Sequence of light microscopic changes in myocardial infarction. A, Changes after around 20 hours of occlusion of the coronary artery, there is loss of eosinophilia of infarcted myocytes and infiltration by a few neutrophils. B, Within 48–72 hours, neutrophilic infiltrate dominates the infracted myocardium. C, At the end of one week after infarction, there is infiltration of macrophages, proliferation of new capillaries and young fibroblasts.

Q17. What are the earliest definitive signs of myocardial necrosis and when do they appear?

i. Cardiac myocytes that have granular eosinophilic cytoplasm devoid of striation are the first signs of necrosis in an infarct.
ii. Their nuclei are pyknotic or have undergone karyolysis.
iii. These signs of necrosis may be seen in some myocytes even 12 hours after coronary occlusion, but are readily identifiable by the end of the first day, i.e. 24 hours after occlusion of the coronary.
iv. Fragments of necrotic myocytes may be seen in the myocardial infarcts until they are phagocytised and removed by inflammatory cells 7–10 days after the onset of infarction.

Q18. When do neutrophils appear within a myocardial infarct?

- Neutrophils start appearing at the margins of the infarct by the end of the first day and then densely infiltrate the necrotic myocardium 48–72 after occlusion.
- Since neutrophils live in tissues up to two days after exudation, they die off and transform into pus cell and start disappearing and are gradually replaced by macrophages.

Q19. When does granulation tissue start forming in a myocardial infarct?

- Macrophages, which start appearing after the neutrophils are disappearing, initiate the formation of the granulation tissue toward the end of the first week.
- Granulation tissue slowly transforms into a fibrous scar composed of collagen fibers.
- A collagenous scar is usually formed by 6 weeks of the onset of infarction (see **Fig. 16.13, C**).

Q20. What is reperfusion injury to the myocardium?

i. Myocardial infarction can be reperfused through several mechanisms:
- Through the initially occluded artery following endogenous plasminogen-mediated lysis of the thrombus.
- Through anastomoses from adjacent branches of the coronary artery.
- Following medical intervention designed to re-establish the blood flow through thrombolysis, angioplasty or coronary artery stenting.

ii. Reperfusion within 30 minutes of the occlusion could salvage many, if not most, cardiac myocytes.

iii. Later attempt at reperfusion result in rapid influx of calcium ions and the generation of toxic oxygen free radicals. Toxic radicals may induce reperfusion injury characterised by *contraction band necrosis* of cardiac myocytes.

Q21. How is myocardial infarction diagnosed clinically?

The diagnosis is based on clinical examination of the patient and the use of ancillary techniques as under:

I. **Clinical features**
i. Sudden, severe crushing substernal and precordial pain, unrelieved by rest or nitroglycerine
ii. Indigestion
iii. Apprehension
iv. Shock
v. Oliguria
vi. Low grade fever

II. **ECG changes** such as under **(Fig. 16.14)**:
i. ST segment elevation (hence the designation STEMI)
ii. T-wave inversion
iii. Deep Q wave

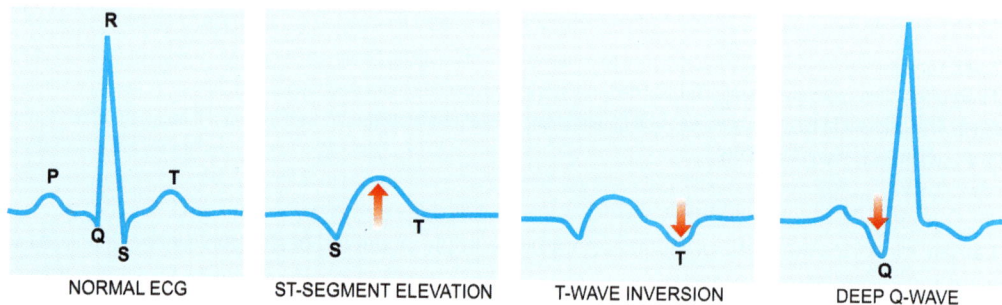

FIGURE 16.14: Some common ECG changes in acute myocardial infarction.

III. **Serum cardiac biomarkers** including myoglobin, cardiac troponins, creatine phosphokinase, CK-MB isoenzyme, and LDH **(Fig.16.15)**. However, only specific and sensitive serum biomarkers used in daily practice are:
i. Cardiac troponins (cTnT and cTnI), and
ii. CK-MB

IV. **Other supportive laboratory tests** which are routinely used are:
i. Neutrophil count (↑)
ii. ESR (↑) and CRP (↑) to monitor inflammation
iii. Tests to monitor renal function
iv. Tests for diabetes control if needed.

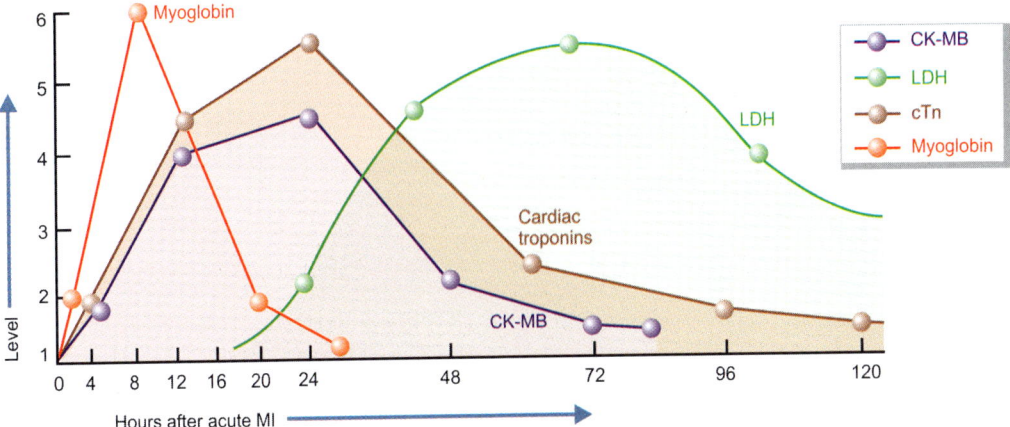

FIGURE 16.15: Time course of serum cardiac markers for the diagnosis of acute MI.

Q22. What are the most important complications of acute myocardial infarction?

Most, i.e. 80–90% of all patients, have one or more complications of acute MI as follows:
i. *Arrhythmia* (most common) due to the irritation of the conduction system.
ii. *Congestive heart failure*, which develops in about 50% of patients, and accounts for 40% of all deaths. It may present as left or right or biventricular failure. The patient may recover, or the clinical problems persist requiring additional treatment.
iii. *Cardiogenic shock* occurs in 10% of acute MI patients requiring intensive treatment to prevent death.
iv. *Thrombosis*, in one form or another, is found in 45% of patients, and accounts for about 10% of all deaths.
- Thrombotic events in the cardiac chambers include atrial thrombi related to arrhythmia and ventricular thrombi overlying myocardial infarcts.
- Prolonged bed rest predisposes to leg vein thrombosis and pulmonary embolism.
v. *Rupture of the necrotic myocardium* of the ventricular wall or papillary muscles occurs in 5% of cases.
- Rupture of left ventricular wall is accompanied by haematopericardium and it is usually lethal due to cardiac tamponade.
- Rupture of mitral papillary muscles causes sudden onset of mitral insufficiency.
- Rupture of the interventricular septum leads to a left to right ventricular shunt.
vi. *Cardiac aneurysm* may occur at the site of fibrous scarring of ventricular MIs.
vii. *Pericarditis* is frequently found in patients with transmural infarcts. It is characterised by exudation of fibrin and usually short lived and of no clinical significance.
viii. *Postmyocardial infarction syndrome (Dressler syndrome)* develops 1–6 weeks after the onset of infarction in 3–4% of all patients. It presents with sterile pericarditis with pleuritis and pneumonitis, which spontaneously disappear on their own in a few weeks. Inflammation in such cases is mediated by autoantibodies to cardiac myocytes.

Q23. What is chronic ischaemic heart disease? Discuss its features in brief.

Definition Chronic ischaemic heart disease (CIHD) is prolonged progressive heart failure related to myocardial fibrosis. It is usually found in the elderly, many of whom have history of angina pectoris or previous MIs.
Pathogenesis and pathology Ischaemia of myocardium is typically related to marked atherosclerotic narrowing of coronary arteries.
i. In most instances, there are functioning anastomoses between major coronary arteries.
ii. Myocardial fibrosis results from ischaemic death of myocytes in the form of microinfarcts which are replaced by fibrous tissue **(Fig. 16.16)**.
iii. The remaining myocardial cells show signs of ischaemia such as myocytolysis and brown atrophy, combined with compensatory hypertrophy of myocytes that have not been affected by ischemia.

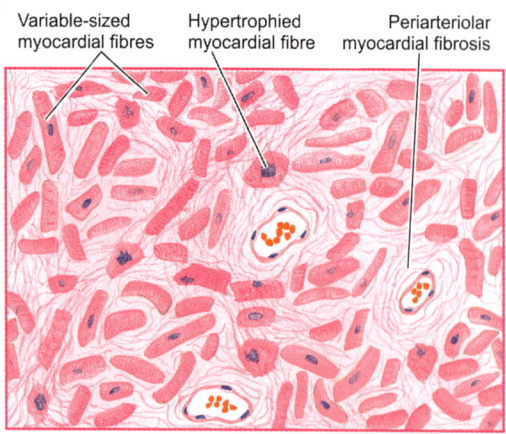

FIGURE 16.16: Chronic ischaemic heart disease. There is patchy myocardial fibrosis, especially around small blood vessels in the interstitium. The intervening single cells and groups of myocardial cells show myocytolysis.

Q24. Tabulate relationship of various coronary lesions in IHD with salient clinicopathologic features.

Lesions in coronary arteries in various forms of IHD are summarised in **Table 16.3**.

TABLE 16.3 Lesions in coronary artery in various forms of IHD.

TYPES OF IHD	CORONARY LESION	MORPHOLOGY*	CLINICAL EFFECTS
1. Stable angina	➤ Critical coronary narrowing (3/4th)	A, Normal	Nil
2. Chronic IHD	➤ Chronic progressive coronary ➤ Atherosclerosis ➤ Plaque rupture, haemorrhage, ulceration ➤ Mural thrombosis with thromboembolism	B, Severe, fixed, 3/4th narrowing	Stable angina, CIHD
3. Unstable (pre-infarction) angina			
4. Myocardial infarction	➤ Plaque haemorrhage ➤ Fissuring and ulceration ➤ Complete mural thrombosis	C, Thrombosis with haemorrhage	Plaque haemorrhage, unstable angina
5. Sudden ischaemic death	➤ Severe multi-vessel disease ➤ Acute changes in plaque ➤ Thrombosis with thromboembolism	D, Occlusive thrombosis	Acute coronary syndromes

(IHD, ischaemic heart disease; CIHD, chronic IHD).
*Figure on left is cross section and on right is longitudinal section of affected coronary artery.

Q25. Briefly describe sudden cardiac death.

Definition Sudden cardiac death is death that occurs within 24 hours of the onset of cardiac symptoms.
Etiology Myocardial ischaemia is most often caused by atherosclerosis.
i. *Atherosclerotic narrowing* of coronaries resulting in fatal arrhythmias, chiefly ventricular asystole or fibrillation.

ii. Less often, it may also be caused by *coronary spasm* of relatively normal coronaries or mildly atherosclerotic coronaries.

iii. *Other non-coronary diseases* may also cause sudden cardiac death as under:
- Calcific aortic stenosis (usually in the elderly)
- Hypertrophic cardiomyopathy (especially in young persons)
- Myocarditis
- Mitral valve prolapse
- Endocarditis
- Hereditary or acquired defects of the conduction system

Pathology In most adults, the autopsy will reveal coronary atherosclerosis.

i. Atherosclerosis with coronary artery stenosis of 75% of more.

ii. Sometimes, there is superimposed thrombosis or hemorrhage into the plaque.

iii. Healed and acute MI are found in many cases.

Q26. Define rheumatic fever. What is geographic prevalence?

Definition Rheumatic fever (RF) is a systemic post-streptococcal, non-suppurative inflammatory disease, principally affecting the heart, joints, central nervous system, skin and subcutaneous tissue.

Epidemiology
- The disease affects predominantly children and adolescents in the 5 to 15 years age group, when the streptococcal infections are most frequent and intense.
- There is a slight female predominance.
- The disease is more common in poor socioeconomic strata and is still prevalent in underdeveloped countries of Asia, Africa and South America.
- In India, Pakistan, Bangladesh and Afghanistan, RF continues to be a major public health problem, with an incidence in India of 1 to 5.5 per 1000 children.

Q27. What is the pathogenesis of rheumatic fever?

Infection with group A β-haemolytic streptococci precedes the development of RF in all cases. The factors that influence the development or RF fall under three headings: i) environmental factors, ii) host susceptibility, and iii) immunologic evidence **(Fig. 16.17)**.

I. **Environmental factors** pertaining to streptococcal infection promote RH. Evidences in support are as follows:

i. The onset of RF follows *2–3 weeks* after streptococcal infection suggesting a period of immunisation.

ii. *Reinfection* with streptococci is associated with recurrent episodes of RH.

iii. Conditions that predispose to epidemics of streptococcal infections in *closed communities* such as children in camps or boarding schools and recruits in barracks also predispose to RF.

iv. *Socioeconomic factors* like poverty and crowding, predispose to the spread of streptococcal infection and thus are associated with higher incidence of RF. The same holds true for geographic distribution of RF, which is more common in poor countries.

v. Administration of *antibiotics* for streptococcal throat infections leads to lowering of the incidence of RF.

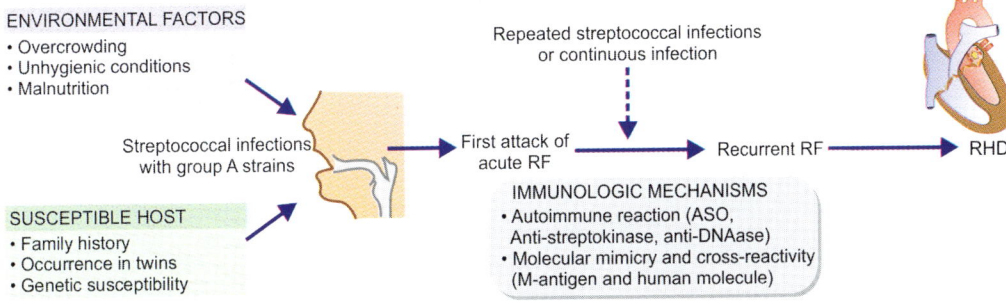

FIGURE 16.17: Pathogenesis of RHD, schematic evolution.

II. **Host susceptibility** seems to have a genetic basis.
i. *Familial cases* of RF and occurrence of RF among *identical twins* suggest a genetic basis of susceptibility.
ii. Some *HLA class II alleles* (HLA-DR7 and HLA-DR4) are strongly associated with RF.
iii. *First-degree relatives* of patients with RF and RHD have increased expression of a particular alloantigen (D8–17) on B cells, which may act as a marker for inherited susceptibility for RF.
III. **Immunologic evidence** supports the notion that the immune response to streptococci may cross-react with human antigens and injure human tissues.
i. Clinical RF is associated with *high titres of antibodies to antigen* on β-haemolytic streptococci, including anti-streptolysin O (ASO) and S, anti-streptokinase, anti-streptohyaluronidase, and anti-DNAse.
ii. *Antibodies against cell wall polysaccharide* of group A *Streptococcus* react against cardiac valves.
iii. Furthermore, patients with valvular involvement have *autoantibodies* that react with valves, in contrast to patients who do not have endocardial involvement.
iv. *Hyaluronate capsule* of group A streptococci is identical to hyaluronate in human joint tissues.
v. *Membrane antigens* of group A streptococci react with sarcolemma of smooth and cardiac muscle cells, dermal fibroblasts and neuron of the caudate nucleus.
Combined proposed pathogenesis based on the above data involves the following events:
- Genetically determined individual *susceptibility to Streptococcus* infection generates *antibodies to streptococcal antigens*.
- *Antistreptococcal antibodies cross-react* with host tissues because several streptococcal antigens, including the streptococcal M proteins, are immunologically identical to human molecules (a phenomenon called *'molecular mimicry'*).
- Cross-reacting antibodies elicited by streptococci act as *autoantibodies damaging human tissues*.

Q28. Enumerate the major anatomic sites of involvement in rheumatic fever.

- The pathologic changes occur in: i) heart, ii) skin, iii) joints, and less often, iv) CNS and v) lungs.
- Most important clinical manifestation of RF is heart involvement called rheumatic heart disease (RHD). Heart is involved in the form of focal inflammation involving the endocardium, myocardium and pericardium, hence presenting as a *pancarditis*.

Q29. Discuss the salient pathologic features of rheumatic endocarditis.

Definition and locations
i. Rheumatic endocarditis most often involves the valves and thus presents as *valvulitis*.
ii. *Mural endocarditis* is less common, typically involving the left atrial endocardium in the form of *MacCallum patch*, a fibrino-inflammatory induration of the endocardium of the left atrium **(Fig. 16.18)**.
iii. Valvulitis may involve all four orifices.
iv. Most often, it presents with inflammation and deformities of the mitral valves, then aortic valves, or in a combination of both mitral and aortic orifice valves. *Mitral valve is involved in almost 80% of all cases*, and in one third of all cases this is the only valve affected.
v. Tricuspid and pulmonary valves are rarely involved.

Pathology The changes depend on the stage of the disease, which may be classified as *i) acute (early), ii) chronic active,* and *iii) healing or late chronic stage*.

I. **Acute stage**
i. Valvulitis begins with slight thickening and a loss of translucency of the valve followed by the formation of small (1–3 mm) fibrin rich *vegetations* or *verrucae*.

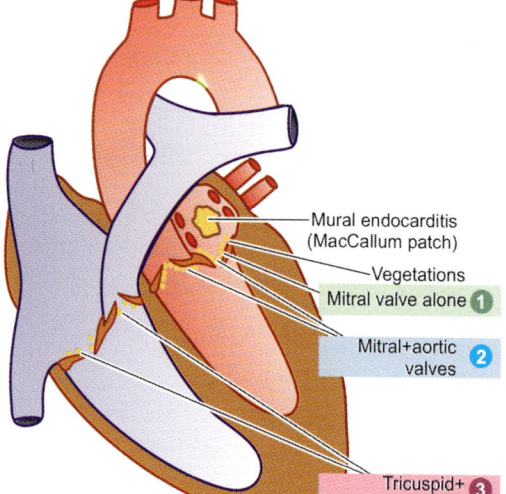

FIGURE 16.18: Schematic representation of the anatomic regions of involvement and location of vegetations in rheumatic endocarditis (both valvular and mural). Serial numbers 1, 2 and 3 are denoted for the frequency of valvular involvement.

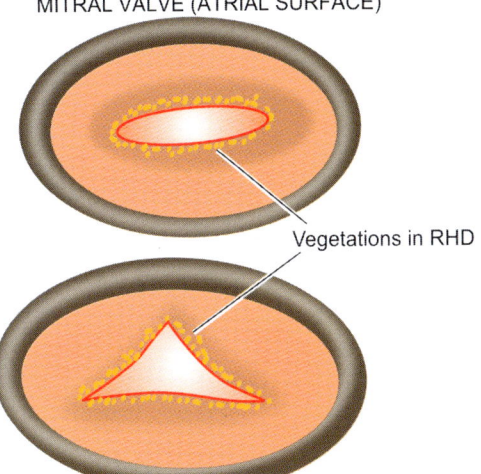

MITRAL VALVE (ATRIAL SURFACE)

Vegetations in RHD

AORTIC VALVE (VENTRICULAR SURFACE)

FIGURE 16.19: Rheumatic valvulitis. Location of vegetations on the valves of the left heart. The location of vegetations on mitral valve (left upper diagram) is shown as viewed from the left atrium, while the vegetations on aortic valve (left lower diagram) are shown as seen from the left ventricular surface.

ii. Verrucae are located along the line of closure of the valves, proximally to the valvular free margins **(Fig. 16.19)**.

iii. The verrucae are made of fibrin and platelets; they are friable and confluent and firmly attached to the valve by acute inflammation permeating the valve itself **(Fig. 16.20)**.

iv. The location of lesions on the valves (on the atrial side of the mitral valve, and the ventricular side of the aortic valve) suggests that the mechanics of blood flow determines the location of valvular injury and subsequent location of the vegetations.

v. The preponderance of vegetations in the left heart, which is operating under higher pressure than the right heart, also supports the notion that the mechanical factors are important and determine the location of vegetations.

vi. The valve is involved by chronic inflammatory cells, which are more prominent at the base rather underneath the vegetations.

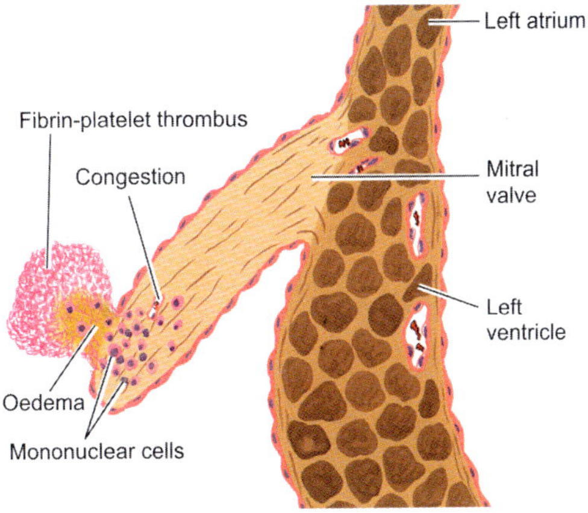

FIGURE 16.20: Rheumatic heart disease. Diagrammatic appearance of rheumatic valvulitis and a vegetation on the cusp of mitral valve in sagittal section.

II. **Chronic active stage**

i. It is characterised by persistent inflammation, prominent formation of the granulation tissue and fibrosis with foci of dystrophic calcification.

ii. All these changes contribute to the thickening of valves and their deformity and narrowing of the ostia ('*stenosis*').

iii. Mitral valve is involved in over 75% of cases and typically it shows '*fish-mouth stenosis*' or '*button-hole stenosis*'.

iv. Mitral valve leaflets fuse with each other, roll up and lose their mobility. At the same time, chordae tendineae become shortened, thickened and tend to fuse with each other.

v. Shortened chordae combined with rigidity of the valves prevents full closure of the mitral valve resulting in reflow of the blood ('*insufficiency*').

III. **Healing or late chronic stage**

i. This stage is characterised by reduced inflammation and the predominance of fibrosis and calcification.

ii. Vegetations may be present, and there is vascularisation of the valves but there are only scant foci of chronic inflammation.

iii. There are almost no Aschoff bodies. Persistence of Aschoff bodies is a sign of activity of RF.

Q30. What is rheumatic myocarditis? Briefly discuss its pathologic features.

Definition Inflammatory involvement of myocardium in rheumatic fever is called rheumatic myocarditis.
Pathology
Gross
i. In early stage of the disease, inflammation makes the myocardium soft and flabby. Later, when fibrosis ensues, the heart muscle becomes stiffer.
ii. On gross examination at autopsy, foci of inflammation and fibrosis can be sometimes recognised as whitish patches or scars in the wall of the left and right ventricle.
Microscopy
i. There is focal inflammation characterised by the formation of pathognomonic lesions called *Aschoff nodules (bodies)*. Most often, they are found in perivascular interstitium of the myocardium and less often in the deeper layers of the endocardium.
ii. Aschoff nodules begin to form approximately four weeks after the onset of rheumatic carditis.
iii. The Aschoff nodules or the Aschoff bodies are spheroidal or fusiform distinct tiny structures, 1–2 mm in size, occurring in the interstitium of the heart in RF and may be visible to naked eye. They are especially found in the vicinity of small blood vessels in the myocardium and endocardium. Lesions similar to the Aschoff nodules may be found in the extracardiac tissues.
iv. *Evolution* of fully-developed Aschoff bodies occurs through three stages all of which may be found in the same heart at different stages of development. These are as follows:
a. *Early (exudative or degenerative) stage* is characterised by *fibrinoid degeneration* in the collagen and mucopolysaccharides in the interstitial tissue.
b. *Intermediate (proliferative or granulomatous) stage* follows fibrinoid change. There is proliferation of cells that includes infiltration by lymphocytes (mostly T cells), plasma cells, a few neutrophils and the characteristic *cardiac histiocytes (Anitschkow cells)* at the margin of the lesion. Some of these modified cardiac histiocytes become multinucleate cells containing 1 to 4 nuclei and are called *Aschoff cells* and are pathognomonic of RHD **(Fig. 16.21)**.
c. *Late (healing or fibrous) stage* is the stage when macrophages are replaced by fibrous tissue that forms spindle shaped scars, usually located in the perivascular interstitium.
v. With passage of months and years, the Aschoff body becomes less cellular and the collagenous tissue is increased.

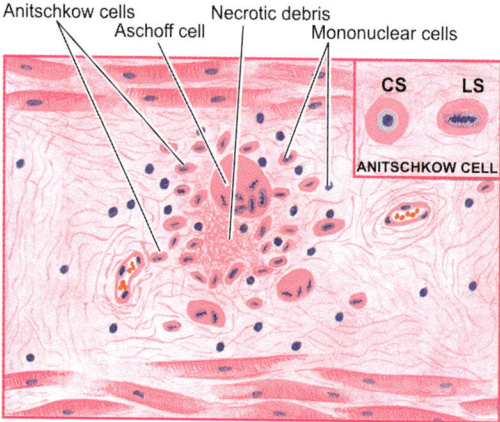

FIGURE 16.21: Aschoff body (granulomatous stage) in the myocardium. *Inbox* shows Anitschkow cell in longitudinal section (LS) with caterpillar-like serrated nuclear chromatin, while cross section (CS) shows owl-eye appearance of central chromatin mass and perinuclear halo.

Q31. Describe the salient features of rheumatic pericarditis.

Definition Involvement of pericardium is common in RF in all stages of the disease.
Pathology
Gross It presents as a *fibrinous inflammation* giving the two layers of pericardium a *'bread and butter'* appearance. This term is used in analogy to two sticky layers of bread in a sandwich with a layer of sticky butter in between. Fibrin strands between the visceral and mural pericardium correspond in this analogy to the sticky but stringing butter preventing complete separation of two opposing slices of bread.

Microscopy
i. Underlying the fibrin exudate, there is an *inflammatory infiltrate* composted of lymphocytes, macrophages, plasma cells and scattered neutrophils. Scanty Aschoff bodies may be found.
ii. With time, granulation tissue invades the fibrin layer organising it and transforming it into fibrous tissue typical of *adhesive pericarditis*.
iii. Less often, pericardial fibrosis may completely obliterate the pericardial cavity and it may progress to *constrictive pericarditis* which may prevent diastolic inflow of blood into the chambers of the heart.

Q32. What are the extracardiac features of rheumatic fever?

RF tends to involve connective tissue of several organs as follows:
I. **Polyarthritis** involving large joints is found in 90% of all cases of RF in adults but is less commonly seen in children.
i. Clinically, it presents as joint swelling and pain.
ii. As swelling and pain subside in one joint, other joints get involved resulting in a clinical picture of *migratory polyarthritis,* involving more than one joint at a time.
iii. Swollen joint often contains serous effusion.
iv. *Microscopy* shows nonspecific acute and chronic inflammation with exudation of fibrin and hyperaemia of the synovial membranes of the joints. Inflammation tends to heal on its own.
II. **Subcutaneous nodules**, which occur more often in children than adults, are usually painless.
i. Nodules tend to be small (< 2 cm) and attached to the underlying structure like tendons or periosteum, thus remaining undetected by the patient. Most often they appear on the extensor surfaces of wrists, elbows, knees and ankles.
ii. *Microscopy* shows changes that resemble large Aschoff bodies, and consist of three zones:
a. a central zone of fibrinoid necrosis,
b. rimmed by a zone of macrophages and fibroblasts arranged in a palisaded manner, and
c. an outer zone containing chronic inflammatory cells and proliferating small blood vessels.
NOTE: RF nodules must be distinguished from subcutaneous nodules in *rheumatoid arthritis*, which are larger, painful and tender, and persist for years, in contrast to the nodules of RF which are relatively short-lived and not painful.
III. **Erythema marginatum** is nonpruritic, involves the trunk and proximal extremities and is characteristic of RF.
i. It tends to clear centrally and has slightly elevated margin.
ii. It is short-lived and migratory.
IV. **Rheumatic arteritis** involves major arteries and their branches. For example, in the myocardium it involves the small branches of the coronary artery.
Microscopy resembles microscopic angiitis or polyarteritis nodosa with focal fibrinoid necrosis.
V. **Chorea minor** is an uncommon delayed manifestation of RF and results from involvement of the CNS. It affects most often younger patients and especially girls.
i. Clinically, it presents with involuntary jerky movements of the trunk and extremities, and some emotional instability.
ii. *Microscopy* shows changes in the brain that includes focal oedema, microscopic haemorrhages and perivascular infiltrates of lymphocytes in the cerebral haemispheres, basal ganglia and brain-stem.
VI. **Pulmonary changes** include:
i. Rheumatic pneumonitis and pleuritis, but these are rare.
ii. Pleural effusion is accompanied by oedema and capillary haemorrhages in the lung, and fibrinous exudate in the alveoli with foci of nonspecific inflammation.

Q33. How is rheumatic fever diagnosed clinically?

It is worth noticing that there is no single diagnostic test that could be used to diagnose RF. The diagnosis is based on *WHO revised Jones criteria* which includes five major criteria and five minor criteria. The diagnosis is established by the presence of any two major criteria, or one major and two minor criteria as follows:

I. **Major criteria**
i. Carditis (50–60%)
ii. Polyarthritis (60–75%)
iii. Chorea (2–3%)
iv. Erythema marginatum (<5%)
v. Subcutaneous nodules (<5%)
II. **Minor criteria**
i. Fever
ii. Polyarthralgia
iii. Previous history of RF
iv. Laboratory findings: ESR (↑), C-reactive protein (↑), leucocytosis
v. ECG changes with prolonged PR interval
III. **Supportive evidence of group A streptococcal infection** in preceding 45 days:
i. Positive throat culture for group A streptococci.
ii. Raised titres of anti-streptococcal antibodies (anti-streptolysins O and S, anti-streptokinase, anti-streptohyaluronidase and anti-DNAase B).

Q34. What are the major causes of death in rheumatic fever?

i. *Cardiac failure* is the most common cause of death. In younger patients death is related to valvular deformities, and in the elderly it is coronary artery disease superimposed of RHD.
ii. *Bacterial endocarditis* (acute of subacute) superimposed on rheumatic endocarditis.
iii. *Thromboemboli* from mural thrombi, most often in the left atrium related to mitral stenosis.
iv. *Ball thrombus* in the left atrium occluding the mitral orifice and causing sudden death.

Q35. How is endocarditis classified?

Endocarditis, an inflammation of the endocardial layer of the heart, can be classified on the basis of several criteria:
i. *Temporal classification* based on duration of the disease: acute or chronic.
ii. *Anatomic classification* depending on the location and extent of inflammation: valvular or mural.
iii. *Etiological classification* based on the causation: infective or non-infective. This classification is given in **Table 16.4**.

TABLE 16.4 Classification of endocarditis.

A. NON-INFECTIVE
1. Rheumatic endocarditis
2. Atypical verrucous (Libman-Sacks) endocarditis
3. Non-bacterial thrombotic (cachectic, marantic) endocarditis
B. INFECTIVE
1. Bacterial endocarditis
2. Other specific infective types (tuberculous, syphilitic, fungal, viral, rickettsial)

Q36. What is atypical verrucous (Libman-Sacks) endocarditis? Discuss its salient features.

Definition Libman-Sacks originally described this sterile endocarditis in patients with systemic lupus erythematosus. Today the same term is also used for sterile endocarditis found in other autoimmune collagen vascular diseases such systemic sclerosis (scleroderma) or thrombotic thrombocytopenic purpura.
Clinicopathologic features
i. Valvular endocarditis is characterised by the appearance of small verrucous vegetations composed of fibrin and platelets. Vegetations are most often found on the mitral and tricuspid valves and may involve both sides of the leaflets.
ii. Underneath the vegetations, there is fibrinoid necrosis of endocardium, chronic inflammation with infiltrates of lymphocytes, plasma cells and macrophages, and proliferation of small blood vessels.
iii. Inflammation and fibrin deposits may also be seen on the chordae and even adjacent atrial or ventricular myocardium.
iv. Coexistent with endocarditis, these patients usually have fibrinous pericarditis with pericardial effusion, which is the most common cardiac lesion in SLE.
v. This sterile endocarditis may heal upon treatment of SLE or other autoimmune diseases that have caused it and usually does not lead to significant destruction or deformity of the valves.

Q37. What is non-bacterial thrombotic endocarditis?

Definition Non-bacterial thrombotic endocarditis (NBTE), also known as cachectic or marantic endocarditis, or terminal endocarditis simplex, is a form of endocarditis characterised by the formation of sterile, fibrin rich, valvular vegetations without local signs of valvular dysfunction.

Etiopathogenesis

i. NBTE is most often found in hypercoagulable states such as DIC or cancer related coagulation disorders.
ii. Often it is also found in terminally ill cachectic patients suffering from a variety chronic debilitating diseases.
iii. Trauma of the valves due to catheterisation or haemodynamic trauma may also cause NBTE.

Clinicopathologic features

i. NBTE is characterised by the formation of small verrucous, sterile vegetations along the line of closure of the valves.
ii. Most often, NBTE affects the mitral valve, but it may involve other valves as well.
iii. NBTE does not cause valvular dysfunction, and thus there are no symptoms.
iv. *Complications*: Most cases of NBTE remain asymptomatic but in some cases the vegetations may be infected (especially in bacteraemia and sepsis), whereupon NBTE transforms into bacterial endocarditis.
v. The vegetations are friable and may give rise to arterial thromboemboli which may cause infarcts in major organs.

Q38. What is infective endocarditis? Briefly discuss its etiology and predisposing factors.

Definition Infective endocarditis (IE), also known as bacterial endocarditis (BE), is a serious disease of the valvular or mural endocardium caused most often by bacteria resulting in the formation of infected vegetations and clinical evidence of a critical infectious disease.

Classification Depending on the severity of the infection, IE can be subdivided into two clinical forms:

I. *Acute bacterial endocarditis (ABE),* a fulminant and destructive acute infection by highly virulent bacteria in a previously normal heart, that almost invariably runs a rapidly fatal course in a period of 2–6 weeks.

II. *Subacute bacterial endocarditis (SABE)* or endocarditis lenta, caused by less virulent bacteria in a previously diseased heart and has a gradual downhill course in a period of 6 weeks to a few months and sometimes years.

The classification of bacterial endocarditis into these two forms has been largely discarded because the clinical course of these diseases has been altered by antibiotic treatment. Yet, there are a few important distinguishing features as listed in **Table 16.5**.

TABLE 16.5 Distinguishing features of acute and subacute bacterial endocarditis.

FEATURE	ACUTE	SUBACUTE
1. *Duration*	<6 weeks	>6 weeks
2. *Most common organisms*	*Staph. aureus*, β-streptococci	*Streptococcus viridans*
3. *Virulence of organisms*	Highly virulent	Less virulent
4. *Previous condition of valves*	Usually previously normal	Usually previously damaged
5. *Lesion on valves*	Invasive, destructive, suppurative	Usually not invasive or suppurative
6. *Clinical features*	Features of acute systemic infection	Splenomegaly, clubbing of fingers, petechiae

Etiology In 90% of cases, BE is caused by streptococci and staphylococci. Infections with other bacteria are uncommon.

i. *ABE* is most often caused by *Staphylococcus aureus*.
ii. *SABE* is most often caused by *Streptococcus viridans*, which forms part of the normal flora of the mouth and pharynx. Other less common etiologic pathogens are *Staphylococcus epidermidis* (a commensal on the skin), and some gram negative bacteria (*Streptococcus bovis*, a normal gastrointestinal bacterium), *Streptococcus pneumoniae*, *E.coli*, *Klebsiella*, etc.).
iii. *Specific etiologic forms* of endocarditis are rare and usually associated with systemic generalised infection with specific pathogens such as fungi, rickettsiae, or *Mycobacterium tuberculosis*.
iv. *Treponema pallidum* may extend to the aortic valves in syphilitic aortitis.

Predisposing conditions

I. *Conditions initiating transient bacteraemia, septicaemia or pyaemia*
i. Severe or persistent bacterial infections (e.g. periodontal infections, GI infections, urogenital infections, skin infections)
ii. Surgery of internal organs, especially involving bowels, hepatobiliary and urogenital tract
iii. Intravenous drug abuse
iv. Cardiac catheterisation and cardiac valvular surgery

II. *Underlying heart disease*
i. Cardiac valvular diseases (e.g. rheumatic heart disease, floppy mitral valve, calcific aortic stenosis, etc.)
ii. Prosthetic heart valves
iii. Congenital heart diseases (e.g. VSD, bicuspid aortic valve, coarctation of the aorta, PDA)

III. *Impaired host defenses*
i. Haematologic diseases, e.g. aplastic anemia, leukaemia, lymphoma
ii. Cytotoxic therapy of various cancers
iii. Congenital or acquired immunodeficiency
iv. Autoimmune diseases treated by corticosteroid and immunosuppressive drugs.

Q39. Discuss pathogenesis and main pathologic findings of acute bacterial endocarditis.

Pathogenesis
i. Bacteria invade the valves causing destruction, acute inflammation and exudation of fibrin which forms the vegetations.
ii. Typically, vegetations involve the atrial side of the mitral and tricuspid valves, and the ventricular surface of the aortic and pulmonary valves **(Fig. 16.22)**.
iii. Damaged valves are more susceptible to bacterial infection.
iv. Pre-existent fibrin vegetations (e.g. in NBTE) are a fertile ground for bacterial growth.

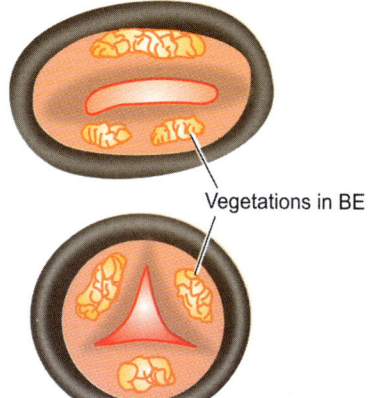

FIGURE 16.22: Infective endocarditis. Schematic location of vegetations on the valves of the left heart. The vegetations are shown on the mitral valve (left upper diagram) as viewed from the left atrium, while those on the aortic valve (left lower diagram) are shown as seen from the left ventricle.

Pathology
i. Florid purulent inflammation and large vegetations with destruction or rupture of valves are typical of ABE.
ii. Vegetations are composed of fibrin admixed with necrotic remnants of the valves and inflammatory cells which may form aggregates of pus **(Fig. 16.23)**.
iii. Bacterial colonies are found in the vegetations or the inflamed valves. Bacteria can be stained with Gram stain and are either bluish (Gram positive) or red (Gram negative).
iv. The underlying valves are oedematous, partially destroyed and inflamed or distorted by granulation tissue and fibrosis.
v. Abscesses may be found inside the valves.

vi. Calcifications are common.
vii. ABE may completely destroy the valves which may show huge defect or rupture.
NOTE: Vegetations and inflammation are less prominent in SABE, which usually develops on previously damaged valves.

Q40. How is bacterial endocarditis diagnosed clinically?

The diagnosis of BE is clinically based on Duke criteria as follows:
I. **Major criteria:**
i. Positive blood culture for virulent pathogens
ii. Evidence of endocardial involvement, as supported by ECG or ultrasound investigation, documentation of valvular masses or destruction of the valves with regurgitation of blood
II. **Minor criteria:**
i. Predisposing heart condition
ii. Fever > 100.4° F
iii. Major vascular embolic phenomena
iv. Immunologic phenomena (e.g. glomerulonephritis, Osler subcutaneous nodes)
v. Microbial evidence of positive blood culture but not meeting major criteria

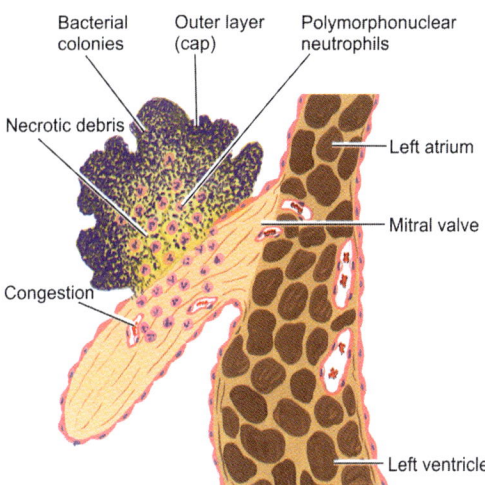

FIGURE 16.23: Infective endocarditis. Diagrammatic appearance of a vegetation of BE on the surface of mitral valve in sagittal section.

Q41. What are the complications of bacterial endocarditis?

Complication can be classified as i) cardiac, and ii) extracardiac.
I. **Cardiac complications (Fig. 16.24, A):**
i. Valvular stenosis or insufficiency
ii. Perforation, rupture or aneurysm of the valves
iii. Abscess of the valve ring
iv. Myocardial abscesses

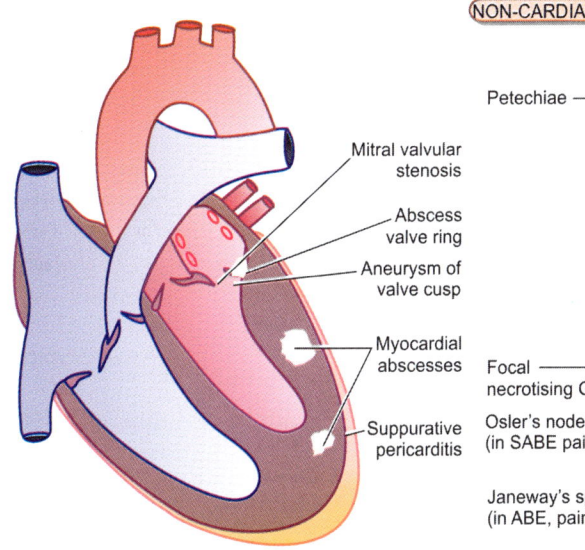 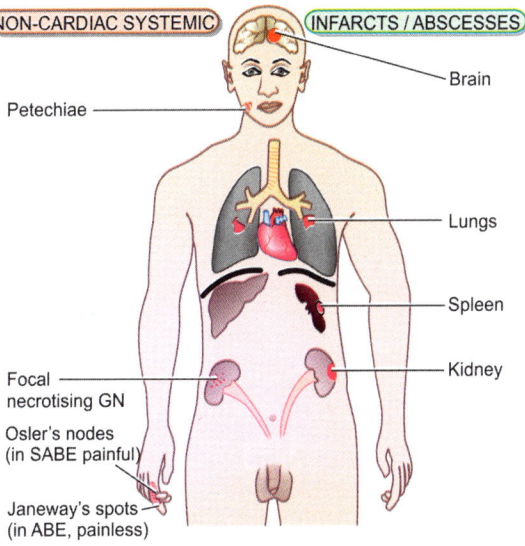

A, CARDIAC SEQUELAE OF INFECTIVE ENDOCARDITIS   B, EXTRA-CARDIAC COMPLICATIONS

FIGURE 16.24: Cardiac and extracardiac complications of infective endocarditis.

v. Suppurative pericarditis
vi. Cardiac failure from one or more of the foregoing

II. **Extracardiac complications (Fig. 16. 24, B)**:
i. Septic emboli leading to infarction of peripheral organs and abscess formation
ii. Petechiae of the skin and conjunctiva due to microemboli
iii. *Osler nodules* as painful lesions on finger tips in SABE
iv. Similar painless non-tender maculopapular lesions on the pulp of the finger in SBE are called *Janeway spots*. In either case, they are due to toxic or immune reactions involving the small blood vessels.
v. Focal necrotising or diffuse glomerulonephritis which is more common in SABE than ABE, and is caused by circulating immune complexes deposited in the glomeruli.

Q42. Tabulate contrasting features of various types of vegetations seen in endocarditis of different etiologies.

Summary of salient distinguishing features of principal types of vegetations in endocarditis of different etiologies is given in **Table 16.6**.

TABLE 16.6 Distinguishing features of vegetations in major forms of endocarditis.

FEATURE	RHEUMATIC	LIBMAN-SACKS	NON-BACTERIAL THROMBOTIC	BACTERIAL (INFECTIVE)
1. *Valves commonly affected*	Mitral alone; mitral and aortic combined	Mitral, tricuspid	Mainly mitral; less often aortic and tricuspid	Mitral; aortic; combined mitral and aortic
2. *Location on valve cusps or leaflets*	Occur along the line of closure, atrial surface of atrioventricular valves and ventricular surface of semilunar valves	Occur on both surfaces of valve leaflets or cusps, in the valve pockets	Occur along the line of closure	SABE more often on diseased valves: ABE on previously normal valves; location same as in RHD
3. *Gross appearance*	Small, multiple, warty, grey brown, translucent, firmly attached, generally produce permanent valvular deformity	Medium-sized, multiple, generally do not produce significant valvular deformity	Small but larger than those of rheumatic, single or multiple, brownish, firm, but more friable than those of rheumatic	Often large, grey-tawny to greenish, irregular, single or multiple, typically friable
4. *Microscopy*	i. Composed of fibrin with superimposed platelet thrombi and no bacteria ii. Adjacent and underlying endocardium shows oedema, proliferation of capillaries, mononuclear inflammatory infiltrate and occasional Aschoff bodies	i. Composed of fibrinoid material with superimposed fibrin and platelet thrombi and no bacteria. ii. The underlying endocardium shows fibrinoid necrosis, proliferation of capillaries and acute and chronic inflammatory infiltrate including the haematoxylin bodies of Gross	i. Composed of degenerated valvular tissue, fibrin platelets thrombi and no bacteria. ii. The underlying valve shows swelling of collagen, fibrinoid change, proliferation of capillaries but no significant inflammatory cell infiltrate	i. Composed of outer eosinophilic zone of fibrin and platelets, covering colonies of bacteria and deeper zone of non-specific acute and chronic inflammatory cells. ii. The underlying endocardium may show abscesses in ABE and inflammatory granulation tissue in the SABE

(ABE, acute bacterial endocarditis; SABE, subacute bacterial endocarditis; RHD, rheumatic heart disease).

Q43. Briefly discusss major types and causes of cardiac valvular deformities.

Key facts:
i. Valvular deformities could be congenital or acquired.
ii. Many of them result in heart failure.
iii. Rheumatic heart disease is the most common cause of acquired valvular deformities.
iv. Left-sided valves are more often involved than the right heart valves.
v. The mitral valve is affected most often, followed in descending frequency by aortic, and combine mitral aortic deformities.
vi. Bicuspid aortic valve is the most common congenital valvular deformity, affecting 1–2% of all people.

Pathophysiology Valvular deformities may result in:
- *Stenosis,* i.e. narrowing causing partial obstruction to blood flow, or
- *Insufficiency* (or incompetence) marked by regurgitation (backward flow) of blood.

Causes The following diseases and pathologic processes could cause valvular deformities:
i. Rheumatic heart disease
ii. Infective endocarditis
iii. Non-bacterial thrombotic endocarditis
iv. Libman-Sacks endocarditis
v. Syphilitic endocarditis
vi. Calcific aortic valve stenosis
vii. Calcification of mitral valve annulus
viii. Myxomatous degeneration (floppy valve syndrome)
ix. Carcinoid heart disease

Q44. What is mitral stenosis? Discuss its salient features and consequences.

Definition Mitral stenosis (MS) is a mitral valve dysfunction resulting from pathologic changes of the mitral valve causing an obstruction of the blood flow from the left atrium to the left ventricle.

Etiopathogenesis MS may be congenital but is more frequently acquired:
i. Rheumatic heart disease
- The most common cause of mitral stenosis
- Found in 40% of patients with RHD (70% of which are women)
- Clinical symptoms appear 20 years after the initial bout of RHD

ii. Congenital parachute mitral valve
iii. Severe mitral valve annular calcification
iv. Libman-Sacks endocarditis

Pathology The extent of stenosis varies from mild to severe:
i. *Mild stenosis*
- Valve remains mobile but the free margins of the leaflets appear thickened and puckered narrowing the lumen ('purse-string puckering').

ii. *Advanced stenosis*
- Diffuse thickening of valves with calcification especial toward the closing margin.
- Fibrous adhesion of mitral commissures.
- Shortening and fusion of chordae tendineae.

iii. *Severe stenosis*
- Leaflets are rigid, fixed and immobile.
- The opening of the orifice is narrow and the valve cannot open during diastole.
- From the atrial side it looks like a narrow slit or rigid oval opening (colloquially called 'button-hole' or 'fish-mouth' like) **(Fig. 16.25, A, B)**.

Consequences of mitral stenosis
i. Dilatation and hypertrophy of left atrium
ii. Normal-sized or smaller than normal left ventricle (due to reduced inflow of blood)
iii. Pulmonary hypertension resulting in:
a. Chronic passive congestions of the lungs

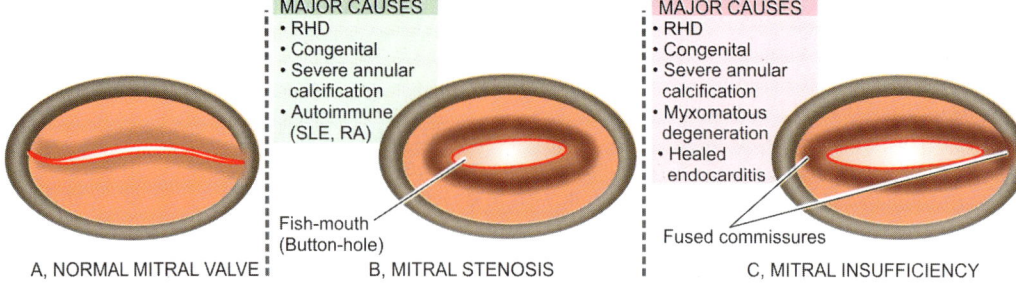

FIGURE 16.25: Mitral valve disease. Normal mitral valve (A) contrasted with mitral stenosis (B) and mitral insufficiency (C). (RHD, rheumatic heart disease; SLE, systemic lupus erythematosus; RA, rheumatoid arthritis)

b. Hypertrophy and dilatation of the right ventricle
c. Dilatation of the right atrium when right heart failure supervenes
Clinical features Symptoms appear 20 years after the initial onset of RHD.
i. Symptoms appear when the mitral orifice is reduced approximately five times, i.e. from its normal size (about 5 cm^2) to about 1 cm^2.
ii. Atrial pressure rises from normal 12 mmHg to 25 mmHg → backpressure in pulmonary veins → exertional dyspnoea (the chief symptom of mitral stenosis!).

Q45. What is mitral insufficiency? Discuss its causes, mechanisms and effects.

Definition Mitral insufficiency (also known as mitral incompetence) is a mitral valve dysfunction resulting from a pathologic changes of the mitral valve causing regurgitation (backflow) of blood from the left ventricle to the left atrium during systole.
Etiopathogenesis It may be congenital but is more frequently acquired **(Fig. 16.25, C)**:
i. Rheumatic heart disease
- The most common cause of mitral insufficiency
- Found in 50% of patients with RHD (75% of which are men)
- May be combined with stenosis

ii. Other causes of mitral stenosis (listed above) may also cause insufficiency (e.g. bacterial endocarditis, annular calcification)
iii. Rupture of mitral valve in endocarditis
iv. Myxomatous transformation of mitral valve (floppy valve syndrome)
v. Rupture of papillary muscle in MI
Pathology The morphology depends on the underlying cause:
i. *Rheumatic endocarditis* leads to calcification, scarring and deformity of leaflets.
- The leaflets are thickened, rigid, retracted and attached to shortened chordae.
- Due to their deformity the valves cannot close the mitral orifice completely during systole.

ii. *Myxomatous degeneration of leaflets* renders the valves 'floppy' and ballooned, prone to aneurysmal protrusion into the left atrium.
- The cause of these changes is not known.
- Some younger patients have Marfan syndrome.
- *Microscopically*, the valves contain mucoid or myxoid material due to abundance of mucopolysaccharides in the extracellular matrix.

iii. *Mitral annulus calcification* is an old age degenerative change of unknown etiology, related to ageing. The annulus is stone-hard and beaded and has lost all its pliability.
Consequences of mitral insufficiency
i. Dilatation and hypertrophy of the left ventricle
ii. Marked dilatation of the left atrium
iii. Pulmonary hypertension the same way as in mitral stenosis.
Clinical features Symptoms are mostly related to decreased cardiac output, and backpressure into the left atrium and pulmonary veins resulting in pulmonary hypertension.
i. Decreased ventricular output causes fatigue and weakness.

ii. Since the left ventricle cannot empty completely, there is also increased end-diastolic volume and pressure, reducing the pump function of the left ventricle.
iii. Backpressure into the left atrium and pulmonary veins leads to pulmonary hypertension and cor pulmonale with right heart failure.
iv. Pulmonary venous backflow leads to pulmonary congestion and oedema, presenting clinically with exertional dyspnoea and orthopnea. These findings are similar to those in mitral stenosis, even though less well marked.

Q46. Define aortic stenosis. What are its causes, mechanisms and effects?

Definition Aortic stenosis is aortic valve dysfunction resulting from pathologic changes of the aortic valve causing an obstruction to blood outflow from the left ventricle into the aorta during systole. It comprises 25% of all patients with chronic valvular heart disease. Approximately 80% of symptomatic patients are males.

Classification and etiology There are two forms of aortic stenosis: i) non-calcific, and ii) calcific.
i. *Non-calcific aortic stenosis* is most often caused by rheumatic heart disease. Other causes such as congenital valvular and subaortic stenosis, congenital bicuspid valve, and radiation exposure are less common.
ii. *Calcific aortic stenosis* is the more common type. Calcification of valves may occur in RHD, bacterial endocarditis, Mönckeberg calcific aortic stenosis, familial hypercholesterolaemia and xanthomatosis.

Pathology
i. Valves are thickened due to fibrosis and rigid, narrowing the lumen of the orifice.
ii. In rheumatic aortic stenosis, the commissures between the valves are fused, whereas in non-rheumatic aortic stenosis there is no commissural fusion.
iii. In calcific aortic stenosis the valves show calcific nodularity of the closing edges and confluent nodules inside the sinus of Valsalva **(Fig. 16.26, A, B)**.

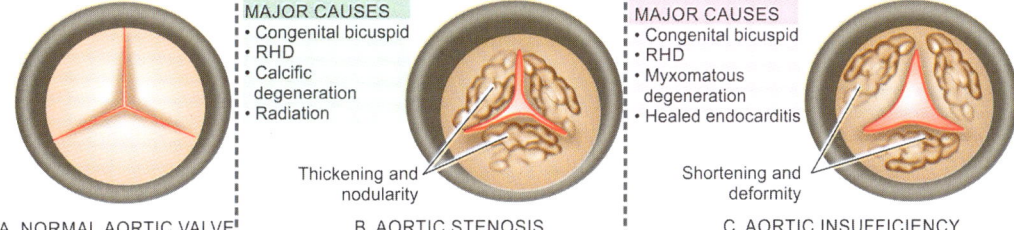

FIGURE 16.26: Aortic valve diseases. Normal aortic valve (A) contrasted with aortic stenosis (B) and aortic insufficiency (C).

Consequences
i. Concentric hypertrophy of the wall of the left ventricle due to the obstruction of the aortic outflow of blood.
ii. Terminal heart failure results in superimposed dilatation of the left ventricle ('eccentric hypertrophy'), and pulmonary congestion due to inefficient emptying of the left ventricle.

Clinical features Symptoms appear when the valve orifice is reduced to 1 cm^2 from its normal 3 cm^2. Three cardinal symptoms of aortic stenosis are as follows:
i. *Exertional dyspnoea* due to increased pulmonary capillary pressure and pulmonary oedema.
ii. *Angina pectoris* due to hypoperfusion of the coronary arteries.
iii. *Syncope* due to sudden coronary insufficiency; it may also result in sudden cardiac death.

Q47. What is aortic insufficiency? Briefly discuss its etiology, effects and clinicopathologic features.

Definition Aortic insufficiency is a aortic valve dysfunction resulting from pathologic change of the aortic valve characterised by regurgitation of blood from the aorta into the left ventricle **(Fig. 16.26, C)**. 75% of patients are male.

Etiopathogenesis Numerous causes as follows:
i. Chronic RHD seen in 75% cases (most common)
ii. Congenital bicuspid valve
iii. Myxomatous degeneration (floppy aortic valve) and Marfan syndrome

iv. Infective endocarditis and syphilis
v. Cystic medial necrosis

Consequences and clinical features
i. Due to regurgitant blood flow through the insufficient aortic valve, there is hypertrophy and dilatation of heart (huge heart >1000 g).
ii. Left ventricular failure leads to pulmonary congestion and ultimately to right heart failure.
iii. Due to additional strain on the left ventricle the patient is typically aware of the heart beat and feels pounding in the head!
iv. Low diastolic pressure and high pulse pressure, rapidly rising and collapsing 'water hammer pulse' (Corrigan pulse), booming 'pistol shot sound' over the femoral artery.
v. Systolic and diastolic murmur heard over the femoral artery when highly compressed (Durozier sign).
vi. Angina pectoris may occur due to coronary insufficiency.

Q48. Briefly discuss carcinoid heart disease.

Definition Carcinoid heart disease is a set of cardiac changes found in patients who have hepatic metastases of carcinoids from the GI tract.
Pathogenesis Not fully understood.
Hypothesis is that the carcinoid secretes serotonin, bradykinin and other vasoactive substances that bypass the liver and are not metabolised. Hence, these substances reach the heart and produce valvular and other changes, most prominently in the right heart.
Clinicopathologic features
i. Found in 50% of patients with carcinoids metastatic to the liver.
ii. Right heart more affected than the left.
iii. Fibrosis of the tricuspid and pulmonary valve and endocardium of right atrium and ventricle, presents as cartilage-like fibrous plaques.
iv. Similar changes may be seen in great veins, and less often on the left side of the heart.
v. Clinically, there is pulmonary stenosis and tricuspid insufficiency and right heart failure.

Q49. What is myocarditis? Briefly discuss its major types.

Definition Myocarditis is inflammation of the myocardium, that often remains unrecognised clinically and is thus more commonly diagnosed at autopsy.
Classification There are many classifications but the most useful is the etiologic classification that divides it into four main groups:
I. Infective myocarditis
II. Idiopathic (Fiedler) myocarditis
III. Myocarditis of connective tissue diseases
IV. Miscellaneous types
I. *Infective myocarditis* may be caused by any of the human pathogens (e.g. viruses, bacteria, protozoa, etc.).
i. *Viral myocarditis* is the most common infectious myocarditis, found in up to 5% of systemic viral infections.
- Most often mild and subclinical, or clinically not recognised, but it may also cause heart failure.
- Most common etiologic viruses are coxsackie A and B and enteroviruses.
- Viruses may invade cardiac myocytes and kill them or elicit a T-cell mediated immune reaction. The myocardium is infiltrated with lymphocytes.
ii. *Bacterial myocarditis* is usually seen in systemic infections and is often a complication of bacteraemia. It may produce microscopic abscesses in the myocardium.
iii. *Borrelia burgdorferi* (bacterial spirochete) may cause myocarditis which is seen in up to 5% of patients with systemic Lyme disease. For some unknown reasons, this myocarditis often affects the conduction system causing irregular heart beat.
iv. *Granulomatous myocarditis* can be caused by *M. tuberculosis*, and is typically seen during miliary dissemination of the disease. In the US and Europe, granulomatous myocarditis is, however, more commonly a feature of sarcoidosis than tuberculosis.

v. *Fungal myocarditis* is usually seen in immunosuppressed and debilitated persons in terminal stages of cancer or chronic systemic disease, often accompanied by systemic dissemination of fungi such as *Candida, Aspergillus, Cryptococcus*, etc.

vi. *Rickettsial myocarditis* is encountered in Rocky Mountain typhus and scrub typhus (caused by R. tsutsugamushi).

vii. *Protozoal myocarditis* is prevalent in endemic areas of the World. For example,
- *Trypanosoma cruzi* myocarditis accounts for most cases of myocarditis of Chagas' disease in Brazil.
- *Toxoplasma gondii* is a cause of myocarditis in immunosuppressed persons and AIDS patients.

II. **Idiopathic (Fiedler) myocarditis** does not have an identifiable cause. Typically, it is limited to the myocardium, and is not associated with any other inflammatory disease of the other layers of the heart or other organs. It usually leads to heart failure and may often cause sudden death.

Pathologic forms are: i) Diffuse and ii) Giant cell type.

i. *Diffuse idiopathic myocarditis* is characterised by infiltrates of chronic inflammatory cells, lymphocytes, macrophages and plasma cells. If the patient survives, it heals with myocardial fibrosis.

ii. *Giant cell myocarditis* also known as granulomatous myocarditis is characterised by infiltrates of epithelioid macrophages and multinucleated giant cells and lymphocytes, which may form granulomas. It has usually a rapidly downhill course and is lethal unless a heart transplantation is performed to save the patient's life.

III. **Myocarditis of connective tissue diseases** may be part of the clinicopathologic spectrum of these systemic autoimmune diseases. It may be found in SLE, dermatomyositis, polyarteritis nodosa, scleroderma.

IV. **Miscellaneous forms of myocarditis** can be caused by a variety of toxic chemical, physical and metabolic injuries. More common causes are as under:
- Physical agents, e.g. irradiation, contusion of the myocardium, cardiac surgery.
- Chemical agents, e.g. arsenic, phosphorus, carbon monoxide.
- Drugs, e.g. cytotoxic drugs, catecholamines.
- Muscle diseases, e.g. muscular dystrophies, myasthenia gravis.
- Metabolic derangements, e.g. uraemia, hypokalaemia.

Q50. Define cardiomyopathy. How is it classified?

Definition Cardiomyopathy is a term which was previously applied to heart diseases of unknown etiology presenting with heart failure. Currently, under this term we include a number of genetic diseases, disease putatively linked to exogenous adverse influences, and others that are still considered to be idiopathic.

Classification Cardiomyopathies are subdivided into three groups: dilated (congestive), hypertrophic and restrictive. Their further subtypes are given in **Table 16.7**.

TABLE 16.7 Classification of cardiomyopathies.

I. DILATED (OR CONGESTIVE) CARDIOMYOPATHY
II. HYPERTROPHIC CARDIOMYOPATHY
i. Obstructive type
ii. Non-obstructive type
III. RESTRICTIVE (OR OBLITERATIVE OR INFILTRATIVE) CARDIOMYOPATHY
i. Cardiac amyloidosis
ii. Endocardial fibroelastosis
iii. Endomyocardial fibrosis
iv. Löeffler endocarditis (fibroplastic parietal endocarditis with peripheral blood eosinophilia)
v. Other forms

Q51. Discuss salient features of dilated (congestive) cardiomyopathy.

Definition Dilated cardiomyopathy is a term applied to a heterogeneous group of myocardial diseases characterised by dilatation of all four chambers and systolic dysfunction leading invariably to death in a few years.

It is the most common cardiomyopathy (90% of all cases).

Etiopathogenesis Many cases are idiopathic, whereas others have an identifiable cause as follows:

i. Genetic basis can be established in 20–50% cases, especially common in younger persons, and those with history of familial inheritance.

ii. It may be related to a mutation of one of more than 50 genes encoding the following proteins:
a. Cytoskeletal proteins (e.g. actin, desmin)
b. Sarcomeric proteins (e.g. titin, the longest protein in the heart muscle)

c. Nuclear proteins (e.g. lamin A and lamin C)
d. Contractile proteins (e.g. myosin)
e. Cell membrane and membrane linked proteins (e.g. dystrophin in Duchenne dystrophy)
f. Mitochondrial proteins (e.g. enzymes involved in oxidative phosphorylation)
g. Conduction system proteins accounting for the 'channelopathies'
iii. Viral myocarditis in healing stages with extensive fibrosis and no signs of inflammation. Molecular biology techniques may identify viral imprints in heart cells.
iv. Alcohol abuse and related vitamin deficiency (e.g. beriberi heart).
v. Cytotoxic drugs (e.g. doxorubicin).
vi. Toxins (e.g. cobalt).
vii. Peripartum cardiomyopathy, a rare but potentially serious complication of late pregnancy or early postpartum period; probably related to pregnancy hormones (reversible in 50% of cases!).

Clinicopathologic features
i. The heart is enlarged (600 to over 1000 g).
ii. Four-chamber dilatation gives the heart a globular appearance **(Fig. 16.27, A, B)**.
iii. The wall of all four chambers is thickened and shows marked scarring.
iv. Mural thrombi may be present in any of the chambers.
v. *Microscopy* reveals collagenous fibrosis replacing myocardial cells with compensatory hypertrophy of the preserved myocytes.
vi. The findings are nonspecific and do not provide clues about the possible cause of heart injury.
vii. Clinical picture is dominated by systolic insufficiency due to inadequate strength of ventricular contraction.
viii. Dilatation of ventricles leads to functional insufficiency of mitral and tricuspid valve.
ix. Fibrosis is accompanied by conduction disorders such as atrial and ventricular fibrillation.
x. Mural thrombi may give rise to thromboemboli to major organs.

Q52. What is hypertrophic cardiomyopathy?

Definition Hypertrophic cardiomyopathy (also known as asymmetrical hypertrophy, hypertrophic subaortic stenosis or Teare's disease) is a congenital heart disease marked by prominent hypertrophy of cardiac myocytes and diastolic dysfunction **(Fig. 16.27, C)**.
Estimated prevalence is 1:500.

Etiopathogenesis
- The disease is based on mutation of one of several *sarcomeric proteins* resulting in hypertrophy and increased contractile strength of cardiac myocytes (gain of function).
- The most common are the mutations of genes encoding *β-myosin heavy chain*. Together with the mutations of *myosin binding protein C* and *troponin T*, it accounts for ¾ of all cases.
- The transmission of mutated genes is usually *autosomal dominant* with variable penetrance.

Pathophysiology Hypertrophy of the myocardium has several possible drawbacks including the following:
i. *Relative ischaemia of hypertrophic myocytes* which requires more oxygen for contraction.

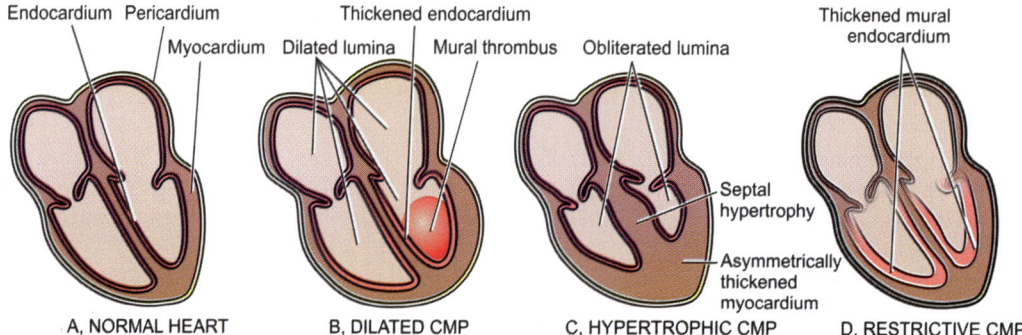

FIGURE 16.27: Three pathophysiologic forms of idiopathic cardiomyopathies.

ii. Reduced size of the ventricles surrounded by hypertrophic myocardial wall which *cannot fully dilate during diastole*. This leads to reduced diastolic filling of ventricle and increased end-diastolic pressure.
iii. Hypertrophy of left ventricular wall provides *resistance to filling of the branches of the coronary arteries*, contributing to ischaemia of the myocytes.
iv. The transmission of electrical impulse through the hypertrophic myocardium and the compression of the intramural branches of the conduction system lead to *irregular ventricular contractions, atrial fibrillation and formation of atrial mural thrombi*.
v. *Asymmetrical hypertrophy of the subaortic septum* (found in 25% of all cases) causes obstruction to ventricular ejection of blood from left ventricle, which may result in *hypotensive angina pectoris, syncope due to cardiac or cerebral hypoperfusion ischaemia, and even sudden cardiac death*.

Q53. What is restrictive cardiomyopathy? Discuss its subtypes and their main features.

Definition Restrictive cardiomyopathy, also known as obliterative or infiltrative cardiomyopathy, is heterogeneous group of heart diseases characterised by diastolic failure due to reduced volume of ventricles which show endomyocardial infiltration that may be fibrillar material, granulomas, or products of abnormal metabolism due to genetic disorders **(Fig. 16.27, D)**.
It accounts for less than 5% of all cardiomyopathies and is thus the rarest of the three recognised forms of cardiomyopathy.

Etiopathogenesis The myocardium is rigid because it is infiltrated with material that restricts the relaxation of cardiac myocytes and the dilatation of ventricles.
The material found infiltrating the cardiac walls includes the following:
i. *Amyloidosis* affecting the heart can be of two types: a) as part of *systemic amyloidosis*, or b) *Isolated cardiac amyloidosis*, as seen in the senile.
ii. *Fibrous scar tissue*, as seen following therapeutic irradiation or chemotherapy, or in endomyocardial fibrosis.
iii. *Fibro-elastotic material* involving endocardium and extending into the myocardium, as in endocardial fibroelastosis.
iv. *Granulomas* in the myocardial interstitium as in sarcoidosis.
v. *Metabolites* accumulating in increased amounts.

Clinicopathologic features Restrictive cardiomyopathy comprises several clinicopathologic entities as under:

I. **Amyloidosis** Cardiac amyloid may be of two types:
i. Part of *systemic AA or AL amyloidosis* involving many other internal organs.
ii. *Senile cardiac amyloidosis*, characterised by deposits of *transthyretin*, the heart is the only organ affected.
In either case, deposits of amyloid destroy and replace the cardiac myocytes, contributing to the rigidity of the myocardium and causing weakening of its pump function.

II. **Endocardial fibroelastosis** In its most common form, this is predominantly a disease of infants living in Africa and other tropical countries. Less often, it may also affect older children as well as young adults. Worldwide it is the most common restrictive cardiomyopathy.
Etiology The cause of the disease is unknown.
i. The more common infantile form may be congenital (due to intrauterine ischaemia) and have a genetic predisposition (affects twins and siblings).
ii. Geographic distribution suggests an environmental effect.
iii. The late onset disease might be caused by ischaemia or could represent a connective tissue disease.
iv. Environmental effects are probably also important.
Clinicopathologic features The left ventricle is most often involved, but the disease may involve other chambers as well.
i. Endocardium is thickened and appears diffusely pearly white.
ii. *Microscopically*, the endocardium contains layers of collagen and elastic fibres.
iii. The valves also show fibroelastosis and occasionally there are mural thrombi.
iv. The wall of the left ventricle is hypertrophic, and yet the volume of the left ventricle is diminished and its function is restricted due to endocardial fibroelastosis.
v. Clinical features include bouts of sudden breathlessness, cyanosis, and progressive cardiac failure with a lethal outcome.

III. **Endomyocardial fibrosis** It is also a tropical disease prevalent in some countries of Africa and Asia. It affects children and young adults, causing congestive heart failure with usually lethal outcome.
Etiology Unknown. The geographic distribution suggests some environmental causes.
Clinicopathologic features
i. Endocardial fibrosis of the ventricles that extends into the inner third of the myocardium.
ii. Atrioventricular valves may be fibrotic, but the semilunar valves are not affected.
iii. Mural thrombi may be present.
iv. *Microscopically*, there is fibrosis that contains scattered chronic inflammatory cells.
IV. **Loeffler endocarditis** It is also known as fibroplastic parietal endocarditis with eosinophilia and is a rare disease of unknown etiology. It may occur at any age and it is not geographically restricted to any particular region.
Etiology Unknown. Molecular biology studies show that at least some of the cases of eosinophilia represent a *clonal haematologic disorder.*
Clinicopathologic features
i. The hallmarks of the disease are *endomyocardial fibrosis* associated with *infiltrates of eosinophils* and *blood eosinophilia.*
ii. The heart failure has all the features of restrictive cardiomyopathy with inadequate diastolic filling of the ventricles and biventricular pump failure.
iii. Eosinophils probably play a significant role in damaging the heart and causing endomyocardial fibrosis.

Q54. What are the causes of pericardial fluid accumulation?

Pericardial fluid accumulations include: pericardial effusions and haemopericardium.
I. **Pericardial effusion** Most often, it is serous fluid accumulation in the pericardial sac. Serous effusions are also called *hydropericardium.*
Pericardial effusions are classified according to the nature and or appearance of the fluid as follows:
i. *Serous effusion* is marked by an accumulation of clear, watery, straw-coloured fluid in excess of the normal pericardial fluid content which is 30–50 ml. It may be transudate or exudate. Most often, it is found in following conditions:
a. Transudate in chronic heart failure
b. Component of generalised oedema due to hypoalbuminaemia in chronic liver or renal disease
c. Serous pericarditis (see later)
ii. *Serosanguinous effusion*, most often caused by blunt chest trauma or cardiac resuscitation. Myocardial infarction and pericardial malignancies could also produce it.
iii. *Chylous effusion* is marked by an accumulation of milky lymph and is usually caused by obstruction of the lymphatic ducts in the mediastinum.
II. **Haemopericardium** It is accumulation of blood in the pericardial sac.
Etiopathogenesis The most common causes of haemopericardium are as under:
i. Rupture of heart through myocardial infarct
ii. Rupture of dissecting aneurysm of the aorta
iii. Bleeding diathesis as in acute leukaemia, thrombocytopenia, or less common causes such as scurvy
iv. Traumatic laceration of the heart, aorta or coronary artery
Clinical features of pericardial fluid accumulation
i. Pericardial fluid can be best detected by X-rays or ultrasound.
ii. On auscultation there is a faint apex beat.
iii. Pericardial fluid effusions and haematopericardium produce symptoms which depend on the *amount* of accumulated fluid and the *rate* at which it has accumulated in the pericardial sac.
- *Slow accumulation* of fluid allows pericardial sac to expand, and accordingly even large quantities of fluid (e.g. 500–1000 ml) could have no serious effect on the heart function. Same is true for chronic pericardial effusions: effusions up to 500 ml usually produce few circulatory problems and do not require interventions.
- *Rapid filling of the pericardial sac* with smaller quantities of fluid (e.g. 250–300 ml) could cause cardiac tamponade with lethal outcome due to the compression of atria and great veins, impeding diastolic filling.

Q55. What is acute pericarditis? Discuss its main types.

Definition Acute pericarditis is an inflammation of the pericardium, most often secondary to inflammation of the heart proper, adjacent organs in the thoracic cavity, or systemic disease involving more than one organ. Primary, isolated pericarditis is rare.

Types The most important forms of acute pericarditis are as follows:

I. **Serous pericarditis** is characterised by a clear straw-coloured exudate that contains more proteins and cells than a transudate. The amount of fluid ranges from 50–200 ml in most cases, and thus the function of the heart is not seriously impaired. The common causes include the following:
i. Viral pericarditis caused by a variety of viruses, such as coxsakie A and B virus, adenoviruses or cytomegalovirus
ii. Autoimmune diseases such as rheumatoid arthritis, SLE
iii. Rheumatic fever
iv. Pericardial malignant tumours, most often metastasis from adjacent organs (e.g. lungs, oesophagus)
v. Tuberculous pericarditis

II. **Fibrinous and serofibrinous pericarditis** is dominated by exudation of fibrin-rich fluid and fibrin deposition on the internal surfaces of the visceral and parietal pericardium, giving it a 'bread and butter' appearance. On physical examination, one can hear a 'pericardial friction rub' as the two surfaces of the pericardium covered with fibrin slide over one another. The inflammation can resolve upon treatment, or the fibrin may become organised and cause adhesions between the visceral and parietal pericardium. The possible causes include the following:
i. Bacterial pericarditis
ii. Transmural myocardial infarction
iii. Rheumatic fever
iv. Uraemia
v. Trauma and open heart surgery

III. **Purulent or fibrinopurulent pericarditis** is usually caused by pyogenic bacteria, such as staphylococci, streptococci, etc. Exudate rich on neutrophils and pus cells is typically seen on microscopic examination. Purulent exudate does not resolve spontaneously or even after treatment and it usually leads to formation of fibrosis and adhesion between the two layers of pericardium. Bacterial infections may reach the pericardium through several routes as under:
i. Direct extension from infection in adjacent organs, such bacterial pneumonia, pleuritis, or mediastinitis
ii. Haematogenous spread
iii. Lymphatic permeation
iv. Direct implantation of bacteria during cardiac surgery

IV. **Haemorrhagic pericarditis** results from admixture of blood with any of the forms of pericarditis mentioned above. The causes are as under:
i. Malignant neoplasms of the pericardium
ii. Haemorrhagic diathesis in a patient that has a pericardial effusion
iii. Severe acute inflammation of any kind
iv. Tuberculosis.

Q56. Discuss chronic pericarditis and its types briefly.

Definition Chronic pericarditis is a term for the prolongation of non-healing acute inflammation or several recurrences of acute pericarditis. Some chronic infectious diseases such as tuberculosis can also cause chronic pericarditis.

Types The most important forms of chronic pericarditis are listed as under:

I. **Tuberculous pericarditis** is the most common granulomatous disease of the pericardium.
- M. tuberculosis can reach the pericardium by direct extension from the foci of pulmonary tuberculosis or by lymphatic spread from tracheobronchial lymph nodes, or foci of pulmonary and pleural tuberculosis.
- The pericardial exudate is turbid caseous or fibrino-haemorrhagic, leading to fibrotic adhesions obliterating the pericardial cavity.
- Caseating granulomas are found in the pericardium on microscopic examination.

II. **Chronic adhesive pericarditis** is characterised by formation of fibrous adhesions that form after an incompletely resolved acute infection **(Fig. 16.28, A)**. Fibrosis may extend into the mediastinum;

such a condition is then called *adhesive medistino-pericarditis*. In contrast to constrictive pericarditis, adhesive pericarditis usually does not embarrass the function of the heart. Compensatory hypertrophy of the heart seen in many cases indicates that heart is nevertheless under stress and must strain to maintain its pump function.

III. **Chronic constrictive pericarditis** is a rare form of chronic pericarditis characterised by formation of dense fibrous or fibrocalcific thickening of the pericardium encasing the heart **(Fig. 16.28, B)**. The fibrotic pericardium obliterates the pericardial cavity thus preventing proper dilatation of the heart chambers during diastole. It also leads to constriction of the great veins preventing the venous blood inflow into the right atrium. All these changes will markedly reduce the cardiac output and lead to heart failure. The heart is not enlarged as in chronic adhesive pericarditis.

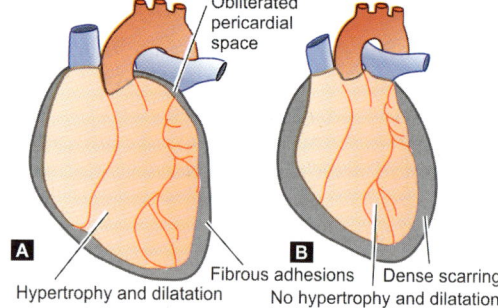

FIGURE 16.28: Appearance of the heart and the pericardium in chronic adhesive (A) and chronic constrictive pericarditis (B).

Chronic constrictive pericarditis can develop from unresolved acute or chronic pericarditis of any kind but most often it results from the following diseases:
i. Tuberculous pericarditis
ii. Purulent pericarditis
iii. Haemopericardium
iv. Concato disease (polyserositis)

Q57. What is the most common primary tumour of the heart?

Primary heart tumours are rare. Most heart tumours are benign, but even benign tumours are rare. *Myxoma* is overall the most common primary heart tumour.

Cardiac myxoma
Clinical and gross Myxoma is typically polypoid, pedunculated and moves back and forth in the blood stream circulation. Most myxomas are located in the left atrium and could act as ball valve obstructing the atrioventricular orifice.
Microscopy Myxomas are composed of myxoid stroma, capillaries and sparse spindle cells, some of which may be multinucleated.

Q58. What are the malignant tumours of the heart?

i. Primary malignant tumours of the heart are rare.
ii. Metastatic tumours are much more common than primary tumours.
iii. Highest on the list of primary tumours are *angiosarcoma and malignant mesothelioma*.
iv. *Metastastic tumours* reach the heart through the lymphatics or haematogenously from other sites.
v. Primary sites of origin, in descending order of frequency, are: carcinoma of the lung, carcinoma of breast, malignant lymphoma, leukaemia and malignant melanoma.
vi. About 10% of all cases of disseminated cancer have metastases in the heart discovered at autopsy.

Q59. Comment on important pathologic findings in transplanted heart.

i. *Transplant rejection* with infiltration of the graft with T-lymphocytes and macrophages.
ii. *Accelerated coronary atherosclerosis.*
iii. *Infections:* Some infections may be related to bacteria accidentally introduced during surgery.
iv. *Immunosuppression* is associated with infections with *Toxoplasma gondii* and cytomegalovirus.

Chapter 16e Supplement: Online Content

Digital content of this chapter available with this book is meant for enhanced learning and self-assessment. In addition, it contains 36 Multiple Choice Questions (MCQs), 05 Clinicopathologic Vignettes, and 07 Image-based Questions; these are followed by their answers along with explanatory notes of correct and incorrect answers.

CHAPTER 17

Respiratory System

LUNGS

Q1. What are the key anatomic features of the respiratory system relevant to understanding pathologic lesions of this system?

- Lungs and the heart form a dual, yet fully integrated, *cardiorespiratory system* whose main function is to supply oxygen the tissues, and to remove carbon dioxide.
- The principal anatomic parts of the respiratory system are the nose and the upper respiratory tracts, trachea and the bronchi and the lungs.
- The right lung comprises three lobes (upper, middle and lower), whereas the left lung has only two lobes.
- The *bronchial tree* begins with left and right main bronchi which divide into smaller bronchi, which in turn divide into bronchioles, visible only by microscopy. Bronchioles undergo several divisions and end in terminal bronchioles, which measure only 2 mm in diameter. The part of the lung distal to the terminal bronchioles is called acinus.
- The *acinus* consists of three parts: a) respiratory bronchioles originating from the terminal bronchiole, b) alveolar ducts originating from the respiratory bronchioles, and c) alveolar sacs (alveoli) **(Fig 17.1)**.
- Lungs have a *dual circulation*. On one hand, they receive venous blood through the pulmonary artery and on the other hand arterial blood through the bronchial arteries. Oxygenated blood leaves the lungs through the pulmonary veins, which drain into the left atrium.

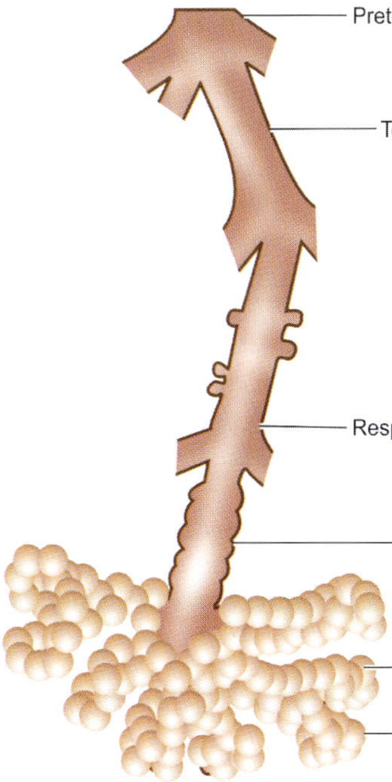

FIGURE 17.1: Structure of an acinus which is part of the lung distal to terminal bronchiole. It shows respiratory bronchiole, alveolar ducts and alveolar sacs.

Q2. What are the key histologic features of the lungs?

- **Bronchi** are lined by pseudostratified columnar epithelium containing ciliated, mucus-secreting and neuroendocrine cells, also called *respiratory epithelium*.
- **Bronchioles** are lined by a single layer of respiratory epithelium **(Fig. 17.2)**. As they divide, they contain fewer and fewer mucus-secreting and neuroendocrine cells. Bronchioles also contain scattered

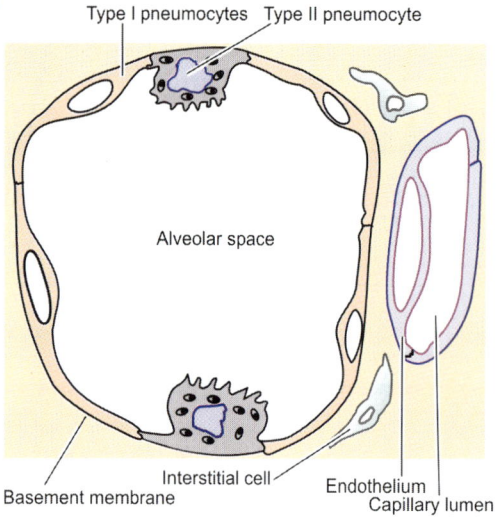

FIGURE 17.2: Histologic structure of alveolar wall (alveolar septa), diagrammatic view. It shows capillary endothelium, capillary basement membrane and scanty interstitial tissue and the alveolar lining cells (type I or membranous pneumocytes and type II or granular pneumocytes).

Clara cells which secrete proteins like lysozyme and immunoglobulins, and some undifferentiated stem cells, which are important for the regeneration of damaged epithelia.
- **Alveoli** are the part of the lung where the exchange of gases between the air and the blood takes place. The alveolar wall is lined on the alveolar surface by type I pneumocyte, covering 90% of its surface and scattered granular type II pneumocytes that secrete surfactant. The blood reaches alveoli through the alveolar capillaries.

Q3. What are the main bronchopulmonary congenital anomalies?

Bronchopulmonary anomalies are uncommon and rarely cause clinical problems. These anomalies include i) pulmonary agenesis and hypoplasia, ii) cysts, iii) bronchopulmonary sequestration.

I. **Pulmonary agenesis**, which may be unilateral or bilateral, and **hypoplasia** (small incompletely developed lungs) are usually seen in severely malformed foetuses and newborn infants that have other congenital anomalies as well.

II. **Pulmonary cysts** may be solitary or multiple. These cysts may be from bronchi or alveoli. They rarely cause clinical problems. Larger cysts may compress the normal parenchyma, become infected or bleed.

III. **Bronchopulmonary sequestration** refers to the presence of pulmonary lobes or segments that are separate from normal lung and are not connected to the bronchial airways system. They appear as a distinct mass on X-rays that will usually compress the normal lung parenchyma. This mass is often resected.

Q4. Define and discuss atelectasis briefly.

Definition Atelectasis is a loss of pulmonary respiratory volume due to inadequate expansion or collapse of alveoli.
Classification Atelectasis may be primary or secondary:
I. **Primary atelectasis** It is typically seen in prematurely born infants.
Etiology/pathogenesis It results from incomplete expansion of neonatal alveoli due to weak respiratory action.
- Additional contributory factor is immaturity of lungs. The alveoli of the immature lungs cannot remain open because the pneumocytes type II do not synthesise enough surfactant that would keep the alveoli open.
- Clinical causes include: prematurity, cerebral birth injury, CNS malformations and intrauterine hypoxia.

II. **Secondary atelectasis** This results from collapse of alveoli in a previously expanded and well-aerated lung.

Etiology/pathogenesis Atelectasis results from compression of alveoli, obstruction of airways, or contraction of pulmonary parenchyma.

i. *Compressive atelectasis* is caused by outside pressure causing the collapse of alveoli. The causes could be: massive pleural effusion, haemothorax, pneumothorax, intrathoracic tumour and deformities of the thoracic cage and vertebral column. Peripheral parts of the lung are more affected than the central parts.

ii. *Obstructive/absorptive atelectasis* is caused by the obstruction of the bronchi followed by absorption of the air from alveoli distal to the obstruction. Bronchial obstruction may be caused by accumulation of mucus in bronchial asthma, chronic bronchitis or bronchiectasis, aspirated fluid or foreign bodies. Atelectasis is usually patchy and less pronounced than in compressive atelectasis.

iii. *Contraction atelectasis* is caused by localised fibrosis and scarring of the lung parenchyma and pleura. It is usually patchy and irreparable.

Q5. Define respiratory distress syndrome. What are its types?

Definition Respiratory distress syndrome (RDS), also known as acute respiratory distress syndrome (ARDS), is a severe, at times life-threatening, progressive respiratory insufficiency with diffuse lung involvement and pathologic changes in the alveolar epithelium, alveolar lumina, and interstitial tissue. Clinically, it presents with dyspnoea and hypoxia.

Classification Two distinct entities that have different etiology and pathogenesis:

i. *Neonatal RDS* which begins a few hours after birth presenting with tachypnoea, hypoxia and cyanosis and possible lethal outcome.

ii. *Adult ARDS* is also known as shock lung, acute lung injury, traumatic wet lungs, post-traumatic respiratory insufficiency. The underlying pathologic changes are known as *diffuse alveolar damage (DAD)*. Clinically it presents with sudden onset of severe respiratory distress, tachypnoea, tachycardia, cyanosis and severe hypoxemia.

Q6. Briefly discuss the etiology, pathogenesis, pathologic changes and outcome of neonatal respiratory distress syndrome.

Etiology Conditions predisposing to neonatal RDS are as follows:

i. Preterm birth, especially those born before the 28th week of gestation (60% will have RDS)
ii. Infants born to mothers who had a previous preterm delivery
iii. Birth by caesarian section
iv. Excessive sedation of the mother during delivery
v. Maternal diabetes
vi. Birth asphyxia (e.g. coils of umbilical cord around the neck)
vii. Male preponderance (M>F= 1.5 to 2 times more likely), probably related to earlier maturation of female baby lungs.

Pathogenesis The basic defect is a deficiency of lecithin-rich pulmonary surfactant resulting in the primary atelectasis of alveoli which leads to hypoventilation and hypoxia **(Fig. 17.3, A)**.

i. Atelectasis is accompanied by intrapulmonary blood shunting away from unventilated alveoli.
ii. Ensuing hypoperfusion of lungs will cause ischaemic injury of alveolar and endothelial cells.
iii. Leaky endothelium allows for exudation of fibrinogen, which will polymerise into fibrin and form hyaline membranes, further impeding entry of oxygen into the blood.

Pathology

Gross Lungs are atelectatic and appear airless at autopsy.

Microscopy

i. Atelectasis of alveoli, most of which do not have a visible lumen.
ii. Some alveoli and dilated alveolar ducts and respiratory bronchiole are lined by hyaline membranes.
iii. Hyaline membranes are composed primarily of fibrin but also contain cell debris from necrotic alveolar cells **(Fig. 17.4)**.

Outcome and consequences

i. Neonatal RDS had a high mortality but today it can be efficiently treated with exogenous surfactant and respirator-assisted oxygen delivery so that most babies survive and recover. Hyaline membranes

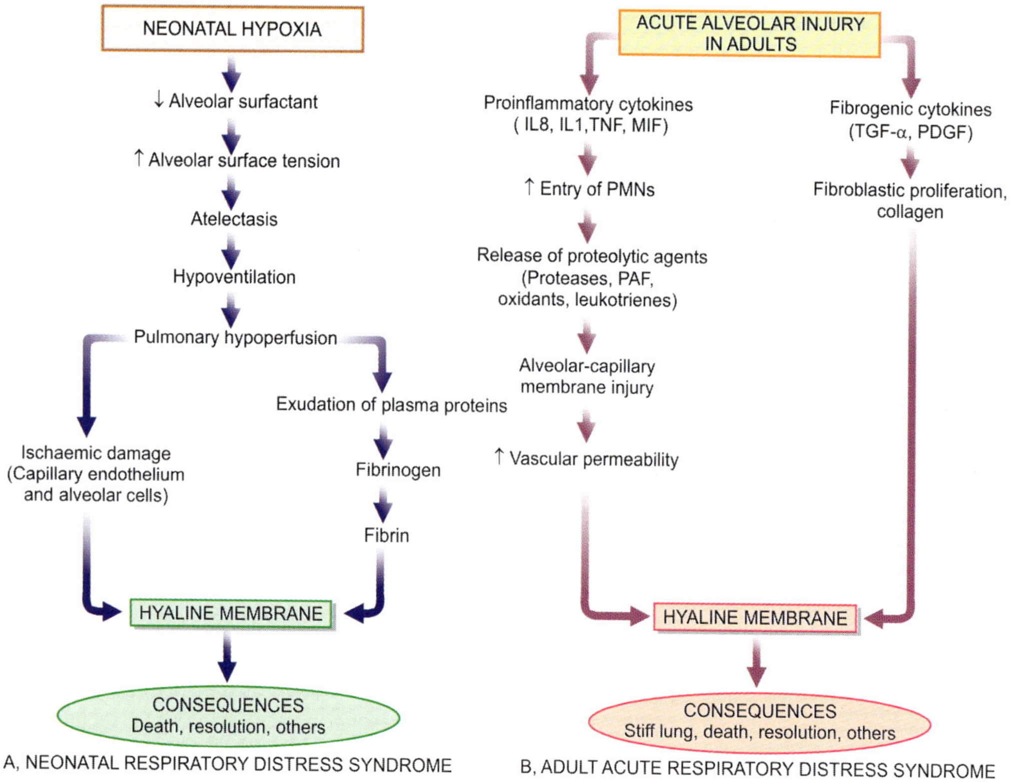

```
                NEONATAL HYPOXIA                    ACUTE ALVEOLAR INJURY
                                                         IN ADULTS

              ↓ Alveolar surfactant          Proinflammatory cytokines      Fibrogenic cytokines
                                              ( IL8, IL1,TNF, MIF)           (TGF-α, PDGF)

              ↑ Alveolar surface tension
                                                 ↑ Entry of PMNs         Fibroblastic proliferation,
                      Atelectasis                                                collagen

                                             Release of proteolytic agents
                    Hypoventilation               (Proteases, PAF,
                                               oxidants, leukotrienes)

                Pulmonary hypoperfusion
                                                 Alveolar-capillary
                                                  membrane injury
                         Exudation of plasma proteins

        Ischaemic damage                        ↑ Vascular permeability
        (Capillary endothelium        Fibrinogen
         and alveolar cells)

                                 Fibrin

                  HYALINE MEMBRANE                         HYALINE MEMBRANE

                    CONSEQUENCES                             CONSEQUENCES
                Death, resolution, others              Stiff lung, death, resolution, others

     A, NEONATAL RESPIRATORY DISTRESS SYNDROME    B, ADULT ACUTE RESPIRATORY DISTRESS SYNDROME
```

FIGURE 17.3: Schematic representation of sequence of events leading to the formation of hyaline membrane in neonatal RDS and adult acute respiratory distress syndrome (ARDS).

may resolve upon treatment and normal pulmonary architecture is restored without any residual damage.

ii. *Incomplete recovery* occurs in some infants who develop *bronchopulmonary dysplasia*. In such cases, the hyaline membranes are not resorbed. Instead, they are organised by granulation tissue and replaced by fibrous tissue, obliterating the alveoli partially and extending into the interstitial spaces. These late pathologic changes in the alveoli are combined with focal obliterating bronchiolitis and peribronchial fibrosis. Some of these changes are probably caused by oxygen radicals generated by the delivery of oxygen in the treatment of RDS.

Q7. Discuss the major features of adult acute respiratory distress syndrome.

Etiology Adults ARDS results from an injury of pulmonary alveolar or capillary cells **(Fig. 17.3, B)**. The injury may be classified as direct or indirect as under:

I. *Direct lung injury* affecting the alveolar cells can occur due to the following:
i. Infection (pneumonia)
ii. Oxygen injury (e.g. respirator assisted breathing)
iii. Inhalation of toxins and irritants (e.g. smoke, war gases, nitrogen dioxide, metal fumes, etc.)

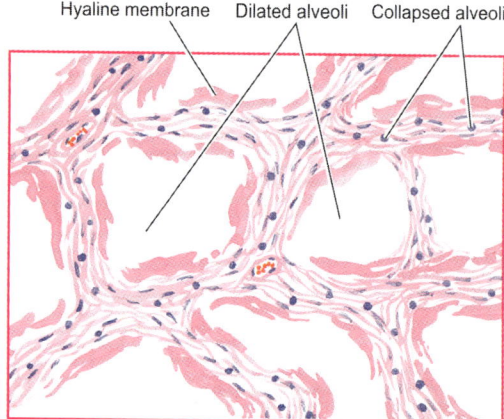

FIGURE 17.4: Histological appearance of neonatal respiratory distress syndrome (hyaline membrane disease). There are alternate areas of collapsed and dilated alveolar spaces, many of which are lined by eosinophilic hyaline membranes.

iv. Aspiration of gastric contents
v. Near drowning
II. *Indirect lung injury* usually affecting the pulmonary capillaries can occur due to the following:
i. Shock related to sepsis, trauma, burns, etc.
ii. Narcotic overdose
iii. Acute pancreatitis
iv. Drug related toxicity
v. Fat embolism
vi. Radiation
vii. Multiple transfusions

Pathology ARDS develops fast in most patients and severe dyspnoea is present usually within three days of the initial lung injury.
Gross At autopsy the lungs are heavy, airless and wet on sectioning.
Microscopy will reveal:
i. Protein-rich oedema and foci of intra-alveolar haemorrhage.
ii. Typically there are prominent fibrin-rich hyaline membranes focally lining the dilated alveoli.
iii. If the patient survives a few days, neutrophils and macrophages will enter focally into the alveoli in an attempt to remove the hyaline membranes.
iv. Massive intra-alveolar exudation of neutrophils is, however, usually a sign of pneumonia, which is often superimposed on ARDS.

Prognosis
- Mortality of ARDS is very high. It varies from 25% up to 50% depending on the severity of disease.
- Patients who survive ARDS may recover and restore their pulmonary function several months later.
- However, pulmonary function may be reduced in many of them for the rest of their lives.

Q8. Define pulmonary hypertension. How is it classified? Briefly discuss its pathogenesis and pathologic changes.

Definition Pulmonary hypertension is increased pulmonary blood pressure over 25 mmHg at rest, which is much higher in magnitude than the normal pressure of 3–8 mmHg.

Classification Pulmonary hypertension may be *primary (idiopathic) or secondary*; the latter is more common and is related to some other cardio-pulmonary or systemic connective tissue disease. This classification has been replaced with WHO classification that divides pulmonary hypertension into five groups as under:
- Group 1, *pulmonary arterial hypertension (PAH)* is a heterogeneous group of diseases caused by changes in pulmonary arteries. Some of the cases are hereditary, some drug-induced, some related to connective tissue disorders, HIV infections and congenital heart diseases.
- Group 2, *pulmonary hypertension due to left heart disease* such as hypertensive heart disease, endocarditis or cardiomyopathy.
- Group 3, *pulmonary hypertension due to chronic lung disease,* such as chronic obstructive pulmonary disease and chronic interstitial pulmonary diseases.
- Group 4, *chronic thromboembolic pulmonary hypertension.*
- Group 5, *pulmonary hypertension with unclear or multifactorial mechanisms.*

Pathogenesis The sequence of events in patients belonging to groups 2, 3, 4 can be theoretically linked to the underlying *cardio-pulmonary diseases* which have produced secondary changes in pulmonary arteries and thus caused pulmonary hypertension.
i. Easiest is to understand the hypertension caused by *thrombi* in small and medium-sized arteries which become organised or recanalised, thus impeding the blood flow through the pulmonary artery branches.
ii. The pathogenesis of other forms of pulmonary hypertension, and most notably hereditary and primary or idiopathic pulmonary hypertension, *remains poorly understood.*
iii. It remains to be determined what initiates and then stimulates the proliferation of endothelial and vascular smooth muscle cells.
iv. Many cases of primary pulmonary hypertension are familial and thus have a *genetic basis*.

- This relatively rare hereditary disease affects preferentially young women, who develop symptoms (e.g. dyspnoea, fatigue) between 20 and 40 years of age. The disease has a relentless down-hill course and is usually lethal in about five years from onset of symptoms.
- *Mutation of bone morphogenetic protein receptors type 2 (BMPR2)* and combined with downregulation of certain related modifying genes, has been discovered in some families. However, since pulmonary hypertension develops in less than 20% of members of these families, the significance of the molecular biology findings is not apparent.

Pathology Pathologic changes are seen in the entire pulmonary artery system, extending from arterioles through small, medium-sized and large pulmonary arterial branches to the main pulmonary artery. The changes include:

i. *Intimal thickening* and medial *proliferation of smooth muscle cells* with marked thickening of the wall and *narrowing of the lumen* of small arteries and arterioles **(Fig. 17.5)**. These changes are more prominent in primary than in secondary hypertension.

ii. *Elastic laminae are reduplicated* and show concentric layering.

iii. *Thrombi* that are present in the lumen of some vessels show signs of *organisation or recanalisation*. In some arteries, albeit rarely, there are intraluminal newly-formed inter-anastomosing capillaries forming so called *plexiform lesions*.

iv. Pulmonary artery and its major branches contain *intimal plaques* and *atheromas* similar to early atheromas of the aorta.

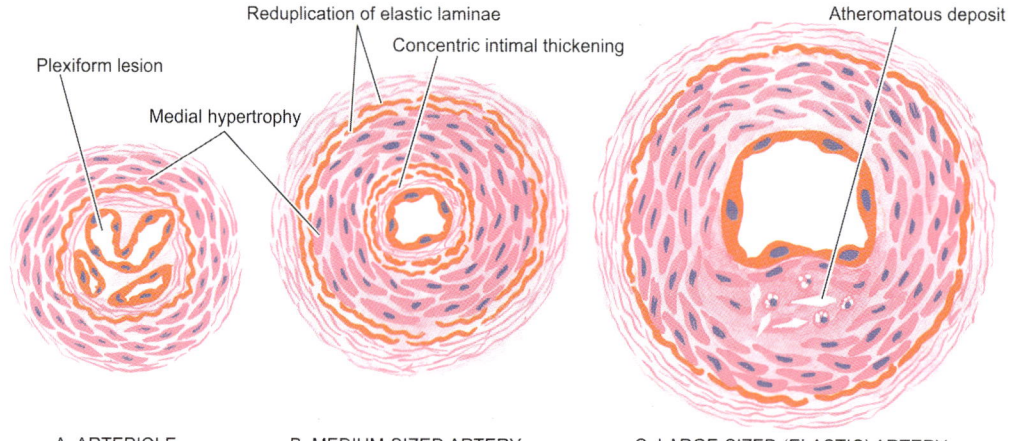

FIGURE 17.5: Histologic changes in the pulmonary arterial branches of different sizes in pulmonary hypertension.

Q9. Define pneumonia. Enumerate the conditions predisposing to it.

Definition Pneumonia is inflammation of pulmonary parenchyma, involving alveoli or interstitium, or both.

Pathogenesis The pathogens can reach the lung by several routes:

i. Inhalation of pathogens present in the air
ii. Aspiration from nasopharynx or oropharynx
iii. Haematogenous spread
iv. Direct spread from an adjacent site of infection

Predisposing conditions and disorders that facilitate infection

i. Altered consciousness (e.g. coma, seizures, cranial trauma)
ii. Depressed cough and glottic reflexes (e.g. intubation and post-tracheostomy states, neuromuscular diseases, weakness due to malnutrition)
iii. Impaired mucociliary transport (e.g. cigarette smoking, viral infection, old age)
iv. Impaired alveolar macrophage function (e.g. cigarettes smoking, starvation, pulmonary oedema, viral respiratory infections)
v. Endobronchial obstruction (e.g. foreign body, tumour, mucus plugs in cystic fibrosis, chronic bronchitis)
vi. Immunocompromised states (e.g. AIDS, immunosuppressive therapy, cancer treatment)

Q10. How are pneumonias classified?
Several approaches can be used as under:
I. **Anatomic classification**
i. Lobar pneumonia
ii. Bronchopneumonia (lobular pneumonia)
iii. Interstitial pneumonia
II. **Etiologic classification**
i. Bacterial
ii. Viral
iii. Mycoplasmal
iv. Fungal
v. Pneumonia of non-infectious etiology
III. **Clinical classification**
i. Community acquired pneumonia
ii. Healthcare-associated pneumonia
iii. Hospital-acquired pneumonia
iv. Ventilator associated pneumonia
v. Pneumonia in immunocompromised host (e.g. fungal pneumonia)
vi. Miscellaneous pneumonias (aspiration pneumonia, hypostatic pneumonia, lipid pneumonia, necrotising pneumonia, chronic pneumonia)

Q11. What is community-acquired pneumonia?
Definition Community-acquired pneumonia is an acute lung infection in a patient who has not been treated or admitted in long-term care facility for ≥ 14 days preceding presentation.
Etiology Most often caused by bacteria, but other pathogens can cause it as well, alone or as co-pathogens. In 10–15% of cases it is polymicrobial.
Pathogens causing this type of pneumonia are divided into two groups:
I. **Typical bacterial pathogens** that are frequently implicated:
i. *Streptococcus pneumoniae* (30–60% of all cases)
ii. *Staphylococcus aureus*, usually by haematogenous spread from some other site
iii. Gram-negative aerobic bacteria such as *Haemophilus influenzae, Klebsiella pneumoniae, Pseudomonas aeruginosa* and *Moraxella catarrhalis*)
II. **Atypical bacterial pathogens** that cannot be cultured or identified on Gram stain of the sputum, such as:
i. *Mycoplasma pneumoniae*
ii. *Chlamydia pneumoniae*
iii. *Legionella pneumoniae*

Q12. Define lobar pneumonia. What are its salient pathologic features?
Definition: Lobar pneumonia is acute pulmonary infection involving the entire lobe or large portions of one or more pulmonary lobes.
Pathology Four stage are recognised as under **(Fig. 17.6)**:
I. *Congestion (Initial stage)*
Gross The lungs appear heavy, and on section are wet and red due to congestion.
Microscopy reveals intra-alveolar oedema fluid with sparse neutrophils, often in the presence of numerous bacteria.
II. *Red hepatisation (Early consolidation)*
Gross The lungs are airless and consolidated, and appear red-brown on cross section resembling the liver.
Microscopy Oedema from the previous stage has been replaced by fibrin which forms an intra-alveolar meshwork encasing inflammatory cells and extravasated red blood cells.
Expectorated exudate gives the sputum a typical rusty red appearance.

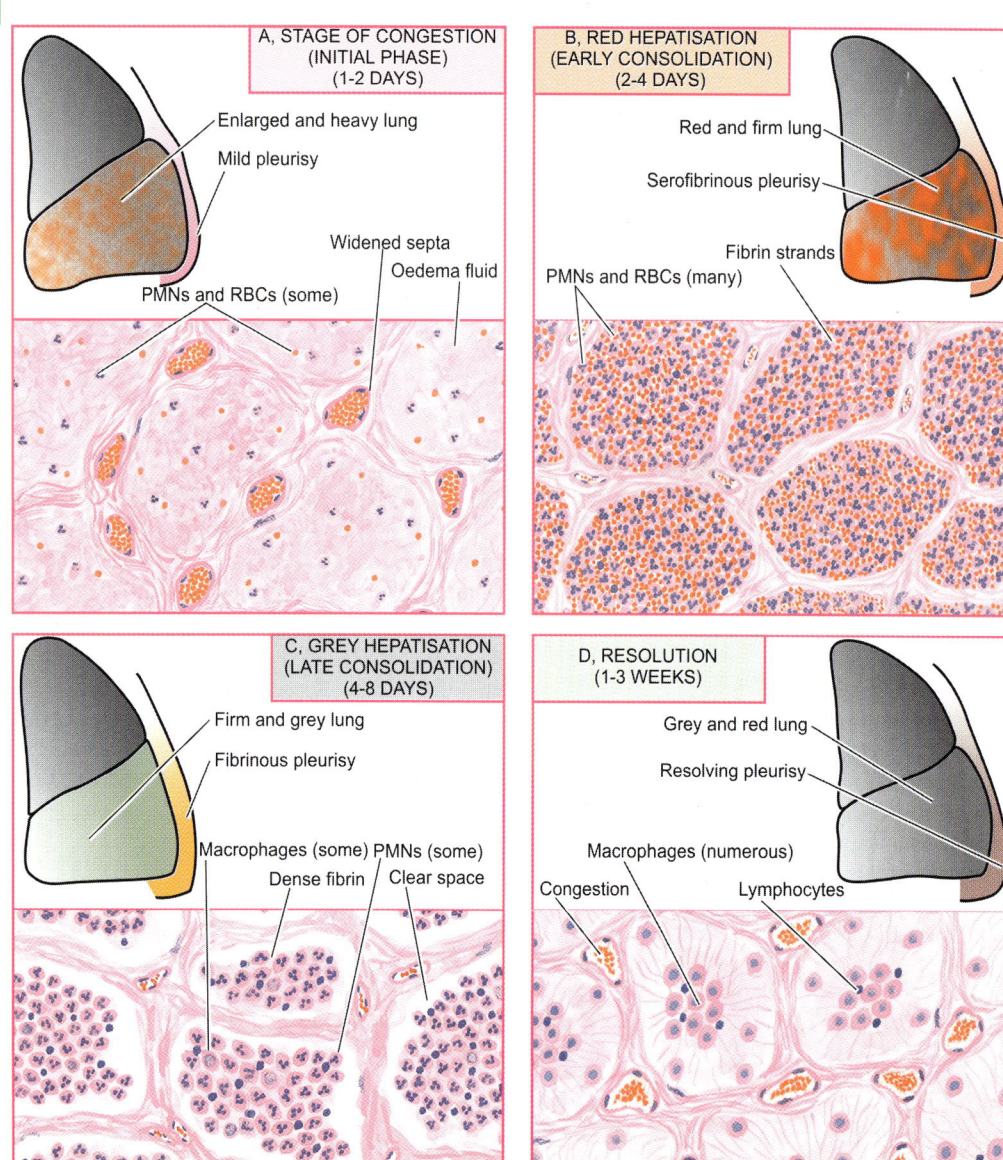

FIGURE 17.6: Stages of lobar pneumonia, showing correlation of gross appearance of the lung with microscopic features in each stage.

III. *Grey hepatisation (Late consolidation)*
Gross The lung are airless and consolidated.
Microscopy The alveoli are filled with neutrophils. Intra-alveolar exudate will compress the alveolar capillaries, reducing the congestion and imparting the cross section a pale greyish-yellow appearance. The sputum has a yellow brown colour due to pus formed from disintegrated neutrophils.

IV. *Resolution*
Microscopy In this final stage of pneumonia, the neutrophils have either disappeared or disintegrated and have been replaced by macrophages which act as scavengers removing the cell debris and fibrin.

Clinical features Typically, lobar pneumonia has a sudden onset.
- *Symptoms* include high fever, chest pain, dyspnoea, tachypnoea, tachycardia, cough with expectoration of sputum which is rusty brown or purulent. Cyanosis is seen in severely hypoxaemic patients.
- *Chest X-rays* show consolidation of the lung parenchyma (a highly diagnostic finding!).

- *Laboratory findings* include leucocytosis. Sputum cultures are positive for bacteria and are also used to determine bacterial sensitivity to antibiotics. Blood cultures are positive in 30% cases.

Q13. What are the complications of lobar pneumonia?

Modern antibiotic therapy has reduced the number of complications of pneumonia. Yet, some 5–10% of treated patients, and even more of those who have not been adequately treated, develop complications that are similar to those in the pre-antibiotic era. These complications include the following:

I. **Organisation** of the exudate and destroyed tissue occurs in patients who have not been able to remove all residues and consequences of inflammation. The remaining exudate and the cell debris and fibrin are invaded by granulation tissue rich in macrophages, imparting the picture of chronic pneumonia **(Fig. 17.7)**. Over time, the granulation tissues will gradually transform into fibrous scars, which affect adversely the gas exchange in the lungs.

II. **Lung abscess**, a cavitary localised purulent inflammation, is seen most often as a complication of pneumonia caused by *Staphylococcus aureus*.

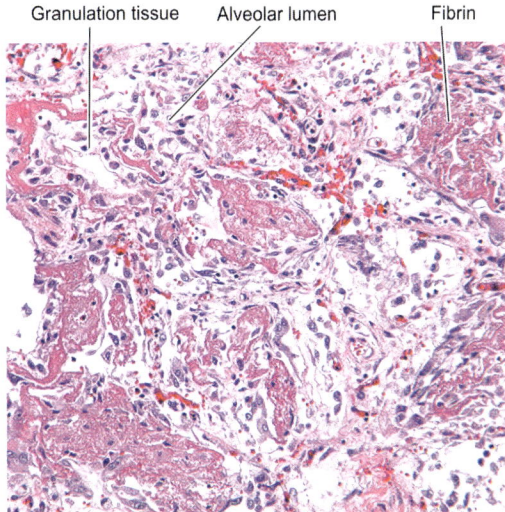

FIGURE 17.7: Chronic organising pneumonia. The alveoli are infiltrated with young granulation tissue replacing the inflammatory infiltrate and fibrin.

III. **Pleural effusion**, which is common in active pneumonia extending to the pleural surface, may persist in some patients for prolonged periods of time.

IV. **Empyema**, i.e. accumulation of pus in the pleural cavity, may be resistant to antibiotics and needs to be drained surgically.

V. **Bacteraemia** due to the entry of bacteria into the blood circulation may result in distant abscesses.

Q14. What is bronchopneumonia? Discuss its salient features.

Definition Bronchopneumonia, also known as lobular pneumonia, is a bacteria-caused bronchocentric acute pulmonary inflammation involving bronchioles and alveoli and resulting in a patchy consolidation of one or both lungs.

Epidemiology Bronchopneumonia is more common than lobar pneumonia.
- It may be community-acquired or hospital-acquired infection.
- It is particularly frequent at the extremes of life (i.e. infancy and old age).
- It is a common terminal event in many chronic debilitating diseases.
- Bacterial infection causing bronchopneumonia is often superimposed on viral pneumonia and systemic viral infections of childhood.

Clinicopathologic features

Gross Macroscopic examination reveals patchy areas of red or grey consolidation. It may involve one or both lungs, most often involving the lower lobes due to gravitation related distribution of bronchial mucus containing inhaled bacteria **(Fig.17.8)**.

Microscopy shows neutrophil-rich exudates filling the bronchi, bronchiole and adjacent alveoli accompanied by congestion and oedema in the zone of surrounding lung parenchyma **(Fig.17.9)**.

Complications are similar to those in lobar pneumonia. Persistent inflammation is common and usually related to the underlying destruction of lung parenchyma.

Clinically, bronchopneumonia is usually preceded by acute bronchitis marked by cough and expectoration, gradually progressing to bronchopneumonia.
- In some cases, it is preceded by a viral infection of the respiratory tracts or systemic viral infection.

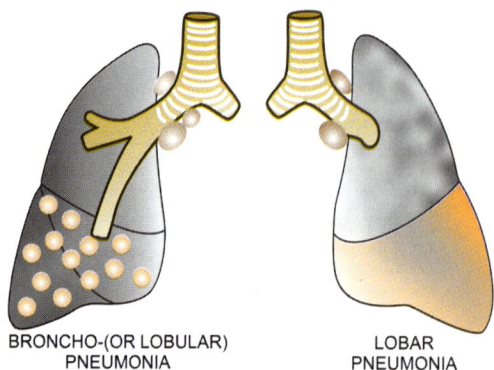

BRONCHO-(OR LOBULAR) PNEUMONIA   LOBAR PNEUMONIA

FIGURE 17.8: Gross appearance of bronchopneumonia contrasted with that of lobar pneumonia.

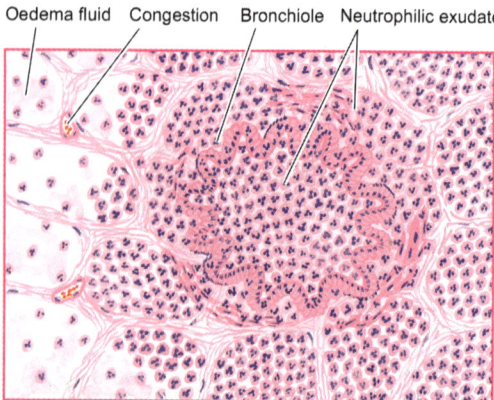

FIGURE 17.9: Microscopic appearance of bronchopneumonia. The bronchioles as well as the adjacent alveoli are filled with exudate consisting chiefly of neutrophils. The alveolar septa are thickened due to congested capillaries and neutrophilic infiltrate.

- It is common in patients with debilitating chronic diseases.
- Once bronchopneumonia develops, the symptoms are similar to those in lobar pneumonia, albeit less debilitating and less likely associated with severe dyspnoea.

Q15. Tabulate the contrasting features of lobar pneumonia and bronchopneumonia.

Salient contrasting features of bacterial lobar pneumonia and bronchopneumonia are outlined in **Table 17.1**.

TABLE 17.1 Contrasting features of lobar pneumonia and bronchopneumonia.

FEATURE	LOBAR PNEUMONIA	BRONCHOPNEUMONIA
1. *Definition*	Acute bacterial infection of a part of a lobe of one or both lungs, or the entire lobe/s	Acute bacterial infection of the terminal bronchioles extending into adjoining alveoli
2. *Age group*	More common in adults	Commoner at extremes of age–infants and old age
3. *Predisposing factors*	More often affects healthy individuals	Pre-existing diseases, e.g. chronic debility, terminal illness, flu, measles
4. *Common etiologic agents*	Pneumococci, *Klebsiella pneumoniae*, staphylococci, streptococci	Staphylococci, streptococci, *Pseudomonas*, *Haemophilus influenzae*
5. *Pathologic features*	Typical case passes through stages of congestion (1–2 days), early (2–4 days) and late consolidation (4–8 days), followed by resolution (1–3 weeks)	Patchy consolidation with central granularity, alveolar exudation, thickened septa
6. *Investigations*	Neutrophilic leucocytosis, positive blood culture, X-ray shows consolidation	Neutrophilic leucocytosis, positive blood culture, X-ray shows mottled focal opacities
7. *Prognosis*	Better response to treatment, resolution common, prognosis good	Response to treatment variable, organisation may occur, prognosis poor
8. *Complications*	Less common; pleural effusion, empyema, lung abscess, organisation	Bronchiectasis may occur; other complications same as for lobar pneumonia

Q16. What is community-acquired viral pneumonia? Discuss its salient features.

Definition Community-acquired viral pneumonia is an interstitial pulmonary inflammation caused by viruses. It is also known as *interstitial pneumonitis,* because it primarily involves the pulmonary interstitium. Also, it is called *primary atypical pneumonia* because it does not have the 'typical' clinical features of bacterial lobar pneumonia, nor does it present with intra-alveolar exudation of neutrophils.
Etiopathogenesis It is caused by viruses. More than 200 viruses have been reported as a potential cause.

i. These pathogens are viruses causing upper respiratory tract infections, colloquially known as the *common cold viruses*:
- Respiratory syncytial virus (RSV) (the most common in children)
- Influenza and parainfluenza virus
- Coronaviruses (CoV) that cause Middle-East Respiratory Syndrome (MERS), Severe Acute Respiratory Syndrome (SARS), and a novel coronavirus identified in Covid-19
- Adenoviruses

NOTE: The conditions favouring the extension of the upper respiratory infection into the lungs include malnutrition, chronic debilitating diseases and alcoholism.

ii. *Childhood systemic viral infections* also may cause pneumonia.

iii. *Cytomegalovirus* is a cause of viral pneumonia in immunosuppressed persons.

iv. Epidemics with newly-identified pathogens have also been reported, such as *severe acute respiratory syndrome (SARS)* caused by corona virus.

Clinicopathologic features

Clinical and gross Lungs may be involved in a patchy or diffuse manner depending on the severity of infection and the virulence of the pathogen.

Microscopy The usual microscopic features include three sets of findings, as under:

i. *Interstitial inflammation* characterised by widening of the alveolar septa and infiltration of interstitial spaces with lymphocytes and macrophages or plasma cells.

ii. *Alveolar changes* such as protein-rich oedema are common. Focal hyaline membranes and detachment of damaged pneumocytes may be seen in some alveoli, admixed to a few inflammatory cells.

iii. *Reactive changes* in epithelial cells of the infected alveolar and bronchiolar cells are rarely seen. In RSV infection and some other viral infections one may see virus induced *multinucleated cells*.

Bacterial superinfection, common in many lethal cases of documented viral pneumonia examined at autopsy, complicates the diagnosis of viral pneumonia even more.

Microscopic differential diagnosis between viral and bacterial pneumonia may be difficult and, in many cases, even impossible.

- Viruses are not visible by light microscopy and a search by electron micrococpy is too time-consuming and often inconclusive to be useful for clinical practice.
- Immunohistochemical identification of viruses is limited by the availability of antibody stains to specific viruses, and in daily pathology practice it is limited to viruses found in immunosuppressed persons (e.g. CMV).

Immunologic and molecular biologic identification of viruses requires special diagnostic techniques, which are available only in highly specialised reference centres and research laboratories.

Q17. What are the common causes of pneumonia in immunocompromised persons?

Pathogens causing pneumonia in immunocompromised persons, such as those infected with HIV, can be classified into three categories: a) fungal, b) viral, and c) bacterial **(Table 17.2)**.

Pneumocystis pneumonia, caused by the fungal pathogen *Pneumocystis jirovecii* is the most common cause of pneumonia in AIDS patients. It is characterised by the presence of fungi in the alveoli and an interstitial inflammation in their walls **(Fig.17.10)**. Special stain (Grocott methenamine silver) is used to demonstrate the oval or crescentic cysts in the alveoli.

Fungal pneumonia may be caused by several fungi listed in **Table 17.2**. These fungi can also be demonstrated by Grocott or Gomory methenamine silver stain **(Fig. 17.11)**.

TABLE 17.2 Common etiologic types of HIV-infection associated pneumonias.

A. FUNGAL
1. *Pneumocystis* pneumonia (PCP)
2. Coccidioidomycosis
3. Invasive aspergillosis
4. Invasive candidiasis

B. VIRAL
1. Cytomegalovirus
2. Idiopathic interstitial pneumonia

C. BACTERIAL
1. *Streptococcus pneumoniae*
2. *Haemophilus influenzae*
3. *Staphylococcus aureus*
4. *Pseudomonas aeruginosa*
5. *Mycobacterium tuberculosis*
6. *Mycobacterium avium-intracellulare*

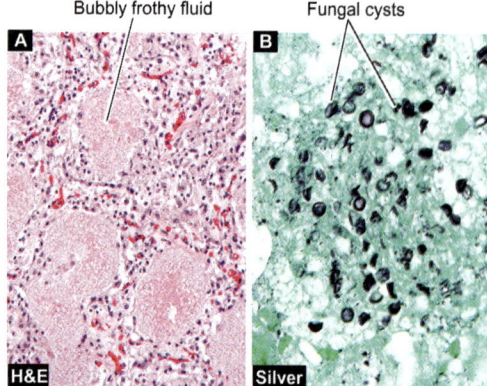

FIGURE 17.10: *Pneumocystis* pneumonia. A, Alveoli are filed with frothy vacuolated exudate containing the organisms in H & E stain. B, It demonstrates fungal cysts in black colour in Grocott silver methenamine stain.

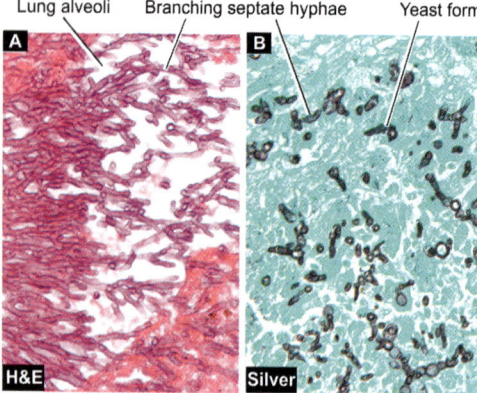

FIGURE 17.11: Aspergillosis lung. A, Acute angled septate hyphae lying in necrotic debris and acute inflammatory exudates in lung abscess. B, Organisms, *Apergillus flavus*, are best identified with a special stain for fungi, Gomory methenamine silver (GMS).

Q18. What is aspiration pneumonia? Discuss its predisposing conditions and pathologic features.

Definition Aspiration pneumonia results from inhalation of various materials into the lungs. Aspirated material may include food, gastric contents, foreign bodies or infected material from the oral cavity.

Predisposing conditions
i. Unconsciousness
ii. Drunkenness
iii. Neurological disorders affecting swallowing
iv. Drowning
v. Necrotic nasopharyngeal tumours
vi. In neonates, trachea-oesophageal fistula

Pathology The right side is affected more often than the left lung since the right bronchus is at lower angle from the trachea and thus allows easier passage of the aspirated material into the lungs. Pathologic changes depend on the nature of the aspirated material and if it is infected or sterile:
i. *Non-sterile aspirated material* contaminated with bacteria cause foci of suppurative and necrotising bronchopneumonia. Particulate vegetable matter will often elicit a foreign body giant cell reaction.
ii. *Aspiration of gastric contents* which is sterile will cause *chemical pneumonitis* with pulmonary oedema and haemorrhage and particulate matters in the bronchi or bronchiole.

Prognosis Massive aspiration may be lethal and such patients develop severe dyspnoea, cyanosis shock and cardiac failure.

Q19. What is hypostatic pneumonia?

Definition Hypostatic pneumonia is the term used for pneumonia that develops on a background of dependent pulmonary oedema and retained bronchial secretions in severely debilitated and bed-ridden patients. It is a common terminal event in debilitated, comatose and very old patients of limited mobility.

Pathology The pathogens usually reach the lungs from the upper respiratory tract and the mouth.
- In sedentary patients it affects the basal part of the lower lobes.
- In bed-ridden patients it affects the posterior parts of the lungs.

Q20. Discuss lipid pneumonia briefly.

Definition Lipid pneumonia is a chemical non-infectious type of pneumonia caused by lipids that have gained access to the alveoli.

Pathology There are two types of lipid pneumonia:

I. *Exogenous lipid pneumonia* results from aspiration of various oily materials, such as salad dressing, oil-containing nasal drops, regurgitated oil-rich capsules given for digestive problems, fat-soluble vitamins droplets, etc.

II. *Endogenous lipid pneumonia* is the more common variant.

i. It results from the release of lipid-rich material from necrotic tissues (e.g. bronchogenic cancer, necrotising granulomas of tuberculosis, resolving bronchopneumonia, etc.).

ii. It most often develops distal to bronchial obstruction preventing expectoration of such cellular debris.

iii. Macrophages take up the lipid-rich material and transform into foamy macrophages.

iv. On gross examination such areas appear consolidated and on cross section they have a golden yellow color due to the high content of lipids.

Q21. What is chronic pneumonia?

Definition Chronic pneumonia is a lung infection that last long time and is characterised pathologically by signs of chronic inflammation.

Etiology Most common causes are *Mycobacterium tuberculosis* and various fungi.

Pathology The features are as under:

i. In tuberculosis and fungal infections, the lungs contain granulomas.

ii. In other cases there is nonspecific chronic inflammation with infiltration of tissues with lymphocytes, macrophages and plasma cells.

iii. The inflammation tends to destroy normal lung architecture and promote fibrosis.

Q22. Discuss lung abscess briefly.

Definition Lung abscess is localised purulent bacterial infections accompanied by secondary liquefaction necrosis of the affected tissue and formation of a pus-filled cavity.

Classification There are two types of lung abscesses: primary and secondary **(Fig. 17.12)**.

I. **Primary abscess** develops in an otherwise normal tissue. The commonest cause is *aspiration* of infected material. It is most often located in the lower part of the right upper lobe or apex of right lower lobe.

II. **Secondary abscess** develops as a *complication of some other pre-existing lung disease* (e.g. pneumonia) or *dissemination of infection* from some other site (e.g. septic emboli). Abscesses complicating preexistent pneumonia or resulting from septic emboli are *frequently multiple*.

Etiopathogenesis Abscesses may have multiple causes, especially under conditions that reduce the gag-reflex such as anaesthesia, coma, alcoholism, generalised debility, etc. These conditions are as under:

i. *Aspiration of foreign infected material*

ii. *Preceding bacterial infection*, e.g. bronchopneumonia, especially in a debilitated patient.

• Certain pathogens, such as *Staphylococcus aureus* and *Klebsiella pneumoniae* are more likely to cause abscesses than others.

iii. *Bronchial obstruction*, e.g. bronchial tumour, or aspirated foreign matter.

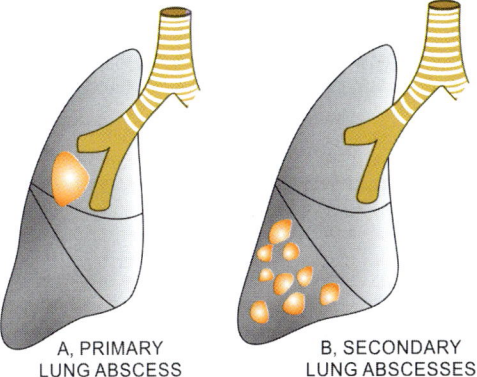

A, PRIMARY LUNG ABSCESS

B, SECONDARY LUNG ABSCESSES

FIGURE 17.12: Common locations of lung abscess. A, *Primary lung abscess*—mostly single, large, commonly due to aspiration, located most frequently in the lower part of right upper lobe or apex of right lower lobe. B, *Secondary lung abscesses*—mostly multiple, small, most commonly post-pneumonic or following septic embolism.

iv. *Septic thromboemboli*, e.g. infected vegetations in endocarditis of the right heart, bacterial thrombophlebitis, thrombosis in a patient who has septicaemia.
v. *Rare causes* include infected pulmonary infarcts, bullet wound or stabbing wound of the lungs. Abscesses in the thorax (e.g. abscess in the mediastinum or thoracic spine or subdiaphragmatic abscess of the liver) may extend into the lungs.

Pathology *Clinical and gross* Lung abscesses may be solitary or multiple.
- Size may vary from a few millimeters (visible only by microscope), to large cavities 5–6 cm in diameter.
- Initially they might not be sharply demarcated from surrounding tissue, which may be normal, oedematous or inflamed but to a lesser extent.
- With time, they acquire a fibroblast-rich collagenous wall, separating the abscess from the adjacent tissue.

Microscopy Dense exudate composed of neutrophils permeates the tissue causing necrosis.
- The exudate also contains pus cells ('dead and dying neutrophils'), cell debris, oedema fluid, strands of fibrin.
- As the process evolves, chronic inflammatory cells start invading the abscess from the periphery, also contributing to the formation of the fibrous wall of the abscess.

Clinical picture may be quite variable.
- In acute cases, the symptoms resemble those of acute pneumonia, or as a prolongation and intensification of a pre-existent infection.
- In chronic cases, it resembles chronic obstructive pulmonary disease or bronchiectasis. Chronic suppuration and persistent inflammation may predispose for AA amyloidosis.

Q23. What is chronic obstructive pulmonary disease? Enumerate its most common forms and tabulate their contrasting features.

Definition Chronic obstructive pulmonary disease (COPD) includes a group of pulmonary diseases characterised by airway limitation due to chronic, partial or complete, obstruction to the airflow at any level from trachea to smallest airways in the lungs.

Types Five most common forms of COPD are:
i. Chronic bronchitis
ii. Emphysema
iii. Bronchial asthma
iv. Bronchiectasis
v. Small airways disease (bronchiolitis)

The contrasting features of these most common forms of COPD are presented in **Table 17.3**.

TABLE 17.3 Contrasting features of major forms of COPD.

FEATURE	CHRONIC BRONCHITIS	EMPHYSEMA	ASTHMA	BRONCHIECTASIS	SMALL AIRWAYS DISEASE
1. *Location*	Bronchus	Acinus	Bronchus	Bronchus	Bronchiole
2. *Age at diagnosis*	Adults	Adults	Extrinsic: children Intrinsic: adults	Adults	Children
3. *Etiology*	Smoking, air pollution	Smoking, air pollution	Extrinsic: allergy Intrinsic: viral infection	Infection, obstruction	Viral infection, smoke
4. *Pathogenesis*	Impaired ciliary movement	Deficiency of α-1 antitrypsin	IgE-sensitised mast cells	Damaged airways	Defect in surfactant
5. *Major gross feature*	Thickened bronchial wall	Distended air sacs	Overdistended lungs	Dilated bronchi and bronchioles	Occluded bronchioles
6. *Main histology*	Hyperplasia of mucous glands	Broken alveolar septa	Mucus plugs in bronchioles	Inflamed bronchi	Fibrous plugs in bronchioles
7. *Major clinical feature*	Persistent cough with expectoration	Exertional dyspnoea	Bronchospasm	Copious foul-smelling expectoration	Cough, dyspnoea

Q24. What is chronic bronchitis? Briefly discuss its etiopathogenesis and clinicopathologic features.

Definition Chronic bronchitis is a common condition defined *clinically* as persistent cough with expectoration on most days for at least three month of the year for two or more consecutive years.

Epidemiology It is a very common disease, affecting middle-aged males more often than females.
- Estimates are that 20% adult men and 5% of adult females are affected to some extent, even though most of them have still manageable respiratory problems.
- Only a minority of affected persons develop disabling pulmonary failure or cor pulmonale.
- Association with emphysema is common.

Etiopathogenesis Most important etiologic factors are as under:

i. *Smoking* is the most important cause and has the following effects:
- Impairs ciliary movement.
- Inhibits the action of alveolar macrophages.
- Causes hypertrophy and hyperplasia and hyperfunction of bronchial mucus-secreting glands.
- Causes obstruction of small airways.
- Stimulates bronchoconstriction directly or through the stimulation of the vagus.

Bronchial infections tend to be common in smokers than nonsmokers.

ii. *Air-pollution* from industry, cars, coal-burning power plants, wood burning, etc. increases the concentration of toxic gases such as sulfur dioxide, nitrogen dioxide, toxic fumes and dust.

iii. *Occupational exposure* to harmful materials (e.g. byssinosis developing on cotton mills workers)

iv. *Familial and genetic factors* play a role, but its significance cannot be determined.

Pathology Bronchi of all sizes and bronchioles are affected.

i. Bronchi are dilated and have thickened walls.
ii. The ratio of enlarged bronchial glands to entire thickness of the bronchial wall (called the Reid index) exceeds the normal (0.4) **(Fig. 17.13)**.
iii. The surface epithelium shows goblet cell metaplasia and focally also squamous cell metaplasia.
iv. There is focal chronic inflammation, but it is usually mild.
v. The bronchial lumen contains mucus plugs with scattered inflammatory cells.
vi. Small bronchi and bronchioles show goblet cell metaplasia and peribronchial fibrosis.

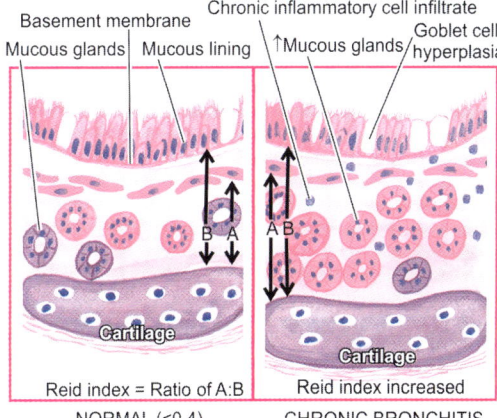

FIGURE 17.13: Diagrammatic representation of increased Reid index in chronic bronchitis.

Clinical features These may vary depending on the extent of pathological changes. Many cases show considerable overlap with emphysema, which often coexists with chronic bronchitis.

The salient symptoms of progressive COPD are as follows:

i. Morning cough ('throat clearing') which becomes gradually worse with time and then lasts in bouts for the rest of the day. Winter and cold weather, in general, aggravate the symptoms.
ii. In patients with progressive disease, there is exertional dyspnoea combined with cyanosis and oedema ('blue bloaters').
iii. Chest X-ray shows enlarged heart and prominent great vessels.
iv. Recurrent pulmonary infections are common.
v. Signs of right heart failure (cor pulmonale) develop as the disease enters its terminal stages with progressive hypoxaemia and hypercapnia.

Q25. Define emphysema. What are its salient features?

Definition Emphysema is permanent dilatation of airspaces distal to terminal bronchioles combined with wall destruction of dilated air spaces. Emphysema is often combined with chronic bronchitis and thus it is common practice to classify the patients as 'COPD, predominantly chronic bronchitis', or 'COPD, predominantly emphysema'.

Etiopathogenesis The most important exogenous etiologic factors are *cigarettes smoking* and *air pollution*. An important genetic predisposition is determined by the genes that encode α-1-antitrypsin (α-1-AT) and *proteases* (predominantly *elastase*). Smoking was found to increase the function of protease and also to decrease the action of α-1-antitrypsin, thus promoting the enzymatic destruction of alveolar walls and promoting the development of emphysema **(Fig. 17.14)**. It has been shown that heavy smokers who have α-1-AT deficiency develop emphysema 15 years earlier than nonsmokers.

Genetics: α-1-antitrypsin gene has several alleles which have autosomal codominant inheritance and are classified as normal (*PiMM*), deficient (*PiZZ*), null type (*Pi nul null*) and dysfunctional (*PiSS*).

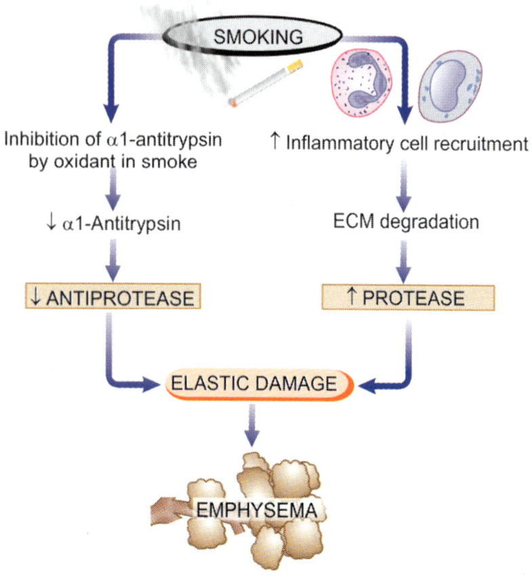

The most common abnormal phenotype is classic α-1-antitrypsin deficiency, *homozygous PiZZ*. Clinically significant deficiency is associated with homozygous *Pi null null* and *Pi null Z*. Heterozygotes *PiMZ* have an intermediate level of deficiency which is not sufficient to produce clinical deficiency. However, in heavy smokers this gene produces a higher risk of emphysema.

FIGURE 17.14: Pathogenesis of alveolar wall destruction in emphysema by protease-antiprotease mechanism. (ECM, extracellular matrix).

Clinical features Clinical signs of emphysema appear in predominantly emphysema patients after *one third* of the pulmonary parenchyma is damaged, most severely in panacinar emphysema. Symptoms occur usually 10 years later (at age of 60 years) than in predominantly bronchitis patients and include the following:

i. Exertional dyspnoea is the most prominent complaint.
ii. The patient is in obvious distress and is using muscles for respiration.
iii. Hacking dry cough and scant expectoration.
iv. 'Pink puffer' since the blood remains oxygenated and the patient is tachypnoeic.
v. Barrel-shaped chest, hyperresonant on percussion.
vi. Evident weight loss.
vii. Cor pulmonale and right heart failure are late events with hypercapnic cardiopulmonary failure.

Q26. What are the clinicopathologic forms of emphysema?

Depending upon the component of respiratory airways involved, there are five forms of emphysema which have distinct pathological and clinical features **(Fig. 17.15)**. Emphysema must, however, be distinguished from overinflation **(Table 17.4)**.

I. Centriacinar (centrilobular) emphysema is one of the common types of emphysema.
i. It is characterised by initial involvement of respiratory bronchioles, i.e. the central or proximal part of the acinus.
ii. It usually coexists with chronic bronchitis and it is commonly found in smokers and coal-miners' pneumoconiosis.
iii. It is most pronounced in upper lobes of the lungs.
iv. It shows distension and destruction of centrally located respiratory bronchioles which are surrounded peripherally by well-

TABLE 17.4 Classification of 'true emphysema' and 'overinflation'.

A. TRUE EMPHYSEMA
1. Centriacinar (centrilobular) emphysema
2. Panacinar (panlobular) emphysema
3. Paraseptal (distal acinar) emphysema
4. Irregular (para-cicatricial) emphysema
5. Mixed (unclassified) emphysema

B. OVERINFLATION
1. Compensatory overinflation (compensatory emphysema)
2. Senile hyperinflation (ageing lung, senile emphysema)
3. Obstructive overinflation (infantile lobar emphysema)
4. Unilateral translucent lung (unilateral emphysema)
5. Interstitial emphysema (surgical emphysema)

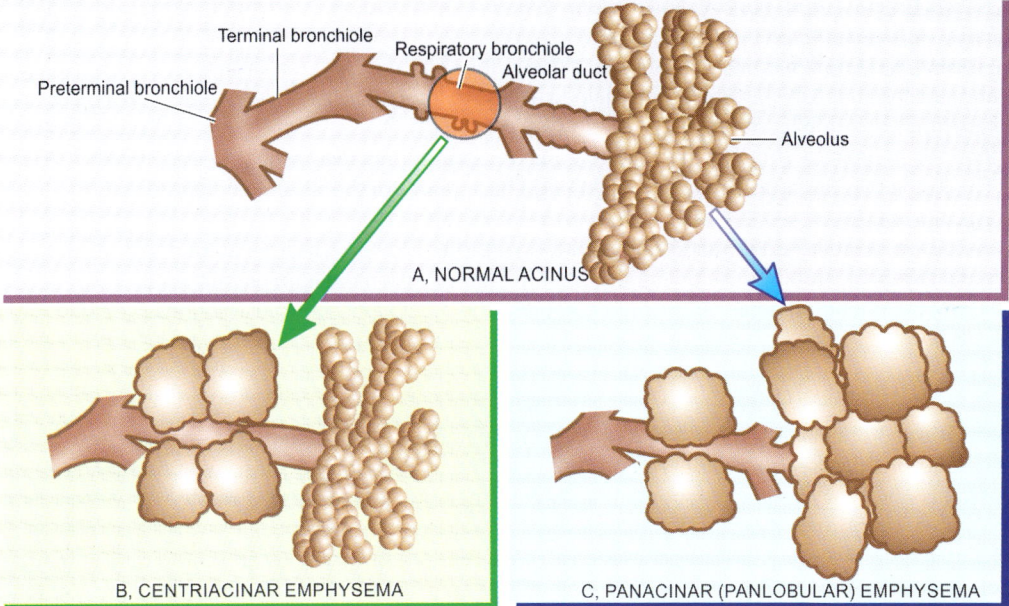

FIGURE 17.15: The anatomic regions of involvement in an acinus in major forms of emphysema.

preserved alveoli. The terminal bronchiole providing the air to the area has a narrowed lumen and shows chronic inflammation in its wall with deposition of black pigment.

II. **Panacinar (panlobular) emphysema** is the other common type of emphysema.

i. As the name implies, this form of emphysema affects all components of the acinus (respiratory bronchiole, alveolar ducts and alveoli) evenly.

ii. It is most often seen in α-1-AT deficiency afflicted middle-aged smokers, but can affect even those α-1-AT deficient persons who are not smokers, albeit at an older age.

iii. The lower parts of the lungs are affected more often than the upper parts.

iv. It does not involve the lungs parenchyma uniformly and in many cases only a few lobules are affected and overinflated.

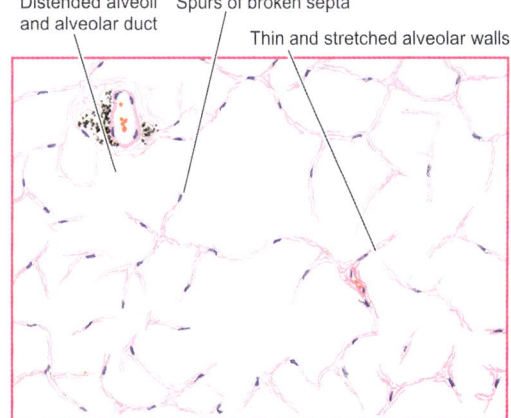

FIGURE 17.16: Panacinar (Panlobular) emphysema showing involvement of the entire lobules and whole of acinus.

v. The affected lobules are all affected to the same extent and show marked distention of the alveoli, alveolar ducts and the respiratory bronchioles with thinning and destruction of their walls. Spurs of broken septa project into their lumina **(Fig. 17.16)**.

vi. There is no evidence of inflammation.

III. **Paraseptal emphysema** is localised underneath the pleura and perilobular septa.

i. Most often, it affect the upper lobes of the lungs and may then present in form of pulmonary or subpleural cysts.

ii. It is not associated with clinical signs of COPD and its clinical significance lies in the fact that it may cause pulmonary rupture and pneumothorax in young adults.

IV. **Irregular (para-cicatricial) emphysema** is the most common form of emphysema, typically surrounding pulmonary fibrous scars of any etiology. It usually does not cause any symptoms and it is diagnosed only at autopsy.

V. **Mixed (unclassified) emphysema** has some features of the above listed emphysema and is hard to classify, and is usually identified at autopsy.

VI. **Interstitial emphysema** is a misnomer since it does not represent real emphysema. It is usually a traumatic lesion in which some air has gained access to interstitial spaces separating the connective tissue fibres one from another.

i. Blebs of air typically show up in the subpleural or septal connective tissue.

ii. This lesion may be caused by violent coughing, chest trauma or the air could enter the tissue through surgical wounds.

iii. Small amount of air does not produce clinical symptoms. However, if larger amounts of air enter the pleural cavity, this could cause pneumothorax with compression the lung parenchyma.

iv. Likewise, pneumomediastinum could compress the great veins and cause serious problems with blood flow.

Q27. What is bronchial asthma? Discuss its major types and their salient features.

Definition Bronchial asthma is a chronic disease characterised by increased responsiveness of the tracheobronchial tree to a variety of stimuli resulting in widespread spasmodic narrowing of air passages which may be relieved spontaneously or by therapy. Clinically it is manifested by paroxysms of dyspnoea, cough and wheezing. Pathologically, it presents as chronic bronchitis with accumulation of mucus in the airways, hypertrophy of bronchial grands and smooth muscles, and chronic inflammation dominated by eosinophils.

Epidemiology Bronchial asthma is a very common and prevalent disease affecting 4% of the population in the United States. Il occurs in all ages but in nearly 50% of all cases the disease has its onset in childhood before the age of 10 years. The male to female ratio is 2:1.

Classification Based on the stimuli initiating the disease, two type are recognised: *extrinsic (allergic, atopic) and intrinsic (idiosyncratic or non-atopic)*. A third type called mixed type asthma also exists and includes the cases that do not completely fit into the principal two categories.

Pathogenesis Two major forms of asthma share some common features but have a completely different pathogenesis as follows:

I. **Extrinsic bronchial asthma** is the most common form of asthma.

i. It begins in *childhood or adolescence*.

ii. *Occupational asthma* stimulated by fumes, dusts or organic substances in air is a variant that usually begins in adulthood.

iii. Most children have a *genetic predisposition* evidenced by a family and personal history of allergies such as allergic rhinitis, infantile eczema or urticaria.

iv. Testing can usually reveal hypersensitivity to *extrinsic allergens* such as house dust, animal dander, pollens, molds, etc.

v. All these patients have *elevated levels of IgE* in serum and have positive skin test for the offending allergen.

vi. The underlying mechanism is a classical *type I hypersensitivity reaction* to allergens initiated by excessive activation of *helper T_H2 cells* and the action of *interleukins* they secrete. These interleukins stimulate plasma cells to secrete IgE, activate eosinophils and attract neutrophils and stimulate mucus secretion. IgE is attached to mast cells and leads to their degranulation upon contact with allergen. All this occur in two phases: acute immediate response and late phase reaction:

a. *Acute immediate response* is initiated by IgE sensitised mast cells on the mucosal surface. Allergic stimulus leads to a degranulation of mast cells and a release of preformed mediators of inflammation such as histamine, prostaglandins and leukotrienes and chemotactic factors for neutrophils and eosinophils. These mediators cause bronchial oedema, bronchoconstriction and mucus hypersecretion.

b. *Late phase reaction* includes mucosal inflammation and is responsible for the prolonged manifestations of asthma. In addition to immune cells like T_H2 and plasma cells it includes the participation of basophils, eosinophils and neutrophils. Repeated episodes of inflammation lead to structural changes in the wall of the bronchi including hypertrophy and hyperplasia of mucous glands and smooth muscles, and increased fibrous tissue. All these changes contribute to the thickening of the bronchial wall and narrowing of its lumen.

II. **Intrinsic (non-atopic) asthma** begins in adulthood and affects people who do not have a history or allergies. IgE is not elevated.
i. Asthmatic attacks usually begin after a viral infection or exposure to some noxious fumes.
ii. Most patients suffer from recurrent upper respiratory tract infections which may lead to formation of nasal polyps and chronic bronchitis.
iii. Pathologic changes in the bronchi are similar to those as seen in extrinsic asthma and thus both forms of asthma are treated the same way.

III. **Mixed asthma** includes forms that cannot be properly classified, even though the patients with childhood onset disease have a strong allergic history. Those with adult onset of disease are most often considered to be variants of non-atopic asthma with no IgE elevation. Aspirin-sensitive asthma is an example of non-IgE related mixed asthma of unknown pathogenesis, probably based on an exaggerated smooth muscle reaction to aspirin.

The pathogenesis of these forms of asthma is not known, but it is assumed that they are based on some type of hypersensitivity causing bronchial smooth muscle overreaction.

Asthmatic attacks, like in all other forms of asthma, can be precipitated by external factors such as exercise, exposure to cold, alcohol, excitement and strong emotions.

Pathology Pathologic changes in the bronchi are the same in all forms of asthma and include the following:
i. Mucus plugs in the bronchus.
ii. Mucus usually contains Curschmann's spirals formed from strips of epithelium eosinophils and Charcot-Leyden crystals formed from the cytoplasmic granules of eosinophils **(Fig. 17.17)**.
iii. Thickening of the bronchial wall which is fibrotic and contains enlarged and hyperplastic mucous glands, and prominent bundles of smooth muscles.
iv. Inflammatory cells permeate all layers of the bronchial wall and include eosinophils, lymphocytes and plasma cells.
v. There is evidence of chronic bronchitis and emphysema, especially in intrinsic asthma.

Clinical features Typically, the disease is characterised by repeated episodes of acute exacerbations and alternating with symptom-free intervals.

Asthmatic attacks, which may be short or last a few hours, are characterised by paroxysmal bronchospasm associated with dyspnoea, cough and wheezing.

If the attacks do not end a more serious condition called *status asthmaticus* develops, which may have a lethal outcome. Patients dying in status asthmaticus have overinflated lung and prominent bronchial mucous plugs. Laboratory findings include prominent eosinophilia. Sputum contains also prominent eosinophils, Curschmann spirals, and Charcot-Leyden crystals.

Q28. Tabulate the salient contrasting features of two main forms of bronchial asthma.

Features of two main types of asthma, extrinsic and intrinsic, are given in **Table 17.5**.

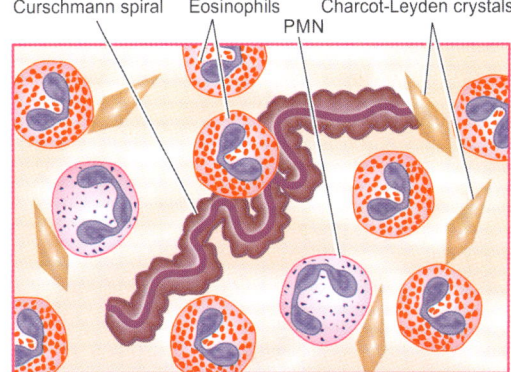

FIGURE 17.17: Diagrammatic appearance of Curschmann spiral and Charcot-Leyden crystals found in mucus plugs in patients with bronchial asthma.

TABLE 17.5 Contrasting features of the two major types of asthma.

FEATURE	EXTRINSIC ASTHMA	INTRINSIC ASTHMA
1. Age at onset	In childhood	In adult
2. Personal/family history	Commonly present	Absent
3. Preceding allergic illness (atopy)	Present (e.g. rhinitis, urticaria, eczema)	Absent
4. Allergens	Present (dust, pollens, danders, etc.)	None
5. Drug hypersensitivity	None	Present (usually to aspirin)
6. Serum IgE level	Elevated	Normal
7. Associated chronic bronchitis, nasal polyps	Absent	Present
8. Emphysema	Unusual	Common

Q29. What is bronchiectasis? Discuss its etiology and salient pathologic features.

Definition Bronchiectasis is abnormal and irreversible dilatation of bronchi and bronchioles, secondary to inflammatory weakening of their walls. Clinical symptoms include chronic cough and expectoration of foul-smelling purulent sputum.

Etiology Two major sets of factors play a pathogenetic role: chronic infections and bronchial obstruction.

I. **Chronic infections** usually affect the entire bronchial system and cause diffuse bronchiectases as under:

i. Congenital developmental defect (congenital bronchiectasis).

ii. Cystic fibrosis with accumulation of viscous mucus in the bronchi and superimposed bacterial infection.

iii. Primary immunodeficiencies.

iv. Immotile cilia syndromes including Kartagener syndrome (immotile cilia with bronchiectasis, chronic sinusitis, *situs viscerum inversus*, and infertility due to immotility of sperm in males).

v. Necrotising pneumonia (most notably caused by *Staphylococcus aureus* or *Klebsiella pneumoniae*) may destroy peribronchial tissue allowing bronchi to dilate.

vi. Postinfectious peribronchial fibrosis (e.g. tuberculosis) may cause bronchiectasis by exerting traction on the bronchi from outside.

II. **Bronchial obstruction** usually results in localised bronchiectasis confined to a part of the bronchial tree. Possible causes include:

i. Tumours inside the bronchus or compressing it from outside.

ii. Compression of bronchi by peribronchial post-inflammatory scarring.

iii. Compression by enlarged hilar lymph nodes (e.g. in tuberculosis).

iv. Aspirated foreign body obstructing a large bronchus.

Pathology Grossly, bronchiectasis may be:

- *Localised* to a single bronchus and its branches, or may be *diffuse* involving the entire bronchial tree.
- According to their shape they can be classified as *cylindrical (tube-like), fusiform (spindle-shaped), saccular (sac-like), varicose (irregularly distended and narrowed)* **(Fig.17.18)**.
- Lower lobes are usually involved more often than upper lobes, especial if infection is the main cause of bronchial dilatation.
- Peribronchial parenchyma is usually fibrotic; atelectatic and the overlying pleura show also fibrosis.
- Multiple bronchiectases surrounded by fibrotic lung parenchyma may impart to the affected lung a honey-comb appearance **(Fig.17.19, A)**.

Microscopy reveals:

i. Chronic inflammation and fibrosis of the bronchial wall, often combined with purulent inflammation and ulceration of the mucosa **(Fig. 17.19, B)**.

ii. Surrounding parenchyma of the lungs usually shows fibrosis, atelectasis and nonspecific chronic inflammation.

iii. Fibrosis may extend to the pleura.

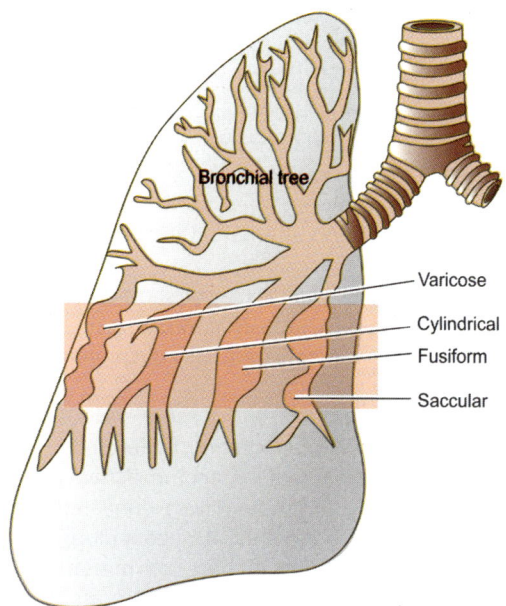

FIGURE 17.18: Types of bronchial dilatations in bronchiectasis.

Q30. Define chronic restrictive lung diseases. How are these classified? Briefly discuss their pathogenesis.

Definition Chronic restrictive lung diseases form a heterogeneous group of more than 200 diffuse lung diseases characterised by reduced expansion of lung parenchyma during inspiration, reduced compliance ('stiff lungs'), and decreased lung capacity.

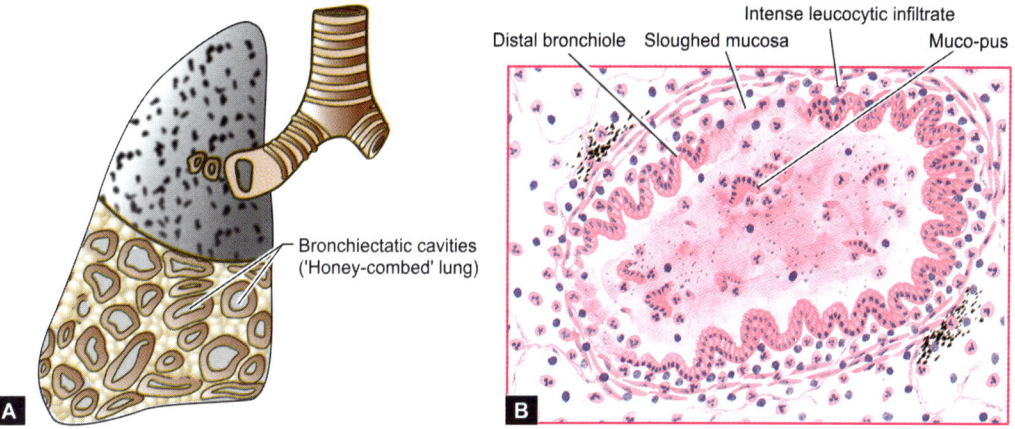

FIGURE 17.19: Bronchiectasis of the lung. A, Sectioned surface shows honey-combed appearance of the lung in the lower lobe where many thick-walled dilated cavities with cartilaginous wall are seen. B, Microscopic appearance of a dilated distal bronchiole in bronchiectasis. The bronchial wall is thickened and infiltrated by acute and chronic inflammatory cells. The mucosa is sloughed off at places with exudate of muco-pus in the lumen.

- Clinically restrictive lung diseases present with exertional dyspnoea, non-persistent productive cough, tachypnoea, cyanosis and sometimes haemoptysis.
- Spirometry is used clinically for the final diagnosis and to distinguish restrictive lung diseases from COPD.
- There is no wheezing that is characteristic of COPD.

Classification Two major groups of restrictive lung disease are recognised depending on the nature and location of the restriction: i) chest wall disorders, and ii) interstitial and infiltrative lung diseases.

I. **Chest wall disorders** include the following:
i. Kyphoscoliosis preventing expansion of the lungs during inhalation.
ii. Polyomyelitis and other muscle diseases affecting the respiratory muscles.
iii. Severe obesity compressing the chest from outside.
iv. Pleural diseases preventing the expansion of the lungs during inhalation.

II. **Restriction due to interstitial and infiltrative diseases**, which include several *non-infectious diseases* with diffuse parenchymal involvement:

- The term *'diffuse'* is used to mean involving all elements of peripheral lung tissue (i.e. alveolar lumina and walls, capillary basement membranes, perivascular pulmonary interstitial space and lymphatics).
- The term *'infiltrative'* is used to denote the radiologic appearance of the lung which radiologically appears in form of *ground glass opacities*.

As a group, these diseases have high morbidity and mortality.

i. *Based on etiology*, two kinds of restrictive disease are recognised:
- *Primary* if limited to the lungs and not related to any other cause.
- *Secondary* if pulmonary involvement occurs in the course of a systemic disorder.

ii. *On the basis of pathology and pathogenesis*, restrictive lung diseases are divided into four groups as follows **(Table 17.6)**:
a. With predominant fibrosis
b. With predominant granulomatous reaction
c. Immunologic lung diseases
d. Smoking associated lung diseases

Pathogenesis of interstitial lung diseases is not fully understood. However, *key features* are as follows:
- An interplay of identifiable or presumed *exogenous stimuli* (e.g. dust, fumes, viral infection, etc.) and *endogenous factors* (e.g. genetic or immune factors) cause an *alveolar cell injury* initiating a *local inflammatory reaction* **(Fig. 17.20)**.
- *Macrophages* attracted to the site of injury secrete chemotactic cytokines which amplify the inflammatory reaction and also stimulate *fibroblasts* to lay down collagen fibres obliterating the alveoli (*'cryptogenic fibrosing alveolitis'*).

TABLE 17.6 Classification of interstitial lung diseases (ILDs).

I. WITH PREDOMINANT FIBROSIS
1. Pneumoconiosis with inorganic minerals: coal, asbestos, fumes, gases
2. Connective tissue disease-associated ILDs
3. Idiopathic pulmonary fibrosis (usual interstitial pneumonia)
4. Cryptogenic organising pneumonia (bronchiolitis obliterans organising pneumonia, i.e. BOOP)
5. Nonspecific interstitial pneumonia
6. Therapy related-ILD (radiation, antibiotics, chemotherapy)
7. Residual effects of ARDS

II. WITH PREDOMINANT GRANULOMATOUS REACTION
1. Sarcoidosis (page 79)
2. Pneumoconiosis with inorganic dusts: silica, beryllium
3. Granulomatous vasculitis (page 328)
4. Wegener granulomatosis (page 327)

III. IMMUNOLOGIC LUNG DISEASES (EOSINOPHILIC PNEUMONIAS)
1. Hypersensitivity pneumonitis: with organic dusts
2. Pulmonary infiltrates with eosinophilia (PIE)
3. Pulmonary haemorrhage syndromes (Goodpasture syndrome)
4. Pulmonary alveolar proteinosis

IV. SMOKING-ASSOCIATED ILDS
1. Desquamative interstitial pneumonia (DIP)
2. Respiratory bronchiolitis-associated ILD
3. Pulmonary Langerhans cell histiocytosis (eosinophilic granuloma of the lung)

- *The sequence of lung destruction and repair* repeats itself for extended periods of time leading to a loss of functioning pulmonary parenchyma, distortion of the remaining parenchyma with formation of cystic spaces ('honey-comb lung'), presenting clinically as progressive lung failure.

Q31. How do chronic restrictive lung diseases differ from COPD?

Features distinguishing restrictive from obstructive pulmonary diseases are given in **Table 17.7**.

Q32. What are pneumoconioses and how are these classified? Briefly discuss their pathogenesis.

Definition and classification Pneumoconioses are lung diseases caused by inhalation of dust and particulate matter. Since many pneumoconioses are related to work place, they are often called *occupational lung diseases*, a term that includes diseases caused by both inorganic and organic dusts **(Table 17.8)**.

Pathogenesis The type of lung disease varies according to the nature of inhaled dust. Some dusts are inert whereas others may become antigenic or promote the formation of cancer. The tissue damage depends upon the physical properties of the inhaled dust as under:

i. *Size and shape of particles*:
a. Large particle measuring more than 10 μm and are trapped in tracheobronchial mucus do not reach the terminal air spaces.

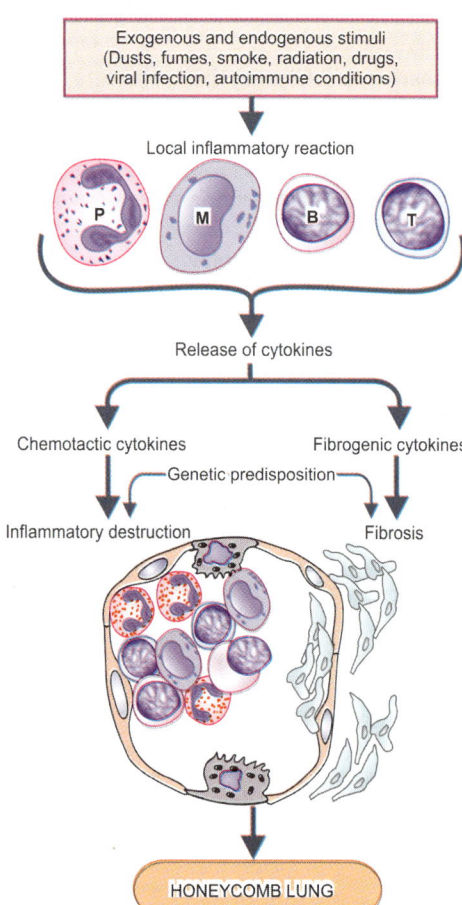

FIGURE 17.20: Schematic evolution of interstitial lung disease (ILD).

TABLE 17.7 Obstructive versus restrictive pulmonary diseases.

FEATURE	OBSTRUCTIVE	RESTRICTIVE
1. *Airways*	Obstructed at any level from trachea to respiratory bronchiole	Reduced expansion of lung parenchyma
2. *Pulmonary function test*	Increased pulmonary resistance and obstruction of maximal expiratory airflow	Decreased total lung capacity
3. *X-ray chest*	Variable appearance depending upon the cause	Typically bilateral infiltrates giving ground-glass shadows
4. *Examples*	• Chronic bronchitis • Emphysema • Bronchial asthma • Bronchiectasis	➢ Chest cage disorders (e.g. kyphoscoliosis, poliomyelitis, severe obesity and pleural disease) ➢ Interstitial lung diseases (ILDs) (e.g. pneumoconioses, idiopathic pulmonary fibrosis, connective tissue diseases, sarcoidosis, immunologic lung diseases, smoking-related ILDs, etc.)

b. Those that measure 5–10 μm are phagocytosed by alveolar macrophages and expectorated in sputum.

c. The very small ones (less than 0.5 μm) are innocuous.

d. However, the particles measuring between *0.5 and 5 μm* reaching the alveoli are potentially the most dangerous dust particles.

ii. *Solubility and physicochemical composition* of particles.

iii. *Amount of dust* inhaled and also retained in the lungs.

iv. Additional effect of other irritants such as *tobacco smoke*.

v. *Host factors* regulating the clearance mechanism and the immune response to some particles.

The tissue response to inhaled dust particles depends on their chemical composition and includes one of the three types:

- *Fibrous nodule formation*, e.g. silicosis and coal-workers pneumoconiosis
- *Interstitial fibrosis*, e.g. asbestosis.
- *Hypersensitivity reaction*, mostly in the form of granulomas, as in berylliosis.

TABLE 17.8 Classification of pneumoconioses.

AGENT	DISEASES
A. INORGANIC (MINERAL) DUSTS	
1. *Coal dust*	Simple coal-workers' pneumoconiosis Progressive massive fibrosis Caplan syndrome
2. *Silica*	Silicosis Caplan syndrome
3. *Asbestos*	Asbestosis Pleural diseases Tumours
4. *Beryllium*	Acute berylliosis Chronic berylliosis
5. *Iron oxide*	Pulmonary siderosis
B. ORGANIC (BIOLOGIC) DUSTS	
1. *Mouldy hay*	Farmer's lungs
2. *Bagasse*	Bagassosis
3. *Cotton, flax, hemp dust*	Byssinosis
4. *Bird droppings*	Bird-breeders' (bird fancier's) lung
5. *Mushroom compost dust*	Mushroom-workers' lung
6. *Mouldy barley, malt dust*	Malt-workers' lung
7. *Mouldy maple bark*	Maple-bark disease
8. *Silage fermentation*	Silo-fillers' disease

Q33. What is coal-workers' pneumoconiosis? Briefly discuss features of its types.

Definition Coal-workers' pneumoconiosis is a chronic lung disease resulting from inhalation of coal dust particles over a period of 20–30 years. It exists in two forms: a milder form called simple coal-workers' pneumoconiosis, and a more advanced form called progressive massive fibrosis. It should be noted that it can be combined with other lung diseases such as rheumatoid lung disease or tuberculosis.

Features of types

I. **Simple coal-miners' pneumoconiosis** It is a milder form that can progress to progressive massive fibrosis in about 5–10 % patients.

- It is characterised by the deposition of coal particles in the lung parenchyma, pleura and bronchial lymph nodes.

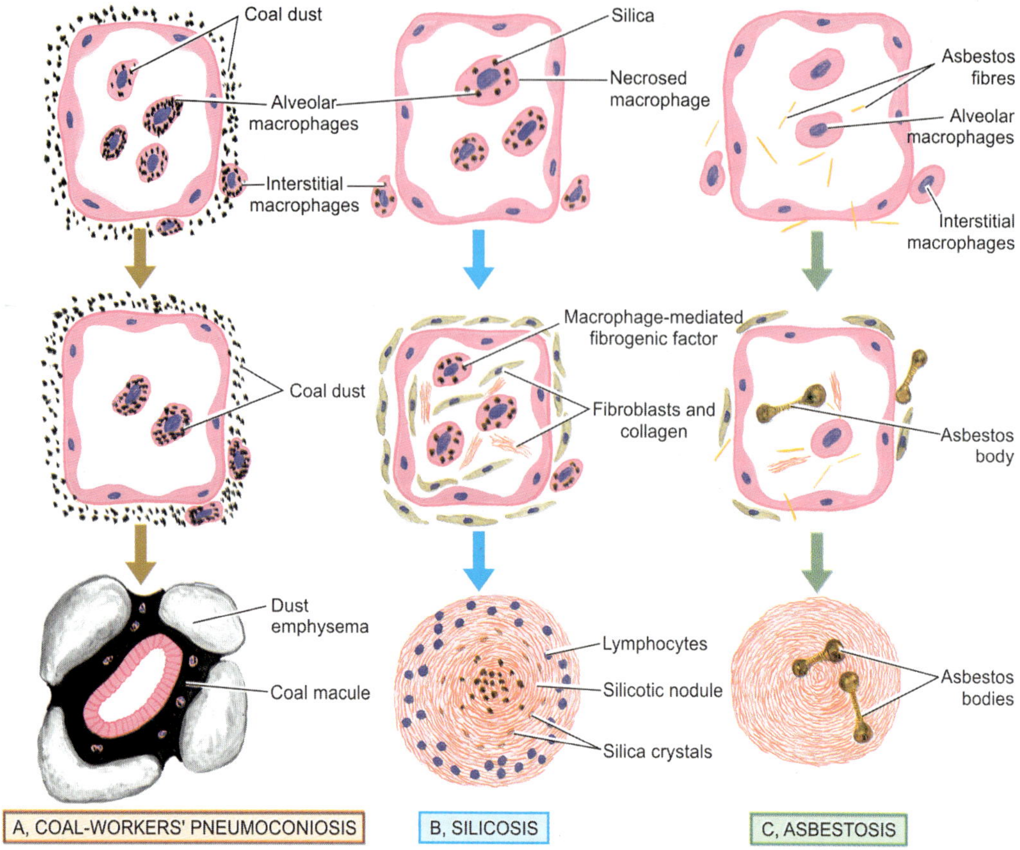

FIGURE 17.21: Pathogenesis of three common forms of pneumoconiosis. A, *Coal-workers' pneumoconiosis*. The macrophages phagocytose large amount of coal dust particles which are then passed into the interstitial tissue of the lung and aggregate around respiratory bronchiole and cause focal dust emphysema. B, *Silicosis*. The tiny silica particles are toxic to macrophages. The dead macrophages release fibrogenic factor and eventually result in silicotic nodule. C, *Asbestosis*. Asbestos fibres initiate lot of interstitial fibrosis and also form asbestos bodies.

- These deposits are similar but less prominent than to those in asymptomatic *anthracosis* seen in smokers and some city dwellers exposed to air pollution rich in coal particles.
- In the lung, the deposits of coal particles form 0.5 cm *coal macules* which may coalesce into palpable black *nodules* **(Fig. 17.21, A)**.
- *Microscopy* reveals that these lesions consist of aggregates of *coal-laden macrophages* in the alveoli and alveolar and bronchiolar walls **(Fig. 17.22)**.
- Exposed coal-miners keep coughing and expectorating black sputum, but otherwise they do not have any serious impairment of lung function.

II. **Progressive massive fibrosis** In addition to the changes seen in simple coal-miners' pneumoconiosis, the lungs of affected coal-miners show prominent fibrosis and black scars measuring more than 2 cm in diameter or more.
- Some larger masses may breakdown due to central ischaemic necrosis and transform into cavities filled with black semifluid material resembling India ink.
- Some of these lesions represent foci of tuberculosis.

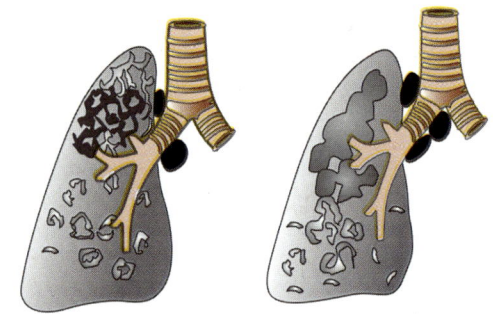

A, SIMPLE COAL-WORKERS' PNEUMOCONIOSIS   B, PROGRESSIVE MASSIVE FIBROSIS

FIGURE 17.22: Gross appearance of the lungs in simple coal-workers' pneumoconiosis (A) and progressive massive fibrosis (B).

- Clinically, there is incapacitating and progressive pulmonary insufficiency, pulmonary hypertension and right heart failure.

III. **Rheumatoid pneumoconiosis (Caplan syndrome)** It includes coal-miners' pneumoconiosis combined with immunologically mediated pulmonary rheumatoid nodules, which may show central necrosis, cavitation or calcification.

Q34. What is silicosis? Discuss its pathogenesis and salient pathologic features.

Definition Silicosis is a form of pneumoconiosis caused by inhalation of silicon dioxide crystals, commonly called silica.

Epidemiology Silica compounds represent one fourth of the earth's crust. They occur in a crystalline form (e.g. quartz) and an amorphous form; only the crystalline form poses health problems.

Workers of several professions are exposed daily to crystalline silica:
- Workers at risk for silicosis include miners, sandstone workers, querry workers, sandblasters, grinders, foundry workers, ceramic workers and several others.
- In India, occupational exposure to pencil, slate, and agate grinding industry carries a high-risk of silicosis. There are three million workers at high-risk for silicosis in India alone.

Pathogenesis Not fully understood, although a following facts are unquestionably established:
- The reaction to silica crystals is mediated by *macrophages*.
- Inhaled silica crystals are phagocytosed by macrophages, which get stimulated to secrete various *cytokines* that promote inflammation, immune response, proliferation of fibroblasts and deposition of collagen fibres.
- Ingested silica tends to kill macrophages which then release from their cytoplasm many of the *biologically active mediators* stored in their granules.
- Silica crystals are *fibrogenic* and stimulate formation of *silicotic nodules*.

Pathology The hallmarks of silicosis are *hard fibrotic nodules* composed of concentric layers of collagen fibres (*see* **Fig. 17.21, B**). Birefringent silica crystals can be seen between the fibres. There are also scattered lymphocytes and pigmented macrophages that contain carbon dust.

i. Similar nodules may be seen underneath the pleura and the regional lymph nodes, which are usually enlarged (**Fig. 17.23**).

ii. Smaller nodules tend to coalesce and form *fibrotic scars* in the pulmonary parenchyma and in the subpleural space (**Fig. 17.24**). These nodular lesions tend to calcify and produce radiologically visible 'egg-shell' shadows.

iii. Large confluent nodules may undergo *necrosis and cavitation*.

iv. *Superimposed tuberculosis* is common and could also cause necrosis and cavitation. Similar changes are seen, albeit less often, in superimposed rheumatoid pneumoconiosis (Caplan syndrome).

v. In a less common but more deadly form called *accelerated silicosis,* pulmonary fibrosis is rapidly

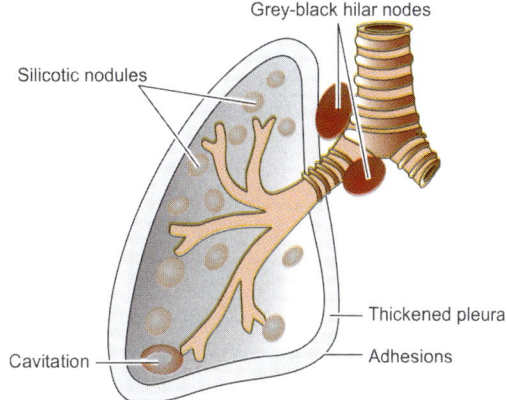

FIGURE 17.23: Gross appearance of the lung in silicosis, diagrammatic appearance.

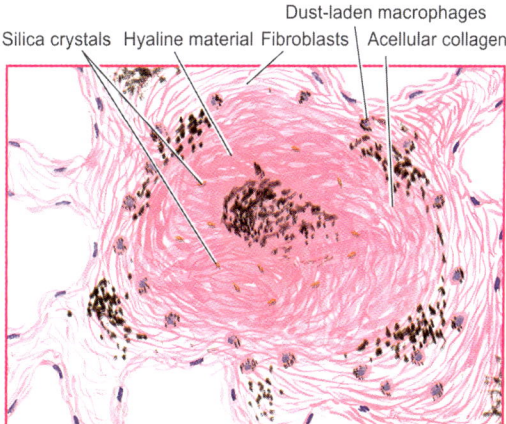

FIGURE 17.24: Microscopic picture of the lung in silicosis. The silicotic nodule consists of hyaline centre surrounded by concentric layers of collagen which are further enclosed by fibroblasts and dust-laden macrophages. Polarising microscopy in photomicrograph on right shows bright fibres of silica.

progressive. It is usually associated with accumulation of lipoportein aceous exudate in the alveoli resembling alveolar proteinosis.

Clinical features Pulmonary silicosis leads to:
- Slowly evolving dyspnoea with features of obstructive lung disease.
- With time pulmonary disease becomes incapacitating.
- Silicosis may increase susceptibility to tuberculosis.

Q35. What is asbestosis? Discuss pathogenesis and salient features of lesions related to asbestosis.

Definition Asbestosis is a pneumoconiosis resulting from exposure to asbestos fibres. In addition to this fibrosing lung disease, prolonged exposure to asbestos may produce non-neoplatic pleural disease and malignant tumours (lung cancer and malignant mesothelioma).

Epidemiology Exposure to asbestos occurs in many industries including mining, ship-building, construction work. Asbestos is found in many industrial products such as pipes, tiles, roof sheets, textiles, insulating boards, sewer and water conduits, automobile and train brake lining, clutches and many others. During the last few decades, an effort has been made to remove as much asbestos as possible from the human habitat and replace it with fibreglass. Still asbestos remains an important health hazard, especially in the less developed and poorer countries.

Physicochemical properties of asbestos Asbestos exists in the form of long fibrils which are fire resistant and can be spun into yarn and fabrics suitable for thermal and electrical insulation. There are two geometric forms of asbestos:

I. *Serpentine form* consists of curly and flexible fibres. It includes the most common chemical form chrysotile (white asbestos) comprising 90% of all commercially used asbestos.

II. *Amphibole form* consists of straight, stiff and rigid fibres. It includes the less common forms such as crocidolite (blue asbestos), amosite (brown asbestos), tremolite, anthophyllite and actinolite. Even though less common, amphiboles (especially *crocidolite*) are more important as they are associated with the induction of malignant pleural tumours.

Pathogenesis Not fully elucidated. The following facts are known to play a potential role (*see* **Fig. 17.21, C**):

- Inhaled asbestos fibres are phagocytosed by alveolar macrophages, which then move to the interstitium or a transported to the pleura and bronchial lymph nodes.
- Macrophages containing asbestos fibres secrete cytokines which attract more macrophages and stimulate fibroblasts to produce collagen rich fibrous tissue.
- Asbestos fibres are coated with glycoprotein and haemosiderin ('ferruginous bodies') and transform into brown, dumbbell-shaped *asbestos bodies* **(Fig. 17.25, B)**.

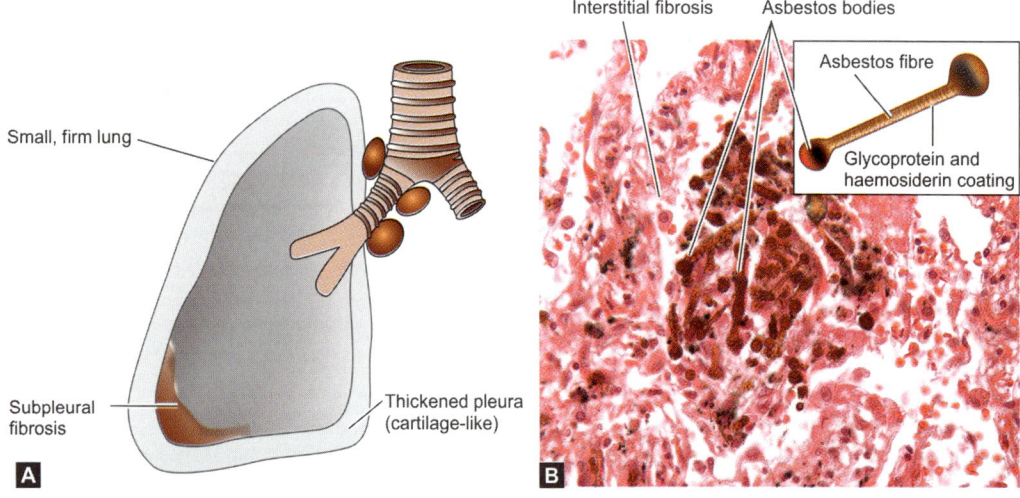

FIGURE 17.25: Asbestosis lung. A, Diagrammatic appearance of the lung in asbestosis. B, The lung parenchyma shows interstitial fibrosis and a few asbestos or ferruginous bodies. These appear dumbbell-shaped and brown in colour due to coating of asbestos fibre with glycoprotein and haemosiderin.

- Pulmonary fibrosis results from the action of cytokines released from macrophages and the action of asbestos fibres, which are considered to be fibrogenic.
- Several forms of asbestos, most notably crocidolite, are carcinogenic producing malignant mesothelioma. They also potentiate the carcinogenic effects of tobacco smoke and contribute to the development of lung cancer.

Pathology Three most important lesions induced by asbestos are: i) pulmonary asbestosis, ii) non-neoplastic pleural disease, and iii) tumours.

I. *Asbestosis* of the lungs is characterised by extensive parenchymal fibrosis.

Grossly, fibrotic lungs are firm and contracted and show fibrous scarring, most prominently underneath the pleura and the bases of both lungs **(Fig. 17.25, A)**.

Microscopy reveals nonspecific interstitial fibrosis and scattered asbestos bodies which stain positively for the Prussian blue reaction due to their content of hemosiderin **(Fig. 17.25, B)**.

Clinically, asbestosis presents with dyspnoea, productive cough and progressive deterioration of pulmonary functions and cor pulmonale.

II. **Non-neoplastic pleural disease** includes the following:
i. Visceral pleural fibrosis which in some cases may encase the entire lung.
ii. White fibrocalcific parietal pleural plaques (most common finding)
iii. Pleural effusion (in 5%).

III. **Tumours** most often associated with exposure to asbestos are: i) bronchogenic carcinoma, and ii) malignant mesothelioma.

i. *Bronchogenic carcinoma* develops due to the carcinogenic effects of asbestos and due to the interaction of asbestos with other carcinogens, such as smoking.
- Carcinoma has an incidence that is 5 times higher in non-smoker asbestos workers than in non-smokers who were not exposed to asbestos.
- The incidence in smokers exposed to asbestos is 10 times higher than in smokers not exposed to asbestos.

ii. *Malignant mesothelioma* of the pleura and peritoneum has been epidemiologically linked to asbestos exposure.
- Tumours develop after a long lag period of 20–30 years and can occur not only in asbestos workers but members of worker's family are also at risk presumably because of exposure to asbestos carried home on worker's garment.

Q36. What is berylliosis? What are the main features of its types?

Definition Berylliosis is a pneumoconiosis caused by heavy exposure to dust or fumes of metallic beryllium or its salts.

Epidemiology Exposure to beryllium or its salts can occur in nuclear and aerospace industry and in manufacture of electrical and electronic equipment.

Classification and features Berylliosis occurs in two forms: acute and chronic.

I. **Acute berylliosis** occurs in individuals who are extremely sensitive or those who are exposed to heavy doses of beryllium for 2–4 weeks.

Microscopy Acute chemical pneumonitis with exudation of protein rich fluid into the alveoli, and focal hyaline membranes.

Clinically, Symptoms include sudden onset of dyspnoea, hyperpnoea, and substernal pain.

Prognosis Most patients recover completely and without sequelae.

II. **Chronic berylliosis** develops in persons who have been sensitised to beryllium for a number of years. Symptoms may appear with a long delay of 20 years or more after exposure.

Microscopy Reaction to beryllium includes formation of *granulomas*, which represent a cell mediated, *type IV hypersensitivity reaction*. Non-caseating granulomas composed of epithelioid macrophages, multinucleated giant cells and lymphocytes resemble those of sarcoidosis, but in contrast to these, they contain birefringent crystals. Noncaseating granulomas may occur in other organs as well such as liver, kidneys, spleen.

Clinically, symptoms include dyspnoea and progressive impairment of lung function.

Q37. How do autoimmune connective tissue/collagen-vascular diseases affect lungs?

A number of connective tissue/collagen vascular diseases can affect lungs as under:

i. **Systemic sclerosis (scleroderma)**—interstitial pulmonary fibrosis with accentuated subpleural fibrosis is found in 80% advanced cases.

ii. **Rheumatoid arthritis**—pleural effusion, interstitial pneumonitis, necrobiotic granulomas similar to those in subcutaneous tissue. It may be combined with anthracosis or silicosis (Caplan syndrome).

iii. **Systemic lupus erythematosus**—pleural effusion and fibrinous sterile pleuritis, and less often interstitial pneumonitis and vasculitis involving lung vessels.

iv. **Sjögren syndrome**—immunological inflammation of bronchial mucous glands similar to the inflammation of salivary gland will cause reduce secretion of mucus and reduced resistance to infection.

v. **Wegener granulomatosis**—necrotising pulmonary granulomas and angiitis of lung vessels. In limited form of Wegener granulomatosis the lungs are the only organ involved.

Q38. What is idiopathic pulmonary fibrosis? Briefly discuss its etiopathogenesis and clinicopathologic features.

Definition Idiopathic pulmonary fibrosis is a chronic restrictive lung disease of unknown etiology characterised by interstitial and replacement fibrosis involving both lungs in a patchy manner. In UK, it is known under the name *cryptogenic fibrosing alveolitis* and the radiologists usually report it as *usual interstitial pneumonia (UIP)*.

Etiopathogenesis Unknown.

- Genetic predisposition and immune reaction to alveolar cell injury are thought to play a role.
- Patients' age and gender are also important, since the disease affects predominantly males in 40–70 years age group.
- The sequence of events is thought to begin with an injury of alveolar lining cells that cannot be repaired.
- Alveolar cell injury is accompanied by nonspecific inflammation and repair involving proliferation of fibroblasts ('fibrosing alveolitis').
- Progressive fibrosis replaces normal pulmonary parenchyma and the remaining terminal bronchioles become cystically dilated because they are 'cut-off' from the more central parts of the bronchial tree.

Clinicopathologic features Destruction of alveoli combined with focal replacement fibrosis and cystic dilatation of terminal bronchioles account for the *alternating honey-comb like zones with zones of broad scarring* **(Fig. 17.26)**.

i. Foci of chronic inflammation are seen in the fibrotic lung parenchyma, and in the mucus filling the cystic spaces suggesting that inflammation plays a pathogenetic role.

ii. Both lungs are involved but the changes are not evenly distributed.

iii. The changes are most prominent along the *interlobular septa and subpleural parts of the lower lobes*.

iv. The diagnosis is made by correlating the clinical and radiologic data, reported as 'usual interstitial pneumonia', with corresponding pathologic findings.

v. Furthermore, it is important to exclude other well-known causes of diffuse pulmonary fibrosis (such as pneumoconiosis, collagen vascular lung diseases, and hypersensitivity pneumonitis), which may present with similar if not identical X-ray and pathologic findings.

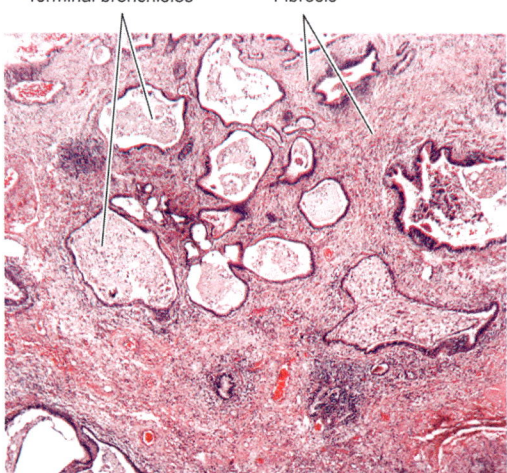

FIGURE 17.26: Idiopathic pulmonary fibrosis. There is destruction of alveoli and replacement with fibrosis. Advanced stage of idiopathic pulmonary fibrosis develops dense fibrosis around terminal bronchioles giving a honey-comb appearance.

Prognosis The clinical course is characterised with progressive deterioration of pulmonary function and death in 3–5 years of onset of symptoms. Treatment includes pulmonary transplantation.

Q39. Define and discuss hypersensitivity (allergic) pneumonitis briefly.

Definition Hypersensitivity pneumonitis is a group of immunologically mediated interstitial lung diseases occurring in workers inhaling a variety of organic antigenic materials.

Pathogenesis Hypersensitivity pneumonitis is based on type III (immune complex-mediated) or type IV (cell-mediated)hypersensitivity reaction in most (80%) cases.
- Skin testing can demonstrate hypersensitivity to specific antigens.
- Bronchoalveolar lavage contains an increased number of CD4+ and CD8+ T cells.
- Deposits of immune complexes can be demonstrated in lung biopsy.

Classification The causative antigens are either part of the inhaled industrial material or are related to fungi and bacteria that grow on it. Various diseases in this group are named according to the work place of exposure and the nature or the antigenic material as under:

i. *Farmers' lung*—exposure to thermophilic actinomyces in humid and warm mouldy hay.
ii. *Bagassosis*—exposure to sugarcane bagasse used for the production of paper and cardboard.
iii. *Byssinosis*—exposure to fibres of cotton, flex and hamp.
iv. *Bird breeders' lung*—exposure to bird droppings and danders from their feathers. It typically affects bird-breeders or fanciers of pigeons and parrots or chicken farmers.
v. *Mushroom-workers' lung*—affects mushroom cultivators exposed to mushroom compost dust.
vi. *Maple-bark disease*—affects workers stripping maple bark and inhaling the mouldy maple bark.

NOTE: These immune mediated diseases must be distinguished from *silo-fillers' disease*, and acute toxic lung injury caused by fumes and nitric oxide inside generated by the fermentation of silo. Upon entering or falling into a silo, the affected person develops acute pulmonary oedema and ARDS with a rapid fatal outcome.

Clinicopathologic features All the above listed diseases have the same underlying pathology and comparable clinical courses.
- *Acute stages* of the disease are characterised by interstitial infiltrates of lymphocytes and noncaseating granulomas.
- *Chronic changes* are marked by interstitial fibrosis causing clinically evident signs of restrictive lung disease.
- Respiratory functional studies (spirometry) are used to document decreased diffusion capacity, lung compliance and total lung volume.

Prognosis These diseases have a slowly progressive course ultimately leading to respiratory failure.

Q40. What are the pulmonary restrictive diseases with pulmonary infiltrates and eosinophilia?

Definition Pulmonary restrictive diseases with pulmonary infiltrates and eosinophilia (PIE) form a heterogeneous group of hypersensitivity lung diseases accompanied by blood and tissue eosinophilia.

Classification The following entities are included in this group:

i. *Löeffler syndrome* which includes eosinophilia with migratory radiologic lung shadows of unknown etiology. Lung infiltrates wax and wane and disappear on their own. The disease has a self-limited benign course.

ii. *Tropical pulmonary eosinophilia* is caused by the passage of worm larvae through the lung during their migration through the human body. This event can occur in several parasitic diseases, such as filariasis, strongyloidosis, ascariasis, toxocariasis, and ancylostomiasis.

iii. *Secondary pulmonary eosinophilia* is encountered in:
- Some adverse immune reactions to drugs and also it may occur in the course of some infections. It may be acute or chronic.
- *Allergic pulmonary aspergillosis* and *infections superimposed on asthma* need to be mentioned because of their clinical significance.

iv. *Idiopathic chronic eosinophilic pneumonia* is diagnosed after one has excluded all other possible causes of eosinophilia. In the differential diagnosis, one must consider the *hypereosinophilic syndrome*, which is defined as blood eosinophilia over 1500/μL for at least 6 months, but unaccompanied by pulmonary or any other organ infiltration.

Q41. Briefly discuss smoking-associated restrictive interstitial lung diseases.

Smoking is primarily linked with COPD and several other obstructive lung conditions. However, smoking can also cause restrictive interstitial lungs diseases such as: i) desquamative interstitial pneumonia, and ii) respiratory bronchiolitis:

I. **Desquamative interstitial pneumonia (DIP)** is an uncommon condition that affects predominantly male smokers in the 4th and 5th decade.
i. It presents with peculiar diffuse hazy opacities typical of ILD.
ii. Cessation of smoking leads to resolution of infiltrates.
Pathology It is a misnomer since there is no real pneumonia
- Instead, there are only intra-alveolar macrophages. Macrophages have with abundant cytoplasm that contains black pigment ("smokers' macrophages").
- In later stages and if the person does not stop smoking, it may progress to interstitial fibrosis.

II. **Respiratory bronchiolitis** is much more common than DIP.
i. It begins as a bronchiolocentric accumulation of macrophages and is considered to be a mild form of DIP.
ii. If the person stops smoking it regresses on its own.
Pathology It is characterised by:
- An accumulation of "smokers' macrophages" and scattered lymphocytes.
- If the person does not stop smoking, it may progress and in advanced cases it is called *respiratory bronchiolitis associated with ILD*.
- Advanced cases may be associated with centriacinar emphysema.

Q42. Classify lung tumours. Comment briefly on epidemiology of lung cancer.

Classification Lung tumours can be benign or malignant and are classified according to their cell of origin as i) epithelial, ii) mesenchymal, iii) lympho-histiocytic, iv) tumours of ectopic origin, and v) metastatic tumours **(Table 17.9)**. Epithelial tumours account for the majority of cancers.

Epidemiology Lung cancer is the most common primary malignant tumour in men.
- It accounts for nearly 30% of all cancer death in both sexes in developing countries.
- The peak incidence is in the 55–65 years age groups, more commonly in males than females.
- The campaign to stop smoking has somewhat reduced the incidence of malignant lung tumours, and yet it remains a major health problem. WHO has predicted 10 million lung cancer deaths by 2030.

Q43. What are the key factors in the etiology and pathogenesis of lung tumours?

Smoking plays a key role in the etiology and pathogenesis of lung tumours, and the role of other factors is secondary.

TABLE 17.9 Abbreviated WHO classification of lung tumours (2015)*.

I. EPITHELIAL TUMOURS
A. BENIGN
1. Papilloma, squamous cell (exophytic, inverted)
2. Adenomas
3. Mixed squamous and glandular papilloma

B. MALIGANT
1. Adenocarcinoma (Major types: lepidic, acinar, papillary, micropapillary, solid, mucinous, pre-invasive)
2. Squamous cell carcinoma (Major types: keratinising, non-keratinising, basaloid, pre-invasive)
3. Neuroendocrine tumours (Major types: small cell, large cell, carcinoid, pre-invasive)
4. Large cell carcinoma
5. Adenosquamous carcinoma
6. Sarcomatoid carcinoma
7. Others and unclassified carcinomas
8. Salivary gland type tumours

II. MESENCHYMAL TUMOURS
1. Pulmonary hamartoma
2. Chondroma
3. PEComas
4. Myofibroblastic tumour (congenital, inflammatory)
5. Rare tumours

III. LYMPHOHISTIOCYTIC TUMOURS
1. MALToma
2. Diffuse large cell lymphoma
3. Pulmonary Langerhans cell histiocytosis

IV. TUMOURS OF ECTOPIC ORIGIN
1. Germ cell tumours
2. Intrapulmonary thymoma

V. METASTATIC TUMOURS

*Adapted from Travis et al (on behalf of WHO Panel). The 2015 WHO classification of lung tumours: Impact of genetic, clinical and radiologic advances since 2004 classification. J Thorac Oncol 2015; 10:1243-60.

I. **Smoking** The following evidence supports that smoking plays a key role in pathogenesis of lung tumours:
i. *Total dose* directly correlates with the death rate from lung cancer.
- An average smoker has a 13 times higher chance of developing cancer than the non-smoker.
- The risk of smokers who smoke 2 packs per day (40 cigarettes) for 20 years is 60–70 times higher than non-smokers. Overall, only 10% of heavy smokers develop cancer.
- Cessation of smoking reduces the risk, but it never comes down to the risk level of non-smokers.
- Pipe smokers who inhale less smoke are at a lower risk level than cigarette smokers.
ii. *Histologic evidence* for the development of squamous cell carcinoma has been well documented and it has been shown that invasive carcinoma is preceded by carcinoma in situ and this in turn has been preceded by squamous metaplasia and dysplasia **(Fig. 17.27)**.
iii. *Biochemical and experimental studies* on animals show that the tobacco smoke contains carcinogens (e.g. polycyclic hydrocarbons, nitrosamines) and tumour promoters (e.g. phenol derivatives) that can produce tumours in experimental animals.
II. **Other factors** Following factors account for approximately 15% of tumours, especially those in women:
i. *Radiation exposure,* especially inhalation of *radon,* that is prevalent in the basements of older houses. Historically, radon has been blamed for lung cancer in uranium miners.
ii. *Atmospheric pollution* contributes to carcinogenicity of smoke, as evidenced by higher incidence of cancer in smoky cities than in rural areas.
iii. *Occupational causes* are known to increase the occurrence of lung cancer in certain industries.
- Exposure to asbestos increases the risk of lung cancer in smokers over 50 times.
- Exposure to nickel beryllium, arsenic, metallic iron has been linked with an increased incidence of lung cancer.
iv. *Chronic scarring* plays a role in the pathogenesis of peripheral lung cancers as in various diseases such as chronic interstitial fibrosis, old infarcts, foci of healed tuberculosis and scleroderma. So called *'scar cancers'* can be peripheral adenocarcinomas or squamous cell carcinomas.

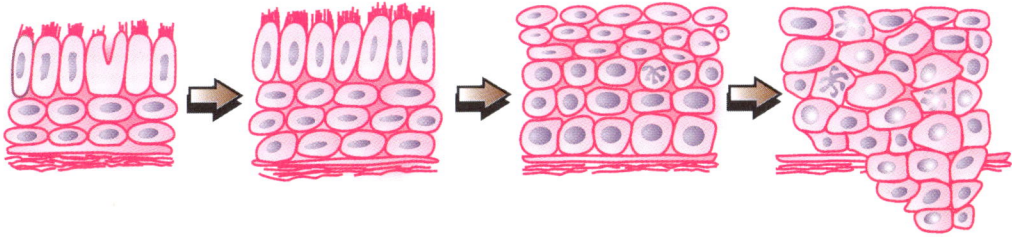

A, NORMAL BRONCHIAL MUCOSA   B, BASAL CELL HYPERPLASIA   C, SQUAMOUS METAPLASIA AND DYSPLASIA   D, CARCINOMA *IN SITU* WITH MICROINVASION

FIGURE 17.27: Schematic representation of sequential development of squamous cell carcinoma of the lung.

Q44. What are the known facts about the molecular pathogenesis of lung tumours?

The most important genetic changes known about lung tumours are as follows:
I. **Inactivation of tumour suppressor genes**
i. Deletion of short arm of chromosome 3 is found in 80–90% of both small cell and non-small cell lung cancers (SCLC and NSCLC). It is an early event and is also found in preinvasive CIS in bronchi.
ii. Many tumour suppressor genes are mutated and inactivated or lost, most notably *TP53* and *RB* gene.
II. **Activation of growth promoting oncogenes**
i. Mutation of *K-RAS* oncogene plays a dominant role in NSCLC, even though it appears to be a late event.
ii. Mutation in the tyrosine kinase domain of *EGFR* oncogene, mutually exclusive with *K-RAS* mutations, plays a role in the pathogenesis of adenocarcinoma of non-smokers, especially those of East Asian origin.
NOTE: Oncogene mutations are not found in small cell carcinomas (SCLC).
III. **Autocrine growth factors** The role of these factors is not fully understood but there is evidence that *nicotine* can act as a promotor and that *certain hormones* have the same effect.
IV. **Genetic predisposition** Only 10% of heavy smokers develop lung cancer indicating that they probably have a genetic predilection.

i. *Some cancer families* have a higher incidence of lung cancer than people in general population.
ii. *Li-Fraumeni syndrome* based on hereditary *TP53* mutation is marked by increased incidence of lung cancer.
iii. *Close relatives of lung cancer patients* are at a 2–3 fold higher risk for lung cancer than general population.

V. Molecular targets for therapy
i. Targeted molecular therapy against mutations of *EGFR in adenocarcinoma* of non-smokers is used in clinical medicine.
ii. Likewise, *inhibitors of anaplastic lymphoma kinase (ALK)* have been used in adenocarcinoma patients with *ALK mutations,* which are unfortunately found only about 5% of NSCLC.

Q45. How are lung cancers classified macroscopically on the basis of their location?

Lung cancers are topographically divided into two groups: hilar type and peripheral type **(Fig. 17.28)**.
I. **Hilar lung cancers** originate from major bronchi.
i. They may narrow or occlude the lumen and cause bronchiectasis and bronchopneumonia.
ii. Frequently, they extend/metastasise to bronchial and hilar lymph nodes.
iii. Necrosis of large masses may result in cavitation.
iv. Irritation of bronchi leads to coughing and may cause haemoptysis.
v. *Microscopically,* they could represent all types of lung cancer, but most often these are squamous cell carcinoma and small cell carcinoma.
II. **Peripheral lung cancers** are located usually in the subpleural region of the lungs.
i. On cut section the tumour is greyish and mucoid and appears as consolidated lung parenchyma of different colour than normal lung tissue.
ii. They originate from bronchioles.
iii. *Microscopically*, most of them are adenocarcinomas.

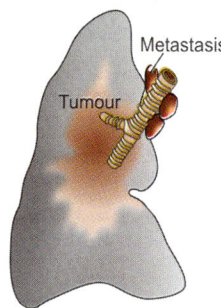
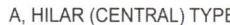
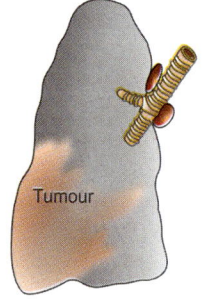

FIGURE 17.28: Two main gross patterns of lung cancer. A, Hilar or central lung cancer. Squamous cell carcinoma shows homogenous grey white appearance with metastasis in the hilar lymph node containing anthracotic pigment. B, Peripheral lung cancer. It shows adenocarcinoma lung in subpleural location developing in dense grey white scar.

Q46. How are lung cancers classified microscopically?

Four major microscopic types of lung cancer are recognised **(Fig. 17.29)**:

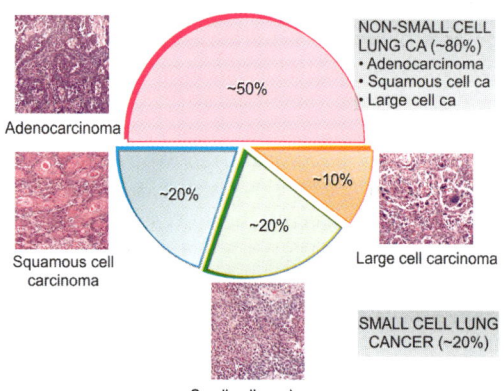

FIGURE 17.29: Four major histologic types of lung cancer and their corresponding average incidence. From therapeutic point of view, lung cancer is divided into small cell (SCLC) and non-small cell lung carcinoma (NSCLC). SCCL comprises ~20%, while NSCLC constitutes remaining ~80% cases and includes three major histologic types: adenocarcinoma ~50%, squamous cell carcinoma ~20%, and large cell carcinoma ~10%). (Adapted from Harrison's Principles of Internal Medicine. 19th edition 2015. Eds Kasper et al. McGraw Hill).

i. Adenocarcinoma (~50%)
ii. Squamous cell carcinoma (~20%)
iii. Small cell carcinoma (~20%)
iv. Large cell carcinoma (~10%)
For therapeutic purposes, lung cancers are divided into two groups:
i. Nonsmall cell lung carcinoma (NSCLC) comprising 70–75% of all cancers
ii. Small cell lung carcinoma (SCLC)

Q47. Tabulate the contrasting features of small cell and non-small cell lung cancers (SCLC and NSCLC).

Major differences between NSCLC and SCLC are shown in **Table 17.10**.

TABLE 17.10 Comparison of features of small cell (SCLC) and non-small cell lung carcinoma (NSCLC).

FEATURE	SCLC	NSCLC
1. *Etiologic relationship*	Strongly related to tobacco smoking	Smoking implicated; other factors: pollution, chronic scars, asbestos exposure
2. *Morphology*		
i. Pattern	Diffuse sheets	Squamous or glandular pattern
ii. Nuclei	Hyperchromatic, fine chromatin	Pleomorphic, coarse chromatin
iii. Nucleoli	Indistinct	Prominent
iv. Cytoplasm	Scanty	Abundant
v. EM: dense-core granules	Present	Absent
3. *Neuroendocrine markers* (e.g. chromogranin, synaptophysin, neuron-specific enolase, CD56, CD57)	Present	Absent
4. *Epithelial markers* (e.g. epithelial membrane antigen, carcinoembryonic antigen, cytokeratin)	Present	Present
5. *Mucin*	Absent	Present in adenocarcinoma
6. *β2 microglobulin*	Absent to low	Present
7. *Peptide hormone production*	Gastrin, ACTH, ADH, calcitonin	Parathormone
8. *Genetic abnormalities*	3p allele loss, *RB* and *p53* mutations	3p allele loss, *EGFR* and *K-RAS* mutations
9. *Treatment type*	Radiotherapy and/or chemotherapy	Surgical resection possible, limited response to radiotherapy and/or chemotherapy
10. *Prognosis*	Poor	Better

Q48. Briefly discuss morphologic features of major histologic types of lung cancer.

I. **Adenocarcinoma** is the most common microscopic type of lung cancer.
Most peripheral cancers are adenocarcinoma, but they may also be hilar.
i. Invasive adenocarcinoma is usually preceded by a *preinvasive stage*, also known as *atypical adenomatous hyperplasia*.
ii. To meet the criteria of the preinvasive neoplasia, the lesion must measure less than 3 cm in diameter and show only intra-alveolar growth (*lepidic growth*), with no signs of invasion.
iii. The next step in progression to higher grade neoplasia is *minimally invasive carcinoma* with less than 5 mm invasion.
iv. *Invasive adenocarcinoma* is diagnosed if there is unquestionable invasion of surrounding tissue exceeding 5 mm. Invasion is usually accompanied by a desmoplastic reaction comprising fibroblasts and myofibroblasts encasing tumour cells.
v. Adenocarcinomas form *gland like structures* (**Fig. 17.30**). Several architectural patterns are recognised, such as acinar, papillary or lepidic (along the preexisting alveolar walls), or it may appear solid with only minimal glandular differentiation.
vi. Some tumour cells may secrete mucus.
vii. Microscopic patterns do not predict the prognosis or influence the therapy; thus, there is no need to classify further adenocarcinomas into additional histopathologic subclasses.

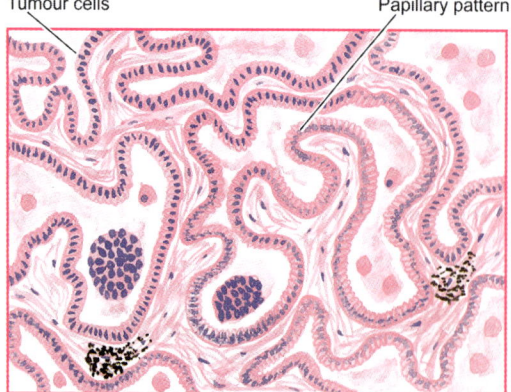

FIGURE 17.30: Adenocarcinoma lung. The tumour cells are seen to grow along alveolar spaces while the alveolar walls are fibrotic.

II. **Squamous cell carcinoma** is found more often in men then women and is usually related to smoking.

i. Most tumours originate from large bronchi and are located in the hilar region.

ii. They tend to metastasise early and are prone to necrosis and cavitation.

iii. *Microscopically*, they are composed of sheets of squamous cells interconnected one with another by intercellular bridges **(Fig. 17.31)**.

iv. Squamous pearls are seen in well differentiated cancers.

v. Poorly differentiated cancer may show less squamous differentiation and may be even composed of spindle shaped cells.

vi. Adjacent to invasive cancer one may find foci of *carcinoma in situ* and other preinvasive precursor lesions such as *high grade squamous dysplasia and metaplasia*.

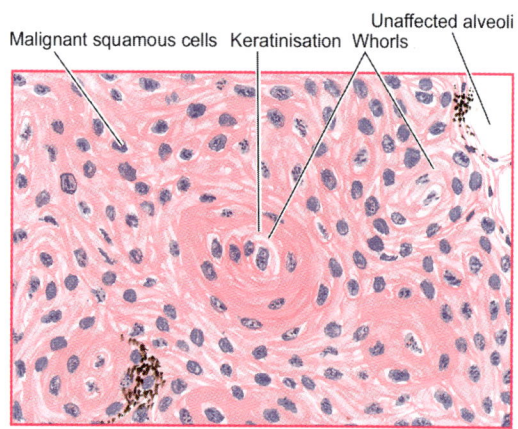

FIGURE 17.31: Squamous cell carcinoma of the lung. A few well-developed cell nests with concentric keratinisation are seen.

III. **Small cell carcinomas** are composed of neuroendocrine cells and are highly malignant tumours.

i. SCLC have a strong etiologic relationship to cigarette smoking.

ii. Most tumours originate from large bronchi and are hilar by location.

iii. Tumour cells have oval nuclei (hence the term 'oat cell carcinoma') and scant cytoplasm, with a high nucleocytoplasmic (N:C) ratio **(Fig. 17.32)**.

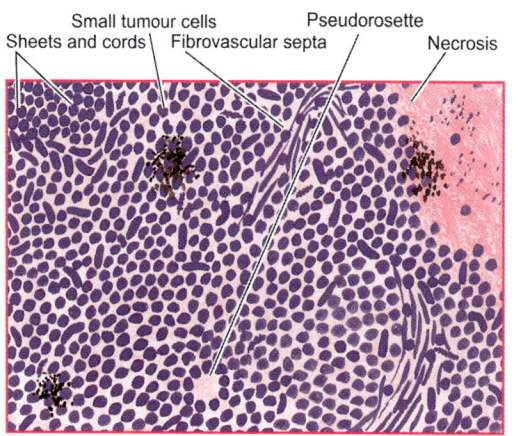

FIGURE 17.32: Small cell carcinoma of the lung. The tumour cells are arranged in sheets, cords or aggregates in a background of necrosis. The individual tumour cells are small, uniform, lymphocyte-like, having diffuse chromatin and scanty cytoplasm.

iv. By electron microscopy, one may see in their cytoplasm scarce *neuroendocrine granules*.
v. By immunohistochemistry, one can demonstrate granular staining of tumour cell cytoplasm with antibodies to *chromogranin* and *synaptophysin* which are contained in neuroendocrine granules.
vi. In addition to pure small cell carcinomas, there are some small cell tumours that also contain other components, like adenocarcinoma. Some are composed of large neuroendocrine cells ('large cell variant of SCLC'). Biologically, these tumours behave like pure small cell carcinomas.
vii. Small cells are often associated with ectopic hormone production causing *paraneoplastic syndromes*.

IV. **Large cell carcinoma** is the least common form of lung carcinoma.
i. These tumours are composed of *undifferentiated large cells* that lack the specific features by which one could diagnose them as squamous cell carcinoma or adenocarcinoma.
ii. They are related to smoking and occur more often in men than women.
iii. They are not curable by present day surgical and medical therapy and have a *poor prognosis*.

Q49. What are the salient clinical features of lung carcinoma?

Symptoms are quite variable but can be considered under several headings as under:

I. **Local symptoms** include cough, dyspnoea, haemoptysis. Other causes of haemoptysis should be considered in the differential diagnosis **(Table 17.11)**.

II. **Bronchial obstructive symptoms** are those related to bronchopneumonia, lung abscess, bronchiectasis, pleural effusion, and include fever, cough, shortness of breath and hypoxia.

III. **Symptoms due to metastases** are common because lung cancer tends to metastasise early. The routes of metastasis include *direct and lymphatic spread in the thoracic cavity* (opposite lung, pleura, mediastinum, lymph nodes); lymph node metastases are seen in the supraclavicular and paraaortic region. Superior vena caval syndrome, paralysis of the recurrent nerve, and chylothorax due to the obstruction of the lymph flow through the thoracic duct are also encountered. Haematogenous metastases (listed in descending order or involvement) occur in the liver, adrenals, bones, pancreas, brain.

TABLE 17.11 Causes of haemoptysis.

A. INFLAMMATORY
1. Bronchitis
2. Bronchiectasis
3. Tuberculosis
4. Lung abscess
5. Pneumonias
B. NEOPLASTIC
1. Primary and metastatic lung cancer
2. Bronchial adenoma
C. OTHERS
1. Pulmonary thromboembolism
2. Left ventricular failure
3. Mitral stenosis
4. Trauma
5. Foreign bodies
6. Primary pulmonary hypertension
7. Haemorrhagic diathesis

IV. **Paraneoplastic syndromes** occur most often with small cell lung carcinoma, but may be found also with other microscopic forms of lung cancer (including carcinoids). Features of paraneoplastic syndrome are as under:
i. *Ectopic hormone production:*
a. ADH—hyponatraemia
b. ACTH—Cushing syndrome
c. PTH—hypercalcaemia
d. Calcitonin—hypercalcaemia
e. Gonadotropins—gynaecomastia
ii. *Neuromuscular:* Polymyositis, myopathy, peripheral neuropathy, cerebellar degeneration.
iii. *Skeletal:* Clubbing of the fingers and hypertrophic osteoarthropathy.
iv. *Cutaneous:* Acanthosis nigricans, dermatomyositis.
v. *Cardiovascular:* Migratory thrombophlebitis (Trousseau syndrome), non-bacteria thrombotic endocarditis.
vi. *Haematologic:* Coagulopathy, leukaemoid reaction.

Prognosis It depends on the *stage and microscopic form* of lung cancer.
- In general, tumours that measure less than 3 cm are stage I.
- Tumours that measure more than 5 cm in diameter have the worst prognosis.
- Stage III tumours are those that involve adjacent structures, irrespective of their size.

- Small squamous carcinomas and adenocarcinoma diagnosed early (i.e. while still small) have the best prognosis, whereas small cell and large cell carcinoma, irrespective of their size, have the worst prognosis.
- The overall prognosis for lung cancer patients is abysmal; only 15% of them survive five years.

Q50. Write briefly on bronchial carcinoids.

Definition Carcinoids are neuroendocrine carcinomas of low-grade malignancy.

Epidemiology Carcinoids account for 5% of lung carcinomas. They occur in young adults under the age of 40 years, uncommon.

Pathology *Gross* Most carcinoids originate in the large bronchi and are diagnosed as relatively small tumours causing bronchial irritation and cough.

Microscopy Carcinoids are composed of:

i. Uniform cells arranged into trabeculae, cords or nests surrounded by thin fibrous septa **(Fig. 17.33)**.

ii. Tumour cells have round nuclei surrounded with well developed cytoplasm that contains *neuroendocrine granules,* seen best by electron microscopy.

iii. The cytoplasm stains with antibodies to *chromogranin and synaptophysin*, which proves their neuroendocrine nature.

iv. Mitoses are rare and there is no necrosis. Nevertheless, tumour cells are locally invasive and may metastasise to local lymph nodes and distant organs.

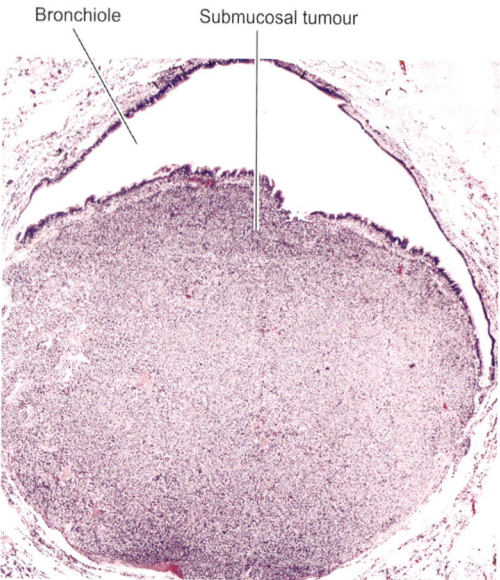

FIGURE 17.33: Bronchial carcinoid. The tumour shows a characteristic submucosal nodule covered by intact bronchial mucosa.

v. Less often, some carcinoids show more mitotic activity and contain foci of necrosis and are, therefore, called *atypical carcinoids.*

Prognosis In contrast to classical carcinoids which have a 10 year survival rate of over 85%, atypical carcinoids have a worse prognosis and such patients survive 10 years in 35% of cases only.

Q51. What are pulmonary hamartomas?

Definition Pulmonary hamartomas are small tumour-like developmental lesions composed of normal bronchial tissues. Clinically they are usually asymptomatic and found accidentally on X-ray examination ('coin lesions').

Pathology They may be solitary or multiple:

I. *Solitary hamartomas* are found in peripheral lung parenchyma. They measure 2–5 cm and are usually composed of cartilage surrounded by fibrous and adipose tissue admixed with bronchial epithelium.

II. *Multiple small hamartomas* are located underneath the pleura, measure 1–2 cm and are most often composed of smooth muscle cells and bronchiolar epithelium.

Q52. Which malignant tumours commonly metastasise to the lungs?

- Secondary/metastatic tumours are more common than the primary lung tumours.
- Both carcinoma and sarcomas can metastasise to the lungs, which reach by haematogenous route, or less often through lymphatics and direct extension.

Pathology Metastases originate from tumour cell emboli which most often lodge in the peripheral parts of the pulmonary arterial circulation.

- Typically, they give rise to multiple nodules which appear radiologically as *round cannon-ball masses* on X-ray examination.

- Metastases may originate from any organ and even lungs themselves. More common malignant tumours for pulmonary metastasis are carcinoma of the intestines or breast.

PLEURA

Q53. What is pleuritis? Discuss salient features of common types.

Definition Pleuritis or pleurisy is inflammation of the pleura, which may be acute or chronic.
Pathology
i. Acute inflammation is usually accompanied by an exudate which may be serous, fibrinous or serofibrinous.
ii. Most often, pleuritis is secondary to pulmonary infections and other pathologic processes.
iii. Common causes are pneumonia, tuberculosis, pulmonary infarcts, lung abscesses and bronchiectasis.
iv. Other less common causes include a few collagen vascular diseases (e.g. rheumatoid arthritis, SLE), uraemia, metastatic tumour, irradiation, and systemic infections caused by viruses and bacteria.
Clinical features
i. Pleuritis causes pain that is accentuated by breathing.
ii. A friction rub may be heard on auscultation.
iii. The exudate is usually minimal and will resorb upon healing of the primary process.
iv. Repeated attacks of pleurisy may result in organisation of the exudate and formation of fibrous adhesion between two layers of the pleura with obliteration of the pleural cavity.

Q54. What is thoracic empyema?

Definition Empyema or suppurative pleuritis is a pleural infection characterised by accumulation of pus in the pleural cavity.
Etiopathogenesis Most often, empyema results from the spread of a pulmonary infection to the pleura. It usually begins with a serofibrinous exudate which becomes purulent. Less common sources of infection are subdiaphragmatic or hepatic abscess, or direct penetrating chest wounds. Haematogenous and lymphatic routes of infection occur occasionally.
Clinicopathologic features
i. Empyema is characterised by accumulation of yellow-green creamy pus accumulating in large a volumes in the pleural cavity.
ii. It is ultimately replaced by granulation tissue which gives rise to fibrous adhesions obliterating the pleural cavity.
iii. Empyema prevents expansion of the lungs during inhalation thus causing respiratory problems. Fibrous obliteration of pleural cavities also causes respiratory problems.

Q55. Discuss salient features of common non-inflammatory pleural effusions.

These include: i) hydrothorax, ii) haemothorax, and iii) chylothorax.
I. **Hydrothorax** is non-inflammatory accumulation of serous fluid within the pleural cavity. It may be bilateral or unilateral. It may fill the entire pleural cavity or it may be limited to part of due to pre-existing pleural fibrous adhesions.
Etiopathogenesis
i. The most common cause of bilateral hydrothorax is *heart failure* resulting in venous congestion and transudation.
ii. Other causes include renal and liver failure with systemic oedema, pulmonary oedema, primary and secondary lung tumours.
iii. Meigs syndrome is a rare but remarkable form of pleural effusion, with or without acites, associated with ovarian fibroma.
Clinicopathologic features Pleural fluid is a transudate. The fluid is straw-coloured, with a specific gravity <1.012, protein content < 1 g, and little cellular content.
- Small effusion (less than 300 ml of fluid) produces usually no clinical symptoms. Fluid can be detected by X-ray examination as obliterating the costo-diaphragmatic angle.

- Larger effusion may be recognised as pleural opacities on X-ray examination.
- If the fluid is one-sided, it may cause deviation of the trachea to the opposite side.
- Large effusions cause respiratory embarrassment and dyspnoea, which are relieved on withdrawal of fluid from the chest.

II. **Haemothorax** is characterised by accumulation of blood in the pleural cavity.
- The most common cause is trauma to the chest wall and thoracic viscera, or rupture of the aortic aneurysm.
- It is important to remove the blood as soon as possible. Otherwise the blood will organise resulting in fibrous adhesions and obliteration of the pleural cavity.

III. **Chylothorax** is an uncommon condition in which there is accumulation of milky fluid of lymphatic origin in the thoracic cavity.
- Most often, it is caused by rupture of the thoracic duct by trauma or obstruction by malignant tumours, usually malignant lymphomas.
- Chylothorax is often confined to the left side.

Q56. What is pneumothorax?

Definition Pneumothorax is accumulation of air in the pleural cavity.
Types It can be i) spontaneous, ii) traumatic, or iii) therapeutic.

I. *Spontaneous pneumothorax* results from spontaneous rupture of alveoli in any form of lung disease.
- Most often, it is associated with emphysema, asthma or tuberculosis.
- In young patients, recurrent spontaneous rupture of subpleural peripheral blebs may occur without any cause resulting in a disabling condition called *spontaneous idiopathic pneumothorax*.

II. *Traumatic pneumothorax* occurs following traumatic rupture of the lungs, oesophagus or stomach, or cardiothoracic surgery.

III. *Therapeutic pneumothorax* used to be employed in the treatment of tuberculosis by introducing air into the pleural cavity and thus collapsing the lungs to limit its respiratory movement.

Q57. What are the most common tumours of the pleura?

Tumours of the pleura can be benign or malignant, primary or secondary.
Secondary malignant tumours are more common than primary tumours. Most common metastases are from the primaries in the lungs and breasts.
Primary pleural tumours include i) solitary fibrous tumour, and ii) malignant mesothelioma.

I. **Solitary fibrous tumour** is a rare benign pleural tumour.
i. It is well circumscribed often protruding into the pleural cavity.
ii. *Microscopically*, it is composed of non-descript fibroblasts encased in dense collagenous matrix.
iii. Tumours of the same histologic appearance occur in many other organs.

II. **Malignant mesothelioma** is an uncommon malignant tumour arising from the mesothelial lining of pleura and other serous cavities, like pericardium and peritoneum.
- Most mesotheliomas are associated with long-term professional exposure to amphibole type of *asbestos,* most often *crocidolite*.
- Asbestos bodies are found microscopically in the pleura and lungs of most patients.

Pathology Grossly, mesotheliomas form thick, white, coating over the pleural surface of the lungs obliterating the pleural cavity **(Fig. 17.34, A)**.
Microscopy Three patterns **(Fig. 17.34, B)**:
i. *Epithelioid resembling adenocarcinoma*: The tumour is distinguished from adenocarcinoma by means of immunohistochemistry. Mesotheliomas are positive for *calretinin, Wilms tumour antigen 1 (WT-1) and cytokeratin CK5/6*.
ii. *Sarcomatoid resembling fibrosarcoma*
iii. *Mixed epithelioid-sarcomatoid*

Clinical features include dyspnoea, thoracic pain, pleural effusion and increased incidence of infections. The tumour has a poor prognosis and most patients die within one year of diagnosis.

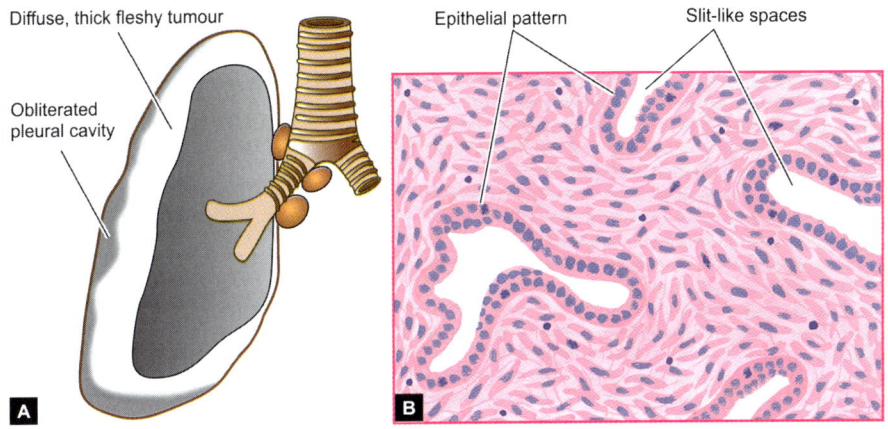

FIGURE 17.34: Malignant (diffuse) mesothelioma. A, Gross appearance. The tumour is seen to form a thick, white, fleshy coat over the parietal and visceral surfaces. B, Microscopy shows epithelial glandular pattern.

> **Chapter 17e Supplement: Online Content**
>
> *Digital content of this chapter available with this book is meant for enhanced learning and self-assessment. In addition, it contains 36 Multiple Choice Questions (MCQs), 05 Clinicopathologic Vignettes, and 08 Image-based Questions; these are followed by their answers along with explanatory notes of correct and incorrect answers.*

CHAPTER 18

Eye, ENT and Neck

■ EYE

Q1. Illustrate the normal structure of the eye.

The eyes are sensory organs transmitting visual information to the brain, thus maintaining visual acuity.
Each eye has a complex structure, which is diagrammatically presented in **Figure 18.1**. The principal parts of the eye are as follows:
Sclera, choroid, iris, uveal tract, retina, lens, anterior chamber, posterior chamber, and vitreous chamber.

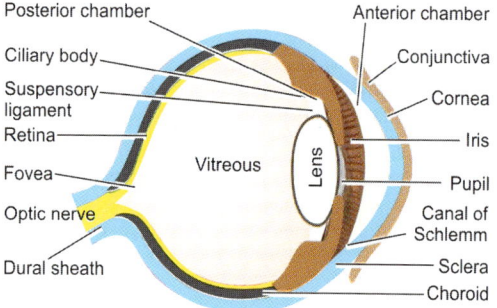

FIGURE 18.1: Schematic diagram of longitudinal section of the eyeball.

Q2. What are the most important congenital lesions of the eyes?

Two of the important congenital lesions are: retrolental hyperplasia and retinitis pigmentosa.
I. **Retrolental hyperplasia**, also known as retinopathy of prematurity (ROP) is a developmental disorder encountered in premature infants who have been given oxygen therapy at birth.
i. The basis lesion lies in the retinal blood vessels which are extremely sensitive to high to exposure to high concentrations of oxygen.
ii. The peripheral retina is incompletely vascularised and exposure to oxygen results in vaso-obliteration.
iii. On cessation of oxygen therapy, vaso-proliferation begins leading to neovascularisation, cicatrisation and retinal detachment resulting in a loss of sight.
II. **Retinitis pigmentosa** is a group of diseases of unknown etiology characterised by degeneration of the retinal pigment epithelium.
i. It may be inherited as an autosomal dominant, autosomal recessive or sex-linked trait.
ii. The earliest clinical finding is night blindness due to loss of rods, gradually progressing to blindness.
iii. *Microscopically*, there is disappearance of rods and cones of the photoreceptor layer of the retina, degeneration of retinal pigment epithelium and ingrowth of glial membrane on the optical disc.

Q3. What are the important inflammatory conditions of the eyes?

Eye inflammations are named according to the tissue affected. The term *uveitis* is used for the ocular inflammation of the uveal tracts, which is the most vascular tissue of the eye. Other inflammatory conditions are as follows:
I. **Sty (hordeolum)** includes two conditions:
- *External hordeolum* is the more common form of acute inflammation involving the sebaceous glands of Zeis, the apocrine glands of Moll and the eyelash follicles.
- *Internal hordeolum* is a suppurative inflammation of the meibomian glands.

II. **Chalazion** is a very common lesion, presenting as a chronic inflammation of meibomian glands.
- It begins with destruction of meibomian glands and duct, subsequently involving the tarsal plate.
- *Microscopically*, it is characterised by formation of lipogranulomas, i.e. granulomas which contain fat globules in their centre.

III. **Endophthalmitis-panophthalmitis** is an acute suppurative intraocular inflammation involving retina, choroid and sclera and extending to the orbit.
- It may be of *exogenous* origin, i.e. caused by pathogens introduced from outside, or be *endogenous*, when the infections reach the eye by a haematogenous route.
- It may be caused by a variety of infectious agent such as bacteria, viruses, fungi, etc.

IV. **Conjunctivitis and keratoconjunctivitis** represent acute or chronic inflammation of the conjunctiva and cornea caused by a variety of microbial, chemical or physical agents.
- In the *acute form*, these layers of eye are infiltrated with neutrophils.
- In the *chronic form*, there are infiltrates of lymphocytes, macrophages, plasma cells and proliferation of small blood vessels and fibroblasts (pannus formation).

V. **Trachoma** is most often caused by *Chlamydia trachomatis*, a pathogen that is quite prevalent in developing countries of the world.
- It is a major cause of blindness on a large scale.
- It begins with an infection of the conjunctival epithelium that can be recognised by the formation of intracytoplasmic inclusion bodies.
- Later, the conjunctiva thickens due to dense chronic inflammation with lymphocytes forming follicles and macrophages, leading to conjunctival cicatrisation and blindness.
- *Inclusion conjunctivitis*, caused by *Chlamydia oculogenitalis* is a similar inflammation, but milder.

VI. **Granulomatous uveitis** can be caused by a numbers of bacteria (e.g. *M. tuberculosis, M. leprae, Treponema pallidum*), fungal diseases (e.g. aspergillosis, blastomycosis, etc.), viral infections (e.g. herpes zoster, CMV), parasitic diseases (e.g. toxoplasmosis, onchocerciasis).

VII. **Sympathetic ophthalmia** is a rare condition in which there is bilateral diffuse granulomatous uveitis following penetrating injury to one eye. Presumably, it is immune-mediated, resulting in blindness, if not treated early after its onset.

Q4. Write briefly on diabetic retinopathy.

Definition Diabetic retinopathy includes complex vascular changes caused by long-lasting and inadequately controlled diabetes mellitus. It is one of the most important causes of blindness.

Epidemiology
- Most patients are over the age of 50 years and have had diabetes for 15–20 years.
- Diabetic retinopathy is seen in more than 60% of chronic diabetics.
- In 2% cases, it is associated with blindness.
- Women are more often affected than men.

Pathogenesis Diabetes affects several parts of the eye including retina, iris, lens and vitreous. The sequence of events that leads to blindness is diagrammatically shown in **Figure 18.2**.

Pathology Changes seen by retinoscopy and microscopy are classified as: non-proliferative (background) changes, and proliferative changes (*retinitis proliferans*).

I. **Non-proliferative (background) retinopathy** includes *capillary microangiopathy* with thickening of the capillary basement membranes with degeneration of vascular cells (endothelial cells and pericytes). These changes, as seen by *retinoscopy*, are as under:

i. *Microaneurysms*
ii. *Waxy exudates*, from accumulation of lipids around the microaneurysms
iii. *'Dot and blot haemorrhages'* in the deeper layers of retina
iv. *'Cotton-wool spots'*, representing microinfarcts of the nerve fiber layers
v. *Degeneration of nerve fibres and ganglion cells* not readily seen on retinoscopy but presenting clinically as *scotomas* (defined as focal loss of visual acuity surrounded by fields of normal vision)

II. **Proliferative retinopathy (retinitis proliferans)** is characterised by neovascularisation of retina, i.e. formation of new blood vessels, and includes following:

i. *Neovascularisation* of the retina at the optic disc
ii. *Vitreous haemorrhage* which is related to the friability of newly-formed blood vessels which rupture easily and are prone to bleeding

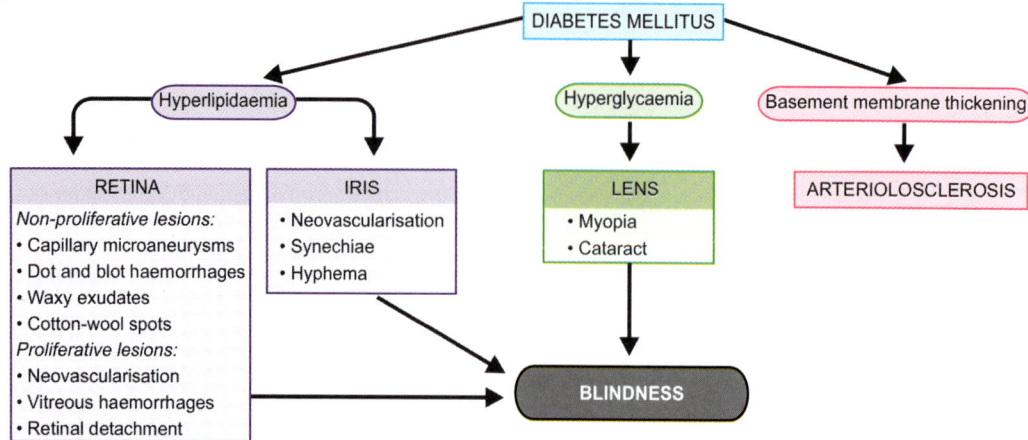

FIGURE 18.2: Schematic illustration showing the effects of diabetes mellitus on eye in causing blindness.

iii. *Proliferation of astrocytes and fibrous tissue* around the blood vessels
iv. *Retinal detachment* and blindness resulting from all the above listed changes
Common ocular complications of diabetes include the following disease processes which are also found in other ophthalmic conditions:
i. Glaucoma
ii. Cataract formation
iii. Corneal disease with formation of adhesions between iris and cornea and iris and lens (*anterior and posterior synechiae*).

Q5. What is hypertensive retinopathy?

Definition Hypertensive retinopathy results from the hypertension-induced arteriolar injury resulting in narrowing and consequent ischaemia of the retina.

Pathogenesis and pathologic features Arteriolosclerosis and spasm of arterioles lead to narrowing of arterioles, ischaemia and haemorrhages. The following changes are seen on *retinoscopy* **(Fig.18.3)**:
i. Arteriolo-venous nicking
ii. Flame-shaped haemorrhages in the retinal nerve fibre layer
iii. Macular star (i.e. exudates radiating from the centre of macula)
iv. Cotton-wool spots (i.e. fluffy white bodies in the superficial layer of the retina)
v. Microaneurysms

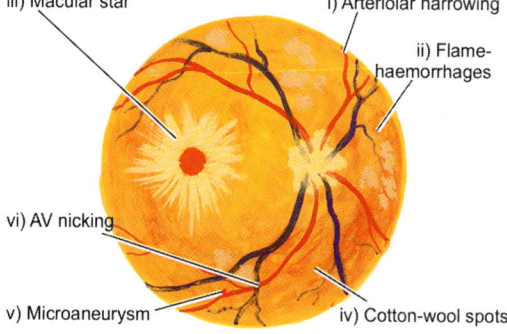

FIGURE 18.3: Schematic diagram of ocular lesions in hypertension.

Q6. Define pinguecula and pterygium.

Pinguecula results from degenerative changes of subepithelial collagen of the bulbar conjunctiva. It presents as a raised yellowish lesion of interpalpebral bulbar conjunctiva in middle-aged or older patients.
Pterygium is closely related to pinguecula but it is located at the limbus and often involves the cornea; hence it may affect vision.

Q7. Comment on age-related (or senile) macular degeneration.

Definition Age-related (or senile) macular degeneration (AMD) is a disease of unknown etiology affecting the elderly, and is characterised by degeneration of the photoreceptor and pigment epithelium of the macular region of the retina.

Epidemiology AMD is the leading cause of legal blindness in the US. The incidence increases with age from 2–3% in those that are 60 years-old to 20–30% in those 80 years of age.
Clinicopathologic features
i. Loss of photoreceptor cells in the macula.
ii. Associated with the irregular thickening of the Bruch membrane that separates the retinal pigment epithelium from the choroid.
iii. Clinically, AMD presents with bilateral loss or marked diminution of central vision.

Q8. What is retinal detachment?

Definition Retinal detachment is the separation of the neurosensory retina from the retinal pigment epithelium. It can result from trauma or it may be spontaneous.
Pathogenesis Normally, the cones and rods of the photoreceptor layer are intertwined with the projections of the retinal pigment epithelium. Under pathologic conditions, these two components of the retina separate from each other. There are three possible mechanisms that may cause it:
i. Pathologic process in the vitreous or anterior segment causing traction on the retina.
ii. Collection of serous fluid in the sub-retinal space from inflammation or tumour of the choroid.
iii. Accumulation of vitreous under the retina through a hole or tear in the retina.

Q9. What is phthisis bulbi?

Definition Phthisis bulbi is the end-stage of advanced degeneration and disorganisation of the entire eyeball in which the intraocular pressure is decreased and the eyeball shrinks.
Etiopathogenesis These are: trauma to the eye, infections, glaucoma.
Pathology
i. Marked atrophy, disruption and disorganisation of all the ocular structures.
ii. Sclera is markedly thickened showing hyalinisation of collagen and even occasionally osseous metaplasia.

Q10. Write briefly on etiopathogenesis of cataract.

Definition Cataract is opacification of a normally crystalline translucent lens, that leads to gradual painless blurring of vision.
Etiopathogenesis
i. Old age ('idiopathic senile cataract', the most common)
ii. Congenital (e.g. Down syndrome, maternal rubella, galactosaemia)
iii. Physical injury (e.g. penetrating eye injury, electrical injury)
iv. Metabolic (e.g. diabetes, hypoparathyroidism)
v. Drug-induced (e.g. long-term corticosteroid injury)
vi. Smoking and chronic alcohol abuse
Pathology Lens fibres undergo degeneration, fragmentation and liquefaction but the central nucleus remains intact and is quite sclerotic.
Treatment includes surgical removal of the lens and its replacement with a plastic one.

Q11. Give a brief description of glaucoma.

Definition Glaucoma is a group of ocular disorders that have in common increased intraocular pressure. It is one of the leading causes of blindness.
Classification and pathogenesis The basic defect is impaired outflow of aqueous humour out of the bulb, which may be classified as congenital, primary or secondary:
i. *Congenital eye malformation-related glaucoma*, diagnosed in infants and children.
ii. *Primary open-angle glaucoma* of unknown cause, also known chronic simple glaucoma. It probably has a genetic predisposition and it is the most common form of glaucoma.
iii. *Primary angle-closure glaucoma* (shallow anterior chamber glaucoma) of unknown cause associated with considerable pain.
iv. *Secondary glaucoma* due to eye injury or haemorrhage, cataract, diabetes, intraocular tumour.
Pathology In all forms of glaucoma, the increased intraocular pressure will cause compression atrophy of retina and optic nerve and cause blindness.

Q12. What is papilloedema?

Definition Papilloedema is oedema of the optic disc resulting from increased intracranial pressure.

Pathogenesis Papilloedema develops because of anatomic continuation of the subarachnoid space of the brain around the optic nerve so that increased intracranial pressure is passed onto the optic disc area.

Pathology Changes can be acute or chronic.
- *Acute papilloedema* is characterised by oedema, congestions and focal haemorrhage.
- *Chronic papilloedema* shows degeneration of nerve fibres, gliosis and optic nerve atrophy.

Q13. How are the tumours and tumour-like lesions of the eye and adnexa classified?

The most important tumours and tumour-like lesions of the eye and adnexa, depending on their location, are divided into five groups as those from i) eyelids, ii) conjunctiva-cornea, iii) lacrimal glands, iv) orbit, and v) intraocular tumours **(Table 18.1)**.
- In each group, there are examples of benign and malignant tumours.
- Besides benign and malignant tumours, there are some important examples of tumour-like lesions in the eye.
- Since the lids are covered externally by squamous epithelium similar the skin surface in other site, it is to be expected that the most common tumour is *basal cell carcinoma*, accounting for 85% of lid tumours.

TABLE 18.1 Tumours and tumour-like lesions of the eye and adnexal structures.

BENIGN	MALIGNANT*
I. EYELID	
Squamous cell papilloma	Squamous cell carcinoma
Basal cell papilloma	Basal cell carcinoma
Sebaceous adenoma	Sebaceous adenocarcinoma
Naevi	Malignant melanoma
II. CONJUNCTIVA-CORNEA	
Squamous cell papilloma	Squamous cell carcinoma
Pseudoepitheliomatous hyperplasia	Mucoepidermoid carcinoma
Naevi	Malignant melanoma
Haemangioma	
III. LACRIMAL GLAND	
Pleomorphic adenoma	Carcinoma in pleomorphic adenoma
IV. ORBIT	
Ectopic glial tissue	Malignant glioma
Inflammatory 'pseudotumour'	Malignant lymphoma
Meningioma	Rhabdomyosarcoma
V. INTRAOCULAR	
Naevi	Malignant melanoma
Neurofibroma	Retinoblastoma

*The list of malignant tumours on right column is not necessarily as corresponding malignant counterparts of benign tumours.

Q14. What are inflammatory pseudotumours of the orbit?

Definition These are a group of inflammatory enlargements, especially in the orbit, which clinically look like tumours but surgical exploration and pathologic examination fail to reveal any evidence of neoplasm.

Pathology *Grossly,* it is a circumscribed lesion which sometimes may have fibrous capsule.

Microscopy
- Many of the lesions can be placed in well-established categories of pseudotumours such as tuberculous, syphilitic, mycotic, parasitic, foreign-body granuloma, etc.
- Others show non-specific histologic appearance having abundant fibrous tissue, lymphoid follicles and inflammatory infiltrate with prominence of eosinophils.

Q15. What is sebaceous carcinoma?

Definition Sebaceous carcinoma is an eyelid tumour originating from the Meibomian glands in the tarsus or Zeis' glands of eyelash follicles.
- Sebaceous carcinomas are rare tumours but on the eyelids they are the *second most common* malignant tumour after basal cell carcinoma (BCC).
- In contrast to BCC which predominantly originates from the lower lid, sebaceous carcinomas preferentially originate from the upper lid.

Pathology *Gross* varies and it may present as localised nodule or diffuse swelling of the tarsus, or ulcerated, nodular or papillomatous tumour at the lid margin.

Microscopy
i. Tumour cells arranged into lobules and basaloid nests showing focal sebaceous differentiation.
ii. Such cells have well-developed foamy cytoplasm containing lipid vacuoles, reminiscent of normal sebaceous glands.
iii. Some tumours are, however, poorly-differentiated requiring specials stains for proper pathologic identification.

Q16. Write briefly on uveal malignant melanoma.

Definition Uveal malignant melanoma (MM) is an intraocular malignant tumour composed of melanocytes. It is the most common primary ocular malignancy in white adults in North America and Europe.

Pathology Most MM originate from the posterior choroid protruding into the vitreous cavity. Less common are MM originating from the ciliary body and the iris **(Fig. 18.4)**.

Microscopy MM are divided into four subgroups:
i. *Spindle A MM* composed of uniform, spindle-shaped cells with spindled nuclei, indistinct nucleoli and rare mitoses.
These tumours have the *most favourable prognosis* (85% 10-year survival).
ii. *Spindle B MM* composed of larger and plump spindle-shaped cells with ovoid nuclei, and conspicuous nucleoli.
These tumours have a somewhat worse prognosis (80% 10-year survival).
iii. *Epithelioid MM* composed of larger, irregular and pleomorphic cells with larger nuclei and abundant eosinophilic cytoplasm.
These tumours have the *worst prognosis* (35% 10-year survival).
iv. *Mixed cell type MM* has features of spindle cell and epithelioid type.
This type has intermediate prognosis (45% 10-year survival).

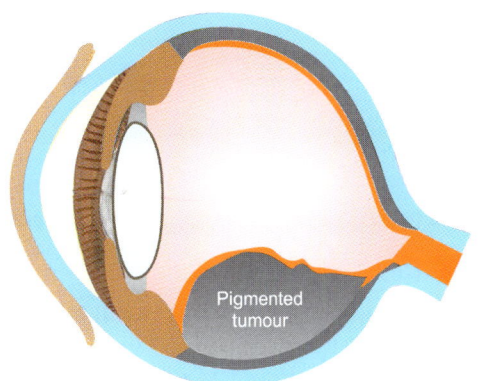

FIGURE 18.4: Malignant melanoma of the eye. Cross sectioned eyeball contains a black tumour attached to the posterior-inferior inner side of the eye.

Clinical features Uveal MM are usually slow growing, late metastasising tumours and have a better prognosis than MM of the skin. Metastases occur by haematogenous route and in 90% of cases are found in the liver. Large tumours of the epithelioid type have the worst prognosis.

Q17. Discuss retinoblastoma briefly.

Definition Retinoblastoma is a malignant eye tumour of infancy and childhood, composed of undifferentiated retinal cells.

Pathogenesis/Classification All retinoblastomas are related to mutations and loss of tumour suppressor function of the *RB* gene (page 162). In 60% of cases, retinoblastomas are *sporadic* and in 40% are *familial*:
i. *Familial tumours* develop in persons who have inherited the germline mutation of *RB* gene.
- The mutated *RB* gene is transmitted as an autosomal dominant trait.
- Retinoblastomas are often bilateral and may be multiple.
- Affected individuals are at risk for developing secondary malignant tumours, particularly osteogenic sarcoma.

ii. *Sporadic cases* have lost both normal alleles due to the somatic cell mutation of the *RB* gene in retinoblasts.

Clinicopathologic features Retinoblastoma may develop in utero and present as a congenital tumour. Most tumours are, however, diagnosed in infancy and early childhood prior to age of 4 years.
I. *Leukocoria* (white pupillary reflex) is a common finding:
- Child has also problems with vision and does not see well.

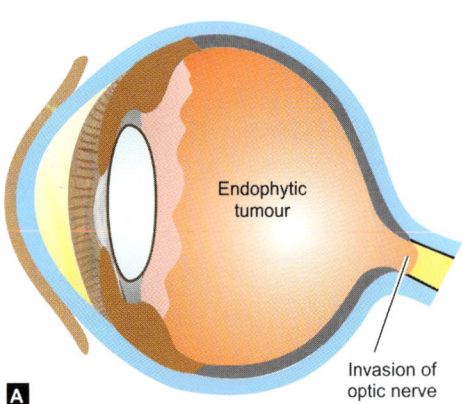
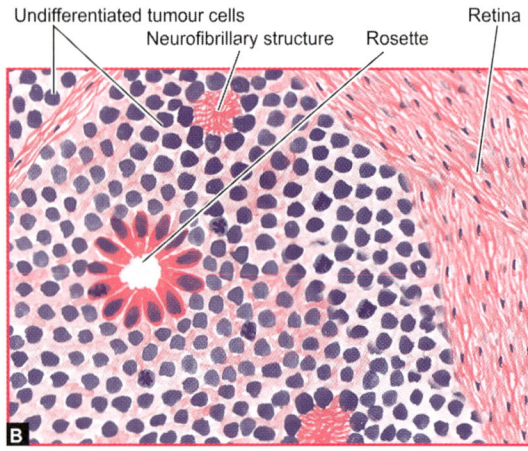

FIGURE 18.5: Retinoblastoma. A, The tumour shows white mass growing extensively within the posterior part of the eye. B, The tumour arising from the retina shows undifferentiated retinal cells and typical rosettes.

- The prognosis depends on the extent of local spread and the presence of metastases, which usually occur by haematogenous route to the lungs.

II. *Gross* **(Fig. 18.5, A)**
i. The tumour is intraocular and appears as a white, partially necrotic mass.
ii. Most often, it is *endophytic* and protrudes into the vitreous cavity.
iii. Less often, the tumour grows in an *exophytic* manner between the retinal and the pigment layer.

III. *Microscopy* **(Fig. 18.5, B)**
i. The tumour composed of undifferentiated cells, resembling embryonic retinal cells ('retinoblasts').
ii. These cells have the appearance of 'small blue cells' with scanty cytoplasm surrounding oval-shaped hyperchromatic nuclei.
iii. Mitoses and foci of necrosis are common.
iv. Tumour cells have a tendency to form rosettes.

Q18. What are the main contrasting clinicopathologic features of uveal malignant melanoma and retinoblastoma?

Salient features of retinoblastoma are contrasted with those of uveal melanoma in **Table 18.2**.

TABLE 18.2 Uveal malignant melanoma versus retinoblastoma.

FEATURE	UVEAL MELANOMA	RETINOBLASTOMA
1. Inheritance	Rarely familial; mostly sporadic	About 40% cases familial; 60% sporadic
2. Age	>50 years	Birth to 4 years
3. Race	Common in Caucasians, uncommon in Africans	No predisposition
4. Location	Most commonly choroid	Retina
5. Bilaterality	Rare	Common (30%)
6. Cell of origin	Melanocytes	Embryonic retinoblasts
7. Colour of tumour	Grey-black	Creamy
8. Spread	Haematogenous route common, rarely via optic nerve	Common via both haematogenous and optic nerve

Q19. What are the most common metastatic tumours in the eyes?

Metastases to the eye are more common than primary malignant eye tumours. The most common primary site for such metastases is:
i. The breast in women
ii. The lung in men
iii. Leukaemia and lymphoma also commonly invade ocular tissues

EAR

Q20. Write briefly on the most important inflammatory ear diseases.

The ear is divided in three parts: external, middle, and internal ear. Inflammatory involvement of the middle ear is termed otitis media. It may be acute or chronic.

I. **Acute otitis media** is the most important inflammatory ear disease, especially common in children. Other forms of otitis are less common, but still important clinically.

Etiopathogenesis Most common causative pathogens found in acute otitis are *Streptococcus pneumoniae, Haemophilus influenzae,* and *β-Streptococcus haemolyticus*, that reach the middle ear through the eustachian tube.

Clinicopathologic features According to the nature of the exudates, otitis media may be purulent, serous or mucoid.

i. *Acute suppurative otitis media* presents clinically with deep ear pain and tenderness to palpation of the entire area. It is the most common form of otitis media in children.
- It is often accompanied by fever and signs of upper respiratory tract infection.
- Otoscopy will typically reveal a bulging, red hyperaemic tympanic membrane.
- Rupture of the tympanic membrane and extension of the inflammation into the mastoid and loss of hearing are common complications in untreated cases.

ii. *Serous otitis media*, also known as *otitis media with serous effusion*, is characterised by an accumulation of serous fluid in the middle ear behind the tympanic membrane.
- It may follow healed suppurative otitis media, or it may precede it in some cases.
- In some cases, it develops spontaneously with no obvious reason, or secondary to obstruction of eustachian tubes unrelated to bacterial infection.

iii. *Mucoid otitis media* is characterised by an accumulation of mucus rich fluid in the middle ear, unrelated to bacterial infection.
- The etiology is not known, but possibly related to serous otitis media.
- Clinically, it presents with hearing loss and bulging tympanic membrane seen on otoscopy.

II. **Chronic otitis media** is caused by repeated bouts of acute infection which becomes chronic.
- The usual findings are tympanic membrane perforation and draining exudate.
- Typically associated with hearing impairment.
- Infection may extend locally and cause mastoiditis or infection of the inner ear and meningitis.

Q21. What are the most common tumours and tumour-like lesions of the ear?

External ear and the earlobe are covered with squamous epithelium which can give rise to the usual skin tumours. These skin tumours are much more common than tumours that are specific for the ear itself. Tumours and tumour-like conditions that are specific for the ear are as under:

I. **External ear canal and middle ear lesions:**

i. *Aural (otic) polyps* are pseudotumours representing exuberant post-inflammatory granulation tissue.

ii. *Cerumen gland adenoma and adenocarcinoma* are rare counterparts of sweat gland tumours of the skin.

iii. *Cholesteatoma (keratoma)* is a pseudotumour.

iv. *Glomus tympanicum and glomus jugulotympanicum* (or paragangliomas), are benign tumours originating from the glomus bodies found along the inferior tympanic nerve and involving the middle ear.

II. **Inner ear lesions:**

Schwannoma of 8th nerve is a benign tumour originating from the 8th cranial nerve (i.e. vestibular nerve). It is located in the internal auditory canal. It has also been loosely called as *acoustic neuroma*, which is a double misnomer since it neither arises from acoustic nerve, nor it is a neuroma.

Q22. What is cholesteatoma?

Cholesteatoma is a post-inflammatory pseudotumour, most often found in the middle ear or mastoid air cells.

i. It is the most common mass surgically removed from the middle ear.

ii. The lesion begins as an invagination of the squamous epithelium through a perforation of the tympanic membrane into the middle ear.
iii. The 'implanted' squamous epithelium forms a cyst-like lesion covered internally with squamous cells.
iv. Squamous cells desquamate into the lumen and often disintegrate causing an inflammatory reaction.
v. The lumen of cholesteatoma is thus filled with desquamated squamous cells, cell debris, lipid material, cholesterol crystals and macrophages **(Fig. 18.6)**.
vi. The mass effect of the cholesteatoma may erode the mastoid bone.

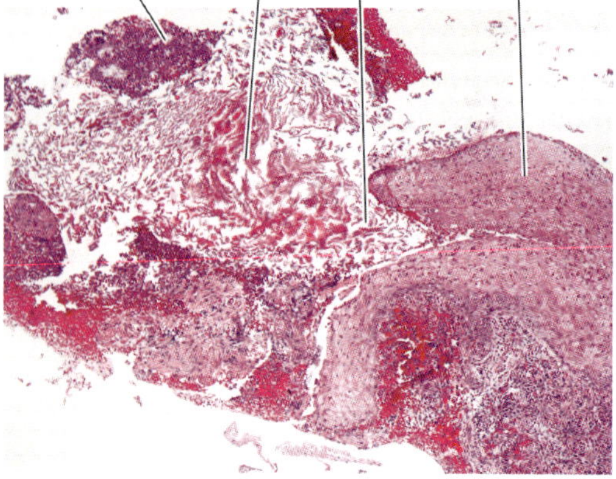

FIGURE 18.6: Cholesteatoma middle ear. There is chronic inflammatory granulation tissue and foreign body giant cells around the cholesterol clefts and pink keratinous material.

■ NOSE AND PARANASAL SINUSES

Q23. What are the most common inflammatory conditions affecting the nose and the paranasal sinuses?

Inflammations of the mucosa of the nose (rhinitis) and paranasal sinuses (sinusitis) are caused by infections, most often viral and bacterial, or allergies. These may be acute or chronic.

i. **Acute rhinitis** ('common cold') is a viral infection presenting with rhinorrhoea, nasal obstruction and sneezing.
- Most often, it is caused by *adenovirus*.
- *Bacterial superinfections* are common.
- The nasal mucosa is oedematous and red and the nose appears obstructed by sero-mucinous fluid.
- *Microscopy* The mucosa is infiltrated with inflammatory cells, including PMNs and lymphocytes and a few plasma cells.

ii. **Allergic rhinitis** (hay fever) is an IgE-mediated type I hypersensitivity reaction.
- Most common *exogenous allergens* are pollen and dust.
- Nasal mucosa is oedematous and infiltrated with acute and chronic inflammatory cells, most prominent of which are eosinophils and basophils.

iii. **Sinusitis** is usually a complication of acute or allergic rhinitis.
- Due to the oedema of ostia, sinuses fill up with *seromucinous exudate*.
- *Mucocele* refers to an accumulation of mucus.
- Exudate becomes *purulent* if a bacterial superinfection occurs.
- *Empyema* is accumulation of pus.
- *Chronic sinusitis* develops due to poor drainage of inflammatory exudate.

iv. **Nasal polyps** which may be *allergic or inflammatory*, are formed from prolonged or recurrent inflammation of the nose and sinuses.
- *Nasal polyps* are most often located on the middle turbinate.
- *Antrochoanal polyps* originate from the mucosa of the maxillary sinus protruding into the nasal cavity.
- They present as fungating gelatinous masses with smooth and shining surface.
- *Microscopy* They represent oedematous folds of nasal mucosa infiltrated with inflammatory cells. In allergic polyps, eosinophils are prominent.

v. **Rhinosporidiosis** is a chronic nasal inflammation caused by a fungus *Rhinosporidium seeberi*.
- It is common in India and Sri Lanka.
- *Microscopy* It involves nasal polyps in form of chronic inflammation and granulation tissue formation.
- Organisms are encapsulated in diagnostic sporangia **(Fig. 18.7)**.
- It may also be found in other parts of the upper respiratory tract and even eye mucosa.

vi. **Rhinoscleroma** is a chronic destructive lesion of the nose and upper respiratory airways, caused by *Klebsiella rhinoscleromatis*.
- It is endemic in parts of Africa, America and South Asia and Eastern Europe.
- It begins as common cold to progress into chronic inflammation with nodular tumour-like submucosal masses occluding the nasal cavity.
- *Microscopy* shows chronic inflammatory cells with prominent foamy macrophages.

vii. **Granulomas** of nasal cavity and paranasal sinuses may be caused by:
- *M. tuberculosis*, usually in patients who have pulmonary tuberculosis.
- Other pathogens causing granulomas are *M. leprae* and various fungi like *Aspergillus fumigatus*, or *Mucor mucosae*.

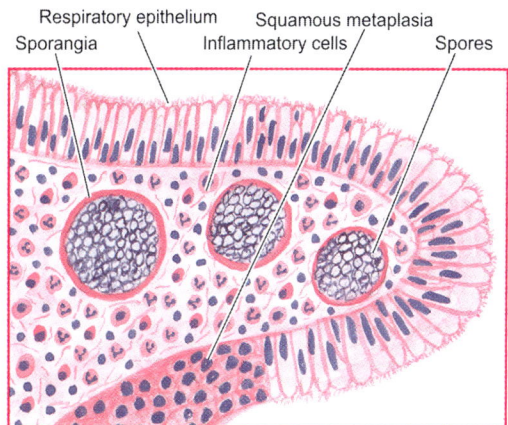

FIGURE 18.7: Rhinosporidiosis in a nasal polyp. The spores are present in sporangia as well as are intermingled in the inflammatory cell infiltrate.

Q24. Discuss briefly important sino-nasal tumours.

Sino-nasal tumours may be benign or malignant. Benign tumours are more common than malignant tumours. They can originate from the epithelium or connective tissues and blood vessels. A few common examples are as under:

i. **Capillary haemangioma** is a small vascular tumour that tends to bleed.
- Some haemangiomas are ulcerated and inflamed and resemble granulation tissue, hence called *granuloma pyogenicum*.

ii. **Nasal papilloma** is a benign tumour which may occur in the nasal vestibule, nasal cavity or paranasal sinuses.
- Papillomas may appear in two forms: *fungiform and exophytic*, or *inverted papilloma* with inverted growth which may be mistaken for carcinoma.

iii. **Sino-nasal carcinomas** are most often *squamous cell carcinomas*.
- Predisposing conditions include smoking and chronic sino-nasal inflammation.
- They occur at an increased frequency in workers of certain occupations, such as nickel refinery and wood workers.
- Besides squamous cell type, other less common microscopic forms of sino-nasal cancer are adenocarcinomas, small cell carcinoma and olfactory neuroblastoma.

■ PHARYNX

Q25. Briefly describe clinicopathologic features of tonsillitis.

Tonsillitis is a very common infection caused by streptococci or staphylococci. Most often, it is acute but it may be chronic as well.

I. **Acute tonsillitis** presents with swollen, red tonsils that are infiltrated with acute inflammatory cells.
- Hyperplastic lymphoid follicles surrounded with crypts that contain pus and cell debris are features of *acute follicular tonsillitis*.
- *Peritonsillar abscess* also known as *quinsy* is rare but very dangerous complication of acute tonsillitis spreading into the peritonsillar space.
- *Retropharyngeal abscess* is a rare but severe throat infection. It occurs in the space between the posterior wall of the pharynx and vertebral column and is related to suppurative infection of retropharyngeal lymph nodes.

II. **Chronic tonsillitis** is caused of repeated attacks of acute tonsillitis.
- Tonsils may remain enlarged due to follicular hyperplasia or they may become small and fibrosed.

NOTE: *Angina* is a generic term used to denote acute inflammation of the throat including the tonsils. In the pre-antibiotic era, there were several forms of severe angina which are nowadays quite rare:

- *Ludwig angina* is a severe acute streptococcal cellulitis involving the neck, tongue and back of the throat. In the pre-antibiotic era, it was a life-threatening complication of dental infection or mandibular fracture.
- *Vincent angina* is a painful ulceration of tonsils, mouth or pharynx caused by *Vincent bacillus*.

Q26. Enumerate the most important tumours of the pharynx.

Three pharyngeal tumours are of clinical importance, one of which is benign and two that are malignant:
- Nasopharyngeal angiofibroma
- Nasopharyngeal carcinoma
- Lymphoma

Q27. Discuss briefly nasopharyngeal angiofibroma.

Definition Nasopharyngeal angiofibroma is a benign vascular tumour found almost exclusively in 10–20 years old adolescent males.

Pathogenesis Its occurrence in adolescent males suggests that it might be related to testosterone stimulation. Androgen receptors are expressed in 75% of all cases.

Pathology Nasopharyngeal angiofibroma is typically found in the nasopharynx. Although benign, it may grow into sinuses, cheek and even orbit.

Microscopy The tumour is composed of numerous thin-walled branching ('staghorn') vessels lined by endothelial cells and surrounded by myofibroblastic stromal cells **(Fig. 18.8)**.

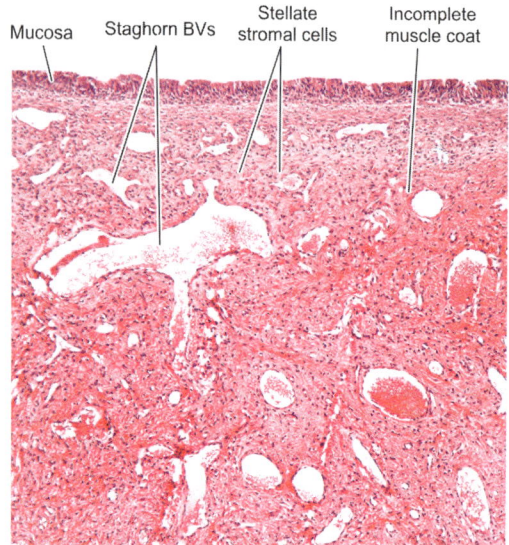

FIGURE 18.8: Angiofibroma nasopharynx. There is admixture of staghorn-shaped blood vessels and spindled stroma. The blood vessels are variable-sized, some having incomplete muscle coat and there is absence of elastic tissue. The stroma has stellate fibroblasts and mast cells.

Q28. What is nasopharyngeal carcinoma?

Definition Nasopharyngeal carcinoma (NPC) is a form of squamous cell carcinoma related to infection with Epstein-Barr virus (EBV), that is most prevalent in South-East Asia and also in other parts of the world among people of Chinese descent.

Pathogenesis EBV genome is found in virtually all tumours, indicating that this virus plays a key role in the pathogenesis of NPC.

Pathology The primary tumour in the nasopharynx is usually small but the metastases in the cervical lymph nodes may be quite large.

Microscopy Three variants:
i. Non-keratinising squamous cell carcinoma
ii. Keratinising squamous cell carcinoma
iii. Undifferentiated carcinoma, composed of cells, grouped together without distinct cell borders and infiltrated with lymphocytes, which is 'lymphoepithelioma'- like pattern.

Prognosis Microscopic subtyping of tumours has no prognostic significance.
- The survival of treated patients is dependent on tumour stage.
- Overall, 5-year survival for all stages of NPC is 60%, but it varies from 70% for stage I, to 40% for stage IV tumours.

■ LARYNX

Q29. What are the important inflammatory conditions of the larynx?

I. **Laryngitis** is an inflammation that may occur in an acute and a chronic form. Most often, it is caused by viral or bacterial infections.

i. *Acute laryngitis* may occur in several forms, such as:
- Localised infection of the larynx (e.g. *Haemophilus influenzae* related acute epiglottitis typical of whooping cough).
- *Diphtheric pseudomembranous laryngitis* was previously an often lethal childhood disease but has been eradicated by immunisation at an early age.
- Part of upper or lower respiratory tract infection, such as parainfluenza caused laryngotracheo-bronchitis presenting with inspiratory stridor known as *croup*.
- Acute laryngitis may be part of systemic infectious diseases, such as measles and influenza or typhoid.
- Excessive smoking, industrial and domestic smoke, or vocal abuse, may facilitate the onset of infections.

ii. *Chronic laryngitis* results from repeated attacks of acute laryngitis, or is related to irritation by cigarette smoking, vocal strain and abuse, and chronic alcoholism.

II. **Acute oedema of the larynx** is a swelling of the larynx causing partial or complete obstruction of airflow. It may be caused by infection, inhalation of irritants, or immune-mediated anaphylactic shock. It requires immediate medical attention because it can cause death by suffocation.

Q30. What is a laryngeal nodule?

Definition Laryngeal nodules, also known as laryngeal polyps, are tumour-like, non-neoplastic protrusions on true vocal cords.
- They are typically found in smokers and person who habitually strain or abuse their voice. Hence, the synonyms for this lesion: singers' node, preachers' node, or screamers' node.
- In all these conditions, the patient complains of progressive hoarseness.

Pathology The lesion appears on vocal cords as a small (<0.5 cm), rounded, smooth, sessile nodule or polypoid protrusion or ill-defined swelling.

Microscopy The nodule consists of oedematous fibrous tissue and dilated thin-walled blood vessels, some of which may be hyalinised.

Q31. Write briefly on carcinoma of larynx.

Definition Carcinoma of the larynx is almost in all instances a squamous cell carcinoma.
Predisposing conditions Cigarette smoking is found in the history of most patients. Less commonly, there is history of cigar or pipe smoking, or exposure to asbestos.
Classification is based on their clinical location as under:
i. *Glottic*, found on the vocal cord and anterior and posterior commissures (the most common).
ii. *Supraglottic*, involving ventricles and arytenoids.
iii. *Subglottic*, in the wall of subglottis.
iv. *Marginal zone*, between the tip of epiglottis and aryepiglottic folds.
v. *Laryngo-(hypo-) pharynx* in the pyriform fossa, postcricoid fossa and posterior pharyngeal wall.
Pathology *Grossly*, the tumour mass appears as a pearly white, plaque-like thickening, that may be ulcerated of fungated. Metastases are often found locally in cervical lymph nodes.
Microscopy shows keratinising or non-keratinising squamous carcinoma similar to that found in the mouth or bronchus, and may vary with regards to its grade of differentiation.
Prognosis It depends on the stage of cancer. Laryngeal carcinomas are grouped as follows: early (stage I), intermediate (stage II) or advanced (stages III and IV) disease.
- Stage I cancers, especially those that are detected early due to their location on the vocal cords, have a cure rate of 80–95%.
- Patients with advanced stage cancer have a 5-year survival of 25% or less.

■ NECK

Q32. Enumerate the cysts of the neck.

Cysts of the neck can be divided by their location into two groups:
i. *Medial (midline) cysts*, e.g. thyroglossal and dermoid cyst.
ii. *Lateral cysts*, e.g. branchial cyst, parathyroid cyst, thymic cyst and cystic hygroma.

Q33. What is a thyroglossal cyst?

Definition Thyroglossal cyst is a midline neck cyst originating from the vestiges of the incompletely involuted thyroglossal duct.

Pathogenesis Thyroglossal duct is a foetal structure connecting the foramen caecum at the base of the tongue with the thyroid. It involutes spontaneously in late pregnancy. Incomplete involution of the thyroglossal duct results in formation of the thyroglossal cyst.

Clinicopathologic features

i. Cyst measures 2.5 cm on average but may be smaller or much larger.

ii. It is usually solitary and located on the anterior midline side of the neck at the level of hyoid bone.

iii. It is soft to palpation and usually loosely attached to adjacent structures and thus mobile.

iv. *Microscopy*

- The cyst is lined by respiratory cuboidal epithelium.
- The lining may undergo focally squamous metaplasia.
- If the squamous metaplasia is extensive, it may be confused with midline dermoid cysts (developmental inclusion cysts).
- In the connective tissue around the cyst, there are atrophic thyroid follicles, which make the diagnosis easier.

Q34. Write briefly on the lateral neck cysts.

Lateral cervical cysts are either developmental or formed within the normal or ectopic organs on the neck. Common examples are given below.

i. **Branchial (lymphoepithelial) cyst** is formed from incomplete closure and involution of the 2nd or 3rd branchial cleft.

- It is usually located anterior to the sternocleidomastoid muscle near the angle of the mandible.
- It is small (1–3 cm) and is filled with serous or mucinous fluid.
- *Microscopy* These cysts are lined by squamous or respiratory epithelium and contain subepithelial lymphoid follicles with germinal centres.

ii. **Parathyroid cyst** is also a small cyst found in one of the four parathyroid glands.

iii. **Thymic cyst** develops from degeneration of Hassall corpuscles in ectopic thymic tissue. Usually it is located on the left lateral side of the neck.

iv. **Cystic hygroma** is a large swelling at the root of the neck behind the sternocleidomastoid muscle.

- It may be found at the time of birth or within the first two postnatal years.
- *Microscopy* It is a multicystic lymphangioma.

Q35. What are carotid body paragangliomas?

i. Paragangliomas of the carotid body originate from chemoreceptor cells of the carotid body at the bifurcation of the common carotid artery into internal and external carotid artery.

ii. In 90% of cases, these relatively rare tumours are benign but recurrences are frequent.

iii. In a minority of cases (5%), they may be multiple and/or familial.

iv. Tumours of the same microscopic type can originate from other paraganglia, such as the glomus jugulare (jugulotympanic bodies) in the middle ear.

> **Chapter 18e Supplement: Online Content**
>
> *Digital content of this chapter available with this book is meant for enhanced learning and self-assessment. In addition, it contains 17 Multiple Choice Questions (MCQs), 03 Clinicopathologic Vignettes, and 06 Image-based Questions; these are followed by their answers along with explanatory notes of correct and incorrect answers.*

CHAPTER 19

Oral Cavity and Salivary Glands

ORAL SOFT TISSUES

Q1. What are the common developmental anomalies of the oral cavity?

I. **Facial clefts** The commonest developmental anomalies of the face are:
- Cleft upper lip (harelip)
- Cleft palate

Harelip is more common than cleft palate:
i. It has an incidence of 1:1000 in Caucasians, but is much higher in Chinese and people of East Asian descent and Native Americans (1:500).
ii. It occurs in an isolated form (70%) or together with cleft palate or as part of a syndrome together with other developmental defects (30%).
iii. It can run in families, indicative of the role of genetic factors.
iv. Males are affected two times more often than females.

II. **Tongue developmental defects** These include:
- Changes of the *size* (macroglossia).
- Changes of the *shape* (fissured tongue, bifid tongue, tongue tie due to short lingual frenulum).

Q2. What are the important mucocutaneous lesions of the oral cavity?

Oral mucosa is involved in many skin diseases and they are similar in morphology, as under:

I. **Lichen planus**, an autoimmune disease affecting primarily the skin, involves oral mucosa in 70% cases.
Microscopy It presents as interlacing network of whitening or keratotic changes, most often on the buccal mucosa.

II. **Vesicular lesions** are found in pemphigus vulgaris, pemphigoid, erythema multiforme, Steven-Johnson syndrome, epidermolysis bullosa.

Q3. What are the important inflammatory diseases involving the mouth?

Inflammation of the oral mucosa is called **stomatitis**. It may occur in many forms as under:

I. **Aphthous ulcers** (cancer sores) are shallow painful mucosal ulcers that may occur on any part of the mouth.
- Etiology of these ulcers is unknown, although it is known that they may be precipitated by emotional factors, stress, allergy, hormonal imbalance, nutritional deficiencies, etc.
- They heal spontaneously.
- Recurrent aphthae may form as part of Behçet syndrome and inflammatory bowel disease.

II. **Herpes labialis** occurs at any age.
- In infants and children, it is the most common manifestation of primary infection with herpes simplex virus 1.

- It presents with grouped vesicles on the lips.
- Recurrent attacks occur due to stressful event such as emotional upset or upper respiratory infections.

III. **Necrotising stomatitis** (noma or cancrum oris) occurs in poorly-nourished children like in kwashiorkor, infectious diseases like measles, immunodeficiencies and emotional stress.
- It presents with necrosis of the gingival margin, often extending into the oral mucosa, and even causing cellulitis of the neck.

IV. **Mycotic infections** may involve oral mucosa.
- Most common is *candidiasis (oral thrush)* which occurs as an opportunistic infection in immunocompromised and debilitated persons, presenting as white plaques on the mucosa.

V. **Glossitis** is inflammation of the tongue, which may be acute or chronic.

i. *Acute glossitis* is characterised by swollen papillae, as seen in common infections caused by streptococci or various viruses (e.g. measles).

ii. *Chronic glossitis* appears raw and red tongue, as seen in various vitamin deficiencies (deficiency of riboflavin and niacin or pellagra).

iii. *Chronic atrophic glossitis* with atrophy of papillae and smooth upper surface of the tongue is seen in iron deficiency and pernicious anaemia and sprue.

VI. **Syphilis** may involve the mouth in all three stages of the disease as well as congenital syphils.

i. *Primary extragenital* syphilitic ulcers are most often seen on the lips.

ii. *Secondary syphilis* may involve the mouth in form of a maculopapular eruption.

iii. *Tertiary syphilis* involves the mouth in form of submucosal fibrosis, most prominently on the hard palate and tongue.

iv. *Congenital syphilis* may present with oral fissures at the angles of the mouth and characteristic peg-shaped notched Hutchinson incisors that appear after the dentition is complete.

VII. **HIV infections** are associated with oral manifestations such as opportunistic infections of fungal, bacterial or viral origin, tumours and other lesions such as hairy leukoplakia; these are listed in **Table 19.1**.

TABLE 19.1 Oral manifestations of AIDS.

A. OPPORTUNISTIC INFECTIONS		
Fungal	:	Candidiasis (oral thrush)
		Histoplasmosis
		Cryptococcosis
Bacterial	:	Dental caries and periodontitis
		Mycobacterial infections
Viral	:	Herpetic stomatitis
		Cytomegalovirus
		Human papillomavirus
B. TUMOURS		
		Kaposi sarcoma
		Squamous cell carcinoma
		Non-Hodgkin lymphoma
C. OTHERS		
		Hairy leukoplakia
		Recurrent aphthous ulcers

Q4. What are the possible causes of oral pigmentation?

i. *Melanotic hyperpigmentation* of the lips and oral mucosa may occur in some systemic and metabolic diseases such as Addison disease, Albright syndrome, Peutz-Jeghers syndrome and haemochromatosis.

ii. *Melanocytic lesions* such as naevi and malignant melanoma may occur in the mouth.

iii. *Exogeneous pigmentation* may occur in lead poisoning which affects the gingiva.

Q5. What are the most common tumour-like lesions of the mouth?

I. **Fibrous growths** of oral soft tissues are very common. They are related to irritation of infection. They are all composed of hyperplastic fibrous tissue and newly formed blood vessels.

In clinical and pathologic practice, they and are known under descriptive names, and often called *polyps or epulis* (Greek word for 'outgrowth or lump'), or simply *hyperplasia* and *fibromatosis* as under:

i. *Fibroepithelial polyp*, a small exophytic protruding outgrowth which most often occurs on the gingiva due to irritation and repeat trauma.

ii. *Fibrous epulis* is a small nodule somewhat larger than polyp, composed of hyperplastic connective tissue and vessels and most often found on the gingiva at the dental socket. It is also related to trauma.

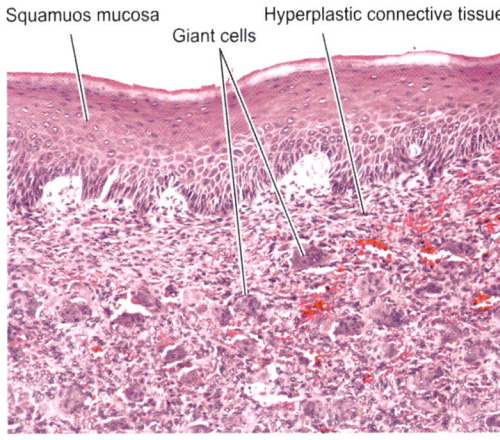

FIGURE 19.1: Epulis in the gingiva. The lesion is covered by squamous mucosa and is composed of vascularised hyperplastic connective tissue containing several multinucleate giant cells.

iii. *Giant cell epulis* is a variant of fibrous polyp seen more commonly in females in response to trauma. Its name stems from the fact that it contains multinucleated giant cells in a vascular stroma **(Fig. 19.1)**.

iv. *Denture hyperplasia* which presents as fibrous thickening of edentulous gingiva, caused by pressure of ill-fitting dentures.

v. *Fibromatosis gingivae*, a diffuse process which presents as connective tissue hyperplasia of the entire gingiva

II. **Pyogenic granuloma** which presents as a bright red swelling often with surface ulceration. It can occur anywhere in the mouth, but most often on the gingiva and the tooth socket. It is a vasoproliferative inflammatory lesion composed of granulation rich in capillaries and inflammatory cells.

- Pyogenic granuloma found during pregnancy on gingiva and other anatomic sites in the mouth is called *pregnancy tumour*.

III. **Mucocele** is a mucus-filled retention cyst formed from obstructed salivary gland ducts, or ruptured small salivary glands in the wall of the mouth.
Extravasated mucus elicits an inflammatory reaction and is taken up by macrophages which have a foamy cytoplasm **(Fig. 19.2)**.

- **Ranula** is a large mucocele located on the floor of the mouth. It is filled with mucus that has accumulated due to the obstruction of sublingual salivary gland duct or a traumatically ruptured salivary gland. The inner surface of ranula may contain remnants of the ductal or acinar epithelium and infiltrates of inflammatory cells with mucin filled macrophages.

IV. **Dermoid cyst** is a developmental cyst formed by inclusion of squamous epithelium. It is found in the midline of the floor of the mouth.

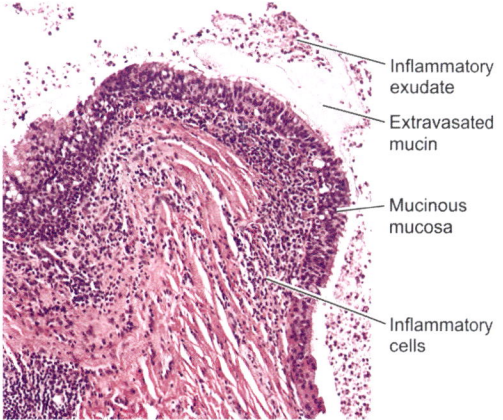

FIGURE 19.2: Mucous retention cyst (mucocele). The cyst is lined by tall columnar mucinous epithelium and contains mucin and inflammatory exudates in the lumen. The cyst wall shows mixed inflammatory reaction.

Q6. What are the common benign tumours of the mouth?

- Benign tumours of the mouth are equivalent to epithelial and mesenchymal tumours of the same name in other parts of the body.
- Mesenchymal tumours include such entities as capillary haemangioma, lymphangioma, fibroma, granular cell tumour (schwannoma), etc.
- Granular cell tumour (schwannoma) is most often localised on the tongue.
- Squamous cell papilloma is the most common epithelial tumour.

- Minor salivary glands are located all over the mouth and can give rise to tumours (benign or malignant) as seen in major salivary glands.

Q7. Define oral leukoplakia. Briefly discuss its etiopathogenesis and clinicopathologic features.

Definition Oral leukoplakia is a white plaque on the oral mucosa, exceeding 5 mm in diameter. It cannot be rubbed off, nor can it be classified into any other diagnosable disease. Microscopically, it represents epithelial thickening which may range from benign reactive hyperplasia with surface hyperkeratosis to atypical proliferation and premalignant cellular changes.

Etiopathogenesis Risk factors are the same as those for oral carcinoma:

i. *Tobacco smoking* in any form such as cigarettes, cigar and pipe-smoking or reverse smoking (hence the name 'smokers keratosis' or *stomatitis nicotina*).

ii. *Chewing tobacco-containing products*, e.g. paan, paan masala, zarda, gutka, etc.

iii. *Chronic friction and irritation* by ill-fitting dentures, or jagged teeth.

iv. *Local irritants* in food and drinks (e.g. alcoholic beverages, hot and spicy foods).

Pathology Biopsy is essential for diagnosis and to exclude invasive carcinoma.

Gross

i. Patches that are white or whitish-yellow (from smoking) are the usual finding.

ii. They are well circumscribed, slightly elevated, smooth or wrinkled.

iii. Sometimes, they may be also speckled or nodular.

iv. *Erythroplasia* appears a red patch, usually showing signs of high degree of dysplasia on microscopic examination.

Microscopy Two types of leukoplakia:

i. *Hyperkeratotic type* characterised by orderly hyperplasia of epithelium with surface keratinisation is a reactive form or low-grade dysplasia **(Fig. 19.3, A)**.

ii. *Dysplastic type* characterised by high grade dysplasia including irregular stratification and focal hyperchromasia, pleomorphism, loss of polarity, single cell keratinisation and mitoses **(Fig. 19.3, B)**.

Clinical features The prognosis depends on the severity of dysplasia.
- Mild dysplasia is reversible and may disappear upon cessation of smoking.
- Severe dysplasia is irreversible and will progress to *carcinoma in situ* and then to invasive squamous cell carcinoma.

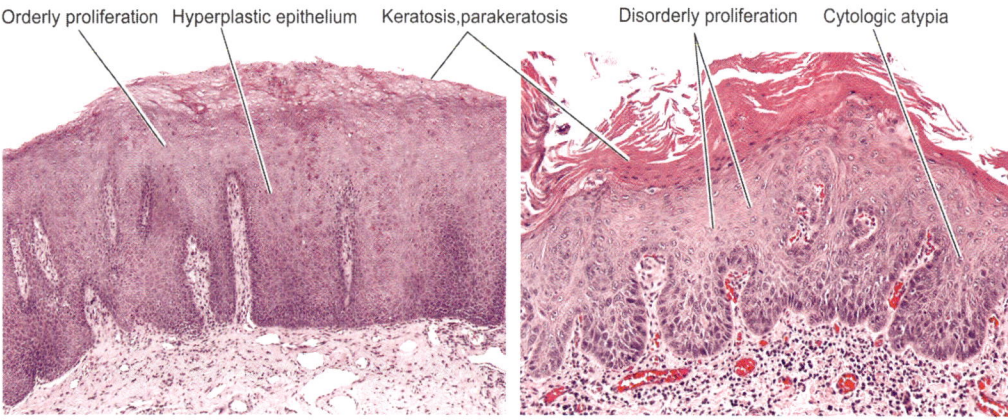

A, HYPERKERATOSIS   B, DYSPLASTIC

FIGURE 19.3: Leukoplakia oral mucosa. A, *Hyperkeratosis type*. There is keratosis and parakeratosis and orderly arrangement of increased number of layers of stratified mucosa and few mitoses. B, *Dysplastic type*. The number of layers is increased and the individual cells in layers show features of cytologic atypia and mitosis but there is no invasion across the basement membrane.

Q8. What are the salient features of oral carcinoma?

Definition Oral carcinoma is a very common invasive malignant epithelial tumour, which is histologically classified in most instances as squamous cell carcinoma.

Epidemiology Oral cancer is a very common malignancy, accounting for 5% of all cancers.
- It is especially common in Asian countries such as India and China.
- It is more common in men than women.
- Peak age incidence 55–75 years in the US and Western Europe, and 40–45 in India, Sri Lanka and Eastern countries.

Etiology Risk factors fall into two groups:

I. *Strong association:*
i. Tobacco smoking.
ii. Alcohol abuse, which combined with smoking, has an additive effect.
iii. Human papilloma virus infection, particularly with HPV 16, 18 and 33 types.

II. *Weak association*:
i. Chronic irritation with ill-fitting denture and jagged teeth.
ii. Poor orodental hygiene.
iii. Submucosal fibrosis from eating excess of chillies.
iv. Nutritional and vitamin deficiencies.
v. Exposure to sunlight (for lip cancer).

Molecular biology Most cancers have the so called 'genetic *tobacco signature*' and commonly carry mutations of *TP53* and *RAS* genes. Human papilloma virus-related cancers carry the *HPV* genes.

Pathology The most common locations are (in descending order): lower lip, tongue, anterior floor of the mouth, buccal mucosa in the region of alveolar lingual sulcus, and palate **(Fig. 19.4)**. Carcinoma of the lip is usually diagnosed earlier than others and thus has a somewhat better prognosis.

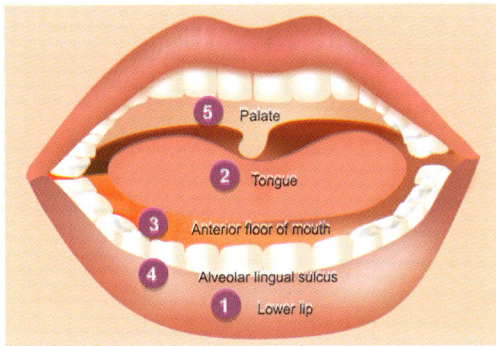

FIGURE 19.4: Frequency of occurrence of squamous cell carcinomas in the oral cavity.

Gross There are four macroscopic forms of oral cancer: *ulcerative, papillary, nodular and scirrhous type* **(Fig. 19.5)**. Adjacent to the invasive cancer there are usually foci of leukoplakia or erythroplasia.

A, ULCERATIVE TYPE   B, PAPILLARY (VERRUCOUS) TYPE   C, NODULAR TYPE   D, SCIRRHOUS TYPE

FIGURE 19.5: Squamous cell (Epidermoid) carcinoma of oral cavity, patterns of gross appearance.

Microscopy Squamous cell carcinoma of the oral cavity could be graded from well-differentiated keratinising squamous cell carcinoma on one end of the spectrum to poorly-differentiated highly undifferentiated on the other. Well-differentiated squamous cell carcinomas predominate and account for 90% of all tumours **(Fig. 19.6)**.

Several microscopic variants must be distinguished from conventional squamous cell carcinoma since they have different prognosis than the classical form of oral cancer.

i. *Verrucous carcinoma* forms differentiated bulbous squamous rete ridges that do not invade surrounding tissue as rapidly as the conventional squamous carcinoma.
This variant has a better prognosis than the conventional squamous cell carcinoma.

ii. *Basaloid squamous carcinoma* is composed of bluish basaloid cells that have scant cytoplasm. These cells are arranged into nests that tend to show central 'comedo-type' necrosis.
These tumours are high grade with a tendency for distant metastases.

iii. *Spindle cell squamous carcinoma* is composed of non-keratinising spindle cells resembling sarcoma. These tumours metastasise to lymph nodes frequently.

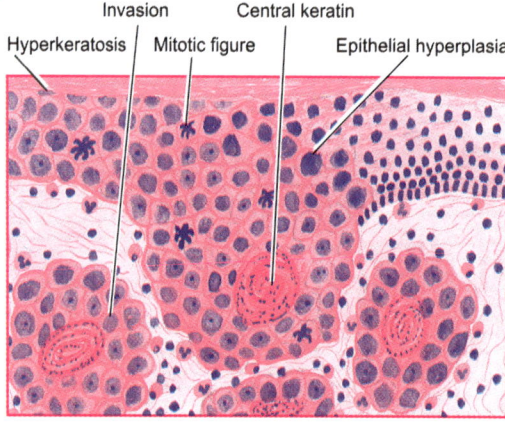

FIGURE 19.6: Invasive oral squamous cell carcinoma. The malignant squamous tumour cells show pleomorphism and are arranged in aggregates of tumour cells invading the subepithelial soft tissues.

iv. *Adenoid-squamous carcinoma* occurs on sun-exposed areas such as lips. It is composed of cells that dissociate one from another thus forming gland like structures.

v. *Adenosquamous carcinoma* is a biphasic tumour showing glandular and squamous differentiation. These tumours tend to form distant metastases.

Prognosis
- For localised carcinoma of the conventional type, the 5-year survival is 75%. The major problem, however, is that most patients present at the time of diagnosis with lymph node metastases.
- Tumours that have metastasised to the lymph nodes, the survival is dramatically reduced to approximately one half of that (35–40%).
- The prognosis of lip carcinoma is excellent (90% 10-years survival) because most tumours are recognised early before they have metastasised.
- Microscopic variant forms of oral cancer, which are prone to early metastases, have worse prognosis.

TEETH AND PERIODONTAL TISSUES

Q9. What are the normal teeth components?

The teeth are part of the odontogenic apparatus which also includes the gingiva and the jawbones, the maxilla and the mandible.

Embryology The odontogenic apparatus develops from the *dental lamina*.
- **The epithelial layer** of dental lamina, the ameloblasts, secrete enamel matrix, also called *enamel organ*.
- **Mesoderm-derived** connective tissue gives rise to *dental papilla*. The outer layer of the dental papilla differentiates into odontoblasts (the counterparts of osteoblasts in the bone), which secrete *dentin* and with ameloblasts form the teeth.
- Nests of odontogenic epithelium are normally present in the jaw and may develop into cysts and tumours.

Anatomy/histology The teeth are composed of enamel, dentin and cementum and the pulp is composed of connective tissue and blood vessels **(Fig. 19.7, A)**:
- *Enamel* forms the outer covering and is composed almost exclusively of inorganic material.
- *Dentin* comprises most of the tooth substance. It is composed of organic material such as collagen, and calcium phosphates produced by odontoblasts.
- *Cementum* is the portion of tooth which covers the dentin at the root of tooth. It is the site where the periodontal ligament is attached to the tooth. Cementum is similar to bone in morphology and composition.
- *Dental pulp* occupies the central pulp cavity. It consists of connective tissue, blood vessels and nerves.

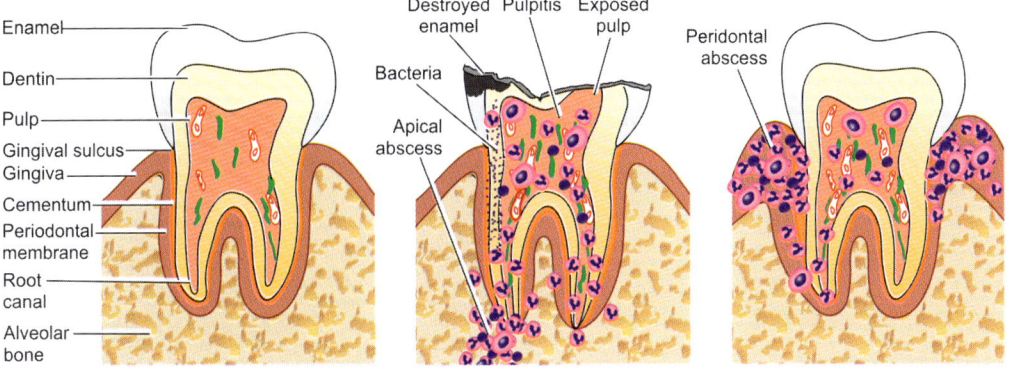

FIGURE 19.7: The normal structure of molar tooth in longitudinal section embedded in the jaw (A) contrasted with dental caries (B) and periodontal disease (C). In caries, there is complete destruction of enamel, deposition of secondary dentine and evidence of pulpitis (B), while there is formation of abscess in the periodontal tissue in chronic marginal gingivitis (C).

Q10. What is dental caries? Discuss salient features in its pathogenesis and pathology.

Definition Dental caries is a multifactorial tooth disease initiated by acidogenic bacteria which ferment carbohydrate-rich food remnants attached to teeth. Bacteria generate organic acids which decalcify dentin and enamel leading to the formation of cavities, destruction and loss of teeth.

Pathogenesis Four elements play a key role in the pathogenesis of dental caries which, in essence, is a disease of modern society : i) carbohydrate-rich diet, ii) oral hygiene, iii) bacterial flora, and iv) the basic chemical structure of teeth components.

I. *Carbohydrate-rich diet* contains large amounts of refined sugars which provide the substrate for the outgrowth of *acidogenic bacteria.*

- *Organic acids* formed from carbohydrates lead to *demineralisation* of dentin and enamel, a key event initiating the formation of caries.

II. *Oral hygiene* is important for removing *sticky food remnants* from occlusal pits and interdental spaces, thus depriving bacteria of their nutrients.

- Brushing and flossing on a regular basis are also essential for removing *bacterial plaques* that form a biofilm on the surface of teeth and lead to the formation of calcified *tartar*.

III. *Bacterial flora,* i.e. *oral microbiome* comprises some 300 bacterial species. Even though we do not know enough about these bacteria, it is obvious that only a few of these bacteria can produce acids and are proteolytic and thus involved in the formation of caries.

- Conditions that favour the growth of *cariogenic bacteria* promote formation of caries.

IV. *Basic chemical structure of dentin and enamel*, that is in part genetically determined, accounts for the fact that some people are more prone to caries than others.

- *Fluoridisation* of drinking water (adding of fluoride one part per million) strengthens the teeth and has been shown to protects against caries in children.

Pathology Caries begins most often in the pits and fissures on the surface of molars and premolars and in the cervical part of other teeth, i.e. areas where food retention occurs **(Fig. 19.8, A)**:

i. First changes appear as *white spots* on the enamel.
ii. White spots enlarge and become yellow or brown, leading to the formation of a *defect* in the enamel layer and underling dentin.
iii. Deepening defects transform into a *cavity or a deep fissure* toward the pulp.
iv. *Secondary dentin* formation ensues as a repair process, but it cannot prevent the invasion of bacteria and subsequent acute inflammation (*see* **Fig. 19.7, B**).

Q11. What are the complications of dental caries?

Most complications are related to persistent bacterial infection, and include the following:
I. **Pulpitis**, which may be acute or chronic, results from the entry of bacteria into the pulp.

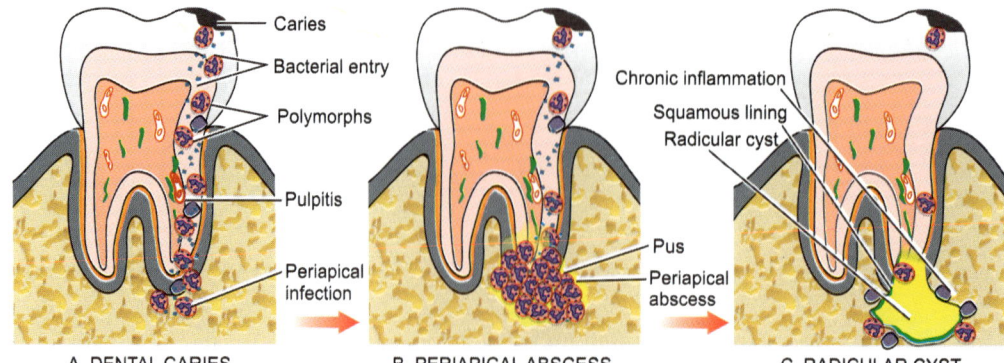

FIGURE 19.8: Pathogenesis of radicular cyst. The sequence involves spread of bacterial infection from dental caries to the pulp, causing pulpitis and periapical abscess. Resident squamous epithelial cells line the inflamed cyst wall.

II. **Apical granuloma** (a misnomer since there are no granulomas—only *granulation tissue*) is formed from the spread of infection from the pulp through the apical foramen into the tissue surrounding the root of the tooth **(Fig. 19.7, C)**. Inflammation is accompanied by formation of inflamed granulation tissue. Inside the granulation tissue, one may see microscopic remnants of odontogenic epithelium normally present in the periodontal membrane.

III. **Apical abscess** results from the lytic action of neutrophils in the inflammatory exudate, forming a pus-filled cavity adjacent to the apical tip of the tooth **(Fig. 19.8, B)**. Cessation of infection leads to resorption of neutrophil-rich exudate and can transform it into a *radicular cyst* **(Fig. 19.8, C)**.

IV. **Extension of the inflammation to adjacent tissues,** resulting in *osteomyelitis* of the mandible or maxilla, *cellulitis* of soft tissues of face and neck, *meningitis* and *cerebral abscess, cavernous sinus thrombosis*.

Q12. Briefly discuss periodontitis.

Definition Periodontitis is a bacterial infection of the tooth-support tissue including the periodontal ligament (membrane), leading ultimately to tooth loss.

Pathogenesis
- The disease begins as *chronic marginal gingivitis* secondary to bacterial plaques and calculus (tartar) on the surface of teeth in the periodontal pockets that contain food residues.
- Predisposing conditions include poor oral-dental hygiene, tooth decay and ill-fitting dentures, or diabetes, pregnancy and drugs like dilantin.
- Altered bacterial oral flora leads to an overgrowth of Gram negative bacteria belonging to several species, which colonise the gingival sulcus causing suppurative inflammation.

Pathology
- Periodontal pockets may contain pus which can be expressed by digital pressure.
- *Periodontal abscess* may form (see **Fig. 19.7, C**).
- In chronic periodontitis, persistent *pyorrhoea* (drainage of pus) leads to absorption and destruction of periodontal bone tissue, loosening of the periodontal ligament, and subsequent loss of loosened up teeth.

Q13. How are dental cysts classified?

Dental cyst also known as *odontogenic cysts*, can be divided into two major groups **(Table 19.2)**:
i. Inflammatory cysts
ii. Developmental cysts; these in turn are divided into odontogenic and non-odontogenic cysts.

TABLE 19.2 The WHO Classification of odontogenic cysts*.

I. Inflammatory odontogenic cysts
Radicular (apical, periodontal, dental) cyst

II. Developmental cysts
A. *Odontogenic cysts*
   1. Dentigerous (follicular) cyst
   2. Eruption cyst
   3. Gingival cyst
   4. Primordial cyst (odontogenic keratocyst, keratocystic odontogenic tumour)
B. *Non-odontogenic and fissural cysts*
   1. Nasopalatine duct (Incisive canal, Median anterior maxillary) cyst
   2. Nasolabial (nasoalveolar) cyst
   3. Globulomaxillary cyst
   4. Dermoid cyst

*Naggar et al. WHO classification of head and neck tumours (4th edition) 2017. Chapter 8, 204-260, IARC, Lyon.

The most common odontogenic cysts are as follows: i) radicular cysts (60%), ii) dentigerous cysts (20%), and iii) primordial cysts (12%), whereas all others are rare.

Q14. What are radicular cysts and how are these formed?

Definition Radicular cysts (also called *apical* or *periodontal cysts*, or simply *dental cysts*) are formed from apical abscesses. They are the most common dental cysts.

Pathogenesis Radicular cyst is a complication of dental caries complicated by purulent pulpitis that leads to the formation of an apical abscess.

- The inflammatory exudate is gradually absorbed whereupon the cavity fills with serous or seropurulent fluid.
- The wall of the cysts contains inflammatory cells, granulation tissue and squamous epithelial nests formed from the remnants of odontogenic epithelium which is normally embedded in the periodontium.
- Ultimately, the cyst might be lined by only squamous epithelium surrounded by fibrous tissue (*see* **Fig.19.8, C**).

Q15. What are the most important developmental cysts of teeth?

Definition These cysts are called developmental because they originate from tooth-forming (dentigerous) epithelium or epithelial odontogenic rests.

- They are often associated with unerupted teeth.
- They are most often diagnosed in children and young adults.

Types These cysts are divided into two groups: odontogenic and no-odontogenic.

I. **Developmental odontogenic cysts** Most important developmental cysts are as under:

i. *Dentigerous (or follicular) cyst* arises from enamel of an unerupted tooth.

- The cyst is most often found in children and young adults.
- It occurs most often in the region of the mandibular third molars and maxillary canines.
- These cysts may predispose to formation of ameloblastomas.

Microscopy The cyst is lined by a layer of stratified squamous epithelium lying on a thin band of fibrous tissue. It may thus resemble radicular cyst, but in contrast to radicular cysts it does not contain inflammatory changes.

ii. *Primordial cyst* (*odontogenic keratocyst,* recently renamed as *keratocystic odontogenic tumour*) originates from the tooth-forming epithelium, like the dentigerous cyst. The common location is mandibular third molar. Some cases that are familial, have multiple cysts.

Microscopy The cyst is lined by a furrowed keratinising squamous epithelium with a prominent basal cell layer.

NOTE: Primordial cysts seem to be locally invasive neoplasms as evidenced by the fact that approximately 50% of them recur after surgery. Furthermore, multiple primordial cysts may occur in association with a hereditary naevoid basal cell carcinoma syndrome (*Gorlin syndrome*) which is related to the mutation of the tumour suppressor gene *PTC* ('patched').

II. **Developmental non-odontogenic and fissural cysts** These are rare cysts of developmental origin.

- They develop from the enlargement of small remnants of embryonic/foetal structures that have not completely involuted during the fusion of the facial bones and have later transformed into cysts.
- Most often, they are located in the maxilla but may also be found in the nasal cavity.
- They are lined by cuboidal respiratory epithelium or squamous epithelium.
- The most common are the *nasopalatine duct cyst* found of the midline in the anterior part of maxilla, and *small dermoid cysts* that develop from mandibular and branchial arches.

Q16. What are odontogenic tumours? Describe salient features of common examples.

Definition Odontogenic tumours are uncommon tumours of the jaws derived from the epithelial or mesenchymal components of the odontogenic apparatus.

Types

- Most *follicular pattern* odontogenic tumours are benign and some of them are actually considered to be hamartomas.

- Malignant odontogenic tumours are exceptionally rare and are classified as carcinoma or sarcomas or carcinosarcomas.

The most common odontogenic tumours are ameloblastoma and odontoma.

I. **Ameloblastoma** is a benign but locally invasive tumour, most often found in the molar ramus of the mandible or maxilla. It originates from the foetal enamel or its residues. Sometimes, it may originate from the epithelium of dentigerous cysts.
Microscopy Several patterns are recognised, but there is no clinical value of subclassifying tumours on the basis of their histopathology. The most common pattern is characterised by the formation of follicles composed of central areas of stellate cells and a peripheral layer of cuboidal or columnar cells **(Fig. 19.9)**.

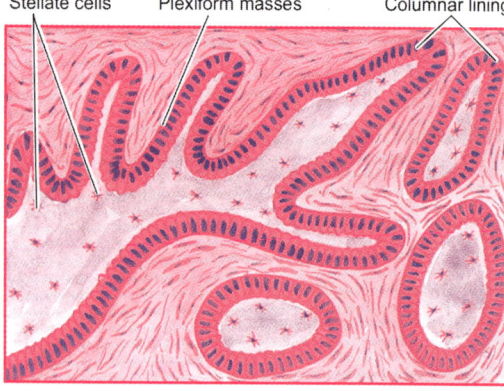

FIGURE 19.9: Ameloblastoma, follicular and plexiform patterns. Epithelial follicles are composed of central area of stellate cells and peripheral layer of cuboidal or columnar cells. Plexiform areas show irregular plexiform masses and network of strands of epithelial cells.

Clinical features These tumours grow in an indolent manner but tend to be locally invasive and destroy bone.
- On X-ray examination, ameloblastoma appears as a bone destructive multilocular cystic mass. Occasionally, it may be unicystic.
- Malignant ameloblastoma with a capacity for to metastasis may occur but it is very rare.

II. **Odontomas** are hamartomatous tumours composed of epithelial and mesodermal dental tissue components. They are composed of a mixture of normal dental tissues such as dentin, enamel or cementum and nonspecific fibrous tissue.

■ SALIVARY GLANDS

Q17. What are the main anatomic and histologic features of salivary glands?

Anatomy The salivary glands are divided in two groups:
i. *Major salivary glands* comprising paired parotid, submandibular and sublingual glands.
ii. *Minor salivary glands* widely distributed in the mucosa of the oral cavity.
- The main duct of the parotid gland drains into the oral cavity on the buccal side.
- The major ducts of the submandibular and sublingual gland drain into the floor of the mouth.

Histology The salivary glands consist of ducts and acini comprising mucinous or serous cells.
- The parotid gland is a purely serous gland; the submandibular gland is a mixed gland, but predominantly serous; the sublingual gland is a mixed gland of the predominantly mucinous type.
- Minor salivary glands are serous, mucinous or mixed type.

Q18. What is sialadenitis? Discuss salient features of its types.

Definition Sialadenitis is an inflammation of salivary glands, which may be acute or chronic; latter is more common form.
Etiology Sialadenitis may be caused by infections (viral and bacterial or mycotic) or it may be an autoimmune disease.
Types Based on etiology and pathogenesis, classification of sialadenitis includes three entities as under:
i. **Viral sialadenitis** most commonly is caused by *mumps virus*. Mumps is a childhood disease and it affects the salivary glands, pancreas and testis **(Fig.19.10)**.
ii. **Bacterial sialadenitis** may be acute or chronic.
a. *Acute sialadenitis* may occur in the course of acute systemic fevers. Ascending bacterial infection from the mouth can occur in postoperative patients, very old people and debilitated or dehydrated persons.
Microscopy It is characterised by infiltrates of neutrophils.

b. *Chronic sialadenitis* may be classified as recurrent obstructive or non-obstructive type.
• *Recurrent obstructive* sialadenitis occurs in people who have salivary stones (sialolithiasis), strictures of the excretory duct, or had surgery in that area. Recurrent attacks of acute inflammation gradually progress to chronic sialadenitis.
• *Recurrent non-obstructive* type occurs due to ascending infection in people who have reduced salivary secretion due to medications (e.g. antihistaminics, antihypertensives, antidepressants), following irradiation or congenital malformations of the excretory duct system. Chronic diseases such as tuberculosis rarely affect salivary glands.
iii. **Autoimmune sialadenitis** Sjögren syndrome is the most important autoimmune disease affecting the salivary glands. *Clinically,* triad of findings includes dry mouth (xerostomia), dry eyes (xerophthalmia) and rheumatoid arthritis.

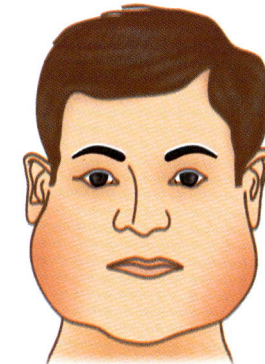
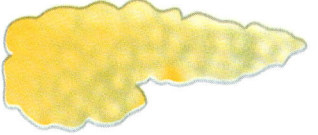
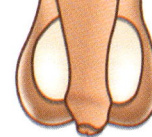

FIGURE 19.10: Lesions in mumps.

Microscopy Chronic sialadenitis due to chronic inflammation or autoimmune diseases is characterised by infiltrates of lymphocyte, plasma cells and macrophages. It is marked by a loss of acinar cells and extensive fibrosis that may contain prominent lymphoid follicles.

Q19. Classify tumours of the salivary glands. What are their key general features?

Classification Salivary gland tumours may be classified as benign or malignant; epithelial or mesenchymal or mixed tumours **(Table 19.3)**. Salivary glands may be involved by lymphomas and rarely by metastases from other sites.

Key features about salivary gland tumours are as follows:
• Parotid gland, the largest salivary gland, is most often affected and contains about 75% of all salivary gland tumours.
• Most salivary gland tumours are benign, but the ratio of benign to malignant tumours decreases proportionately with the decreasing size of the glands (parotid (75%) > submandibular (60%) > sublingual (20%). Approximately 50% of minor salivary gland tumours are malignant.
• The most common salivary tumour is pleomorphic adenoma, accounting for 65% of major and 50% of minor salivary gland tumours. It is benign but tends to recur if not excised completely. Malignant transformation occurs in 2–3% of these tumours.
• Overall, the most common malignant tumour is mucoepidermoid carcinoma, accounting for 15% of all tumours.
• Adenoid cystic carcinoma is the most common malignant tumour of minor salivary glands.

TABLE 19.3 The WHO classification of salivary gland tumours (2017).

I. Benign epithelial tumours
1. Pleomorphic adenoma (50%)
2. Warthin tumour (8%)
3. Oncocytoma (1%)
4. Others (myoepithelioma, basal cell adenoma, sebaceous adenoma)

II. Borderline epithelial tumours
Sialoblastoma

III. Malignant epithelial tumours
1. Mucoepidermoid carcinoma (15%)
2. Adenocarcinoma (polymorphous, basal cell, and NOS) (10%)
3. Carcinoma ex pleomorphic adenoma (5%)
4. Adenoid cystic carcinoma (5%)
5. Acinic cell carcinoma (3%)
6. Squamous cell carcinoma (1%)
7. Others (secretory carcinoma, intraductal carcinoma, salivary duct carcinoma, epithelial-myoepithelial carcinoma, clear cell carcinoma, carcinosarcoma)

IV. Mesenchymal tumours
1. Haemangioma
2. Lipoma

V. Haematolymphoid tumours
Extranodal marginal zone MALT lymphoma

*Naggar et al. WHO classification of head and neck tumours (4th edition) 2017. Chapter 8, 204-260, IARC, Lyon.

- Molecular biology testing is useful for subclassifying malignant salivary gland tumours in order to distinguish those with good prognosis from those that have worse prognosis.

Q20. Discuss major features of pleomorphic adenoma.

Definition Pleomorphic adenoma(PA, also known as *mixed tumour*)is a benign tumour of salivary glands that has an epithelial and a mesenchymal stromal component. It is the most common salivary gland tumour.

Pathology PAs occur most often in the parotid gland but can involve other glands as well.

Gross The tumour is usually solitary, smooth surfaces and sometime nodular. It measures 2–5 cm in largest diameter **(Fig. 19.11)**.

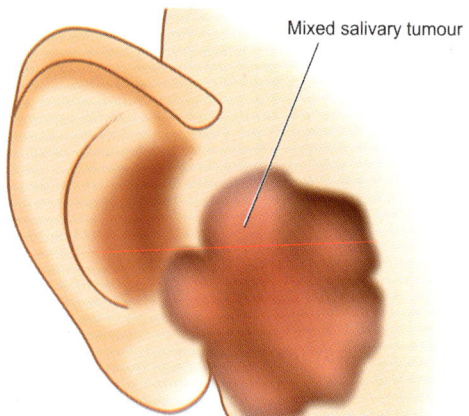

FIGURE 19.11: Pleomorphic adenoma (mixed salivary tumour) of the parotid gland, diagrammatic location.

Microscopy It is a mixed tumour comprising an epithelial and a stromal component **(Fig. 19.12)**.
- The epithelial cells form glands, ducts, tubules, acini sheets and strands.
- Mesenchymal stromal component appears loose, myxoid containing myoepithelial cells or forming cartilage like areas.

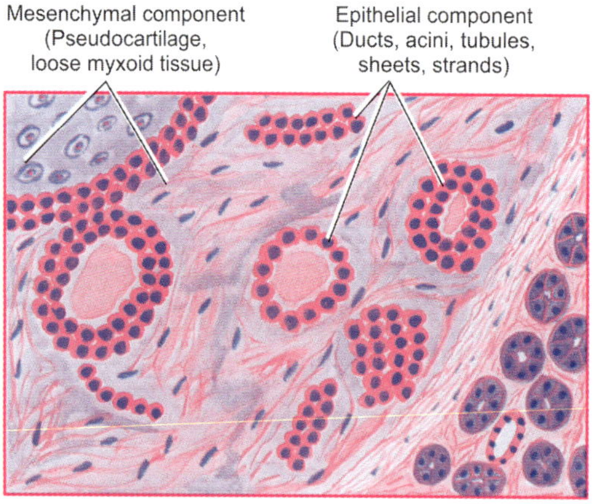

FIGURE 19.12: Pleomorphic adenoma. The epithelial element is comprised of ducts, acini, tubules, sheets and strands of cuboidal and myoepithelial cells. These are seen randomly admixed with mesenchymal elements composed of pseudocartilage which is the matrix of myxoid, chondroid and mucoid material.

Clinical features
i. PAs have a peak incidence in 3rd and 4th decade, and affect more often women than men.
ii. Due to its vicinity to the facial nerve crossing through the parotid gland, it might be difficult to resect it completely and, therefore, many tumours recur.
iii. Malignant transformation (carcinoma ex pleomorphic adenoma) occurs in 2% but it is higher in tumours that have not been removed, or those that have recurred after surgery. Malignant tumours have a high mortality, up to 50% at 5 years after surgery.

Q21. Briefly discuss Warthin tumour.

Definition Warthin tumour, also known as papillary cystadenoma lymphomatosum, is a benign salivary gland tumour that occurs almost exclusively in the parotid gland. It accounts for approximately 10% of parotid gland tumours.

Pathology
Gross The tumour is encapsulated, round or oval and has a smooth external surface.
Microscopy It is composed of columnar epithelium resembling ducts of the salivary gland, and lymphoid tissue forming follicles in the stroma **(Fig. 19.13)**.

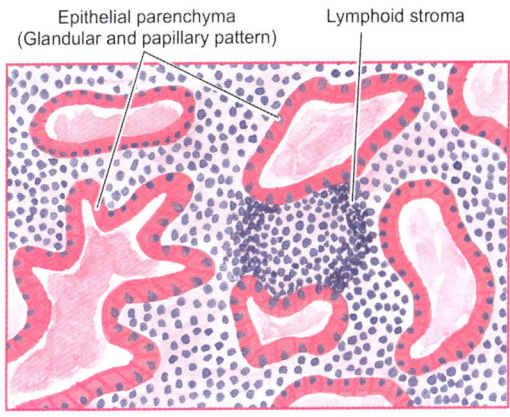

FIGURE 19.13: Warthin tumour, showing eosinophilic epithelium forming glandular and papillary, cystic pattern with intervening stroma of lymphoid tissue.

Q22. What is mucoepidermoid carcinoma?

Definition Mucoepidermoid carcinoma is a the most common malignant tumour of salivary glands composed of squamous and mucin producing or intermediate cells.

Pathology Mucoepidermoid carcinoma can be classified as low grade, intermediate and high grade carcinomas. The *CRTC1-MAML2* fusion gene resulting from a t(11;19) (q21;p13) translocation, is a feature of both low-grade and high-grade mucoepidermoid carcinomas.

Clinical features Mucoepidermoid carcinoma can occur at any age, including childhood. Most of them are in the parotid gland, but they can occur in other salivary glands and minor salivary glands in the mouth.

Prognosis depends on the degree of differentiation of tumour.
- Low grade tumours recur in 15% of cases and have a 5-year survival of 95%.
- High grade tumours recur in up to 30% of cases and have a 5 year survival of 50%.

Q23. What are other malignant salivary gland tumours besides mucoepidermoid carcinoma?

Several malignant salivary gland tumours can be recognised microscopically, but overall these tumours are rare, each accounting for 2–5% of all salivary gland tumours. A few examples are as under:

I. **Adenocarcinomas**, including adenocarcinoma NOS (not otherwise specified) and salivary duct carcinoma (resembling invasive breast duct carcinoma) occur in 50–60 years old persons. They are mostly high grade malignant tumours and have a poor prognosis.

II. **Adenoid cystic carcinoma** occurs in 50–60 years old persons as a slow growing tumour that has a predilection for local invasion and spread along the nerve sheaths.

III. **Acinic cell carcinoma** is a low grade carcinoma that occurs in all age groups, including childhood. It is composed of cells resembling serous cell of normal glands. After resection of these slow growing tumours, at least one third of all will recur.

> **Chapter 19e Supplement: Online Content**
>
> *Digital content of this chapter available with this book is meant for enhanced learning and self-assessment. In addition, it contains 23 Multiple Choice Questions (MCQs), 05 Clinicopathologic Vignettes, and 06 Image-based Questions; these are followed by their answers along with explanatory notes of correct and incorrect answers.*

CHAPTER 20

Gastrointestinal Tract

■ OESOPHAGUS

Q1. What is the basic structure of the tubular part of the gastrointestinal tract?
The tubular GI tract includes oesophagus, stomach, small intestine and the large intestine. All these anatomic parts have the same basic structure and consist of four layers:
i. Mucosa
ii. Submucosa
iii. Muscularis propria
iv. Adventitia/serosa

Q2. What is congenital oesophageal atresia?
Definition *Oesophageal atresia,* usually associated with *tracheo-oesophageal fistula,* is the most important congenital anomaly of the oesophagus.
Features It occurs at a rate of 1:3,000 to 1:5,000 births.
• It may be an isolated anomaly but in 60% of cases it is associated with some other developmental anomaly.
• It is lethal if not corrected surgically within the first 48 hours after birth.
• Atresia of the oesophagus (complete obliteration of the lumen) prevents the entry of ingested fluid and food into the stomach, and thus the baby would die of thirst and hunger.
• Oesophageal-tracheal fistula allows the passage of ingested material into the trachea, where it obstructs the air-passage causing asphyxia. Food entering the lungs may also cause aspiration pneumonia.

Q3. What is achalasia of the esophagus? What are its types?
Definition Achalasia is a neuromuscular dysfunction of the oesophagus caused by incomplete relaxation of the lower esophageal sphincter resulting in progressive dysphagia and dilatation of the esophagus above the sphincter.
Etiologic classification Achalasia may be:
• *Idiopathic,* i.e. congenital, or
• *Secondary* due to a loss of intramural ganglion cells and neurons from some other causes such as Chagas disease (*Trypanosoma cruzi* infection), viral infection (e.g. CMV or herpes) or neurodegenerative diseases, and tumours.
Pathology The lowermost portion of the oesophagus is contracted and the oesophagus above that contracture is dilated (*megaoesophagus*). The dilated oesophagus may show a variety of secondary changes such as ulcerations and infection.

Q4. Define hiatus hernia. What are its major types?
Definition Hiatus hernia is the herniation or protrusion of the proximal part of the stomach through the oesophageal hiatus of the diaphragm into the thoracic cavity.

Etiopathogenesis The basic defect is the failure of diaphragmatic muscle fibres to maintain the regular margins of the hiatus so that it does not dilate. It could be:
i. *Primary* in childhood due to a 'short oesophagus' pulling the stomach up into the hiatus, or
ii. Much more often *secondary,* which is acquired.
The real reasons for herniation are not known but it is known that following factors favour it:
a. *Ageing,* as it weakens diaphragmatic muscles and reduces their resilience.
b. *Increased intra-abdominal pressure* in pregnancy, abdominal tumors, etc.
c. *Obesity* which will decrease the elasticity of diaphragm and increase intra-abdominal pressure.

Classification Three patterns are recognised as follows **(Fig. 20.1)**:
i. *Sliding or oesophagogastric hernia* is the most common occurring in 85% of cases. In this, the cardia portion of the stomach slides up into the thorax.
ii. *Rolling or paraoesophageal hernia* is seen in 10% of cases. Here, the cardia part of the stomach rolls up next to the oesophagus, producing an intrathoracic sac.
iii. *Mixed or transitional hernia* is a combination of sliding and rolling, and is found in 5% of cases.

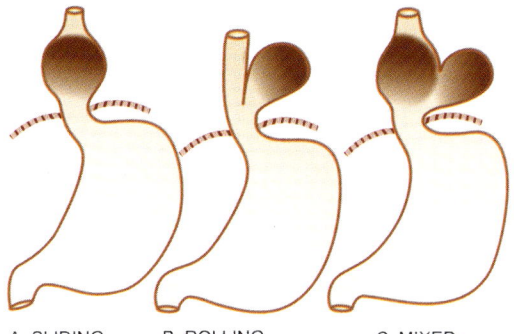

A, SLIDING (OESOPHAGO-GASTRIC) TYPE B, ROLLING (PARAOESOPHAGEAL) TYPE C, MIXED (TRANSITIONAL) TYPE

FIGURE 20.1: Patterns of hiatus hernia.

Q5. What are oesophageal diverticula? Briefly discuss their types and pathogenesis.

Definition Diverticula are the outpouchings of the oesophageal wall at point of their weakness.
Pathogenesis and classification They may be congenital or acquired:
I. *Congenital diverticula* can occur at any level along the oesophagus but they are rare.
II. *Acquired diverticula* are of two types:
i. *Pulsion (Zenker) type* diverticula are found in the hypopharynx and develop secondary to oesophageal obstruction, as in cancer or inflammatory fibrosis or a defect in the muscularis propria and the cricopharyngeal muscle. The mucosa and submucosa herniate through the weakened wall forming a sac-like outpouching.
ii. *Traction type diverticula* are found in the lower third of the oesophagus due to fibrous tissue outside of oesophagus (e.g. pleural scars, healed tuberculosis of hilar lymph nodes, etc.), which pulls the oesophageal wall into a protrusion.
Clinical features Diverticula may cause:
i. Oesophageal obstruction.
ii. Painful swallowing (*dysphagia*).
iii. Bad breath (*halitosis*) due to retention of food, which will predispose to infections.
iv. Perforations require surgery.

Q6. What are oesophageal webs and rings?

Definition Webs and rings are mucosal protrusions in persons with dysphagia best seen by oesophagoscopy or X-ray examination after barium swallow.
• **Webs** are mucosal folds in the upper oesophagus most often seen in women who have iron deficiency anaemia.
• **Rings** are semicircular fibrous strands in the wall in the lower oesophagus **(Fig. 20.2)**.

Q7. What is the etiology of oesophagitis?

Four main causes of oesophagitis are as follows:
I. **Reflux** of gastric juice, causing a sterile, chemical oesophagitis (the most common form, often associated with oesophageal hernia).

II. **Infections**, most often by viruses (e.g. herpes simplex and CMV), or fungi (e.g. *Candida albicans*), usually in debilitated persons, immunosuppressed persons or those treated for cancer.

III. **Secondary oesophagitis** related to some other GI disease (e.g. Crohn disease of the ileum and colon), skin diseases (e.g. pemphigus), or systemic immune mediated diseases (e.g. graft versus host disease, scleroderma).

IV. **Eosinophilic oesophagitis** is an immune mediated form of oesophagitis, especially common in children who have other allergic diseases such as atopic dermatitis and asthma.
- It is characterised by distinct rings and fissure and plaques visible on endoscopy.
- The diagnosis is made by oesophageal biopsy which typically contains numerous eosinophils and eosinophilic abscesses in the oesophageal mucosa.
- It responds well to corticosteroid treatment.

V. **Iatrogenic oesophagitis** related to medical and surgical procedure (e.g. endoscopy), irradiation (e.g. lung cancer treatment), or various drugs (e.g. anticholinergic drugs, tetracycline, doxycycline).

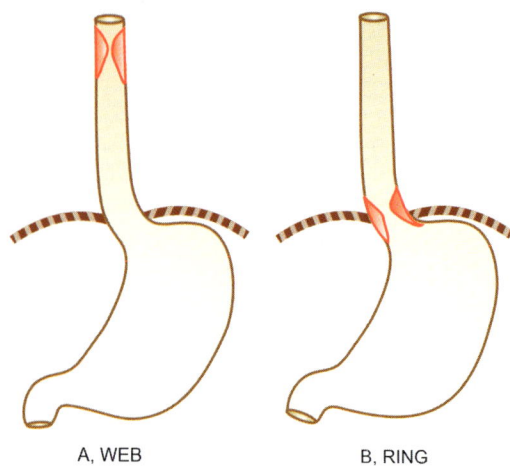

FIGURE 20.2: Oesophageal webs and rings.

Q8. What is reflux oesophagitis?

Definition Reflux oesophagitis is an inflammation of the oesophagus caused by reflux of gastric juice into the oesophagus. In the US, it is also called gastroesophageal reflux disease (GERD).

Etiopathogenesis Reflux can occur occasionally in normal healthy individuals, and is especially common during pregnancy. Recurrent or excessive reflux will, however, cause oesophagitis which requires treatment. Conditions that predispose to reflux and oesophagitis include the following:
i. Sliding oesophageal hernia
ii. Chronic gastritis and peptic ulcer disease
iii. Persistent vomiting
iv. Chronic alcoholism and diabetes mellitus
v. Medical interventions such as gastroscopy, nasogastric tubes, oesophagogastrostomy

Clinicopathologic features Reflux oesophagitis is a very common disease. The diagnosis is made by correlating the clinical findings with endoscopy and microscopy findings.
i. *Oesophagoscopy* reveals inflamed mucosa which appears different from the normal whitish grey oesophageal mucosa. It is usually red and friable and may bleed on touch.
ii. *Microscopy* Biopsy reveals:
- Microscopic changes in the squamous epithelium, such as basal cell hyperplasia, and elongation of the papillae.
- Infiltrates of inflammatory cells vary depending on the duration of the disease including initially eosinophils and neutrophils.
- Later on, lymphocytes predominate and there is subepithelial fibrosis.

iii. *Symptoms* typically include:
- Heartburn, especially if lying down.
- Nocturnal reflux is common causing distressful regurgitation.
- Difficulty in swallowing, especially hard food may be painful (*odynophagia*).

iv. *Complications* of reflux oesophagitis are:
- Barrett oesophagus
- Oesophageal bleeding accompanied by melaena
- Ulceration
- Oesophageal stricture due to healing by fibrosis.

Q9. What is Barrett oesophagus? Discuss its pathologic changes.

Definition Barrett oesophagus is intestinal metaplasia involving the squamous mucosa of the lower oesophagus affected by chronic oesophagitis, most often caused by gastric reflux.

Pathology Biopsy shows:
i. Intestinal (columnar) metaplasia with or without dysplasia.
ii. The intestinal epithelium replacing the normal squamous epithelium contains prominent goblet cells **(Fig. 20.3)**.
iii. The stroma contains chronic inflammatory cells.
iv. Metaplastic intestinal epithelium is prone to dysplasia which may be classified microscopically as low grade or high grade. High grade dysplasia may progress to adenocarcinoma in situ and invasive adenocarcinoma.

Prognosis Overall, malignancy develops in Barrett oesophagus at a rate of 0.5% per year after diagnosis, mandating careful follow-up of all cases with periodic repeat endoscopic biopsies.

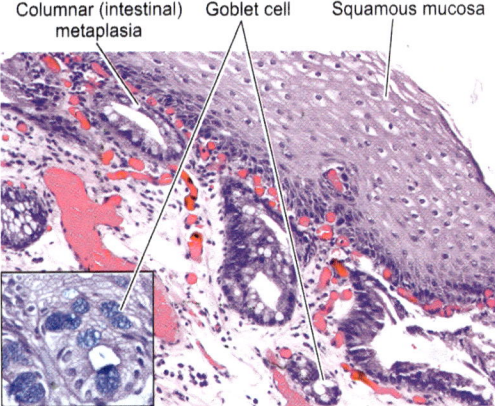

FIGURE 20.3: Barrett oesophagus. Under the squamous mucosa, glands lined by metaplastic columnar epithelium are seen. Inbox shows goblet cells in the metaplastic epithelium (alcian blue stain).

Q10. Enumerate the most important tumours of the oesophagus.

- As in other organs, tumours of the oesophagus may be epithelial or mesenchymal, benign or malignant, solitary or multiple, primary or metastatic.
- Benign tumours, both epithelial (such as squamous cell papilloma) or mesenchymal (such as leiomyomas) are rare and clinically not so significant.
- Most tumours are solitary, and the malignant tumours are more often primary than metastatic.
- Oesophageal cancer is clinically the most important tumour of the oesophagus.
- Sarcomas occur but are rare.

Q11. What are the main epidemiological and etiologic risk factors in oesophageal cancer?

Epidemiology It is ranked third in the tubular part of the GI tract (after colon and stomach). However, it contributes disproportionally much more to GI cancer mortality due to its poor prognosis.

i. *Age and sex* Peak incidence is in the 45–65 years age group, more common in males than females (M:F=4:1).
- Adenocarcinomas occur in somewhat younger men than squamous cell carcinomas.

ii. *Geographic and racial variation* The incidence varies, showing significant geographic and racial differences:
- More common in parts of Asia (e.g. China and Japan) and Africa than in Europe and North America.
- More common in African Americans than in other races in the US.
- The incidence of adenocarcinoma versus squamous cell carcinoma has increased in Western Europe and North America, where it accounts now for almost 50% of all oesophageal cancers.

Etiologic risk factors These can be divided into three groups: i) diet and person habits, ii) oesophageal disorders, and iii) other factors.

I. ***Diet and personal habits*** are most important and include:
i. Foremost are heavy smoking and alcohol consumptions.
ii. Dietary habits play a role and include intake of food contaminated with fungus (e.g. pickled vegetables), foods containing nitrates that convert to nitrites.
iii. Nutritional deficiencies of vitamins and trace elements (e.g. iron deficiency).
iv. High fat diet and low intake of fresh fruits also may be important.

II. ***Oesophageal disorders*** include: primarily Barrett oesophagus (predisposing to adenocarcinoma) and to a lesser extent achalasia, diverticula, herniation.

III. ***Other factors*** include poorly understood contributing data such as family history, genetic factors and HPV infection.

Q12. Discuss salient clinicopathologic features of oesophageal cancer?

Pathology There are two microscopic subtypes of oesophageal cancer: squamous cell carcinoma and adenocarcinoma.

I. **Squamous cell carcinoma** It comprises 90% of all oesophageal carcinomas world-wide and is especially common in parts of world with high prevalence of oesophageal cancer in Asia and Africa.
- Approximately 50% of tumours occur in the middle third, 30% in the lower and 20% in the upper third of the oesophagus **(Fig. 20.4, A)**.
- *Grossly,* three types of growth are seen: polypoid, ulcerating, and diffuse infiltrating **(Fig. 20.4, B)**.
- *Microscopy* shows the usual features of squamous cell carcinoma, which can be classified as well, moderately or poorly differentiated.

II. **Adenocarcinoma** occurs mostly in the lower third.
Tumours grow as nodular elevated masses and invade through the wall of the oesophagus or into the cardia portion of the stomach.
Microscopy shows the usual features of mucin producing adenocarcinomas arising in Barrett oesophagus, which is still present at its margins.

Spread of cancer and metastases Irrespective of it microscopic appearance,
i. Carcinoma of the oesophagus *invades rapidly* through the relatively thick wall of the oesophagus. Thus, it may *extend locally* into the adjacent thoracic and abdominal organs, such as trachea and stomach.
ii. Abundant lymphatics in the wall of the oesophagus allow for early *lymphatic metastases* to local lymph nodes.
iii. The direction of lymphatic spread depends on the location of the tumour, because the lymph drainage from each segment of the oesophagus (upper, middle or lower third) is anatomically distinct.
iv. *Haematogenous spread* to the liver and lungs occur as well but these metastases are of lesser clinical significance since most patients die before metastases become apparent.
v. If *distant metastases* are found during the staging (in consideration of surgical resection), most surgeons do not recommend the resection of the primary cancer in the oesophagus because the disease has advanced too far for effective treatment.
vi. *Prognosis* Overall 5-year survival is only 15%.

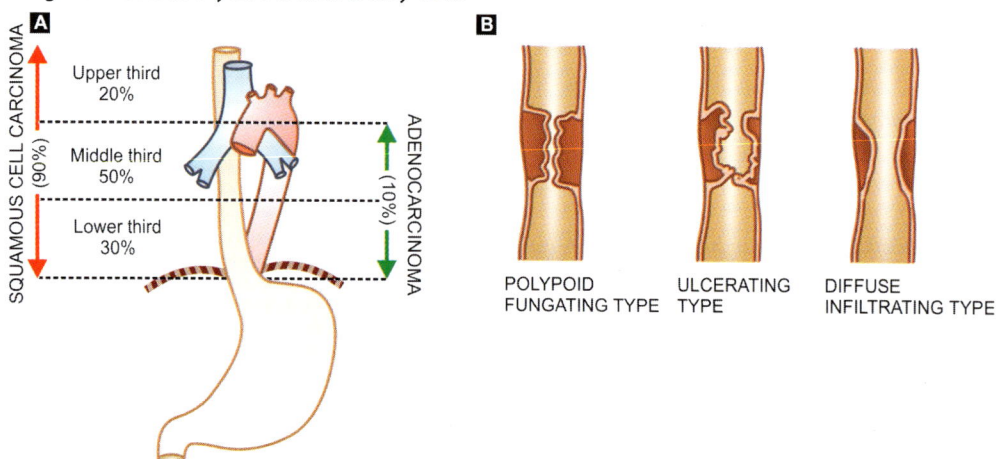

FIGURE 20.4: A, Carcinoma oesophagus—sites of predilection for squamous cell carcinoma and adenocarcinoma. B, Gross patterns of squamous cell carcinoma of the oesophagus.

■ STOMACH

Q13. What are the main anatomic parts of the stomach?

i. The stomach can be divided into five regions: cardia, fundus, body of the stomach, pyloric antrum and pylorus **(Fig. 20.5)**.
ii. These regions contain glands that are classified into three groups:
a. Short tubular glands of cardia

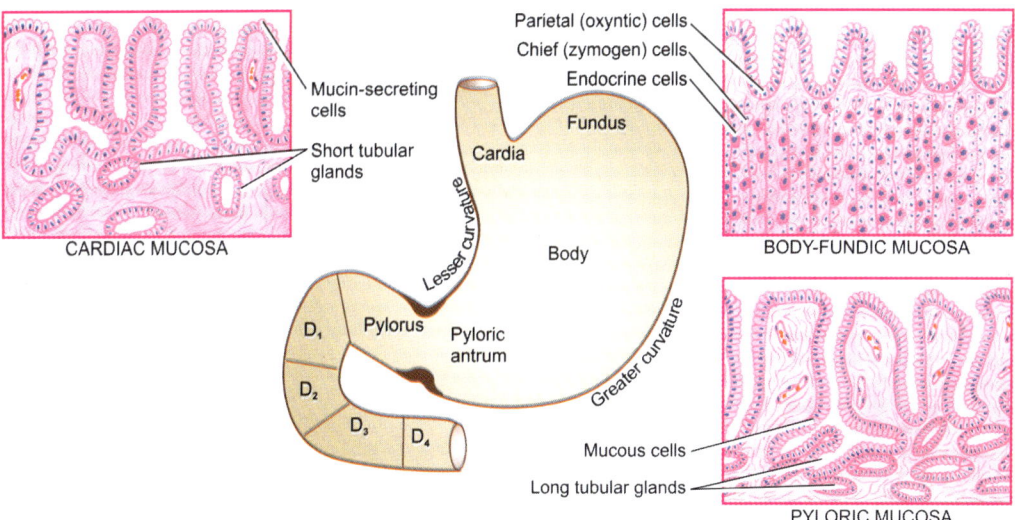

FIGURE 20.5: Anatomical subdivisions of the stomach correlated with histological appearance of gastric mucosa in different regions. D_1, D_2, D_3 and D_4 are the first to fourth parts of the duodenum.

b. Glands of the oxynthic mucosa in the fundus and the body
c. Pyloric glands in the pyloric antrum and pylorus.
iii. The surface layer of all glands is composed of mucin-secreting cells.
iv. The oxynthic mucosa has the most complex structure. The deeper layer glands of this region comprise four cell types:
a. Parietal cells producing hydrochloric acid and intrinsic factor
b. Chief (peptic) cells producing pepsin
c. Mucin secreting neck cells
d. Endocrine cells, secreting polypeptide hormones like gastrin.

Q14. What is the most important developmental disorder of the stomach?

It is *congenital hypertrophic pyloric stenosis* that affects 1 in 400–600 newborn infants.
Genetics This disorder has a *multifactorial inheritance*, which is supported by some observations as under:
i. It shows familial clustering, but no distinct Mendelian inheritance.
ii. It has a very high concordance rate among monozygotic twins.
iii. It predominantly affects male infants (4:1), suggesting that females have a higher threshold for the penetrance of the trait.
iv. Some chromosomal disorders, such as Turner syndrome, are often associated with this disorder, most likely lowering the threshold for expression of the trait in females.

Clinicopathologic features
i. It presents as marked narrowing of the pyloric canal due to hyperplasia and hypertrophy of the smooth muscle cells in the muscularis propria of the pylorus **(Fig. 20.6)**.
ii. The disease presents clinically with *projectile vomiting* approximately 2–4 weeks after birth.
iii. Visible peristalsis from the left to the right side of the abdomen can be noticed.

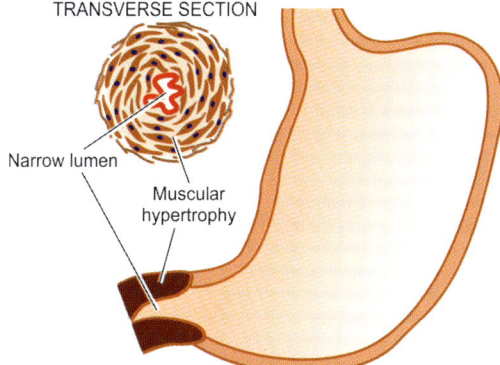

FIGURE 20.6: Pyloric stenosis, infantile type. Longitudinal and transverse section of the stomach showing hypertrophy of the circular layer of the muscularis in the pyloric sphincter.

iv. A nodular mass corresponding to thickened pylorus can be palpated through the infant's thin abdominal wall.
v. There is also constipation and weight loss due to reduce food intake.
vi. Myotomy, i.e. surgical incision of the thickened pyloric muscle will usually resolve the obstruction.

Q15. What is acute gastritis? Briefly discuss its etiopathogenesis and clinicopathologic features.

Definition Acute gastritis is an inflammation of sudden onset and limited duration.
Etiology A variety of causes have been implicated as under:
i. *Diet and personal habits* include highly spices food, excess of alcohol, heavy smoking.
ii. *Infections* such as:
- *Bacterial infection* with *Helicobacter pylori* (albeit usually asymptomatic in most cases!) or *Salmonella typhi*, staphylococcal food poisoning.
- *Viral infections,* e.g. viral hepatitis, influenza, infectious mononucleosis.

iii. *Drugs,* such as non-steroidal anti-inflammatory drugs (NSAIDs), aspirin, cortisone, chemotherapeutic agents.
iv. *Chemicals and physical agents,* such as caustic soda, phenol, lysol, gastric irradiation, gastric freezing.
v. *Severe stress* which may be based on strong emotions (e.g. fear, rage) or caused by burns, trauma, surgery, etc.

Pathogenesis Mucosal injury by any of the above listed agents could cause inflammation by one of the following mechanisms:
i. *Reduced blood flow* and mucosal hypoperfusion will lead to ischaemic cell necrosis eliciting an acute inflammatory reactions to chemotactic substances released from dead cells.
ii. *Increased acid secretion* combined with reduced protection against its deleterious effects on gastric cells, best illustrated by the effects of *H. pylori* on gastric mucosa.
iii. *Decreased production of bicarbonate buffer* which protects the gastric cells from the adverse effects of hydrochloric acid.

Pathology *Macroscopic features* include oedema and hyperaemia of the mucosa with multiple focal pin point haemorrhages.
Microscopy
- Infiltration of neutrophils into the oedematous lamina propria mucosae.
- Mucosa may be focally sloughed off and such defects are filled with extravasated blood, which may become black due to the action of hydrochloric acid.

Clinical features The patient complains of epigastric pain which may be aggravated by certain events like feeding or potentially noxious influences (e.g. intake of NSAIDs) or emotional upheaval. Gastric bleeding may cause melaena.

Q16. Define chronic gastritis. What are its major types? Discuss their salient features.

Definition Chronic gastritis is an inflammation of gastric mucosa accompanied by its infiltration with lymphocytes, plasma cells and macrophages.
- Microscopic diagnosis of chronic gastritis does not necessarily mean that the patient under observation will also have clinical symptoms of gastritis.
- It has been shown that 35% of biopsies of endoscopically normal mucosa of normal asymptomatic persons contain infiltrates of chronic inflammatory cells.
- Clinical symptoms of chronic gastritis are not specific and may vary in intensity.
- Most often, symptoms include vague complaints, or upper abdominal pain, nausea and urge to vomit.

Etiology Chronic gastritis with pathologic evidence of chronic inflammation and clinical symptoms supporting that diagnosis could be caused by the following:
i. Repeated bouts of acute gastritis
ii. *Helicobacter pylori* infection
iii. Autoimmune gastritis caused by antibodies to parietal cells
iv. Reflux of duodenal juice and or bile
v. Associated with gastric peptic ulcer or gastric cancer
vi. Associated with chronic hypochromic anaemia and atrophic gastritis.

Classification It is based on the location of inflammation in the stomach and etiology/pathogenesis as follows:

I. ***Type A gastritis (autoimmune gastritis):***
i. It involves mainly body-fundic mucosa.
ii. It accounts for only 10% of chronic gastritis patients and it is age dependent, i.e. affects older persons, more commonly women than men.
iii. It is often associated with other autoimmune diseases such as Hashimoto thyroiditis.
iv. Affected patients typically have autoantibodies to parietal cells or intrinsic factor.
v. Autoantibodies will reduce the number of parietal cells in the glands and cause gastric atrophy with intestinal metaplasia.
vi. Reduced acid secretion results ultimately in achlorhydria and reactive hyperplasia of gastrin-producing G cells in the antrum causing hypergastrinaemia.
vii. Reduced secretion of intrinsic factors may lead to B_{12} hypovitaminosis and pernicious anaemia in some patients.

II. ***Type B gastritis (H. pylori-related gastritis):***
i. It involves predominantly the antral mucosa.
ii. It is more common than type A gastritis.
iii. *H. pylori* stimulate secretion of hydrochloric acid and therefore it is also called hypersecretory gastritis.
iv. It may be associated with peptic ulcer.
v. It is not associated with any autoimmune disease and there are no autoantibodies in patients' blood.

III. ***Type AB gastritis (mixed gastritis, environmental gastritis):***
i. It is the most common symptomatic gastritis.
ii. It affects the antral-body mucosa.
iii. It can occur at any age and affect both sexes equally.
iv. It is also called atrophic gastritis because it leads to atrophy of the mucosa and intestinal or pseudopyloric metaplasia.

Q17. What is *Helicobacter pylori* gastritis? Briefly discuss its pathogenesis and consequences.

Definition *H. pylori*-related chronic gastritis is an infectious superficial gastritis involving predominantly the antral mucosa.
Pathogenesis *H. pylori* infection usually occurs in childhood but it remains asymptomatic and or quiescent until it becomes active chronic gastritis in adulthood. Following features are important for understanding the pathogenesis of *H. pylori* gastritis:
i. The pathogenic bacteria are identified in the biopsies as lying in the mucus on the surface of foveolar surface cells.
ii. *H. pylori* do not invade the mucosa.
iii. *H. pylori* secrete toxins which damage the mucosal cells attracting neutrophils which invade the glands and the surrounding lamina propria.
iv. Lymphocytes are recruited and some of them transform into plasma cells, which contribute to the mixed inflammatory infiltrate containing PMNs, lymphocytes and plasma cells *('active chronic gastritis')*.
v. Lymphocytes also form *lymphoid aggregates* with germinal follicles.
vi. Damage of epithelial cells leads to glandular atrophy (*atrophic gastritis*) and also *intestinal metaplasia* and the appearance of goblets cells **(Fig. 20.7)**.
vii. Metaplastic cells are prone to malignant transformation and could give rise to *adenocarcinoma* (estimated risk is 3–6 times).
viii. Proliferation of lymphocytes in the mucosa may give rise to lymphoma (*MALToma*) (estimated risk is 6–50 times).
ix. *H. pylori* infection also may cause *peptic ulcer* (estimated risk 3–6 times) **(Fig. 20.8)**.
Diagnosis *H. pylori* gastritis can be diagnosed by the following techniques:
i. Endoscopic biopsy examined in standard H&E stained sections, supplemented by special bacterial stains (Giemsa, Steiner silver impregnation) or immunohistochemistry with antibodies to *H. pylori*.
ii. Serologic tests for antibodies to *H. pylori* antigens performed on patients' blood.
iii. Urea ^{14}C breath test.

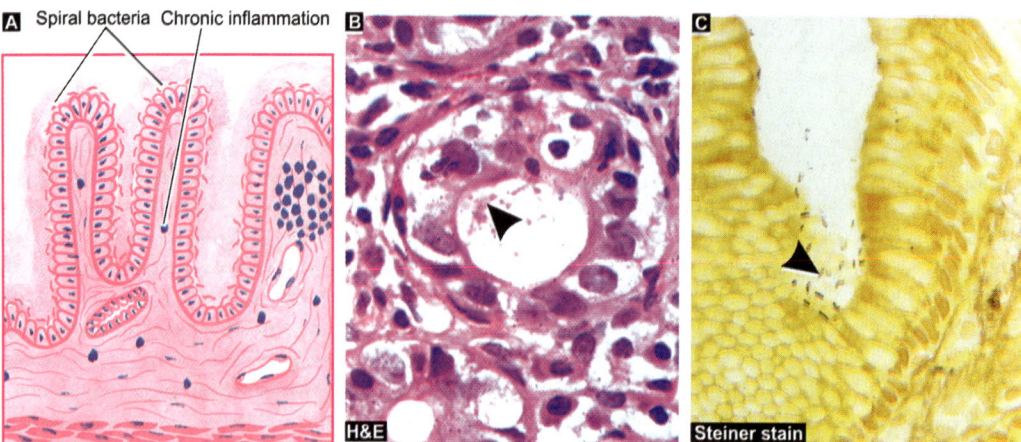

FIGURE 20.7: Histologic appearance of *H. pylori* chronic gastritis. A, Diagrammatic representation. B, H&E stained section shows lamina propria infiltrated by neutrophils and plasma cells. C, *H. pylori* in Steiner stain shows spiral or wavy organisms on the surface of faveolar mucosal cells.

Q18. What is chronic hypertrophic gastritis (Ménétrier disease)?

Definition Chronic hypertrophic gastritis is a rare disease of unknown etiology characterised pathologically by enormous foveolar hyperplasia leading to thickening of gastric rugal folds.

Clinicopathologic features
- *Clinically and grossly,* gastric mucosa of the fundus and body is transformed into huge folds resembling cerebral convolutions. Antrum is spared.
- *Microscopy* shows the folds containing an increased number of mucus-secreting foveolar cells due to excessive stimulation by transforming growth factor alpha (TGF-α).
- Excessive secretion of mucus which is rich in proteins cause '*protein loosing enteropathy*' and diarrhoea with digestive problems ('*dyspepsia*'), weight loss and generalised oedema due to hypoproteinaemia.
- Treatment is symptomatic and also includes surveillance because there is an increased incidence of adenocarcinoma.

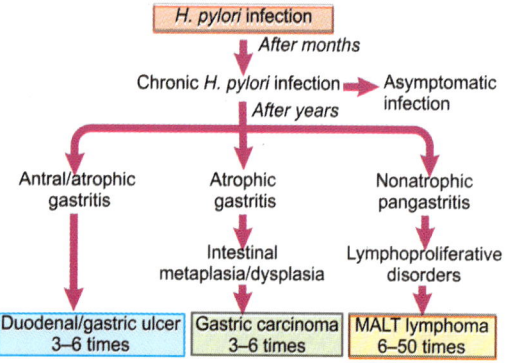

FIGURE 20.8: Consequences of long-term *H. pylori* gastritis.

Q19. What are acute peptic (stress) ulcers? Discuss their salient features.

Definition Acute peptic ulcers are small mucosal erosions seen most commonly in the stomach in conditions of severe stress, which render the mucosa more susceptible to damaging effects of gastric juice acid and pepsin.

Etiology Acute peptic ulcers develop under stress, which may be *psychological* or *pathophysiological* as under:
i. Psychological stress in severe anxiety
ii. Physiological stress
iii. Circulatory shock
iv. Sepsis
v. Severe trauma
vi. Extensive burns (Curling ulcers in the posterior aspect of the first part of duodenum)
vii. Intracranial lesions like tumours, brain trauma, intracranial surgery (Cushing ulcers developing from hyperacidity following excessive vagal stimulation)

viii. Drugs (e.g. aspirin, steroids, NSAIDs such as indomethacine, ibuprophen, etc.)
Pathogenesis Not fully elucidated.
- Except for Cushing ulcers that are related to hyperacidity, the gastric acidity is not increased in other forms of acute ulceration.
- Most likely theory concentrates on the possible *ischaemic hypoxic injury* of mucosal cells and a loss of *mucus barrier*, which render the mucosa more susceptible to injury by the *acid-peptic action of gastric juice*.

Pathology
i. Acute peptic ulcers are multiple, small (< 1 cm), shallow and found in any part of the stomach.
ii. Duodenum is less often involved than stomach, except in burns (Curling ulcer in duodenum).
iii. They affect only the mucosa and do not penetrate into the muscularis.
iv. They bleed and are filled with blood which, in contact with the hydrochloric acid, may become black.
v. There is minimal inflammation at the margins.
vi. They heal without consequences.

Q20. What is chronic peptic ulcer (peptic ulcer disease)? Discuss factors in its etiology and pathogenesis.

Definition Peptic ulcer or peptic ulcer disease is a multifactorial disease affecting the stomach or duodenum, resulting from a imbalance between noxious influences that damage the mucosa and protective mechanisms that keep its integrity intact.

Etiopathogenesis Key components of this multifactorial disease are i) peptic digestion of mucosa, ii) ulcerogenic action of *H. pylori*, and iii) action of other risk factors that increase the vulnerability of the gastric and duodenal mucosa and impair the protective mechanisms.

I. *Peptic digestion* The name 'peptic ulcer' could serve as a reminder that peptic digestion is essential for the development of such ulcers.
i. Ulcers develop only in parts of the GI tract that are exposed to peptic juices, primarily stomach and duodenum, but also Barrett oesophagus or ectopic gastric mucosa in Meckel diverticulum, or mucosa of the small intestine on the margins of gasto-jujunal anastomosis.
ii. Patients with pernicious anaemia-related achlorhydria never develop peptic ulcers.
iii. *Excess of acid secretion* is crucially important for the pathogenesis of duodenal ulcer, and the proton pump inhibitor drugs have a beneficial effect on the course of the disease.
iv. *Gastrin-secreting pancreatic tumours* in the Zollinger-Ellison syndrome have peptic ulcers related to tumor derived hypergastrinaemia.
v. In gastric ulcer patients, there is no hyperacidity, and one must assume that other factors play a local role such as chronic gastritis, bile reflux, cigarettes smoking, etc.

II. *H. pylori infection* It plays a key role in the pathogenesis of both gastric and duodenal ulcers (60% in the US and 90% in other parts of the world). Ulcerogenic activity of *H. pylori* is based on several mechanisms:
i. By reducing mucosal defense mechanism through the secretion of bacterial enzymes (urease, protease, catalase, phospholipase)
ii. By stimulating the host mucosal and inflammatory cells to release proinflammatory cytokines.
iii. By direct mucosal epithelial cell injury with cytotoxic proteins, e.g. cytotoxin-associated gene protein A (CogA) and vacuolating cytotoxin A (VacA)

III. *Other risk factors* These are too numerous to list, and thus only some of the most important ones are listed as under:
i. NSAIDs, which may cause mucosal injury in the stomach and duodenum and inhibit synthesis of prostaglandins which play an important role in mucosal protection.
ii. Old age (>70 years).
iii. Chronic gastritis, which is usually found in the gastric mucosa adjacent to gastric peptic ulcer.
iv. Local irritants like alcohol, smoking, spiced foods, non-buffered aspirin.
v. Psychological factors.
vi. Hormonal and metabolic factors that account for the appearance of peptic ulcers in patients with cirrhosis of the liver, chronic renal failure, hyperparathyroidism, COPD and chronic pancreatitis.

vii. Genetic predisposition, as evidenced by familial occurrence of duodenal peptic ulcers, concordance in monozygotic twins, and association with HLA-B5 haplotype.

Q21. What are the main pathologic features of chronic peptic ulcers?

Location Duodenal ulcers are more common than gastric (4:1). Uncommon locations include ulcer in the cardia, marginal ulcer on the gastro-jejunal anastomosis and Meckel diverticulum **(Fig. 20.9)**.

- *Gastric ulcers* are most often located along the lesser curvature in the region of the pyloric antrum, usually on the posterior wall.
- *Duodenal ulcers* are most often found in the first part of the duodenum, immediately past the pylorus.
- Most ulcers are *solitary* but in about 10–20% cases gastric and duodenal ulcers are coexistent.
- Multiple ulcers, ulcers in unusual locations and ulcers that are resistant to standard therapy are found in association with gastrin-secreting tumours (Zollinger-Ellison syndrome).

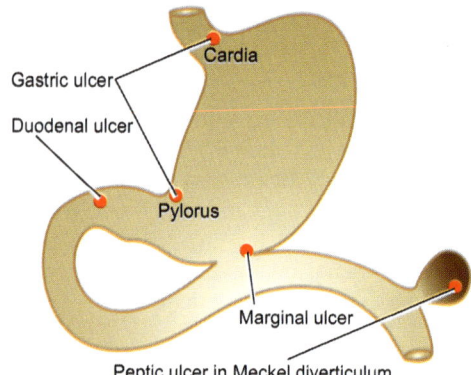

FIGURE 20.9: Distribution of peptic ulcers.

Macroscopic features
i. Small size (<2.5 cm).
ii. Round or oval in shape, quite regular.
iii. Punched out appearance, flat margins, haemorrhagic at its base.
iv. In contrast to them, ulcerated gastric carcinomas are larger and of irregular shape, bowl-like, and have rolled-up indurated margins **(Fig. 20.10)**.

Microscopy There are four distinct zones **(Fig. 20.11)**:
i. Necrotic zone
ii. Superficial exudative zone
iii. Granulation tissue zone
iv. Zone of fibrosis and cicatrisation

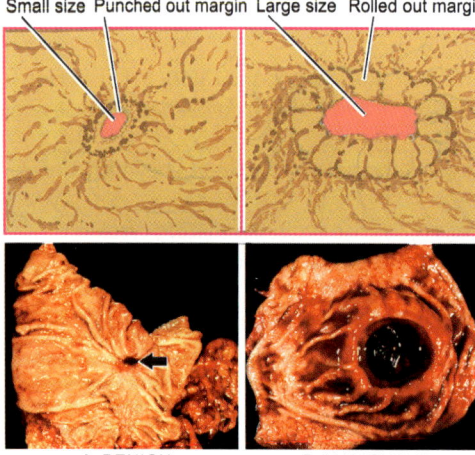

FIGURE 20.10: Chronic gastric ulcer (A) contrasted with malignant gastric ulcer (B). A, Sharp punched out oval small benign ulcer on the mucosa, about 1 cm in diameter (arrow). B, Ulcer which is large with haemorrhage at the base and overhanging margins, likely to be malignant.

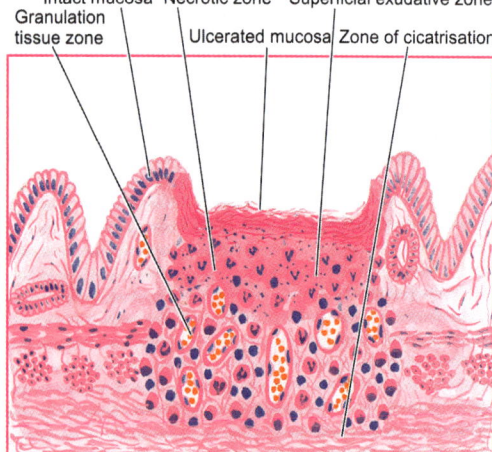

FIGURE 20.11: Chronic peptic ulcer. Histologic zones of the ulcer are illustrated in the diagram. The photomicrograph on right shows necrotic debris, ulceration and inflammation on the mucosal surface.

Q22. What are the major complications of peptic ulcers?

With modern therapy, complications of peptic ulcers have become uncommon. Besides haemorrhage which is found in one out of 6 patients, all other complications listed here occur in only 2–5% of all peptic ulcer patients.

I. **Haemorrhage** is a common symptom and also, in a massive form, it may be a major complication.
- Gastric ulcers cause more often haematemesis with black 'coffee ground' material in it, whereas duodenal ulcers cause more often melaena.
- A penetrating chronic ulcer may erode a major artery and cause massive bleeding, which may be even lethal.
- Chronic bleeding will cause iron deficiency anaemia.

II. **Obstruction** results due to oedema or scarring and stenosis of the pyloric canal, but can occur in the duodenum as well.
- Scarring of gastric ulcer along the lesser curvature may produce 'hourglass deformity' seen by X-rays due to fibrosis and contracture.

III. **Perforation** occurs rarely and is seen more often in duodenal than gastric ulcers.
- It is recognised radiologically by detecting air under the diaphragm.
- Contamination of the peritoneal cavity by food and bacteria through the perforation leads to peritonitis.

IV. **Penetration into the pancreas** is a rare complication of deep chronic posterior wall duodenal ulcers. It is accompanied by deep pain and an elevation of pancreatic enzymes in serum.

NOTE: *Malignant transformation* of gastric ulcer occurs in less than 1% of cases and it never occurs in duodenal ulcers. It is, however, quite possible that even in these cases the early gastric cancers were misdiagnosed as ulcers, and that no 'malignant transformation' ever took place. The time-proven dictum is: *'cancers ulcerate but ulcers rarely cancerate'*.

Q23. What are the major clinical features of peptic ulcers?

I. **Age:** 5th decade for duodenal ulcers and a decade later for gastric ulcers.
II. **People at risk**: Duodenal ulcers in high stress profession (e.g. executives, doctors), whereas gastric ulcers are more common in labouring groups.
III. **Periodicity:** The attacks of gastric ulcers last 2–6 weeks with quiescent intervals of 1–6 months.
IV. **Pain** is epigastric.
- In gastric ulcer patients, it occurs immediately or within 2 hours after food intake, and never at night.
- In duodenal ulcer, pain is severe, occurs at night ('hunger pain') and associated with 'water brash' (burning fluid into the mouth). Heart-burn (retrosternal pain) is common.

V. **Vomiting** that relieves the pain is a conspicuous feature in gastric ulcer patients. Vomiting is not seen in duodenal ulcer patients.
VI. **Haematemesis** and melaena occur more often in duodenal than gastric ulcer patients. The ratio of haematemesis to melaena is 60:40 in gastric and 40:60 in duodenal ulcer patients.
VII. **Appetite** is good but gastric patients are afraid to eat, in contrast to duodenal ulcer patients who are not afraid to eat. Gastric cancer patients get used to bland diet, whereas duodenal ulcer patients eat normal food.
VIII. **Weigh loss** is a common finding in gastric ulcer patients but is not seen in those with duodenal ulcers.
IX. **Deep tenderness** on palpation is demonstrable in both peptic ulcer types.

Q24. Tabulate the salient contrasting features of two major forms of peptic ulcer (duodenal *versus* gastric ulcer).

Major features distinguishing duodenal from gastric ulcers are presented in **Table 20.1**.

Q25. Classify the main gastric tumours and tumour-like lesions.

The WHO classification of benign and malignant gastric tumours and premalignant lesions is given **Table 20.2**.

TABLE 20.1 Distinguishing features of two major forms of peptic ulcers.

FEATURE	DUODENAL ULCER	GASTRIC ULCER
1. *Incidence*	i. Four times more common than gastric ulcers ii. Usual age 25–50 years iii. More common in males than in females (4:1)	Less common than duodenal ulcers Usually beyond 6th decade More common in males than in females (3.5:1)
2. *Etiology*	i. Most commonly as a result of *H. pylori* infection ii. Other factors—hypersecretion of acid-pepsin, association with alcoholic cirrhosis, tobacco, hyperparathyroidism, chronic pancreatitis, blood group O, genetic factors	i. Gastric colonisation with *H. pylori* asymptomatic but higher chances of development of duodenal ulcer ii. Disruption of mucus barrier most important factor iii. Association with gastritis, bile reflux, drugs, alcohol, tobacco
3. *Pathogenesis*	i. Mucosal digestion from hyperacidity most significant factor ii. Protective gastric mucus barrier may be damaged	Usually normal-to-low acid levels; hyperacidity if present is due to high serum gastrin Damage to mucus barrier significant factor
4. *Pathologic changes*	i. Most common in the first part of duodenum ii. Often solitary, 1–2.5 cm in size, round to oval, punched out iii. Histologically, composed of four layers—necrotic, superficial exudative, granulation tissue and cicatrisation	Most common along the lesser curvature and pyloric antrum Grossly similar to duodenal ulcer Histologically, indistinguishable from duodenal ulcer
5. *Complications*	Commonly haemorrhage, perforation, sometimes obstruction; malignant transformation never occurs	Perforation, haemorrhage and at times obstruction; malignant transformation in less than 1% cases
6. *Clinical features*	i. Pain-food-relief pattern ii. Night pain common iii. No vomiting iv. Melaena more common than haematemesis v. No loss of weight vi. No particular choice of diet vii. Deep tenderness in the right hypochondrium viii. Marked seasonal variation ix. Occurs more commonly in people at greater stress	Food-pain pattern No night pain Vomiting common Haematemesis more common Significant loss of weight Patients choose bland diet devoid of fried foods, curries, etc. Deep tenderness in the midline in epigastrium No seasonal variation More often in labouring groups

Q26. What are gastric polyps? Discuss salient features of the main types.

Definition Polyps are tumour-like mucosal protrusions, which could represent tumour-like benign lesions or true neoplasm; these cannot be distinguished from one another without microscopic examination.

Types On microscopy, they can be classified as i) hyperplastic and/or reactive, ii) fundic gland, iii) inflammatory fibroid polyp, and iv) neoplastic/adenomatous polyps.

I. **Hyperplastic or inflammatory polyps** are reactive non-neoplastic lesions, accounting 30–40% of gastric polyps.
Clinical and gross They may be pedunculated or sessile, and show surface ulceration or haemorrhage.
Microscopy They are mostly composed of irregular hyperplastic mucus-secreting foveolar glands, which are often dilated. The stroma surrounding the glands usually contains chronic inflammatory cells.

II. **Fundic gland polyps** are the most common gastric polyps seen in clinical practice.
Clinical and gross They are usually small (<0.5 cm), and do not cause symptoms but are discovered incidentally during endoscopy.
In a minority of cases, they are part of adenomatous polyposis syndrome or the Zollinger-Ellison syndrome.
Microscopy They are composed of dilated oxynthic glands lined by parietal and chief cells.

III. **Inflammatory fibroid polyps** are small mucosal polyps of the stomach composed of benign spindle cells and inflammatory cells including prominent eosinophils. Similar polyps occur in the intestines.

IV. **Adenomatous polyps** (also called **gastric adenomas**) are true benign neoplasms similar to colonic adenomatous polyps, but less common. They account for only 10% of gastric polyps but are clinically the most important since they can undergo malignant transformation in about 30% cases.

Q27. What are gastrointestinal stromal tumours (GISTs)? Discuss their pathogenesis and morphologic features.

Definition GISTs are mesenchymal tumours of the GI tract composed of spindle cells that have acquired proliferation promoting gain-of-function mutations of *KIT* gene; less often the gene encoding *platelet derived growth factor receptor-α (PDGFRA)*, and rarely genes for *BRAF* or *succinate dehydrogenase (SDH) complex*.

Molecular biology KIT, a transmembrane receptor protein kinase is normally activated by its ligand called stem cell factor or Steel factor. Stem cell factor binding results in homodimerisation of the inactive KIT and autophosphorylation of the intracellular tyrosine residues, exposing it to the action of intracellular transduction molecules. All this results in transmission of pro-mitotic signals to the nucleus, initiating cell division and proliferation.

- In GISTs, the mutation of *KIT* gene leads to *constitutive phosphorylation* tyrosine kinase that does not require the stem cell factor binding.
- This *ligand-independent activation* of KIT drives the GIST cell proliferation, which can be inhibited by *tyrosine kinase inhibitors* such as imatinib.
- Similar pro-mitotic signal are generated by other mutations in GIST cells.
- *KIT* gene mutation is found in 75–85% of GISTs, 8–10% have *PDGFRA* mutations, whereas other genes are mutated rarely.
- Most tumours are sporadic but a few originate in families affected by neurofibromatosis type 1 and in association with paragangliomas related to a loss of SDH complex function.
- Tumours that occur in these genetically predisposed persons occur before the age of 40 years, in contrast to sporadic GISTs which are most often diagnosed around the 60 years of age.

Pathology GISTs have an overall incidence of 15 per million.

Location They are most often (60%) found in the stomach. Other parts of the GI tract and mesentery give rise to the rest, and some tumours occur even outside of the abdominal cavity.

Clinical and gross The tumours begin as small microscopic nodules in the submucosa or muscularis propria.

- Most of these nodules, which are often seen in resected stomachs, remain small and only less than 0.5 per 1000 continue proliferating to form visible tumours.
- At the time of diagnosis, the tumours are typically submucosal varying in size from one to several centimetres in diameter.
- Tumours typically protrude underneath the mucosa, which remains intact but stretched over the small tumours **(Fig. 20.12)**. Larger tumours cause mucosal ulceration or obstruct the lumen.

TABLE 20.2 The WHO classification of gastric tumours*.

A. Epithelial benign/premalignant lesions
1. Adenoma
2. Intraepithelial neoplasia (low-grade, high-grade)

B. Epithelial malignant tumours

I. *Carcinomas (90%)*
   1. Adenocarcinoma
      i. Intestinal type
      ii. Diffuse type
   2. Papillary adenocarcinoma
   3. Tubular adenocarcinoma
   4. Mucinous adenocarcinoma
   5. Signet-ring adenocarcinoma
   6. Adenosquamous carcinoma
   7. Squamous cell carcinoma
   8. Small cell carcinoma
   9. Undifferentiated carcinoma

II. *Carcinoid tumour (3%)*

C. Non-epithelial tumours (6%)
1. Leiomyoma
2. Schwannoma
3. Granular cell tumour
4. Glomus tumour
5. Leiomyosarcoma
6. Gastrointestinal stromal tumour (GIST)
7. Kaposi sarcoma
8. Malignant lymphomas

D. Secondary tumours (1%)

*Bosman et al. WHO classification of tumours of the digestive system. 4th edition. IARC Lyon, 2010;48-58.

- Large tumours metastasise to other parts of the GI tract, mesentery and peritoneum or the liver. Extra-abdominal metastases are uncommon.

Microscopy GISTs are composed of:

i. *Spindle cells* resembling smooth muscle cells.

ii. Their nuclear features vary from well differentiated to highly anaplastic. The mitotic activity also varies.

iii. Typically, these cells show immunohistochemical reactivity with antibody to *CD117* (another name for the *KIT*).

Clinical features GISTs are quite often asymptomatic or produce nonspecific abdominal complaints.

- Many are discovered incidentally during the work-up for such nonspecific gastrointestinal symptoms.
- Some may cause bleeding with haematemesis or melaena.
- Large tumours and those that have spread through the abdominal cavity cause mass effects such as compression, obstruction or pain.

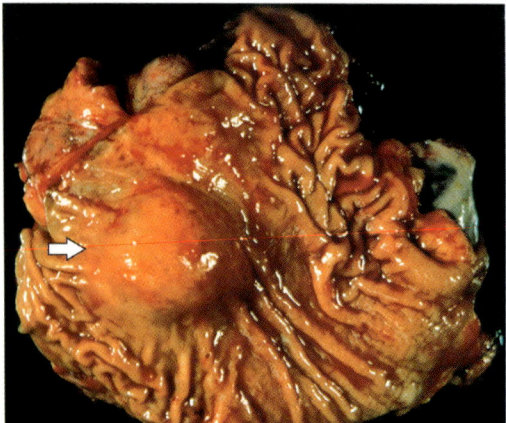

FIGURE 20.12: Gastrointestinal stromal tumour (GIST). Submucosal tumour protruding into lumen of the stomach shown with an arrow. The surface of the tumour is covered by intact mucosa.

Prognosis depends on the size of the tumour, mitotic activity and the site of origin.

- Tumours that are large and have high mitotic activity are more likely to recur or to metastasise than the smaller tumours.
- Gastric tumours have a better prognosis than intestinal GISTs.
- Most tumours respond to the treatment with tyrosine kinase inhibitor, but after some time many develop resistance to treatment.

Q28. What are the main clinicopathologic features of gastric carcinoma?

Definition Gastric carcinoma is in most instances (90%) an adenocarcinoma and is the second most common cause of cancer mortality worldwide.

Etiology Not fully elucidated and most likely multifactorial. The following are the risk factors identified in epidemiologic studies:

i. *Infection with Helicobacter pylori* is associated with 3–6 time higher risk.

ii. *Dietary factors* play an important role as evidenced by higher incidence in populations eating dried, salted and smoked fish and red meat, possibly related to high content of nitrates which are converted in human body to carcinogenic nitrites. Consumption of fresh green leafy vegetables reduces the risk of gastric cancer.

iii. *Alcohol and smoking* increase the risk.

iv. *Geographic differences* in the incidence of gastric cancer suggest possible effects of environmental factors in countries with high incidence (Japan, Korea, Italy, Chile).

- Japanese immigrants to North America have a much lower incidence of gastric cancer than in Japan.
- Decreased incidence of gastric cancer since 1930s in highly developed countries like the US and Western Europe could be related to the changing eating habits and refrigeration of food.

v. *Genetic factors* play a role as evidenced by racial differences: high incidence of gastric cancer in American Blacks, Chinese in Indonesia and in Indians.

- Familiar incidence of gastric cancer is noted only in 4% of patients, suggesting a minor role for the genetic factors. Families with mutation of *E-cadherin* gene have a genetic predisposition for gastric cancer.

vi. *Association with certain pathologic conditions* in the stomach indicates that gastric cancer is at least sometimes preceded by premalignant changes such as under:

- Atrophic gastritis with intestinal metaplasia and hypochlorhydria.
- Chronic gastric ulcer in association with achlorhydria.
- Adenomatous polyps of the stomach.

- Stump carcinoma in patients who have undergone partial gastrectomy.

Pathology

Location Gastric cancers are not evenly distributed in all parts of the stomach. They most often develop in the pyloric canal and least often in the fundus **(Fig. 20.13)**.

Two basic forms of gastric carcinoma are recognised developing from carcinoma in situ:

I. ***Early gastric carcinoma*** is limited to mucosa and submucosa. In countries like Japan, systematic search for early carcinoma has significantly reduced the incidence of invasive gastric cancer, and 35% of all cancers are in the early stage. Resection of early cancer is associated with a survival of 93–99%.

II. ***Advanced gastric carcinoma*** is the term used for cancers that have invaded into the muscularis propria or deeper.

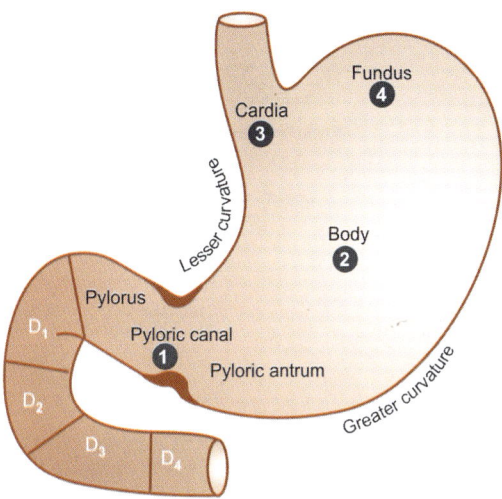

FIGURE 20.13: Distribution of gastric carcinoma in the anatomical subdivisions of the stomach. The serial numbers in the figure indicate the order of frequency of occurrence of gastric cancer.

Gross Various forms of advanced carcinoma are as follows **(Fig. 20.14)**:

i. *Ulcerative carcinoma,* which is the most common form. It appears as a prepyloric ulcer which has a necrotic base and raised margins.

ii. *Fungating carcinoma (polypoid)* is the second most common pattern, presenting as a cauliflower growth projecting into the lumen. It is more often seen in the cardia and fundus.

iii. *Scirrhous carcinoma (linitis plastica)* in which the tumour cells infiltrate the gastric wall diffusely giving it the appearance of a 'leather bottle'.

iv. *Colloid (mucoid) carcinoma* containing large amounts of gelatinous mucus, is usually found in the fundus.

Microscopy Four types are recognised by WHO **(Fig. 20.14)**:

i. *Tubular carcinoma,* the most common form, composed of tubular glands.

ii. *Papillary carcinoma* formed of cells lining the protruding papillae with fibrovascular cores.

iii. *Signet ring carcinoma* composed of dissociated cells filled with mucus, which is pushing the nucleus in a signet ring form.

iv. *Mucinous carcinoma* which is rich in extracellular mucus surrounding the signet ring cells in >50% of tumour tissue.

Spread of gastric carcinoma occurs locally (most often), or in form of distant metastases as under:

i. *Lymphatic spread* to local lymph nodes along the lesser or greater curvature.

ii. *Distant metastases* to the supraclavicular lymph node (*Virchow node* or *Troisier sign*) may sometimes be a presenting sign of gastric carcinoma.

iii. *Transcoelomic spread* in the abdominal cavity and often involving the ovaries bilaterally (*Krukenberg tumours*)

iv. *Haematogenous spread* most often to the liver and lungs, may involve other organs as well.

Clinical features vary and include the following:

i. Abdominal pain

ii. Gastric distention and vomiting

iii. Weight loss (cachexia) and loss of appetite (anorexia)

iv. Anaemia, weakness and malaise

Complications include: haemorrhage with haematemesis and melaena, obstruction, perforation and obstructive jaundice.

Prognosis for advanced gastric carcinomas is abysmal, with a 5-year survival rate in the range of 5–15%.

Q29. What are gastric lymphomas?

Definition Gastric lymphomas can originate as *primary* gastric neoplasms or as *secondary* lymphomas that originate in the lymph nodes and spread to the stomach thereafter.

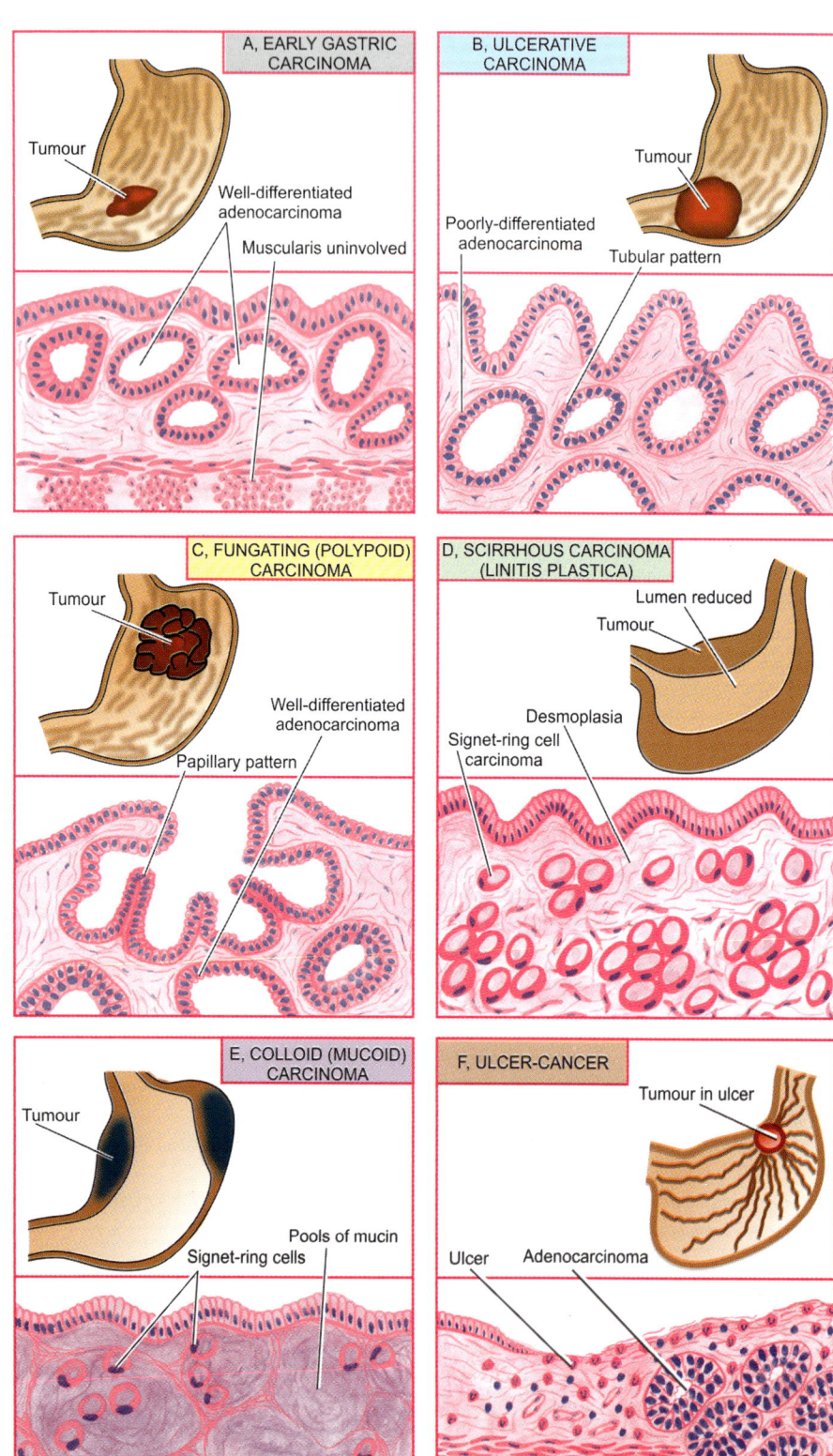

FIGURE 20.14: Gastric carcinoma, gross appearance of subtypes and their corresponding dominant histological patterns.

- Overall, lymphomas do not account for more than 5% of all gastric neoplasms. Yet, the stomach harbours 60% of all GI tract lymphomas and is thus the most commonly involved part of the GI tract.

Pathology

Gross Gastric lymphoma may infiltrate the wall of the stomach diffusely or it may present in form of a solitary or multiple polyps.

Microscopy There are two types of lymphoma :
- Low grade extranodal marginal zone B-cell lymphomas (MALToma) arising from the mucosa associated lymphoid tissue, related to *H. pylori* infection.
- High grade diffuse large B cell lymphoma (DLBCL)

MALTomas represent the most common form of lymphoma.

Prognosis MALTomas respond well to treatment of *H. pylori* infection. DLBCL requires aggressive chemotherapy.

Q30. Tabulate the differences between benign and malignant gastric ulcer.

Differences between benign and malignant gastric ulcer are summarised in **Table 20.3** (*also see* **Fig. 20.10**).

TABLE 20.3 Differences between benign and malignant gastric ulcers.

FEATURE	BENIGN ULCER	MALIGNANT ULCER
1. *Age*	Younger age	Older age
2. *Sex*	Markedly common in males	Slightly common in males
3. *Duration of symptoms*	Weeks to years	Weeks to months
4. *Location*	Commonly lesser curvature of pylorus and antrum	Commonly greater curvature of pylorus and antrum
5. *Gross features*		
a. *Size*	Small	Large
b. *Shape*	Regular	Irregular
c. *Mucosal folds*	Radiating	Interrupted
d. *Ulcer bed*	Haemorrhagic	Necrotic
6. *Barium studies*	Punched out ulcer	Irregular filling defect
7. *Acidity*	Usually normal-to-low	May be normal-to-even achlorhydria
8. *Therapy*	Responds well to medical therapy	Usually does not respond to medical therapy

SMALL INTESTINE

Q31. What are cells of the intestinal mucosa?

Intestinal mucosa forms *plicae* which extend into *villi* to increase the absorptive surface of the intestine. In the basal portion or deeper part of the mucosa, there are invaginations called *crypts*.

Intestinal villi contain three types of cells:

i. *Simple columnar cells* which have an absorptive function.

ii. *Goblet cells* that secrete mucus.

iii. *Endocrine cells* that secrete polypeptide hormones.

In the intestinal crypts, there are also *Paneth cells* and intestinal *stem cells* which are capable of differentiating into other cell types to replace other cells, which are regularly deleted by apoptosis.

Q32. Briefly describe the features of Meckel diverticulum.

Definition Meckel diverticulum is a congenital outpouching on of the ileum representing an incompletely involuted foetal vitellointestinal (omphalomesenteric) duct.

Clinicopathologic features Meckel diverticulum is found in 2% of population. On an average, it is 3–6 cm long. In most instances, there are no symptoms, but in 2% of those who have Meckel diverticulum it is symptomatic.

Location It is located 1 metre proximally from the ileocaecal valve on the antimesenteric border of the ileum **(Fig. 20.15)**. This location of Meckel diverticulum is important for the following reasons: if an *acute diverticulitis* develops, the symptoms will resemble those of acute appendicitis, except that the pain is centered on the left side of the lower abdomen.

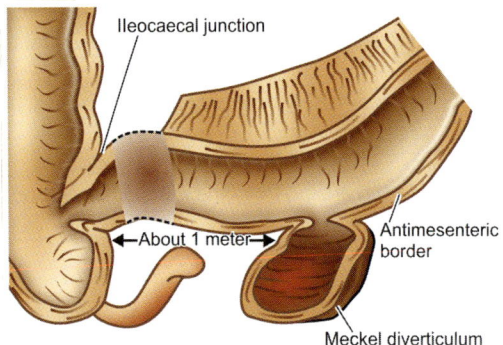

FIGURE 20.15: Meckel diverticulum. Common location and gross appearance.

Microscopy It is lined by intestinal mucosa, but it may contains islands of ectopic pancreatic or gastric mucosa, which may undergo *peptic ulceration*, resulting in *bleeding and haematochezia*. Other less common complications include volvulus and perforation with peritonitis.

Q33. What is intestinal obstruction? Discuss various etiologic factors in its pathogenesis. What are its common clinical features and complications?

Definition Intestinal obstruction is a mechanical or functional pathologic process that prevents the normal passage of intestinal contents.

Etiopathogenesis Obstruction can involve the small or the large bowel. The causes can be classified as mechanical, or functional as under:

I. **Mechanical obstruction** can be either internal or external:

i. *Internal obstruction (intraluminal or intramural)*:
- Congenital stenosis, atresia or imperforate anus
- Meconium in cystic fibrosis
- Inflammatory strictures (e.g. Crohn disease)
- Roundworms (*Toxocara canis*)
- Tumours
- Foreign bodies, faecaliths, gallstones
- Ulcerations caused by potassium chloride tablets to counter hypokalaemia

ii. *External compression*:
- Peritoneal adhesions and bands; most often they are residues of healed inflammation of the peritoneum.
- Strangulated hernia
- Intussusception
- Volvulus
- Intra-abdominal tumour (e.g. pseudomyxoma peritonei, peritoneal metastases of ovarian cancer)

II. **Functional obstruction:**

i. Paralytic ileus due to neuro-muscular paralysis of intestines after abdominal surgery or in peritonitis.

ii. Intestinal infarction following vascular obstruction of the superior mesenteric artery, caused by thrombi, thromboemboli or accidental ligation during surgery.

Complications i) Bowel ischaemia and necrosis, ii) perforation with peritonitis, iii) sepsis, and iv) shock.

Clinical features Signs and symptoms of intestinal obstruction include:

i. Abdominal pain increasing in intensity, with or without colics
ii. Vomiting and dehydration
iii. Abdominal bloating and inability to pass gas
iv. X-ray examination in upright position reveals multiple fluid levels, but CT is more informative

Prognosis Treatment depends on the etiology of obstruction and may be conservative or surgical. There is high mortality.

Q34. What is hernia?

Definition Hernia is protrusion of portion of a viscus through an abnormal opening in the wall of its natural cavity.

Clinicopathologic features
i. Inguinal hernia is the most common and it occurs through the inguinal canal.
ii. Less common are femoral and umbilical hernias.
iii. The hernial sac is composed of connective tissue which is usually internally lined with a mesothelial layer.
iv. Mechanical irritation or infection of the content may cause acute and chronic inflammatory changes and fibrous adhesions.

Clinical classification Hernias can be classified as follows:
i. *Reducible hernia* is one where the contents of the hernial sac can be repositioned into the abdominal cavity.
ii. *Irreducible hernia* is one where the contents of the hernia cannot be returned into the abdominal cavity because of their bulky size or because there are adhesions that prevent repositioning.
iii. *Strangulated hernia* is one with a constricted neck or fibrous adhesions obstructing the arterial or venous blood flow. Ischaemia is typically accompanied by infarction or gangrene of the strangulated intestine.

Q35. Discuss intussusceptions briefly.

Definition Intestinal intussusception is invagination, also known as telescoping, of a segment of intestine into the segment below due to the propulsive effects of peristalsis **(Fig. 20.16)**.

- The segment protruding into the distal intestinal lumen is called *intussusceptum* and the segment receiving it is called *intussuscipiens*.
- External compression of the arteries providing the blood to the intussusceptum may cause its infarction or gangrene, perforation and peritonitis.

Clinical features Intussusception may occur at an early age or in adulthood.
i. Intussusception occurs more often in infants and young children.
- Typically, it occurs in the ileocaecal region with distal ileum invaginating into the colon.
- The cause is not known, but it is presumed that it results from lymphoid hyperplasia of terminal ileums which serves as the leading edge for the propulsion of ileal loops into the caecum.
- Ileo-ileal and colic-colic intussusceptions are less common.
ii. In adults, the tip of the intussusceptum may contain a tumour or a foreign body wedged into the intestinal loop.

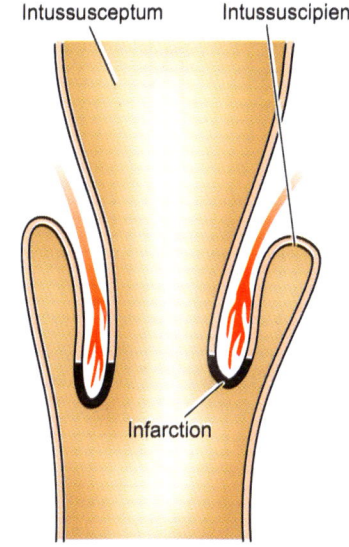

FIGURE 20.16: Ileocaecal intussusception.

Q36. What is volvulus?

Definition Volvulus is twisting of loop of intestine upon itself through 180 degree or more.
Pathogenesis Intestinal rotation leads to obstruction of the intestine and compromise of blood supply.
- Twisting of the mesentery which contains the blood vessels will cut-off the blood supply for the affected loop.
- The usual causes are peritoneal adhesions and bands (congenital or acquired) and congenitally long mesenteric attachment.
- Sigmoid colon is the most often affected intestinal segment and it occurs more often than the volvulus of small intestinal loops.

Clinicopathologic features Ischaemia will cause necrosis or gangrene of the intestinal loop, rupture of intestinal wall and peritonitis.
- Clinically, it presents with intensive pain of sudden onset and rapid development of shock due to sepsis.

Q37. What is ischaemic bowel disease? What are its main types?

Definition Ischaemic bowel disease is an acute or chronic disease resulting from inadequate blood supply to the small or large intestine. The anatomic features of the GI tract, including a generous blood supply through anastomosing blood vessels, accounts for the fact that ischaemia involves the small and large intestine, whereas the stomach, duodenum and anus are spared.

Classification Depending upon the extent and severity of ischaemia, three pathological patterns are recognised **(Fig. 20.17)**:
i. Mucosal ischaemia.
ii. Mural involving the inner part of the intestine including the inner part of the muscularis propria.
iii. Transmural involving the full thickness ischaemic necrosis and gangrene of the bowel.

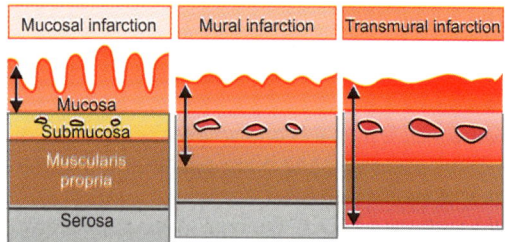

FIGURE 20.17: Schematic diagram to show the three types of ischaemic bowel disease depending upon the extent of involvement.

Q38. Discuss main features of transmural intestinal infarction.

Definition Transmural infarction is a full-thickness necrosis of the bowel wall, most often caused by arterial or venous thrombi.

Etiopathogenesis Following are the common causes in development of full-thickness intestinal infarction:

i. *Mesenteric arterial thrombosis* usually superimposed on mesenteric artery atherosclerosis. It may be a complication of aortic aneurysm. Other causes of arterial obstruction (e.g. polyarteritis or invasions of artery by tumours) are less common.

ii. *Mesenteric artery embolism* may originate from mural thrombi overlying a left ventricular infarct of the heart, endocarditis, or aortic mural thrombi overlying ulcerated atheromas.

iii. *Mesenteric venous occlusion* may be a complication of abdominal inflammation (e.g. appendicitis or peritonitis), portal vein thrombosis in cirrhosis, or mesenteric tumours.

iv. *Miscellaneous causes* affecting more than one type of mesenteric vessels, such as strangulated hernia, volvulus.

Pathology Necrosis of any segment of the small or large intestine may be found depending on the artery involved.

Grossly, the resected specimen or at autopsy may reveal thrombi in the major arteries or veins.

- If the patient survives the thrombotic event for a few days, thrombi may get lysed and may be difficult to find them at autopsy.
- Irrespective of the causes, infarctions of the intestine are always haemorrhagic (red) **(Fig. 20.18)**.
- The wall of the infarcted segment is oedematous and haemorrhagic, and thus initially red, moist and thickened.
- Thereafter, it becomes purple and covered with a fibrinous layer on the serosa, whereas the content of the intestinal loop is suffused with blood.
- In arterial occlusion, the margin between the infarcted area and the normal intestines is sharp, whereas in the venous occlusion the infarcted area merges imperceptibly with the normal.

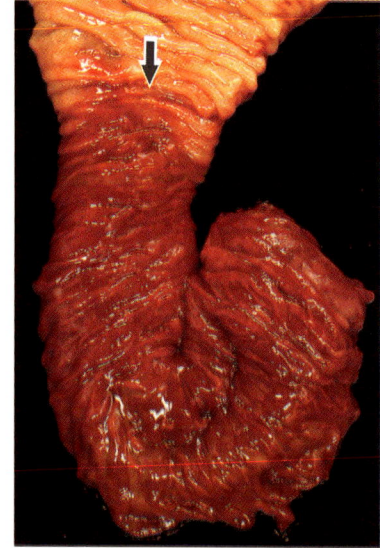

FIGURE 20.18: Haemorrhagic infarct. Small intestine shows swollen, dark tan coloured serosa while the adjacent viable intestine is light brown in colour (arrow).

Microscopy
i. Necrosis of all layers, sloughing off of the necrotic mucosa and haemorrhage into the infarcted tissue.
ii. Small intramural and mesenteric blood vessels may contain thrombi.
iii. Serosal surface is covered with a fibrin-rich haemorrhagic layer.
iv. In colonic infarcts, the most common site is the splenic flexure, corresponding to the area at the border between the supply area of the superior and inferior mesenteric arteries.
Clinical features Intestinal transmural infarction is a catastrophic event requiring surgical resection of the infarcted segment. It presents with severe abdominal pain and prostration and an early onset of hypotensive shock.
Prognosis It has a high mortality due to progressive shock, and major complications such as intestinal rupture with peritonitis or sepsis.

Q39. What are salient features of intestinal mural and mucosal infarction?

Definition Intestinal mural and mucosal infarction is necrosis caused by non-occlusive hypoperfusion and limited to superficial layers of the bowel sparing the external layers and the serosa. Clinically, it presents as haemorrhagic gastroenteropathy.
Etiopathogenesis: Non-occlusive hypoperfusion can be caused by several conditions as under:
i. Shock
ii. Cardiac failure
iii. Infections
iv. Drugs that cause vasoconstriction (e.g. digitalis, norepinephrine, etc.)
Pathology *Grossly,* any segment of the small or large bowel may be affected. The length of these segments varies.
- On the mucosal side, the affected intestinal segment appears red but there is no serosal involvement.
- There is no fibrin exudation on the serosa.

Microscopy
- Foci of ischaemic necrosis of the mucosa, submucosa and inner muscularis propria.
- Bacterial infection may supervene leading to pseudomembranous enterocolitis.
- Ischaemia involving splenic flexure of the colon may heal by fibrosis and mucosal atrophy, which is typical of *chronic ischaemic colitis.* It may cause colonic stricture.

Clinical features Symptoms include:
i. Vague abdominal pain, nausea, vomiting and diarrhoea, but these are reversible and mostly disappear on their own.
ii. Normal mucosal architecture is restored in superficial lesions, but the deeper lesions may heal by fibrosis.
iii. In chronic ischaemic colitis, vague abdominal pain and problems such as alternating constipation and mild diarrhoea may persist for long time.

Q40. What is necrotising enterocolitis of preterm infants?

Definition Necrotising enterocolitis (NEC) is an acute inflammation of unknown origin, occurring primarily in premature and low-weight infants within the first week of life.
Epidemiology NEC is the most common surgical emergency in premature infants.
Etiopathogenesis It is considered to be an ischaemic bowel disease, probably of multifactorial origin and yet incompletely understood pathogenesis. The following *risk factors* play a role:
i. *Prematurity and low-birth weight* are the major risk factors and 90% of cases are premature or low weigh babies.
ii. *Diseases of prematurity,* such as respiratory distress syndrome and patent ductus arteriosus.
iii. *Congenital malformations* such as congenital heart disease and genetic/chromosomal syndromes.
iv. *Enteric alimentation,* as related to the fact that the onset of symptoms coincides with the introduction of feeding with formula milk substitutes; it correlates with the amount of formula given.
v. *Bacterial infection and sepsis* as documented by positive blood cultures in one third of all cases.
vi. *Maternal cocaine abuse and infections during pregnancy* are also risk factors.

Pathology *Grossly,* NEC preferentially involves the terminal ileum and ascending colon. In the fully developed form, the affected segment of the intestines is dilated, necrotic, haemorrhagic and friable.

Microscopy The changes vary depending on the stage of the disease:
- *Initial changes* are confined to the mucosa which shows oedema, focal haemorrhage and necrosis.
- Necrotic epithelium is then covered with fibrin-rich *pseudomembranes* containing acute inflammatory cells and cell debris.
- Ultimately, necrosis becomes transmural and the intestines may rupture and give rise to *peritonitis*.

Clinical features The disease presents with vomiting, abdominal distention, blood-stained faeces and signs of impending shock.

Prognosis The untreated disease has a very high mortality.
- Surgical resection of necrotic bowel segment is indicated and could have life-saving results.
- Infants that survive develop may develop fibrotic intestinal strictures and so called *short bowel syndrome* with nutritional deficiencies.

Q41. What is inflammatory bowel disease? Discuss main features in its etiopathogenesis.

Definition The term inflammatory bowel disease (IBD) is commonly used to include two idiopathic bowel disease, having many similarities but also quite distinctive morphological and clinical features:
- *Crohn disease or regional enteritis* is characterised by transmural chronic granulomatous inflammation affecting most commonly segments of the terminal ileum and caecum or ascending colon with interposed skip areas; other parts of the GI tract may be affected but less commonly.
- *Ulcerative colitis (UC)* is an idiopathic acute and chronic ulcero-inflammatory colitis. It affects chiefly the mucosa and submucosa of the rectum extending proximally into the descending colon, and sometimes continuously involving the entire length of the large bowel.

Both Crohn disease and ulcerative colitis are primarily bowel disease but also may have systemic involvement in the form of polyarthritis, uveitis, ankylosing spondylitis, skin lesions and hepatic involvement.

Epidemiology Both diseases can occur at any age but begin most often in second or third decades of life, with a smaller peak in the fifth decade.
- IBD shows differences in geographical distribution, with higher prevalence in economically more advanced countries of North America and Western Europe.
- In countries with high prevalence, there are also ethnic and racial differences, with predominance in whites, as compared with other races, and especially in those of Ashkenazi Jewish origin.
- The prevalence if IBD is increasing worldwide, mostly in countries that had lower prevalence before.

Etiopathogenesis IBD is multifactorial. Current clinical and experimental studies point to several possible leads that include: i) genetic predisposition, ii) immunologic factors, iii) microbial factors, and iv) environmental factors **(Fig. 20.19)**.

I. **Genetic predisposition** evidenced by higher prevalence among first-degree relatives of the affected person.

i. Concordance among *monozygotic twins* is 60% for Crohn disease and 15% for UC.

ii. HLA studies show a link with certain *HLA-DRB* haplotypes.

iii. Some *susceptibility genes* have been identified from the study of more than 200 genes, but most of them occur in a minority of patients.

iv. Most commonly mentioned genes are: *NOD2* (nucleotide oligomerisation domain 2) and *CARD 15* (caspase-associated recruitment domain containing protein 15), but their pathogenetic role has not been established.

II. **Immunologic factors** seem to play a role but there is no consensus about the role of various components and the key immune defects.

i. Epidemiologic and clinical studies point to an increased prevalence of IBD in persons with *autoimmune diseases*.

ii. Immunologic testing of patients with IBD often reveals *defects in cell mediated and humoral immunity*.

iii. *Intestinal mucosal immunity* has a role in IBD but no key pathogenetic elements have been identified so far.

iv. Treatment of IBD patients with *immunomodulatory agents* has proven to be clinically useful.

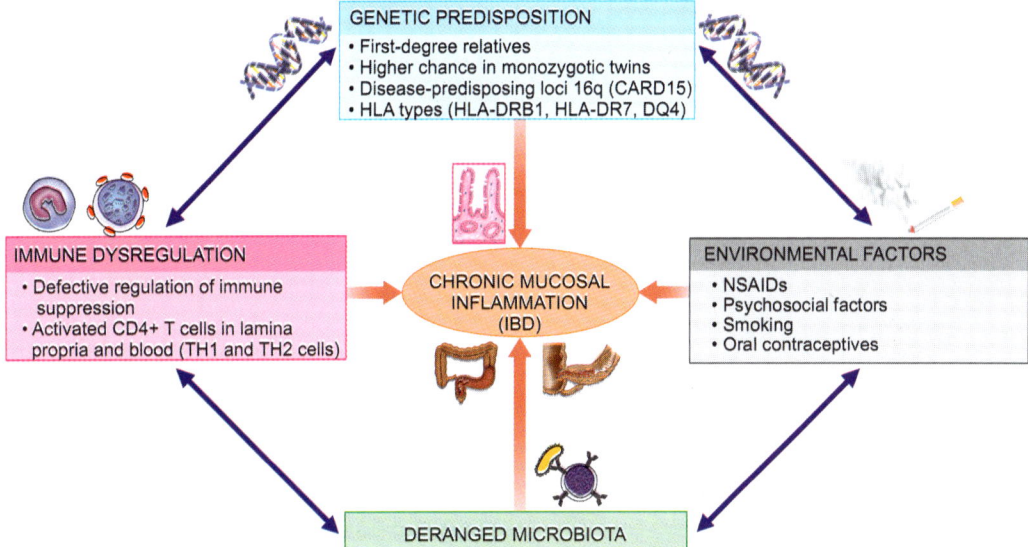

FIGURE 20.19: Schematic pathogenesis of inflammatory bowel disease. In a genetically predisposed individual, derangement of commensal flora and target by environmental factors, result in dysregulation of mucosal immune function that incites chronic inflammation.

III. **Microbial factors** probably play an important role, but so far no definitive evidence has emerged for any particular pathogen to be crucially involved.

IV. **Environmental factors** that could play a role include the use of NSAIDs, psychosocial factors, and paradoxically, the beneficial effects of smoking in UC, compared with the adverse effects of smoking in Crohn disease.

Q42. Discuss salient pathologic features and complications of two forms of inflammatory bowel disease.

There are major differences in pathologic features between Crohn disease and ulcerative colitis. However in 10% cases, there is an overlap between these two diseases and such cases are called 'IBD, indeterminate'

I. **Crohn disease** Involves most often 15–25 cm of terminal ileum often extending into the caecum **(Fig. 20.20, A)**.

Gross Involvement of the intestine is:

i. *Discontinuous* and the affected areas are separated from one another by uninvolved skip areas.
ii. The wall of the affected bowel segment is thick and hard, resembling a '*hose pipe*', narrowing the lumen.
iii. The mucosa has *serpiginous ulcers* with fine granularity of the swollen adjacent mucosa which gives the mucosa a '*cobble-stone*' appearance.
iv. *Deep fissuring* may extend into the deeper layers of the intestine.

Microscopy Shows the following main features **(Fig. 20.20, B)**:

i. Transmural chronic infiltration involving all layers of the intestine.
ii. Noncaseating granulomas found in 60% cases.
iii. Patchy ulceration of the mucosa that may be superficial or deep and is usually associated with chronic inflammation.
iv. Widening of the submucosa due to oedema and prominent lymphoid aggregates.
v. Fibrosis of the muscularis, most prominently intersecting the muscle fibres in chronic cases.

Complications These include structural and functional changes as under:

i. Malabsorption due to impaired absorption of fat, vitamin B_{12}, proteins and electrolytes from the diseased small bowel.
ii. Fistula formation following adhesions of intestinal loops.
iii. Stricture formation.

II. **Ulcerative colitis** Typically begins in the rectum and in continuity extends upwards, so that it may involve the entire large intestine **(Fig. 20.21, A)**.

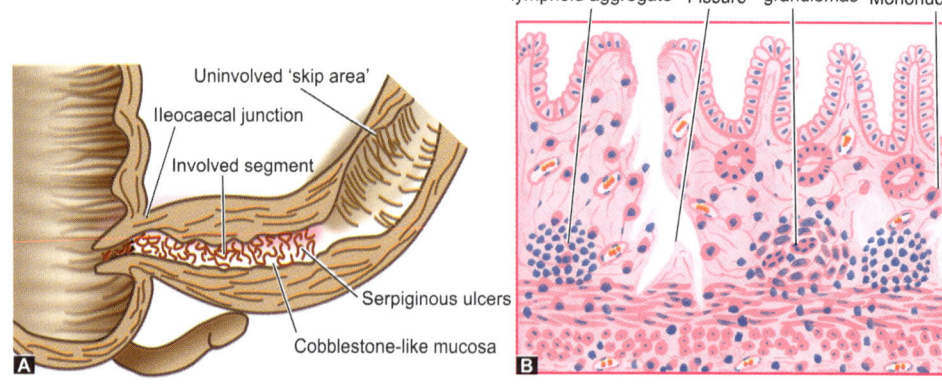

FIGURE 20.20: Crohn disease of the terminal ileum. A, The lesions are characteristically segmental with intervening uninvolved 'skip areas'. The bowel wall is thickened and the lumen narrowed, giving hose-pipe appearance. Serpiginous ulcers, some deep fissures and swollen intervening surviving mucosa giving 'cobblestone appearance', are present. B, The histological features present are: transmural chronic inflammatory cell infiltration, deep fissures into the bowel wall, submucosal widening due to oedema, some prominent lymphoid follicles and a few non-caseating epithelioid cell granulomas in the bowel wall.

Gross Features include:
i. Thickening of the muscle layer due to contraction with a loss of haustral folds leading to a foreshortening the large intestine with smooth external surface (*'garden-hose appearance'*).
ii. Mucosa shows *superficial linear ulcers* not penetrating into the muscularis.
iii. The intervening preserved mucosa forms small protrusions called *'inflammatory pseudopolyps'*.

Microscopy Includes alternating areas of 'active disease' marked by and 'resolving colitis' marked by the following **(Fig. 20.21, B)**:
i. Invasion of colonic crypt epithelium by PMNs *('cryptitis')* is an early event, followed by accumulation of PMNs in the crypts (*crypt abscess*).
ii. Superficial *mucosal ulcerations* not penetrating into the muscle layer and surrounded by dense chronic inflammatory cell infiltrates and scattered groups of PMNs.

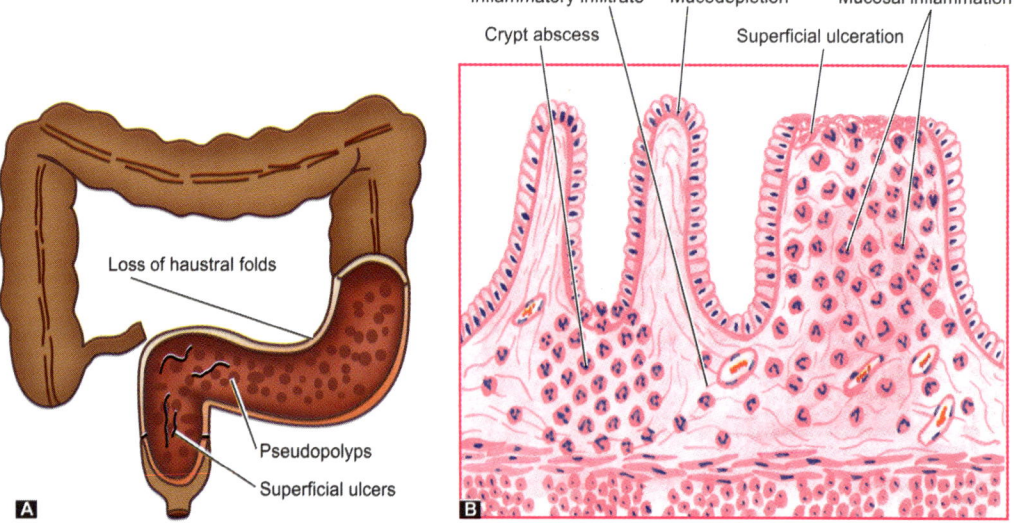

FIGURE 20.21: Ulcerative colitis. A, Continuous involvement of the rectum and colon without any uninvolved skip areas. The ulcers are superficial with intervening inflammatory pseudopolyps. The lumen is narrow and the haustral folds are lost giving 'garden-hose appearance'. B, The microscopic features seen are mucosal infiltration by acute inflammatory cells, mucodepletion, cryptitis and a 'crypt abscess'.

iii. Reduced number of goblet cells in the remaining intact or regenerating epithelium, which may form *'pseudopolyps'* protruding above the surrounding ulcerated mucosa.
iv. Mucosal regeneration is accompanied by *muco-depletion* of lining cells.
v. During colonoscopy, the most visible finding is the *congestion of the mucosa* which looks dark blue-red due to dilation of small mucosal vessels and foci of haemorrhage making the mucosa *friable to touch* and prone to *bleeding.*
vi. In chronic less active cases, there is only *crypt distortion* and *irregular branching* along with chronic inflammation of lamina propria, predominantly lymphocytes.
vii. *Epithelial atypia* ranging from mild to severe and evolving into adenocarcinoma in situ is a feature of long-standing UC (>10 years duration), with numerous bouts of active inflammation.

Complications Major ones are:
i. *Toxic megacolon (fulminant colitis)* with marked dilatation of colon, prone to perforation and faecal peritonitis.
ii. *Perianal fistula*, which develops rarely.
iii. *Carcinoma*, with risk factors as follows: Onset of UC at an early age, pancolitis involving the entire length of the colon, and duration of colitis for more than 10 years.

Q43. Tabulate the major contrasting features of two forms of inflammatory bowel disease.

The distinguishing features of Crohn disease and UC are presented in **Table 20.4**.

TABLE 20.4 Distinguishing features of Crohn disease and ulcerative colitis.

FEATURE	CROHN DISEASE	ULCERATIVE COLITIS
A. MACROSCOPIC FEATURES		
1. *Distribution*	Segmental with skip areas	Continuous without skip areas
2. *Location*	Commonly terminal ileum and/or ascending colon	Commonly rectum, sigmoid colon and extending upwards
3. *Extent*	Usually involves the entire thickness of the affected segment of bowel wall	Usually superficial, confined to mucosal layers
4. *Ulcers*	Serpiginous ulcers, may develop into deep fissures	Superficial mucosal ulcers without fissures
5. *Pseudopolyps*	Rarely seen	Commonly present
6. *Fibrosis*	Common	Rare
7. *Shortening*	Due to fibrosis	Due to contraction of muscularis
B. MICROSCOPIC FEATURES		
1. *Depth of inflammation*	Typically transmural	Mucosal and submucosal
2. *Type of inflammation*	Non-caseating granulomas and infiltrate of mononuclear cells (lymphocytes, plasma cells and macrophages)	Crypt abscess and non-specific acute and chronic inflammatory cells (lymphocytes, plasma cells, neutrophils, eosinophils, mast cells)
3. *Mucosa*	Patchy ulceration	Haemorrhagic mucosa with ulceration
4. *Submucosa*	Widened due to oedema and lymphoid aggregates	Normal or reduced in width
5. *Muscularis*	Infiltrated by inflammatory cells	Usually spared except in cases of toxic megacolon
6. *Fibrosis*	Present	Usually absent
C. IMMUNOLOGIC FEATURES		
1. *Lymphocyte type*	CD4+ T_{H1}	CD4+ T_{H2}
2. *Cytokines*	INF-γ, TNF, IL-12	TGF-β, IL-4, IL-5, IL-13
3. *ANCA-P antibodies*	Positive in a few	Positive in most
D. COMPLICATIONS		
1. *Fistula formation*	Internal and external fistulae in 10% cases	Extremely rare
2. *Malignant changes*	Rare	May occur infrequently in disease of more than 10 years' duration
3. *Type of malignancy*	Lymphoma more often than carcinoma	Carcinoma more often than lymphoma
4. *Fibrous strictures*	Common	Never

Q44. Enumerate common types of infective enterocolitis.

Definition Infective enterocolitis includes a number of inflammatory intestinal diseases caused by bacteria, viruses, fungi, protozoa, or helminths. Some of the most important infective intestinal diseases are listed in **Table 20.5**.

Q45. What is intestinal tuberculosis? Briefly discuss its various forms.

Definition Intestinal tuberculosis is today most often caused by *M. tuberculosis*, in contrast to previous time, i.e. before widespread pasteurisation of milk was introduced, it was caused by *M. bovis*.

Types It occurs in several forms as under (**Fig. 20.22**):
Primary tuberculosis which includes a small intestinal lesion (Ghon focus) and prominent regional lymph node enlargement that contains numerous confluent granulomas showing caseous necrosis. Similar caseating granulomas are found in other forms of tuberculosis as well.

TABLE 20.5 Infective enterocolitis.

A. BACTERIAL ENTEROCOLITIS
1. Entero-invasive bacteria
   i. *M. tuberculosis*
   ii. *Salmonella*
   iii. *Campylobacter jejuni*
   iv. *Shigella*
   v. *Escherichia coli*
   vi. *Yersinia enterocolitica*
2. Enterotoxin-producing bacteria
   i. *Vibrio cholerae*

B. VIRAL ENTEROCOLITIS

C. FUNGAL ENTEROCOLITIS
   i. Candida
   ii. Mucor

D. PROTOZOAL AND METAZOAL INFESTATIONS
   i. *Giardia lamblia*
   ii. *Entamoeba histolytica*
   iii. *Balantidium coli*
   iv. *Taenia solium*
   v. *Ascaris lumbricoides*
   vi. *Ancylostoma duodenale*
   vii. *Strongyloides stercoralis*

Secondary intestinal tuberculosis results from swallowing of infected sputum in patients with pulmonary tuberculosis. It begins in the Peyer patches or mucosal lymphoid follicles of the ileum leading to the formation of ulcers which enlarge laterally forming a larger transverse ulceration. Healing may result in fibrosis casing strictures of obstruction of the intestine.

Hyperplastic ileocaecal tuberculosis is a variant of secondary tuberculosis involving terminal ileum and caecum. The lesion is characterised by mucosal ulceration and thickening of the intestinal wall and external fibrous adhesion with surrounding structures. This form of tuberculosis may resemble colonic carcinoma, from which it must be distinguished.

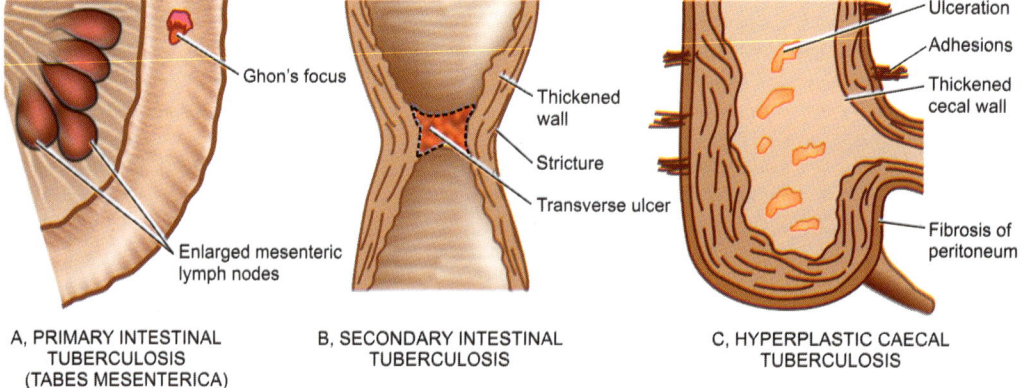

A, PRIMARY INTESTINAL TUBERCULOSIS (TABES MESENTERICA)
B, SECONDARY INTESTINAL TUBERCULOSIS
C, HYPERPLASTIC CAECAL TUBERCULOSIS

FIGURE 20.22: Intestinal tuberculosis, three patterns.

Q46. Discuss salient features of enteric fever.

Definition Enteric fever is an acute infectious intestinal disease caused by *Salmonella typhi* (typhoid fever) or *Salmonella paratyphi* (paratyphoid fever).
NOTE: *Salmonella typhimurium* does not cause enteric fever. It is, however, an important cause of food poisoning.

Pathogenesis Salmonellae are ingested in food or contaminated water. After an asymptomatic incubation period of two weeks, bacilli invade the mucosa of the jejunum and ileum. From here, they enter the Peyer patches and regional lymph nodes where they proliferate causing haemorrhagic lymphadenitis.

Bacteraemia with fever ensues and other many other organs are affected including the skin which shown 'rose spots'.

Pathology In the intestines, the features are:

i. An inflammatory response that includes lymphocytes, plasma cells and macrophages which show erythrophagocytosis. Neutrophils are absent and in the blood there is neutropenia with relative lymphocytosis.

ii. Breakdown of the mucosa overlying the enlarged Peyer patches results in oval longitudinal ulcers **(Fig. 20.23)**.

iii. There is no significant fibrosis and thus the lesions do not cause stricture. Rupture of intestine is more common.

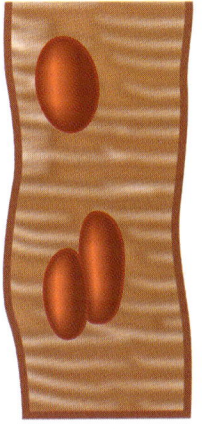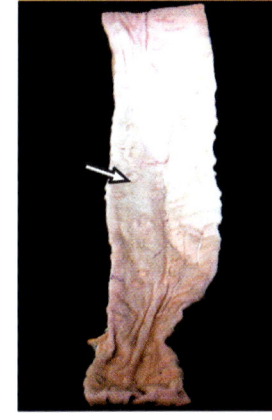

FIGURE 20.23: Typhoid ulcers in the small intestine appear characteristically oval with their long axis parallel to the long axis of the bowel.

Q47. What are the major distinguishing features of intestinal ulcers in intestinal tuberculosis and enteric fever?

Major contrasting features of tuberculous and typhoid ulcers of small intestine are given in **Table 20.6**.

TABLE 20.6 Salient contrasting features of tuberculous and typhoid ulcers of small intestine.

FEATURE	TUBERCULOUS ULCERS	TYPHOID ULCERS
1. Etiology	M. tuberculosis	Salmonella typhi, S. paratyphi
2. Common site	Ileum and caecum	Terminal ileum and jejunum
3. Orientation	Perpendicular to long axis	Parallel of long axis
4. Gross appearance	i. Transverse ulcers, along the direction of lymphatics ii. Fibrous scarring common iii. Intestinal stricture and obstruction common	i. Longitudinal oval ulcers, over Peyer patches ii. Bowel wall thin iii. Intestinal perforation common
5. Microscopy	Caseating epithelioid cell granulomas	Infiltrate of lymphocytes, plasma cells and histiocytes; erythrophagocytosis in some histiocytes
6. Major complications	Intestinal obstruction	Intestinal perforation

Q48. What is dysentery? Discuss its major forms.

Definition Term 'dysentery' is a clinical term used for diarrhoea with cramps, tenesmus and passage of mucus in stools.

Types Dysentery can be bacterial or amoebic:

I. **Bacterial dysentery** is caused by infection with *Shigella* species (*S. dysenteriae, S. flexneri, S. boydii, S. sonnei*) transmitted by faeco-oral route in contaminated food and water. The common housefly also spreads the infection.

Pathogenesis/pathology Pathologic changes are usually seen in the colon and only rarely in the small intestine.

• Infection results in acute mucosal inflammation with necrosis of surface epithelium resulting in ulcerations, which are transverse to the longitudinal axis and usually overlying mucosal lymphoid follicles.

• Some ulcers are covered with fibrin-rich pseudomembranes. Ulcers heal spontaneously without consequences.

II. **Amoebic dysentery** is caused by *Entamoeba histolytica*. This infection is more prevalent in tropical countries. It primarily affects the large intestine.

Pathogenesis/pathology Infection begins with the ingestion of cyst form of the parasite.

- The cyst wall is dissolved in the small intestine and liberated amoebae pass into the large intestine where, usually in the caecum they invade the mucosa, reach the submucosa and form typical *flask-shaped ulcers*.
- *Microscopy* of the inflammatory exudate from the bottom of the ulcers reveals numerous amoebic *trophozoites* which typically contain ingested erythrocytes in their cytoplasm.
- *Clinically,* amoebic colitis presents with diarrhoea and colic or ano-rectal haemorrhage.
- *Complications* include: *Amoebic abscesses* in the liver, rupture of the intestine followed by formation of a tumour-like mass called *amoeboma*.

Q49. What is pseudomembranous colitis?

Definition Pseudomembranous colitis is an acute inflammation of the colon characterised by formation of fibrin-rich pseudomembranes over the site of mucosal injury.

Etiology *Clostridium difficile* (abbreviated commonly *C. diff* and recently renamed *Clostridioides difficile*) is the most common cause, and it acts usually in context of treatment with broad spectrum antibiotics which changes the bacterial flora of the intestines. Other bacteria that could cause pseudomembranous colitis include *Staphylococcus, Shigella, Candida albicans*, but these infections are less common in routine clinical practice.

Pathogenesis/pathology *C. diff* secretes a toxin, which has the capacity to kill colonic mucosal cells.
i. Toxin-induced cell necrosis results in an erosion or shallow mucosal ulceration which is then covered with a layer of fibrin admixed to other blood components exuded from the opened-up mucosal capillaries.
ii. Fibrin is the principal component of the pseudomembranes, which also contain exudated neutrophils, cell debris and mucus released from damaged intestinal cells.
iii. The term '*pseudomembrane*' is used to describe this layered, fibrin-rich exudate which resembles membranes that cover many organs (e.g. serous membranes like pleura or peritoneum).
iv. Like true membrane, pseudomembranes form a covering layer but they do not have the structure and biochemical composition of true membranes: they do not have an epithelial surface layer, and do not contain extracellular basement membrane components like collagen type IV or laminin.
v. These 'fake membranes' in the colon can be scraped away with a metal instrument during endoscopy, revealing the underlying bleeding ulceration.
vi. Eradication of *C. diff* infection leads to disappearance of pseudomembranes and healing of mucosal ulcers without any consequences.

NOTE: Besides colon, the mucosa of most, if not all other organs of the tubular GI tract, could form pseudomembranes.

- For example, mucosal infections of small intestine, oesophagus, mouth and even in the respiratory tract may present with pseudomembranes.
- In previous times, pharyngeal and laryngeal pseudomembranes were a feature of diphtheria, a disease that has lost its clinical significance due to widespread early childhood immunisation.

Q50. What is malabsorption syndrome? Discuss its main clinicopathologic features and laboratory diagnosis.

Definition Malabsorption syndrome is characterised by impaired intestinal absorption of nutrients, especially of fats, but also of proteins, carbohydrates, vitamins and minerals.

Classification There are two major groups as under:
- *Primary* due to a deficiency of mucosal absorptive surfaces and the associated enzymes.
- *Secondary* due to other diseases, e.g. post-surgery states, trauma, drugs and other conditions that impair digestions or absorption of nutrients **(Table 20.7)**.

Clinical findings include the following:
i. Steatorrhoea, the hallmark of malabsorption syndrome characterised by pale, bulky foul-smelling greasy stools
ii. Diarrhoea
iii. Abdominal distention
iv. Borborygmi and flatulence

v. Anorexia
vi. Weight loss and muscle wasting
vii. Dehydration
viii. Hypotension
ix. Specific malnutrition and vitamin deficiencies depending upon the cause
x. Retarded growth and development in children

Laboratory tests include testing for malabsorption of specific groups of nutrients such as follows:

I. *Fat malabsorption*
i. Faecal analysis of fat content
ii. Microscopic analysis for faecal fat
iii. Blood lipid levels after a fatty meal
iv. Tests for absorption of radioactive labelled fat
v. Prothrombin time (vitamin K deficiency)
vi. Bile acid malabsorption

II. *Protein malabsorption*
i. Radioactive-labelled glycine breath test
ii. Secretin and other functional pancreatic tests

III. *Carbohydrate malabsorption*
i. D-xylose tolerance test
ii. Lactose tolerance test
iii. Hydrogen breath test
iv. Bile acid test

IV. Vitamin B_{12} malabsorption
i. Schilling test

TABLE 20.7 Classification of malabsorption syndrome.

I. PRIMARY MALABSORPTION
1. Coeliac sprue
2. Collagenous sprue
3. Tropical sprue
4. Whipple disease
5. Disaccharidase deficiency
6. Allergic and eosinophilic gastroenteritis

II. SECONDARY MALABSORPTION
1. *Impaired digestion*
   i. Mucosal damage, e.g. in tuberculosis, Crohn disease, lymphoma, amyloidosis, radiation injury, systemic sclerosis
   ii. Hepatic and pancreatic insufficiency
   iii. Resection of bowel
   iv. Drugs, e.g. methotrexate, neomycin, phenindione, etc.
2. *Impaired absorption*
   i. Short or stagnant bowel (blind loop syndrome) from surgery or disease resulting in abnormal proliferation of microbial flora
   ii. Acute infectious enteritis
   iii. Parasitoses, e.g. Giardia, Strongyloides, hookworms
3. *Impaired transport*
   i. Lymphatic obstruction, e.g. in lymphoma tuberculosis, lymphangiectasia
   ii. Abetalipoproteinaemia

Intestinal mucosal biopsy of the duodenum performed by endoscopy is essential for the diagnosis and in the follow-up of treated patients. The biopsy could reveal several patterns as follows **(Fig. 20.24)**:

Normal mucosa has slender, tall finger-shaped villi lined by tall columnar absorptive epithelium and few scattered lymphocytes in the lamina propria.

Partial villous atrophy results from fusion of villi which become shorter and broad, forming convolutions and irregular ridges. The stroma contains an increased number of lymphocytes and

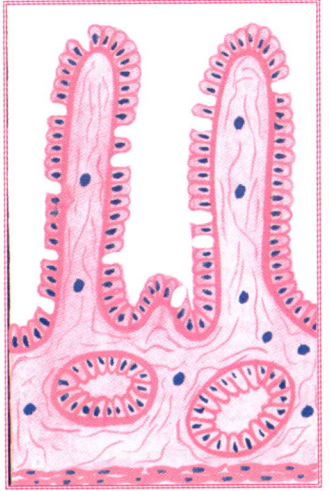
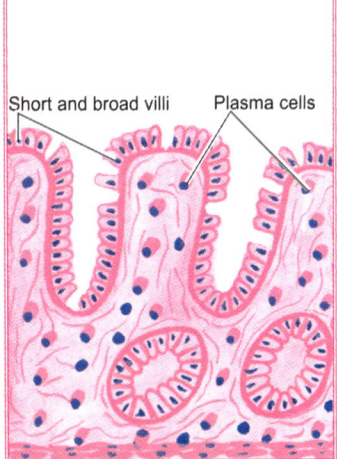
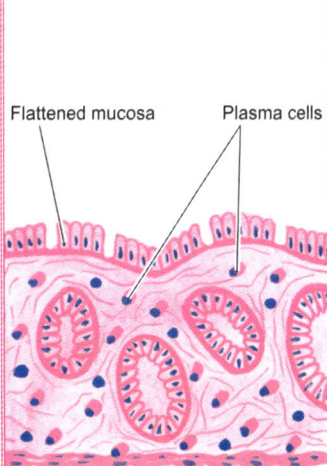

A, NORMAL VILLOUS B, PARTIAL VILLOUS ATROPHY C, SUBTOTAL VILLOUS ATROPHY

FIGURE 20.24: Jejunal biopsy diagrammatic appearance in malabsorption syndrome.

plasma cells. These changes are found in adults and children with diarrhoea, parasitic infestations, Crohn disease, ulcerative colitis and malabsorption due to drugs and irradiation.

Subtotal/total villous atrophy is the severe form of atrophy marked by flattening of mucosa due to advance villous fusion. The stroma contains an increased number of lymphocytes and plasma cells. This form of atrophy is seen in coeliac sprue, tropical sprue, intestinal lymphoma, protein-calorie malnutrition and a few other conditions.

Q51. Discuss salient features of coeliac sprue.

Definition Coeliac sprue is a malabsorption disease of uncertain etiology associated with sensitivity to gluten and its derivative gliadin, presenting pathologically with atrophy of small intestinal mucosa.

Etiopathogenesis Coeliac sprue has a genetic basis as it runs in families.

i. It is associated with specific HLA haplotypes: HLA-DQ2 or HLA-DQ8.

ii. All patients exhibit sensitivity to *gluten/gliadin*, and removal of this carbohydrate from the diet improves the symptoms.

iii. The pathogenesis is not clear. There are two hypotheses:

a. *Immunologic:* According to this hypothesis sensitivity to gluten/gliadin is immunologically mediated.
- Circulating antibodies like those to *tissue transglutaminase*, or *IgA to deamidated gliadin* and *IgA to anti-endomysial antigen* favour the immune explanation.
- These antibodies are useful for diagnostic purposes.

b. *Toxicity of gluten:* According to this hypothesis, gluten may be toxic in context of some underlying enzyme deficiency in certain patients.

Pathology Duodenal biopsy will reveal:

i. Partial or subtotal mucosal atrophy, which also extends deeper into the jejunum, sometimes affecting the entire small intestine.

ii. Loss of villi is accompanied by elongation and hyperplasia of crypt and an increased number of intraepithelial lymphocytes and stromal plasma cells and lymphocytes.

iii. Intraepithelial lymphocytes include T helper (CD4+) and cytotoxic (CD8+) cells, which probably damage the surface epithelial cells and allow the entry of gluten into the tissue where it is deaminated by tissue transglutaminase.

Clinical features Sprue can affect children at an early age (first year), older children and even adults.

i. In small children, it is commonly called *coeliac disease*.

ii. The symptoms start a few months after birth upon introduction of gluten-containing cereals and bread, and include diarrhoea, abdominal bloating and pain, failure to thrive and muscle wasting.

iii. In older children and adults, the disease may vary in intensity from mild diarrhoea with vague abdominal complaints to *massive malabsorption and diarrhoea*.

iv. Some patients with sprue have skin bullae in the form of a full-blown *dermatitis herpetiformis*, an immune mediated disease characterised by deposits of IgA along the dermal-epidermal junction.

v. Most patients do well on gluten-free diet. They need long-term supervision since they are at risk for developing *intestinal T-cell lymphoma*, and even *adenocarcinoma* of the intestines.

Variants of sprue and closely related diseases Two closely related conditions are tropical sprue and collagenous sprue:

- *Tropical sprue* is a disease of unknown etiology that affects people living in or visiting tropical countries. Most likely, it is caused by some bacterial enterotoxin. Clinically, it resembles coeliac sprue, but it is not affected by dietary gliadin.
- *Collagenous sprue* is a characterised by villous atrophy and fibrosis of the mucosa. It is considered to be the end-stage of untreated or treatment resistant coeliac sprue.

Q52. What is Whipple disease?

Definition Whipple disease is an uncommon multisystemic infectious disease caused by the bacillus *Tropheryma whipplei*.

Features

i. Among many other systemic symptoms, malabsorption and diarrhoea are common presenting findings.

ii. Duodenal biopsy reveals mucosal infiltrates of macrophages which have PAS-positive cytoplasm.

iii. Cytoplasm also contains ingested bacteria (*Tropheryma whipplei*), best recognised by electron microscopy.
iv. The disease responds well to antibiotic treatment.

Q53. What are the most important small intestinal tumours?

- Tumours of the small intestine are rare, which is paradoxical, since the small intestine is the longest part of the tubular GI tract.
- The most common benign tumours in descending order of incidence are: small gastrointestinal stromal tumours (GIST), leiomyoma, adenomas, and vascular tumours (haemangiomas and lymphangiomas).
- The most common malignant tumours are: carcinoid tumours, lymphomas, adenocarcinoma and large GISTs.

Q54. Discuss salient features of carcinoid tumours of GI tract.

Definition Carcinoid tumours are low grade malignant tumours composed of neuroendocrine cells, which are also known as enterochromaffin cells, argentaffin cells, Kulchitsky cells.

Classification Carcinoid tumours of the GI tract are divided according to their *site of origin* into three groups:
- *Midgut carcinoids* seen in terminal ileum and appendix are the most common (60–80%).
- *Hindgut carcinoids* occur in rectum and colon (10–20%).
- *Foregut carcinoids* (10–20%) are found in the stomach, duodenum and oesophagus.

NOTE: Carcinoids may occur outside the GI tract, most often in the respiratory tract, or in some germ cell tumours like teratomas of the ovary. Microscopically, they are closely related to islet cell tumours.

Pathology *Grossly*, carcinoids present as submucosal or deep mucosal nodules protruding into the lumen, but covered with an intact mucosa **(Fig. 20.25, A)**.

Microscopy Tumour nests are mostly located in the submucosa and the lamina propria mucosae, focally invading the muscle layer.

i. Irrespective of their site of origin, all carcinoids are composed of uniform neuroendocrine cells.
ii. Tumour cells have round nuclei with granular finely dispersed chromatin ('salt and pepper').
iii. There are no mitoses and there is no necrosis **(Fig. 20.25, B)**.
iv. Immunohistochemically, carcinoids stain with antibodies to chromogranin (proteins of neuroendocrine granules) and synaptophysin, confirming their neuroendocrine nature.

Grading is important for carcinoids. It is performed microscopically using a scale from 1 to 3. It is based on the following criteria:
- Microscopic assessment of nuclear uniformity

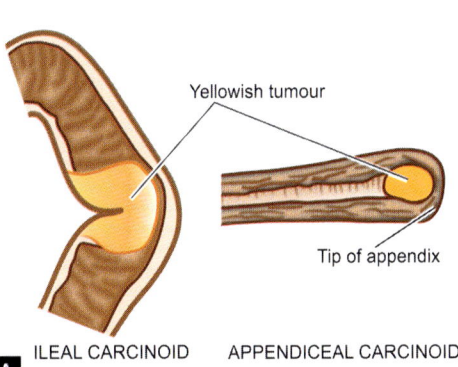
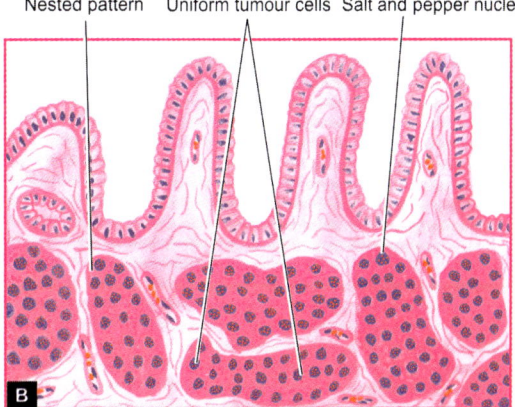

FIGURE 20.25: Carcinoid tumour. A, Gross appearance at common locations in longitudinal section. B, Microscopic appearance shows tumour infiltrating in the ileal wall. It is composed of solid nests and trabeculae of uniform, monotonous, small cells with palisading of the peripheral cells.

- Nuclear features, such as lack or presence of anaplasia and hyperchromasia
- Presence or absence of necrosis
- Presence or absence of mitoses and positive immunohistochemical staining with a marker for proliferation (Ki-67).

i. Most carcinoid are small (<2.5 cm) with 'classic' microscopic features described above and thus *grade I*.

ii. Despite the fact that they invade locally, most of them do not form distant metastases and have an indolent clinical course.

iii. Less often, carcinoids show focal nuclear anaplasia, hyperchromasia and higher mitotic activity with foci of necrosis and are considered to represent *grade 2 and grade 3* tumours. These carcinoids have a higher propensity for metastases and have a worse prognosis.

Clinical features Carcinoids are usually solitary except for the gastric and ileal tumours which may be multiple.

- Midgut carcinoids tend to metastasise, except appendiceal carcinoids which are usually locally invasive. Similarly, the fore-gut and hind-gut are also usually locally invasive.
- Carcinoids secrete serotonin (5-hydroxytryptamine, or 5-HT) which is metabolised to *5-hydroxyindolacetic acid* excreted in urine. It is a useful biochemical marker for the diagnosis of carcinoids.
- Bioactive substances secreted by carcinoid tumours usually do not produce symptoms except in the carcinoid syndrome (discussed below).

Q55. What is carcinoid syndrome?

Definition Carcinoid syndrome is a clinical condition caused by carcinoid tumours which have metastasised to the liver and are thus discharging their bioactive secretory product into the systemic circulation bypassing the liver, which would normally degrade and neutralise them.

Pathogenesis Carcinoids secrete a number of bioactive substances, which may be degraded and excreted in urine, such as under:

- 5-Hydroxytryptamine (5-HT, serotonin)
- 5-Hydroxytryptophan
- 5-Hydroxyindoleacetic acid (5- HIAA)
- Kallikrein
- Bradykinin

i. Normally, these bioactive substances enter the liver through the portal vein from their primary site in the small intestine, and are degraded and inactivated by liver cells.

ii. However, if the carcinoid metastasises to the liver, their secretory products are excreted into the branches of the hepatic veins and, therefore, bypass the liver, so as to enter the systemic circulation.

iii. Thus, serotonin and other products of metastatic carcinoid tumours in the liver reach many organs producing pathological and functional changes.

Clinicopathologic features Heart damage by serotonin and related compounds is prototypical of carcinoid syndrome. Other organs are, however, also affected.

i. Consequences are most prominent in the right ventricle and include endocardial fibrosis and tricuspid and aortic valve fibrosis leading to tricuspid or aortic insufficiency and stenosis, and rigidity and progressive failure of the overstrained right ventricle.

ii. Facial skin experiencing attacks of flushing.

iii. Bronchial tree experiencing attacks of bronchospasm with coughing and dyspnoea.

iv. Abdominal pain and spastic bowel movement and watery diarrhoea.

■ APPENDIX

Q56. Discuss salient features of acute appendicitis.

Definition Acute appendicitis is an inflammation of the appendix, a vestigial organ attached to the caecum. It is the most common abdominal condition requiring surgery.

Etiology
I. *Obstructive causes*
i. Faecolith

ii. Calculi, e.g. biliary
iii. Foreign body in food
iv. Tumour
v. Worms, especially *Enterobius vermicularis*
vi. Diffuse lymphoid hyperplasia, especially in children

II. **Non-obstructive causes (less common)**
i. Haematogenous spread of generalised infection
ii. Vascular occlusion
iii. Inappropriate diet lacking roughage

Pathogenesis Most commonly, the sequence in inflammation of the appendix and its spread is as under:
- *Obstruction* of the narrow lumen of the appendix → *smooth muscle contraction* in the wall of appendix → increased *intraluminal pressure* → *compression of intramural blood vessels* in the appendix → *ischaemic necrosis* of the surface layer of mucosal epithelium → *bacteria* invade the ulcer → deeper extension the infection through the wall (*transmural appendicitis*) and extending to the serosal surface (*fibrinopurulent serositis*).
- *Ischaemia and bacterial infection* → *gangrene* of the appendix → may lead to *rupture* and entry of pus and bacteria into the abdominal cavity → *perityphlitic abscess*, which if not contained → *peritonitis*.
- Entry of bacteria into the blood stream → *bacteraemia*.
- Entry of bacteria into the branches of the portal vein → *pylephlebitis* → *hepatic abscesses*.

Pathology Acute inflammation, most often transmural, and accompanied by fibrinopurulent serositis (**Fig. 20.26**).

Clinical features Attack of acute appendicitis presents with the following symptoms:
i. Colicky pain, initially around the umbilicus but later localised to right iliac fossa
ii. Nausea and vomiting
iii. Abdominal tenderness to palpation
iv. Pyrexia of mild grade and increased pulse rate
v. Neutrophilic leukocytosis

Complications
i. Peritonitis
ii. Appendix abscess
iii. Adhesions
iv. Portal pylephlebitis with infected thrombi in the tributaries of portal vein and extending into the liver to form liver abscesses.

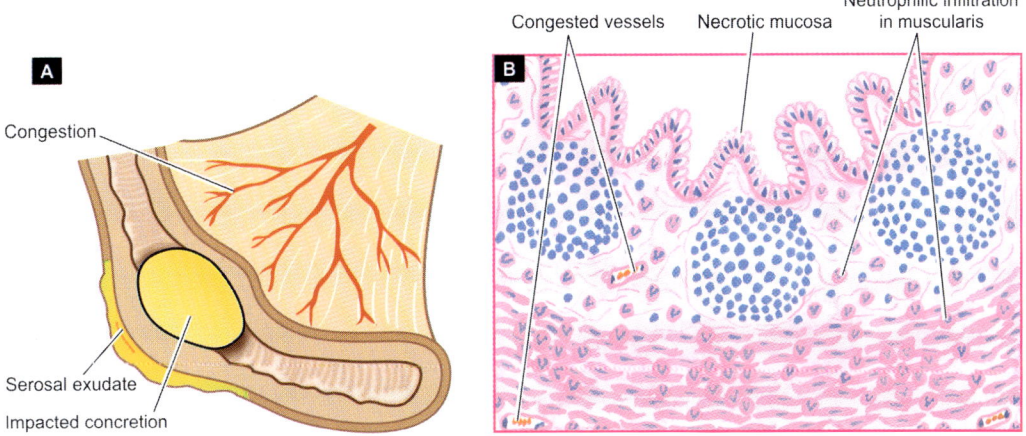

FIGURE 20.26: Acute appendicitis. A, Gross appearance of longitudinally opened appendix showing impacted faecolith in the lumen and exudate on the serosa. B, Microscopic appearance showing diagnostic neutrophilic infiltration into the muscularis.

Q57. What are the most important tumours of the appendix?

Two most important tumours of the appendix are:
- Carcinoid tumour, and
- Mucinous tumours, although non-mucinous tumors like those in the colon also may occur.

I. **Carcinoid tumour** of the appendix is a low grade neuroendocrine malignancy, most frequently located on the tip of the appendix.

II. **Mucinous tumours** may be benign (cystadenoma), borderline malignant (low grade mucinous tumour) or malignant (mucinous cystadenocarcinoma).
- These tumours secrete mucus which distends the appendix producing a *mucocele*.
- Rupture of mucocele or the invasion of borderline or frankly malignant tumours through the wall of the appendix produces widespread peritoneal dissemination of mucin producing cells filling the abdominal cavity with mucus.
- *Pseudomyxoma peritonei,* colloquially called *'jelly-belly',* resulting from peritoneal dissemination of mucus-secreting tumours is hard to cure and has usually a lethal outcome.

LARGE INTESTINE

Q58. What are the anatomic features of the large intestine that are most important for the understanding of its pathology?

Gross The large intestine can be divided into caecum, ascending colon, transverse colon, descending colon and rectum, terminating in the anus.

Microscopy The large intestine has four layers like the rest of the GI tract.
- The mucosa lacks villi and is composed of crypts only.
- Mucosa and submucosa contain abundant lymphoid cells, which are forming follicles, most prominently in caecum and rectum.
- The muscularis propria consists of a circular layer and a longitudinal layer; the latter forms three muscle band externally called taeniae coli.
- External surface underneath the serosa is sacculated forming haustra.

Blood supply of the small intestine and most of the large intestine:
- Comes from the *superior mesenteric artery*.
- The remaining blood supply of the colon comes through the *inferior mesenteric artery*.
- The lower rectum is supplied by the haemorrhoidal branches.

Innervation of the large bowel consists of three plexuses of ganglion cells:
- *Auerbach* or myenteric plexus lying between the two layers of muscularis.
- *Henle* plexus in the deep submocosa inner to the circular muscle layer.
- *Meissner* plexus that lies in the superficial mucosa just beneath the muscularis mucosae.

Q59. Discuss Hirschsprung disease briefly.

Definition Hirschsprung disease is a congenital megacolon, i.e. dilatation of the large intestine, that develops due to its defective innervation resulting in aganglionosis of its distal part.

Epidemiology Incidence is 1:5,000 newborns, affecting more often males than female, even though if found in females it is more severe. In about 4% cases, it is familial. It is commonly found in Down syndrome.

Genetics The disease has a heterogeneous genetic background.
- Autosomal dominant inheritance with variable penetrance in familial cases is related to loss of function mutations of receptor tyrosine kinase *RET* gene, which is also found in 1 of 6 sporadic cases.
- A dozen of other genes contributing to aganglionosis have been identified. Most of their gene products regulate the migration of foetal ganglion cells and formation of the intestinal neural plexuses.

Pathology The basic defect is aganglionosis in which the ganglion cells are missing from all three plexuses of the colorectal segment of the large intestine.

i. The aganglionic segment is narrow and contracted, whereas the large intestine proximal to it is normally innervated and dilated **(Fig. 20.27)**.

ii. In the classical most common form of Hirschsprung disease, the aganglionic segment is only 2–3 cm long.
iii. However, the length of aganglionosis may vary from one case to another and sometimes it extends into sigmoid or it may involve most of the colon.
iv. Pathologic diagnosis is made by examining the biopsy of the stenotic segment and demonstrating the absence of ganglion cells.
v. Immunohistochemical stain for acetylcholinesterase may be useful for proving the absence of ganglion cells and concomitant prominence of non-myelinated nerve fibres.

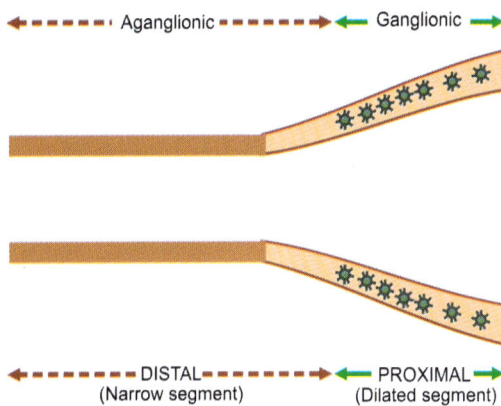

FIGURE 20.27: Hirschsprung disease, diagrammatic representation of the pathologic changes.

Clinical features The neonate does not discharge meconium during or after birth and appears constipated.
- Obstructed defaecation leads to fluid and electrolyte disturbances, and if the conditions is not corrected the colon may rupture and produce peritonitis.
- Surgical resection of the stenotic segment and anastomosis with the normally innervated colon is the treatment of choice.

Q60. What is diverticulosis coli?

Definition Diverticulosis is an outpouching (herniation) of the mucosa and submucosa into the subserosal space between the taeniae coli.
Etiopathogenesis Colonic diverticula are an age-related disorder and are rare under 30 years of age, unless the patient has also some congenital connective tissue disorder like Marfan syndrome.
- They develop due to a weakness of the colonic wall, and are typically located at thinnest part of intestinal wall between the longitudinal taeniae coli containing striated muscle cells.
- Increased intraluminal pressure due to strain caused by constipation and the low-fibre Western diet predispose to formation of diverticula.
- Age contributes to weakening of the colonic wall.

Pathology Diverticula are a feature of ageing and are uncommon under the age of 30 years.
Location They occur most often in the left colon (90%) and are most often located in the sigmoid colon.
Gross Diverticula are usually small (< 1 cm), flask-shaped protrusions connected with main colonic lumen through a narrow neck. They bulge under the serosa and extending into the plicae epiploicae so that they can be recognised on gross examination of the colon during surgery or at autopsy.
Microscopy Usually reveals atrophy of the protruding mucosa, submucosa and muscle layer.
Clinical features Mostly, diverticula are asymptomatic and found only accidentally during colonoscopy. They may retain inspissated faecal material which may cause pain or bleeding, or irregular bowel movements.
Complications Most common complication is *diverticulitis*. Inflammation is usually related to retention of faecalith or particulate material in the faeces stuck inside the diverticulum.
- Inflamed sigmoid diverticula are the most common cause of haematochesia in the elderly. Bleeding is usually light and stops spontaneously because of healing fibrosis which obliterates the vessels.
- Inflammation may extend into the adjacent fat tissue or the mesentery and form a mass-like lesion.
- Inflamed diverticula may cause adhesions with other intestinal loops and contribute even to fistula formations.
- Diverticula may perforate and cause peritonitis, but that occurs rarely.

Q61. What are colorectal polyps? How are they classified?

Definition Polyps are finger-like or wart-like protrusions on the colorectal mucosa.
Classification They may be neoplastic or non-neoplastic, benign or malignant, solitary or multiple (**Table 20.8**).

Q62. Briefly discuss the most common non-neoplastic colorectal polyps.

Non-neoplastic polyps can be classified as i) hyperplastic, ii) hamartomatous, or iii) inflammatory. Common examples are discussed below.

I. **Hyperplastic polyps** are the most common epithelial polyps found on endoscopy.
Clinical and gross They are small (<0.5 cm) and may be solitary or multiple.
- They are sessile and round with a smooth surface, resembling a dew drop on colonoscopy.
- These innocuous polyps are of no clinical significance and have no malignant potential.

Microcopy On their surface, hyperplastic polyps are lined by mucus-secreting normal colonic cells arranged into serrated ('saw-toothed') crypts.

NOTE: Microscopically, hyperplastic polyps must be distinguished from sessile serrated polyps/adenomas, which are somewhat larger and may be clinically more ominous.

II. **Juvenile polyps** Juvenile polyps also known as retention polyps, are hamartomatous developmental polyps composed of mucus-secreting glands embedded in an inflamed stroma. Most often, they are *solitary,* but they may also be multiple in a rare (1:100,000) hereditary *juvenile polyposis syndrome.*

Clinical and gross Solitary juvenile polyp presents as a rectal small round and usually pedunculated mass measuring around 2 cm in diameter.

Microscopy It consists of dilated glands lined by mucus-secreting cells enclosed in an inflamed, frequently oedematous stroma **(Fig. 20.28)**.
- Surface of the polyp is usually ulcerated and covered with inflamed stroma.
- Solitary juvenile polyp occurs most often as rectal bleeding in children under the age of 5 years, but may be seen in older children and young adults.

Prognosis It has no malignant potential, in contrast to *hereditary juvenile polyposis* patients who are at risk of developing cancer.

III. **Peutz-Jeghers polyps** Peutz-Jeghers (P-J) syndrome is a genetic syndrome characterised by mucocutaneous hyperpigmentation and formation of hamartomatous gastrointestinal polyps. It has an incidence estimated to be in the range from 1:25,000 to 1:250,000.

Genetics Approximately 50% percent of patients diagnosed with P-J syndrome have a family history and thus have the hereditary autosomal dominant form of disease.
- Only 50% the hereditary cases and some spontaneous cases have a loss-of-function mutation of the tumour suppressor gene *STK11,* which means that other genes must have a pathogenetic role.
- *STK11* gene encodes the serum threonine kinase 11, which is important metabolic enzyme involved also in the maintenance of cell polarity, regulation of cell growth and apoptosis.

TABLE 20.8 The WHO classification of colorectal polyps and tumours*.

I. **Colorectal polyps**
A. *Non-neoplastic polyps*
1. Hyperplastic (metaplastic) polyps
2. Juvenile (Retention) polyps and polyposis
3. Peutz-Jeghers polyps and polyposis

B. *Neoplastic polyps (Adenomas)*
1. Tubular adenoma
2. Villous adenoma
3. Tubulovillous adenoma
4. Serrated polyps

II. **Epithelial malignant tumours**
A. *Carcinoma*
1. Adenocarcinoma
2. Other carcinomas (Mucinous adenocarcinoma, signet-ring cell carcinoma, small cell carcinoma, adenosquamous carcinoma, undifferentiated carcinoma)

B. *Carcinoid tumour*

III. **Benign non-epithelial tumours** (GIST, leiomyomas, leiomyoblastoma, neurilemmoma, lipoma and vascular tumours)

IV. **Malignant non-epithelial tumours** (Leiomyosarcoma, malignant lymphoma, malignant melanoma, angiosarcoma, Kaposi sarcoma)

V. **Secondary tumours**

*Adapted from Bosman et al. WHO classification of tumours of the digestive system. 4th edition. IARC Lyon, 2010;48-58.

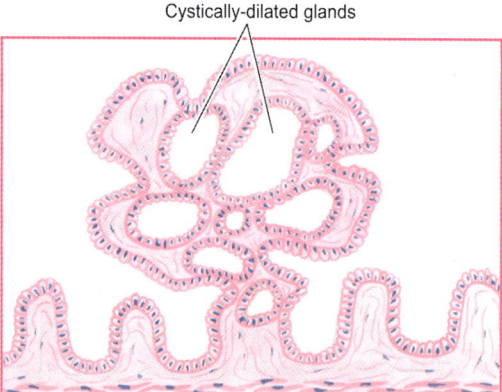

FIGURE 20.28: Juvenile polyp. The surface of the polyp is ulcerated. The polyp is composed of dilated glands and inflamed stroma.

Clinical and gross Peutz-Jeghers syndrome presents with mucocutaneous hyperpigmentation and gastrointestinal polyposis. Melanotic pigmentation is seen on the lips, buccal and nasal mucosa and the skin of palms, genitalia and perianal region.
• Hamartomatous polyps may occur in the stomach and intestines, most frequently involving the ileum.
• These polyps are often multiple, vary in size and may be large enough to cause obstruction and intussusception of intestine, or haemorrhage.
Microscopy P-J polyps are composed of normal cells lining prominent tree-branching muscularis mucosae **(Fig. 20.29)**. Epithelial cells may show focal hyperplasia and form cystic spaces but there is no atypia or dysplasia and they have no malignant potential.
Clinical features The syndrome is usually diagnosed in childhood because of prominent mucosal pigmentation.
i. P-J polyps, which may be solitary or more often multiple, involve the small intestine and may cause obstruction, intussusception or present with bleeding.
ii. Adult patients with P-J syndrome are at increased risk of developing cancers of the GI tract (most often in the colon, stomach, then small intestine and pancreas), and in other organs such as breast or uterus. Benign or low grade malignant tumours also occur in ovaries or testes.

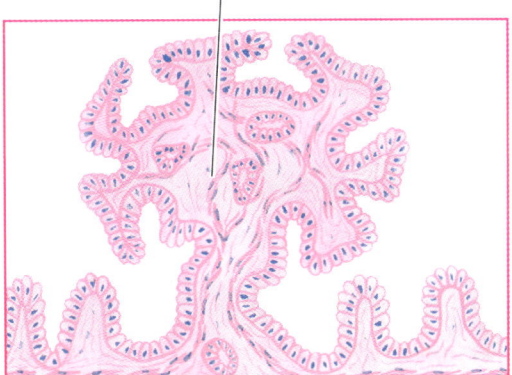

FIGURE 20.29: Hamartomatous polyps—Peutz-Jeghers polyp. The polyp shows a tree-like branching of muscularis mucosae into villi.

Q63. What are the neoplastic polyps? Discuss features of common examples.

Definition Neoplastic polyps are benign colonic adenomas that have a potential for malignant transformation. They can be solitary or multiple, spontaneous or syndromic, and appear in several microscopic forms. Several microscopic types are recognised such as i) tubular adenoma, ii) villous adenoma, iii) tubulovillous adenoma, and iv) serrated polyp and adenoma.
I. **Tubular adenomas** are the most common colorectal neoplastic polyps (75%).
Clinical and gross Most of them are small sessile spherical masses rising just above the surface of the mucosa and measuring less than 1 cm.
• The larger ones, 2–4 cm in diameter have a recognisable fibrous stalk and appear pedunculated.
• Most often they are seen in the left colon and rectum.
Microcopy Tubular adenomas are composed of simple and interanastomosing tubular glands.
• Glands are lined by pseudostratified columnar epithelium showing mild to moderate dysplasia **(Fig. 20.30, A)**.
Prognosis Most of them are benign.
• Malignancy occurs in 5% of tubular adenoma, most of which are larger than average.
• Carcinoma is first preinvasive (*carcinoma in situ*) and then becomes invasive adenocarcinoma invading the stroma of the stalk.
II. **Villous adenomas** are less common than tubular adenomas.
Clinical and gross They account for 20–30% of all intestinal neoplastic polyps.
• They occur in somewhat older patients than tubular adenomas and are most often located in the distal colon and rectum.
• They form exophytic usually sessile masses, varying in size from 1 to 10 cm or even more in diameter.
Microscopy They are composed of cuboidal, mucus-secreting cells lining finger-like villi.
• Tumour cells may show minimal nuclear atypia, but in some cases atypia may be quite prominent **(Fig. 20.30, B)**.
• Invasive carcinoma is found in 30% of cases.
Prognosis These tumours are invariably symptomatic especially if located in the rectum when they produce excess mucus, bleeding or cause constipation or diarrhoea.

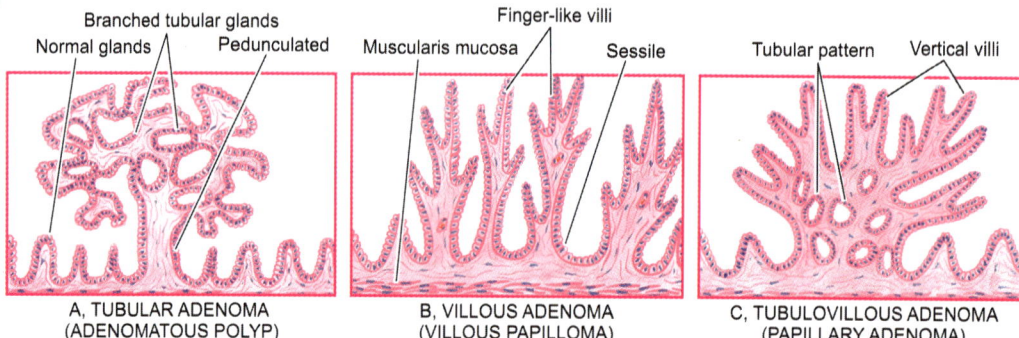

A, TUBULAR ADENOMA (ADENOMATOUS POLYP)   B, VILLOUS ADENOMA (VILLOUS PAPILLOMA)   C, TUBULOVILLOUS ADENOMA (PAPILLARY ADENOMA)

FIGURE 20.30: Adenomas (neoplastic polyps)—three main varieties. A, Tubular adenoma is composed of simple tubular glands. B, Villous adenoma shows finger-like projections on the surface. C, Tubullovillous adenoma having villifrom surface while the core contains tubular glands. The lining epithelium shows high-grade dysplasia.

- The presence of severe atypia, carcinoma *in situ* and invasive carcinoma are seen more frequently.
- Invasive carcinoma has been reported in 30% of villous adenomas.

III. **Tubulovillous adenomas** have features intermediate between pure tubular and villous adenomas **(Fig. 20.30, C)**.

IV. **Serrated polyps/adenomas** These account for 10–15% neoplastic polyps. These newly recognised polyps appear in two forms: i) sessile serrated polyp, and ii) traditional serrated adenoma.

i. *Sessile serrated polyps*, as the name implies, are sessile and broad-based.

- They are composed of crypts which show serration along their entire length, in contrast to hyperplastic polyps which are serrated only on the upper superficial part of their crypts **(Fig. 20.31)**.

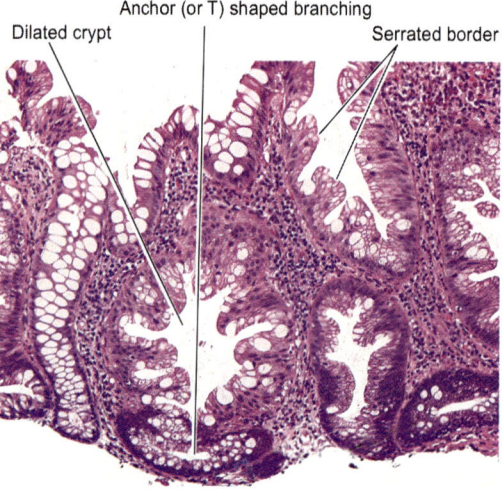

FIGURE 20.31: Sessile serrated adenoma/polyp. The polyp consists of dilated crypts lined by mucinous epithelium having serrated border. (Reproduced with permission from Atlas of Histopathology by Ivan Damjanov 2012, Jaypee Brothers Medical Publishers Pvt Ltd, New Delhi).

- Furthermore, the crypts are often dilated at the base and characteristically show lateral extension assuming a boot-like appearance.
- Sessile serrated polyps are bigger than hyperplastic polyps (> 0.6 cm) and mostly occur in the right colon.
- In contrast to hyperplastic polyps, these polyps can show *dysplasia* and may also transform into adenocarcinomas.

ii. *Traditional serrated adenomas* are pedunculated and larger polyps that occur more often in the left colon than on the right side.

- Their surface is villiform.
- There is prominent serration of the epithelium including the lower parts of the crypts.
- The cells lining the crypts have pseudostratified nuclei and abundant eosinophilic cytoplasm.
- Nuclear atypia may be prominent, correlating with the propensity of these polyps to transform into adenocarcinoma.

Q64. Tabulate the contrasting features of non-neoplastic and neoplastic polyps (adenomas).

The contrasting features of non-neoplastic and neoplastic polyps are given in **Table 20.9**.

TABLE 20.9 Contrasting features of non-neoplastic and neoplastic colorectal polyps.

FEATURE	NON-NEOPLASTIC POLYPS	NEOPLASTIC POLYPS (ADENOMAS)
Frequency	More common	Less common
Number	Often sporadic	Sporadic as well as multiple
Familial predisposition	No	Yes, in sporadic cases
Types	Hyperplastic (90%) Others: hamartomatous (Peutz-Jeghers, juvenile) inflammatory, lymphoid	Tubular, villous, tubulovillous and serrated adenomas
Familial syndromes	Juvenile polyposis syndrome	Familial polyposis coli, Gardner, Turcot
Biologic behaviour	Always benign	Variable malignant potential: Tubular adenoma 5%, villous 30%, tubulovillous and serrated adenomas intermediate

Q65. What are the most important risk factors for colorectal carcinomas?

Two major risk factors are i) diet, and ii) genetic susceptibility, to which third can be added as iii) high-risk conditions.

I. **Diet** that contains few *vegetable fibres* leading to a low stool bulk is associated with higher risk. Excessive consumption of *refined carbohydrates* will lead to the changes in the intestinal microbiome and also contribute to cancerogenesis.

II. **Genetic susceptibility** is important as evidenced by an increased incidence of colorectal cancer in family members of the affected patient. There are also well known preneoplastic familial syndromes with a high incidence of colorectal cancer:

i. *Familial adenomatous polyposis* (FAP), an autosomal dominant disease characterised by the formation of numerous colorectal polyps which invariably transform into adenocarcinoma. It is related to the germ line mutations of the *APC* (adenomatous polyposis coli) gene.

ii. *Gardner syndrome* is a variant of FAP combined with osteomas of the mandible and maxilla, epidermoid cysts and desmoid tumour.

iii. *Turcot syndrome* is another variant of FAP combined with medulloblastoma, a brain tumour.

iv. *Hereditary non-polyposis colonic cancer (HNPCC or Lynch syndrome)* is an autosomal dominant condition characterised by common occurrence of colorectal carcinoma and primary cancers in other organs such as endometrium and ovary.

III. **High-risk conditions** that increase the risk colorectal cancer are as follows:
i. Inflammatory bowel disease, especially ulcerative colitis of long duration
ii. Diverticular disease of long duration
iii. Tobacco smoking, especially in younger patients

Q66. Briefly discuss the pathogenesis of colorectal carcinoma.

There are two main pathways from normal colorectal mucosa to development of invasive adenocarcinoma: i) mutation pathway, and ii) microsatellite pathway.

I. **Mutation pathway,** also called **APC/ β-catenin pathway,** is characterised by a sequence of molecular changes paralleled with morphologic changes in the colorectal mucosa **(Fig. 20.32)**.

i. The sequence of *morphological changes* begins with the formation of adenoma, which becomes dysplastic and transforms into an invasive carcinoma.

ii. *Molecular events* in adenoma-adenocarcinoma sequence parallel the normal-to-adenoma and *begin with a loss of APC* (in 80% cases).

iii. Next step is translocation of β-catenin (encoded by the *CTNNB1* gene) into the nucleus followed by activation of transcription of *MYC* and *cyclin D* genes.

iv. *K-RAS* point mutation occurs as a relatively late event and is found only in 10–50% cases.

v. It is followed by deletion of *DCC* gene ('deleted in colonic carcinoma') (60–70% cases), and finally a loss of *TP53* found in 70–80% cases.

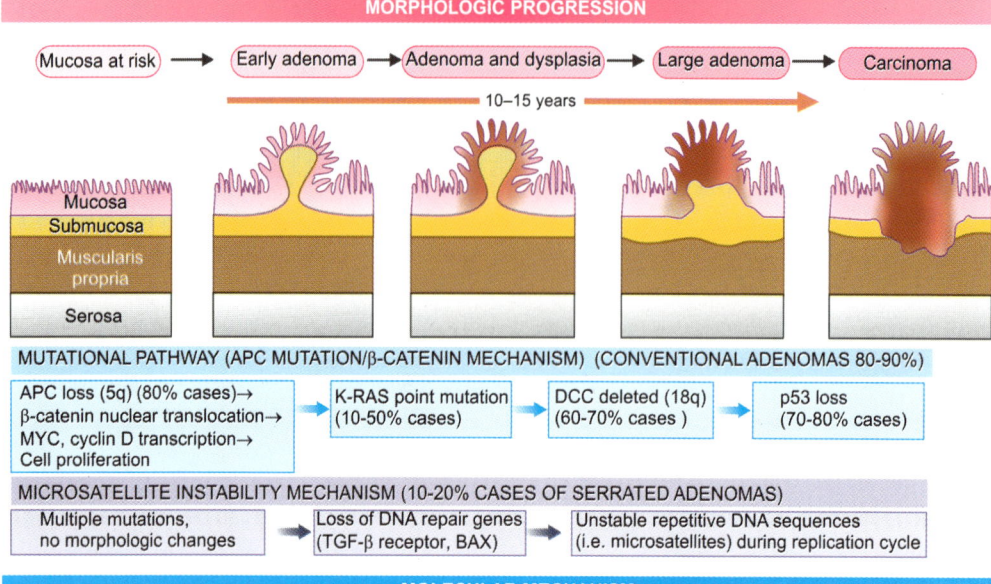

FIGURE 20.32: Adenoma-carcinoma sequence—schematic diagram of molecular and morphologic evolution.

Adenoma-carcinoma sequence plays a key role in the pathogenesis of most colorectal carcinomas (85%), as supported by the following evidence:
i. Incidence of adenomas in the colon is directly proportionate to the prevalence of colorectal carcinoma.
ii. The risk of adenocarcinoma declines upon endoscopic removal of adenomas.
iii. Peak incidence of adenomas precedes a few years the peak incidence of adenocarcinoma.
iv. Long-term continuous intake of low dose aspirin or NSAIDs reduces the incidence of adenomas and in parallel reduces the incidence of invasive adenocarcinomas.
v. Adenoma-related factors may increase the risk of adenocarcinoma as under:
- *Number of adenomas* as in FAP, where their number correlates with increased risk.
- *Size of adenomas* since the size of polyps increases the chance of malignant transformation.
- *Type of adenoma*—villous adenoma are more likely to give rise to cancer than tubular adenomas.

II. **Microsatellite instability pathways** is characterised by several distinct molecular changes but these changes are *not paralleled by any morphological changes.*
i. The key molecular event is the *loss of DNA repair genes,* such as human MutL homologue2 *(hMLH2).*
ii. Repetitive DNA sequences (i.e. microsatellites), therefore, become unstable during replication cycle. This *microsatellite instability* is the hallmark of the entire pathway, as under:
- *TGF-β receptor* which normally inhibits cell proliferation is mutated and thus allows uncontrolled proliferation of cells.
- *BAX* gene which causes apoptosis is defective allowing cells to escape apoptosis.

Q67. What are the major clinicopathologic features of colorectal carcinoma?

Distribution of tumours in the large intestine shows that left-sided tumours are more common (85%) than those on the right side **(Fig. 20.33)** as under:

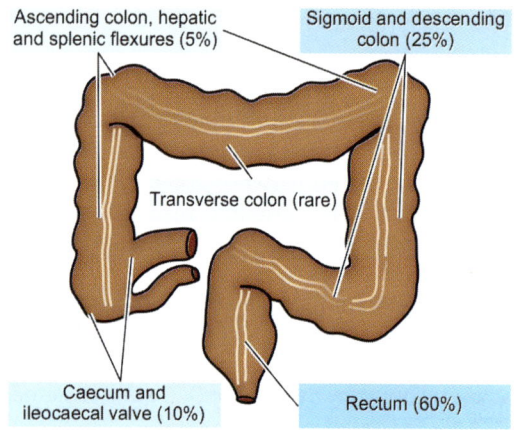

FIGURE 20.33: Distribution of the primary colorectal cancer.

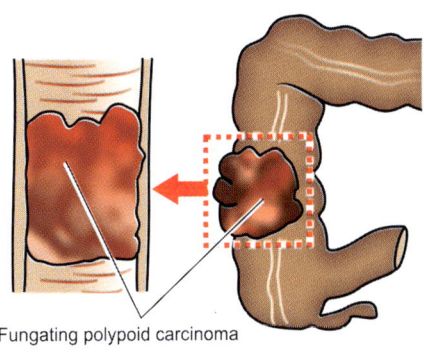
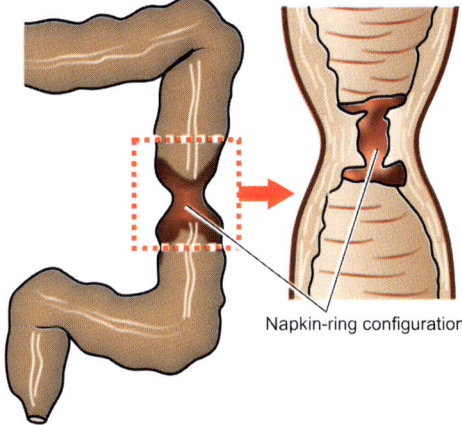

A, RIGHT-SIDED GROWTH   B, LEFT-SIDED GROWTH

FIGURE 20.34: Gross appearance of colorectal carcinoma. A, *Right-sided growth*—fungating polypoid carcinoma showing cauliflower-like growth projecting into the lumen. B, *Left-sided growth*—napkin-ring configuration with spread of growth into the bowel wall.

- Rectum 60% (the most common site)
- Sigmoid and descending colon (25%)
- Caecum and ileocaecal valve (10%)
- Colonic flexures (hepatic and splenic) and ascending colon (5%)

Gross Right-sided tumours differ from those in the left colon as under **(Fig. 20.34)**:
- Carcinoma of caecum and ascending colon form a large cauliflower-like soft fungating and friable mass.
- Carcinomas of the left colon have a napkin-ring appearance, circumferentially encircling and narrowing the lumen. These carcinomas are firm, invade the wall of the intestine and often show surface ulceration.
- On X-ray examination with barium enema, left colon growth has an 'apple-core' appearance.

Microscopy Both left and right-sided colorectal cancers are adenocarcinomas, which show varying degree of differentiation **(Fig. 20.35)**:
- Classical adenocarcinomas account for 90–95% of all colorectal carcinomas.
- Colloid, mucin-rich carcinomas, showing focally signet ring features account for 10% of tumours.

Spread of tumours Local invasion into the fat tissue of the mesentery or the pericolic fat tissue is the most common extension of cancer.
- Lymphatic spread to regional lymph nodes is common, followed by involvement of other abdominal lymph nodes.

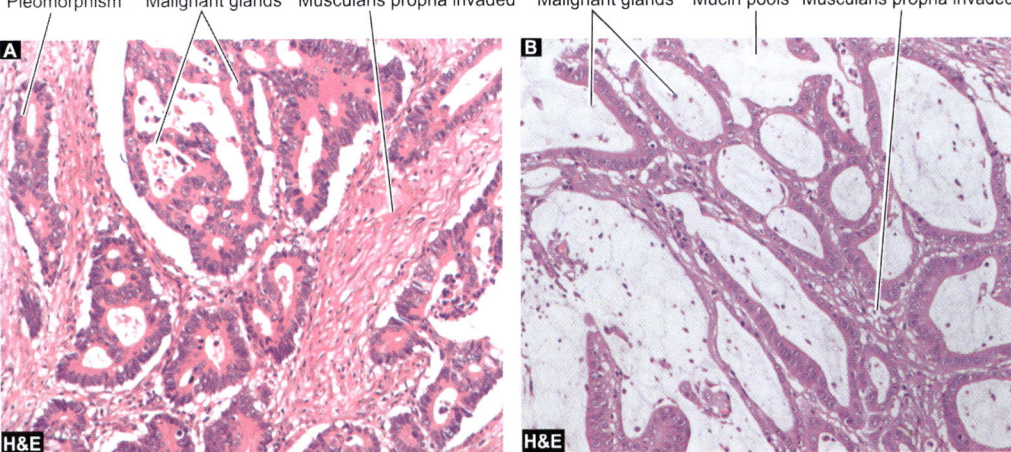

FIGURE 20.35: Colonic adenocarcinoma. A, Moderately differentiated. B, Mucin-secreting adenocarcinoma.

- Haematogenous spread leads through the portal vein to the liver, but also to the lungs, bones and other organs.
- Peritoneal transcoelomic spread may be associated with pseudomyxoma peritonei.

Clinical features Blood in the stool, which is best detected by testing for occult blood. Left-sided tumours are more likely to cause visible haematochesia.

i. Change in the bowel habits, such as constipation in left-sided tumours (pencil-like faeces).
ii. Loss of weight, cachexia, weakness, anaemia are seen in advanced cases.
iii. Early diagnosis is essential and is accomplished by colonoscopy.
iv. Carcino-embryonic antigen (CEA) test is not good for screening and early diagnosis, but it is useful for follow-up for recurrence after the resection of the primary tumour.

Staging is done according to the TNM system, but traditional approaches such as Astler-Coller modification of the original Dukes system, are still used.

Prognosis It depends primarily on the size and stage of the tumour (depth of invasion and the presence of metastases in the lymph nodes or distant organs).

Five-year survival depends on the TNM stage and varies as follows:
- Stage I tumours 90%
- Stage II tumours 70–85%
- Stage III tumours 20–65%
- Stage IV tumours 5%

Q68. What are the main contrasting features of right-sided and left-sided colonic cancer?

Contrasting features of right-sided and left-sided colon cancer are shown in **Table 20.10**.

TABLE 20.10 Contrasting features of right-sided and left-sided colon cancer.

FEATURE	RIGHT-SIDED COLON CANCER	LEFT-SIDED COLON CANCER
1. Location	Caecum, ascending colon	Descending and sigmoid colon
2. Gross appearance	Fungating, large, polypoid, growing into lumen	Ulcerative with elevated margins, napkin-ring like, annular constriction, growing into the bowel wall
3. Possible pathogenesis	Grows intraluminally due to liquid luminal content in right colon	Grows intramurally due to semisolid content in the lumen of left colon
4. Clinical presentation	Mass right iliac fossa, bleeding per rectum	Change in bowel habit, often constipation, occult bleeding
5. Diagnosis and prognosis	Late symptoms, remains undiagnosed until late, worse prognosis	Early symptoms, easy access to endoscopy/biopsy, diagnosed early, better prognosis

Q69. What is the most common malignant tumour of the anal canal?

It is squamous cell carcinoma. Some of these tumours may be preceded by high-grade dysplasia and carcinoma-in-situ related to HPV infection. HPV-related warts, called condyloma accuminatum, are the only anal benign lesions of note.

PERITONEUM

Q70. What is peritonitis? What are its main types?

Definition Peritonitis is an inflammation of the peritoneum, which may be acute or commonly chronic. It may be caused by bacteria or it may be sterile and caused by chemicals. Bacterial peritonitis may be primary (rare) or secondary, usually related to an infection spreading from an infected abdominal organ or due to organ perforation.

Classification

I. **Chemical peritonitis** may be caused by following:
i. Bile leaking from the gallbladder or following gallbladder trauma or surgery
ii. Pancreatic enzyme in acute pancreatitis
iii. Gastric juice due to perforation of gastric ulcer
iv. Barium sulfate leaking during contrast enhanced X-ray examination

II. **Bacterial peritonitis** is usually secondary and related to the following:
i. Acute appendicitis
ii. Acute cholecystitis
iii. Salpingitis
iv. Gangrene of the bowel
v. Rupture of peptic ulcer
vi. Tuberculosis following military dissemination

Q71. What are the common malignant tumours of the peritoneum?

- The most common malignancy of peritoneum are **metastases** from a variety of primary carcinomas of abdominal organs (e.g. ovarian cancer or colorectal carcinoma), and less often malignant tumours from other sites, such as lung or breast.
- Mucin-producing tumours, most often originating from the gastrointestinal tract, may produce **pseudomyxoma peritonei**.
- **Mesothelioma** of peritoneum is a rare primary malignancy, typically developing after chronic exposure to asbestos. It has the same microscopic features as the more common pleural mesothelioma.

Q72. Enumerate the major causes of bleeding from upper GI, small intestine and large intestine.

GI bleeding from upper (haematemesis), middle (small intestinal) and lower (melaena) part is a major presenting clinical feature of a variety of gastrointestinal diseases. A summary of its major causes is tabulated in **Table 20.11**.

TABLE 20.11 Causes of gastrointestinal (GI) bleeding.

UPPER GI BLEEDING	SMALL INTESTINAL BLEEDING	LOWER GI BLEEDING
1. Oesophageal varices	Vascular ectasias	Inflammatory bowel disease (IBD)
2. Mallory-Weiss tear	Tumours (adenocarcinoma, lymphoma, leiomyoma)	Carcinoma colon
3. Haemorrhagic/erosive gastritis	NSAIDs	Carcinoma rectosigmoid
4. Duodenal ulcer	Meckel diverticulum	Haemorrhoids
5. Gastric ulcer	Intussusception	Anal fissure
6. Cancer stomach	Crohn's disease	Diverticulosis

Chapter 20e Supplement: Online Content

Digital content of this chapter available with this book is meant for enhanced learning and self-assessment. In addition, it contains 36 Multiple Choice Questions (MCQs), 05 Clinicopathologic Vignettes, and 15 Image-based Questions; these are followed by their answers along with explanatory notes of correct and incorrect answers.

CHAPTER 21

Liver, Biliary Tract and Exocrine Pancreas

LIVER

Q1. What are the key facts about the normal anatomy, histology and physiology of the liver that are important for understanding liver pathology?

Anatomy The liver is the largest organ in the body weighing 1400 to 1600 g in males and 1200 to 1400 in females. It has a large right lobe and a smaller left lobe **(Fig. 21.1)**. It is covered by the Glisson capsule.

Porta hepatis is the part of the liver in which the large bile ducts exit the liver and the hepatic artery and the portal vein enter the liver, providing its dual blood supply.

Histology The liver is composed of numerous hexagonal or pyramidal lobules, each with a diameter of 0.5 cm. Functionally, these lobules correspond to acini and have three zones **(Fig. 21.2)**.

- The blood flows from the portal tract at the periphery of the lobule or the centre of the acinus (*zone 1*), toward the centre of the lobule through the sinusoids in between the liver cells.
- The blood leaves the lobules/acini through the central vein (hepatic venule) in *zone 3*, from where it drains into the tributaries of the hepatic vein.

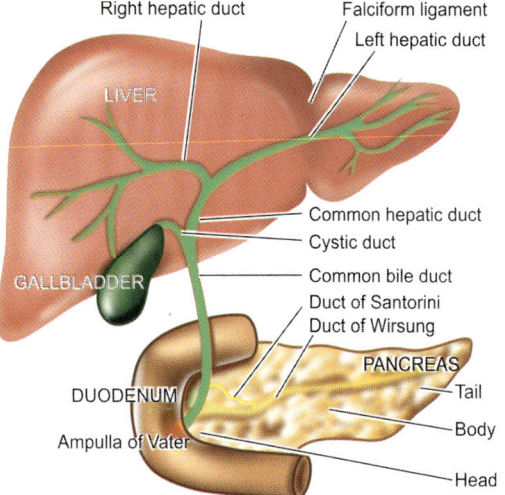

FIGURE 21.1: Anatomy of the liver and its relationship to the gallbladder, pancreas and duodenum.

- The transition of hepatic arterial blood into venous blood from zone 1 to zone 3 is accompanied by the reduction of oxygen content; that is why the centrolobular zone 3 receives the least amount of oxygen and is most susceptible to hypoxia.

Cell of the liver parenchyma The hepatic lobules/acini are composed of liver cells arranged into cords.

- The liver cells are *polygonal* and have a sinusoidal surface as well as a biliary (lateral) surface.
- On the *sinusoidal surface*, the liver cells face the sinusoids, from which they are separated by the *space of Disse* that contains the *interstitial cells of Ito*. Sinusoids have fenestrated wall composed of endothelial cells with interspersed fixed macrophages called *Kupffer cells*.
- The biliary system begins with the *bile canaliculi* on the lateral side of the hepatocytes, that provides the route for the flow of bile into the bile ductules located in the portal tracts.

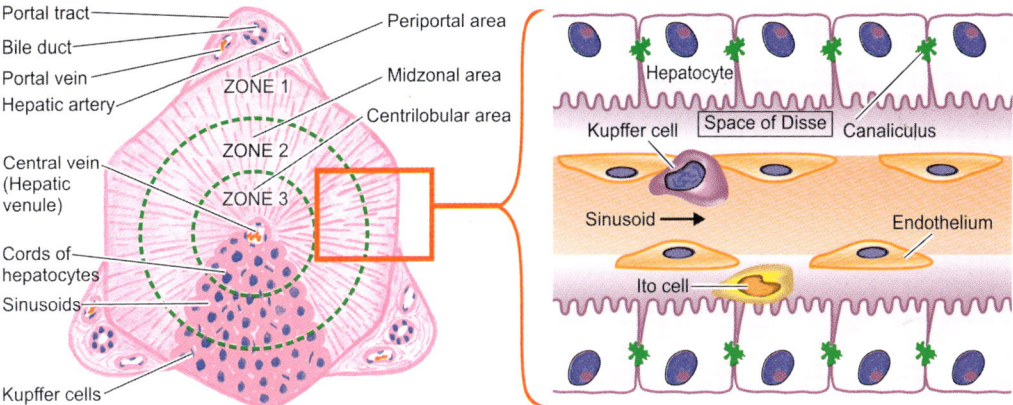

FIGURE 21.2: Histology of hepatic lobule. The hexagonal or pyramidal structure with central vein and peripheral 4 to 5 portal triads is termed the classical lobule. The figure on left shows functional divisions of the lobule into 3 zones shown by circles. The figure on right shows hepatic sinusoid perisinusoidal space and cords of hepatocytes.

- From bile ductules the blood flows into the bile ducts and ultimately leaves the liver through the right and left hepatic ducts, which form the *common bile duct*.
- The common bile duct is linked to the gall bladder through the *cystic duct*.

Physiology The liver has numerous functions which could be summarised under following headings:
i. Formation and excretion of bile.
ii. Synthesis of most plasma proteins.
iii. Metabolism of proteins, carbohydrates and lipids.
iv. Storage of vitamins (A, D and B_{12}) and iron.
v. Detoxification of toxins, alcohol and drugs.

Q2. What are the different forms of liver cell necrosis?

Liver cell necrosis may result from microbiologic, toxic, circulatory and traumatic injury. Depending on the extent of involvement of hepatic lobule, there are three forms of necrosis: i) diffuse, ii) zonal, and iii) focal.
I. **Diffuse (submassive or massive) necrosis** is characterised by extensive necrosis involving all the cells in groups of lobules. It is most often caused by viral hepatitis or drug toxicity.
II. **Zonal necrosis** affects differentially three zones of the lobule and thus can be classifies as under:
i. *Centrilobular necrosis* is the commonest type involving hepatocytes in zone 3 in the centre of the lobule. It is characteristic of ischaemic injury and occurs in shock and congestive heart failure. It also occurs in certain forms of poisoning, such as those caused by chloroform, carbon tetrachloride and certain drugs.
ii. *Midzonal necrosis* involves zone 2 and is uncommon. It is seen in yellow fever and viral hepatitis and is marked by the formation of acidophilic rounded hepatocytes called Councilman bodies.
iii. *Periportal (peripheral) necrosis* involves liver cells in zone 1, which is most vulnerable to the effects of hepatotoxins in circulating blood, entering the lobule from the branches of hepatic artery and portal vein, as in phosphorus poisoning or eclampsia.
III. **Focal necrosis** involves single hepatocytes or small groups of hepatocytes irregularly distributed in the hepatic lobules. Focal necrosis is most often caused by infections which may be viral, bacterial or fungal. Drug-induced hepatitis is also characterised by focal necrosis.

Q3. Tabulate the battery of liver function tests.

Since the liver has complex functions, they can be adequately assessed only by a battery of tests which can be grouped under following headings:
i. Tests for manufacture and excretion of bile
ii. Serum enzyme assays
iii. Tests for metabolic functions of the liver
iv. Immunologic tests

v. Ancillary diagnostic tests

Various common tests in these groups along with their significance are summed up in **Table 21.1**.

TABLE 21.1 Liver function tests.	
TESTS	SIGNIFICANCE
I. TESTS FOR MANUFACTURE AND EXCRETION OF BILE	
1. *Bilirubin:*	
i. Serum bilirubin (0.3–1.3 mg/dL)	Increased in hepatocellular, obstructive and haemolytic disease, Gilbert's disease
ii. In faeces	Absent in biliary obstruction
iii. In urine	Conjugated bilirubinuria in patients of hepatitis
2. *Urobilinogen:*	Increased in hepatocellular and haemolytic diseases, absent in biliary obstruction
3. *Bile acid (Bile salts):*	Increased in serum and detectable in urine in cholestasis
II. SERUM ENZYME ASSAYS	
1. *Alkaline phosphatase* (33–96 U/L)	Increased in hepatobiliary disease (highest in biliary obstruction), bone diseases, pregnancy
2. *γ-Glutamyl transpeptidase (γ-GT)* (9–58 IU/L)	Rise parallels alkaline phosphatase but is specific for hepatobiliary diseases
3. *Transaminases:*	
i. SGOT (AST) (12–38 U/L)	Increased in tissue injury to liver as well as to other tissues like in myocardial infarction
ii. SGPT (ALT) (7–41 U/L)	Increase is fairly specific for liver cell injury
4. *Other enzymes:*	
i. 5′-Nucleotidase	Rise parallels alkaline phosphatase but more specific for diseases of hepatic origin
ii. Lactate dehydrogenase (115–221 U/L)	Increased in tumours involving the liver
iii. Cholinesterase	Decreased in hepatocellular disease, malnutrition
III. TESTS FOR METABOLIC FUNCTIONS	
1. *Amino acid and protein metabolism:*	
i. Serum proteins (total=6.7–8.6 g/dL; A/G ratio=1.5–3:1)	Hypoalbuminaemia in hepatocellular diseases; hyperglobulinaemia in cirrhosis and chronic active hepatitis
ii. Immunoglobulins	Nonspecific alterations in IgA, IgG and IgM
iii. Clotting factors	Prothrombin time and partial thromboplastin time prolonged in patients with hepatocellular disease
iv. Plasma ammonia (19–60 µg/dL)	Increased in acute fulminant hepatitis, cirrhosis, hepatic encephalopathy
v. Aminoaciduria	In fulminant hepatitis
2. *Lipid and lipoprotein metabolism:* Blood lipids (total serum cholesterol <200 mg/dL; triglycerides < 150 mg/dL; and lipoprotein fractions)	Increased in cholestasis, decreased in acute and chronic diffuse liver disease and in malnutrition
3. *Carbohydrate metabolism:* Blood glucose and GTT	Decreased in hepatic necrosis
IV. IMMUNOLOGIC TESTS	
1. *Nonspecific immunologic reactions:*	
i. Smooth muscle antibody	In autoimmune hepatitis
ii. Mitochondrial antibody	In primary biliary cirrhosis
iii. Antinuclear antibody and LE cell test	In chronic active hepatitis
2. *Antibodies to specific etiologic agents:*	
i. Antibodies to hepatitis B (HBsAg, HBc, HBeAg)	In hepatitis B
ii. Amoeba antibodies	Amoebic liver abscess
V. ANCILLARY DIAGNOSTIC TESTS	
1. *Ultrasound examination*	Cholestasis of various etiologies; SOLs, US-guided-FNAC/liver biopsy
2. *FNAC and/ or percutaneous liver biopsy*	Unknown cause of hepatocellular disease, hepatomegaly and splenomegaly; long-standing hepatitis; PUO and SOLs of the liver

Q4. What are the test for production and excretion of bile?

Bile is produced by liver cells, stored in the gallbladder, and excreted via the bile ducts into the duodenum. Bile consists of bilirubin, bile acids and bile phospholipids. Following tests are used to assess how these substances are produced and excreted:

I. **Bilirubin** is a yellow pigment that can be detected in serum, urine and faeces.

i. *Serum bilirubin* occurs in two forms: unconjugated (indirect), and conjugated (direct).
- The normal serum of adults contains less than 1 mg/dL, 0.25 mg of which is unconjugated.
- Conjugation of bilirubin occurs in the liver.
- Hyperbilirubinaemia due to obstruction is caused by an elevation of conjugated bilirubin, whereas haemolysis and other causes of 'prehepatic jaundice' lead to an elevation of unconjugated bilirubin. Hepatitis and other forms of liver cell injury cause a mixed form of hyperbilirubinaemia.

ii. *Urinary bilirubin* can be detected by a dipstick method. Normal urine does not contain bilirubin. Bilirubinuria accounts for the deep yellow or brown colour of urine.
- In contrast to unconjugated bilirubin which circulates in serum bound to serum proteins, conjugated bilirubin is not protein-bound and can be excreted in urine.
- Bilirubinuria is, thus, seen only in jaundice caused by obstruction of bile ducts or hepatitis.

Faecal bilirubin is not measured chemically but its presence can be estimated by naked eye inspection of faeces.
- Normally, bilirubin imparts a brown colour to faeces. In obstructive jaundice, no bile will reach the intestines and, therefore, faeces will be *acholic*, i.e. pale-yellow, 'clay-coloured'.

II. **Urobilinogen** is normally excreted in urine.
- In obstructive jaundice, urobilinogen disappears from urine.
- In other forms of jaundice, urine contains increased amounts of urobilinogen.

III. **Bile salts** are formed from cholesterol in liver cells and excreted in bile.
- Most bile acids are reabsorbed in the intestine, and only 10% is lost in faeces in form of toxic lithocholic acid.
- In all forms of jaundice other than obstructive jaundice, the faeces contain increased amounts of bile salts.

Q5. Which enzyme assays are commonly used for assessing liver injury?

Several serum enzymes are used to determine if the liver injury is hepatocellular or cholestatic:

I. **Alkaline phosphatase** in serum is mostly derived from the bones and it is also elevated in pregnancy. If bone disease and pregnancy are excluded, marked elevation of alkaline phosphatase (3–10 times the normal) is related to obstructive jaundice.

II. **γ-glutamyl transpeptidase (GGT)** in serum is mostly of hepatic origin and it is used to confirm that elevated levels of alkaline phosphatase are of hepatic origin. GGT is elevated in serum in cholestatic and hepatocellular diseases.

III. **Transaminases** include serum aspartate transaminase (AST) and serum alanine transaminase (ALT).
- ALT (*mnemonic L*=liver) is a cytosolic enzyme found mostly in the liver.
- AST is a mitochondrial enzyme found in liver cells but also in many other tissues, and thus less specific for the liver.

Transaminases are elevated in serum in various diseases that cause acute liver cell injury and necrosis.

Q6. Discuss briefly common tests for assessing metabolic liver functions.

Liver is the principal organ for the synthesis of plasma proteins and amino acids, lipid and lipoproteins, carbohydrates and vitamins. The following tests are used for evaluating these functions:

I. **Aminoacid and plasma protein metabolism** Aminoacids derived from diet and tissue breakdown are metabolised in the liver. Several plasma proteins and immunoglobulins are synthesised in the hepatocytes.

i. *Serum proteins* Liver injury will decrease the blood levels of all proteins that are synthesised in the liver.
- In would not be practical to measure plasma concentration of all these proteins, and in routine clinical practice it is customary to measure only the following: albumin, fibrinogen, prothrombin

α-1-antitrypsin, haptoglobin, ceruloplasmin, transferrin alpha-foetoprotein, and acute phase reactant proteins such as C-reactive protein.
- *Hypoalbuminaemia* is the most common sign of reduced plasma protein synthesis in chronic liver diseases.

ii. **Immunoglobulins** are produced by plasma cells and lymphocytes and thus their concentration in plasma is increased in inflammatory chronic liver diseases, such as chronic viral hepatitis and cirrhosis. The albumin to globulin (A:G) ratio which is 1.5 to 3:1 is decreased.

iii. **Clotting factors** synthesis is decreased in chronic liver disease. The best approach to estimating the clotting factors production is by performing the coagulation tests, such as prothrombin time and partial thromboplastin time. These tests measure the activity of several clotting factors and are prolonged in chronic liver diseases, such as cirrhosis.

iv. **Serum ammonia** is elevated in blood in severe liver injury, preventing normal conversion of ammonia to urea which is then excreted in urine.

II. **Lipid and lipoprotein metabolism** can be monitored by measuring serum lipid, cholesterol and cholesterol esters, lipoproteins and triglycerides.
- In chronic cholestasis, there is an increased concentration of cholesterol which is excreted normally in bile. Triglycerides are also elevated.
- Values of blood lipids are lowered in acute and chronic diffuse liver diseases and in malnutrition.

III. **Carbohydrates** are actively metabolised and stored in the liver.
- Blood glucose level is lowered in fulminant acute liver necrosis.
- In chronic liver disease, there is impaired glucose tolerance and relative insulin resistance.

Q7. What are the immunologic tests for the diagnosis of specific liver diseases?

Immunologic tests can be divided into two groups: i) nonspecific immunologic tests, and ii) antibodies to specific etiologic agents.

I. **Nonspecific immunologic tests** include the search for antibodies to cell components as under:
i. *Anti-smooth muscle actin antibody*, which is found in autoimmune hepatitis.
ii. *Anti-mitochondrial antibody*, which is found in primary biliary cirrhosis.
iii. *Antinuclear antibody* which is found in SLE involving the liver and some forms of chronic hepatitis.

II. **Antibodies to specific etiologic agents** include various antibodies to hepatitis B virus (e.g. hepatitis B surface antigen, hepatitis B core antigen), hepatitis C virus, *Entamoeba histolytica*, etc.

Q8. What are the main indications for liver biopsy?

The following are the main indications for liver biopsy that can be performed as a percutaneous needle biopsy, or surgical laparoscopic, or intraoperative targeted, or random wedge biopsy:
i. Hepatocellular disease of unknown etiology
ii. Suspected chronic hepatitis
iii. Hepatomegaly of unknown etiology
iv. Splenomegaly of unknown cause
v. Fever of unknown cause
vi. Liver tumours
vii. Liver nodule or mass found on radiologic examination

Q9. What is jaundice? Comment on its classification.

Definition Jaundice (Latin *icterus*) is yellow discoloration of skin and mucosae by hyperbilirubinaemia. Normal serum bilirubin concentration is 0.3–1.3 mg/dL; jaundice becomes visible when the concentration exceeds 2 mg/dL. Elevation above 1.3 mg/dL but below 2 mg/dL, not associated with visible jaundice is called latent jaundice.

Classification Jaundice may result from one or more of the following mechanisms **(Fig. 21.3)**:
i. Increased bilirubin production
ii. Decreased hepatic uptake of unconjugated bilirubin
iii. Decreased conjugation
iv. Decreased excretion of conjugated bilirubin into bile

Pathophysiologic classification recognises three types of jaundice: i) pre-hepatic, ii) hepatic, and iii) posthepatic (cholestatic).

Clinical classification of jaundice is more practice-oriented and it takes into account the predominance of conjugated or unconjugated bilirubin. In clinical practice, this is done by measuring total bilirubin and direct (conjugated) bilirubin; subtracting the latter from total is calculated and expressed as indirect (unconjugated) bilirubin. Thus, based on pathogenesis, there are two groups of hyperbilirubinaemia:

I. Predominantly unconjugated hyperbilirubinaemia

II. Predominantly conjugated hyperbilirubinaemia

Q10. What are the differences between unconjugated and conjugated bilirubin?

Major differences between unconjugated (or indirect) and conjugated (or direct) bilirubin are summarised in **Table 21.2**.

Q11. Briefly discuss etiopathogenesis of unconjugated and conjugated hyperbilirubinaemia.

Major causes of the two groups are listed in **Table 21.3**.

I. **Predominantly unconjugated bilirubinaemia** is the condition when conjugated bilirubin accounts for less than 20%. This may result from three sets of conditions: i) increased bilirubin production, ii) decreased hepatic uptake, and iii) decreased bilirubin conjugation.

i. **Increased bilirubin production** occurs in various haemolytic conditions, such as haemolytic anaemia or spherocytosis.

ii. **Decreased hepatic uptake** as in sepsis, due to drugs and prolonged starvation.

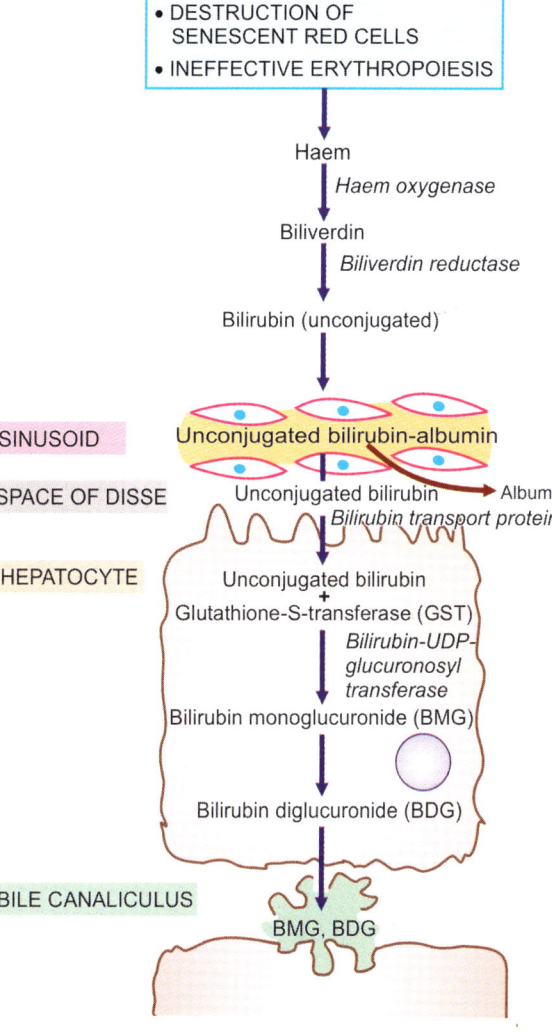

FIGURE 21.3: Schematic representation of hepatic phase of bilirubin transport.

TABLE 21.2 Major differences between unconjugated and conjugated bilirubin.

FEATURE	UNCONJUGATED BILIRUBIN	CONJUGATED BILIRUBIN
1. Normal serum level	More	Less (less than 0.25 mg/dL)
2. Water solubility	Absent	Present
3. Affinity to lipids (alcohol solubility)	Present	Absent
4. Serum albumin binding	High	Low
5. van den Bergh reaction	Indirect (Total minus direct)	Direct
6. Renal excretion	Absent	Present
7. Bilirubin albumin covalent complex formation	Absent	Present
8. Affinity to brain tissue	Present (Kernicterus)	Absent

iii. **Decreased conjugation** such as defective function of UDP-glucuronosyltransferase that conjugates bilirubin to glucuronic acid. Defective conjugation is seen in certain genetic disorders such as Gilbert disease and Crigler-Najjar syndrome, in hepatitis and drug induced liver injury.

Physiologic neonatal jaundice that occurs during the first week after delivery is in part due to relative deficiency of UDP-glucuronosyltransferase and in part due to increased haemolysis of red blood cells containing foetal haemoglobin.

II. **Predominantly conjugated hyperbilirubinaemia** is defined as failure of normal amounts of bile to reach the duodenum. It may be caused by i) intrahepatic cholestasis or ii) extrahepatic cholestasis.

i. **Intrahepatic cholestasis** may develop due to:
- *Hereditary causes*, also called pure cholestasis, e.g. Rotor syndrome, Dubin-Johnson syndrome, cystic fibrosis.
- *Acquired causes*, e.g. in viral hepatitis, drug-induced hepatitis or alcoholic hepatitis.

Clinical and laboratory features of intrahepatic cholestasis include:
a. Predominantly conjugated hyperbilirubinaemia due to regurgitation of conjugated bilirubin into the blood
b. Elevated bile acid and consequent pruritus
c. Elevated alkaline phosphatase
d. Hyperlipidaemia
e. Vitamin K deficiency resulting in prolonged prothrombin time.

Liver biopsy shows **(Fig. 21.4, A)**:
- Bile plugs in the dilated intercellular canaliculi.
- Bile stagnation in the hepatocytes leads to clearing up of the cytoplasm, a feature of feathery degeneration.

ii. **Extrahepatic cholestasis** develops due to obstruction of bile ducts outside the liver at the porta hepatis: The causes include:
- Gallstones
- Tumours of the biliary ducts or the head of the pancreas

TABLE 21.3 Pathophysiologic classification of jaundice.

I. PREDOMINANTLY UNCONJUGATED HYPERBILIRUBINAEMIA

1. *Increased bilirubin production (Haemolytic, acholuric or prehepatic jaundice)*
   i. Intra- and extravascular haemolysis
   ii. Ineffective erythropoiesis

2. *Decreased hepatic uptake*
   i. Drugs
   ii. Prolonged starvation
   iii. Sepsis

3. *Decreased bilirubin conjugation*
   i. Hereditary disorders (e.g. Gilbert syndrome, Crigler-Najjar syndrome)
   ii. Acquired defects (e.g. drugs, hepatitis, cirrhosis)
   iii. Neonatal jaundice

II. PREDOMINANTLY CONJUGATED HYPERBILIRUBINAEMIA (CHOLESTASIS)

1. *Intrahepatic cholestasis (Impaired hepatic excretion)*
   i. Hereditary disorders or *'pure cholestasis'* (e.g. Dubin-Johnson syndrome, Rotor syndrome, fibrocystic disease of pancreas, benign familial recurrent cholestasis, intrahepatic atresia, cholestatic jaundice of pregnancy)
   ii. Acquired disorders or *'hepatocellular cholestasis'* (e.g. viral hepatitis, drugs, alcohol-induced injury, sepsis, cirrhosis)

2. *Extrahepatic cholestasis (Extrahepatic biliary obstruction)*
   Mechanical obstruction (e.g. gallstones, inflammatory strictures, carcinoma head of pancreas, tumours of bile ducts, sclerosing cholangitis, congenital atresia of extrahepatic ducts)

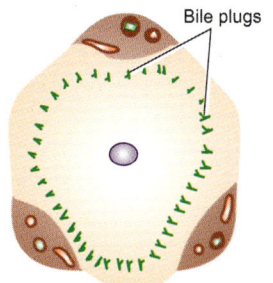 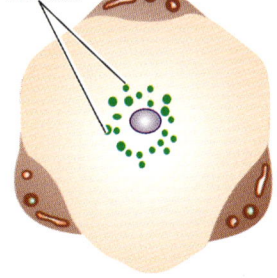

A, INTRAHEPATIC CHOLESTASIS   B, EXTRAHEPATIC CHOLESTASIS

FIGURE 21.4: Salient features in morphology of liver in intra- and extrahepatic cholestasis. A, Intrahepatic cholestasis is characterised by elongated bile plugs in the canaliculi of hepatocytes at the periphery of the lobule. B, Extrahepatic cholestasis shows characteristic bile lakes due to rupture of canaliculi in the hepatocytes in the centrilobular area.

- Sclerosing cholangitis
- Congenital atresia of extrahepatic bile ducts

Clinical and laboratory features are similar to those in intrahepatic cholestasis. However, the two are distinguished by the following additional features:

a. There is steatorrhoea and malabsorption of fat soluble vitamins (A, D, K, E).
b. Prolonged prothrombin time can be ameliorated by parenteral administration of vitamin K, in contrast to giving vitamin K to patients with intrahepatic cholestasis who do not respond to such treatment.
c. The stools are acholic and the urobilinogen has disappeared from the urine.
d. These patients often develop fever, usually due to ascending cholangitis.

Liver biopsy shows **(Fig. 21.4, B)**:
- Prominent cholestasis and rupture of canaliculi with formation of *bile lakes*.
- Bile is chemotactic for neutrophils and the necrosis of hepatocytes around the bile lakes contributes to the accumulation of *neutrophils* at their periphery.
- Neutrophils are seen in dilated, small and medium-sized bile ducts, usually reflecting the appearance of ascending cholangitis, which is a common complication.
- If the cholestasis and bile duct injury persist, there will be reactive proliferation of bile ducts, which are also surrounded by neutrophils because they leak bile, which is chemotactic.

Q12. Define neonatal jaundice. What are its major causes?

Definition Neonatal jaundice is appearance of jaundice in neonates when the total serum bilirubin is more than 3 mg/dL.

Causes It can be *physiologic* that develops in all babies, and *pathologic* which affects only some of the neonates:

Physiologic neonatal jaundice develops due to an increased supply of unconjugated bilirubin liberated from haemolysed RBCs exceeding the capacity of the immature liver to conjugate it. It is characterised by unconjugated hyperbilirubinaemia. In general terms, physiologic jaundice is more prominent in premature infants than in term babies.

Pathologic neonatal jaundice All other forms of neonatal jaundice (beside the physiologic jaundice) are pathologic and can be classified as unconjugated and conjugated hyperbilirubinaemia; the former being more common.

Important causes of neonatal jaundice are listed in **Table 21.4**.

TABLE 21.4 Causes of neonatal jaundice.

A. UNCONJUGATED HYPERBILIRUBINAEMIA
1. Physiologic and prematurity jaundice
2. Haemolytic disease of the newborn and kernicterus (page 270)
3. Congenital haemolytic disorders (page 243)
4. Perinatal complications (e.g. haemorrhage, sepsis)
5. Gilbert syndrome
6. Crigler-Najjar syndrome (type I and II)

B. CONJUGATED HYPERBILIRUBINAEMIA
1. Hereditary (Dubin-Johnson syndrome, Rotor syndrome)
2. Infections (e.g. hepatitis B, hepatitis C or non-A non-B hepatitis, rubella, coxsackievirus, cytomegalovirus, echovirus, herpes simplex, syphilis, toxoplasma, gram-negative sepsis)
3. Metabolic (e.g. galactosaemia, alpha-1-antitrypsin deficiency, cystic fibrosis, Niemann-Pick disease)
4. Idiopathic (neonatal hepatitis, congenital hepatic fibrosis)
5. Biliary atresia (intrahepatic and extrahepatic)
6. Reye syndrome

Q13. Discuss salient features of hereditary non-haemolytic hyperbilirubinaemias.

Definition Hereditary non-haemolytic hyperbilirubinaemias are a small group of uncommon familial disorders. The group includes:

- *Hereditary unconjugated hyperbilirubinaemias* like Gilbert disease (the commonest) and Crigler-Najjar syndrome.
- *Hereditary conjugated hyperbilirubinaemias* like Dubin-Johnson syndrome, Rotor syndrome, recurrent intrahepatic cholestasis, and progressive familial intrahepatic cholestasis.

Salient features These are briefly discussed below and their contrasting features are presented in **Table 21.5**.

I. **Gilbert syndrome** affects up to 5% of the total population, and is four times more common in males than females.

i. It is an autosomal dominant disorder related to mutations of *UGT1A1* gene which encodes the UDP-glucuronosyl transferase in liver cells.

TABLE 21.5 Contrasting features of major hereditary non-haemolytic hyperbilirubinaemias.

FEATURE	GILBERT SYNDROME	TYPE 1 CRIGLER-NAJJAR SYNDROME	TYPE 2 CRIGLER-NAJJAR SYNDROME	DUBIN-JOHNSON SYNDROME
1. *Inheritance*	Autosomal dominant	Autosomal recessive	Autosomal dominant	Autosomal recessive
2. *Predominant hyperbilirubinaemia*	Unconjugated	Unconjugated	Unconjugated	Conjugated
3. *Intensity of jaundice*	Mild (< 5 mg/dL)	Marked (>20 mg/dL)	Mild to moderate (<20 mg/dL)	Mild (<5 mg/dL)
4. *Basic defect*	↓ UDP-glucuronosyl transferase activity	Absence of UDP-glucuronosyl transferase	↓ UDP-glucuronosyl transferase	Defect in canalicular excretion (Prolonged BSP excretion test)
5. *Hepatic morphology*	Normal (except slightly increased lipofuscin)	Normal (except mild canalicular stasis)	Normal	Greenish-black pigment
6. *Prognosis*	Excellent	Poor (due to kernicterus)	Good	Excellent

ii. Reduced activity of this enzyme causes periodic mild jaundice marked by unconjugated hyperbilirubinaemia and no other liver abnormality.

iii. Onset of jaundice, which is accompanied by mild constitutional symptoms, may be precipitated by exertion, mental stress, infection or alcohol.

iv. There is no liver pathology and no treatment is required.

II. **Crigler-Najjar syndrome** is a rare hereditary jaundice, also related to *UGT1A1* gene mutations and is associated with severe unconjugated hyperbilirubinaemia. It occurs in two forms:

• *Autosomal recessive* form due to complete absence of UDP-glucuronosyl transferase with early death during first year of life mostly due to kernicterus.

• *Autosomal dominant* milder form due to reduced activity of the same enzyme, that has a good prognosis since the infants do not develop kernicterus.

III. **Dubin-Johnson syndrome** is an autosomal recessive disorder associated with mild conjugated hyperbilirubinaemia due to defective canalicular excretion of bilirubin from liver cells.

• It is caused by one of several possible mutations of the *ABCC2* gene encoding the MRP2 (multidrug resistance protein 2), a bile transporter, involved in the export of bile from liver cells.

• In contrast to other congenital hyperbilirubinaemia, Dubin-Johnson syndrome is accompanied by changes in the liver, which appears black on gross examination and histologically shows black cytoplasmic granules unrelated to bilirubin.

IV. **Rotor syndrome** is associated with mild jaundice with conjugated hyperbilirubinaemia. It is thus similar to Dubin-Johnson syndrome but the liver shows no black pigment accumulation.

Q14. What is neonatal hepatitis? Discuss its features briefly.

Definition Neonatal hepatitis, also known as giant cell hepatitis, is a term used for a variety of neonatal diseases presenting during the first postnatal week of life with conjugated hyperbilirubinaemia

Etiology The cause of neonatal hepatitis may be identified in approximately 50% of infants, whereas the others are idiopathic (*see* **Table 21.4**). Estimates are that α-1-antitrypsin deficiency accounts for at least one half of all identifiable causes.

Pathology *Microscopy* shows:

i. Loss of lobular architecture

ii. Presence of multinucleated giant cells derived from hepatocytes

iii. Mononuclear infiltrate in the portal tracts with some fibrosis, haemosiderosis and cholestasis

Clinical features These include:

i. Jaundice that appears during the first week of life

ii. Conjugated hyperbilirubinaemia

iii. High alkaline phosphatase in serum

iv. Acholic stools

Neonatal hepatitis must be distinguished from intrahepatic or extrahepatic biliary atresia, which requires surgical treatment.

Q15. What is biliary atresia? Discuss salient features of its major types.

Definition Congenital biliary atresia is a term used for neonatal disorders presenting as obstructive jaundice during the first three months after birth due to abnormal development of the biliary system, resulting in obliteration and destruction of bile ducts, or a loss of intrahepatic bile ducts and portal ductules (*ductopenia*).

Classification Two forms are recognised: i) extrahepatic biliary atresia, and ii) intrahepatic biliary atresia.

I. ***Extrahepatic biliary atresia*** involves the major extrahepatic bile ducts and is often associated with other developmental anomalies. Two forms are recognised:
- *Perinatal form* is more common (80%); in these cases the biliary tree is normally developed but manifestations appear days or weeks after birth.
- *Foetal form* (20%) accounts for cases in which extrahepatic tree is abnormally developed and the infant presents at birth.

Pathology Microscopic features are:
i. Obliteration of extrahepatic bile ducts, with or without concomitant inflammation.
ii. Cholestasis and bile plugs in periportal ducts associated with periductal fibrosis.
iii. Portal tract bile ductular proliferation and periductular inflammation.
iv. Changes progress to secondary biliary cirrhosis in advanced stages and those that have not been treated.

Clinical features Obstructive jaundice appears during first three month after birth, and often it becomes evident even in the first week of postnatal life. Surgical repair of the bile ducts may be attempted but often the defects cannot be corrected and liver transplantation is the only possible treatment.

II. ***Intrahepatic biliary atresia*** is characterised by:
i. Intrahepatic bile duct hypoplasia and a paucity of bile ducts.
ii. Cholestatic jaundice with conjugated hyperbilirubinaemia appears clinically during the first week of postnatal life.
iii. Some cases are related to giant cells neonatal hepatitis, and may have the same causes.

Q16. What is Reye syndrome? What are its main causes and salient features?

Definition Reye syndrome is an acute post-viral syndrome of childhood presenting with encephalopathy, fatty liver and fatty change in other viscera.

Etiopathogenesis The exact pathogenesis is not known but it is assumed that the underlying cause is mitochondrial injury caused by one of the following:
- Viral infection, most often influenza A or B and varicella.
- Drugs such as salicylates, and toxins such as aflatoxin or insecticides may aggravate the clinical symptoms.

Clinicopathologic features Salient features are:
i. *Grossly*, the liver is enlarged and appears fatty.
ii. *Microscopy* shows microvesicular fatty change of hepatocytes, cardiac and skeletal myocytes and renal tubules.
iii. *Brain* shows oedema and focal necrosis of nerve cells.
iv. Most patients are 6 months to 15 years of age.
v. *Clinically*, they present with sudden onset of intractable vomiting and psychiatric and neurologic signs of encephalopathy leading to stupor, coma and death.

Q17. What is hepatic failure? Discuss its types and their salient features.

Definition Liver failure is characterised by a loss of all or most liver functions. It may be:
- *Acute* due to a massive loss of hepatocytes, or
- *Chronic* due to a loss of normal hepatic architecture preventing the normal functioning of hepatocytes.

Etiology

Acute (fulminant) hepatic failure Major causes are:
- *Viral hepatitis:* most frequent.
- *Other causes*: drugs taken in large doses (e.g. acetaminophen), toxins such as carbon tetrachloride or mushroom poisoning, alcohol and eclampsia of pregnancy.

Chronic hepatic failure is most often caused by cirrhosis.

Clinicopathologic features Major manifestations of acute or chronic liver failure are presented diagrammatically in **Figure 21.5** and are as under:

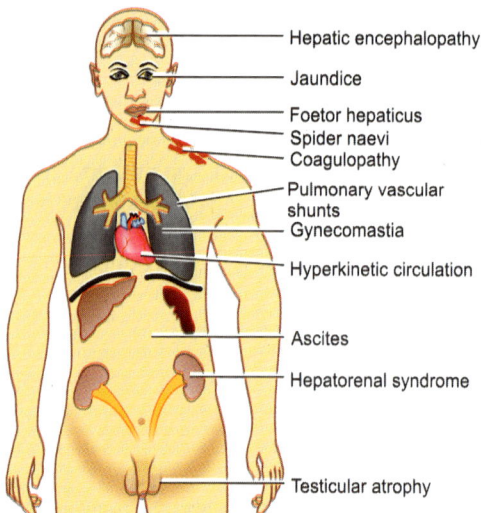

FIGURE 21.5: Complications of hepatic failure.

i. **Jaundice** which is related to a loss of capacity to process and excrete bilirubin. The extent of jaundice usually reflects the severity of liver failure.

ii. **Hepatic encephalopathy** which includes personality changes, intellectual deterioration, low slurred speech, flapping tremors, and ending up in hepatic coma and death. These changes are related to ammonia in blood and probably other metabolic byproducts that fail to get neutralised by the ailing liver.

iii. **Foetor hepaticus**, a pungent smell of the breath, is related to the presence of sulphur-containing substances of intestinal origin that could not be eliminated from blood by the diseased liver.

iv. **Hyperkinetic circulation** characterised by splanchnic vasodilatation, increased splanchnic blood pooling, and increased cardiac output, combined with renal hypoperfusion. It results in tachycardia, low blood pressure and reduced renal function.

v. **Hepatorenal syndrome** which develops in about 10% of both acute and chronic liver failure due to effective hypovolaemia. It presents with oliguria, uraemia but good preservation of tubular function and it is reversible after recovery from liver failure.

vi. **Hepatopulmonary syndrome** due to intrapulmonary vasodilatation and arteriovenous shunting, leading to ventilation-perfusion inequality. It presents with dyspnoea and deterioration of pulmonary function, hypoxaemia and cyanosis.

vii. **Coagulation defects** as evidenced by prolonged prothrombin time, thrombocytopenia due to sequestration of platelets in the enlarged spleen, predisposing to uncontrollable bleeding. On the other hand, DIC is also common with consumption coagulopathy and the appearance of fibrin split products in urine.

viii. **Ascites and oedema**, in part due to hypoalbuminaemia and hyperaldosteronism, and in part due to portal hypertension and circulatory disturbances.

ix. **Endocrine changes** such as hyperestrinism due to reduced catabolism of oestrogen in male patients.
- **Gynecomastia** is a common sign of hyperestrinism which also plays a role in testicular atrophy.
- In females, inadequate removal of androgens could cause *atrophy of the ovaries and breasts*.

x. **Skin changes** like *arterial spiders* and *palmar erythema* reflect vascular and circulatory changes in the body, and could also be related to hormonal changes.

Q18. What is Budd-Chiari syndrome? Discuss its main features.

Definition Budd-Chiari syndrome is thrombotic occlusion of the hepatic vein and adjacent inferior vena cava obstructing the venous outflow from the liver.

Etiology In 30% cases, the cause is not known (idiopathic) and the others are associated with increased thrombotic tendencies as under:
i. Polycythaemia vera
ii. Paroxysmal nocturnal haemoglobinuria
iii. Oral contraceptives
iv. Pregnancy and postpartum state

v. Intra-abdominal cancer involving the liver (e.g. hepatocellular carcinoma)
vi. Chemotherapy and radiation therapy of cancer
vii. Myeloproliferative diseases
viii. Formation of membranous webs in the suprahepatic portion of inferior vena cava (congenital or acquired due to organizing mural thrombi)
Pathology *Grossly,* The liver is enlarged, markedly congested and has a tense capsule.
- Upon cross-sectioning at autopsy, the blood is pouring from the dark red cut surface.
Microscopy
- Centrolobular congestion and extravasation of blood from ruptured sinusoids.
- Peripheral to the blood-filled centrolobular area, the compressed hepatocytes undergo necrosis.
- Longer lasting congestion leads to perivenular fibrosis which may progress in chronic cases to cardiac cirrhosis.
Clinical features It is a rare disease with an incidence of 1:1 million. It may develop in an acute or chronic form:
i. *Acute Budd-Chiari syndrome* presents with acute abdominal pain, most intense over right upper quadrant, with vomiting, ascites and mild jaundice.
- Liver failure develops in a matter of days.
ii. *Chronic Budd-Chiari syndrome* presents with pain over the progressively enlarging liver, ascites and other features of portal hypertension.
- Patients may live for several months or years.
NOTE: *Hepatic veno-occlusive disease* involving the central lobular venules and small tributaries of the hepatic vein may produce the same symptoms as chronic Budd-Chiari syndrome.
Etiology This syndrome is caused by high dose chemotherapy given before bone marrow transplantation.
- In India, Africa and tropical countries, it may be related to consumption of medicinal tea ('bush tea') and it may be related to tea alkaloids.

Q19. What are the causes of portal vein obstruction?

Etiology This obstruction could be i) intrahepatic, or ii) extrahepatic:
I. *Intrahepatic obstruction of portal vein*
- Most often caused by cirrhosis.
- Other less common causes are: hepatic carcinomas, congenital hepatic fibrosis and polycystic liver disease, or parasitic infections such as schistosomiasis.
II. *Extrahepatic obstruction of portal vein*
- Thrombi in hypercoagulable states
- Sepsis
- Local malignancy
- Postsurgical changes.
Pathogenesis
- Thrombi that have formed in portal vein tributaries could extend into the portal tract, especially if they are infected with bacteria.
- Obstruction of portal veins will cause portal hypertension and all the consequence of this event.
- Acute obstruction could result in venous infarction of the bowel.
- Pylephlebitis is a complication of thrombosis complicated with infection, typically occurring due to some acute bacterial infectious process, such as acute appendicitis.

Q20. What is viral hepatitis? Tabulate salient features of main types of hepatitis viruses.

Definition Viral hepatitis is a term used to designate liver infection with one of the five hepatotropic viruses: hepatitis A, B, C, D and E viruses.
The key facts about viral hepatitis are summarised in **Table 21.6**.

Q21. Discuss the main features of viral hepatitis A.

Virology Viral hepatitis A is a mild acute infection caused by HAV, *an RNA virus*.
i. Infection occurs usually by faecal-oral route; water and food contaminated by human sewage account for most cases (80%).

TABLE 21.6 Salient features of various types of hepatitis viruses.

FEATURE	HEPATITIS A	HEPATITIS B	HEPATITIS C	HEPATITIS D	HEPATITIS E
1. *Agent*	HAV	HBV	HCV	HDV	HEV
2. *Year identified*	1973	1965	1989	1977	1980
3. *Viral particle*	27 nm	42 nm	30–60 nm	35–37 nm	32–34 nm
4. *Genome*	RNA, ss, linear	DNA, ss/ds	RNA, ss, linear circular	RNA, ss, circular	RNA, ss, linear
5. *Morphology*	Icosahedral non-enveloped	Double-shelled, enveloped	Enveloped	Enveloped, replication defective	Icosahedral, non-enveloped
6. *Spread*	Faeco-oral	Parenteral, close contact	Parenteral, close contact	Parenteral, close contact	Water-borne
7. *Incubation period*	15–45 days	30–180 days	20–90 days	30–50 days (In superinfection)	15–60 days
8. *Antigen(s)*	HAV	HBsAg HBcAg HBeAg HBxAg	HCV RNA C 100-3 C 33c NS5	HBsAg HDV	HEV
9. *Antibodies*	Anti-HAV	Anti-HBs Anti-HBc Anti-HBe	Anti-HCV	Anti-HBs Anti-HDV	Anti-HEV
10. *Severity*	Mild	Occasionally severe	Moderate	Occasionally severe	Mild
11. *Chronic hepatitis*	None	Occasional	Common	Common	None
12. *Carrier state*	None	<1%	<1%	1–10%	Unknown
13. *Hepatocellular carcinoma*	No	+	+	±	None
14. *Prognosis*	Excellent	Worse with age	Moderate	Acute good; chronic poor	Good

(ss, single-stranded; ss/ds, partially single-stranded partially double-stranded)

ii. Travellers to underdeveloped countries are at high-risk.
iii. It is the second most common viral hepatitis reported in the US.
iv. At least 30% of the US population has antibodies to HAV by the age of 50 years indicating that many Americans have had the infection that was unrecognised.

Clinicopathologic aspects There is no chronic infection and no carrier state.

i. Virus replicates in human liver cells eliciting a CD8+ T-cell reaction resulting in mild acute hepatitis which heals without consequences.

ii. IgM anti-HAV develops approximately four weeks after infection and persists for 12 weeks **(Fig. 21.6)**.

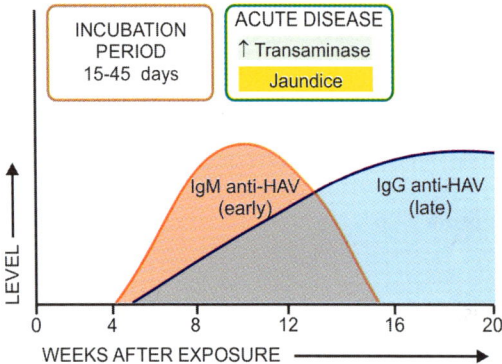

FIGURE 21.6: Sequence of appearance of antibodies to HAV.

iii. IgG antibody titre rises slowly but it persists at high level and provides long-term immunity.
iv. The vaccine against HAV will also induce IgG antibodies and is highly effective.
v. Clinical symptoms are mild and a complete recovery is to be expected in most patients, with minimal mortality.
vi. Jaundice is found in 70% infected person (the most common form of hepatitis to cause jaundice!).

Q22. What are the key features of hepatitis B virus (HBV)?

It is most commonly reported form of viral hepatitis in the US.
Virology Infection occurs by:
i. Viral hepatitis B is caused by HBV, a double stranded *DNA virus*.
ii. Exposure to blood and blood products (transfusions, sharing of needles in drug addict, health care persons).
iii. Additional routes of transmission are sexual contact, close contact with the infected person (virus is in saliva, tears, and breast milk)
iv. Transplacental transmission infects the foetus in utero.
Clinicopathologic aspects Viraemia and virus in body fluids may persist in chronic cases and account for their infectivity.
i. Antibodies to components of the virus can identify those who have been infected, those that have persistent infection, and those who are persistently infectious.
ii. HBV is not directly cytopathic. It elicits production of antibodies and a cellular immune response which then destroys hepatocytes.
iii. CD8+ T-cytotoxic cells kill hepatocytes and the T cell response determines if the infection will be mild or severe, and if chronic disease will develop.
iv. Newborns and immunodeficient persons are most likely groups to develop chronic hepatitis (>90%).
v. Immunisation against HBV is very efficient.

Q23. Enumerate the clinical forms of disease by HBV infection.

Clinically, HBV infection may produce several forms of disease as under:
i. Subclinical acute hepatitis (asymptomatic or clinically unrecognised)
ii. Acute icteric hepatitis, which may be fulminant in a very small number of cases (5%)
iii. Chronic hepatitis
iv. Cirrhosis
v. Cirrhosis with hepatocellular carcinoma
Outcome of the acute infection is unpredictable but most cases (80–90%) will recover completely.

Q24. What are the serologic and viral markers of viral hepatitis B?

The appearance of serologic and viral markers and their persistence following an acute infection is outlined in **Figure 21.7**. These are as follows:

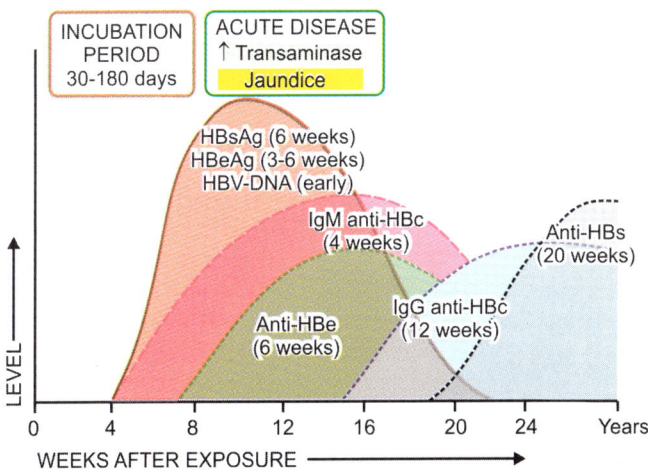

FIGURE 21.7: Sequence of serologic and viral markers in acute hepatitis B.

i. **Hepatitis B surface antigen (HBsAg)** appears in blood approximately 6 weeks after infection and usually disappears after 3–6 months. Its persistence for more than 6 months indicates a carrier state or chronic hepatitis.

ii. **Anti-hepatitis B surface antigen (anti-HBs)** appears in serum late, about 3 months after infection. It persists for life and provides permanent immunity. It is also found in immunised persons who have good immunity.

iii. **Hepatitis B core antigen-derived e antigen (HBeAg)** is present transiently (3–6 weeks) during an acute attack. Its persistence beyond 10 weeks is indicative of chronic disease and carrier state.

iv. **Antibody to HBe antigen (anti-HBe)** appears after the disappearance of HbeAg at 8–12 weeks after infection and is a sign of resolution of the infection.

v. **Hepatitis B core antigen (HBcAg)** *cannot be detected in serum*. It can be demonstrated in the nuclei of hepatocytes in chronic carriers, and chronic hepatitis cases, but it is not seen in acute stages of the disease.

vi. **Antibody to HBc (anti-HBc)** can be detected in the pre-icteric stage of the disease and later on. It is first IgM, which means acute infection, and then it persists as IgG which is indicative of an infection in the past.

vii. **Hepatitis virus B DNA (HBV-DNA)** by Southern blotting is the most sensitive technique for diagnosing HBV infection.

Q25. What is hepatitis D virus infection?

HDV accounts for <1% viral hepatitis in the US.

Virology HDV is a single-stranded, incomplete RNA that requires HBsAg to replicate, and thus the infection can occur as coinfection or superinfection of a HBV infected person.

i. HDV has a direct cytopathic effect on hepatocytes, although this effect is not obvious in all cases.
ii. Infection is transmitted by blood, sexual intercourse, and vertically.

Clinicopathologic aspects The outcome depends on the mode of infection **(Fig. 21.8)**:

i. *In coinfection*, majority of cases recover and develop immunity (90%), whereas chronicity is rare.
ii. *In superinfection*, most cases develop chronic viral disease and cirrhosis (80%); recovery occurs only in 10% cases.
iii. Fulminant and acute severe hepatitis develop in a minority of cases, but have high mortality.
iv. Fulminant hepatitis is more common in coinfection.
v. Prevention includes immunisation against HBV.

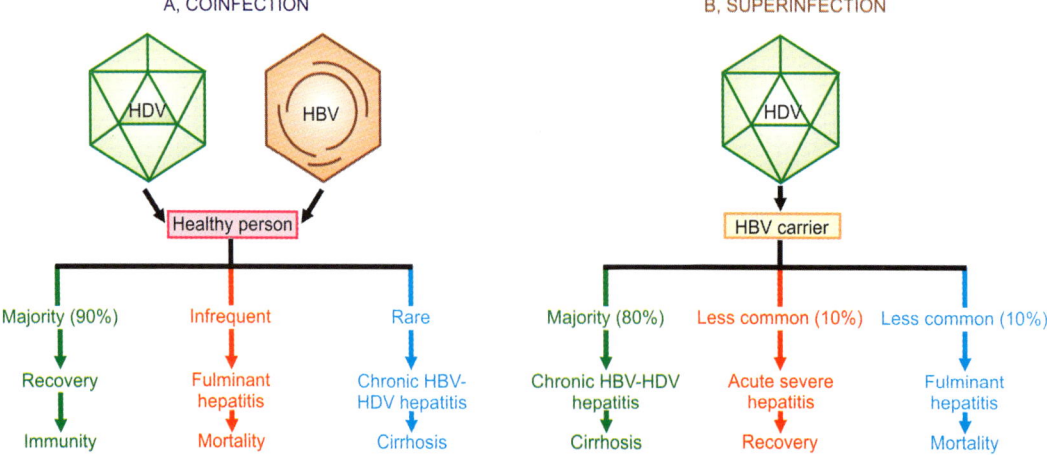

FIGURE 21.8: Consequences of coinfection *versus* superinfection in combined HDV-HBV infection.

Q26. What is hepatitis C virus infection?

HCV is the most common chronic blood-borne infection in the US (~ 4–5 million) and the most common indication for liver transplantation.

Virology HCV is a single-stranded RNA flavivirus which is inherently unstable, thus giving rise to numerous subtypes. Infection can occur through several routes as under:
i. Transmission is most often by blood: 60% cases are intravenous drug abusers/needle sharing persons. Blood transfusions are safe now due to better screening for HCV.
ii. Other risk factors are past surgical operations, needle sticks, close contact with HCV infected persons, including multiple sex partners.
iii. Perinatal transmission accounts for 5% of cases and has much lower rate of infection than HBV.
iv. In 30% of cases, no risk factors can be identified.
Pathogenesis HCV is hepatotropic but not directly hepatotoxic.
- Acute infection results in relatively mild hepatitis which is often subclinical, and 80% cases are unicteric.
- It will induce a T-cell mediated immunological injury of the liver which results in chronic hepatitis in 85% infected persons.
- Cirrhosis develops in 20%, and the risk for hepatocellular carcinoma in these patients is 2% per year (about 10% overall).
- Genotype 3 HCV results in fatty liver and steatohepatitis, often accompanied by the metabolic syndrome and insulin resistance.

Diagnosis is based on virologic and serologic evidence, and clinical/pathologic signs of chronic hepatitis or cirrhosis.
i. Viral RNA can be detected in blood of most infected persons.
ii. Antibodies to HCV can be detected in 50% of cases in acute phase, while others develop anti-HCV antibodies within a few weeks **(Fig. 21.9)**.
iii. Antibodies may cause immunologically mediated complications such as:
a. Cryoglobulinaemia found in 30% patients.
b. Vasculitis involving small vessels due to deposition of cryoglobulins, resulting in purpura and is associated with Raynaud phenomenon.
c. Membranoproliferative glomerulonephritis, a rare complication.

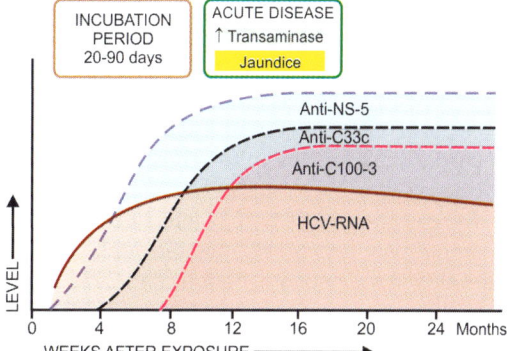

FIGURE 21.9: Sequence of serologic and viral markers of HCV infection.

Prognosis No vaccine is available. Excellent results have been achieved with new drugs targeting viral enzymes.

Q27. What is hepatitis E?

Virology Hepatitis E virus infection occurs mostly in underdeveloped countries and tourists visiting them.
- HEV is a single stranded RNA virus belonging to the Hepevirus genus that can be isolated from stools, bile and liver of infected persons.
- Its main reservoirs are animals like monkeys, dogs and cats.

Clinicopathologic aspects
i. Transmission is faecal-oral, mostly through contaminated water.
ii. Diagnosis is based on serology/virology: Antibodies that are IgM in acute phase and IgG thereafter.
iii. HEV RNA can be detected in blood.
iv. Clinically, it presents as mild acute viral hepatitis, which heals on its own. Chronic hepatitis does not develop.
v. Fulminant acute form may develop in pregnant women and has a high mortality (20%).

Q28. List the spectrum of clinicopathologic features of the viral hepatitis.

Various etiologic types of hepatotropic viruses produce viral hepatitis that includes several clinicopathologic entities as under:
i. Carrier state
ii. Asymptomatic infections

iii. Acute hepatitis
iv. Chronic hepatitis
v. Fulminant hepatitis
Chronic hepatitis can progress to cirrhosis and liver cancer (discussed later).
- Evidence linking HBV and HCV infection with the spectrum of clinicopathologic changes is stronger than with other hepatotropic viruses.
- Besides, HAV and HEV do not have a carrier stage nor cause chronic hepatitis.

Q29. What is carrier state of viral hepatitis?

Definition Carrier state is characterised by a persistent infection with a hepatotropic virus that can be transmitted to another person, even though the original carrier of the virus has no clinical manifestations of that viral disease.

Features of carrier state

i. *Types of carrier state* Two forms:
- As *asymptomatic healthy carrier* who does not suffer from ill-effects of the viral infection, but he is able to transmit. Liver biopsy shows no or only minimal inflammatory change.
- As *asymptomatic carrier with chronic disease*, which can be documented on clinical or pathologic examination.

ii. *Type of viral hepatitis* Carrier state cannot develop after HAV and HEV infection because these infections heal after some time. Coinfection of HDV and HBV will usually cause progressive HBV infection rather than a carrier state.
- As per WHO, estimated global prevalence of carrier state for HCV is 2–3%.
- Carrier state for HBV in the US and Western Europe is 0.5% while it is 5–20% in Asia and tropical countries.
- The early age at the time of infection and impaired immunity influence the rate of carrier state. For example, only 10% of HBV infected adult persons cannot clear the HBV, while 90% of infants infected with HBV in the neonatal period cannot clear it in 6 months.

Q30. What are the clinical phases of acute viral hepatitis?

Clinically, acute hepatitis is categorised into 4 phases: i) incubation period, ii) pre-icteric phase, iii) icteric phase, and iv) post-icteric phase.

I. **Incubation period** varies among different hepatotropic viruses as under:
- Hepatitis A → 4 weeks (15–45 days)
- Hepatitis B →10 weeks (30–180 days)
- Hepatitis C → 7 weeks (20–90 days)
- Hepatitis E → 2–8 weeks (15–60 days)

i. From these data, we can see that the incubation period varies considerably.

ii. It is shortest for hepatitis A and hepatitis E (transmitted by the faeco-oral route).

iii. It shows the highest range of variation for hepatitis B and hepatitis C (transmitted by parenteral route).

iv. The patients remain asymptomatic during the incubation period, but infectivity is the highest during the last days of this period.

II. **Pre-icteric phase** is marked by:

i. Prodromal constitutional symptoms, like nausea, vomiting, malaise, headache and arthralgia.

ii. Laboratory studies show elevation of transaminases.

III. **Icteric phase** is heralded by:

i. Appearance of jaundice, whereas the constitutional symptoms diminish.

ii. Hyperbilirubinaemia is accompanied by abnormal liver function tests, and hypergammaglobulinaemia.

iii. Serologic tests for viral hepatitis become positive.

IV. **Post-icteric phase** covers the 2–12 weeks period after cessation of jaundice.

i. It is marked by recovery except in lethal cases due to fulminant hepatitis (1%) and those that progress to chronic hepatitis (10%).

ii. The outcome of acute viral hepatitis varies from complete recovery to subclinical disease and persistent infection to fulminant hepatitis **(Fig. 21.10)**.

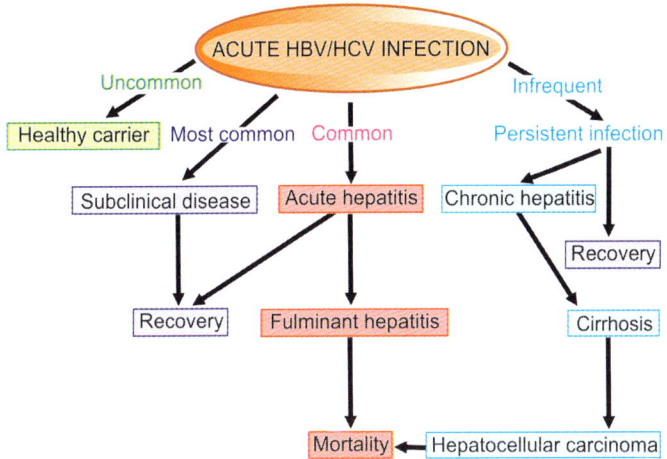

FIGURE 21.10: Clinicopathologic course of HBV and HCV infection.

Q31. What are the histopathologic features of acute viral hepatitis?

I. **Hepatocellular injury**, which is most pronounced in the centrolobular zone 3. These changes are:
i. *Ballooning degeneration* (reversible swelling of hepatocytes).
ii. *Apoptosis* of single liver cells resulting in acidophilic, rounded, anuclear bodies (also called *Councilman bodies*) **(Fig. 21.11)**.
iii. *Dropout necrosis* in which groups of cells lyse and disappear collapsing the size of the lobule.
iv. *Bridging necrosis* presenting as bands of necrotic cells extending from portal tracts to central hepatic venules; it is a sign of severe hepatitis or its progression to chronic hepatitis.
II. **Inflammatory infiltrates** in portal tracts and inside the lobules composed predominantly of lymphocytes, but also scattered macrophages and plasma cells. Inflammatory infiltrates are most prominent in hepatitis A.
III. **Kupffer cell hyperplasia** with cytoplasmic accumulation of cell debris fragments, bile pigment or lipofuscin granules.
IV. **Cholestasis,** which is usually mild, may present as feathery degeneration of liver cells or accumulation of bile in the cytoplasm of swollen hepatocytes.
V. **Regeneration of hepatocytes** recognised by mitotic figures or crowding of liver cells leading to a disarray of the lobular architecture.

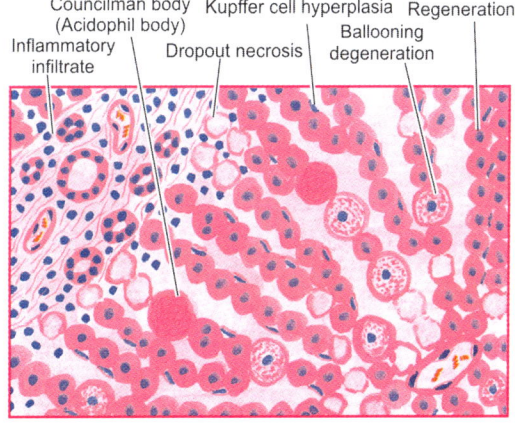

FIGURE 21.11: Acute viral hepatitis. The predominant histologic changes are: variable degree of necrosis of hepatocytes, most marked in zone 3 (centrilobular); and mononuclear cellular infiltrate in the lobule.

Q32. Briefly discuss the clinicopathologic features of chronic viral hepatitis.

Definition Chronic viral hepatitis is defined as an inflammation that lasts more than 6 months with persistent symptoms, along with biochemical, serologic and histopathologic evidence of persistent viral infection, i.e. inflammation, and necrosis of liver cells.
Etiology Chronic viral hepatitis is caused by HBV, HCV and combined HBV with HBD infection.
Same morphologic findings can be seen in some chronic non-infectious forms of hepatitis, such as drug-induced hepatitis, immune and genetic forms of hepatitis.
Pathology Similar microscopic changes are seen in all cases of chronic hepatitis as follows **(Fig. 21.12)**:
i. *Interface hepatitis,* also called *piecemeal necrosis* which includes periportal destruction of hepatocytes along the limiting plate between the portal tract and the lobule. The limiting plate is eroded due to

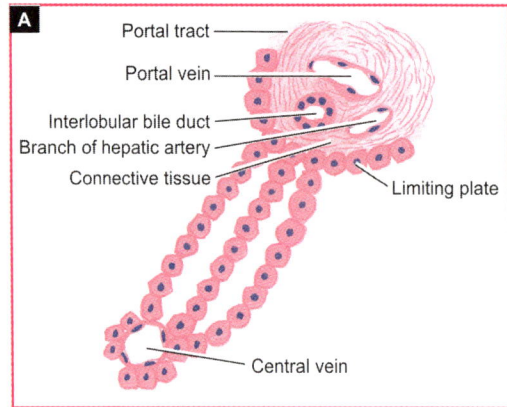
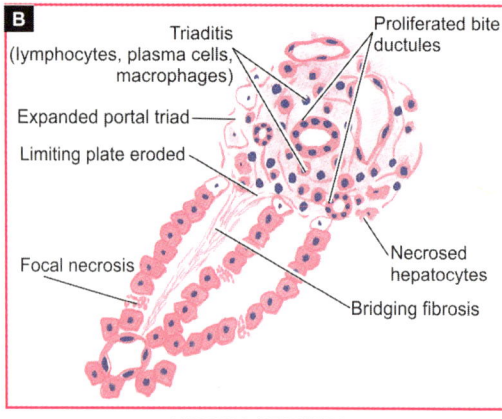

FIGURE 21.12: Chronic hepatitis. Diagrammatic representation of pathologic changes in chronic hepatitis (B) contrasted with normal morphology (A).

necrosis of hepatocytes and extension of inflammation from the expanded portal tract into the lobules.

ii. *Portal tract changes* include expansion of the portal tracts that contain inflammatory cells (lymphocytes, plasma cells, macrophages), proliferating bile ductules. In HCV infection, there are also lymphoid follicles with germinal centre formation and infiltrates of lymphocytes into the damaged bile ductules.

iii. *Intralobular lesions* which include foci of necrosis of hepatocytes, scattered acidophilic bodies, Kupffer cell hyperplasia, more severe bridging necrosis and regenerative changes. Immunostains to HBc and HBs antigens can be used to identify certain viruses such as HBV.

iv. *Bridging fibrosis* extending from areas of interface hepatitis into the lobule. Early changes give portal tracts a stellate appearance, and later the fibrous strands become thicker and more pronounced, progressing to cirrhosis.

NOTE: All these microscopic changes can be graded numerically to determine if the disease is progressing or stationary.

Clinical and laboratory findings are variable and depend on the activity or the disease process and the extent of fibrosis. However, often the clinical findings do not correlate with the pathology findings.

Q33. What is fulminant hepatitis leading to submassive or massive liver necrosis?

Definition Fulminant hepatitis leading to submassive or massive liver necrosis is the most severe form of acute hepatitis leading to a rapidly progressive liver failure.

Etiology Two groups of causes, each accounting for 50% of cases, are as follows:
- *Viral hepatitis*, most often HBV and HCV.
- *Non-viral causes*, such as drug toxicity (e.g. acetaminophen, NSAIDs, anti-depressants), poisoning, hypoxic liver injury, massive hepatic tumors.

Pathology *Grossly*, The liver is small and reduced to less than one half of its normal side, weighing 500–700 g. It appears shrunken and is covered by a loose and wrinkled capsule.

Microscopy

i. Broad areas of necrosis and loss of hepatocytes from the lobules with collapsed reticulin framework **(Fig. 21.13)**.

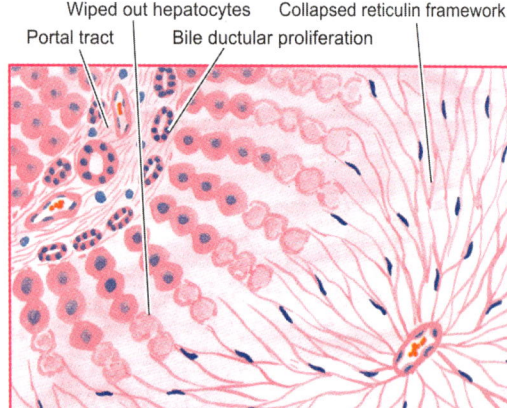

FIGURE 21.13: Fulminant hepatitis. There is wiping out of several liver lobules appearing pale as compared to pink colour in intact hepatocytes. There is no significant inflammation or fibrosis.

ii. A narrow zone of hepatocytes around the portal tracts may remain preserved and could serve as the starting point for regeneration if the patient survives.

Prognosis Mortality is, however, very high, and the only treatment that could save life is urgent liver transplantation.

Q34. Discuss main features of liver abscesses.

Definition Liver abscess is a localised infection of the liver characterised by accumulation of pus in a cavity formed through the lytic action of neutrophils inside the liver parenchyma.

Etiopathogenesis Liver abscesses are most often caused by bacteria.
- Most common are mixed bacterial infections dominated by *E. coli* and gram-negative aerobes, such as *Klebsiella* and *Proteus*.
- Less common are amoebic abscess, more prevalent in tropical countries, and hydatid (*echinococcal*) cyst transforming into an abscess, typically seen in sheep-raising countries of South America or New Zealand.

Routes of infection Bacteria may enter the liver through several routes as follows:

i. *Ascending cholangitis* in which the bacteria gain access to the liver through the bile ducts, which are usually obstructed by gallstones, cancer or some chronic bile duct diseases.
ii. *Portal pyaemia* that develops from bacterial infections of the gastrointestinal tract or pelvic organs. For example acute appendicitis, empyema of the gallbladder, diverticulitis, IBD, pancreatitis, etc.
iii. *Septicaemia and bacteriaemia.*
iv. *Hepatic surgery complications.*
v. *Direct extension from adjacent organs,* infected haematoma, or perihepatic and subdiaphragmatic suppurative lesions.
vi. *Penetrating wound of the liver,* e.g. gunshot or stabbing wounds.

Pathology Liver abscesses may present as a *solitary* mass or they may be *multiple*.

i. **Pyogenic liver abscesses** usually have a *fibrous capsule* enclosing a cavity filled with pus and necrotic cell debris. The capsule consists of inflamed granulation tissue and fibrous tissue **(Fig. 21.14,A)**.
ii. **Amoebic abscess** is usually solitary and its content is brown resembling anchovy paste or melted chocolate **(Fig. 21.14,B)**.
iii. **Hydatid cyst** is a cystic lesion caused by *Echinococcus granulosus* or *E. multilocularis*. These tapeworms are transmitted to humans from dogs and sheep. They form cysts in the liver which may be unilocular or multilocular **(Fig. 21.15,A)**. The cyst wall is composed of 3 distinguishable zones—outer *pericyst*, intermediate characteristic *ectocyst* and inner *endocyst* **(Fig. 21.15,B)**. If infected by bacteria, they transform into abscesses.

Complications of bacterial hepatic abscesses are due to spread of infection by two ways:
- *Direct extension* of purulent infection, leading to formation of a subphrenic abscess peritonitis or purulent pleuritis.

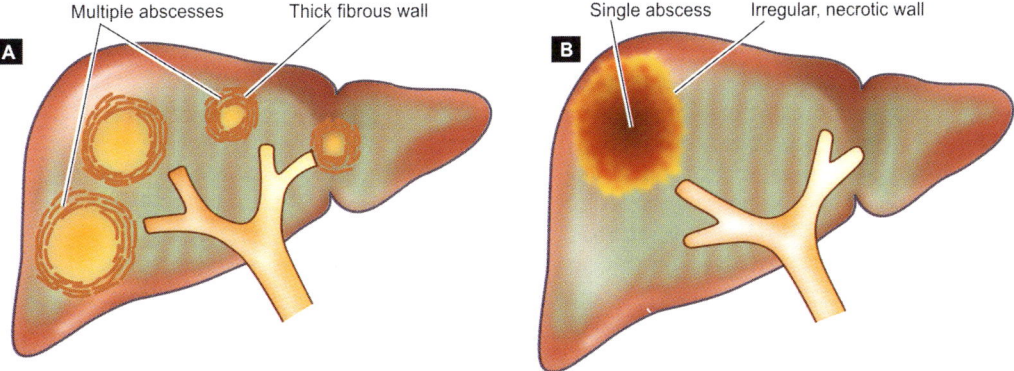

FIGURE 21.14: A, Gross appearance of pyogenic abscesses in the liver. B, Amoebic liver abscess is commonly solitary and its wall is irregular and necrotic.

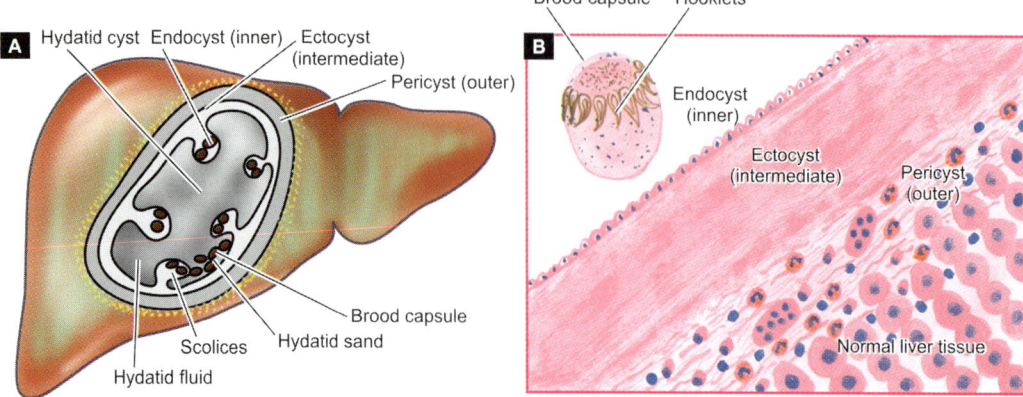

FIGURE 21.15: Hydatid cyst in the liver. A, The cyst wall is composed of whitish membrane resembling the membrane of a hard boiled egg. B, Microscopy shows three layers in the wall of hydatid cyst.

- *Haematogenous dissemination* which leads to the formation of metastatic pyaemic abscesses in many organs.

Q35. What are the most important features of drug-induced liver injury?

Classification Drug injury of the liver may be classified as:
- *Direct or predictable*, and dose dependent hepatotoxic
- *Indirect or unpredictable*, and considered to be idiosyncratic. This is often related to an immune response to the offending drug.

Pathology The changes in the liver can be acute or chronic **(Table 21.7)**:
- *Acute changes* present microscopically in many forms such as necrosis, inflammation, cholestasis, or circulatory changes.
- *Chronic changes* include fibrosis-cirrhosis, focal nodular hyperplasia, adenoma and hepatocellular carcinoma.

Q36. Define cirrhosis. Comment on its etiopathogenesis and classification.

Definition Cirrhosis is the term used for the pathological changes underlying the end-stage of irreversible chronic liver failure. Pathologic features of cirrhosis include diffuse loss of normal liver architecture, which has been replaced by liver cell nodules surrounded by fibrous tissue containing restructured blood vessels.

Pathogenesis Cirrhosis is a combination of a few processes such as:
- Liver cell injury and necrosis,
- Healing by fibrosis,

TABLE 21.7 Classification of hepatic drug reactions.

PATHOLOGIC CHANGES	AGENTS
A. ACUTE LIVER DISEASE	
1. *Zonal necrosis*	Carbon tetrachloride Acetaminophen Halothane
2. *Massive necrosis*	Halothane Acetaminophen Methyldopa
3. *Fatty change*	Tetracycline Salicylates Methotrexate Ethanol
4. *Hepatitis*	Methyldopa Isoniazid Halothane Ketoconazole
5. *Granuloma formation*	Sulfonamides Methyldopa Quinidine Allopurinol
6. *Cholestasis*	Sex hormones (including oral contraceptives) Chlorpromazine Nitrofurantoin
7. *Veno-occlusive disease*	Cytotoxic drugs
8. *Hepatic/portal vein thrombosis*	Oral contraceptives
B. CHRONIC LIVER DISEASE	
1. *Fibrosis-cirrhosis*	Methotrexate
2. *Focal nodular hyperplasia*	Vinyl chloride Vitamin A Sex hormones
3. *Adenoma*	Sex hormones
4. *Hepatocellular carcinoma*	Sex hormones

- Formation of compensatory regenerative nodules, and
- Changes in vascular pattern in the hepatic parenchyma.

Classification Two types:
- On the basis of *macroscopic examination* of the liver nodules, cirrhosis can be classified as: micronodular or macronodular or mixed.
- Much more important clinically is the *etiologic classification* based on underlying cause **(Table 21.8)**.

Q37. What is alcoholic liver disease? Discuss its pathogenesis.

Definition Alcoholic liver disease includes a spectrum of changes associated with alcohol abuse such as alcoholic steatosis (fatty liver), alcoholic hepatitis, and alcoholic cirrhosis.

TABLE 21.8 Classification of cirrhosis.

A. MORPHOLOGIC
1. Micronodular (nodules less than 3 mm)
2. Macronodular (nodules more than 3 mm)
3. Mixed

B. ETIOLOGIC
1. Alcoholic cirrhosis (the most common, ~50%)
2. Post-necrotic cirrhosis
3. Biliary cirrhosis
4. Pigment cirrhosis in haemochromatosis
5. Cirrhosis in Wilson disease
6. Cirrhosis in α-1-antitrypsin deficiency
7. Cardiac cirrhosis
8. Indian childhood cirrhosis (ICC)
9. Cirrhosis in autoimmune hepatitis
10. Cirrhosis in non-alcoholic steatohepatitis
11. Miscellaneous forms of cirrhosis (metabolic, infectious, GI, infiltrative)
12. Cryptogenic cirrhosis

Metabolism of alcohol is important for the formation of potentially toxic metabolites and a reduction of the protective redox system elements. It occurs in two compartments of hepatocytes: i) cytosol, and ii) mitochondria **(Fig. 21.16)**:

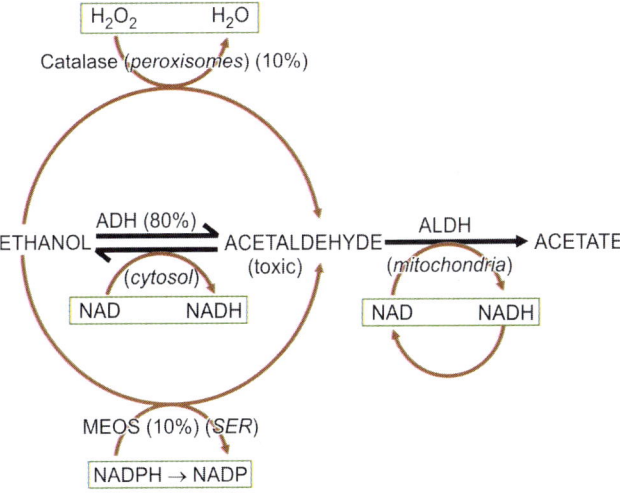

FIGURE 21.16: Metabolism of ethanol in the liver. Thickness and intensity of colour of arrows on left side of figure corresponds to extent of metabolic pathway followed.
(ADH, alcohol dehydrogenase; ALDH or ACDH, hepatic acetaldehyde dehydrogenase; NAD, nicotinamide adenine dinucleotide; NADH, reduced NAD).

I. Cytosolic alcohol metabolism:
- It begins through the action of *alcohol dehydrogenase (ADH)*, a rate-limiting pathway. It results in the formation of *acetaldehyde*, which is a toxic substance and may damage membranes. This process will also reduce the level of *nicotinamide adenine dinucleotide (NAD)* which serves as hydrogen receptor.
- *Microsomal ethanol oxidising system (MEOS, microsomal P-450 oxidising enzymes)* and peroxisomal enzymes play a minor role in this process. MEOS are genetically determined and may play role in the genetic sensitivity to alcohol.

II. Mitochondrial alcohol metabolism:
- It begins with the action *acetaldehyde dehydrogenase (ALDH)* which converts acetaldehyde into acetate, to be metabolised to carbon dioxide and water.
- In this process NAD is reduced to NADH and the critical *NADH:NAD ratio* critical for its redox potential is increased.

Hepatotoxicity of alcohol Exact mechanism is still under study but several important facts are well established as follows **(Fig. 21.17)**:
i. Alcohol itself and its metabolites like acetaldehyde have *direct hepatotoxic effects*.

ii. *Increased redox ratio* of NADH:NAD, and the formation of oxygen radicals have damaging effects.

iii. Alcohol intake has significant *metabolic consequences*: It increases oxygen demand for hepatocytes, leads to retention of water and proteins, and favours accumulation of lipids in liver cells.

iv. Alcohol causes *ill-effects on intestinal epithelium*, favouring the absorption of endotoxin, proinflammatory cytokines and various potentially toxic metabolites.

v. There are *adverse effects of alcohol on the immune system*, Kupffer cells and the promotion of repair by fibrosis contribute to the pathogenesis of cirrhosis.

Key factors determining the adverse effects of alcohol are as follows:

i. *Drinking patterns and quantity of alcohol consumed* Chronic consumption of large quantities has adverse effects. Fatty liver occurs in 90% of chronic alcoholics, and in 10–20% it will progress to alcoholic hepatitis and eventually to cirrhosis over the period of 10 years.

ii. *Gender* Women are more sensitive to alcohol and are affected more than men.

iii. *Genetic factors* Susceptibility to the effects of alcohol is genetically determined.

iv. *Malnutrition* Lack of proteins and vitamins has adverse effects.

v. *Infections* Especially with hepatotropic viruses like HBV and HCV.

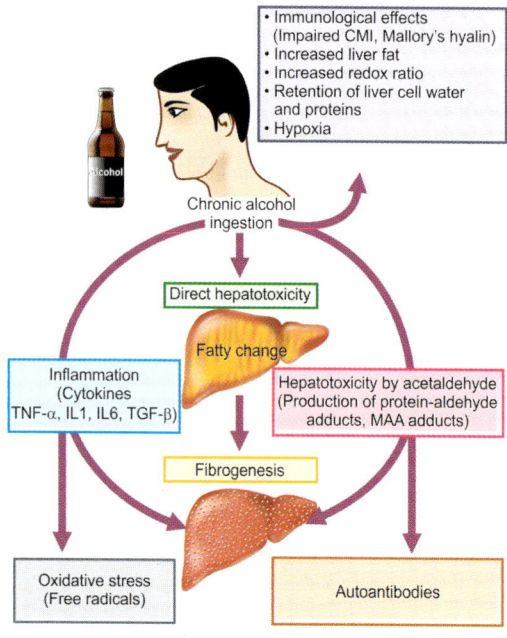

FIGURE 21.17: Pathogenesis of alcoholic liver disease.

Q38. Discuss spectrum of pathologic features of alcoholic liver disease.

Three pathologic changes are related to alcohol intake are: i) fatty change (steatosis), ii) alcoholic hepatitis, and iii) cirrhosis.

I. **Fatty liver** leads to hepatomegaly.

Grossly, the liver appears fatty and yellow.

Microscopy reveals mostly macrovesicular fatty change, sometimes associated with fat cysts from ruptured hepatocytes and lipogranuloma composed of foamy macrophages that have ingested lipid droplets **(Fig. 21.18)**.

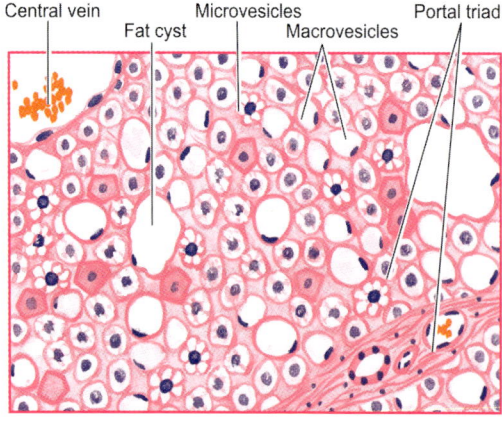

FIGURE 21.18: Fatty liver (alcoholic steatosis). Most of the hepatocytes are distended with large lipid vacuoles with peripherally displaced nuclei.

II. **Alcoholic hepatitis (steatohepatitis)** is characterised by three sets of microscopic changes **(Fig. 21.19)**:
i. *Hepatocellular changes* such as widespread macrovesicular steatosis, ballooning degeneration, formation of Mallory bodies (alcoholic hyaline) in their cytoplasm, and foci of hepatocellular necrosis.
ii. *Acute inflammation* characterised by foci of neutrophils surrounding liver cells.
iii. *Fibrosis* which is pericellular and perivenular producing a web-like 'chicken wire' appearance, also known as creeping collagenosis.

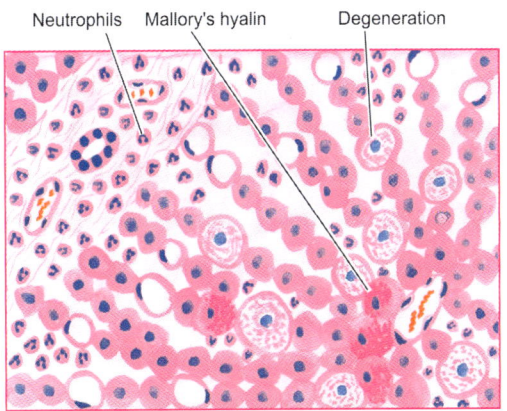

FIGURE 21.19: Alcoholic hepatitis (Steatohepatitis). Liver cells show ballooning degeneration and fatty change. Clusters of chronic inflammatory cells are also present.

III. **Alcoholic cirrhosis** which is most often micronodular and characterised by widespread fatty change of hepatocytes. Increased haemosiderin accumulation may be noted. There is also bile stasis, but Mallory's bodies are hard to find **(Fig. 21.20)**.

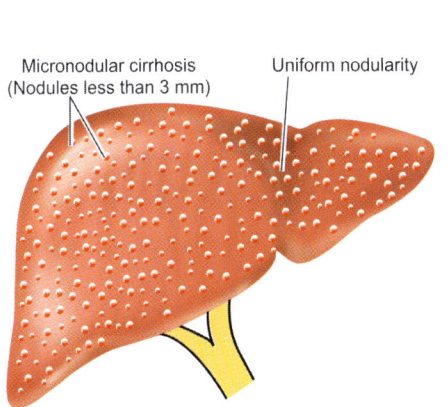
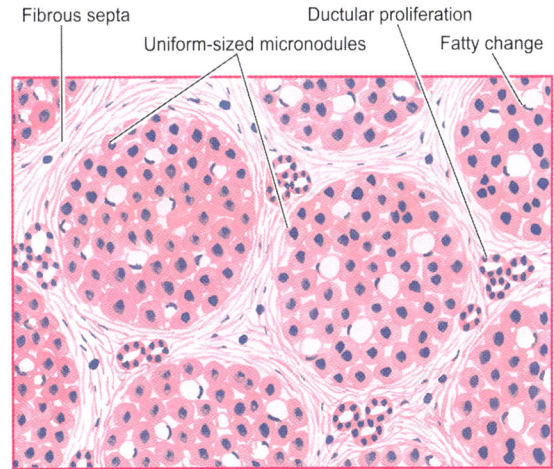

FIGURE 21.20: Alcoholic cirrhosis. A, It shows the typical micronodular pattern (uniform-sized micronodules less than 3 mm diameter) and pale yellow colour. B, Microscopy shows nearly uniform-sized micronodules, devoid of central veins and having thick fibrous septa dividing them. There is minimal inflammation and some reactive bile duct proliferation in the septa.

Q39. What is post-necrotic cirrhosis? Briefly discuss its main features.

Definition Post-necrotic cirrhosis, also termed *post-hepatitic cirrhosis or macronodular cirrhosis,* is characterised by large and irregular nodules with broad bands of connective tissue and occurring most commonly after previous viral hepatitis.

Etiology Following factors have been implicated:
i. *Viral hepatitis* Most common association is with hepatitis B and C; hepatitis A is not known to evolve into cirrhosis. It is estimated that about 20% cases of HBV chronic hepatitis and about 20–30% cases of HCV chronic hepatitis progress to cirrhosis over 20–30 years.

ii. *Drugs and chemical hepatotoxins* A small percentage of cases may have origin from toxicity due to chemicals and drugs such as phosphorus, carbon tetrachloride, mushroom poisoning, acetaminophen and α-methyl dopa.

iii. *Others* Certain infections (e.g. brucellosis), parasitic infections (e.g. clonorchiasis), metabolic diseases (e.g. Wilson disease or hepatolenticular degeneration) and advanced alcoholic liver disease may produce a picture of post-necrotic cirrhosis. Some cases, however, remain idiopathic in which the etiology is unknown.

Pathology Although etiologic and morphologic diagnosis of cirrhosis is attempted by pathologists, invariably it is difficult to reconstruct the course of events which led to end-stage cirrhosis, especially in a liver biopsy. However, typically post-necrotic cirrhosis is macronodular type.

Grossly, the liver has distorted shape with irregular and coarse scars and nodules varying in diameter from 3 mm to a few centimetres (*macronodules*) **(Fig. 21.21,A)**.

Microscopy **(Fig. 21.21,B)**

i. *Nodular pattern* The normal lobular architecture of hepatic parenchyma is replaced by nodules larger than those in alcoholic cirrhosis. However, uninvolved portal tracts and central veins in the hepatic lobules can still be seen in some parts of surviving parenchyma.

ii. *Fibrous septa* The fibrous septa dividing the variable-sized nodules are generally thick.

iii. *Necrosis, inflammation and bile duct proliferation* Active liver cell necrosis is usually inconspicuous. Fibrous septa contain prominent mononuclear inflammatory cell infiltrate which may even form follicles, especially in cases following HCV chronic hepatitis. Often there is extensive proliferation of bile ductules derived from collapsed liver lobules.

iv. *Regenerating hepatic parenchyma* Liver cells vary considerably in size and multiple large nuclei are common in regenerative nodules.

Clinical features Besides the general clinical features of cirrhosis, splenomegaly and hypersplenism are other prominent features. Out of the various types of cirrhosis, post-necrotic cirrhosis, especially when related to hepatitis B and C virus infection in early life, is more frequently associated with development of hepatocellular carcinoma later.

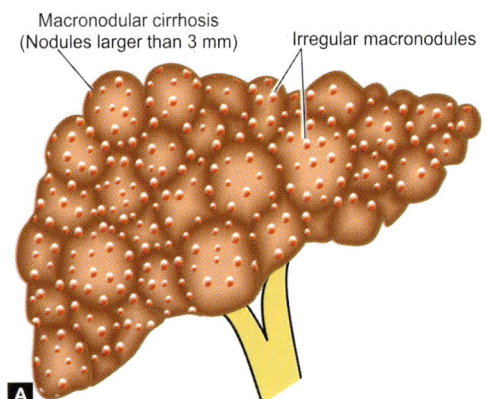
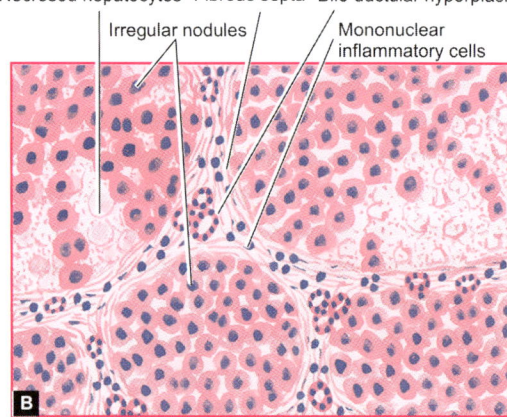

FIGURE 21.21: Post-necrotic cirrhosis. A, Gross appearance show irregular macronodular pattern (nodules larger than 3 mm diameter). Externally the liver is small, distorted and irregularly scarred. B, Microscopy shows fibrous septa dividing the hepatic parenchyma into nodules contain prominent mononuclear inflammatory cell infiltrate and bile ductular hyperplasia.

Q40. Discuss salient features of biliary cirrhosis and its main types.

Definition Biliary cirrhosis is a form of cirrhosis caused by longstanding cholestasis.

Classification Biliary cirrhosis can be caused by intrahepatic or extrahepatic obstruction of bile flow and thus three distinct clinicopathologic entities are recognised:

i. *Primary biliary cirrhosis,* an autoimmune disease of unknown etiology characterised by intrahepatic destruction of bile ducts.

ii. *Secondary biliary cirrhosis* resulting from prolonged mechanical obstruction of the extrahepatic biliary passages.

iii. *Primary sclerosing cholangitis* caused by autoimmune destruction of extrahepatic and intrahepatic bile ducts.

Q41. Discuss main features of primary biliary cirrhosis.

Definition Primary biliary cirrhosis (also known as *primary biliary cholangitis*) is an autoimmune disease of unknown etiology characterised by the destruction of small and medium-sized bile ducts, invariably leading to cirrhosis.

Etiopathogenesis Clinical and laboratory data indicate that it is an autoimmune disease but the basic events which elicit the autoimmune reaction in the liver are not known. The following findings provide support to the view that it is an autoimmune disease, with additional genetic and hormonal influences:
i. Circulating antibodies to mitochondria (>90%) and some other cellular components.
ii. Elevated levels of immunoglobulins in circulation, especially IgM.
iii. Presence of autoreactive T cells in the liver.
iv. Non-caseating granulomas found in 25% cases.
v. Common association with other autoimmune diseases such as autoimmune thyroid diseases and gastritis, Sjögren syndrome, scleroderma, etc.
vi. Association with certain HLA types and the familial occurrence of some cases suggest a genetic predisposition.
vii. Predominance among women (F:M=9:1) suggests that oestrogen plays a role.

Pathology The changes are described as non-suppurative, destructive intrahepatic cholangitis which evolves through four stages:
- *Stage I,* marked by portal infiltrates of T cells destroying the bile ducts (*'florid duct bile duct lesion'*), forming follicles or granulomas in some cases, with evidence of cholestasis in the lobules.
- *Stage II,* marked by a destruction of bile ducts and reactive proliferation of bile ductules and the expansion of the inflammation beyond the limits of the portal tract, and signs of cholestasis in the lobules.
- *Stage III* is marked by fibrous scarring, reduced inflammation and a loss of bile ducts, with more prominent cholestasis in the lobules.
- *Stage IV* is cirrhosis marked by extensive fibrosis and formation of regenerating liver nodules.

Clinical features Most women may be asymptomatic for a long time. Symptoms develop insidiously usually in the 30–50 years age period.
Clinical findings may include the following: persistent pruritus, dark urine, pale stools, jaundice, steatorrhoea with consequences of malabsorption. Xanthomas develop on the skin.
Laboratory findings include conjugated hyperbilirubinaemia, increased levels of alkaline phosphatase, elevation of serum lipids.
Prognosis Ultimately, there is evidence of cirrhosis and hepatic failure. Treatment at that stage is liver transplantation.

Q42. What is primary sclerosing cholangitis?

Definition Primary sclerosing cholangitis is an autoimmune disease leading to fibrosis and a loss of extrahepatic and intrahepatic bile ducts, ultimately progressing to cirrhosis and liver failure.

Etiopathogenesis Unknown, but considered to be of autoimmune origin, with a genetic predisposition and hormonal influences. The following data support these views:
i. Lymphocytic infiltrates in the wall of the bile ducts with their obliteration and periductal fibrosis.
ii. Strong association with ulcerative colitis (70%) and chronic fibrosing diseases such as retroperitoneal fibrosis and chronic pancreatitis.
iii. MPO-ANCA (pANCA) positive in 65% cases, but the pathogenetic role of these antibodies is unknown.
iv. Genetic predisposition linked to certain HLA types.
v. Male predominance (70%) suggests possible hormonal influence.

Pathology Main features are:
i. Chronic inflammation and fibrosis and loss of extrahepatic and with periductal fibrosis of intrahepatic bile duct leading to their obliteration and loss.
ii. Cholestasis leading to portal fibrosis with portal to portal bridging, resulting in biliary cirrhosis.

Clinical features Patients are mostly males, 30–50 years of age.
i. Initially they may be asymptomatic for long time and then develop signs of obstructive jaundice, slowly progressing to cirrhosis and liver failure.
ii. Radiologic findings with contrast aided retrograde cholangiography shows diagnostic '*beading*' due to alternating narrowing and dilatation of large intrahepatic and extrahepatic bile ducts.
iii. Liver transplantation is the only effective treatment.

Q43. Discuss main features of secondary biliary cirrhosis.

Definition Secondary biliary cirrhosis is a form of cirrhosis that develops due to obstruction of major extrahepatic bile ducts.
Etiopathogenesis Obstruction of extrahepatic bile ducts may be caused by the following:
i. Gallstones (most common)
ii. Biliary atresia (most common in children)
iii. Cancer of extrahepatic bile ducts and head of pancreas
iv. Postoperative strictures of the extrahepatic bile ducts
Pathology Obstruction of bile ducts is usually associated with dilatation of ducts proximal to the obstruction.
i. Portal tracts are expanded, show fibrosis and reactive bile duct proliferation **(Fig. 21.22)**.
ii. Bile accumulation in dilated and in bile canaliculi between the hepatocytes in the lobules ('bile plugs').
iii. Rupture of canaliculi and necrosis of liver cells leads to the formation of bile lakes.
iv. Obstruction of bile ducts may be complicated by infection which presents as suppurative cholangitis.
v. Bridging fibrosis from one expanded portal tract to another leads to cirrhosis.

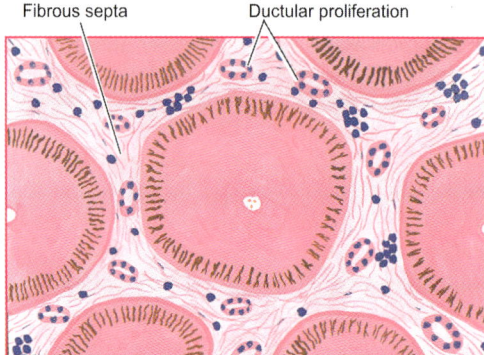

FIGURE 21.22: Biliary cirrhosis. The fibrous septa contain prominent lymphoid infiltrate and proliferation of bile ductules. Many of the hepatocytes contain elongated bile plugs (cholestasis).

Q44. Tabulate salient contrasting features of primary and secondary biliary cirrhosis and primary sclerosing cholangitis.

Contrasting features of these three clinicopathologic entities of that lead to biliary cirrhosis are presented in **Table 21.9**.

TABLE 21.9 Contrasting features of major forms of biliary cirrhosis.			
FEATURE	PRIMARY BILIARY CIRRHOSIS	SECONDARY BILIARY CIRRHOSIS	PRIMARY SCLEROSING CHOLANGITIS
1. *Etiology*	Possibly autoimmune; association with other autoimmune diseases	Extrahepatic biliary obstruction; biliary atresia	Possibly autoimmune; association with inflammatory bowel disease
2. *Age and sex*	Middle-aged women Male: Female = 1:9	Any age and either sex	Middle age Male: Female = 2:1
3. *Laboratory tests*	↑ Alkaline phosphatase ↑ Conjugated bilirubin Autoantibodies present	↑ Alkaline phosphatase ↑ Conjugated bilirubin	↑ Alkaline phosphatase ↑ Conjugated bilirubin Hypergammaglobulinaemia
4. *Pathologic changes*	Chronic destructive; cholangitis of intrahepatic bile ducts	Bile stasis in bile ducts, and sterile or pyogenic cholangitis	Fibrosing cholangitis with periductal fibrosis

Q45. What is hereditary haemochromatosis? Discuss salient features of its epidemiology, etiopathogenesis and clinicopathologic aspects.

Definition Hereditary haemochromatosis is a relatively common genetic autosomal recessive iron-storage disorder in which iron accumulates in various tissues causing functional insufficiency of several organs such as the liver, pancreas, heart and pituitary gland.

Classification Haemochromatosis may be *primary, genetic* and *secondary* due to iron overload in several forms of anaemia, alcoholic cirrhosis or multiple blood transfusions. Here, we discuss only the primary hereditary haemochromatosis (HH).

Epidemiology Clinically apparent HH is encountered in the US and Western Europe at a rate of 1:200–400. Approximately 10% of the general population is heterozygous for the most common mutation causing HH.

Etiopathogenesis of hereditary haemochromatosis This genetic disease may be caused by one of several known genetic mutation which all *decrease the secretion of hepcidin,* a protein that plays a key role in the absorption of iron in duodenal enterocytes:

i. Hepcidin is synthesised by liver cells and transported by blood to enter the enterocytes.
ii. In the enterocytes, it binds to *ferroportin,* an iron transporter protein.
iii. Hepcidin-ferroportin complex inhibits the release of iron that has entered the enterocytes from the intestinal lumen and thus the iron from food never reaches the circulation.
iv. Due to depressed synthesis of hepcidin in HH, the blocking hepcidin-ferroportin complex is not formed, resulting in *uncontrolled entry of iron into the circulation*.
v. The most common cause of reduced synthesis of hepcidin, is the mutation of *HFE* (hemochromatosis gene), which is located close by to the *HLA-I* genes on chromosome 6.
vi. HFE protein regulates the activity of hepcidin gene and all mutations of the *HFE* gene that reduce hepcidin synthesis will cause HH.
vii. The most common mutation causing HH in 70% of patients is a cysteine to tyrosine substitution at amino acid position 282 *(C282Y)*.
viii. Other mutations, including the mutation of hepcidin gene itself, are less common.

Pathology Normal body absorbs 1 mg of iron per day in men and 1.5 mg in women.

i. In HH, the body absorbs 4 mg/day and the extra iron is deposited in the form of ferritin and haemosiderin in parenchymal organs such as the liver, pancreas, heart and endocrine glands.
ii. Iron overload results in production of oxygen radicals which are cytotoxic and destroy cells that have stored the iron.
iii. In the liver, HH leads to cirrhosis and ultimately liver failure, which together with heart failure is the most common cause of death in these patients.
iv. The cirrhotic liver of HH has a brown colour due to increased amounts of ferric iron and it is commonly called 'pigmentary cirrhosis'.
v. Liver biopsy shows accumulation of haemosiderin granules in the cytoplasm of hepatocytes, and less commonly in Kupffer cells and bile ducts. Haemosiderin granules stain blue in the Prussian blue reaction with ferri-ferro cyanide.
vi. Hepatocellular carcinoma is a late complication of HH cirrhosis.

Clinical features Most often, presenting features are:

i. Cirrhosis, diabetes mellitus and brown hyperpigmentation of the skin, traditionally known as *bronze-diabetes*.
ii. *Laboratory findings* include increased serum concentration of iron, ferritin and a high saturation of transferrin.

Q46. What is Wilson disease? Discuss its major features.

Definition Wilson disease, also known as hepatolenticular degeneration, is a rare autosomal recessive genetic disorder of copper metabolism resulting in copper toxicity which affects primarily the liver, brain and eyes, but also other organs.

Epidemiology 1:30,000 persons, even though the carrier of the gene mutation occurs in less than 1: 200 persons. Most patients are mixed heterozygotes.

Etiopathogenesis Wilson disease is caused by a mutation of *ATP7B* gene which may be mutated in more than 200 forms.

i. This gene encodes an adenosine triphosphatase involved in the *excretion of copper in bile* and the *incorporation of copper* into aceruloplasmin to form *ceruloplasmin*.
ii. Aceruloplasmin that is not bound to copper cannot be secreted into the circulation which accounts for the *low level of aceruloplasmin in serum*.

iii. Since copper cannot be secreted into the blood nor excreted into bile, it *accumulates in liver cells*. Intrahepatic copper generates oxygen radicals which are cytototoxic and ultimately kill the liver cells, releasing free copper into circulation.

iv. Free copper released into the blood is loosely attached to albumin and partially excreted in urine or *deposited in extrahepatic tissue* causing cell injury in various organs and also causing haemolysis or red blood cells.

Clinicopathologis features Liver plays the key role in pathogenesis of Wilson disease and it is also the most commonly affected organ; other organs are also affected.

I. **Liver disease** presents in at least 50% of affected persons by the age of 20 years, whereas others develop symptoms in early adulthood.
- Liver may show a variety of microscopic changes that vary from fatty change, to chronic hepatitis, to cirrhosis.
- Increased amounts of copper in hepatocytes can be demonstrated by special stains (rhodamine or rubeanic acid).
- In most instances, the liver changes progress to cirrhosis.
- Clinically, most often it presents as chronic hepatitis, leading to cirrhosis, which often develops at an early age.

II. **Brain** is most often damaged in the basal ganglia. Clinically, brain injury present with movement disorders, progressing to disabling dystonia and spasticity.

III. **Eye** changes accompany neurologic disease and typically include the formation of the Kayser-Fleischer ring. It consists of brown discoloration around the edge of the iris.

IV. **Bone** lesions include ostomalacia and osteoporosis with fractures and arthropathies.

V. **Kidney** may show dysfunction of renal tubules and proteinuria.

VI. **Blood** shows episodes of haemolytic anaemia due to toxic effects of copper on RBCs.

Laboratory findings include:
- High levels of copper in urine and liver biopsy, and
- Low levels of aceruloplasmin in serum.

Q47. What is α-1-antitrypsin deficiency-related liver disease?

Definition α-1-antitrypsin deficiency is an autosomal recessive genetic disease caused by a mutation of gene encoding this serine protease inhibitor (Pi, or serpin), presenting with emphysema and chronic liver disease progressing to cirrhosis.

Epidemiology Homozygotes are found at a rate of 1:2,000 but only 15% of them develop liver disease. Of the 24 alleles labelled alphabetically, the most common normal is PiMM and the most common abnormal PiZZ in a homozygous form. Two additional phenotypes with liver disease are PiSS and Pi-null, characterised by complete deficiency of serpin.

Clinicopathologic features

i. α-1-antitrypsin deficiency may present with liver disease or emphysema. These diseases develop because serpin deficient organisms cannot inhibit elastase on PMNs, which leads to tissue injury.

ii. The abnormal protein accumulates in the liver, inside the cisterns of the rough endoplasmic reticulum.

iii. Protein aggregates form PAS-positive granules that can be seen by light microscopy in liver cells.

iv. In 10% of patients, serpin deficiency may cause neonatal giant cell hepatitis which subsides in most patients spontaneously, but in 10% it may progress to cirrhosis in early life. This genetic disease is the most common cause of cirrhosis in children.

v. Alternatively, the first signs of chronic hepatitis begin in adolescence and early adulthood, also leading to cirrhosis. Cirrhosis is often complicated by hepatocellular carcinoma.

vi. Liver transplantation is curative.

Q48. What is cardiac cirrhosis?

Definition Cardiac cirrhosis is a rare form of cirrhosis caused by chronic passive congestion of liver in patients who have severe right heart failure, tricuspid insufficiency or constrictive pericarditis.

Pathology *Grossly,* the liver is enlarged, congested and the Glisson capsule is tense and stretched.

Microscopy
i. Fibrosis, replacing the necrosed centrolobular hepatocytes.
ii. Bridging fibrosis, interconnecting the centrolobular areas of adjacent lobules leads to a loss of normal architecture, formation of regenerative nodules and cardiac cirrhosis.

Q49. What is Indian childhood cirrhosis?

Definition Indian childhood cirrhosis is a rare form of cirrhosis of unknown etiology developing in children between the age of 6 months and 3 years.
Epidemiology In addition to India, this form of liver disease occurs in South-East Asia and the Middle East. No etiologic factors have been identified.
Epidemiologic data show that the liver contains an increased amount of copper, which might suggest copper toxicity related to copper containing utensils.
Pathology Several microscopic subtypes of liver injury have been described.
i. Most common microscopic changes include ballooning degeneration of hepatocytes, with prominent Mallory bodies, and infiltrates of PMNs and lymphocytes.
ii. Creeping pericellular fibrosis will typically progress to cirrhosis.
iii. These pathologic changes resemble alcoholic hepatitis except for the fact that there is no steatosis.
iv. Chemical analysis of liver tissue will usually reveal increased amounts of copper which is probably not excreted adequately in bile.

Q50. What is autoimmune hepatitis? Discuss its salient features.

Definition Autoimmune hepatitis is an immune-mediated liver disease that primarily affects women.
Epidemiology Autoimmune hepatitis has an incidence of 2 per 100,000 in the US and Europe. Cirrhosis caused by it accounts for 5% of all liver transplants. Approximately 75% of patients are females, and in many cases are linked to a specific HLA haplotype, suggesting a genetic predisposition.
Pathogenesis There are two types of autoimmune hepatitis:
Type I (80% of all cases) affects predominantly women under the age of 40 years, who often have other autoimmune diseases such as autoimmune thyroid disorders, and also HLA-DRB1 haplotype. These women typically have the following *autoantibodies* in serum:
i. Antinuclear antibodies (ANA),
ii. Anti-smooth muscle antibodies (>85%), and
iii. Anti-soluble liver antigen that has high specificity but low sensitivity.
Type II affects children and it is also associated with some other autoimmune diseases. The serum of these children contains antibodies against the liver and kidney microsomes (*anti-LKM*).
Clinicopathologic features Main features of autoimmune hepatitis are:
i. It is a progressive *chronic hepatitis* leading to cirrhosis.
ii. In many women, it presents as *cirrhosis* suggesting that the disease must have been subclinical for some time prior to the onset of symptoms.
iii. The diagnosis is made by correlating the *clinical and laboratory findings*, which typically include signs of active hepatitis, hypergammaglobulinaemia and the specific antibodies listed above.
Prognosis Early forms of disease respond well to corticosteroid treatment.
- Cirrhosis requires liver transplantation.
- Recurrence of autoimmune hepatitis is common and is seen in 1 out of 5 transplant recipients.

Q51. Discuss non-alcoholic steatohepatitis briefly.

Definition Non-alcoholic steatohepatitis (NASH), also called non-alcoholic fatty liver disease (NAFLD), is a common form of chronic hepatitis resembling alcoholic hepatitis found in patients who have metabolic syndrome (dyslipidaemia, diabetes type 2, central obesity and hypertension).
Clinicopathologic features Patients are most often asymptomatic and are diagnosed during routine laboratory surveillance.
i. The liver shows essentially the same changes as in alcoholic steatohepatitis, such as fatty change and ballooning degeneration of hepatocytes, Mallory bodies, liver cell necrosis with prominent pericellular and perivenular centrolobular fibrosis.
ii. Progression to cirrhosis is found in 10–20% of cases.

Q52. What is portal hypertension? Discuss its causes.

Definition Portal hypertension is elevation of blood pressure in the portal vein above 30 mm saline (normal 10–15 mm saline) caused by obstruction of the portal venous blood flow.

Classification Portal hypertension can be classified depending on the site of obstruction as i) intrahepatic, ii) posthepatic, and iii) prehepatic **(Table 21.10)**.

I. *Intrahepatic portal hypertension* is most often caused by cirrhosis (30–60% cases) which may obstruct the blood flow by fibrous bands, compression by hepatic nodules or fatty transformation, granulomas or metastatic tumours from outside, or thrombosis. Hepatocellular carcinoma which usually originates in cirrhotic liver, may physically compress the portal vein or invade into the lumen of its intrahepatic branches.

II. *Posthepatic portal hypertension* is an uncommon event usually related to congestive heart failure or constrictive pericarditis. However, it can be also caused by veno-occlusive disease and as part of the Budd-Chiari syndrome.

III. *Prehepatic portal hypertension* is most often caused by neoplastic occlusion or thrombosis of the portal vein before it enters into the liver.

TABLE 21.10 Major causes of portal hypertension.

A. INTRAHEPATIC
1. Cirrhosis
2. Metastatic tumours
3. Budd-Chiari syndrome
4. Hepatic veno-occlusive disease
5. Diffuse granulomatous diseases
6. Extensive fatty change

B. POSTHEPATIC
1. Congestive heart failure
2. Constrictive pericarditis
3. Hepatic veno-occlusive disease
4. Budd-Chiari syndrome

C. PREHEPATIC
1. Portal vein thrombosis
2. Neoplastic obstruction of portal vein
3. Myelofibrosis
4. Congenital absence of portal vein

Q53. What are the most important clinicopathologic consequences of portal hypertension and cirrhosis?

The most important consequences of portal hypertension are i) ascites, ii) varices, iii) splenomegaly, and iv) hepatic encephalopathy **(Fig. 21.23)**.

I. **Ascites** is an accumulation of excess fluid in the abdominal cavity.

i. In most instances, it is a transudate that has a specific gravity of 1.010, protein content below 3 g/dL and electrolyte contents like other extracellular fluids. The serum-to-ascites albumin ratio is ≥ 1.1 g/dL.

ii. It contains a few mesothelial cells and mononuclear white blood cells. There are no neutrophils, which are found only in infected ascites. There are no erythrocytes; their presence is usually a sign of malignant cells in the peritoneal cavity.

Pathogenesis Clinicopathologic features of ascites result from the interaction of:
- Several *systemic factors* (decreased plasma colloid oncotic pressure, hyperaldosteronism, and impaired renal excretion of sodium and water), and
- *Local hydrodynamic factors* (increased portal venous pressure, and increased hepatic lymph formation).

These factors are as under:

i. *Decreased plasma oncotic pressure* is caused by impaired hepatic synthesis of albumin and other plasma proteins. Since albumin is the main oncotic protein of the plasma, hypoalbuminaemia impairs the capacity of the plasma to retain water and allows it to move into the peritoneal cavity **(Fig. 21.24)**.

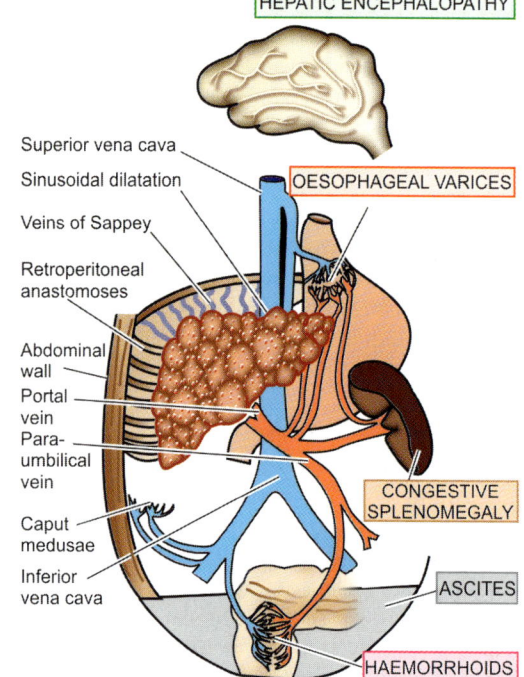

FIGURE 21.23: Major clinical consequences of portal hypertension.

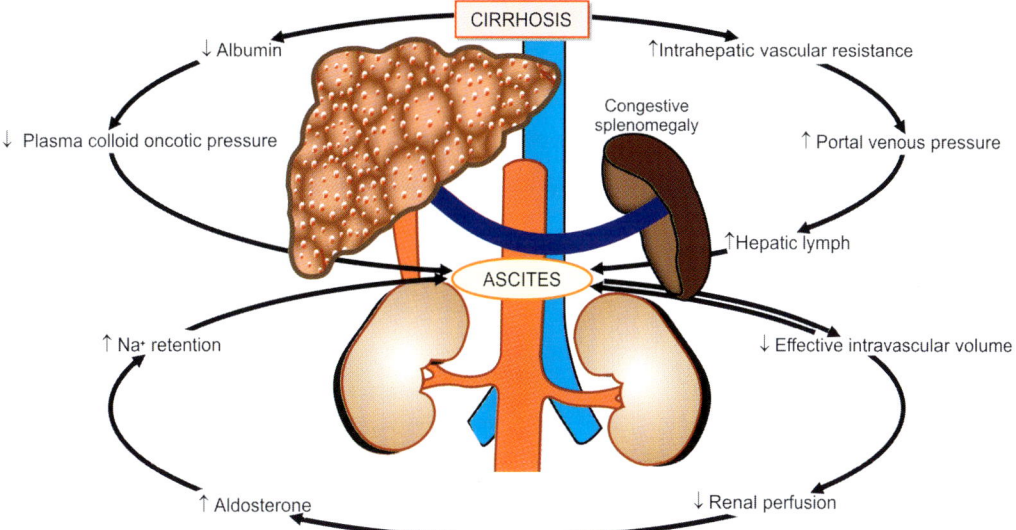

FIGURE 21.24: Mechanisms of ascites formation in cirrhosis.

ii. *Hyperaldosteronism* is related to its increased production in the adrenal cortex, probably related to decreased renal blood flow. Impaired catabolism of aldosterone by the cirrhotic liver and it excretion are contributory factors.

iii. *Impaired renal excretion of water and sodium* is a consequence of reduced renal blood flow and increased release of antidiuretic hormone.

iv. *Increased portal pressure* is typically combined with splanchnic arterial dilatation and compensatory secretion of vasoconstrictors of the renin-angiotensin system. These events will increase the pressure in interstitial capillaries in the splanchnic area and cause transudation of fluid and water retention in the abdominal cavity.

v. *Increased hepatic lymph formation and flow* due to increased sinusoidal pressure in the liver. The fluid from the blood in sinusoids enters under pressure into the spaces of Disse in large quantities, and from there it drains into the lymphatics leading into the thoracic duct. Lymph formation in the normal liver is less than 1 litre per day but in cirrhotic patients it might be 20 times higher, thus exceeding the capacity of the thoracic duct to drain it.

II. **Varices** are dilated tortuous veins that form the venous complexes connecting the portal system with the systemic circulation in a shunt-like manner. Three sites that are most prominently involved by portosystemic venous shunts are as follows (*see* **Fig. 21.23**):

i. *Oesophageal varices* at the oesophageal-gastric junction that may rupture and cause haematemesis.

ii. *Haemorrhoids* at the ano-rectal junction between the superior, middle and inferior haemorrhoidal veins.

iii. *Caput medusae* that are formed from paraumbilical venous plexus and abdominal wall veins which are connected with the portal veins in the hilum of the liver.

III. **Splenomegaly** is a term used for enlargement of the spleen, which weighs 500–1000 g (normal is <150 g). It is full of blood that cannot flow out of the spleen due to back pressure from the cirrhotic liver; hence the designation of *congestive splenomegaly*. Increased sequestration of blood cells in the spleen most often presents with thrombocytopenia.

IV. **Hepatic encephalopathy** is a term for the complex functional disturbances of the central nervous system related to the metabolic changes of cirrhosis. The most prominent changes are disturbed consciousness leading to coma, neurologic signs and flapping tremor of the hands (*asterixis*).

Causes of death in portal hypertension due to cirrhosis are most often from the following:

i. Hepatic coma
ii. Massive gastrointestinal haemorrhage from oesophageal varices.
iii. Intercurrent infection such as pneumonia or peritonitis due to infection of the ascites.

iv. Hepatorenal syndrome and kidney failure.
v. Hepatocellular carcinoma.

Q54. Classify common tumours and tumour-like conditions of the liver.

Benign tumours of the liver may originate from liver cells, bile duct or blood vessels and connective tissue cells **(Table 21.11)**.

Q55. Briefly discuss common benign tumours and tumour-like conditions.

Most benign tumours of the liver are small and of no clinical significance, requiring no treatment.
A few benign tumours and tumour-like condition of clinical significance are as follows:

I. **Haemangioma**, a tumour most often composed of capillaries is the most common benign tumour of the liver **(Fig. 21.25)**. It is found in 5–7% of adults, usually during routine radiologic examination or surgery. It may be solitary or multiple, and in most instances, causes no clinical symptoms.

II. **Focal nodular hyperplasia (FNH)** is a tumour-like mass composed of hyperplastic hepatocyte nodules arranged around a central stellate scar.

i. The hepatocyte nodules are surrounded by fibrous bands that contain bile ducts, vessels and lymphocytes resembling 'localised cirrhosis', a term often used to describe FNHs.

ii. The pathogenesis of FNH is not known. The most likely explanation is that thick-walled arteries with narrow lumina in the central scar are the cause of local ischaemia that has been compensated by subsequent liver cell hyperplasia.

iii. FNH is usually solitary but may be also multiple.

iv. It may vary in size, and some of them are quite large.

v. Because of its size and the fact that it cannot be distinguished from other liver cell tumours with absolute certainty, it is often surgically resected.

vi. FNH is actually more common than hepatocellular adenomas.

III. **Hepatocellular (liver cell) adenoma** is a rare benign tumour composed of liver cells. It is more common in women than men.

i. Tumour cells resemble normal liver cell but are not arranged into lobules that have portal tracts.

ii. Most adenomas are solitary but occasionally some are multiple. If there are more than 10 adenomas in one liver, the condition is called *hepatic adenomatosis*.

iii. There are several microscopic types of adenoma, each linked to a different oncogene.

- The most common type that occurs most often in women and is considered to be induced by

TABLE 21.11 WHO classification of tumours of the liver and intrahepatic bile ducts*.

BENIGN	MALIGNANT
A. Epithelial tumours	
I. *Hepatocellular tumours*	
1. Hepatocellular (liver cell) adenoma	1. Hepatocellular (liver cell) carcinoma
2. Focal nodular hyperplasia	2. Hepatoblastoma (Embryoma)
II. *Biliary epithelial tumours*	
1. Intrahepatic bile duct adenoma (Cholangioma)	1. Intrahepatic cholangiocarcinoma (peripheral bile duct carcinoma)
2. Intrahepatic bile duct cystadenoma	2. Bile duct cystadenocarcinoma
3. Biliary papillomatosis	3. Combined hepatocellular and cholangiocarcinoma
B. Non-epithelial tumours	
1. Angiomyolipoma	1. Epithelioid haemangioendothelioma
2. Haemangioma	2. Angiosarcoma
3. Lymphangioma	3. Embryonal sarcoma
4. Solitary fibrous tumour	4. Rhabdomyosarcoma
5. Mesenchymal hamartoma	5. Kaposi sarcoma
	6. Germ cell tumours (yolk sac tumour, teratoma)
	7. Rhabdoid tumour

*Bosman et al. WHO classification of tumours of the digestive system. 4th edition. IARC Lyon, 2010;48-58.

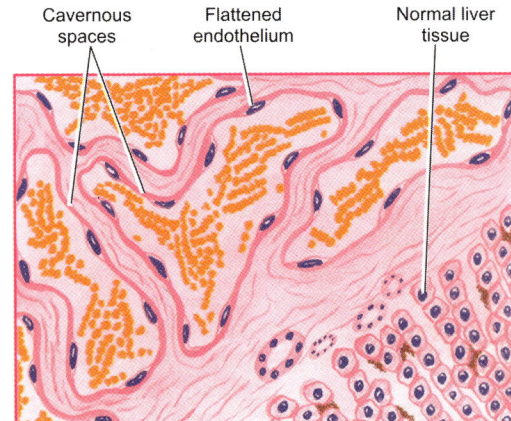

FIGURE 21.25: Cavernous haemangioma of the liver.

oestrogens and contraceptive hormones, contains dilated thin-walled blood vessels ('telangiectasia') and is prone to bleeding.
• Another type (fortunately the rarest) has distinct genetic changes that make it more prone to malignant transformation into hepatocellular carcinoma.
iv. However, most hepatocellular adenomas are benign tumours and the rate of malignant transformation is only 10%.
IV. **Bile duct adenoma** is a benign small tumour (~2 cm) composed of bile ducts. It is of no clinical concern.

Q56. Discuss salient features of hepatocellular carcinoma.

Definition Hepatocellular carcinoma (HCC), also known as liver cell carcinoma or hepatoma, is a malignant tumour composed of liver cells.
Epidemiology It is the most common primary malignant tumour of the liver.
• The incidence of HCC shows significant *geographic variations*, from relatively low in the US and Western Europe (1%), to very high in sub-Saharan Africa and South-East Asia (particularly China) (2–8%).
• Overall, liver cancer is one of the most common cancers in the world and globally it is now the fastest-growing cause of cancer death.
• HCC is more common in males than females (M:F=4:1). In 70–80% of cases, it supervenes on cirrhosis of all kinds but most often related to viral hepatitis HBV and HCV.
Etiology and pathogenesis
i. Most HCC develop on the background of *cirrhosis*.
a. HCC is most often linked to cirrhosis caused by HBV and HCV.
• HCC can develop in HCV and HBV chronic hepatitis without cirrhosis, but less often than in those with cirrhosis.
• Patients who have antibodies to both HBV and HCV have a three-time higher chance of developing HCC than those with either HBV or HCV.
• Alcohol abuse increases the risk in HBV and HCV related cirrhosis.
b. Other forms of cirrhosis, especially those related to genetic diseases (e.g. haemochromatosis, Wilson disease, α-1-antitrypsin deficiency) and steatohepatitis, are also documented precursors of HCC.
ii. *Mycotoxins* such as aflatoxin produced by *Aspergillus flavus,* play a role especially in underdeveloped countries of Africa and Asia.
iii. A number of *carcinogenic chemicals* can induce HCC in experimental animals, but it is not known if they play a role in human cancerogenesis.
iv. Invasive HCC is frequently preceded by *dysplastic nodules* in cirrhotic livers and adenomatous hyperplasia.
Pathology *Grossly,* three macroscopic types of HCC are recognised **(Fig. 21.26)**:
i. Expanding solitary nodule or mass
ii. Multifocal type
iii. Diffusely infiltrating type
Microscopy Several patterns are recognised but there is no clinical significance in histologically subclassifying HCC based on pattern.

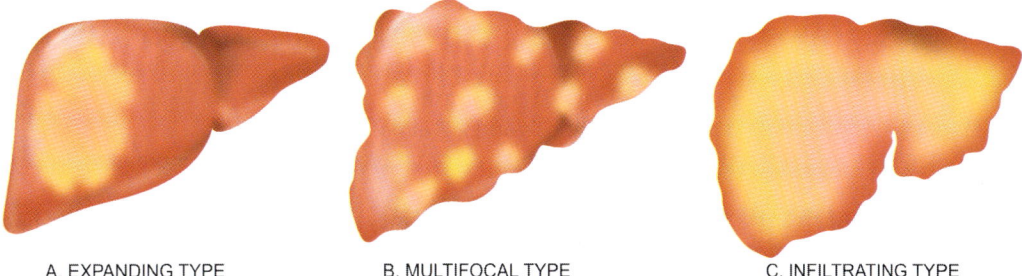

A, EXPANDING TYPE   B, MULTIFOCAL TYPE   C, INFILTRATING TYPE
FIGURE 21.26: Macroscopic patterns of hepatocellular carcinoma.

i. The *common patterns* are trabecular **(Fig. 21.27)** and pseudoglandular but there are many other patterns such as compact and scirrhous pattern.

ii. *Cytologic features* of HCC are characteristic and allow for fine needle aspiration cytologic diagnosis. These include: hyperchromatic vesicular nuclei with prominent nucleoli, basophilic cytoplasm and common pleomorphism in form of giant cells, spindle cells, etc. Tumour cells often have clear cytoplasm and contain Mallory bodies or bile in their cytoplasm or the intercellular canaliculi.

iii. *Immunohistochemical stains* supporting the diagnosis are performed with antibodies to arginase 1, glypican 3 and an antibody called HepPar1. Many HCC secrete alpha-foetoprotein (AFP) which may also be demonstrated immunohistochemically in tumour cells.

Variant forms of HCC do not deserve to be mentioned except for **fibrolamellar HCC** which is found in non-cirrhotic livers of younger persons and thus has a better prognosis than classical HCC. *Microscopically,* it is composed of polygonal cells with abundant eosinophilic cytoplasm. Tumour cells form nests surrounded by abundant fibrous bands.

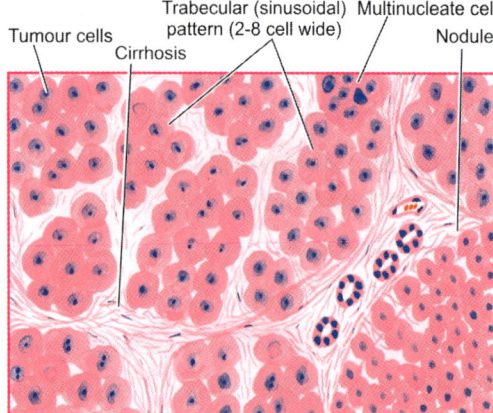

FIGURE 21.27: Hepatocellular carcinoma, typical microscopic pattern. The tumour cells form a few cell thick trabeculae separated by endothelium-lined sinusoidal spaces. The tumour cells resemble hepatocytes but have pleomorphism, increased N:C ratio and prominent nucleoli.

Spread of HCC includes haematogenous intrahepatic spread through the sinusoids, and extrahepatic spread to the lungs and local lymph nodes. Distant metastases to other organs are seen in advanced disease.

Clinical features include those of cirrhosis complicated by progressive hepatomegaly, with a peak incidence in the 50–60 years age group.

i. Enlargement of the liver may be associated with right upper abdominal quadrant tenderness and pain, and even a palpable liver mass.

ii. HCC may aggravate oesophageal varices and ascites, which may become haemorrhagic in 50% patients.

iii. Paraneoplastic syndromes may appear, even though not too often. The features include hypoglycaemia, hypercalcaemia, acquired porphyria and gynaecomastia.

iv. Tumour growth and spread are accompanied by progressive liver failure, jaundice, cachexia and impending hepatic coma that often precedes death.

v. *Laboratory findings* include anaemia, elevated alkaline phosphatase and AFP in serum. An abnormal prothrombin, des-γ-carboxy prothrombin is found in plasma, and this correlates with the elevation of AFP.

vi. Ultrasound examination is very useful, and is most suitable for following the growth of the tumours.

Q57. What are the important malignant liver tumours other than HCC?

I. **Cholangiocarcinoma** is an adenocarcinoma originating from intrahepatic bile ducts.
- It develops in non-cirrhotic livers mostly in men older than 60 years of age.
- In South-East Asia, it may be related to chronic infestation with *Clonorchis sinensis*, but in other parts of the world it is usually unrelated to some presumptive risk factors such as radioactive thorotrast or anabolic steroids which have been implicated in some cases.
- Cholangiocarcinoma has a very poor prognosis and it is almost invariably lethal.
- Pathologists must distinguish cholangiocarcinoma from metastatic adenocarcinomas, which are much more common.

II. **Hepatoblastoma** is a rare highly malignant tumour of infancy and childhood, clinically presenting usually before the end of the third year.
- It may be associated with developmental disorders and some hereditary cancer gene.

- It is composed of immature liver cells resembling embryonic and foetal liver cells, often adjacent to a mesenchymal component comprising immature connective tissue, cartilage and osteoid and foci of extramedullary haematopoiesis.
- Hepatoblastoma grows fast and spreads extensively, which accounts for the poor prognosis in most cases.
- Therapy includes complete hepatectomy with liver transplantation.

III. **Metastatic tumours** are the most common malignant neoplasms of the liver.
- Metastases reach the liver through the haematogenous route.
- In decreasing order of frequency, primary tumours metastasising to the liver include: carcinomas of the stomach, breast, lungs, colon, oesophagus, pancreas, malignant melanoma and haematopoietic malignancies.

■ BILIARY TRACT

Q58. What are the key facts about the normal anatomy, histology and physiology of the biliary tract that are important for understanding of biliary tract pathology?

Anatomy and histology The biliary tract includes the gallbladder and the bile ducts, which can be intrahepatic and extrahepatic.
- The extrahepatic bile ducts comprise the right and left hepatic duct which fuse to form the common bile duct.
- Common bile duct is connected with the gallbladder by the cystic duct.
- The common bile duct ends in the duodenum; in 70% cases it joins the main pancreatic duct and enters into the lumen of the duodenum at the papilla of Vater.
- The intraduodenal part of the common duct is enclosed in the sphincter of Oddi, composed of smooth muscle cells that are in continuity with the muscle layer of the duodenum.
- Histology of the extrahepatic bile ducts includes layers that are similar to those of the tubular part of the GI tract. Gallbladder lacks the muscle layer of the lamina propria but otherwise resembles the bile ducts.

Physiology The gallbladder serves to store and concentrate the bile secreted by the liver and then deliver it into the intestine for digestion and absorption of lipids. Normally, the liver secretes about 500 ml of bile, and the gallbladder concentrates it 5–10 times. The motility, capacity to concentrate and release the bile are under the control of a peptide hormone, cholecystokinin.

Q59. What are the risk factors for formation of gallstones (cholelithiasis)?

Definition Gallstones are solid concretions in the gallbladder or biliary ducts that are composed of bile (viz. cholesterol, bile pigment and calcium salts along with some organic components).

Risk factors It is common to group the risk factors for gallstones under four words beginning with four 'fs': female, forty (over the age of forty), fat and fertile (multiparous). The established risk factors are listed as follows:

i. *Age* is a risk factor because with advancing age the bile contains more cholesterol.

ii. *Geography and population genetic* play a role as evident from the geographic difference in the incidence of gallstones. Gallstones are prevalent in the entire Western world. The highest prevalence has been recorded among American Indians. Black Americans and the entire population in the Eastern world are relatively free of cholelithiasis.

iii. *Familial genetic factors* are important as evidenced by an increased incidence of gallstones in first-degree relatives of a patient with gallstones. Carrier of a mutated gene, CYP7A1, resulting in a deficiency of an enzyme, *cholesterol 7-hydrolase,* develops hypercholesterolaemia and gallstones.

iv. *Sex* is important as evidenced by the predominance of gallstones in women. By the age of 40 years, 20% of American women have gallstones in comparisons with only 6% of men.

v. *Drugs* that have a cholestatic effect, such as hormonal contraceptives, produce a more lithogenic bile. Similar is the effect of cholesterol-lowering drugs like clofibrate.

vi. *Obesity* is associated with increased synthesis of cholesterol and its excretion in bile.

vii. *Diet* that is low of dietary fibres is linked to a higher prevalence of gallstones.

viii. *Gastrointestinal diseases* associated with an increased incidence of gallstones include Crohn disease, ileal resection, ileal bypass surgery, etc. All these conditions interrupt the *enterohepatic circulation of bile*, thus favouring gallstone formation.

ix. *Factors that favour the formation of pigment gallstones* are various forms of chronic haemolytic anaemias resulting in hyperbilirubinaemia. Cirrhosis and various forms of chronic hepatitis are also associated with an increased incidence of pigment stones.

Q60. What is the pathogenesis of gallstones?

Gallstone formation (*lithogenesis*) differs for cholesterol and mixed stones on one hand from that for pigment stones on the other.

I. Pathogenesis of cholesterol and mixed stones, and biliary sludge

Cholesterol is insoluble in water, but can be solubilised by adding another lipid. This cholesterol is secreted in bile with phospholipids (lecithin) as bilayered vesicles but a converted into mixed micelles by addition of bile acids, the third constituent. If this process is disturbed, gallstones will form in several steps that include: i) formation of lithogenic bile, ii) cholesterol nucleation, and iii) gallbladder hypomotility **(Fig. 21.28)**:

i. *Formation of lithogenic bile* is favoured by the following events, each of which is illustrated by abnormal function of an enzyme involved information of bile, as follows:

a. *Supersaturation of bile* (the most common cause of lithogenic bile formation) occurs due to several mechanisms that favour excretion of cholesterol mentioned above. These factors enhance the activity of *HMG-CoA reductase* that normally regulates cholesterol synthesis and its hepatic uptake.

b. *Reduced bile acid pool* with a loss of bile acid in the small intestine, with supersaturation of the remaining bile acid with cholesterol as it occurs following the defective action of *cholesterol 7-hydroxylase*.

c. *Increased conversion of cholic acid to deoxycholic acid*, resulting in increased secretion of deoxycholate in bile, that is associated with hypersecretion of cholesterol into the bile, as seen in *multidrug resistance protein 3 (MDR3)* gene mutation, resulting in defective secretion of phospholipid (lecithin).

ii. *Cholesterol nucleation* involving cholesterol monohydrate crystals, which may occur due to the action of *pronucleation factors* (mucin and non-mucin secretory products of gallbladder epithelial cells) or a deficiency of *anti-nucleation factors* (apolipoprotein AI and AII and some glycoproteins).

iii. *Gallbladder hypomotility* which allows accumulation of debris and sludge. Emptying of the gallbladder is under the regulation of cholecystokinin and the hypomotility is probably related to a loss or defective function of cholecystokinin receptors on gallbladder smooth muscle cells.

II. Pathogenesis of pigment stones

Events that promote pigment gallstone formation include the following:
i. Chronic haemolysis accompanied by unconjugated hyperbilirubinaemia
ii. Alcoholic cirrhosis
iii. Chronic biliary tract infections, e.g. parasitic infestation with *Clonorchis sinensis* and *Ascaris lumbricoides*.
iv. Demographic and genetic factors, e.g. in rural setting and prevalence in Asian countries.

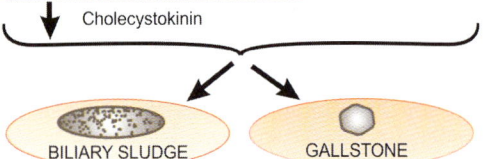

FIGURE 21.28: Schematic pathogenesis of gallstone formation. (HMG-CoAR, hydroxy methyl glutaryl-coenzyme A reductase; 7α-OHase, cholesterol 7α-OHase hydroxylase; MDR3, multidrug resistance- associated protein 3).

Q61. Describe and compare the salient features of the three main types of gallstones.

Key features
- Gallstones contain cholesterol, bile pigment and calcium carbonate in various proportions, and according to their composition they can be classified into three groups: pure, mixed and combined gallstones.
- Mixed gallstones account to 80%, whereas other two forms account for 10% each.
- Gallstones most often originate in the gallbladder and are associated with chronic cholecystitis, but on occasion they can be formed in the bile ducts.

I. **Pure gallstones** can be subdivided into three groups: i) pure cholesterol stone, ii) pure pigment stones, and iii) pure calcium carbonate stones

i. **Pure cholesterol gallstones** are usually solitary and fairly large (3 cm or more).
- Hard, whitish-yellow with a smooth external surface.
- Cut section shows radiating glistening crystals.
- The mucosa of the gallbladder often shows cholesterolosis, but there is generally no cholecystitis.
- Most of them are radiolucent, but 10–20% contain calcium salts and are thus radiopaque.

ii. **Pure bile pigment gallstones** are usually multiple and small.
- Composed of bile pigment, calcium bilirubinate, and contain less than 20% of cholesterol.
- Mulberry-like external surface.
- Soft and can be crushed easily.
- Gallbladder mucosa uninvolved.

iii. **Pure calcium carbonate gallstones** are rare.
- Multiple, small, grain-like, grey-white and faceted, radio-opaque.
- Gallbladder mucosa uninvolved.

II. **Mixed gallstones** are the most common gallstones (80%).
- Composed of cholesterol monohydrate (>50%) admixed to calcium salts, pigment and fatty acids.
- Multiple, multifaceted, moderately firm, varying in size and shape.
- On cross section, laminated displaying alternating dark and light layers.
- Gallbladder mucosa invariably shows signs of chronic cholecystitis.

III. **Combined gallstones** are usually solitary, large and smooth surfaced.
- They have a pure gallstone nucleus and a shell made of mixed stone, or vice versa, i.e. a central mixed stone nucleus and a pure external shell.
- Mucosa of the gallbladder shows sign of chronic cholecystitis.

Contrasting features of these types of gallstones are summarised in **Table 21.12** and illustrated in **Figure 21.29**.

TABLE 21.12 Contrasting features of gallstones.

TYPE	FREQUENCY	COMPOSITION	GALLBLADDER CHANGES	APPEARANCE
1. *Pure gallstones*	10%	i. Cholesterol	Cholesterolosis	Solitary, oval, large, smooth, yellow-white; on C/S radiating glistening crystals
		ii. Bile pigment	No change	Multiple, small, jet-black, mulberry-shaped; on C/S soft black
		iii. Calcium carbonate	No change	Multiple, small, grey-white, faceted; C/S hard
2. *Mixed gallstones*	80%	Cholesterol, bile pigment and calcium carbonate in varying combination	Chronic cholecystitis	Multiple, multifaceted, variable size, on C/S laminated alternating dark-pigment layer and pale-white layer
3. *Combined gallstones*	10%	Pure gallstone nucleus with mixed gallstone shell, or mixed gallstone nucleus with pure gallstone shell	Chronic cholecystitis	Solitary, large, smooth; on C/S central nucleus of pure gallstone with mixed shell or vice versa

CHOLESTEROL (YELLOW-WHITE)   PIGMENT (MULBERRY-SHAPED)   CALCIUM CARBONATE (HARD)   MIXED GALLSTONES (MULTIFACETED)   COMBINED GALLSTONES (SMOOTH-SURFACED)

FIGURE 21.29: Gallstones of various types. A, Three types of pure gallstones. B, Mixed, and C, Combined gallstones.

Q62. What are the clinical manifestations and complications of cholelithiasis?

Gallstones are asymptomatic in 50% of cases and are discovered incidentally. The clinical manifestations and complications pertaining to the remaining cases include the following **(Fig. 21.30)**:

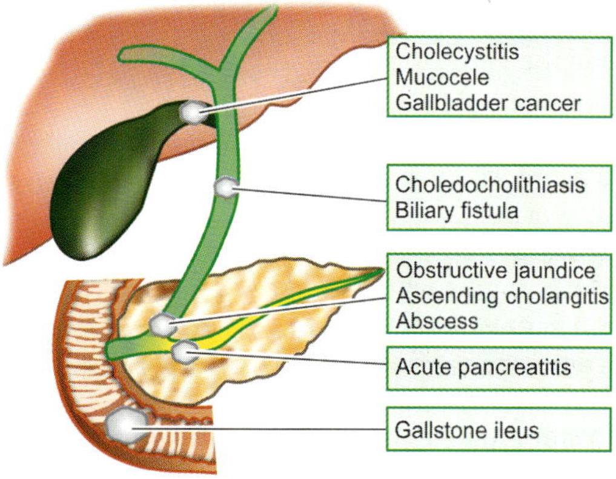

i. **Cholecystitis**, which is mostly chronic but may be exacerbated by fatty meals or overeating and become acute.

ii. **Mucocele** results from an obstruction of the gallbladder neck followed by an accumulation of mucus in the distended gallbladder.

iii. **Empyema** is accumulation of pus in the gallbladder obstructed by a stone. Often, it represents an infected mucocele.

iv. **Choledocholitiasis** with obstructive jaundice and possible cholangitis.

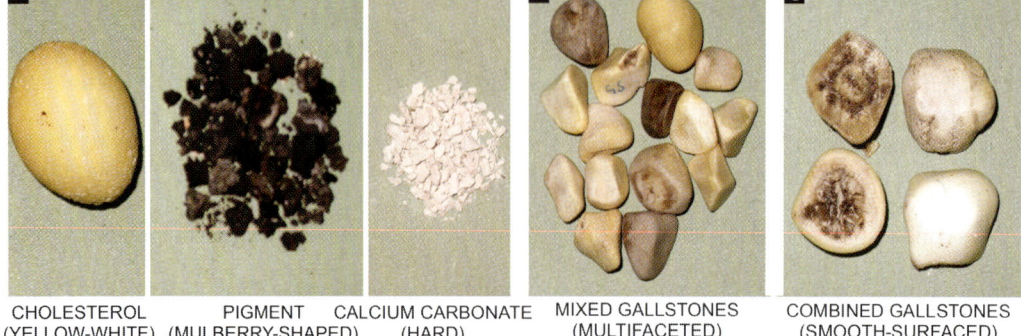

FIGURE 21.30: Major clinical effects and complications of gallstones.

v. **Biliary fistula** is a rare complication in which a fistulous tract connects the inflamed gallbladder with an intestinal loop that has adhered to it.

vi. **Gallstone ileus** is an obstruction of the small intestine by a gallstone that has entered into the intestinal lumen through a dilated common bile duct or a fistula tract. It is a rare event since most gallstones that reach the intestine are small and are passed in faeces without any complications.

vii. **Acute pancreatitis** may develop from the obstruction of the common bile duct by an impacted gallstone and the retrograde pressure into the pancreatic duct caused by that obstruction.

Q63. Discuss main features of acute cholecystitis.

Definition Acute cholecystitis is an inflammation of the gallbladder which is most often caused by a bacterial infection superimposed on obstruction of the neck of gallbladder by a gallstone.

Etiopathogenesis There are two types of acute cholecystitis: calculous and acalculous.

I. *Acute calculous cholecystitis* initiated by a stone obstructing the neck of the gallbladder accounts for 90% of cases of acute cholecystitis. The obstruction of the bile flow leads to an ascending infection, most often by *E.coli* and *Streptococcus faecalis*.

II. *Acalculous acute cholecystisis* is rare accounting for only 10% of cases. It could develop in a variety of situations such as sepsis, post-surgical infection, multiple injuries, burns, recent childbirth, torsion of the gallbladder and diabetes mellitus, or primary infections with *Salmonella* or parasites.

Pathology

Gross

- The gallbladder is distended and tense; its external serosal surface is congested and red, reflecting the underlying inflammation in the gallbladder wall.

- The gallbladder is filled with pus admixed with green bile partially attached to the congested and oedematous mucosal surface.
- An impacted gallstone is typically seen in the neck of the gallbladder.

Microscopy
i. Acute purulent inflammation of the gallbladder wall combined with haemorrhage and necrosis which may be transmural (*gangrenous cholecystitis*).
ii. Massive pus accumulation inside the gallbladder is called *gallbladder empyema*.
iii. The severe form of infection may spread to the liver where it may form a *pericholecystic abscess*.
iv. Rupture of the gallbladder may cause *purulent peritonitis*.
v. In acalculous cholecystitis, there are no gallstones but most other features may be present.

Clinical features
- Severe colicky pain in the right upper quadrant of the abdomen, which may be tense and sensitive to palpation.
- In some cases, the gallbladder may be palpable.
- Fever, leucocytosis with neutrophilia are typically present and may be accompanied by slight jaundice.

Complications are, in essence, the same as listed above under the complications of cholelithiasis.

Prognosis Early cholecystectomy is curative and such an energetic approach has reduced the mortality and the rate of complications of acute cholecystitis to 0.5%.

Q64. Discuss salient features of chronic cholecystitis.

Definition Chronic cholecystitis is a chronic inflammation of the gallbladder, usually presenting in several pathologic forms and associated with gallstones and ill-defined symptoms pertaining to the hepatobiliary tract.

Etiopathogenesis The causes for the chronic infection are not known.
- It is possible that the infection reflects bouts of recurrent acute cholecystitis or an incompletely healed acute inflammation that has progressed to a chronic form.
- Metabolic changes predisposing to gallstones, such as supersaturation of bile with cholesterol, and the mechanical irritation of the bladder mucosa by gallstones, may play a role.

Pathology The gallbladder is generally contracted and has a thickened wall with signs of chronic inflammation. There is usually fibrosis of the mucosa and the muscle layer **(Fig. 21.31)**.

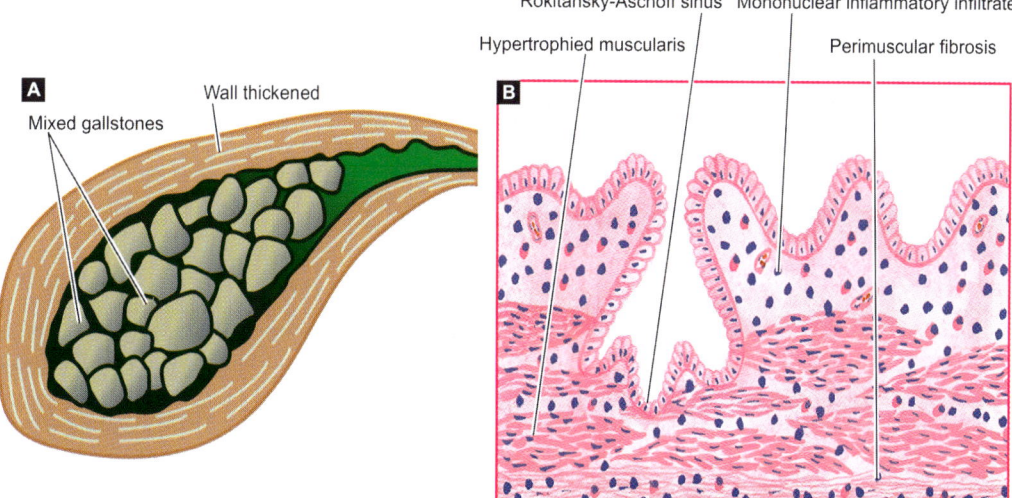

FIGURE 21.31: A, Chronic cholecystitis with cholelithiasis (mixed gallstones). The wall of the gallbladder is thickened and the lumen is packed with well-fitting, multiple, multi-faceted, mixed gallstones. B, Microscopy shows penetration of epithelium-lined spaces into the gallbladder wall (Rokitansky-Aschoff sinus) in an area. There is subepithelial and subserosal fibrosis and hypertrophy of muscularis. Mononuclear inflammatory cell infiltrate is present in subepithelial and perimuscular layers.

Variants of chronic cholecystitis are as follows:

i. *Chronic cholecystitis glandularis* This is the most common form characterised by thickened mucosa that contains scattered infiltrates of chronic inflammatory cells. Typically, the mucosa is also thickened and forms glandular extensions penetrating into the muscle layer (*Rokitansky-Aschoff sinuses*).

ii. *Acute on chronic cholecystitis* in which there are acute inflammatory cells focally in the mucosa that shows chronic inflammation.

iii. *Porcelain gallbladder* is a form of chronic cholecystitis in which the wall of the gallbladder is thickened, calcified and rigid, cracking like an egg-shell.

Clinical features are nonspecific and overshadowed by those produced by the coexistent gallstones.

Q65. Discuss carcinoma of the gallbladder, in brief.

Definition Carcinoma of the gallbladder is a rare form of adenocarcinoma, yet it is the most common malignant tumour of the extrahepatic biliary tract (**Fig. 21.32**).

Epidemiology Like cholelithiasis, it is more common in women than in men (F:M= 4:1). Its peak incidence is in the 7th decade of life. There is a considerable geographic variation in the incidence of gallbladder cancer which is more common in parts of South-East Asia, South and Middle America including Mexico.

Etiopathogenesis As is the case with most cancers, the etiology is not known. Several possible etiologic factors have been implicated on the basis of epidemiologic data, such as:

i. *Cholelithiasis and cholecystitis*, which are coexistent in 75% of cases of gallbladder cancer. On the other hand, only 0.5% patients with gallstones develop cancer, and the role of gallstones as potential carcinogens is thus questionable. Porcelain gallbladder has been often implicated but that is a rare and unusual form of chronic cholecystitis.

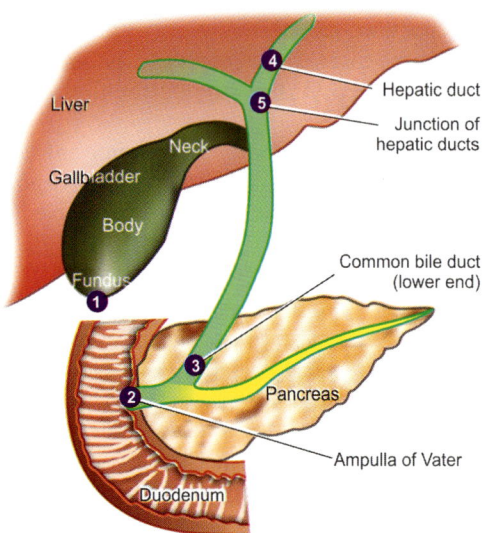

FIGURE 21.32: Frequency of cancer in the biliary system.

ii. *Genetic factors* may play a role as suggested by epidemiologic data on a higher rate of incidence of cancer in Mexicans and Native American Indians, who also have a tendency to form gallstones.

Pathology Most of the cancers of the gallbladder are adenocarcinomas. About 5% are squamous cell carcinomas, preceded by squamous metaplasia of mucosal glands due to chronic inflammation.

Clinical features Clinical diagnosis of gallbladder cancer is usually delayed. Most patients have gallstones and usually ignore the early signs of cancer thinking that they are related to the gallstones.

Prognosis In most patients who have been finally diagnosed with gallbladder cancer, there is extensive local spread of the tumour into the liver and adjacent organs, local lymph nodes or even to the lungs. The prognosis is poor and the five year survival is 5%.

Q66. What is carcinoma of the extrahepatic bile ducts and ampulla of Vater?

Definition Carcinoma of the extrahepatic bile ducts and ampulla of Vater is a relatively rare form of adenocarcinoma that originates most often in the lower part of the common bile duct and ampulla of Vater (*see* **Fig. 21.32**).

In most instances, carcinoma of the lower third of the common bile duct cannot be distinguished from carcinoma of the ampulla of Vater, duodenum and the head of pancreas and, therefore, it is included under the term of **periampullary carcinoma**. Adenocarcinomas of the upper part of the common bile duct and hepatic ducts are somewhat less common.

Etiopathogenesis In contrast to carcinoma of the gallbladder, this cancer is not linked to gallstones.
- Epidemiologic studies show an increased incidence in patients suffering from several diseases such as ulcerative colitis, sclerosing cholangitis and parasitic infestations with *Fasciola hepatica* and *Clonorchis sinensis*.

- These parasitic infestations account for the higher incidence of carcinoma of the extrahepatic bile duct in South-East Asia, especially in China.

Pathology These tumours are all adenocarcinomas which may show intraductal papillary and invasive growth or just invasive growth with narrowing of the lumen.

Clinical features Obstructive jaundice develops early and this fact accounts for a somewhat better prognosis than for carcinoma of the gallbladder. Overall, the prognosis is still very bad because these cancers tend to spread locally and metastasise early.

EXOCRINE PANCREAS

Q67. What are the key facts about the normal anatomy, histology and physiology of pancreas that are important for understanding of pathology of this organ?

Anatomy and histology The pancreas is located in the retroperitoneal space and on the anterior surface only covered with the peritoneum. It lies obliquely in the concavity of the duodenum as an elongated structure divided into three topographic zones: the head, the body and the tail (see **Fig. 21.1**).
- *The exocrine pancreas* is composed of acini arranged into lobules that are linked to the minor and major excretory ducts. The major duct of Wirsung ends at the ampulla of Vater in the duodenum. A minor duct of Santorini is present in a significant number of persons and it also ends in the duodenum in an ampulla located dorsally from the ampulla of Vater.
- *The endocrine pancreas* is discussed in Chapter 27.

Physiology Most of the exocrine pancreatic parenchyma is composed of acinar cells which secrete more than 20 different enzymes. Most enzymes are secreted in the form of proenzymes which are activated upon their entry into the duodenum. Two major enzymes, *lipase and amylase*, are, however, secreted in an active form. Ductal cells secrete bicarbonates which are important for neutralising the acidity of the gastric juices.

Q68. What are the salient features of cystic fibrosis?

Definition Cystic fibrosis (CF) is a very common autosomal recessive genetic disease caused by mutations of *CFTR* gene. It is characterised by viscid mucous secretion in all exocrine glands of the body (*mucoviscidosis*) and increased concentration of electrolytes in the eccrine glands of the skin.

Currently, CF is the most common lethal autosomal recessive disease worldwide, showing no sex predilection.

Genetics/pathogenesis The basic defect in cystic fibrosis are the mutations of *CFTR* gene encoding the protein called *cystic fibrosis transmembrane conductance regulator*.

i. Numerous mutations have been identified affecting the synthesis, folding or regulation of *CFTR* protein and its other functions.

ii. The most common is the mutation coding for phenylalanine at the position 508 ($\Delta 508$) which prevents normal folding of the CFTR protein. It is found in approximately 70% of patients.

iii. CFTR is a cAMP-regulated anion channel protein expressed on the apical surface of epithelial cells of the airways, pancreatic ducts and other tissues.

iv. When it is absent or its activity is reduced, the transport of chloride and bicarbonate is reduced, affecting the function of many organs.

v. Clinical manifestations depend on the type of genetic mutations, which may be classified as mild or severe. The first signs of disease may appear at birth or later on in childhood and adolescences.

Clinicopathologic features Pathological changes vary and depend on the severity of the disease and its duration. Clinicopathologic findings reflect the malfunction of several major organs such as pancreas, intestines, liver, and lungs.

I. **Pancreas** is almost invariably involved.

i. The most prominent finding is the accumulation of inspissated secretions in dilated small and medium-sized ducts accompanied by atrophy and loss of acinar cells, which are replaced by fibrous tissue **(Fig. 21.33)**. After prolonged time, there is *extensive fibrosis* of the pancreas with cystic dilatation of ducts, accounting for the name of the disease.

ii. Atrophy and fibrosis of the pancreas result in pancreatic insufficiency leading to *malabsorption* of fats, proteins and carbohydrates.

iii. Pancreatic fibrosis will ultimately damage the islets or pancreas and their capacity to produce enough insulin, resulting in *diabetes mellitus*.

II. **Gastrointestinal tract** related symptoms appear in 10–15% CF neonates.

i. Most common is in form of *meconium ileus*. Instead of normal evacuation of the intestinal contents (meconium), the affected children have thick viscid meconium obstructing the intestines and causing an ileus. Ileus results from the inability of the pancreatic and intestinal enzymes to digest and liquefy the viscid meconium. If untreated, the obstructed intestines may rupture and cause meconium peritonitis.

ii. In the upper alimentary tract, the salivary glands may be obstructed and this might cause *xerostomia*.

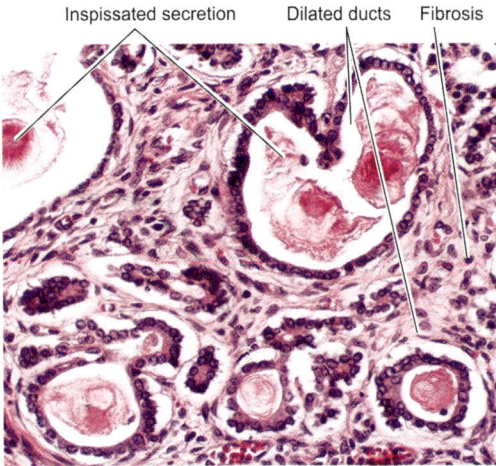

FIGURE 21.33: Cystic fibrosis pancreas. The ducts are dilated and contain inspissated eosinophilic secretions. The intervening pancreatic acinar parenchyma shows fibrous replacement.

III. **Liver** develops inspissated viscid mucus secretions in the small and medium-sized bile ducts in the liver.

i. This may cause biliary obstruction that will typically present as mild obstructive jaundice which over time may progress to secondary biliary cirrhosis.

ii. Liver-related symptoms usually evolve around puberty and may slowly progress.

IV. **Respiratory tract** is invariably affected and the respiratory infections are the most troublesome and life threatening complication of CF. Viscid mucus accumulates in the airways and is readily infected.

i. Pathologic changes include chronic, often purulent, bronchitis and bronchiolitis, bronchiectasis, peribronchiolar pneumonia and inflammatory sino-nasal polyps.

ii. The most common pathogens are *Pseudomonas aeruginosa*, which may be isolated from most patients with pulmonary symptoms, and *Staphylococcus aureus*. Repeated positive sputum cultures for *Pseudomonas* are almost diagnostic of CF.

iii. *Burkholderia cepacia*, found in a minority of cases is also important because it may cause a fulminant infection *('cepacia syndrome')* that is often resistant to antibiotics.

V. **Infertility** due to bilateral loss of parts of vas deferens is found in over 95% CF males resulting in obstructive azoospermia.

VI. **Sweat gland malfunction** with hypersecretion of sodium and chloride in sweat.

i. Children have a 'salty skin' noticed by mothers who kiss them.

ii. Loss of salt in hot weather and following strenuous exercise may lead to salt depletion and physical exhaustion.

iii. Increased sweat chloride was previously used as a diagnostic test for CF.

Clinical manifestations depend on the age of the patient and the severity of the disease.

• Most prominent are symptoms pertaining to pancreatic insufficiency (malabsorption) and pulmonary infections, which are the most common cause of death in CF patients.

Prognosis With therapeutic advances of modern medicine, the life expectancy of CF patients has been prolonged from 1 year to 40 years of age.

Q69. Briefly discuss acute pancreatitis.

Definition Acute pancreatitis is a disease of sudden onset, mediated by intrapancreatic activation of pancreatic enzymes which cause necrosis and subsequent inflammation of pancreatic parenchyma and surrounding fat tissue. Severe acute pancreatitis, also known as acute pancreatic necrosis, or massive haemorrhagic pancreatitis, accounts for 20% of cases of acute pancreatitis and is discussed here.

Etiology
- *Leading causes* of acute pancreatitis are alcoholism and cholelithiasis which account for 80% of all cases.
- *Other less common causes* include: viral infection, extension of bacterial infection from adjacent organs to pancreas, trauma, shock, ischaemia, drugs and some metabolic disorders such as hyperlipoproteinaemia, hypercalcaemia and hyperparathyroidism.

Pathogenesis Injury to the pancreas and surrounding fat tissue is mediated by the interaction of numerous pancreatic enzymes, the most important of which are the following:
i. *Proteases* such as trypsin or chymotrypsin, cause proteolysis of tissues and also activate the clotting and complement system by converting prekallikrein to kallikrein.
ii. *Lipases* degrade lipids in the cytoplasm and phospholipids in cell membranes.
iii. *Elastases* cause destruction of elastic tissue in blood vessels.

Activation of pancreatic enzymes is brought about by the following mechanisms:
- Pancreatic acinic cell damage
- Duct obstruction
- Blocking of exocytosis of enzymes from acinar cells and their intracellular activation.

Pathology *Grossly,* the features of acute pancreatitis are highly variable and include the following:
i. Swelling of the entire organ with focal haemorrhage.
ii. Areas of necrosis of the pancreatic parenchyma which appear muddy brown and softened, or showing bile-tinged discoloration.
iii. Necrosis of peripancreatic fat tissue, which appears chalky-white.
iv. The peritoneal cavity usually contains fluid that is murky and haemorrhagic, accompanied by white flecks of fat necrosis on the peritoneum, mesentery and peripancreatic fat tissue.

Microscopy
i. Necrosis and fragmentation of arterial wall accompanied by haemorrhage.
ii. Necrosis of pancreatic parenchyma surrounded by acute inflammatory cells.
iii. Fat necrosis of peripancreatic fat tissue with deposition of calcium salts due to saponification of fatty acids released from triglycerides.

Clinical features
- Severe upper abdominal pain, progressing rapidly to a clinical picture of acute abdomen, with fever, nausea, vomiting, feeling of distress, guarding and sensitivity to palpation of the abdomen.
- *Laboratory findings* include signs of infection (e.g. leucocytosis with neutrophilia) and elevation of pancreatic enzymes in serum, primarily *amylase* and *lipase*. Amylase rises during the first 24 hours and lipase 3–4 days after the onset of the disease. As the fat necrosis binds calcium, there will be hypocalcaemia, which is usually a poor prognostic finding suggesting severe necrosis.

Complications develop fast and are listed as under:
i. Peritonitis with ascites, which is initially chemical and sterile, but may become infected due to the transmigration of bacteria from the lumen of paralysed intestines into the peritoneal cavity.
ii. Shock, DIC and acute renal failure.
iii. Intestinal obstruction due to the mass effect of enlarged head of the pancreas on the duodenum, and paralytic ileus of the small intestines due to peritonitis.
iv. Pancreatic abscess due to bacterial superinfection.
v. Pancreatic pseudocyst due to the lytic action of pancreatic enzymes.
vi. Chronic pancreatitis due to destruction of pancreatic parenchyma and subsequent pancreatic fibrosis.

Prognosis Mortality is still high and in the range of 20–30%.

Q70. Discuss main features of chronic pancreatitis.

Definition Chronic pancreatitis, also known as chronic relapsing pancreatitis, is a disease resulting from progressive destruction of the pancreas due to repeated, mild and subclinical attacks of acute pancreatitis.

Etiopathogenesis Most cases of chronic pancreatitis are caused by the same factors as acute pancreatitis, and are thus related to either alcoholism or cholelithiasis.

- *Chronic pancreatitis* is a common feature of IgG4 disease with fibrosis that may selectively involve pancreas or present in a multi-organ systemic disease.
- Non-alcoholic cases of chronic pancreatitis seen in tropical countries result most likely from *protein-calorie malnutrition*.
- *Genetic* chronic pancreatitis is a rare form of disease; yet, more often clinically recognised than acute genetic pancreatitis.

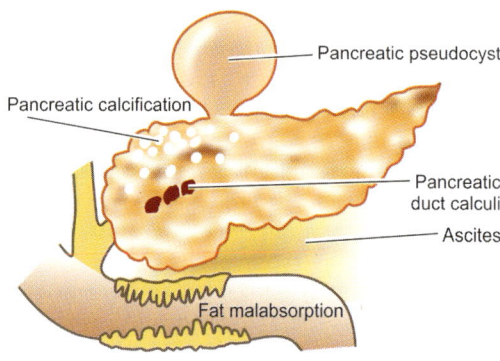

FIGURE 21.34: Complications of chronic pancreatitis.

Pathology Gross and microscopic features vary depending on the stage of disease.
Grossly, initially the pancreas is enlarged, but with time fibrosis prevails and it becomes smaller, firm and gritty on sectioning. Foci of calcification and intraductal calculi are common and visible by X-rays examination. Pseudocysts inside the pancreas or protruding from its surface are common **(Fig. 21.34)**.
Microscopy
i. Extensive fibrosis replacing the acini and surrounding the dilated ducts.
ii. There are scattered foci of atrophic acini and ducts, as well as islets of Langerhans, which are initially spared.
iii. In later stages, there is indiscriminate loss of all pancreatic elements due to extensive fibrosis accompanied by foci of calcification.
Clinical features include progressive pancreatic insufficiency with malabsorption, as under:
i. Steatorrhoea associated with a deficiency of lipids and fat soluble vitamins A, D, K and E.
ii. Protein and carbohydrate deficiency results in malnutrition-related emaciation, muscle weakness and general loss of energy.
iii. Diabetes mellitus develops in later stages of the disease and it is related to the loss of islets of Langerhans.
iv. Fibrosis of the pancreas extending into the peripancreatic nerve plexuses causing pain radiating into the back on the left side.

Q71. What are the major features of carcinoma of the pancreas?

Definition Carcinoma of the pancreas is an adenocarcinoma, originating most often from the cells lining the ducts of the pancreas.
Epidemiology In the United States, carcinoma of the pancreas is the second most common carcinoma of the GI tract (after colon cancer), and the third most common cause of cancer death. It is more common among African Americans than in other races. Most patients are older than 50 years. Global incidence is increasing.
Etiology No dominant causative agents has been identified.
- Among the potential risk factors, the most important are heavy cigarette smoking, diet/obesity and familial genetic factors.
- The incidence of pancreatic cancer is remarkably increased in hereditary cancer syndromes such as Peutz-Jeghers syndrome, in which it is increased more than 100 times over the normal.

Molecular pathogenesis Invasive carcinoma evolves from pancreatic intraepithelial neoplasia (PanIN). Genetic changes that occur during the formation of invasive carcinoma are complex, but can be best analysed by concentrating on early and late changes.
- *Early events,* seen in PanIN and early invasive adenocarcinoma, are shortening of telomeres and activation of the oncogene *K-RAS* (>90% of cases*).*
- *Late events* that occur toward the end of cancerogenic sequence include deletions or inactivating mutations of tumour suppressor genes *p16/CDKN2A, TP53*, and *SMAD4/DPC4* (*depleted in pancreatic carcinoma*). SMAD4/DPC4 is located on chromosome 18, which is lost in >90% of invasive carcinomas.

Pathology

Location Most carcinomas are located in the head of the pancreas **(Fig. 21.35)**.

i. *Tumours of the head of pancreas* are usually small (2–4 cm in diameter), hard, grey-white, without sharp demarcation between the tumour and the surrounding pancreatic parenchyma.
- They cause obstructive jaundice early in the course of the disease.

ii. *Tumours of the body and tail* have more time to grow before they are discovered.
- In contrast to tumours of the head they do not cause jaundice and by the time of diagnosis they form larger masses.
- Larger tumours may be found invading adjacent organs, such as the colon, stomach spleen.
- Metastases to regional lymph nodes occur early and even small carcinomas may have metastases in the liver.

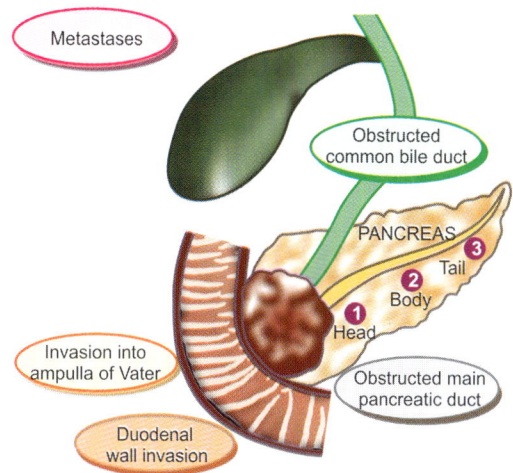

FIGURE 21.35: Distribution of carcinoma of the pancreas (numbered serially) and its major effects.

Microscopy Most tumours are adenocarcinomas arising from ductal cells. Adjacent to invasive carcinoma one may find foci of PanIN which has preceded invasive carcinoma.

i. *PanIN* may have the features of intraductal papillary mucinous neoplasm (IPMN) or intraductal tubulopapillary neoplasm (ITPN), mucinous cystic neoplasm (MCN) and intra-ampullary papillary-papillary tubular neoplasm.

ii. *Invasive adenocarcinomas* are composed of mucus-secreting columnar cells, lying in a desmoplastic fibrous stroma. Perineural invasion is common.

iii. *Acinar carcinomas* account for only 1% of all carcinomas of the pancreas.

iv. *Other microscopic subtypes* are less common and the subdivision of tumour by histologic subtypes is not warranted clinically.

Clinical features

- These are most diagnostic in patients with *carcinoma of the head of pancreas* which present early with painless obstructive jaundice. The jaundice is accompanied with dark brown urine and clay-coloured stools, elevation of serum conjugated bilirubin and alkaline phosphatase.
- *General systemic signs* of malignancy are usually present and include anorexia, weight loss, cachexia, weakness and malaise, nausea and vomiting.
- Migratory thrombophlebitis, GI bleeding and splenomegaly and upper abdominal pain are present in *advanced cases*.

Prognosis for pancreatic carcinoma is poor: median survival is 6 months after diagnosis and only 10% of patients survive one year or more.

Chapter 21e Supplement: Online Content

Digital content of this chapter available with this book is meant for enhanced learning and self-assessment. In addition, it contains 23 Multiple Choice Questions (MCQs), 06 Clinicopathologic Vignettes, and 09 Image-based Questions; these are followed by their answers along with explanatory notes of correct and incorrect answers.

CHAPTER 22

Kidney and Lower Urinary Tract

KIDNEYS

Q1. Describe briefly key facts about the applied aspects of normal anatomy, histology and physiology of the kidney that are important for understanding kidney pathology.

Anatomy Kidneys are paired organs located in the retroperitoneal space of the abdomen. On cross section through each kidney, one may see 3 main parts of each kidney **(Fig. 22.1)**:
i. *Cortex* which contains 85% of renal tubules and all the glomeruli.
ii. *Medulla* which consists of medullary rays ending on the tip of the papilla.
iii. *Renal pelvis* which consist of *calyces* and serves for collecting the urine.
The arterial blood reaches the kidneys through the *renal arteries* which arise on each side from the aorta at the level of the 2nd lumbar vertebra. Renal arteries enter the kidney at the hilum and then divide sequentially into smaller and smaller branches, until they reach the glomeruli through the *afferent arterioles*. From the glomeruli, the blood leaves through the *efferent arterioles*, which lead the blood to the renal venous system.

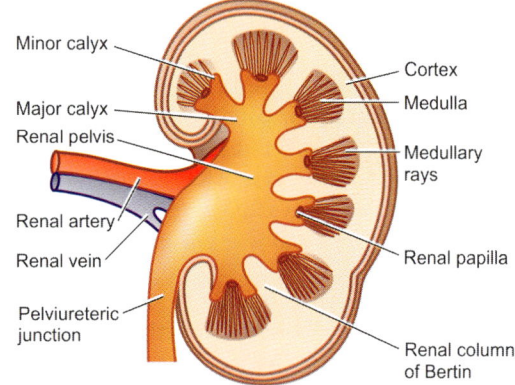

FIGURE 22.1: Cross-section of the kidney showing gross structures.

Histology Kidneys are composed of 1 million *nephrons* which form their basic functional units. Each nephron has five parts **(Fig. 22.2)**: glomerulus, proximal convoluted tubules, the loop of Henle, distal convoluted tubules, and collecting ducts. Besides, there is interstitium and blood vessels.
i. **Glomerulus** consists of an invagination of proximal tubules, which is externally lined by the *Bowman capsule* **(Fig. 22.3)**.
• Inside the glomerulus, there is a *capillary tuft* formed by the branching of the afferent arterioles. Glomerular capillaries form *lobules*, which consist of a centrilobular stalk (*mesangium*) containing mesangial cells.
• Mesangial matrix extends into the hilum where it surrounds the lacis cells of the *juxtaglomerular apparatus (JGA)* essential for the maintenance of the normal blood pressure. The JGA secretes renin in response to the stimuli from *macula densa,* a segment of the distal tubule juxtaposed to the glomerular hilum.
• Each lobule consists of capillaries that have an inner *fenestrated cell layer* composed of *endothelial cells*, and an outer layer composed of *epithelial cells* (*podocytes*) separated one from another by the *glomerular basement membrane (GBM)*. Basement membrane of the capillaries is in continuity with the mesangial matrix, which surrounds the third important cell, the mesangial cell.

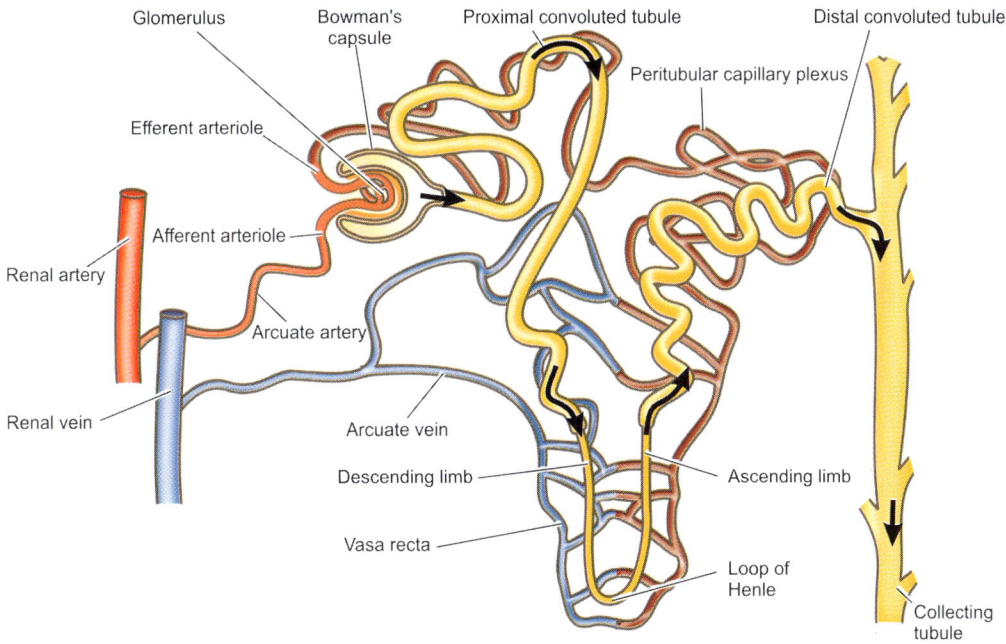

FIGURE 22.2: Structure of a nephron.

- By electron microscopy, one may see that the glomerular basement membrane has a central *lamina densa* and two outside *laminae rarae*. The outer side of the glomerular basement membrane is covered with cytoplasmic extensions of the epithelial cells called *foot processes* (**Fig. 22.4**).

ii. **Tubules** account for the greatest amount of the renal parenchyma and play a key role in the formation of urine by reabsorbing the filtered minerals, amino acids, glucose and water from the primary filtrate formed in the glomeruli. They also add water, organic material and some minerals to urine and contribute to the acidification of urine and its concentration. Collecting ducts also reabsorb water under the control of ADH and secrete H^+ and K^+ ions.

iii. **Interstitium** is the connective tissue component of the kidney providing support to

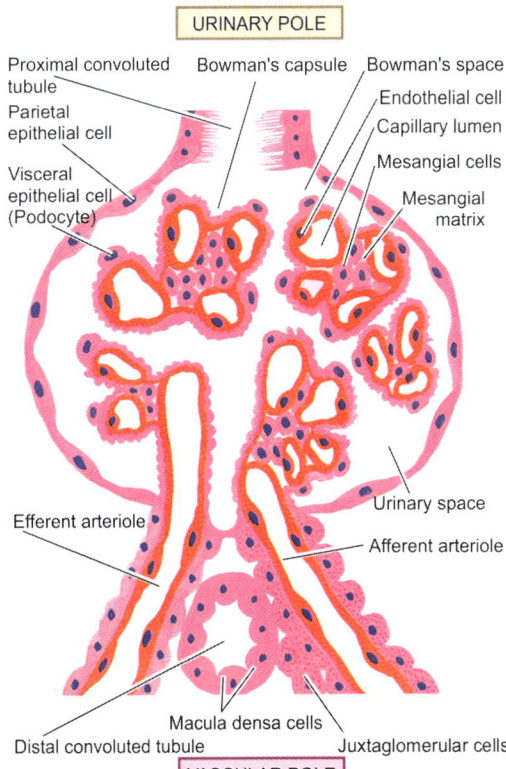

FIGURE 22.3: A schematic illustration of the structure of a nephron (in longitudinal section) and associated blood supply.

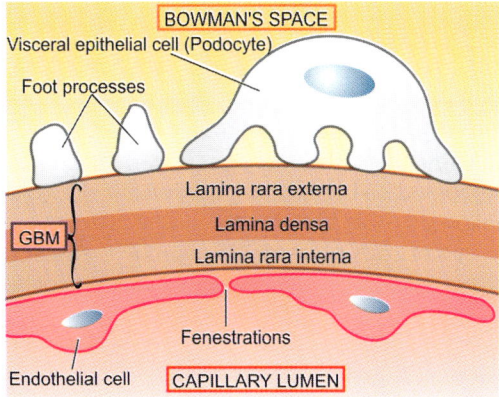

FIGURE 22.4: Ultrastructure of glomerular filtration barrier.

glomeruli, tubules and blood vessels. It consists predominantly of fibroblasts and collagenous stroma, and a few migratory bone marrow and lymphoid tissue-derived cells such as macrophages and lymphocytes.

Physiology Kidneys perform the following main functions:

i. Excretion of waste products from protein metabolism.

ii. Regulation of acid base balance by excretion of H^+ and bicarbonate ions.

iii. Regulation of salt-water balance.

iv. Secretion of renin and erythropoietin, thus regulating the blood pressure and erythropoiesis.

Q2. List the tests for study of renal function.

I. **Renal function tests (RFT)** These are laboratory tests which are broadly divided into 4 groups **(Table 22.1)**:

i. Urine analysis
ii. Concentration and dilution tests
iii. Blood chemistry
iv. Renal clearance tests

II. **Kidney biopsy** In addition to these laboratory tests, renal biopsy is performed to confirm the diagnosis, or to provide the final diagnosis in complicated cases:

i. The tissue obtained percutaneously by a needle biopsy or surgically by a wedge incision, is stained for *light microscopy* using the following stains:
- Routine haematoxylin and eosin stain
- Periodic acid Schiff (PAS)
- Silver impregnation

ii. Additional tissue (fresh unfixed, without formalin fixation) is submitted for *immunofluorescence microscopy* studies with fluorescein isothiocyanates (FITC)-labeled antibodies.

iii. For *electron microscopic* studies, tissue fixed in 4% glutarladehyde is submitted.

TABLE 22.1 Renal function tests.

1. URINE ANALYSIS
i. Physical examination (output, colour, specific gravity, pH, osmolality)
ii. Chemical constituents (protein, glucose, ketones, red cells, haemoglobin)
iii. Bacteriologic examination
iv. Microscopy
2. CONCENTRATION AND DILUTION TESTS
i. Concentration test (fluid deprivation test)
ii. Dilution test (excess fluid intake test)
3. BLOOD CHEMISTRY
i. Urea
ii. Blood urea nitrogen (BUN)
iii. Creatinine
iv. Beta-trace protein
4. RENAL CLEARANCE TEST
i. Inulin or mannitol clearance test
ii. Creatinine clearance
iii. Urea clearance
iv. Para-aminohippuric acid (PAH) clearance

Q3. Discuss briefly common analytes in urine examination.

Urine analysis is the simplest renal function test and it includes physical, chemical, bacteriologic and microscopic examination of urine.

i. **Physical examination** includes 24-hour urinary output, colour, specific gravity and osmolality. Normally, urine is clear, pale or straw-coloured due to pigment urochrome. On an average, 1200 ml (range is 700–2500 ml) of urine is passed in 24 hours, mostly during day hours. Specific gravity is used to measure the concentrating and diluting power of the kidneys.

ii. **Chemical tests** are performed to determine the presence of protein, glucose, ketones, red blood cells and haemoglobin to assess the permeability of GBM. A number of dipstick tests are available for testing these chemical substances and pH of urine.

iii. **Bacteriologic examination** is performed on urine collected aseptically in midstream.

iv. **Urine microscopy** is undertaken on a fresh, unstained sample with the purpose of detecting red blood cells, pus cells, epithelial cells, crystals and urinary casts. The casts are classified as follows:

a. *Hyaline casts* are made up of proteins entering the tubules in the primary filtrate in the glomeruli or normally secreted by the cells of the loop of Henle and ascending loop of the distal tubule (Tamm-Horsfall protein).

b. Cast containing blood cells are classified as *leucocyte casts* (found in inflammatory conditions), or *red blood cell casts* (in haematuria).

c. *Brown muddy casts* are found in acute tubular necrosis; they are made of tubular cell debris.

Q4. What are concentration and dilution tests?

These tests are designed to evaluate the functional capacity of the tubules, as regulated by antidiuretic hormone (ADH).

i. Traditionally, this is done by determining the specific gravity of urine which varies in the range from 1.003 to 1.030.

ii. Additional tests are *water deprivation (concentration)* or *water excess (dilution)*. Upon water deprivation, the kidneys excrete less urine, and it has high specific gravity.

iii. The opposite effect is achieved by giving large amount of water. If the kidneys are diseased, the amount of urine and its specific gravity will not change but will remain constant.

Q5. What are the most important blood chemistry tests for RFT and the renal clearance test?

i. The loss of renal function results in elevation of end-products of protein metabolism, resulting in *azotaemia*. The reactants reflecting the loss of renal function are *blood urea nitrogen* (BUN, normal range 20–40 mg/dL) and *creatinine* (normal range 0.6–1.2 mg/dL).

ii. *Renal clearance test* is used to assess the rate of glomerular filtration and the renal blood flow. It is calculated by the following equation:

$C = UV/P$

where C is the clearance of the substance in ml/minute,
U is concentration of the substance in urine,
V is the volume of urine passed per minute, and
P is the concentration of the substance in the plasma.

The substances that are used for the clearance test are inulin, mannitol, creatinine and urea. Because of the *creatinine clearance test,* that substance is most often used in clinical medicine.

Q6. How are medical renal diseases broadly classified?

Traditionally renal diseases have been classified depending on the primary involvement of one of the four tissue compartments of the kidney: glomerular, tubular, interstitial and vascular. In clinical practice, however, it is common that more than one compartment is involved, and this classification is used for didactic purposes only.

I. *Glomerular diseases*, which are mostly immunological in origin, and can be acute or chronic.

II. *Tubular diseases*, which are more likely caused by toxic or infectious agents and are most often acute. They are usually associated with interstitial diseases and thus called *tubulo-interstitial diseases*.

III. *Vascular diseases* which are associated with hypertension or changes in the blood supply of the kidney, usually involve the glomeruli and tubules as well, which is understandable since the glomeruli are composed of vascular tissue and the function of tubules critically depends on appropriate blood supply through the renal vessels.

Q7. What is acute renal failure? Discuss its etiopathogenesis and clinicopathologic features in brief.

Definition Acute renal failure (ARF) is a syndrome characterised by rapid onset of renal insufficiency presenting as oliguria or anuria and sudden increase of waste products (urea and creatinine) in the blood with consequent development of uraemia.

Etiopathogenesis ARF can be classified as pre-renal, intra-renal, and post-renal.

I. **Pre-renal causes** are those which cause sudden decrease of blood flow to the nephron, with a loss of glomerular and tubular functions. Three most common causes are:

i. inadequate cardiac output due to heart failure,
ii. hypovolaemia due to blood loss, and
iii. vascular diseases obstructing the renal blood flow.

II. **Intra-renal causes** include various renal diseases involving:

i. renal arteries and arterioles,
ii. glomeruli, or
iii. tubules and interstitial tissue.

III. **Post-renal causes** are due to an obstruction to the flow of urine distal to the terminal part of the renal collecting ducts, i.e.

i. diseases involving the ureters, bladder and the urethra, or
ii. pathologic processes compressing those structures from outside.

Clinicopathologic features Three syndromes of ARF are recognised:

I. *Syndrome of acute nephritis* is most often seen in:
i. acute post-streptococcal glomerulonephritis, and
ii. rapidly progressive glomerulonephritis.

Glomerular inflammatory reaction in these conditions will usually markedly reduce the glomerular filtration rate and blood supply to the tubules, resulting in retention of salts and water.

II. *Syndrome accompanying tubular pathology* is seen in acute tubular necrosis (ATN). ARF in ATN occurs in three phases:

i. *Oliguric phase* that lasts 7 to 10 days, characterised by urinary output of less than 400 ml/day and urine of low specific gravity. There is sudden onset of azotaemia, metabolic acidosis, hyperkalaemia, hypernatraemia and hypervolaemia due to circulatory overload and pulmonary oedema.

ii. *Diuretic phase* corresponding to the initial healing of tubular injury with an improvement of urinary output. Since the regenerating tubules cannot concentrate the urine, it has a low or fixed specific gravity.

iii. *Recovery phase* occurs in about 50% of all cases and corresponds to healing of tubular injury marked by tubular regeneration. The process of healing is usually prolonged and may last up to a full year. The patients who do not recover need a renal transplant, or end up on dialysis.

III. *Pre-renal syndrome* occurs due to:
i. renal ischaemia due to various causes,
ii. hypovolaemia, and
iii. cardiac insufficiency causing hypoperfusion of the kidneys.

These processes lead to reduced GFR causing oliguria, azotaemia and possible fluid retention and oedema. Since the tubular cells are functioning normally, the kidneys can concentrate the urine according to the adaptive needs.

Q8. Discuss etiopathogenesis and clinicopathologic features of chronic renal failure.

Definition Chronic renal failure (CRF) is a syndrome characterised by progressive and irreversible deterioration of renal function due to the progressive destruction of renal parenchyma, resulting in death when sufficient number of nephrons have been damaged or lost.

Etiopathogenesis All chronic nephropathies eventually lead to CRF. These include glomerular and tubular (or tubulointerstitial) diseases.

I. *Glomerular diseases* often have immune causes and present in two forms:
i. *Primary glomerular diseases* limited to the glomeruli like membranous glomerulonephritis, membranoproliferative glomerulonephritis, lipoid nephrosis and anti-glomerular basement membrane nephritis.
ii. *Glomerulonephropathies that are part of a systemic diseases* such as systemic lupus nephritis, serum sickness, or diabetes mellitus.

II. *Tubulointerstitial diseases* causing alterations in reabsorption and secretion of important constituents leading to large volumes of undiluted urine. These diseases can be classified according to initiating etiology into 4 groups: vascular, infectious, toxic, and obstructive.

i. *Vascular causes* include longstanding essential hypertension affecting renal arteries and arterioles referred to as nephrosclerosis, which leads to ischaemia and necrosis of renal tissue.

ii. *Infectious causes* such as pyelonephritis which destroys nephrons.

iii. *Toxic causes* include drugs such as phenacetin, acetaminophen and aspirin, various heavy metals such as lead, cadmium and mercury, which cause slow tubular injury culminating in CRF.

iv. *Obstructive causes* resulting in tubular injury by fluid backpressure, such as urinary stones, blood clots, strictures, tumours, etc.

Clinicopathologic features Regardless of the initiating cause, CRF evolves progressively through 4 stages:

i. **Decreased renal reserve**, an early stage in which the kidneys still function normally but the GFR is reduced to 50% of normal. BUN and creatinine values in serum are normal and the patient is usually asymptomatic except at times of stress.

ii. **Renal insufficiency,** a stage characterised by significant loss of parenchyma, which has been reduced by 75%. The GFR is 25% of normal accompanied by elevations of BUN and serum creatinine. Polyuria and nocturia occur due to tubulointerstitial damage. Sudden stress may precipitate uraemic syndrome.
iii. **Renal failure,** a stage characterised by a loss of 90% of functional parenchyma and a GFR reduced to 10% of normal. Tubular cells are essentially nonfunctional and the regulation of water and sodium is lost resulting in oedema, metabolic acidosis, hypocalcaemia and signs and symptoms of uraemia.
iv. **End-stage (chronic kidney disease),** with a GFR of 5% of normal resulting in uraemia with progressive primary (renal) and secondary (extra-renal) manifestations.

Q9. What are the main clinical manifestations of chronic renal failure (or uraemic manifestations)?

Chronic renal failure culminates in uraemic syndrome (colloquially defined as 'intoxication with urine'), which has primary (renal) and secondary (extra-renal) manifestations.
I. **Primary uraemic (renal) manifestations** are the end-result of progressive deterioration of renal functions and include the following:
i. *Metabolic acidosis* caused by an excess of hydrogen ions and reduced amount of bicarbonates in serum.
• Clinical findings include Kussmaul breathing, hyperkalaemia and hypercalcaemia.
ii. *Hyperkalaemia* caused by reduced excretion of potassium. It is worsened by acidosis.
• Clinical consequences include cardiac arrhythmia, weakness, nausea, intestinal colics and diarrhoea, muscular irritability and flaccid paralysis.
iii. *Sodium and water imbalance* due to retention caused by reduced GFR and subsequent renin release.
• Clinical consequences are circulatory overload with congestive heart failure.
iv. *Hyperuricaemia* resulting from reduce GFR and uric acid retention.
• Uric acid can be deposited in joints and produce symptoms of gout.
v. *Azotaemia* due to inadequate excretion of end-products of protein metabolism, such as urea, BUN and creatinine.

II. **Secondary (extra-renal) manifestations** result from fluid-electrolyte and acid-base imbalance, and include the following **(Fig. 22.5)**:
i. *Anaemia* results from reduced renin production affecting the erythropoiesis adversely. Mucosal bleeding from the mucosal ulcerations in the GI tact is a contributory factor.
ii. *Skin changes* are related to urochrome deposition imparting the skin a sallow-yellow colour. Uric acid crystal deposition accounts for the fine powdery appearance of the skin ('uraemic frost').
iii. *Cardiovascular symptoms* result from fluid overload leading to cardiac failure.
iv. *Respiratory system changes* result from fluid overload and heart dysfunction and include pulmonary oedema, and congestion resulting in shortness of breath and dyspnoea.
v. *Digestive system changes* include mucosal ulcerations of the stomach and intestines with nausea, vomiting, diarrhoea and contributing to anaemia.
vi. *Skeletal system changes* are collectively called renal osteodystrophy. These changes include osteomalacia and reduced intestinal absorption of calcium due to vitamin D deficiency and osteitis cystica fibrosa due to parathyroid hormone excess caused by retention of phosphate and reduced calcium levels in serum.

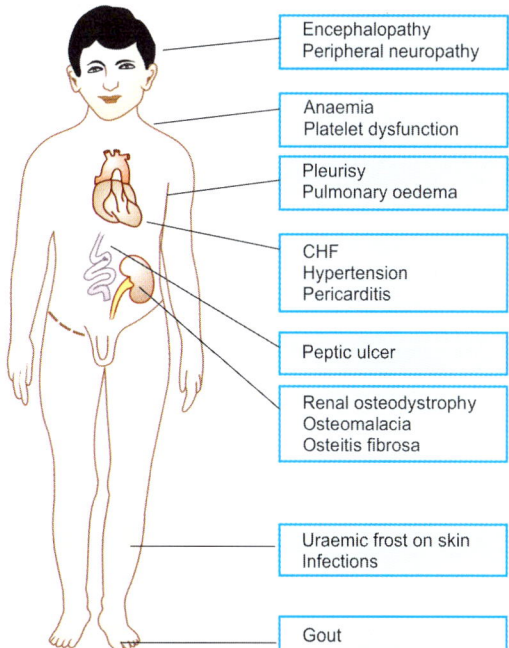

FIGURE 22.5: Clinical manifestations in chronic kidney disease.

Q10. How are congenital malformations of the kidneys classified?

Approximately 10% of persons are born with potentially significant malformations of the kidneys and the lower urinary system. Approximately, one half of those malformations are associated with some anomalies of the urinary system or other organs. These congenital malformations can be classified into three broad groups:

I. **Abnormal amounts of renal tissue** For example: unilateral or bilateral renal hypoplasia or aplasia, or the opposite of it, e.g. renomegaly, supernumerary kidney.

II. **Abnormalities of position, form and orientation** These anomalies include renal ectopia, renal fusion (e.g. horseshoe kidney).

III. **Anomalies of differentiation** These include very important and common conditions under the heading of *cystic diseases of the kidneys*. These cystic diseases include the following:
i. Renal multicystic dysplasia
ii. Polycystic kidney disease, adult, autosomal dominant type
iii. Polycystic kidney disease, infantile, autosomal recessive type
iv. Medullary sponge kidney
v. Nephronophthisis-medullary cystic disease

Q11. What are the most important congenital cystic lesions of the kidneys? Discuss their salient features.

The following developmental cystic lesions are of clinical significance **(Fig. 22.6)**:

I. **Renal multicystic dysplasia** involving just one kidney is found in 1 out of 3500 neonates, typically presenting as a palpable flank mass.
- It is the most common clinically significant renal lesion in neonates and infants.
- Bilateral lesions are less common and usually cause intrauterine foetal or neonatal death.
- Most often, there is no family history of malformation, but in some rare cases the disease may be familial or part of some developmental syndromes.

Pathology The lesion presents as a mass that is composed of multiple fluid-filled cysts that look a bunch of grapes replacing the normal kidney or a part of it.

It is commonly associated with obstructive abnormalities of the ureter and bladder, such as obstruction of pelvic-ureteric junction with megaureter formation or ureteral atresia.

Microscopy
- The cysts are dilated tubules lined by flattened epithelium.
- Stroma is composed of undifferentiated mesenchymal tissue.
- Foci of cartilage or smooth muscle cells and foetal glomeruli may be included.

Clinical features The abnormal kidney may be discovered as a palpable flank mass.
i. Often, it is associated with malformations of other organs or developmental syndromes like Down syndrome.
ii. Removal of the affected kidney is curative, unless there are major malformations of the remainder of the urinary tract.
iii. Bilateral lesions are incompatible with life.

II. **Adult (or autosomal dominant) polycystic kidney disease (ADPKD)** is a common familial genetic disease that has an incidence of 1:400 to 1:1000. It accounts for 4% of patients requiring dialysis for CRF.

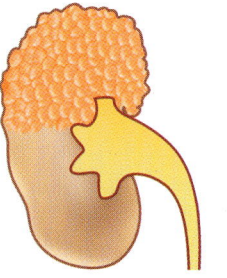

A, RENAL MULTICYSTIC DYSPLASIA

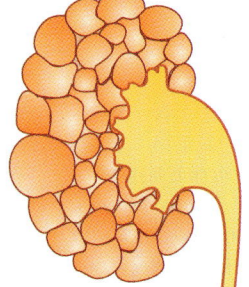

C, ADULT POLYCYSTIC KIDNEY DISEASE (APKD)

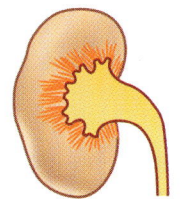

B, MEDULLARY SPONGE KIDNEY (MSK)

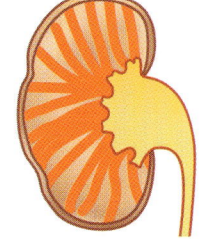

D, INFANTILE POLYCYSTIC KIDNEY DISEASE (ARPKD)

FIGURE 22.6: Cystic diseases of kidney.

Genetics ADPKD is caused by a mutation of *PKD-1* gene, encoding *polycystin* 1, that accounts for 85% of cases, whereas the remaining 15% cases are caused by mutation of *PKD-2* gene.

Pathology Both kidneys are involved diffusely and appear very large.

i. The normal renal parenchyma is usually replaced by fluid-filled cysts enlarging the kidneys; often the kidneys become 20–30 times larger than normal, each weighing 3–4 kg.

ii. The cysts arise from all parts of the nephron and are usually lined by flattened cuboidal epithelium.

iii. The cysts are surrounded by fibrous tissue and do not communicate with the renal pelvis, in contrast to hydronephrosis which also is composed of cystic spaces that are, however, open towards the pelvis.

iv. Foci of acute and chronic pyelonephritis are commonly superimposed.

Clinical features appear in adulthood after the age of 30 years and include:

i. Pain in the lumbar area
ii. Haematuria
iii. Colic
iv. Urinary infections
v. Slowly progressive CRF which usually develops 15- 20 years after the onset of symptoms.
vi. Cysts may be found in other organs including the liver, pancreas and the spleen.
vii. In 15% of patients, there are berry aneurysms of the circle of Willis at the base of the brain.

Treatment requires renal transplantation.

III. **Infantile (or autosomal recessive) polycystic kidney disease (ARPKD)** is much less common (incidence of 1:20,000).

Genetics It is caused by the mutation of *PKHD1* (polycystic kidney and hepatic disease) gene.

Clinicopathologic features

i. Both kidneys are enlarged but of normal shape and a smooth external surface.

ii. On cross section, the kidneys appear sponge-like due to numerous small cylindrical cysts replacing the normal parenchyma and extending radially from the medulla into the cortex.

iii. These cysts are derived from dilated collecting ducts lined by cuboidal to low cylindrical epithelium.

iv. The liver invariably contains cysts made up of dilated portal bile ductules surrounded by fibrous tissue which contains other proliferating ductules. Progressive fibrosis develops with time around the cysts and extending into liver lobules causing portal hypertension and splenomegaly.

IV. **Medullary cystic diseases** include several rare diseases. One of them is a relatively innocuous disease called *medullary sponge kidney,* which usually does not affect renal functions. Two more serious, but fortunately rare diseases, are called *nephronophthisis and medullary cystic disease*.

i. **Nephronophthisis** has several genetic and clinical variants, all of which are rare but present with formation of cysts and progressive fibrosis replacing the tubules at the corticomedullary junction.

- Nephronophthisis is classified depending on the age at presentation as: infantile, juvenile (most common) and adolescent form.
- All forms are inherited as autosomal recessive traits.
- Several mutations of the *NPHP* gene encoding a primary ciliary protein called *nephrocystin* have been identified. In all of them, the disease presents with polyuria and polydipsia, progressing to end-stage renal disease over a 5–10 year period.
- Nephronophthisis is considered to be the most common form of genetic cause of end-stage renal disease in children and young adults.

ii. **Medullary cystic disease** is a rare autosomal dominant kidney disease characterised by formation of medullary cysts.

- It begins in adolescence and leads to end-stage renal disease in 5–10 years.
- It is caused by a mutation of MCKD1 or 2 which code for a protein called *uromodulin*.

Q12. Tabulate the contrasting features of adult and infantile polycystic kidney disease.

The contrasting features of the two main forms of the polycystic kidney disease are presented in **Table 22.2**.

Q13. How are glomerular diseases classified?

Glomerular diseases are classified into two groups:
I. Primary glomerular diseases

TABLE 22.2 Contrasting features of autosomal dominant (adult) and autosomal recessive (infantile) polycystic kidney disease (ADPKD versus ARPKD).

FEATURE	ADPKD	ARPKD
1. *Inheritance*	Autosomal dominant	Autosomal recessive
2. *Cytogenetic defect*	Chromosome 16 (85%): ADPKD-1 Chromosome 4 (15%): ADPKD-2	Chromosome 6
3. *Mutations*	*PKD 1* gene (85%) *PKD 2* gene (15%)	6p21 PKHD1
4. *Incidence*	1:400 to 1:1000	1:20,000
5. *Age at presentation*	Adults (3rd to 5th decades)	Infancy, perinatal
6. *Gross*	Symmetric bilateral enlargement Macrocysts	Micro- and macrocysts radiating from medulla to outer cortex Enlarged, sometimes asymmetric, sponge-like
7. *Microscopy*	Cysts derived from all parts of nephron (glomeruli, tubules)	Cysts from dilated collecting ducts
8. *Other manifestations*	Intracranial berry aneurysms, cysts of the liver	Cysts in the liver progressing to cirrhosis

II. Secondary glomerular diseases that occur as part of some systemic disease

Various types under each category are listed in **Table 22.3**.

Q14. What are the clinical manifestations of glomerular diseases?

Four principal clinical features of glomerular diseases are:
i. proteinuria,
ii. haematuria,
iii. hypertension, and
iv. disturbed excretory functions.

On the basis of these findings, all of which are not found in all cases, or if present are not expressed to the same extent, one can recognise following clinical syndromes:
I. Acute nephritic and nephrotic syndrome
II. Acute and chronic renal failure
III. Asymptomatic proteinuria and haematuria

I. **Acute nephritic syndrome**

Definition Acute nephritic syndrome presents with microscopic haematuria, mild proteinuria, hypertension, oedema of face and extremities, and oliguria, usually following an infective disease 10–20 days earlier.

TABLE 22.3 Classification of glomerular diseases.

I. PRIMARY GLOMERULONEPHRITIS
1. Acute GN
    i. Post-streptococcal
    ii. Non-streptococcal
2. Rapidly progressive GN
3. Minimal change disease
4. Membranous GN
5. Membrano-proliferative GN
6. Focal and diffuse proliferative GN
7. Focal segmental glomerulosclerosis (FSGS)
8. IgA nephropathy
9. Chronic glomerulonephritis
10. C3 glomerulopathy

II. SECONDARY SYSTEMIC GLOMERULAR DISEASES
1. Lupus nephritis (SLE)
2. Diabetic nephropathy
3. Amyloidosis (page 114)
4. Polyarteritis nodosa (page 326)
5. Wegener granulomatosis (page 327)
6. Goodpasture syndrome (page 540)
7. Henoch-Schönlein purpura (page 258)
8. Systemic infectious diseases (*bacterial,* e.g. bacterial endocarditis, syphilis, leprosy; *viral,* e.g. HBV, HCV, HIV; *parasitic* (e.g. falciparum malaria, filariasis)
9. Idiopathic mixed cryoglobulinaemia

(GN, glomerulonephritis; SLE, systemic lupus erythematosus; HBV, hepatitis B virus; HCV, hepatitis C virus).

i. *Haematuria* is mild, but could give the urine a brownish colour ('tea' or 'bouillon soup like'). The urinary sediment contains red blood cell casts.
ii. *Proteinuria* is nonselective and mild (< 3 g/24 hours, '*nephritic range proteinuria*').
iii. *Hypertension* is variable and depends on the severity of the glomerular disease.
iv. *Oedema* is mild, presenting as a puffy face and periorbital swelling, related to retention of sodium and water.
v. *Oliguria* is variable and reflects the severity of the disease.

The underlying disease is acute post-streptococcal glomerulonephritis or some systemic disease (**Table 22.4**).

II. **Nephrotic syndrome**

Definition Nephrotic syndrome presents with heavy proteinuria, hypoalbuminaemia, oedema, hyperlipidaemia, lipiduria and hypercoagulability.

i. *Heavy proteinuria* exceeding 3 g/24 hours ('*nephrotic-range proteinuria*') is the chief characteristic of nephrotic syndrome. It is selective and characterised by urinary loss of low molecular weight proteins like albumin (M.W.= 66,500 daltons).

ii. *Hypoalbuminaemia* due to urinary loss of albumin. Serum level of albumin is reduced from the normal 3.5–5.5 g/dL to 1–3 g/dL.

iii. *Oedema* is related to a fall in colloid osmotic pressure of the plasma due to hypoalbuminaemia. Oedema is usually peripheral. It is more pronounced in children than in adults.

iv. *Hyperlipidaemia* is marked by increased plasma levels of total lipids, cholesterol and all lipoproteins, except HDL which is lost in urine. The exact mechanism is not fully understood but it is assumed that the liver might be releasing more lipoproteins to compensate for hypoalbuminaemia.

v. *Lipiduria* is a consequence of hyperlipidaemia and increased permeability of GBM.

vi. *Hypercoagulability,* which has multiple causes such as a loss of anticoagulant proteins (e.g. antithrombin III), increased synthesis of fibrinogen in the liver, decreased fibrinolysis, altered levels of protein C and S, increased aggregation of platelets.

Etiopathogenesis Primary glomerular diseases are the cause in most nephrotic syndrome cases of childhood (lipoid nephrosis accounts for 65% of cases). In adults, on the other hand, systemic diseases (diabetes, amyloidosis and SLE) predominate, even though the most common cause of nephrotic syndrome is focal segmental glomerulosclerosis. Other causes of nephrotic syndrome are listed in **Table 22.5**.

III. **Acute renal failure (ARF)** is characterised by rapid decline in renal function. ARF may have many causes including rapidly progressive GN and acute diffuse proliferative GN.

IV. **Chronic renal failure** results from many chronic glomerular diseases, causing azotaemia, hypertension, and variable amounts of haematuria and proteinuria. Such patients have small contracted kidneys showing extensive fibrosis, loss of glomeruli and tubules.

TABLE 22.4 Causes of acute nephritic syndrome.

I. PRIMARY GLOMERULONEPHRITIS
1. Acute GN
i. Post-streptococcal
ii. Non-streptococcal
2. Rapidly progressive GN
3. Membranoproliferative GN
4. Focal and diffuse proliferative GN
5. IgA nephropathy
II. SYSTEMIC DISEASES
1. SLE
2. Polyarteritis nodosa
3. Wegener granulomatosis
4. Henoch-Schönlein purpura
5. Cryoglobulinaemia

(GN, glomerulonephritis; SLE, systemic lupus erythematosus)

TABLE 22.5 Causes of nephrotic syndrome.

I. PRIMARY GLOMERULONEPHRITIS
1. Minimal change disease (*most common in children*)
2. Membranous GN
3. Membranoproliferative GN
4. Focal segmental glomerulosclerosis
5. Focal and diffuse proliferative GN
6. IgA nephropathy (*most common in adults*)
II. SYSTEMIC DISEASES
1. Diabetes mellitus
2. Amyloidosis
3. SLE
III. SYSTEMIC INFECTIONS
1. Viral infections (HBV, HCV, HIV)
2. Bacterial infections (bacterial endocarditis, syphilis, leprosy)
3. Protozoa and parasites (*P. falciparum* malaria, filariasis)
IV. HYPERSENSITIVITY REACTIONS
1. Drugs (heavy metal compounds like gold and mercury, other drugs like penicillamine, trimethadione and tolbutamide, heroin addiction)
2. Bee stings, snake bite, poison ivy
V. MALIGNANCY
1. Carcinomas
2. Myeloma
3. Lymphoma
VI. PREGNANCY
Toxaemia of pregnancy
VII. CIRCULATORY DISTURBANCES
1. Renal vein thrombosis
2. Constrictive pericarditis
VIII. HEREDITARY DISEASES
1. Alport disease
2. Fabry disease
3. Nail-patella syndrome

(GN, glomerulonephritis; SLE, systemic lupus erythematous; HBV, hepatitis B virus; HCV, hepatitis C virus; HIV, human immunodeficiency virus).

V. **Asymptomatic proteinuria** may be found in some persons without symptoms, but if associated with haematuria it may be indicative of renal disease.

VI. **Asymptomatic microscopic haematuria** is common in children and adolescents and could have many causes. It may be associated with proteinuria.

Q15. How do we differentiate nephrotic from acute nephritic syndrome?

Contrasting features of nephrotic and acute nephritic syndrome are presented in **Table 22.6**.

TABLE 22.6 Contrasting features of nephrotic and acute nephritic syndromes.

FEATURE	NEPHROTIC SYNDROME	ACUTE NEPHRITIC SYNDROME
1. *Proteinuria*	Heavy (> 3 g per 24 hrs)	Mild (< 3 g per 24 hrs)
2. *Hypoalbuminaemia*	Present	Mild
3. *Oedema*	Marked, generalised peripheral	Mild, in loose tissues
4. *Mechanism of oedema*	↓ plasma osmotic pressure, Na$^+$ and water retention	Na$^+$ and water retention
5. *Haematuria*	Absent	Present, microscopic
6. *Hypertension*	Present in advanced disease	Present
7. *Hyperlipidaemia*	Present	Absent
8. *Lipiduria*	Present	Absent
9. *Oliguria*	Present in advanced disease	Present
10. *Hypercoagulability*	Present	Absent

Q16. List various mechanisms in the pathogenesis of glomerular injury.

Most forms of primary GN and many of the secondary glomerular diseases have an immunologic pathogenesis. These immunologic and other non-immunologic mechanisms are listed in **Table 22.7**.

Pathologic consequences of glomerular injury are best assessed by separately analysing each component of the glomerulus, namely the endothelial, mesangial, visceral and parietal epithelial cells, and the glomerular basement membrane (GBM).

TABLE 22.7 Mechanisms in the pathogenesis of glomerular diseases.

MECHANISM	RELATED GLOMERULAR DISEASE
I. IMMUNOLOGIC MECHANISMS	
A. *Antibody-mediated glomerular injury*	
1. Immune-complex disease	Immune-complex mediated GN (Acute diffuse proliferative GN, membranous GN, membranoproliferative GN, IgA nephropathy; secondary glomerular disease in SLE, malaria, etc.)
2. Anti-glomerular basement membrane (Anti-GBM) disease	Goodpasture disease
3. Alternative pathway disease	Membranoproliferative GN type II
4. Other mechanisms (anti-neutrophil cytoplasmic antibodies or ANCA, anti-endothelial cell antibodies or AECA)	Vasculitis
B. *Cell-mediated glomerular injury*	Pauci-immune GN (type III RPGN)
C. *Secondary pathogenetic mechanisms*	Mediate glomerular injury in various primary and secondary glomerular diseases
II. NON-IMMUNOLOGIC MECHANISMS	
1. Metabolic	Diabetic nephropathy, Fabry disease
2. Haemodynamic	Hypertensive nephrosclerosis, FSGS
3. Deposition	Amyloid nephropathy
4. Infectious	HIV-nephropathy, immune-complex GN in SABE
5. Drugs	NSAIDs-associated minimal change disease
6. Inherited	Alport syndrome, nail-patella syndrome

(GN, glomerulonephritis; GBM, glomerular basement membrane; ANCA, antineutrophil cytoplasmic antibodies; AECA, anti-endothelial cell antibodies; RPGN, rapidly progressive GN; FSGS, focal segmental glomerulosclerosis; SABE, subacute bacterial endocarditis).

Q17. How are various normal cells of the glomerulus related to different mechanisms in causing glomerular injury?

The effect of glomerular injury in different clinical consequences that dominate various diseases, can be correlated with physiologic function of each of components comprising the glomerulus (i.e. cells or GBM) **(Table 22.8)**.

TABLE 22.8 Relationship of physiologic role of glomerular components with consequences in glomerular injury.

COMPONENT	PHYSIOLOGIC FUNCTION	CONSEQUENCE OF INJURY	RELATED GLOMERULAR DISEASE
1. *Endothelial cells*	i. Maintain glomerular perfusion ii. Prevent leucocyte adhesion iii. Prevent platelet aggregation	Vasoconstriction Leucocyte infiltration Intravascular microthrombi	Acute renal failure Focal/diffuse proliferative GN Thrombotic microangiopathies
2. *Mesangial cells*	Control glomerular filtration	Proliferation and increased matrix	Membranoproliferative GN
3. *Visceral epithelial cells*	Prevent plasma protein filtration	Proteinuria	Minimal change disease, FSGS
4. *GBM*	Prevents plasma protein filtration	Proteinuria	Membranous GN, MPGN
5. *Parietal epithelial cells*	Maintain Bowman's space	Crescent formation	RPGN

(GN, glomerulonephritis; FSGS, focal segmental glomerulosclerosis; MPGN, membranoproliferative glomerulonephritis; RPGN; rapidly progressive GN; GBM, glomerular basement membrane).

Q18. Briefly discuss the immunologic mechanisms of glomerular injury.

As listed in **Table 22.7,** immunologic glomerular injury may be classified as:
I. Antibody-mediated
II. Cell-mediated
III. Related to secondary pathogenetic mechanisms.
These mechanisms are briefly considered below.

I. **Antibody-mediated glomerular injury** may occur through following mechanisms:

i. **Immune complex disease** results from the activation of complement by the antigen-antibody complexes deposited in the glomeruli.

Immune complexes are formed either *locally* in the glomerulus, or they are deposited from immune complexes *circulating* in the plasma:

a. *Local immune complex formation* may occur due to:
- Interaction of the antibodies circulating in blood with an endogenous antigen (e.g. phospholipase A2 receptor on podocytes called PLA2R; majority of cases have this antibody).
- An antigen that has been implanted on the GBM from outside (e.g. streptococcal antigens in post-streptococcal GN).

b. *Circulating immune complex deposition* may occur in diseases as follows:
- Mediated by type 3 hypersensitivity reactions such as SLE, which are characterised by circulating antibody-*endogenous antigen* complexes.
- In some infectious diseases, such as hepatitis caused by HBV, circulating immune complexes are formed between the antibody and *exogenous viral antigen*, such as HBS.
- Intraglomerular deposits of such circulating immune complexes activate complement, which can directly injure the glomerulus or initiate an inflammatory reaction.
- Immune complexes may be located in the mesangial areas, and subepithelial or subendothelial sides of the GBM. Pathologists use electron microscopy or immunofluorescence microscopy to precisely localise the deposits of immune complexes which have different locations in different forms of GN **(Fig. 22.7)**.

ii. **Anti-GBM diseases** account for only 5% of all human GN. The prototype disease based on this mechanism is the *Goodpasture syndrome* mediated by antibodies to collagen type IV, a component of the GBM.

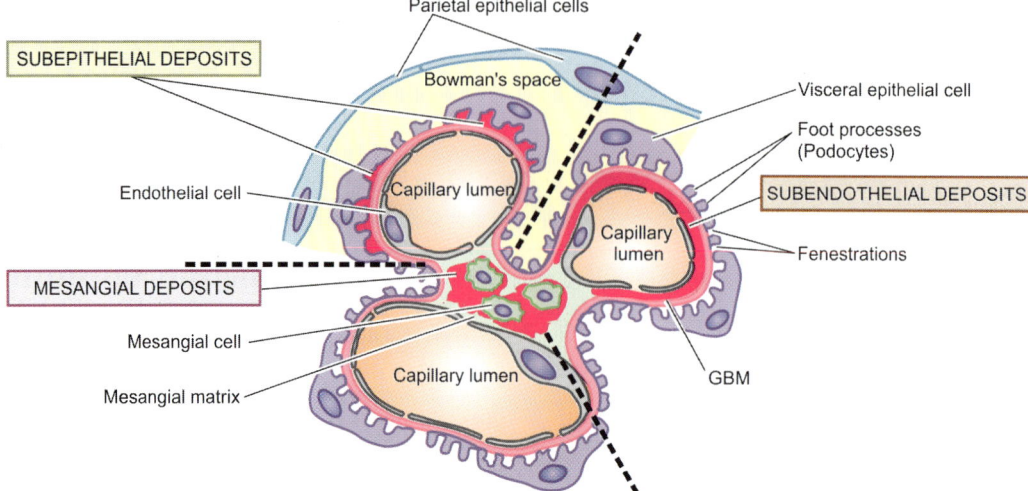

FIGURE 22.7: Diagrammatic representation of ultrastructure of a portion of glomerular lobule. Red colour at three locations (subendothelial, subepithelial and mesangial) denotes the glomerular deposits identified by immunofluoresecence microscopy in immune-complex disease.

iii. **Alternative pathway complement activation** related diseases are associated with deposits of C3 complement and properdin without deposits of immunoglobulins.
a. In most instances, complement activation is related to the presence of *C3NeF* (C3 nephritic factor), an antibody that inhibits C3 convertase, allowing for permanent alternative activation of the complement system without antibodies.
b. *Dense electron-dense deposits* of complement without immunoglobulin are seen in *C3 glomerulopathy* in the mesangium or the subendothelial side of the GBM. In the so called *dense deposit disease* (type II membranoproliferative disease), these deposits are intramembranous and appear like dense smudging of the GBM.
c. *Alternative complement activation* occurs more often than it was previously assumed, and it is found in some patients with rapidly proliferating GN, acute diffuse proliferative GN, IgA nephropathy and some cases of SLE.
iv. **Other mechanisms of antibody-mediated injury** are not fully understood but it is assumed that they play a role in some cases of focal segmental glomerulonephritis and a few other forms of GN:
a. *Anti-neutrophil cytoplasmic antibodies (ANCA)* probably play a role in some forms of pauci-immune crescentic glomerulonephritis as seen in Wegener granulomatosis. It is known that ANCA may damage the endothelial cells, but it is not known if they cause crescentic GN.
b. *Anti-endothelial antibodies (AECA)* have been found in patients with several forms of inflammatory vasculitis. It has been hypothesised that they also may damage glomeruli and cause GN.
II. **Cell-mediated glomerular immune injury** has been proposed as a possible mechanism of glomerular injury such as in crescentic glomerulonephritis, but the evidence supporting this hypothesis is not convincing.
III. **Secondary pathogenetic mechanisms of glomerular injury** include the activation of non-immune inflammatory cells such as neutrophils or macrophages, platelets, coagulation system and other components. These cells and systems amplify the immune mediated tissue reaction and probably can cause glomerular injury on their own, but many details about their role in GN remain unknown.

Q19. Name various non-immunologic mechanisms of glomerular injury with corresponding examples.
The following are examples of non-immunologic glomerular injury:
i. *Metabolic glomerular injury* is seen in diabetic glomerulopathy, due to the adverse effects of hyperglycaemia) and Fabry disease (genetic sulfatidosis).
ii. *Haemodynamic injury*, as in systemic hypertension.
iii. *Infectious diseases* such as HBV, HCV, HIV infection, or *E. coli*-derived nephrotoxin.

iv. *Drugs* such as NSAIDs causing minimal change disease.
v. *Hereditary glomerular diseases* such as Alport syndrome, or nail patella syndrome.

Q20. What is acute glomerulonephritis? Describe its salient features.

Definition Acute glomerulonephritis is an immunologically mediated renal disease of sudden onset that follows an infection and clinically presents with signs and symptoms of acute nephritic syndrome.
Types and salient features Acute GN includes two groups: post-streptococcal GN, and non-streptococcal GN.

I. **Acute post-streptococcal GN** is a common childhood disease in developing countries but is uncommon in highly developed countries like the US and Western Europe.
Etiopathogenesis There is good scientific evidence that the streptococcal infections is of paramount importance, as under:
i. Infection with nephritogenic streptococci belonging to type 12, 4, 1 and Red Lake of A β -haemolytic streptococci, which can be identified by throat culture.
ii. GN develops 2–4 weeks after streptococcal throat or skin infection, consistent with a latent period needed for the immunisation.
iii. Antibodies to streptococcal antigens such as anti-streptolysin O (ASO), anti-deoxyribonuclease B (anti-DNAase B, also included in the *Streptozyme test*), and anti-streptokinase are detected in the blood.
iv. Hypocomplementaemia develops in active disease indicating that complement is used and depleted by binding to antigen-antibody complexes.
v. The most important pathogenic streptococcal antigen seems to be *streptococcal exotoxin B (SpeB)*.
Pathology *Grossly,* both kidneys are enlarged, swollen and appear 'flea-bitten' due to numerous petechiae.
Microscopy shows predominance of the changes in the glomeruli; other part of the nephron show reactive changes **(Fig. 22.8)**:
i. Glomeruli are enlarged and hypercellular due to the diffuse *proliferative* and *exudative* lesions: proliferation of endothelial and mesangial cells, and infiltration with neutrophils and monocytes, which narrow the lumen and impede the normal blood flow through the glomerular capillaries.
ii. Inflammatory cells are anchored to the endothelial cells obstructing the lumina of the capillaries which contain a few RBCs.
iii. Some of the RBCs might have passed through the damaged GBM and enter the Bowman space on their route to the lumen of proximal tubules where they will form *RBC casts*.
Electron microscopy shows *immune complex deposits* in the form of electron dense irregular 'humps' on the epithelial side of the GBM. These humps are obviously just the biggest immune complexes.
Immunofluorescence (IF) microscopy shows that there are many smaller *irregular granular immune deposits* in various locations.

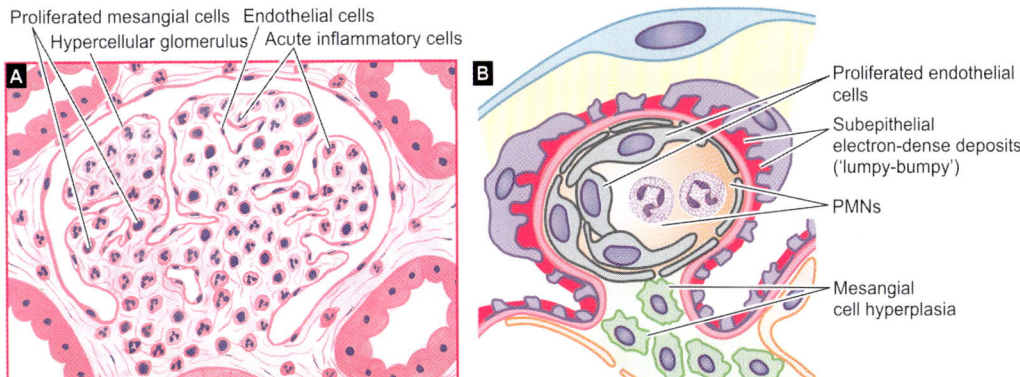

FIGURE 22.8: Acute post-streptococcal GN. A, Light microscopy shows glomerular hypercellularity due to proliferation of mesangial cells, endothelial cells and some epithelial cells and infiltration by numerous neutrophils and some monocytes. B, Diagrammatic representation of deposits in acute glomerulonephritis. Ultrastructure of a portion of glomerular lobule showing location of characteristic electron-dense irregular deposits or 'humps' on the epithelial side of the GBM.

Clinical features Typical clinical features include a sequence of events that begins with a childhood strep throat infections or skin infection, followed 2–4 weeks later by the onset of nephritic syndrome:
i. Oedema develops most prominently on the face and extremities.
ii. The child is sleepy, short of breath, and feels sick and obtunded.
iii. There is mild hypertension.
iv. Urinary output is reduced (oliguria) and the urine is brown from oxidation of haemoglobin to methaemoglobin. It is described as 'smoky' and 'tea-like' or 'bullion soup like'.
v. Urinalysis reveals proteinuria (>150 mg, but < 3000 mg/day) and microscopic haematuria with detectable amount of haemoglobin by stick test.
vi. The urinary sediment contains dysmorphic red blood cells, RBC casts and a few white blood cell casts.
vii. Blood analysis reveals elevation of BUN and creatinine (azotaemia), and mild hypoalbuminaemia.
Prognosis for children is excellent and 95% recover without any consequences. In adults, the prognosis is more guarded due to a protracted course and the possible transition to chronic glomerulonephritis.
II. **Acute non-streptococcal glomerulonephritis** may develop following many other infectious diseases, including bacterial, viral, parasitic diseases. Non-streptococcal GN has the same pathologic and clinical features as the post-streptococcal form, but in general it has a worse long-term prognosis.

Q21. Discuss briefly rapidly progressive (crescentic) glomerulonephritis.

Definition Rapidly progressive glomerulonephritis (RPGN), also known as crescentic GN or extracapillary glomerulonephritis, is an acute form of glomerulonephritis resulting in acute renal failure in a matter of several weeks or months. It is characterised by formation of crescents in the Bowman extracapillary space compressing the glomerular capillary loops, resulting in a loss of glomerular function.

Etiopathogenesis Three pathogenetic groups are identified as under **(Table 22.9)**:

Type I RPGN mediated by *anti-GBM antibodies* with linear deposits of Ig along the GBM. Prototypical disease of this type of RPGN is *Goodpasture syndrome*, a rare form of RPGN (incidence of 1:1 million) characterised by RPGN and pulmonary haemorrhages. It is mediated by autoantibodies to the globular part of collagen type IV in glomerular basement membrane, which also attack the basement membranes in the lungs. Treatment includes dialysis for removing the toxic antibodies from circulation.

Type II RPGN mediated by *immune complexes*, which are deposited in a granular manner on the GBM. This group includes many forms of severe acute glomerulonephritis such as post-streptococcal GN, Henoch-Schönlein purpura, SLE and some other diseases. It is the most common RPGN in children and young adults under the age of 20 years.

TABLE 22.9 Distinguishing features of three main categories of rapidly progressive glomerulonephritis.

FEATURE	TYPE I RPGN (ANTI-GBM DISEASE)	TYPE II RPGN (IMMUNE COMPLEX DISEASE)	TYPE III RPGN (PAUCI-IMMUNE GN)
1. *Clinical syndrome*	Nephritic	Nephritic	Nephritic
2. *Pathogenetic type*	Anti-GBM	Immune-complex	Pauci-immune
3. *Immunofluorescence*	Linear Ig and C3	Granular Ig and C3	Sparse or absent Ig and C3

4. *Serologic markers*
   i. *Serum C3 level*
   ii. *Anti-GBM antibody*
   iii. *ANCA*
	
	Normal
	Positive
	Negative
		
		Low-to-normal
		Negative
		Negative
			
			Normal
			Negative
			Positive

5. *Underlying cause*	Idiopathic Goodpasture syndrome, SLE, vasculitis, Wegener granulomatosis, Henoch-Schönlein purpura	Idiopathic secondary forms: Post-infectious (post-streptococcal GN), MPGN, SLE, IgA nephropathy	Idiopathic polyarteritis nodosa, Wegener granulomatosis

(GBM, glomerular basement membrane; RPGN, rapidly progressive glomerulonephritis; SLE, systemic lupus erythematosus; MPGN, membranoproliferative glomerulonephritis; ANCA, antineutrophil cytoplasmic antibodies; Ig, immunoglobulin; C, complement).

Type III RPGN, called *pauci-immune,* because the glomeruli do not contain deposits of immunoglobulins. Typically, these patients are positive for ANCA, implying a defect in humoral immunity. The best examples of a pauci-immune RPGN are:
- Wegener granulomatosis that involves the kidneys, lungs and upper respiratory tract.
- Microscopic polyarteritis nodosa, which may involve many organs.
- Churg-Strauss syndrome which involves kidneys, lungs and presents with eosinophilia.

Pathology All forms of RPGN present with the same microscopic changes, dominated by obliteration of glomeruli with crescents, that form inside the Bowman space, compressing the capillary loops **(Fig. 22.9)**:

i. The crescents form from macrophages that enter into the Bowman space through the damaged and ruptured glomerular capillaries.

ii. Macrophages are subsequently replaced by fibroblasts which lead to sclerosis and hyalinisation of the glomeruli and irreparable loss of nephrons.

iii. Tubules contain red blood cells and RBC casts reflecting the glomerular injury.

iv. The interstitial spaces contain chronic inflammatory cells and increased amount of fibrous tissue and fibroblasts (*fibrocellular crescents*), which slowly replace the damaged nephrons.

v. *Electron microscopy (EM) and IF findings* vary depending on the etiopathogenesis of RPGN:
- In anti-GBM RPGN, there is linear staining by IF and by EM there are no visible deposits.
- In immune complex mediated RPGN, there are granular electron dense and IF positive deposits of immunoglobulins and complement in various parts of the glomerulus.
- In pauci-immune RPGN, there are no visible immune complexes.

Prognosis The outcome depends on the type of RPGN and the initiation of treatment. All patients must be treated intensely with immunosuppressive drugs, with very good results.
- The sooner the diagnosis is made and the treatment started, better is the prognosis.
- Without treatment, most patients develop end-stage renal disease within a year or two.
- In general, patients with pauci-immune RPGN have the worst prognosis due to recurrence of the disease in 20% after an initial good response to immunotherapy.

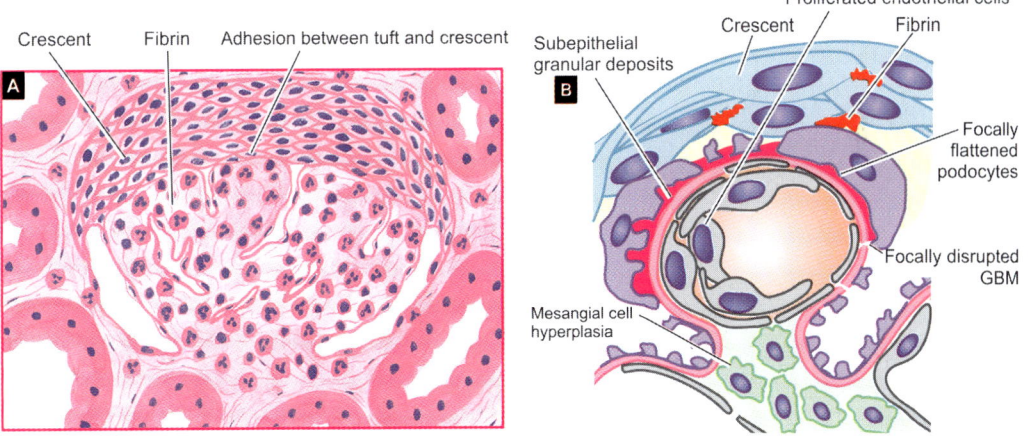

FIGURE 22.9: Crescentic GN (RPGN). A, Light microscopy shows cellular crescents in Bowman's (urinary) space, composed of epithelial cells admixed with inflammatory cells and fibrin, and forming adhesion between the collapsed glomerular tuft and Bowman's capsule. B, Diagrammatic representation of ultrastructure of a portion of glomerular lobule showing epithelial crescent formation and sub-epithelial granular deposits.

Q22. Write briefly on minimal change disease.

Definition Minimal change disease (MCD, also known as lipoid nephrosis and foot process disease or nil deposit disease) is the most common cause of nephrotic syndrome in children (80%), characterised by a lack of microscopic changes in the glomeruli, and flattened podocyte foot processes seen by EM.

Etiopathogenesis Unknown (idiopathic) in most instances.
i. A good response to steroid therapy and an increased suppressor T cell activity with secretion of interleukin suggest an immunologic mechanism.
ii. Some cases are associated with systemic disease (Hodgkin disease, HIV infection) or drugs (e.g. NSAIDs, interferon-α).
iii. Mutation of *nephrin* gene has been detected in some rare hereditary cases.

Pathology
i. Glomeruli appear normal by light microscopy.
ii. By IF, there are no immune deposits.
iii. By EM, there is flattening of fusion of podocyte foot processes **(Fig. 22.10)**.

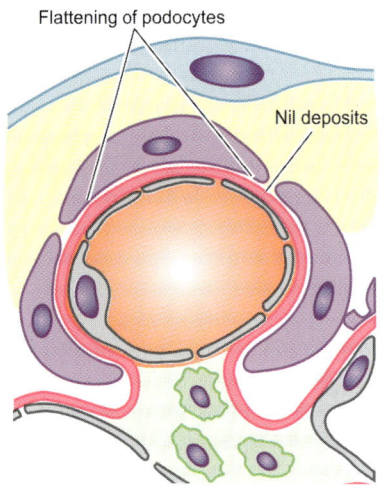

FIGURE 22.10: Minimal change disease. Diagrammatic representation of ultrastructure of a portion of glomerular lobule showing diffuse fusion or flattening of foot processes of visceral epithelial cells (podocytes), normal GBM and no deposits.

Clinical features
i. Most patients are children and the peak incidence is in the 6–8 years age group. The onset of symptoms may be preceded in some cases by an upper respiratory infections, immunisation or allergy.
ii. Most common feature is generalised oedema.
iii. There is nephrotic range highly selective proteinuria limited to albuminuria, associated with lipiduria and hypoalbuminaemia.
Treatment with steroids is curative in most instances, but in some cases the symptoms may recur.
The *prognosis* is very good even for those that have recurrences.

Q23. What is membranous nephropathy? Discuss its salient features.

Definition Membranous nephropathy (MN, also known as membranous glomerulonephritis or MGN) is an immunologically mediated glomerular disease characterised by the formation of immune complexes on the subepithelial surface of the GBM, reflecting a reaction of antibodies with endogenous glomerular antigens or antigens planted into the GBMs.

Classification
- Most cases (85%) of MN are *idiopathic or primary* without an apparent known cause. Primary MN patients, in most instances, have antibodies to *phospholipase A2 receptor* (PLA2R), an antigen expressed in podocytes. However, it is yet unknown if this protein is actually the antigen that is culpable for the pathologic change in the glomeruli in these patients.
- In 15% cases, MN is classified as *secondary* due to an underlying condition such as SLE, malignant tumour, viral hepatitis B or C, syphilis, malaria or some adverse drug reactions.

Pathology
i. By light microscopy, the GBM appear thickened **(Fig. 22.11, A)**.
ii. By IF and EM, one may see that this thickening is due to the numerous subepithelial granular deposits of immunoglobulins and complement in such a way that basement material protrudes as 'spikes' between deposits **(Fig. 22.11, B)**. Immune complexes deposited along the GBM activate complement, which slowly damages the glomeruli.

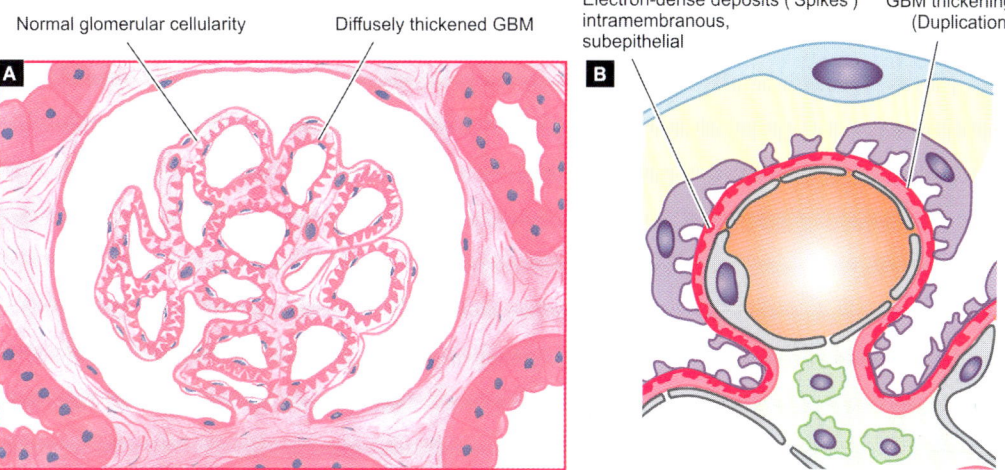

FIGURE 22.11: Membranous GN. A, Light microscopy shows that the glomeruli are normocellular but the capillary walls in the tuft have diffuse thickening of the GBM. B, Diagrammatic representation of ultrastructure of a portion of glomerular lobule showing subepithelial deposits of electron-dense material so that the basement membrane material protrudes between these deposits.

iii. With time, the immune complexes become incorporated into the GBM and the glomeruli lose their capacity to selectively filter substances from plasma, which leads to ESRD over a period of 10 years on an average.

Clinical manifestations The disease is one of the common glomerulopathy in adults than children, but may occur at any age.
i. There is severe non-selective proteinuria causing membranous nephropathy.
ii. In a small number of patients, nephrotic syndrome will heal on its own but most of the others will continue having proteinuria for many years.
iii. Some patients also develop haematuria and hypertension.
iv. ESRD develops in 50% of patients over a period that varies from 2 to 20 years.
v. Renal vein thrombosis is a well-known complication due to increased coagulability of the blood.
vi. Most of the treatment regimens, including those based on corticosteroids, have been inefficient.

Q24. What is membranoproliferative glomerulonephritis?

Definition Membranoproliferative (MPGN) is a chronic proliferative GN of unknown etiology caused by immune complexes, presenting with nephrotic syndrome, and less often with nephritic syndrome.

Classification Previous classification of MPGN into 3 subtypes has become obsolete:
i. It has become customary to include under this heading only *type I MPGN*.
ii. *Type II MPGN* has been reclassified as a *C3 disease* that is not caused by deposits of complement and is not caused by immune complexes.
iii. *Type III MPGN* resembles type I MPGN but it is secondary to an underlying systemic disease (e.g. SLE).

Thus, currently MPGN can be classified into two major forms:
- *Primary or idiopathic* (of unknown etiology), accounting for 70% of all cases.
- *Secondary*, which develops on the background of a systemic immunologic disease or is clearly related to drugs.

Pathology
i. MPGN presents with *enlargement and hypercellularity* of glomeruli, which is related to an increased number of endothelial and mesangial cells and infiltration of the glomeruli with macrophages and PMNs **(Fig. 22.12, A)**.
ii. Sometimes, even the epithelial cells proliferate forming *small crescents* in the Bowman spaces.

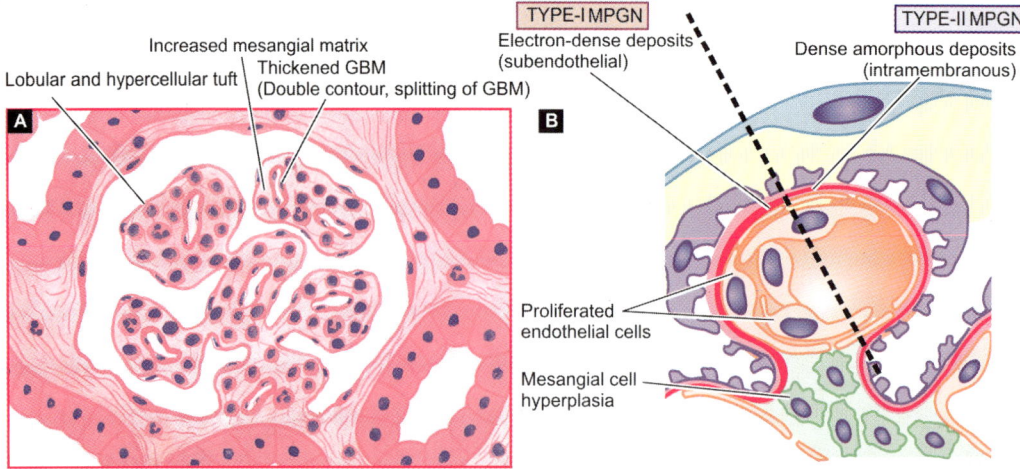

FIGURE 22.12: Membranoproliferative GN. A, Light microscopic appearance. The glomerular tufts show lobulation and mesangial hypercellularity. There is increase in the mesangial matrix between the capillaries. There is widespread thickening of the GBM. B, diagrammatic representation of ultrastructure of a portion of glomerular lobule showing features of type I or primary (left half) and type II or secondary (right half) MPGN. Primary MPGN shows the characteristic subendothelial electron-dense deposits, while secondary (dense deposit disease) is characterised by intramembranous dense deposits.

iii. Proliferation of glomerular cells is accompanied by a production of additional mesangial matrix and glomerular basement membranes which are deposited in parallel with the preexisting membranes contributing to their double contours *('tram-track' appearance)*.

iv. The glomeruli contain prominent *deposits of immune complexes*, mostly in the subendothelial, mesangial and intramembranous locations **(Fig. 22.12, B)**.

Clinical features vary. Most patients are young adolescents and young adults 15–20 of age.
- The disease presents as nephrotic syndrome in 50% cases, asymptomatic proteinuria in 30% and nephritic syndrome in 20% cases.
- Proteinuria is nonselective, and often combined with microscopic haematuria and hypertension.

The *prognosis* is generally poor and half of all patients develop ESRD over a period of 10 years, whereas others continue to have renal dysfunction and none recover completely.

Q25. What is focal proliferative glomerulonephritis?

Definition Focal proliferative glomerulonephritis is a pathologic diagnosis used descriptively for several forms of GN that present with an increased number of mesangial cells in parts of the lobules.

Etiopathogenesis Focal proliferative glomerulonephritis occurs under following three clinical settings:

i. As an early manifestation of a number of systemic diseases, such as SLE or Henoch-Schönlein purpura, bacterial endocarditis, or Wegener granulomatosis.

ii. As a component of a known renal disease like IgA nephropathy.

iii. As a primary idiopathic glomerular disease unrelated to systemic or other renal diseases.

Clinicopathologic features

i. *Light microscopic changes* are mild and include focal and segmental mesangial widening with a slightly increased number of mesangial cells. It means that only some glomeruli are involved, and those that are involved show the changes only in parts of their lobules **(Fig. 22.13, A)**.

ii. Depending on the etiology of the disease, the *IF and EM findings* may be either negative, or as is the case with immunologically mediated diseases, may have mesangial deposits of immune complexes. In IgA nephropathy, these deposits predominantly consist of IgA.

iii. Clinical findings are also highly variable.

iv. In some cases focal proliferative GN will progress to *diffuse proliferative GN*.

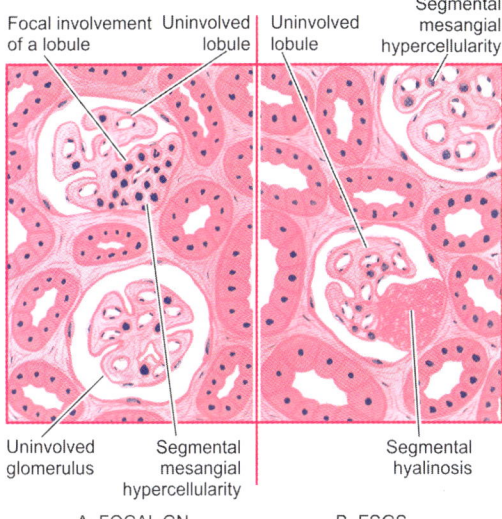

FIGURE 22.13: A, *Focal GN*. The characteristic feature is the cellular proliferation in some glomeruli and in one or two lobules of the affected glomeruli, i.e. focal and segmental proliferative change. B, *Focal segmental glomerulosclerosis*. The features are focal and segmental involvement of the glomeruli by sclerosis and hyalinosis and mesangial hypercellularity.

Q26. Write briefly on focal segmental glomerulosclerosis.

Definition Focal segmental glomerulosclerosis (FSGS) is chronic renal disease characterised by focal and segmental consolidation of the glomerular tufts with deposition of hyaline material, presenting as a nephrotic syndrome.

Etiopathogenesis Three forms of FSGS are recognised:

i. *Idiopathic*, which comprises most of the cases, is a disease of unknown origin. It presents with nephrotic syndrome, heavy non-selective proteinuria resistant to steroid treatment, progressing to chronic renal failure.

ii. *FSGS superimposed on another primary glomerular disease* such as MCD or IgA nephropathy.

iii. *Secondary FSGS* related to an underlying systemic disease, such as HIV infection, diabetes mellitus, reflux nephropathy, heroin abuse or analgesic nephropathy.

Pathology

i. *Light microscopy* The basic lesion is considered to be an injury of visceral epithelial cells of the glomerulus leading to focal collapse and consolidation of the glomerular capillary tufts. The segmental lesion is then permeated by plasma proteins and lipids which give it a hyaline amorphous appearance. These changes are usually accompanied by some mesangial hypercellularity **(Fig. 22.13, B)**. Glomerular changes are progressive and lead to global sclerosis and tubular atrophy with interstitial fibrosis.

ii. *EM* shows diffuse loss of foot processes in addition to areas of hyalinosis composed of finely granular material.

iii. *IF* shows deposits of IgM and C3 in the sclerotic areas, probably due to the trapping of the high molecular weight IgM.

Clinical features include nephrotic syndrome resistant to steroid therapy progressing to ESRD which develops in at least 50% of patients in 10 years.

Q27. Discuss salient features of IgA nephropathy.

Definition IgA nephropathy is a common disease of unknown etiology, usually presenting as recurrent periodic microscopic haematuria. World-wide, it is the most common primary glomerulopathy and the most common cause of microscopic haematuria. Its incidence shows geographic variation, from 10% of all GN in the US to 40% in East Asia.

Etiopathogenesis Unknown, although all the evidences indicate that it is related to abnormal glycosylation of IgA1 as under:

i. IgA which is part of the mucosa-associated immune system is apparently secreted in large amounts and abnormally glycosylated in some genetically predisposed persons.

ii. The onset of IgA nephropathy after some upper respiratory tract infection suggests that such infections may play a pathogenetic role.

iii. If the IgA1component is not properly glycosylated in predisposed persons, it may evoke the production of IgG autoantibodies which form circulating immune complexes with the IgA to be deposited in the mesangial areas of the glomeruli.

iv. IgA immune complexes deposited in the glomeruli contain C3 and less IgG and properdin. They do not contain early components of the complement system, indicating that complement activation occurs through the alternative pathway.

v. IgA deposits in the mesangium of the glomeruli are also seen in some other diseases, such as Henoch-Schönlein purpura, which some authorities consider to be a systemic variant of IgA nephropathy.

vi. IgA is normally cleared from circulation by the liver, and accordingly the patients with cirrhosis have high levels of circulating IgA, which may be deposited in the glomeruli.

vii. IgA deposits in the glomeruli are also seen in patients suffering from certain chronic diseases such as inflammatory bowel disease, interstitial pneumonitis and ankylosing spondylitis.

Pathology
- In most patients, IgA nephropathy presents with mesangial deposits of IgA and C3 and mild mesangial hypercellularity.
- In a proportion of cases, there is diffuse GN progressing to ESRD, and rarely there may even be crescentic glomerulonephritis.

Clinical symptoms and findings depend on the severity of the disease.

i. The disease most often presents in children and young adults, who are diagnosed in 80% cases with microscopic haematuria. In one half of them, it is accompanied by periodic bouts of gross haematuria.

ii. Of the remaining 20%, one half have nephrotic syndrome and the other half have ESRD.

Q28. What is chronic glomerulonephritis? Discuss its main features.

Definition Chronic glomerulonephritis is not a single disease but rather the final outcome of many renal diseases. In 20% cases, it is considered to be idiopathic because no renal disease could be identified preceding it.

Etiopathogenesis Glomerular diseases that progress to chronic glomerulonephritis at a rate given in brackets are listed below:
i. Rapidly progressive GN (90%)
ii. Membranous GN (50%)
iii. Membranoproliferative GN (50%)
iv. Focal segmental glomerulosclerosis (50%)
v. IgA nephropathy (40%)
vi. Acute post-streptococcal GN in children (1%)

Pathology
Grossly, Both kidneys are small and symmetrically shrunken, with a finely granular external surface. On cross section, the cortex is narrow while the medulla is usually still preserved **(Fig. 22.14, A)**.

Microscopy
- Loss of glomeruli and global hyalinisation of the remaining ones. The glomeruli that have a preserved structure may show signs of the underlying disease.
- Most tubules have been replaced by extensive interstitial fibrosis with foci of calcification. The remaining ones are atrophic and may contain inspissated protein casts or crystals of calcium oxalate.
- There is arterial and arteriolar sclerosis with concentric intimal and medial fibrosis causing narrowing of vascular lumina **(Fig. 22.14, B)**.

Clinical features Chronic glomerulonephritis presents with ESRD and hypertension, uraemia, azotaemia and loss of renal functions. Renal dialysis and/or transplantation are the only viable therapeutic approach.

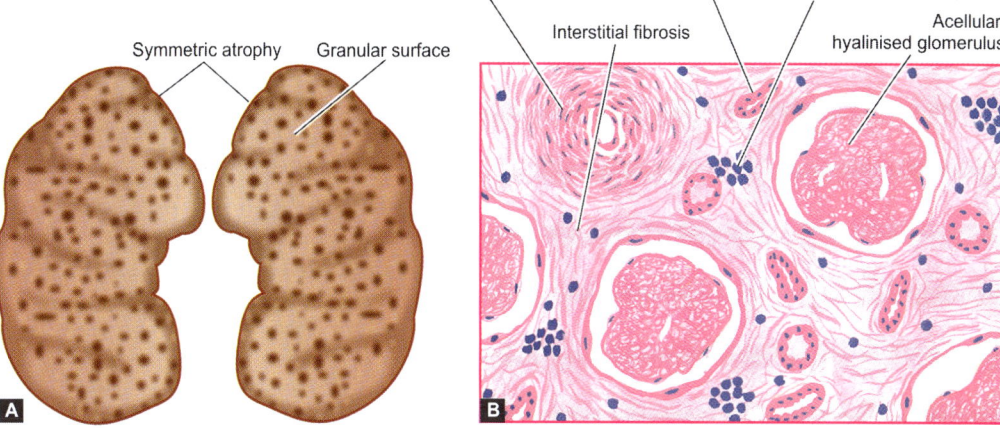

FIGURE 22.14: End-stage kidney. A, Gross appearance of bilaterally small contracted kidneys in chronic glomerulonephritis. The kidneys are symmetrically atrophied, the capsule is adherent to the cortex and has diffusely granular cortical surface. B, Light microscopic appearance in chronic GN. Glomerular tufts are acellular and completely hyalinised. Blood vessels in the interstitium are hyalinised and thickened while the interstitium shows fine fibrosis replacing most of the tubules and a few chronic inflammatory cells.

Q29. Tabulate the salient contrasting features of common forms of primary glomerulonephritis.

The salient features of various forms of primary glomerulonephritis are summarised in **Table 22.10**.

TABLE 22.10 Comparative features of major forms of primary glomerulonephritis.

TYPE	CLINICAL FEATURES	PATHOGENESIS	PATHOLOGY		
			LM	EM	IFM
1. *Acute GN*	Acute nephrotic syndrome	Immune complex disease (local or circulating)	Diffuse proliferation, leucocytic infiltration	Subepithelial deposits ('humps')	Irregular IgG, C3
2. *RPGN*	Acute renal failure	i. Type I: Anti-GBM type ii. Type II: Immune complex type iii. Type III: Pauci-immune RPGN	Proliferation, crescents	i. Linear deposits along GBM ii. Subepithelial deposits iii. No deposits	i. Linear IgG, C3 ii. Granular IgG, C3 iii. Negative
3. *Minimal change disease*	Nephrotic syndrome (highly selective proteinuria)	Reduction of normal negative charge on GBM ?Cell-mediated Mechanism	Normal glomeruli, lipid vacuolation in tubules	Loss of foot processes, no deposits	Negative
4. *Membranous GN*	Nephrotic syndrome	Immune complex disease (local)	Diffuse thickening of capillary wall	Subepithelial deposits ('spikes')	Granular IgG, C3
5. *Membrano-proliferative GN*	Nephrotic syndrome	Type I: Immune complex disease Type II: Dense deposit disease (alternative pathway activation) Type III: Rare, with systemic diseases and drugs	Lobular proliferation of mesangial cells, increased mesangial matrix, double contour of GBM	Type I: Subendothelial deposits Type II: Dense intra-membranous deposits Type III: Subendothelial and subepithelial deposits	Type I: IgG, C3 Type II: C3 properdin Type III: C3, IgG, IgM
6. *Focal GN*	Variable, haematuria common	Variable, possibly immune complex disease	Focal and segmental proliferation	Mesangial deposits	IgA ± IgG, C3 and fibrin

Contd...

Contd...

TYPE	CLINICAL FEATURES	PATHOGENESIS	PATHOLOGY		
			LM	EM	IFM
7. Focal segmental glomerulo-sclerosis	Nephrotic syndrome	i. Idiopathic ii. With superimposed primary glomerular disease iii. Secondary type	Focal and segmental sclerosis and hyalinosis	Loss of foot processes, electron dense deposits in regions of sclerosis and hyalinosis	IgM, C3
8. IgA nephropathy	Recurrent haematuria, mild proteinuria	Unknown, possibly alternate pathway disease	Variable, commonly focal proliferative GN	Mesangial electron-dense deposits	IgA ± IgG, C3, properdin
9. Chronic GN	Chronic renal failure	Variable	Hyalinised glomeruli	Variable	Variable

(GN, glomerulonephritis; LM, light microscopy; EM, electron microscopy; IFM, immunofluorescence microscopy; RPGN, rapidly progressive glomerulonephritis; GBM, glomerular basement membrane; Ig, immunoglobulin; C, complement).

Q30. What is lupus nephritis? Briefly describe its classification and main clinicopathologic features.

Definition Lupus nephritis represents renal involvement in systemic lupus erythematosus (SLE), that occurs in 40–75% of all cases of SLE.

Pathology and classification Primary pathologic lesions in lupus nephritis are immunologically mediated glomerulonephritis, although the disease may involve other parts of the kidney as well. Glomerular changes are used to microscopically classify lupus nephritis into six classes as under:

Class I: Minimal lesions
- By light microscopy, there are almost no changes.
- But by EM and IF, one may detect mesangial immune complexes composed of IgG and C3 complement.

Class II: Mesangial lupus nephritis
- Marked by mesangial widening and hypercellularity.
- Mesangial deposits of immune complexes, which usually contain all three immunoglobulins (IgG, IgA, IgM) and complement (C3).

Class III: Focal segmental lupus nephritis
- Marked by proliferation of mesangial and endothelial cells in segmental parts of some glomeruli.
- Mesangial, subendothelial and subepithelial deposits of immune complexes which contain all immunoglobulins and C3 complement.
- There are also foci of capillary loop necrosis and acute inflammatory cell infiltrates.

Class IV: Diffuse proliferative lupus nephritis
- This is the most severe and the most common form of lupus nephritis.
- There are massive deposits of immune complexes on the subendothelial side of the GBM accounting for the thickening of the GBMs colloquially called *'wire loop lesions'*.
- There are also mesangial, intramembranous and subepithelial deposits.
- Besides, there are foci of fibrinoid necrosis of capillary loops with acute inflammatory cells.
- Proliferation of endothelial, mesangial and epithelial cells contributes further to the hypercellularity of the glomerulus.
- Epithelial cells may even produce crescents in the Bowman capsular space.

Class V: Membranous lupus nephritis
- It resembles idiopathic membranous glomerulopathy.
- It is characterised by diffuse thickening of the GBM due to subepithelial deposits of immune complexes.

Class VI: Sclerosing lupus nephritis
- It is characterised by global glomerulosclerosis and thus it resembles other forms of chronic glomerulonephritis.
- Few glomeruli that are not totally sclerosed may show signs of lupus nephritis.

Clinical features of lupus nephritis depend on the class of the glomerulonephritis.
- In most instances, there are signs of nephritic syndrome, except for class V lesions which present with a nephrotic syndrome.
- Immunotherapy will usually give excellent results except in patients with class V lesions and those that have end-stage class VI lupus nephritis.

Q31. Discuss salient features of diabetic nephropathy.

Definition Diabetic nephropathy is a complication of diabetes mellitus that may include glomerular, tubular, vascular lesions clinically contributing to renal dysfunction in various proportions.

Types of lesions It includes 4 types of renal lesions: diabetic glomerulosclerosis, vascular lesions, diabetic pyelonephritis and tubular lesions (Armanni-Ebstein lesions):

I. **Diabetic glomerulosclerosis** This is very common and accounts for most of the renal findings.
Pathogenesis is based on the following sequence of events that leads to glomerulosclerosis:
- Diabetes mellitus → hyperglycaemia → non-enzymatic glycosylation of the glomerular matrix → advance glycation end product (AGEs) → increased resistance to filtration → glomerular hypertension → renal hyperperfusion against a pressure gradient → insudation of plasma proteins into the mesangial areas and glomerular basement membranes → thickening of hyperperfused areas → glomerulosclerosis.
- Various cytokines such as transforming growth factor-β also contributes to glomerulosclerosis.

Microscopy Two forms of glomerulosclerosis are recognised:
i. *Diffuse glomerulosclerosis,* the more common form, includes thickening of the GBM and diffuse widening of the mesangial area **(Fig, 22.15, A)**.
ii. *Nodular glomerulosclerosis*, also known as Kimmelstiel-Wilson lesion of intercapillary glomerulosclerosis, is characterised by formation of hyaline nodules in the mesangium and variable thickening of the GBM **(Fig. 22.15, B)**.

II. **Vascular lesions** These include:
i. Atherosclerosis of renal arteries.
ii. Hyaline arteriolosclerosis leading to renal ischaemia and inability to regulate the blood flow.

III. **Diabetic pyelonephritis** It is 10–20 times more common than bacterial renal infections in non-diabetic persons.

IV. **Tubular lesions** Also called Armanni-Ebstein lesions, these include reversible vacuolisation of proximal tubules due to the accumulation of glucose in their cytoplasm.

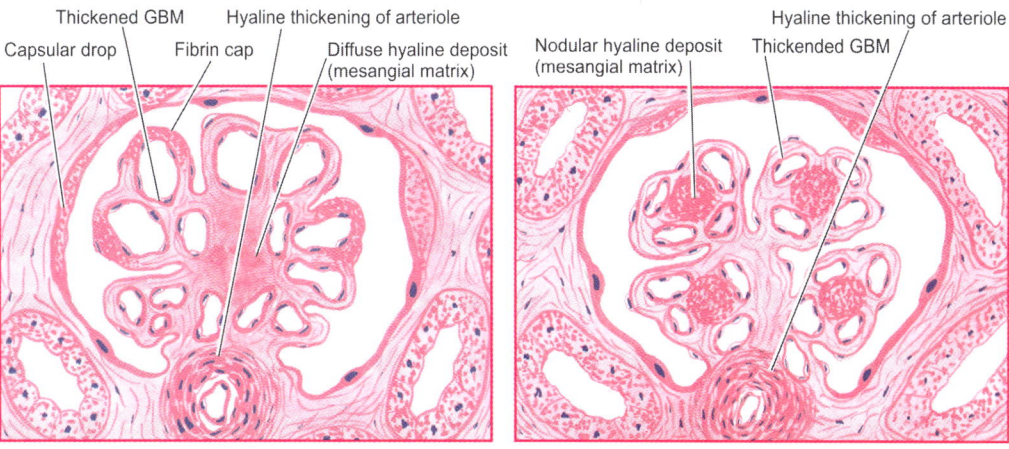

A, DIFFUSE GLOMERULOSCLEROSIS   B, NODULAR GLOMERULOSCLEROSIS

FIGURE 22.15: Diabetic glomerulosclerosis. A, *Diffuse lesions.* The characteristic features are diffuse involvement of the glomeruli showing thickening of the GBM and diffuse increase in the mesangial matrix with mild proliferation of mesangial cells and exudative lesions (fibrin caps and capsular drops). B, *Nodular lesion (Kimmelstiel-Wilson lesion).* There are hyaline nodules within the lobules of glomeruli, surrounded peripherally by glomerular capillaries with thickened walls.

Q32. What is hereditary nephritis?

Definition Hereditary nephritis is a term used for several genetic disorders causing glomerular or tubular lesions affecting the renal function. This group includes more than 60 diseases, each of which has been mapped to a specific gene. Among these genetic disorders, the most important is Alport syndrome, which has a prevalence of 1:5,000 in USA.

Alport syndrome It accounts for 80% of hereditary nephropathies. It is caused by mutations of genes coding for one of the three chains of collagen IV—a_3 and a_4 on chromosomes 2 and 13, and a_5 on X-chromosome.

i. In 85% of cases, Alport syndrome is an X-linked dominant disorder affecting males. It is caused by the large deletions of portions of the gene *COL4A5* which codes for a_5 chain of type IV collagen located on X-chromosome.

ii. In males, progressive renal disease is associated with sensori-neural deafness and ophthalmic complications (cataracts and corneal dystrophy), whereas heterozygote females have only haematuria.

iii. Renal disease presents in late childhood or adolescence with microscopic haematuria, hypertension and late onset of proteinuria, progressing slowly to ESRD, which usually develops by the age of 35 years in most males.

iv. Glomerular changes are initially recognised by EM, which show irregular thickening of the GBM with lamination of the lamina densa which seems interrupted by finely granular rarefied areas. With time these changes progress in males to focal segmental and global sclerosis and ESRD.

Q33. What is acute tubular necrosis and what are its types? Briefly discuss their pathogenesis.

Definition Acute tubular necrosis (ATN) is the pathologic term used for acute renal failure resulting from destruction of tubular epithelium.

Types and pathogenesis There are two forms of ATN: ischaemic and toxic **(Fig. 22.16)**:
- *Ischemic ATN* is initiated by arteriolar vasoconstriction induced by renin-angiotensin system.
- In *toxic ATN*, injury is due to a direct damage of tubules by a toxic agent.

i. Desquamated epithelial debris causes obstruction, increasing tubular pressure and ultimately leading to tubular rupture and leakage of tubular fluid into interstitium, where it raises the pressure and elicits an inflammatory reaction.

ii. All this leads to an increased interstitial pressure, compressing the tubules and blood vessels from outside, thus reducing the inflow of the blood and accentuating ischaemia.

iii. The final outcome is reduced GFR and oliguria.

Q34. Briefly discuss ischaemic ATN.

Definition Ischemic or anoxic ATN (also known as tubulorrhectic ATN, or lower/distal nephron nephrosis, or shock kidney) occurs due to hypoperfusion of the kidneys resulting in focal damage to the distal part of the convoluted tubules. It is more common than toxic ATN, accounting for more than 80% of all cases.

Etiology The most common causes of ischaemic ATN are as follows:
i. Shock (post-traumatic, surgical, obstetrical and septic or due to burns and dehydration).

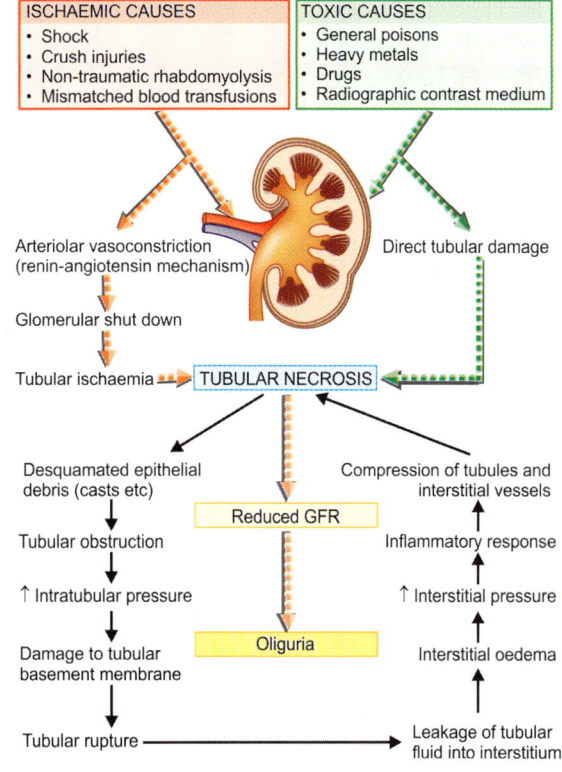

FIGURE 22.16: Pathogenesis of ATN.

ii. Crush injuries.

iii. Non-traumatic rhabdomyolysis induced by alcohol, coma, muscle injury or extensive exertion ('myoglobinuric nephrosis').

iv. Mismatched blood transfusion, black water fever ('haemoglobinuric nephrosis').

Pathology

Grossly, the kidneys are swollen; on cross section the cortex appears pale while the medulla is dark red.

Microscopy **(Fig. 22.17, A)**

i. Tubules are dilated and show focal areas of tubular necrosis with sloughing off of the cellular debris, which accumulates in the lumen and may be admixed to protein rich casts.

ii. In haemoglobinuric ATN, the lumen contains haemoglobin-tinged casts, while in the myoglobinuric ATN, the debris is dark red from myoglobin.

iii. Disruption of tubular basement membranes may be seen focally next to the casts.

iv. After 2–3 days, the tubules are lined by flat epithelium containing dividing cells, suggesting early regeneration.

Prognosis The outcome depends on the extent of injury but in general, extensive trauma with myoglobinuria, surgical shock and burns have a worse prognosis than other forms of shock.

Q35. What is toxic acute tubular necrosis?

Definition Toxic ATN (also called nephrotoxic ATN, or toxic nephrosis, or upper/proximal nephron nephrosis) occurs as a result of direct damage to tubules, more marked in proximal portion of the nephron caused by ingestion, injection or inhalation of toxic agents.

Etiology Toxic agents causing ATN include the following:

i. General poisons such as mercuric chloride, carbon tetrachloride, ethylene glycol, mushrooms, insecticides.

ii. Heavy metals (e.g. mercury, lead, arsenic, phosphorus, gold).

iii. Drugs such as sulphonamides, antibiotics (e.g. gentamycin, cephalosporin), anaesthetic agents (e.g. halothane, methoxyflurane).

iv. Radiographic contrast material.

Pathology

Grossly, the kidneys look like those in ischaemic necrosis.

Microscopy **(Fig. 22.17, B)**

i. Cell necrosis of proximal tubules, which have desquamated into the lumen and may undergo dystrophic calcification.

ii. Tubular membranes of necrotic tubules are intact.

iii. Regeneration starts a few days after ATN and is marked by the appearance of mitotic cells in the tubules lined by flat epithelium.

Prognosis is generally better than for ischaemic necrosis.

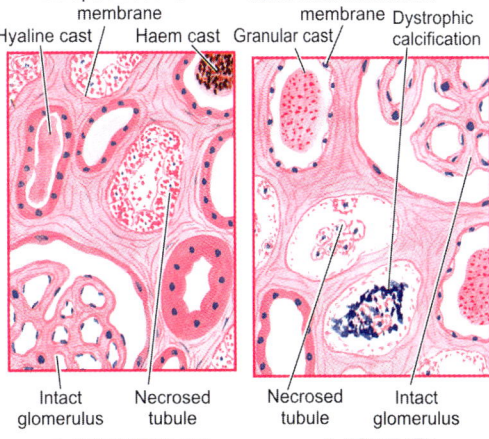

FIGURE 22.17: Two types of ATN. A, *Ischaemic ATN*. There is focal necrosis along the nephron involving proximal convoluted tubule (PCT) as well as distal convoluted tubule (DCT). The affected tubules are dilated, their lumina contain casts (hyaline or pigmented haem) and the affected regions are lined by regenerating thin and flat epithelium. In between, there are preserved tubules and glomeruli having intact nuclei. B, *Toxic ATN*. There is extensive necrosis of epithelial cells involving predominantly proximal convoluted tubule (PCT) diffusely. The necrosed cells are desquamated into the tubular lumina and may undergo dystrophic calcification. The tubular lumina contain casts (granular) and the regenerating flat epithelium lines the necrosed tubule.

Q36. Write briefly on acute pyelonephritis.

Definition Acute pyelonephritis is a suppurative kidney disease caused by bacteria.

Etiopathogenesis Infections can reach the kidneys by two routes, and accordingly they can be classified as *ascending or haematogenous*. Most often, these infections are caused by *Escherichia coli* (90%), followed in decreasing frequency by *Enterobacter, Klebsiella, Pseudomonas* and *Proteus*.

I. *Ascending infections* follow lower urinary tract infection (UTI) which is related to contamination of lower urethral orifice with faecal bacteria. They are more common than haematogenous infections.

i. UTI is more common in females than males for several reasons, which include the following:

a. Anatomic location of the opening of the female urethra which is more accessible to bacteria and is easily traumatised during intercourse.

b. Female urethra is shorter than male urethra.

c. Female sex hormones facilitate the adhesion of bacterial to urethral mucosa.

d. Finally, one should not neglect the fact that the prostatic secretions provide chemical protection against bacterial infections in men.

ii. Susceptibility to bacterial infections of the lower urinary tract is increased by certain diseases such as diabetes, urinary obstruction and instrumentation, and pregnancy.

iii. Initially, these conditions are most often accompanied by asymptomatic bacteriuria, which may transform into a local infection. This progresses into an ascending infection, which will ultimately reach the upper urinary tract and kidneys.

II. *Haematogenous infection* results from blood-borne spread of bacteria from some other site. Such kidney infections occur most often in persons who have urinary tract obstructions, those who are debilitated or immunosuppressed.

Pathology

Grossly, the kidneys are enlarged, swollen and enclosed by a tense capsule. Below the capsule, one may see small yellow-white abscesses. On cross section of the kidney, pus may form streaks extending from the cortex into the medulla.

Microscopy shows aggregates of neutrophils and pus cells expanding the collecting ducts and tubules and forming microscopic abscesses in the interstitial spaces.

Clinical features

i. Sudden onset of fever, chills, loin pain, lumbar tenderness.

ii. The urine is turbid and contains bacteria and pus.

iii. Microscopic examination of the urinary sediment reveals numerous neutrophils, pus cells, pus cell cast and bacteria.

iv. Bacteriologic studies are used to determine antibiotic susceptibility and select the appropriate antibiotics.

Complications are more common in neglected cases or in patients who have diabetes and other debilitating chronic diseases. Important complications of acute pyelonephritis are as follows:

i. *Papillary necrosis,* also known as *necrotising papillitis*, develops due to ischaemic necrosis of renal papilla which has been shut off from the blood supply by the inflammatory exudate at its base. Similar papillary necrosis is seen in patients with sickle cell anaemia and analgesic abuse nephropathy.

Microscopy shows that necrosis of the tubules and ducts forming the papilla; the border between necrotic papillae and the viable cortical renal tissue is infiltrated with neutrophils.

ii. *Pyonephrosis (or pyonephros)* is a term describing accumulation of pus in the dilated renal calices and pelvis due to an obstruction of the upper ureter. It usually develops from purulent pyelonephritis destroying renal tissue followed by a discharge of pus into the renal collecting system. Since the pus cannot flow into the ureter due to ureteral obstruction, it will accumulate above the obstruction and dilate the renal pelvis and calyces into cystic cavities filled with pus.

iii. *Perinephric abscess* develops due to the extension of the suppurative pyelonephritis into the perinephric space.

Q37. What is chronic pyelonephritis? Discuss its salient features.

Definition Chronic pyelonephritis is a chronic tubulointerstitial disease resulting from repeated attacks of inflammation and scarring.

Etiopathogenesis Based on etiopathogenesis, there are two types of chronic pyelonephritis: reflux nephropathy and obstructive pyelonephritis:

I. *Reflux nephropathy* develops due to the reflux of urine from the bladder into the ureter, often extending into the upper urinary tracts **(Fig. 22.18)**.

a. Vesicoureteric reflux may develop in girls due to congenital absence or shortening of the intravesical portion of the ureter so that it is not compressed during micturition, allowing the urine to flow back into the ureters.

b. Reflux of urine may cause increased pressure in the renal pelvis which is then transmitted into the renal parenchyma, damaging the nephrons.

c. Furthermore, reflux predisposes to infections which cause chronic pyelonephritis and further damage the kidneys.

II. *Obstructive pyelonephritis* is caused by urinary stones or other causes of obstruction which predispose the kidneys to chronic infection.

Pathology

Grossly, kidneys are small, contracted and covered with a thick fibrous capsule. Stripping the capsule reveals an unevenly scarred external surface due to U-shaped indentations of the fibrotic parenchyma and thinned cortex. The calyces are dilated (calyectasis) and the pelvis is dilated **(Fig. 22.19,A)**.

Microscopy **(Fig. 22.19,B)**

i. Extensive chronic inflammation in the widened and fibrotic interstitium which is infiltrated with lymphocytes, plasma cells and macrophages.

ii. In some cases, foamy macrophages predominate and the conditions is called *xanthogranulomatous pyelonephritis*.

iii. The tubules are mostly lost and replaced by fibrous tissue, and those that are left behind are atrophic, dilated and filled with proteinaceous casts, resembling thyroid follicles.

iv. Blood vessels entrapped in the fibrous tissue show obliterative endarteritis and the arterioles show hyaline arteriolosclerosis.

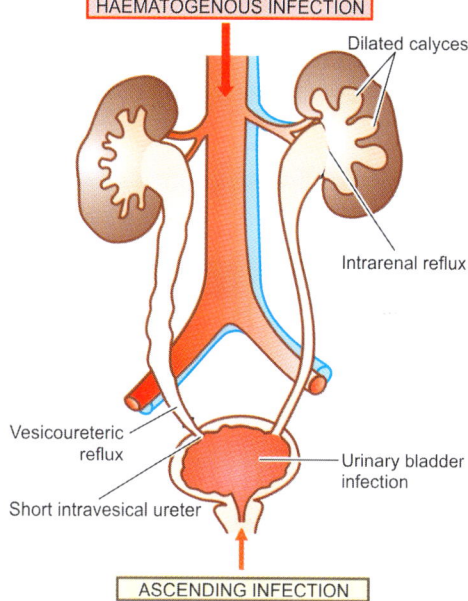

FIGURE 22.18: Pathogenesis of reflux nephropathy.

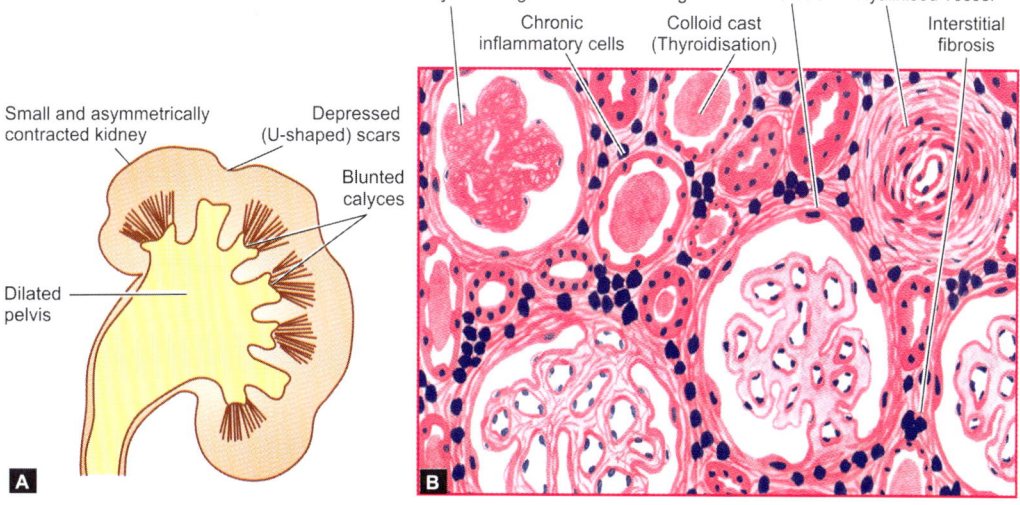

FIGURE 22.19: Chronic pyelonephritis with calyectasis. A, Diagrammatic representation of small contracted kidney. There is asymmetry and irregular scarring. B, Microscopy shows atrophy of some tubules and dilatation of others which contain colloid casts (thyroidisation). The tubules are surrounded by abundant fibrous tissue and chronic interstitial inflammatory reaction. The blood vessels included are thick-walled and the glomeruli show periglomerular fibrosis.

v. Glomeruli are intact and usually show periglomerular fibrosis. Ultimately, they will also undergo hyalinisation as the rest of the nephron has been destroyed.

Clinical features

i. Chronic pyelonephritis usually has an insidious onset and often present with renal insufficiency and hypertension.

ii. Local symptoms may include loin pain, low grade fever, lumbar tenderness, dysuria, pyuria and bacteriuria and frequent micturition.

iii. Intravenous pyelography may reveal small shrunken kidneys.

Q38. What are the distinguishing pathologic features between chronic pyelonephritis and chronic glomerulonephritis?

Features that distinguish chronic pyelonephritis from chronic glomerulonephritis are summarised in **Table 22.11**.

TABLE 22.11 Distinguishing features between chronic glomerulonephritis and chronic pyelonephritis.

FEATURE	CHRONIC GLOMERULONEPHRITIS	CHRONIC PYELONEPHRITIS
1. *Underlying disease*	Primary glomerulonephritis	Tubulointerstitial inflammation
2. *Proteinuria*	+++	+
3. *Urine microscopy*	Casts, epithelial cells	Pus cells, bacteria
4. *Gross appearance*	i. Bilateral involvement ii. Symmetrically small, contracted iii. Granular scars externally iv. Cut surface granular scar v. Calculi absent	i. Bilateral or unilateral involvement ii. Asymmetrically small, contracted iii. Irregular, uneven scars externally iv. Cut surface dilated or distorted pelvicalyceal system, fat infiltration v. Calculi frequent
5. *Histologic features*	i. Glomerulosclerosis (>50%) ii. Interstitial fibrosis+ iii. Periglomerular fibrosis+ iv. Tubular atrophy+ v. Thyroidisation-	i. Glomerulosclerosis occasional ii. Interstitial fibrosis+++ iii. Periglomerular fibrosis+++ iv. Tubular atrophy+++ v. Thyroidisation++

Q39. What is tuberculous pyelonephritis?

Definition Tuberculous pyelonephritis develops as a secondary infection due to the haematogenous spread of *M. tuberculosis*, usually from the primary infection in the lungs. Less commonly, it may also occur as an ascending infection from the fallopian tubes or the testis.

Pathology Renal tuberculosis usually involves the medulla and papillae that are replaced by necrotic caseous material. Necrotic material may gradually slough off and obstruct the ureter causing dilatation of the pelvis and calices.

Microscopy shows caseating epithelioid cell granulomas.

Clinical features are variable and usually include dysuria, microscopic haematuria and 'sterile pyuria' (considered to be sterile because *M. tuberculosis* cannot be cultured on standard bacteriologic media).

Q40. What is obstructive uropathy? Discuss its types, causes and complications.

Definition Obstructive uropathy is a collective term for all the diseases that impede the outflow of urine from the urinary system.

Classification Obstruction of urinary outflow may be classified according to several criteria as under:

I. It may be bilateral or unilateral, complete or partial, and may have a sudden or an insidious onset.

II. Obstruction can be classified as intraluminal, intramural and extramural obstruction **(Table 22.12)**.

III. Anatomic locations of obstruction vary and may involve the ureters, the neck of the bladder or the urethra **(Fig. 22.20)**.

Etiopathogenesis Obstructive uropathy may occur due to many causes, the most important of which are urinary stones (nephrolithiasis). Other causes are listed in **Table 22.12**.

TABLE 22.12 Causes of obstructive uropathy.

A. INTRALUMINAL
1. Calculi
2. Tumours (e.g. cancer of kidney and bladder)
3. Sloughed renal papilla
4. Blood clots
5. Foreign body

B. INTRAMURAL
1. Pelviureteric junction (PUJ) obstruction
2. Vesicoureteric obstruction
3. Urethral stricture
4. Urethral valves
5. Inflammation (e.g. phimosis, cystitis, etc.)
6. Neuromuscular dysfunction

C. EXTRAMURAL
1. Pregnant uterus
2. Retroperitoneal fibrosis
3. Tumours (e.g. carcinoma of cervix, rectum, colon, caecum, etc.)
4. Prostatic enlargement, prostatic carcinoma and prostatitis
5. Trauma

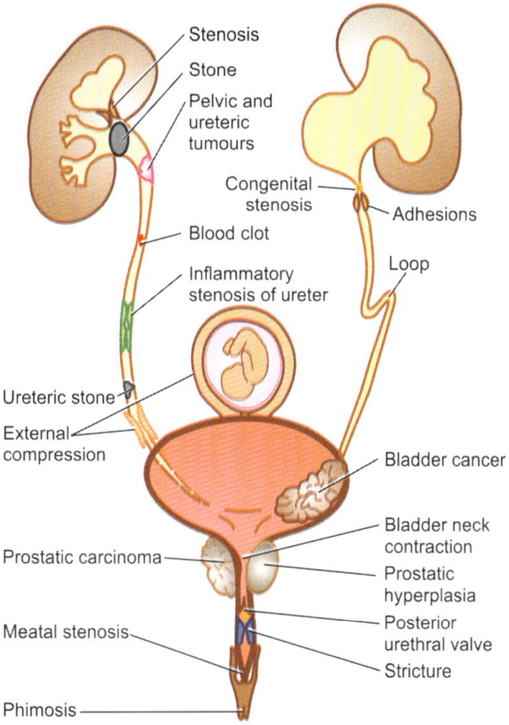

Complications
- *Superimposed infection* is the most common complication, and it may cause various forms of inflammation including urethritis, cystitis, ureteritis and acute and chronic pyelonephritis.
- Other important complications reflect changes in the shape and size of urinary organs such as *hydronephrosis, hydroureters, hypertrophy of the bladder*.

FIGURE 22.20: Causes of obstructive uropathy at different levels in the urinary tract.

Q41. What is urolithiasis? Comment on its epidemiology.

Definition Urolithiasis is formation of urinary calculi (stones) at any level of the urinary tract while nephrolithiasis is formation of stones in the kidney.

Epidemiology The estimates are that 2% of the total world population has urinary stone disease.

i. By the age of 70, approximately 10% of males and 5% of females in the United States have had clinical signs of urinary stone disease.
ii. Urolithiasis is more common in some parts of the World like southern parts of the United States, South Africa, India and South-East Asia.
iii. Males are affected two times more often than females.
iv. The peak incidence of first symptom is in the 2nd and 3rd decade of life.

Q42. Discuss salient features of various types of urinary calculi.

There are four types of urinary calculi: calcium containing, struvite (or mixed), uric acid and cystine stones **(Table 22.13)**:

I. **Calcium stones (75%)** They are the most common of all urinary calculi. They may be composed of:
- calcium oxalate (50%),
- calcium phosphate (5%), or
- mixture of calcium oxalate and calcium phosphate (45%).

Etiology Highly variable; following are predisposing conditions:
i. *Idiopathic hypercalciuria* without hypercalcaemia, which is found in 50% cases.
ii. *Hypercalciuria due to hypercalcaemia,* which is found in 10% cases related to hyperparathyroidism, or a defect in the bowel (i.e. absorptive hypercalciuria) or the kidneys (i.e. renal hypercalciuria).
iii. *Hyperuricosuria* with a normal blood uric acid level and any abnormality of calcium metabolism, which is found in 15% cases.

TABLE 22.13 Salient features of urinary calculi.

TYPE	INCIDENCE	ETIOLOGY	PATHOGENESIS
I. Calcium stones	75%	Hypercalciuria with or without hypercalcaemia; idiopathic	Supersaturation of ions in urine, alkaline pH of urine; low urinary volume, oxaluria and hyperuricosuria
II. Mixed (struvite) stones	15%	Urinary infection with urea-splitting organisms like *Proteus*	Alkaline urinary pH produced by ammonia from splitting of urea by bacterially produced urease
III. Uric acid stones	6%	Hyperuricosuria with or without hyperuricaemia (e.g. in primary and secondary gout)	Acidic urine (pH below 6) decreases the solubility of uric acid in urine and favours its precipitation
IV. Cystine stones	2%	Genetically-determined defect in cysteine transport	Cystinuria containing least soluble cysteine precipitates as cystine crystals
V. Other types	< 2%	Inherited abnormalities of amino acid metabolism	Xanthinuria

iv. *Idiopathic calcium stone disease* with no metabolic or renal excretory abnormalities, which is found in 25% cases.

Pathogenesis The formation of calcium stones reflects an imbalance between supersaturation of urine with ions forming the stones and a low concentration of inhibitors.
- The process of stone formation begins with the deposition of calcium oxalate or phosphates crystals in renal tubules around a nidus of organic debris and cell fragments.
- Additional deposits of crystals form more layers contributing to the growth of initial calcification.
- The growth of calculi is facilitated by alkaline urine, low volume of filtered fluid in the tubules and the presence of oxalates and uric acid.

Morphology Calcium stones are usually small (less than 1 cm), hard, ovoid with a granular external surface. Their surface turns brown from secondary deposits of haemosiderin derived from haemorrhage caused by sharp edges of the stones.

II. **Mixed (struvite) stones (15%)** They are made up of magnesium-ammonium-calcium phosphate (or *triple phosphate stones*), also known as struvite.

Etiopathogenesis of struvite stones is related to infection with urea-splitting organisms that produce urease, such as *Proteus,* and less often *Klebsiella, Pseudomonas* and *Enterobacter. E. coli*, the most common uropathogen is, however, not involved in their pathogenesis.

Morphology Struvite stones are yellow white or grey, soft and friable and of irregular shape. 'Staghorn stone' which is a solitary large stone that takes the shape of the renal pelvis, is a typical examples of struvite stones **(Fig. 22.21)**.

III. **Uric acid stones (6%)** They are made up of uric acid crystals. They are radiolucent, in contrast to calcium-containing stones which are radio-opaque.

Etiopathogenesis Uric acid stone are frequently formed in persons who have hyperuricaemia and hyperuricosuria, such as in primary gout or secondary gout (e.g. in leukaemia, especially after chemotherapy, or due to an intake of uricosuric drugs such as salicylates or probenecid).

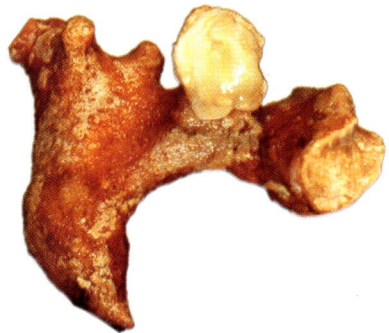

STAGHORN STONE
FIGURE 22.21: A staghorn stone.

- Hyperuricosuria is the most important factor in the pathogenesis of uric acid stones, but it is associated with hyperuricaemia only in 50% of cases.
- Formation of uric acid stones is promoted by acidic urine (pH<6) and low urinary volume. Acidic urine will typically reduce the solubility of uric acid and promote crystallisation.
- Low urine volume promotes supersaturation.

Morphology Uric acid stones are smooth, yellowish-brown, hard and often multiple.

IV. **Cystine stones (2%)** These are rare and found only in patients with cystinuria.
Etiopathogenesis
- Cystinuria is a genetic disease marked by abnormal transport of cystine and other amino acids across the cell membrane of renal tubules and small intestinal mucosal cells.
- Excess of cystine excreted in urine favours the formation of stones, because cystine is the least soluble of the naturally-occurring amino acids.

Morphology Cystine stones are small, rounded, often multiple, yellowish and waxy.

V. **Other calculi (2%)** Besides, calculi may be found in patients afflicted by hereditary enzyme abnormalities, such as hereditary xanthinuria.

Q43. What is hydronephrosis? Briefly discuss its types.

Definition Hydronephrosis is dilatation of renal pelvis and calyces due to partial or intermittent obstruction of the outflow of urine.

Classification It may be unilateral or bilateral, and it is typically associated with hydroureter.

I. **Unilateral hydronephrosis** is usually caused by an obstruction at the level of pelviureteric junction (PUJ). The causes are as under:

i. *Intraluminal,* e.g. calculus in the ureter or pelvis.

ii. *Intramural,* e.g. congenital PUJ obstruction, atresia of ureter, inflammatory stricture, trauma, neoplasm of ureter or bladder.

iii. *Extramural,* e.g. obstruction by inferior renal arty or vein, pressure on the ureter from outside such as carcinoma of cervix, prostate or large intestine and retroperitoneal fibrosis.

II. **Bilateral hydronephrosis** is usually caused by some form of urethral obstruction which may be:

i. *Congenital,* e.g. atresia of urethral meatus or posterior urethral valves.

ii. *Acquired,* e.g. bladder tumour involving both ureic orifices, prostatic enlargement due to prostatic hyperplasia or carcinoma, inflammatory or traumatic urethral stricture and phimosis.

Pathology The changes vary depending upon whether the obstruction is *sudden and complete,* or *incomplete and intermittent.*

i. Initially, there is only *extrarenal hydronephrosis* marked by dilatation of the renal pelvis **(Fig. 22.22)**.

ii. In prolonged obstruction, the dilated pelvi-caliceal system extends into the renal cortex compressing it into a narrow band of atrophic tissue, typical of *intrarenal hydronephrosis.*

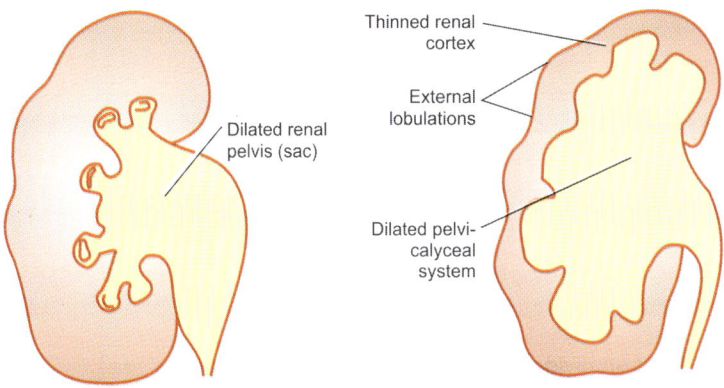

A, EXTRARENAL HYDRONEPHROSIS B, INTRARENAL HYDRONEPHROSIS

FIGURE 22.22: Hydronephrosis. A, Extrarenal hydronephrosis. B, Intrarenal hydronephrosis.

iii. *Microscopy* There is severe interstitial fibrosis with atrophy or tubules and hyalinisation of glomeruli.
iv. Stasis of urine predisposes to infections and the entire kidney may transform into a sac filled with pus (*pyonephrosis*).

Q44. What is hypertensive vascular disease? What are its types?

Definition Hypertension is elevation of systolic blood pressure above 120 mmHg and diastolic blood pressure above 80 mmHg, as defined by American Heart Association and American College of Cardiology **(Table 22.14)**.

TABLE 22.14 Categories of BP in adults*.

BP CATEGORY	SBP		DBP
Normal	<120 mmHg	and	<80 mmHg
Elevated	120–129 mmHg	and	<80 mmHg
Hypertension			
Stage 1	130–139 mmHg	or	80–89 mmHg
Stage 2	≥140 mmHg	or	≥90 mmHg

Individuals having SBP and DBP in 2 categories should be designated to the higher BP category.
BP indicates blood pressure (based on an average of ≥2 careful readings obtained on ≥2 occasions); DBP, diastolic blood pressure; SBP, systolic blood pressure.

*Whelton et al. 2017 ACC/AHA guidelines for the prevention, detection, evaluation and management of high blood pressure in adults. *J Am Coll Cardiol*. 2018. 71:19; e138.

Classification
I. **Based on etiopathogenesis**, hypertension may be of two types:
- *Primary*, i.e. hypertension of unknown cause, also called *essential hypertension*, accounts for 80–95% of cases.
- *Secondary*, which is related to endocrine or renal diseases or some other identifiable causes such as atherosclerosis and neurogenic causes.

II. **According to the clinical course**, either type of hypertension (primary or secondary) may be benign or malignant.
- *Benign hypertension* is moderate elevation of blood pressure and the rise is slow over the years. About 90–95% of all patients have benign hypertension.
- *Malignant hypertension* is marked elevation of blood pressure over 200 mmHg for the systolic and 140 mmHg for the diastolic blood pressure. Less than 5% of patients develop this type of hypertension.

Q45. What is essential hypertension? Briefly discuss its etiopathogenesis.

Definition Essential hypertension is a disease of unknown etiology, influenced by genetic and environmental factors and many modifying risk factors.
Etiopathogenesis Essential hypertension is a multifactorial disease and thus it has many potential causes and modifiers as follows:
i. *Genetic factors,* as evidenced by familial occurrence of hypertension, studies in twins and the identification of hypertension susceptibility genes.
ii. *Racial and environmental factors,* such as higher incidence of hypertension among the African Americans than other races; obesity, salt intake and diet, skilled occupations, higher living standards.
iii. *Risk factors modifying the course of essential hypertension,* such as age of onset (younger onset is linked to worse prognosis), sex (females have better prognosis), incidence of atherosclerosis, smoking, excessive alcohol intake, diabetes mellitus, etc.
iv. *Humoral and circulatory factors that control blood pressure,* such as catecholamines, renin, aldosterone and the reactivity of arterioles, cardiac output, cardiac pacing and rhythm, renal excretion of mineral, etc.

Q46. What is secondary hypertension? Discuss its various causes and mechanisms.

Definition Secondary hypertension has underlying identifiable causes such as renal, endocrine, aortic and neurogenic causes.
Causes
I. **Renal hypertension** is subdivided into two groups:
i. *Renal vascular hypertension,* e.g caused by occlusion of a major renal artery, fibromuscular dysplasia of renal artery, polyarteritis nodosa, etc.

ii. *Renal parenchymal hypertension,* e.g. various forms of glomerulonephritis, pyelonephritis, interstitial nephritis, diabetic nephropathy, polycystic kidney disease, renin-producing tumours.

Pathogenesis of renal hypertension is related to 3 interrelated processes as follows:

i. *Activation of renin angiotensin system* which is activated by renal ischaemia, sympathetic nervous system stimulation, depressed sodium concentration, fluid depletion, decreased potassium intake. Renin acts on angiotensinogen transforming it to angiotensin I, which is converted angiotensin II, which in turn, leads to arteriolar vasoconstriction and also stimulates secretion of aldosterone that promotes the reabsorption of sodium and water in the kidneys **(Fig. 22.23)**.

ii. *Sodium and water retention* which determines the blood volume and cardiac output. Sodium concentration of blood is regulated by 3 mechanisms:
a. Release of aldosterone from activation of the renin angiotensin system.
b. Reduction of GFR which results in increased sodium reabsorption in the kidneys.
c. Release of atriopeptin hormone from atria in response to volume expansion.
iii. *Release of vasodepressor material* counteracting the effects of angiotensin. These include prostaglandins released from interstitial cells of renal medulla, kallikrein-kinin system and platelet activating factor (PAF).

II. **Endocrine hypertension** which is mediated by several hormones:
i. *Adrenal gland*—e.g. in primary hyperaldosteronism, Cushing syndrome, adrenal virilism and pheochromocytoma.
ii. *Thyroid*—e.g. hyperthyroidism and hypothyroidism.
iii. *Parathyroid gland*—e.g. hypercalcaemia in hyperparathyroidism.
iv. *Oral contraceptives* which stimulate the liver to produce the renin substrate.
III. **Coarctation of aorta** causing hypertension in upper part of the body.
IV. **Neurogenic**, which includes psychogenic causes, increased intracranial pressure section, spinal cord section, etc.

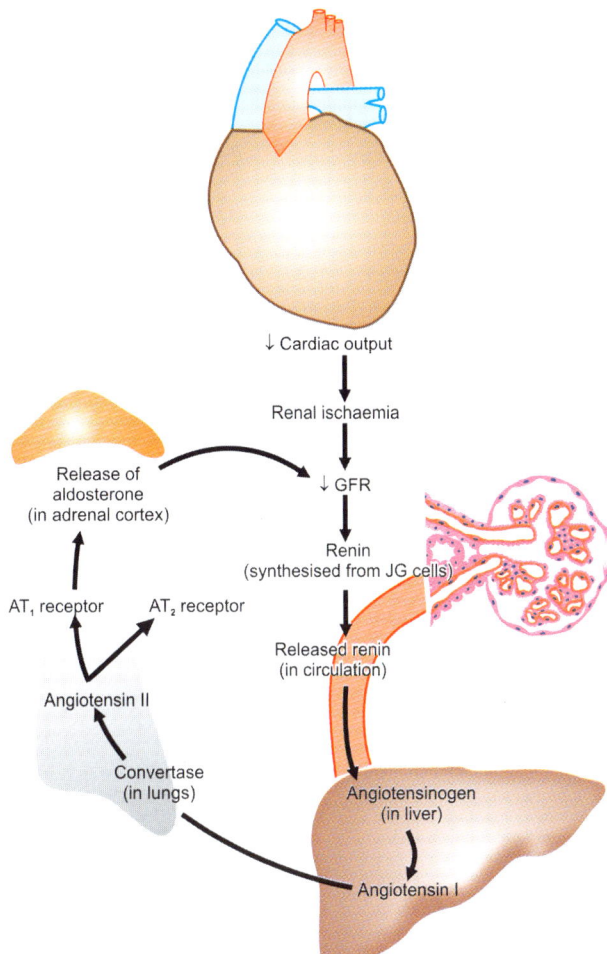

FIGURE 22.23: The renin-angiotensin mechanism.
(JG cells, juxtaglomerular cells; GFR, glomerular filtration rate; AT, angiotensin).

Q47. List the various consequences of hypertension on major target organs.

Systemic hypertension has major effects on the following five main organs:
I. Blood vessels—atherosclerosis and arteriolosclerosis
II. Heart—hypertensive heart disease
III. Kidneys—nephrosclerosis
IV. Nervous system—stroke
V. Eyes—hypertensive retinopathy

Q48. What is nephrosclerosis? Describe its types and their salient features.

Definition Nephrosclerosis is a term used to describe the renal consequences of hypertension.

Types It occurs in two forms: Benign nephrosclerosis and malignant nephrosclerosis.

I. **Benign nephrosclerosis** is characterised by gradual loss of renal parenchyma due to ischaemia.

Pathology Grossly, kidney size and weight are reduced bilaterally. The symmetrically shrunken kidneys have a finely granular external surface and shows V-shaped areas of scarring **(Fig. 22.24, A)**. On cross section, the cortex is thinner than normal.

Microscopy shows vascular changes with secondary results of ischaemia:

i. *Vascular changes* include hyaline arteriolosclerosis, and intimal and medial proliferation of smooth muscle cells in arterioles and arteries.

ii. *Parenchymal changes* include various consequences of ischaemia. These include: glomerular sclerosis, deposition of collagen in the Bowman capsular space and periglomerular fibrosis, tubular atrophy and interstitial fibrosis **(Fig. 22.24, B)**.

Clinical features include:

i. Those of hypertension such as: headaches, dizziness, palpitation, nervousness,

ii. Eye ground changes may be found but papilloedema is absent.

iii. Loss of glomeruli and tubules results in a loss of renal functions, but renal failure is uncommon.

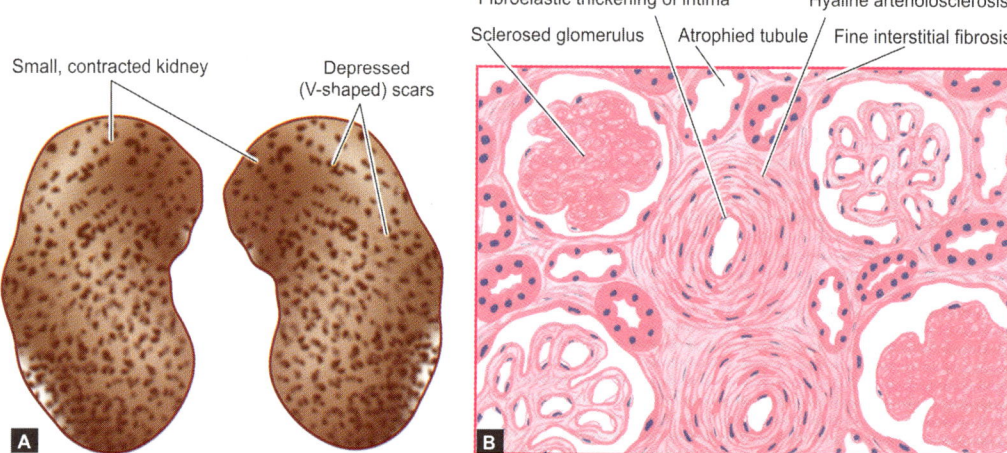

FIGURE 22.24: *Benign nephrosclerosis.* A, Small, contracted kidney in chronic hypertension (benign nephrosclerosis). The kidneys are small and contracted. The capsule is adherent to the cortex and has granular depressed scars on the surface. B, Microscopy shows vascular changes of hyaline arteriolosclerosis and intimal thickening of small blood vessels in the glomerular tuft. The parenchymal changes include sclerosed glomeruli, tubular atrophy and fine interstitial fibrosis.

II. **Malignant nephrosclerosis** occurs in malignant or accelerated hypertension. It is uncommon, accounting for less than 5% of cases, in which malignant hypertension is superimposed on long-standing benign hypertension.

Pathology Grossly, kidneys are similar to those in benign hypertension, and are small and granular on their external surface. If there is no pre-existent benign hypertension, kidneys may be normal in size or even enlarged and show petechial haemorrhages ('flea bitten') **(Fig. 22.25, A)**.

Microscopy shows **(Fig. 22.25,B)**:

i. Proliferative arteriolitis with concentric layering of smooth muscle cells around a narrowed lumen.

ii. Foci of fibrinoid necrosis.

Clinical features reflect sudden onset of high pressure (over 200/140 mmHg).

i. Headache and dizziness common.

ii. Impaired vision frequently found.

iii. Eye background examination will typically show papilloedema.

iv. There is rapid deterioration of renal functions, and urinalysis reveals proteinuria and haematuria.

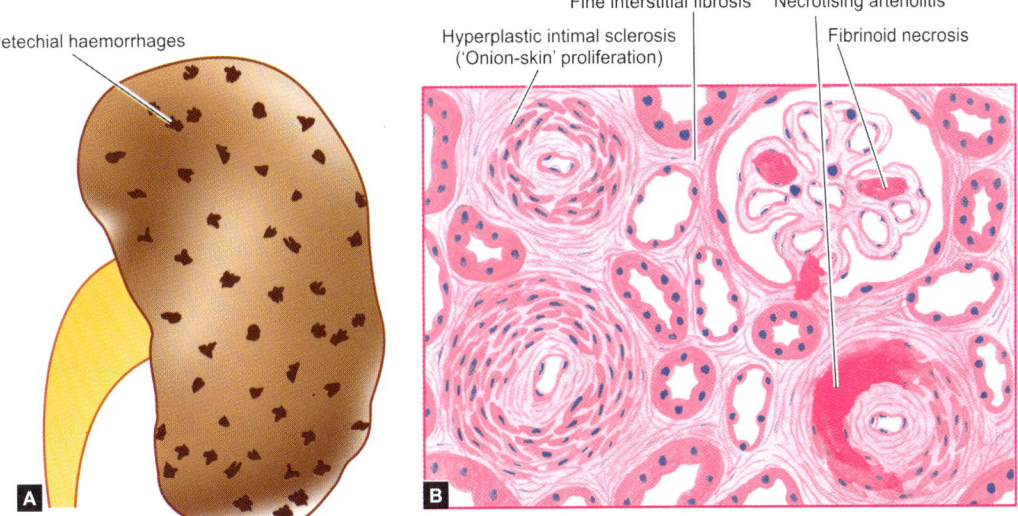

FIGURE 22.25: *Malignant nephrosclerosis.* A, The kidney is enlarged in size and weight. The cortex shows characteristic *'flea bitten kidney'* due to tiny petechial haemorrhages on the surface. B, Microscopy shows concentric proliferation and arteriolitis of small blood vessel, giving onion-skin appearance. A few areas in the vessel wall show fibrinoid necrosis identified as brightly eosinophilic hyalinised material.

Q49. What are the most important renal tumours? Discuss an example of a common benign renal tumour.

Classification Kidney tumours can be classified as benign or malignant. Tumours that are of clinical significance include oncocytoma, a benign tumour, and two malignant tumours (renal cell carcinoma and Wilms tumour). All others are either uncommon or of lesser clinical significance.

Oncocytoma is an example of benign renal tumour arising from the collecting ducts.

Grossly, sectioned surface of the tumour has a mahogany brown colour and usually a central scar, allowing the radiologic diagnosis of this tumour.

Microscopy The tumour is composed of tubular cells that have abundant eosinophilic cytoplasm, filled with numerous mitochondria, best seen by electron microscopy. The tumour cells have round uniform nuclei and show no proliferative activity.

Q50. What is renal cell carcinoma? Discuss its salient features.

Definition Renal cells carcinoma (RCC) is a malignant tumour accounting for 80–85% of all renal malignant tumours in adults.

Etiopathogenesis

I. **Risk factors** These include:
i. Smoking (2 times higher than in nonsmokers)
ii. Obesity
iii. Unopposed oestrogen therapy in women
iv. Hypertension
v. Polycystic kidney disease and acquired polycystic disease in end-stage kidney disease associated with an increased incidence

II. **Genetic predisposition** is found in families of patients diagnosed with RCC, which are at 5–6 times higher risk than the population at large.

Genetic basis of RCC can be demonstrated only in 5% of all cases but the study of these cases has contributed significantly to the better understanding of molecular pathology of RCC in general, as under:
i. Approximately one half of patients with *von Hippel-Lindau syndrome* develop RCC. This fact has led to the discovery of deletion or mutation of the *VHL gene* on 3p chromosome in most (89%) clear cell RCCs.

ii. Familial cases of papillary RCC have a mutation of *MET*, a protooncogene encoding a tyrosine kinase, which has also been found in some sporadic cases of papillary RCC.

iii. *Germ-line mutation* of genes encoding succinate dehydrogenase (SDH) or fumarate dehydrogenase have been found in rare syndromic forms of RCC. It is not known how these gene mutations contribute to the pathogenesis of RCC.

Pathology Three most common and clinically most important histopathologic forms of RCC are: clear cell RCC (75%), papillary RCC (15%) and chromophobe RCC (5%).

I. **Clear cell RCC** is the most common type and it originates from the proximal tubules.

Grossly, it usually presents as a solid mass that appears yellow on the cut surface. Large tumours often show areas of necrosis and haemorrhage and invade into the perinephric fat tissue or the hilum and the renal vein **(Fig. 22.26, A)**.

Microscopy

i. Composed of clear cells forming tubules or solid nests **(Fig. 22.26, B)**.

ii. The cytoplasm is clear because it contains large amounts of glycogen and lipids.

iii. The nuclei may be relatively uniform or show anaplasia, which is used to grade the tumours into four categories of increasing malignancy.

II. **Papillary RCC** originates from distal tubules.

Grossly, it may present as a solitary, well-encapsulated mass but often there are multifocal and even may be bilateral masses.

Microscopy

i. Tumour composed of cells lining papillae that have a fibrovascular core.

ii. Twisting of papillae may cause haemorrhage which accounts for two common microscopic findings:

a. deposits of haemosiderin, and

b. foamy macrophages containing lipids derived from haemolysed RBC.

III. **Chromophobe RCC** has a better prognosis than other RCC.

Microscopy

i. Composed of polygonal cells arranged into solid sheets.

ii. The cells have sharply outlined contours due to raisinoid nuclei and perinuclear halo.

Clinical features

i. Microscopic or macroscopic *haematuria* found in 50% of patients.

ii. The so called *classical triad* of yesteryears, that includes haematuria, flank pain and a palpable mass, is rarely encountered in clinical practice and is found in only 10% of patients.

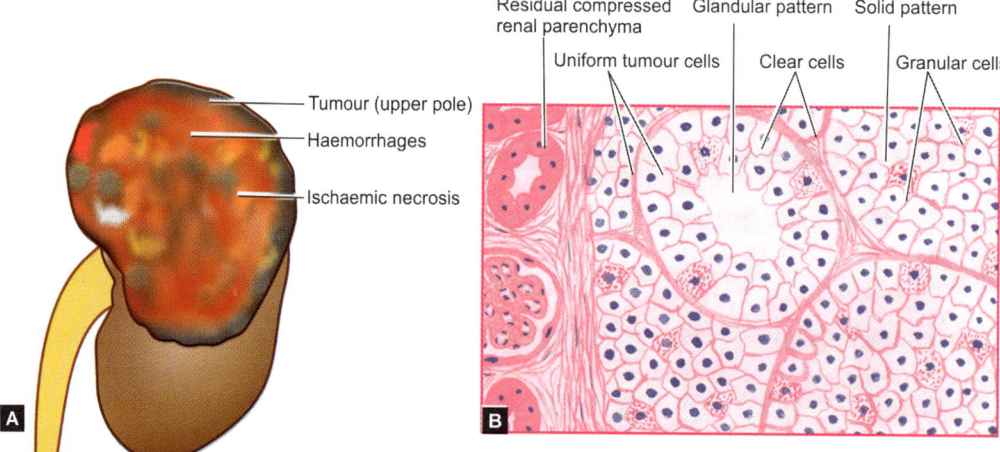

FIGURE 22.26: Renal cell carcinoma. A, The upper pole of the kidney shows a large mass while the kidney retains its reniform contour. Sectioned surface shows irregular, circumscribed, yellowish mass with areas of haemorrhages and necrosis. B, *Clear cell RCC* is composed of sheets of clear cells having hyperchromatic nuclei.

iii. In developed countries of North America and Europe, most RCCs are diagnosed by imaging studies while they are still asymptomatic, and the tumour is diagnosed when patient was examined by CT scan or MRI for some other medical problem.
iv. A number of *paraneoplastic syndromes* have been described in RCC patients. These include:
a. Polycythaemia (excess of erythropoietin)
b. Hypercalcaemia (parathyroid hormone)
c. Signs of feminisation or masculinisation (gonadotropins)
d. Cushing syndrome (glucocorticoids)
Prognosis depends on the stage of the tumour at the time of diagnosis. The overall 5-year survival is 70%. Papillary and chromophobe RCCs have a better prognosis than clear cell RCC.

Q51. What is nephroblastoma (Wilms tumour)? Discuss its salient features.
Definition Nephroblastoma (Wilms tumour) is an embryonic tumour composed of undifferentiated, primitive renal epithelial and mesenchymal components, resembling renal embryonic blastema.
Epidemiology
i. Nephroblastomas have an incidence of 1:10,000.
ii. Most of the patients are 1–3 years of age, and almost all tumours are diagnosed before the age of 10 years. It is the most common renal tumour in children under the age of 10 years and also the most common abdominal malignant tumour of infancy and childhood.
iii. Tumours are sporadic in approximately 90% of cases. The remaining cases are either familial (5%), or are components of several developmental syndromes (5%).
Etiopathogenesis The study of syndromic cases (e.g. *WAGR syndrome*) has contributed to the identification of Wilms tumour predisposing genes. WAGR syndrome comprises of:
i. *W*ilms tumour,
ii. *a*niridia (absence of iris),
iii. *g*enitourinary abnormalities, and
iv. mental *r*etardation (or *Denys-Drash syndrome*) comprising Wilms tumour, intersexual disorders, and glomerular mesangial sclerosis.
The most important of these genes is *WT1*, a tumour suppressor gene, which also plays a role in the normal embryonic/foetal development of the genitourinary system:
• WT1 gene protein product interacts with several other genes, such as β-catenin gene from the wingless signaling pathway and imprinted genes such as *IGF2*, linking Wilms tumour pathogenesis to abnormal development of the kidney.
• WT1 deletion or inactivating mutation are found in most cases of WAGR and Denys-Drash syndrome but only in 10% of sporadic cases of Wilms tumour, indicating that other genes must be also involved.
Pathology *Grossly,* most tumours present as a large mass **(Fig. 22.27, A)**. In 5% of sporadic and 20% of hereditary/syndromic cases, tumours are bilateral or multifocal.
Microscopy shows three components that are intermixed one with another **(Fig. 22.27, B)**:
i. *Blastemal*: composed of small blue cells.
ii. *Epithelial*: composed of abortive tubular and foetal glomeruli-like structures.
iii. *Stromal:* composed of spindle cells.
iv. In 5% of tumours, there are *anaplastic large cells* with irregularly shaped hyperchromatic nuclei and abnormal mitoses; these changes are considered to predict poor prognosis and resistance to chemotherapy.
Clinical features
i. Usually presents as a palpable abdominal mass.
ii. Often associated with pain, haematuria, hypertension and fever.
iii. Some cases present with distant metastases, usually in the lungs.
Prognosis Following surgical resection of the tumour, all children receive chemotherapy, sometimes combined with radiation therapy. Overall, 5-year survival rate is over 90%, but it is somewhat less in patients who have metastases and those with tumours that have anaplastic histopathology.

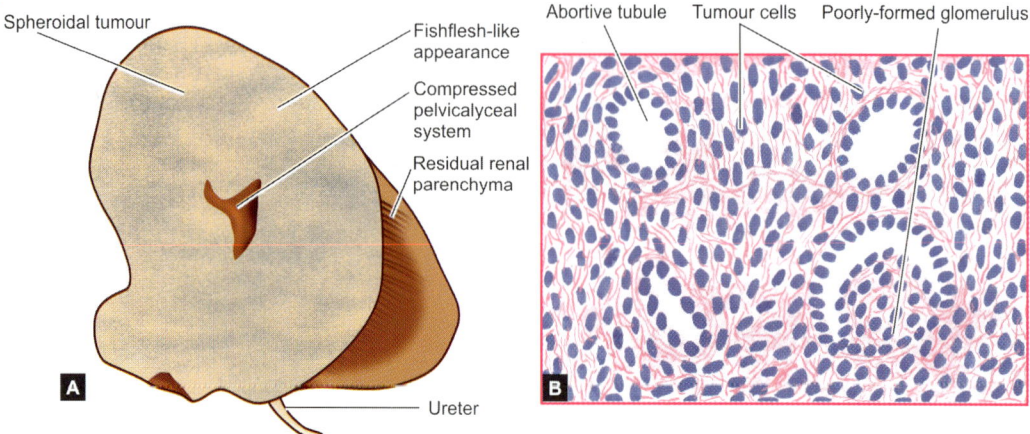

FIGURE 22.27: Wilms tumour (nephroblastoma). A, The kidney is enlarged and has ovoid and nodular appearance. The sectioned surface shows replacement of almost whole kidney by the tumour leaving a thin strip of compressed renal tissue at upper end. Cut section of the tumour is grey white, homogeneous and fleshy and has small areas of haemorrhages and necrosis. B, Microscopy shows predominance of small, immature round to oval epithelial tumour cells having hyperchromtic nuclei. A few immature and abortive tubules are present in it.

LOWER URINARY TRACT

Q52. Briefly describe normal structure of the lower urinary tract.

i. Lower urinary tracts consists of *ureters, urinary bladder and urethra*, which serve as a conduit for the discharge of urine. Bladder also stores urine and it has a capacity of 400–500 ml without overdistention.

ii. Lower urinary tract has the same *features in men and women* except for the terminal part which has its orifice in the vulva in women and on the tip of the penis in men. It is also important to note that women's urethra is shorter and easier injured due to its anatomic location which exposes it to potential trauma during intercourse.

iii. The components of the lower urinary tract have a very *prominent muscular layer* that is important for the dilatation and contraction of these organs and the propulsion of urine. The muscle layer also acts as sphincter at critical sites such as the ureterovesical valves at the entry of the ureter into the urinary bladder.

iv. *Microscopy* shows minor local variation but, in general, the entire lower urinary tract has the same layers, i.e. mucosa, muscularis and adventitia. There is no serosa except on the superior surface of the bladder which is covered with a retroflexion of the peritoneum.

v. On the luminal side, the lower urinary tract is covered with *urothelium*, also known as transitional epithelium, except for the terminal part of the urethra which is covered with *squamous epithelium*. The urothelium is 6–7 layers thick. It consists of a basal layer, intermediate zone and a superficial layer made up of umbrella cells which are resistant to moisture.

Q53. What are the most important congenital anomalies of the lower urinary tract?

Developmental anomalies of the lower urinary tract are relatively common, and found in 2–3% persons. Fortunately, these are usually minor anomalies, like *double ureters,* or *abnormally positioned ureters,* or *diverticula*, that are of limited clinical significance. Clinically more significant anomalies are as under:

I. **Congenital vesicoureteral valve incompetence** is the most important and most common anomaly.
- It is found in 1–2% children and in 30% of adults who have recurrent urinary tract infections (UTI).
- This anomaly is more common in female children and it reflects abnormal positioning of the terminal, intramural part of the ureter as it passes through the wall of the urinary bladder.

- Since the muscle layer of the bladder acts as sphincter preventing the back-flow of urine from the bladder into the ureters, anomalous positioning of the ureters results in cysto-ureteric reflux.
- It may lead to dilatation of ureters (*congenital megaureters*) and quite often to recurrent ureteritis.

II. **Ectopia vesicae (exstrophy)** is a rare anomaly of the bladder and anterior wall of the abdomen.
- It is characterised by incomplete formation of the anterior wall of the urinary bladder.
- It is usually associated with *epispadias*, i.e. incomplete closure of the posterior wall of the urethra on the dorsal side of the penis.

III. **Urachal anomalies** involve the remnants of the urachus, an embryonic structure derived from allantois that is connects the dome of the bladder with the umbilicus.
- Urachus normally involutes but if the involution is incomplete, it may give rise to a congenital bladder diverticulum, vesico-umbilical fistula, or cysts in the dome of the bladder or above it toward the umbilicus.
- Urachal columnar epithelium may give rise to adenocarcinoma of the bladder.

Q54. Write briefly on features of cystitis and its types.

Definition Cystitis is inflammation of the urinary bladder, which may be acute or chronic, infectious or sterile.

Etiopathogenesis Cystitis is a common form of UTI, affecting more often women than men, because of the anatomic positioning of the urethra in women and its short length.

i. Conditions that predispose to infections are urinary stones, prostatic hyperplasia and cancer, urinary tract manipulations (e.g. cystoscopy, resection of tumours), pregnancy.

ii. Most often, cystitis is caused by:
- Enteric bacteria such as *E. coli, Enterobacter, Proteus, Klebsiella* and *Pseudomonas*.
- *Chlamydia, Ureaplasma* and *Mycoplasma* are also pathogens.
- In immunosuppressed persons, fungal infections such as candidiasis are common.
- *Schistosoma haematobium* is a common pathogen in Egypt.

Pathology

I. **Acute cystitis** *Grossly,* the mucosa is oedematous and red from congestion and focal petechiae.
Microscopy It is infiltrated with neutrophils and macrophages and lymphocytes.

II. **Chronic cystitis** It may develop due to repeated attacks of acute cystitis. Thus, the wall of the bladder is thickened and permeated by fibrous bands which prevent its full expansion during the filling of the bladder and thus reducing the volume of the cavity.

Grossly, the mucosa is granular and rough, often suffused with blood and even focally calcified giving rise to polypoid protrusions.

Microscopy There is chronic inflammation, ulceration and granulation tissue with fibrosis. Large lymphoid follicles are sometimes prominent and the lesion is then called *follicular cystitis*.

III. **Clinicopathologic variants** Several subtypes of chronic cystitis are recognised as follows:

i. *Cystitis cystica* is a form of chronic inflammation characterised by the invagination of the surface epithelium which forms cystic Brunn nests in the lamina propria of the mucosa. These epithelial nests composed of urothelium may undergo intestinal metaplasia, and should not be mistaken for adenocarcinoma.

ii. *Malakoplakia* is a form of chronic cystitis with markedly thickened mucosa which is infiltrated with lymphocytes, plasma cells and macrophages. Macrophages have abundant cytoplasm that contains calcific round bodies (Michaelis-Gutmann bodies), formed on the nidus of phagocytosed bacteria. The pathogenesis of malakoplakia is not clear, but it probably represents an unusual response to bacterial infection. It is more common in immunosuppressed persons and following organ transplantation.

iii. *Polypoid cystitis* is characterised by submucosal oedema which leads to the formation of papillary projections and folds of the mucosa that may be mistaken for cancer. It shows microscopic signs of chronic inflammation. Typically, it is most often seen in persons with indwelling catheter inside the bladder.

iv. *Interstitial cystitis* is a form of cystitis of unknown etiology, mostly affecting middle-aged women. Clinically, it is characterised by recurrent bouts of excruciating pain, frequent painful micturition, and reduced capacity of the bladder. The mucosa is swollen and focally inflamed and often ulcerated

(Hunner ulcer). In the United States, the condition has an incidence of 2.5 per 100,000 and affects several thousand women. Currently, there is no effective treatment for this form of cystitis.

v. *Haemorrhagic cystitis* is usually a complication of cytotoxic cancer therapy. Bleeding results from urothelial cell necrosis caused by cytotoxic drugs or their metabolites excreted in urine.

Q55. What is urethritis?

Definition Urethritis is inflammation at the entry portion of the lower urinary tract and is the usual entry for the ascending infections. Thus, it frequently precedes cystitis in evolving UTI.

Etiologic types Isolated urethritis is usually a sexually-transmitted disease, which in clinical practice is divided etiologically in two groups:

i. *Gonococcal urethritis* caused by *Neisseria gonorrhoeae*.

ii. *Non-gonococcal urethritis,* most often caused by *Mycoplasma* or *Ureaplasma*.

iii. *Non-infectious urethritis* is also a part of *Reiter syndrome,* which includes a triad of urethritis, arthritis, and uveitis.

Q56. What are the tumours of the urinary bladder? Discuss their epidemiology and etiologic factors.

Definition Most urinary bladder tumours are urothelial (transitional cell) carcinomas of varying degree of malignancy.

Epidemiology

i. Urinary bladder carcinomas represent 7% of all newly diagnosed malignancies in men and 3% in women.

ii. Overall, this cancer account for 3% of all human malignant tumours.

iii. Urothelial carcinomas are 3-times more common in men than women.

iv. Most tumours originate in the elderly and are rare in persons younger than 50 years.

Etiopathogenesis A number of environmental and host factors are associated with an increased risk of urothelial carcinoma, as under:

i. *Smoking* is the most important risk factor. It is associated with a 2–5 times increased risk, probably related to urinary excretion of metabolites derived from carcinogens in the tobacco smoke.

ii. *Industrial occupations* account still for many cases of urothelial carcinoma, even though improved industrial hygiene has reduced the importance of these factors. At increased risk are the industrial workers exposed for prolonged periods of time (>20 years) to aniline dyes, rubber, plastic and textile components.

iii. *Schistosomiasis* is a risk factor in endemic areas such as Egypt and Sudan. *Schistosoma haematobium* has a predilection for invading the bladder and laying eggs in its wall. These events cause chronic inflammation associated with squamous metaplasia of the urothelium, that leads ultimately to formation of squamous cell carcinoma of the bladder.

iv. *Dietary factors* have been implicated in the pathogenesis of urothelial carcinoma, but there is no definitive proof that any of the suspected food ingredients are really carcinogenic.

v. *Certain drugs*, such as cyclophosphamide and analgesics have been implicated as potential carcinogens, but the evidence is controversial.

vi. *Local factors* that are associated with an increased incidence of cancer are diverticula, extrophied bladder urinary diversion. These conditions are associated with an increased incidence of bladder cancer, but these conditions are rare. Previous irradiation is also a risk factor.

Q57. Discuss salient features of urothelial carcinomas.

General features

i. Urothelial tumours can be solitary or multiple.

ii. In 90% of cases, early tumours are papillary, whereas the remaining 10% present as flat indurated lesions.

iii. In both categories, tumours may be invasive and non-invasive **(Fig. 22.28)**.

iv. Most often, they are located on lateral wall, followed by posterior wall and trigone.

v. Urinary bladder tumours are often *multicentric*, i.e. they arise in several location in the lower urinary tract. They are also *polychronotropic*, i.e. may develop one after another over a period of time. These observations support the theory of *field effect*, which implies that the entire lower urinary tract epithelium is at an increased risk to respond unfavourably to potential carcinogens.

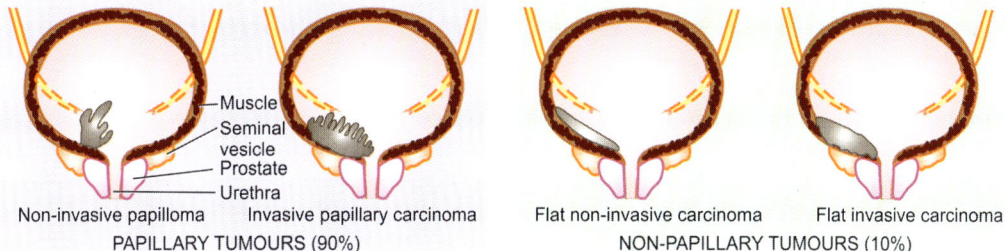

FIGURE 22.28: Gross patterns of epithelial bladder tumours.

Pathology

Most tumours (90%) are urothelial, while others such as squamous cell carcinomas, adenocarcinomas, small cell carcinomas and mixed tumours or sarcomas are less common.

Urothelial tumours are classified as benign (urothelial papilloma) or malignant, which are further subclassified according to the degree of their malignancy **(Table 22.15)**:
- carcinoma in situ (CIS),
- papillary urothelial neoplasm of low malignant potential (PUNLMP), and
- urothelial carcinoma (low grade and high grade)

I. **Papilloma** is a rare benign tumour (1% of all bladder tumours).

Grossly, it may be solitary or multiple, exophytic or inverted (endophytic). Most urothelial papillomas are exophytic, papillary and small (< 2 cm).

Microscopy Papillomas are composed of papillae that have a fibrovascular core and are lined by transitional cells arranged in a normal number of layers (up to 6–7). Tumour cells resemble normal urothelium with surface umbrella cells and well preserved basal cell polarity. Mitoses are not evident and there is no necrosis.

TABLE 22.15 Histologic criteria for classifying urothelial tumours as per WHO/ISUP.

FEATURE	PAPILLOMA	PUNLMP	LOW-GRADE UC	HIGH-GRADE UC
I. ARCHITECTURE				
1. Papillae	Delicate	Delicate	Fused, branching	Fused, branching
2. Cellular organisation				
i. Resemblance to normal	Yes	Generally yes	Orderly	Mainly disordered
ii. Thickness	Normal	Any thickness	Any thickness	Any thickness
iii. Loss of polarity	No	No	Minimal	Frequent
iv. Cohesiveness	Yes	Yes	Yes	Often lost
v. Crowding	No	No	Minimal	Yes
II. CELLULAR FEATURES				
1. Nuclear size	Normal	May be uniformly enlarged	Enlarged with variation in size	Enlarged with variation in size
2. Nuclear shape	Normal	Elongated, uniform	Round-to-oval, slight pleomorphism	Moderate to marked pleomorphism
3. Nuclear chromatin	Fine	Fine	Mild variation	Moderate to marked variation
4. Nucleoli	Absent	Rare	Inconspicuous, small, regular	Conspicuous, multiple
5. Mitosis	Absent	Rare, basal	Occasional, any level	Frequent, any level
6. Umbrella cells	Present	Present	Usually present	May be absent

[WHO/ISUP, WHO-International Society for Urologic Pathology, 2004; PUNLMP, papillary urothelial neoplasm of low malignant potential; UC, transitional cell (urothelial) carcinoma].

Prognosis Although benign, papillomas may recur, but do not progress to cancer.

II. **Papillary urothelial neoplasm of low malignant potential (PUNLMP)** is a rare lesion that has some features of papilloma but show increased cellularity.
- Furthermore, they also show some cytologic changes that are 'worrisome', such as uniform nuclear enlargement of their elongated nuclei and loss of cellular cohesiveness.
- Mitoses may be found but are limited to the basal layer.

Prognosis PUNLMP may recur, but does not require extensive surgery.

III. **Carcinoma in situ**, also known as **flat urothelial carcinoma,** is characterised by microscopic features of high grade malignancy limited to a thickened part of bladder epithelium. The basement membrane underlying the lesion is intact and there is no invasion.

Microscopy These features include: disorderly arrangement of atypical cells that have lost polarity and do not show regular layering. The tumour cells are pleomorphic, lack cohesiveness and usually have enlarged hyperchromatic nuclei which have lost polarity. Mitoses are found in all layers and may be atypical.

Prognosis Carcinoma in situ is treated by injecting attenuated *Mycobacterium tuberculosis* (BCG), into the bladder but if the tumour does not respond, or if it becomes invasive, cystectomy must be performed. If left untreated, most cases (up to 70%) will progress to invasive cancer.

IV. **Low grade papillary urothelial carcinoma** is the most common form of urothelial cancer.
Microscopy
i. It shows mild architectural and cytologic atypia.
ii. Papillae vary in size and may be fused. Papillae have an increased number of layers which retain their ordinary layering and polarity of cells, and the surface is covered with umbrella cells. The cells have enlarged nuclei that slightly vary in size and shape. Nucleoli are inconspicuous and the mitotic figures are rare and limited to the lower half.
iii. Most tumours are noninvasive, or invade only the lamina propria mucosae. Invasion of the muscularis propria is seen in a minority of cases.

Prognosis Tumours tend to recur but have a good prognosis. Progression to high grade tumours may occur but is uncommon (<10%); mortality is low, 2–3%.

V. **High grade papillary urothelial carcinomas** are usually invasive but may be also non-invasive.
Microscopy Features of high grade tumours include: marked architectural disorganisation and cytologic atypia **(Fig. 22.29)**.
- Normal layering is lost and the cells show crowding, loss of polarity and cohesiveness.
- There is nuclear enlargement, hyperchromasia and pleomorphism.
- Nucleoli are prominent and the mitoses are seen in all layers and may be atypical.
- High grade papillary urothelial carcinomas include several *histologic subtypes*, which are almost all associated with adverse prognosis. These microscopic subtypes include entities such as micropapillary, plasmacytoid, sarcomatoid, giant cell type and poorly-differentiated carcinomas.

Prognosis These tumours account for most invasive urothelial carcinomas and consequent mortality which is in the range of 25–35%. The prognosis depends primarily on the stage of the malignancy and its stage, i.e. the extent of its spread.

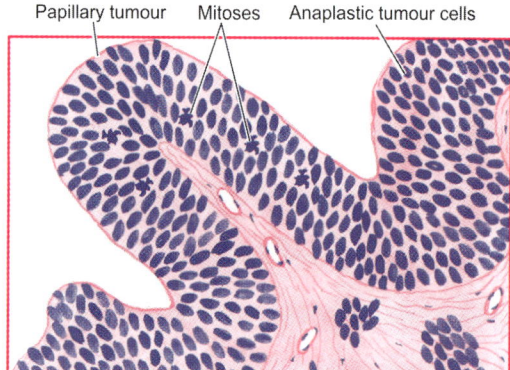

FIGURE 22.29: Urothelial (Transitional cell) carcinoma, high grade. The tumour shows papillae covered by cells having pleomorphism, nuclear enlargement and mitosis.

Q58. Briefly comment on urinary bladder malignant tumours other than urothelial carcinomas.

Urinary bladder tumours, other than urothelial carcinomas, are rare but some of the clinically significant ones are as under:

I. **Squamous cell carcinoma** is a rare highly malignant cancer accounting for only 5% of all bladder malignancies. It is, however, a common form of bladder cancer in some African countries like Egypt and Sudan where it is related to chronic infection with *Schistosoma haematobium*.
- In contrast to urothelial carcinoma which is mostly papillary, squamous cell carcinoma presents as an invasive mass with surface ulceration and deep invasion into the muscularis propria.
- It has a poor prognosis.

II. **Adenocarcinoma** is an invasive tumour composed of gland-like structures. It originates from urachal remnants in the dome of the bladder, metaplastic glands of cystitis cystica, periurethral and periprostatic glands.

III. **Small cell carcinoma** is a neuroendocrine carcinoma similar to the small cell lung carcinoma. It is a rapidly growing tumour that tends to metastasise widely with a rapid downhill clinical course.

IV. **Sarcomas** of the bladder are most often classified as rhabdomyosarcomas or undifferentiated pleomorphic sarcomas.
- Most sarcomas are diagnosed in persons who are older than 40 years and all of them have a poor prognosis.
- Rhabdomyosarcoma of urinary bladder may also occur in children and is classified as *embryonal rhabdomyosarcoma*. It is also known as *sarcoma botryoides* because of its intravesical growth in form of grape-like myxoid multivesicular tumours. Childhood sarcomas are treated quite successfully by combined approach that includes surgical resection followed by chemotherapy.

Q59. What are the tumours and tumour-like lesions of the urethra?

i. *Caruncle* is the only clinically significant tumour-like lesion of the female urethra. It presents as a small nodule, 1–2 cm in diameter in the female urethra. It is composed of inflamed granulation tissue, resembling pyogenic granuloma of the mouth.

ii. *Carcinomas* of the urethra are uncommon. Most of these tumours are urothelial carcinomas similar to those in the urinary bladder.

> **Chapter 22e Supplement: Online Content**
>
> *Digital content of this chapter available with this book is meant for enhanced learning and self-assessment. In addition, it contains 35 Multiple Choice Questions (MCQs), 06 Clinicopathologic Vignettes, and 09 Image-based Questions; these are followed by their answers along with explanatory notes of correct and incorrect answers.*

CHAPTER 23

Male Genital System

■ TESTIS AND EPIDIDYMIS

Q1. What are the key facts about the normal anatomy, histology and physiology of the testis that are important for understanding its pathology?

- *Testicles* (enclosed in tunica albuginea), *epididymis* and the *spermatic cords* are paired organs enveloped by tunica vaginalis and located in the scrotum.
- Testis is the main reproductive organ producing the *spermatozoa*, while the epididymis contributes the fluid to the sperm.
- *Additional fluid* is added by seminal vesicles and the prostate as the spermatozoa pass through the terminal excretory part of the urogenital system on their way to the tip of the urethra.
- Spermatozoa are produced by the *germinal epithelium* in the seminiferous tubules of the testis. Seminiferous tubules are lined by germ cells maturing in a sequence: from spermatogonia (lying on the basement membrane), to spermatocytes, to spermatids, and finally spermatozoa (on the luminal side).
- *Sertoli cells* provide support to spermatogenesis, and also secrete inhibin, which inhibits the secretion of pituitary gonadotropin.
- The peritubular interstitium contains *Leydig cells*, also known as *interstitial cells*, which produce androgens, the male sex hormones like testosterone **(Fig. 23.1, A)**.

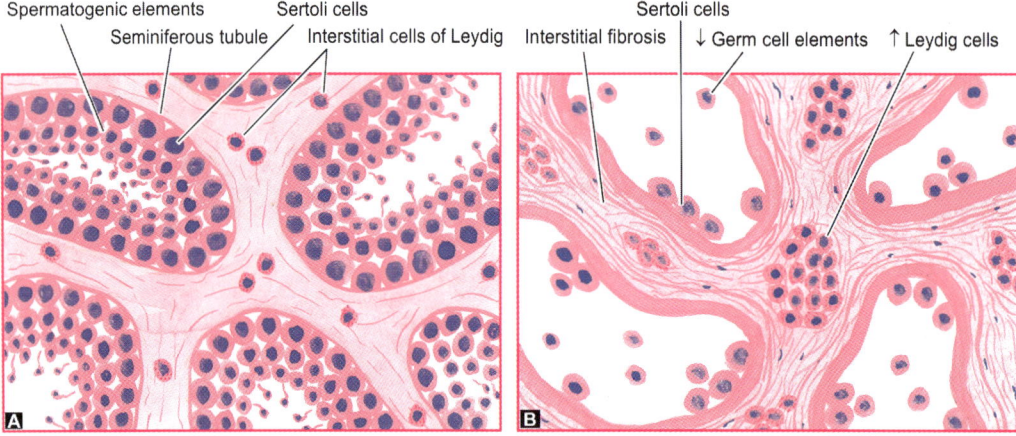

FIGURE 23.1: A, Microscopy of normal testis. It shows seminiferous tubules lined by spermatogenic cells and Sertoli cells while the interstitium contains a few Leydig cells. B, Histology of cryptorchid testis (testicular atrophy). The seminiferous tubules show hyalinisation, thickened basement membrane and interstitial fibrosis. There is no spermatogenic activity. Clusters of Leydig cells are seen in the interstitium.

- The seminiferous tubules drain into *collecting ducts* which form the *rete testis* that connects to *vasa efferentia*, which are part of the epididymis.
- Epididymis conducts the sperms into the *vas deferens* that connects with the *urethra*.

Q2. Write briefly on cryptorchidism.

Definition Cryptorchidism or undescended testis is a congenital abnormality in which the normal descent of the testis from the abdominal cavity through the inguinal canal to the scrotum is arrested. Cryptorchidism is found in 1% of the entire male population. In most cases, the testis is located in the inguinal canal, but in some cases it may be retained in the abdominal cavity. Quite rarely, it is truly hidden, as the name implies (in Greek *cryptos*=hidden), and outside of the normal descent route of the foetal testis. In 10% of cases, cryptorchidism is bilateral.

Etiopathogenesis Cryptorchidism, in most instances, is an isolated abnormality unrelated to any defined risk factor which could include the following:

i. *Mechanical factors* that prevent the descent of the testis, like narrow inguinal canal, short spermatic cord or connective tissue strands obstructing the inguinal canal.

ii. *Genetic and chromosomal abnormalities*, as it has been shown that cryptorchidism may be associated with several developmental syndromes, such as Down syndrome, trisomy 13 and intersex conditions such as gonadal dysgenesis or androgen insensitivity syndrome affecting the development of genital organs.

iii. *Hormonal factors* during pregnancy, such as maternal intake of diethylstilbestrol or oestrogens.

Pathology

Gross The cryptorchid testis is initially of normal size. If retained for longer periods of time outside the scrotum, it becomes smaller, firm and fibrotic.

Microscopy

i. The seminiferous tubules of such testes have thickened basement membranes and are surrounded by interstitial fibrosis.

ii. The number of germ cells is usually reduced and in more than 50% of cases there are only some Sertoli cells and no spermatogenesis **(Fig. 23.1, B)**.

iii. There is prominence of Leydig cells in the interstitium.

iv. In neglected cases there is hyalinisation of tubules.

Clinical features

i. *Infertility* with azoospermia in persons who have *bilateral cryptorchidism*.

ii. Men with *unilateral cryptorchidism* in 60% of cases are normally fertile and have a normal sperm count. In the remaining 40% there is *oligospermia*, defined as 20 million sperms per ml. Despite reduced sperm count, most of them will, however, remain fertile.

iii. *Orchidopexy* does not improve the sperm counts. All persons with cryptorchidism, including those who have had orchidopexy, are at 5–6 times higher risk for testicular germ cell neoplasia than men without cryptorchidism.

Q3. Define male infertility. Based on etiology, how is it classified?

Definition Infertility is defined empirically as an inability to conceive after 1 year of coital activity with the same sexual partner without contraception. The male partner is infertile in 20% couples, the female in 40%, and both partners in 20% instances. In 20% of infertile couples, no cause can be identified.

Classification Male infertility can be classified into three groups: i) pre-testicular, ii) testicular, and iii) post-testicular.

i. *Pre-testicular causes* include several chronic conditions as:

a. Endocrine conditions, e.g. hypopituitarism, oestrogen excess, glucocorticoid excess, hypothyroidism, diabetes mellitus

b. Systemic diseases interfering with fertility, e.g. metabolic syndrome, end-stage liver and renal disease

c. Chronic debilitating infections, e.g. tuberculosis and AIDS

d. Drugs and substance abuse

ii. *Testicular causes* form the largest group of infertility in males. This group comprises diseases that reduce or completely abolish spermatogenesis as under:

a. Bilateral cryptorchidism, hypospermatogenesis, maturation arrest, Sertoli-only syndrome with complete absence of spermatogenesis
b. Developmental chromosomal disorders such as Klinefelter syndrome
c. Orchitis due to mumps infection or autoimmune causes
d. Irradiation damage
iii. *Post-testicular causes* leading to an obstruction to the outflow of sperm from the testis, or sperm motility disorders, as under:
a. Congenital block of the vas deferens as in cystic fibrosis
b. Acquired block in the epididymis due to infections (e.g. gonorrhoea or tuberculosis), or trauma
c. Surgical intervention, e.g. voluntary vasectomy for contraception
d. Impaired sperm motility, e.g. immotile cilia syndrome

Q4. What are the etiologic types of orchitis? Give their salient clinicopathologic features.

Definition Orchitis is an inflammations of the testis. Since the testis is closely linked to the epididymis, it is often associated with epididymitis, presenting as *epididymo-orchitis*.
Etiologic types and clinicopathologic features Following three main types are recognised:
i. **Non-specific epididymitis and orchitis** may be acute or chronic.
a. Most often, it is *secondary* to urethritis, cystitis, prostatitis. Infections of these organs spread to the testis and epididymis via the vas deferens or lymphatics.
b. *Haematogenous infections* occur in viral infections (e.g. mumps, chickenpox or influenza), bacterial sepsis or parasitic infections (e.g. filariasis).
c. The most *common pathogens* in sexually active young adults are *Neisseria gonorrhoeae* and *Chlamydia trachomatis*. In older men, the infection is most often caused by uropathogens such as *E. coli* and *Pseudomonas*.
Clinical and pathologic features
- Acute epididymo-orchitis is characterised by congestion, oedema and swelling, redness and pain.
- Both organs are infiltrated with acute inflammatory cells.
- Gonorrhoea is frequently accompanied by formation of multiple confluent abscesses in the testis and/or epididymis.
- Acute inflammation may resolve or progress to a chronic form with destruction of seminiferous tubules and their replacement by fibrous connective tissue.

ii. **Granulomatous orchitis** is an uncommon autoimmune disorder affecting middle-aged men.
Etiology is not known, but the presence of non-caseating granulomas suggests an immune reaction against the germ cell and sperm.
Gross It presents with enlargement of the testis resembling tumours.
Microscopy In addition to granulomas, the testis contains infiltrates of lymphocytes and plasma cells, causing destruction of seminiferous tubules with replacement fibrosis.

iii. **Tuberculous epididymo-orchitis** results from secondary spread of *M. tuberculosis* from the lungs or genitourinary tuberculosis.
a. It is rare in the Western world but it still can be seen in underdeveloped countries having widespread tuberculosis.
b. Infection begins with an induration and enlargement of the epididymis extending then to the testis.
c. *Microscopy* It is characterised by caseating granulomas which contain *M. tuberculosis*.
d. Destruction of epididymis and testis may be accompanied by the formation of discharging sinuses leading to the scrotal skin.

Q5. Write briefly on torsion of the testis.

Definition Torsion of the testis involves a sudden rotation of the testis around the spermatic cord resulting in a sudden interruption of arterial and venous flow to the testis.
Clinicopathologic features
i. It occurs most often in children and young adults and may involve a fully-descended or an undescended testis.
ii. It is caused by a sudden muscular effort, an unusual movement during sport events or trauma.
iii. Cessation of blood flow leads to haemorrhagic ischaemic necrosis of the testis.

iv. Testis is usually lost since the torsion cannot be reversed fast enough to prevent widespread ischaemic necrosis.

Q6. What is varicocele?

Definition Varicocele is tortuous dilatation of testicular veins in the pampiniform plexus. Varicocele may cause infertility.

Types and clinicopathologic features Varicocele may be primary (or idiopathic) and secondary due to some obstruction of venous outflow from the testis:

i. *Primary varicocele*, the more common variant, almost always involves the left side because the left spermatic vein enters the vena cava at a right angle, in contrast to the right spermatic vein which enters the vena cava obliquely. Furthermore, the left spermatic vein is much longer and can be compressed externally.

ii. *Secondary varicocele* is usually caused by obstruction of venous outflow from the testis, as in pelvic tumours or after surgery. It can be one-sided or bilateral, with no predilection for the left side.

Q7. What is hydrocele?

Definition Hydrocele is an accumulation of serous fluid in the virtual space lined by the tunica vaginalis. It may be acute or chronic, congenital or acquired.

Etiology Two types with distinct causes:

i. *Congenital hydrocele* is seen in infants and small children due to persistence of the space between the layers of tunica vaginalis that fill with serous fluid.

ii. *Acquired hydrocele* may be due to trauma, systemic oedema (e.g. cardiac failure and renal disease), or fibrosis due to scrotal infections (e.g. gonorrhoea, tuberculosis, syphilis).

Pathology Hydrocele contains serous fluid which is clear and yellowish.

- The wall of hydrocele sac is made up of fibrous tissue, which gets infiltrated with lymphocytes in long lasting lesions.
- Secondary haemorrhage due to trauma may transform it into *haematocele*.

NOTE: Haematocele may develop even without pre-existing hydrocele, usually due to traumatic rupture of testicular veins and bleeding into the cavity lined by tunica vaginalis.

Q8. How are testicular tumours classified? Give broad principles of classification.

Testicular tumours can be classified into several groups as listed in **Table 23.1**. Broad principles of this classification are as under:

i. *Germ cell tumours (GCT)* account for 90% of tumours (group I and II in the Table), and must be distinguished from *non-germ cell tumours* (groups III-VI in the Table), most importantly sex cord-stromal cells (e.g. Sertoli and Leydig cells tumours).

TABLE 23.1 The WHO classification of testicular tumours (2016)*.

I. Germ cell tumours derived from germ cell neoplasia in situ

A. *Noninvasive germ cell neoplasia*
 1. Germ cell neoplasia in situ
 2. Specific forms of intratubular germ cell neoplasia
B. *Tumours of single histological type (pure forms)*
 1. Seminoma
 2. Non-seminomatous germ cell tumours
  i. Embryonal carcinoma
  ii. Yolk sac tumour, postpubertal
  iii. Trophoblastic tumours (choriocarcinoma)
  iv. Teratoma, postpubertal type
C. *Non-seminomatous germ cell tumours of more than one histological type*
 1. Mixed germ cell tumours

II. Germ cell tumours unrelated to germ cell neoplasia in situ

1. Spermatocytic tumour
2. Teratomas, prepubertal type
3. Yolk sac tumour, prepubertal type

III. Sex cord-stromal tumours

A. *Pure tumours*
1. Leydig cell tumour
2. Sertoli cell tumour
3. Granulosa cell tumour
B. *Mixed sex cord-stromal tumour*

IV. Combined tumours (Germ cell-sex cord stromal tumours)

Gonadoblastoma

V. Miscellaneous tumours

1. Epithelial tumours
2 Haemangioma

VI. Haematolymphoid tumours

*Adapted from Moch et al. The 2016 WHO classification of tumours of the urinary system and male genital organs—Part A: Renal, penile and testicular tumours. *European Urology*. 2016; 70:93-105.

ii. GCT group is further into two subgroups:
- Group I GCT: Tumours which *originate from germ cell neoplasia in situ (GCNIS),* such as seminoma and non-seminomatous germ cell tumours (NSGCT).
- Group II GCT: Tumours which develop directly from germ cells and *do not originate from GCNIS*, such as spermatocytic tumour, prepubertal teratoma and prepubertal yolk sac tumour.

iii. The group originating from GCNIS contains the most important tumours, such as *seminomatous* (i.e. seminoma) and *non-seminomatous GCT* (NSGCT).

iv. NSGCT comprise several histologic entities such as embryonal carcinoma, yolk sac tumour, trophoblastic tumour (choriocarcinoma), and post-pubertal teratoma.

v. Each of these histologic components may grow as part of a NSGCT, or form tumours composed exclusively of that subtype (e.g. pure embryonal carcinoma, yolk sac tumour, or pure choriocarcinoma).

vi. Tumours that *do not originate from GCNIS* are relatively rare and are mentioned only because some of them (e.g. yolk sac tumour and teratoma) account for most common germ cell tumours in children.

Q9. What are key general features of testicular tumours? Comment on common factors in their etiology and general pathogenesis.

Common general features

i. The *incidence* of testicular tumours shows geographic variation:
- It is the highest in Northern parts of Europe but less common in Africa and Asia, indicating that some environmental and/or genetic factors play a role.
- In the US, testicular tumours have an incidence of 6 per 100,000 and its incidence rates are slowly rising.

ii. *Age profile* Over 90% tumours are found in the men who are 25 to 45 years of age. Two small age peaks are also registered—one in infants and children under that age of 5 years, and the second in the elderly, comprising mostly non-germ cell tumours.

iii. *Histologic types and behaviour*
- Over 90% of testicular tumours are of germ cell origin.
- Over 90% of testicular tumours are malignant, but with modern chemotherapy more than 90% of them can be cured.
- All malignant testicular tumours metastasise first to the periaortic lymph nodes.

iv. *Serologic tumour markers* are found in the blood of 50% of testicular tumour patients and these are useful for diagnosis.
- Common markers are: human chorionic gonadotropin (hCG) and alfa-foetoprotein (AFP).
- Lactate dehydrogenase (LDH) is also elevated in serum of patients with testicular tumours but is not specific for testicular tumours. It is used only as rough estimate of the tumour mass—it correlates with the size of tumour in the testis or in the metastatic sites.

Etiology Unknown, even though there are some well-known risk factors such as:

i. Cryptorchidism, with 5–6 times higher risk than in non-cryptorchid men.

ii. Gonadal dysgenesis and intersex conditions, with 25 times higher risk than normal.

iii. Familial testicular cancer: father-to-son 4 times higher, brother-to-brother 2 times higher risk.

Pathogenesis Histogenesis of testicular tumours is schematically shown in **Figure 23.2**.

i. Most germ cell tumours develop from preinvasive *intratubular germ neoplasia in situ (GCNIS)* which carry a marker *isochromosome [i(12p)]* made of the short arm of the chromosome 12, formed after the deletion of the 12q (the long arm).

ii. *Hyperdiploidy* is a constant feature of all GCNIS-derived tumours. As the tumour becomes invasive seminoma or embryonal carcinoma, it starts losing chromosomes but still remain hyperdiploid.

iii. 10–20% of testicular GCTs *originate directly from spermatogonia* and do not pass through the GCNIS stage at all.

iv. Oncogenes are not involved in tumorigenesis, except *KIT* which is mutated in 25% tumours.

Q10. What is seminoma? Write briefly on its etiopathogenesis, pathology and salient clinical features.

Definition Seminoma is a malignant germ cell tumour composed of a single cell type that has some common features with foetal gonocytes. It is the most common testicular tumour accounting for approximately 50% of all GCTs.

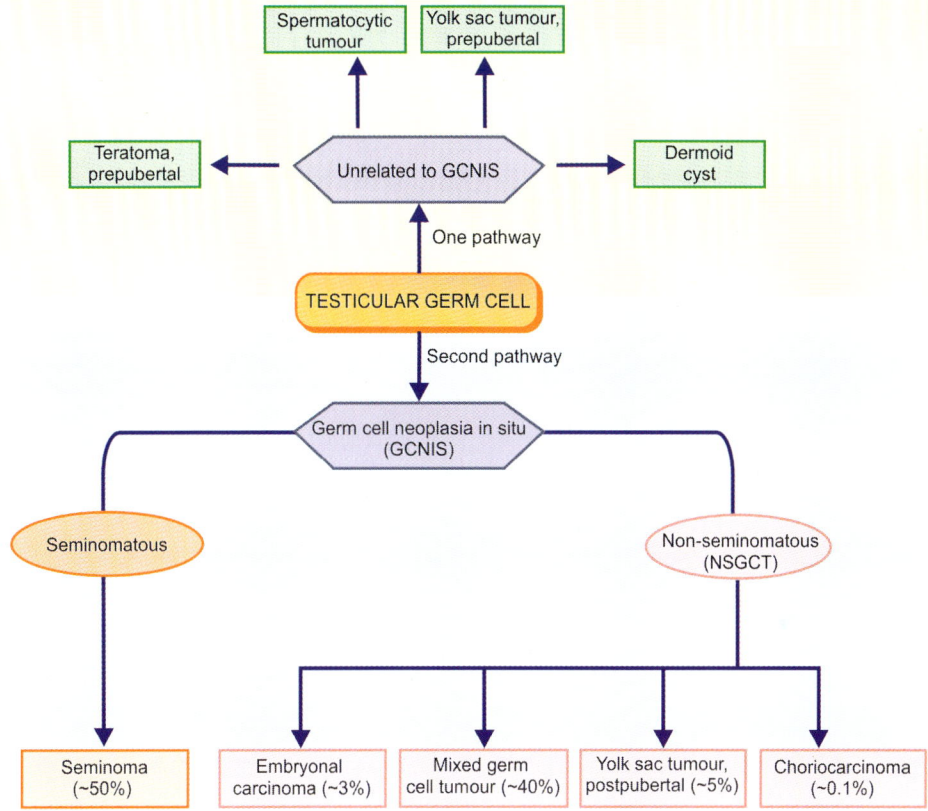

FIGURE 23.2: Schematic illustration on histogenesis of the WHO 2016 classification of testicular tumours.

Etiopathogenesis Incompletely known.
i. Seminomas originate from GCNIS and are the most common germ cell tumours found in cryptorchid testes and dysgenetic gonads, indicating that the tumour is somehow linked to abnormal testicular development.
ii. Like GCNIS, seminoma also has a marker chromosome i(p12).

Pathology
Gross Most tumours measure 3–5 cm in diameter. Typical tumours present as a nodule, sharply demarcated from the normal testis. On cross section, it is multilobulated, fleshy or firm, and homogeneously tan-creamy **(Fig. 23.3,A)**.
Microscopy **(Fig. 23.3,B)**:
i. Arrangement of tumour cells into solid lobules, surrounded by fibrous connective tissue strands infiltrated with lymphocytes.
ii. The tumour cells are polygonal, having abundant clear cytoplasm rich on glycogen and lipids.
iii. The cell membranes are sharply outlined, and there is no cell-to-cell overlapping.
iv. Tumour cells have vesicular nuclei with prominent nucleoli. Mitotic figures are infrequent.
v. Immunohistochemistry is used to confirm the light microscopic diagnosis and to distinguish seminoma from embryonal carcinoma (page 577).
vi. Some tumours (10%) contain scattered syncytiotrophoblastic multinucleated giant cells which account for the slight elevation of hCG in the blood of some seminoma patients.
vii. Most seminomas are composed of a single cell type but in about 10% cases they may be admixed to NSGCT. Such mixed tumours are considered to be variants of NSGCT and are grouped with them for treatment purposes.

Clinical features
i. Seminomas are found in young and middle aged men and have their peak incidence in the 25–45 years age group.

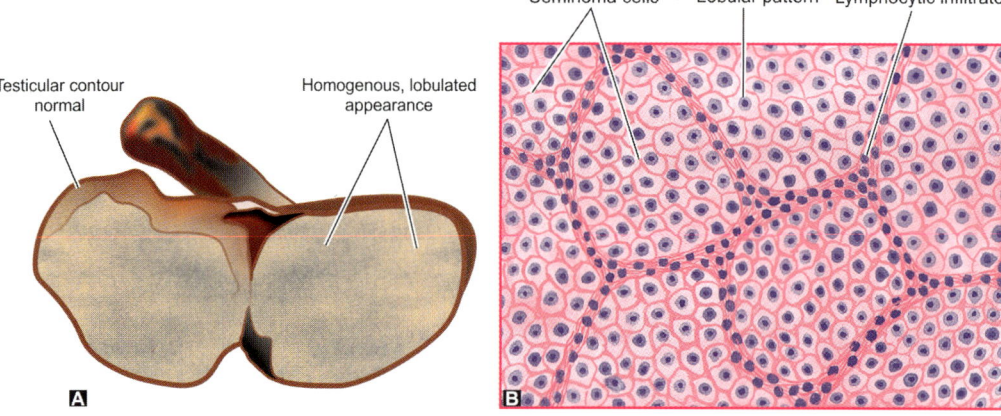

FIGURE 23.3: Seminoma testis. A, The testis is enlarged but without distorting its contour. Sectioned surface shows replacement of the entire testis by lobulated, homogeneous, grey-white mass. B, Microscopy of the tumour shows lobules of monomorphic seminoma cells separated by delicate fibrous stroma containing lymphocytic infiltration.

ii. Retroperitoneal lymph node metastases are found in approximately 30% cases at the time of diagnosis.

iii. Seminomas do not produce diagnostic serologic tumour markers, even though in some cases there is slight elevation of hCG in blood.

iv. Orchidectomy is the treatment of choice for cases that do not have metastases. In more advanced cases, surgery must be supplemented with radiation therapy and even chemotherapy. Seminomas can be cured in over in over 90% of cases. Due to their radiosensitivity, seminomas had a better prognosis than NSGCT even before the era of modern chemotherapy.

Q11. Briefly discuss etiopathogenesis and clinicopathologic features of common non-seminomatous germ cell tumours (NSGCT).

Definition NSGCT, also known as *mixed germ cell tumours*, are malignant germ cell tumours composed of malignant stem cells called embryonal carcinoma cells, and their differentiated derivatives, which may include somatic tissues forming teratoma, and extra-embryonic tissues like yolk sac or placental chorionic epithelium.

Tumours composed of each of these malignant components (i.e. *pure* embryonal carcinoma, choriocarcinoma, and post-pubertal yolk sac tumour) are also included for clinical and treatment purposes under the heading of NSGCT.

NSGCT occur in the same age group (25–45 years) as seminomas, although most patients are 10 years younger.

Etiopathogenesis Following features of NSGCTs are similar to seminomas:

a. They too develop from GCNIS

b. They are hyperdiploid

c. They have a marker chromosome i(p12)

Tumours equivalent to NSGCT may develop in the ovaries and extragonadal sites. The latter tumours probably develop from germ cells which have been misplaced during foetal development and not having reached the foetal gonads during their migration.

Clinicopathologic features Most NSGCT are composed of malignant stem cells called embryonal carcinoma cells and somatic tissues formed of teratoma, as well extraembryonic tissues corresponding to yolk sac and choriocarcinoma.

I. **Embryonal carcinoma** In 10% of NSGCTs, the tumours are composed only of embryonal carcinoma cells.

i. *Microscopy* The tumour is composed of undifferentiated *highly malignant anaplastic cells* with scanty cytoplasm and a high nucleocytoplasmic ratio, resembling embryonic cells from early stages of development. Mitoses are prominent and typically admixed to apoptotic bodies. These cells are arranged in solid nests, tubulo-papillary or glandular structures, and occasionally may form embryoid bodies resembling early stage embryos.

ii. *Immunohistochemistry* is useful for differentiating embryonal carcinoma from seminoma cells. Like seminoma, embryonal carcinoma cells are positive for germ cell markers such as Oct-3/4, SALL4 and PLAP but they differ from seminoma by expressing cytokeratins, CD30, and SOX2 (page 575).

iii. Embryonal carcinoma cells are highly malignant and *metastasise* widely. Early metastases are to retroperitoneal lymph nodes, and from there to other organs in the body.

iv. Since embryonal carcinoma cells are developmentally pluripotent like the normal embryonic cells from early embryos, they can *differentiate into other cells* found in somatic tissues of the body. These include: neural tissue, squamous epithelium, cartilage, etc. These tissues may be intermixed with each other and form *benign teratomas*.

v. *Prognosis* Malignant cells of embryonal carcinoma are very sensitive to modern platinum-based chemotherapy and the tumours can be cured in most cases. Following chemotherapy of primary or metastatic NSGCT, the embryonal carcinomas are wiped out and the remaining tumour tissues composed of only teratoma do not grow, and thus do not endanger the patient's life. Chemotherapy based on that principle has increased the cure rate of NSGCT, even those with distant metastases, to 90%.

II. **Yolk sac and choriocarcinoma** elements are malignant components of NSGCT derived from embryonal carcinoma cells. These components correspond to *extraembryonic structures* called yolk sac and chorionic trophoblast of the placenta.

Extraembryonic derivatives in these tumours are important for two reasons:

i. They produce *tumour markers* that are detectable in blood. Choriocarcinoma elements produce *human chorionic gonadotropin (hCG)*, whereas yolk sac components produce *alpha-foetoprotein (AFP)*.

ii. The second reason of importance for identifying yolk sac and choriocarcinoma elements is that these tissues usually *retain their malignancy* and may be resistant to chemotherapy. Yolk sac elements (more appropriately called yolk sac carcinoma) remaining after chemotherapy, represent actually the most common cause for 'chemotherapy-failure' of NSGCT.

Q12. Tabulate the contrasting features of seminomatous and non-seminomatous germ cell tumours.

Table 23.2 sums up the major distinguishing features of the two main groups of testicular germ cell tumours (GCT).

TABLE 23.2 Distinguishing features of seminomatous (SGCT) and non-seminomatous (NSGCT) germ cell tumours of testis.

FEATURE	SGCT	NSGCT
1. *Tumour type*	Seminoma (pure form)	Embryonal carcinoma, yolk sac tumour (postpubertal), choriocarcinoma, teratomas (postpubertal and with somatic malignancy), mixed GCTs
2. *Primary tumour*	Larger, confined to testis for sufficient time; testicular contour retained	May be smaller, at times indistinct; testicular contour may be distorted
3. *Metastasis*	Generally to regional lymph nodes	Haematogenous spread common and early
4. *Response to radiation*	Radiosensitive	Radioresistant
5. *Serum markers*	hCG; generally low levels	hCG, AFP, and LDH elevated
6. *Prognosis*	Better	Poor

Q13. What is spermatocytic tumour?

Definition Spermatocytic tumour is a very rare benign germ cell testicular tumour, usually found in older adults (average age approximately 50 years).

Clinicopathologic features

i. Spermatocytic tumour originates only in the testes and does not occur at extragonadal sites nor does it have a counterpart in the ovary.

ii. The tumour is bilateral in 10% cases.

iii. In the testis, it is not preceded by a GCNIS.
iv. *Microscopy* It is composed of a mixture of small and larger cells arranged in solid sheets. These cells do not show the usual immunohistochemical markers of seminoma or embryonal carcinoma and do not produce serologic tumour markers. There is a gain of chromosome 9.
v. *Prognosis* Surgery is curative and most tumours have an excellent prognosis.

Q14. Comment briefly on yolk sac tumour of prepubertal testis.

Definition Yolk sac tumour of prepubertal testis is composed of structures that microscopically resemble those found in the yolk sac, a temporary extra-embryonic foetal structure that involutes spontaneously around 16th week of intrauterine life. It is a rare tumour, yet it represents the most common testicular tumour of childhood.
Clinicopathologic features
i. Yolk sac tumour presents as a small, 1–2 cm intratesticular mass typically found in boys, usually younger than 4 years of age.
ii. *Microscopy* The tumour shows several growth patterns such as reticular, papillary, glandular and solid. It often contains glomeruloid structures called Schiller-Duval bodies and eosinophilic hyaline globules.
iii. Essentially, all tumours secrete AFP, which is a useful serologic marker.
iv. *Prognosis* Treatment is surgical and most patients survive with no adverse consequences.
NOTE: Yolk sac tumour of prepubertal testis must be distinguished from yolk cell tumour components that are usually found as AFP-producing components of adult NSGCT. These yolk sac components may be found in the metastases and are usually resistant to chemotherapy.

Q15. Briefly discuss testicular choriocarcinoma.

Definition Choriocarcinoma is a rare germ cell tumour composed of malignant trophoblastic cells that secrete hCG. Most often, they are one of the components of NSGCT but in rare cases they may appear as pure choriocarcinoma, a highly malignant primary testicular or extragonadal tumour.
Clinicopathologic features
i. Most patients are young adults, younger than 30 years of age.
ii. Pure choriocarcinoma presents as a haemorrhagic and mostly necrotic mass invading the testis.
iii. *Microscopy* It is composed of mononuclear cytotrophoblastic and multinucleate syncytiotrophoblastic cells, which secrete hCG.
iv. Serum contains high levels of hCG.
v. *Prognosis* Tumours tend to metastasise early and have a poor prognosis.

Q16. Give a short description of testicular teratomas.

Definition Teratoma is a germ cell tumour composed of various somatic tissue derived from all three germ layers. Testicular teratomas may be present as a component of the NSGCT, or may occur in an isolated form. The latter includes two distinct tumour types: prepubertal and postpubertal teratomas.
Clinicopathologic features Teratomas are composed of somatic tissues derived from all three embryonic germ layers:
- *Ectoderm* which gives rise to skin-like structures and neural tissue or eye.
- *Mesoderm* that gives rise to connective tissue, fat cells, smooth and striated muscle cells, cartilage, bone.
- *Endoderm* which produces gastrointestinal and bronchial tissue and various endocrine glands like thyroid.

Clinicopathologic classification of testicular teratomas includes the following entities:
I. **Prepubertal teratomas** are unrelated to GCNIS and are found in infants and children prior to puberty. These tumours are composed of diploid, well-differentiated tissues and are clinically benign. This group of tumours also includes dermoid and epidermoid cysts which are quite uncommon in testis compared to ovarian counterparts.
II. **Postpubertal teratomas** are derived from GCNIS and are grouped clinically under the heading of NSGCT. These tumours are malignant and composed of mature and immature tissues **(Fig. 23.4)**. The immature embryonic tissues account for their malignancy and their capacity to metastasise.

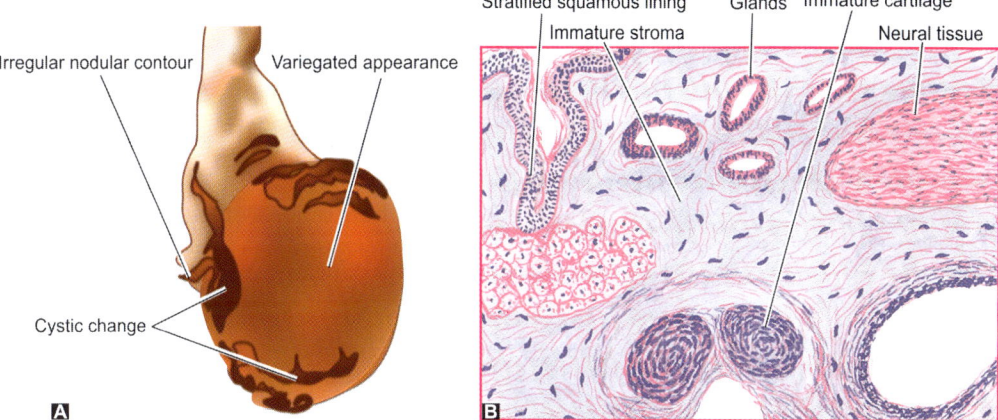

FIGURE 23.4: Post-pubertal testicular teratoma. A, The testis is enlarged and nodular distorting the testicular contour. Sectioned surface shows replacement of the entire testis by variegated mass having grey-white solid areas, cystic areas, honey-combed areas and foci of cartilage and bone. B, Microscopy shows a variety of incompletely differentiated somatic tissue elements (bone, cartilage, neural tissue, and squamous epithelium).

III. *Teratomas with somatic malignancies* are also derived from GCNIS and are grouped under the heading of NSGCT. In addition to teratoma tissues, these tumours contain carcinoma or sarcoma similar to these malignant tumours originating in various organs. Examples of such malignancy are rhabdomyosarcomas, leiomyosarcoma, glioblastoma, nephroblastoma, etc.

Q17. What are sex cord-stromal tumours of the testis?

Definition Sex cord-stromal tumours are composed of cells of the specialised gonadal stroma.
Clinicopathologic features The group of sex-cord-stromal tumours account for less than 5% of all primary testicular tumours. The most important tumours in this group are Leydig cell tumour and Sertoli cell tumour.

I. **Leydig cell tumour** is the most common sex-cord stromal tumor accounting for approximately 3% of all testicular tumours.
i. *Gross* They usually present as a testicular mass, on an average 3–5 cm in size. The tumour is usually solid, brown or yellow on cross section.
ii. *Microscopy* They are composed of solid nests and sheets of Leydig cells, which have round uniform nuclei and well developed eosinophilic cytoplasm. Tumour cells may be lipid-rich and vacuolated or contain lipofuscin and diagnostic *Reinke crystals*.
iii. *Immunohistochemistry* They react with antibodies to inhibin-α, calretinin, androgenic hormones and vimentin.
iv. *Clinical features* Leydig cell tumours occur at any age, including prepubertal boys and very old men. Some tumours produce hormonal symptoms related to their capacity to secrete androgens or oestrogen. In boys, it can cause macrogenitosomia or premature puberty, and in adult men may cause loss of libido and gynaecomastia.
v. *Prognosis* Most Leydig cell tumours are benign, but 10% are malignant. Microscopically, it is not possible always to distinguish benign from malignant tumors and the only definitive sign of malignancy are metastases.

II. **Sertoli cell tumours** account for 1–2% of all testicular tumours.
i. *Gross* The testis contains a mass that may vary in size and appears form and gray-white on cross section.
ii. *Microscopy* Features are variable but most often tumour cells form tubules that have a basement membrane and are lined by cells resembling foetal Sertoli cells. Several rare microscopic variants are recognised by experts who classify the Sertoli cell tumours into subtypes such as: microcystic, retiform, sclerosing, calcifying and large cell. Due to the rarity of these tumours, this subclassification is of limited clinical value.

iii. *Immunohistochemistry* It is similar to Leydig cell tumours, but these tumour cells are cytokeratin positive and androgen negative.
iv. *Clinical* Sertoli cell tumours can be found in any age group: approximately 30% are found in children under the age of 10 years. Most tumours are sporadic but some occur as part of syndromes, such as Peutz-Jeghers and Carney syndrome, or androgen insensitivity syndrome. Majority of tumours are hormonally inactive but some cause hyperestrinism and gynecomastia.
v. *Prognosis* Most tumours are benign but 10% are malignant.
III. **Granulosa cell tumours** resembling those of the ovary may be occasionally found in infants younger than 6 months. Although rare, they are still the most common sex-cord tumour in that age group.

Q18. What do you know about lymphoma of the testis?

i. Lymphoma is the most common testicular tumour in elderly men.
ii. Bilaterality is seen in half the cases.
iii. Most cases represent *secondary spread* to the testis in patients who have primary lymph node involvement or leukaemia.
iv. In rare cases, testis is the only sign of lymphoma (*primary lymphoma of the testis*).
v. Diffuse large cell lymphoma is the most common form of lymphoma involving the testis.

■ PENIS

Q19. What is balanoposthitis?

Definition Balanoposthitis is an inflammation of the glans penis (balanitis) accompanied by the inflammation of the prepuce (posthitis).
Etiopathogenesis Several forms of balanoposthitis can be recognised, such as acute and chronic, non-specific or related to a specific sexually-transmitted disease. In some cases, it may be a disease of unknow etiology.
Clinicopathologic features
I. **Nonspecific balanoposthitis** is related to poor hygiene and accumulation of secretion and smegma. It is a common complication in phimosis. It may be caused by a variety of bacteria such as *E.coli, Staphylococci* and *Streptococci*.
II. **Sexually-transmitted diseases** may cause balanoposthitis combined with urethritis, as seen in gonorrhoea or lymphopathia venereum caused by *Chlamydia trachomatis.*
a. *Genital herpes*, most often caused by HSV II, presents with grouped small vesicles on the penis.
b. *Syphilis* presents with penile ulceration with indurated margins, known as *hard chancre.*
c. Infection with *Haemophilus ducreyi* presents in form of *chancroid* or soft ulcer.
d. *Condyloma acuminatum* is a human papilloma virus-related genital wart.
III. **Balanitis xerotica obliterans** is the penile equivalent of vulvar *lichen sclerosus et atrophicus*. This disease of unknown etiology presents with atrophy of the squamous epithelium of the glans and prepuce and hyaline sclerosis of the underlying connective tissue.

Q20. What is phimosis and paraphimosis?

Definition Phimosis is a condition seen in uncircumcised men in whom the opening of the prepuce is too small to permit its full retraction over the glans penis.
Clinicopathologic features
i. Phimosis may be congenital as seen in newborns or acquired, usually following an infection of the prepuce.
ii. Phimosis predisposes to infections of the penis, and in the long-term may also contribute to development of penile carcinoma.
iii. *Paraphimosis* results from forceful retraction of a phimotic prepuce, which then constricts the glans penis causing circulatory disturbances and its swelling.

Q21. What do you know about carcinoma in situ of penis? How does it differ from bowenoid papulosis?

Definition Carcinoma in situ of the penis (or penile intraepithelial neoplasia (PeIN) is a non-invasive precursor or invasive squamous cell carcinoma.

Etiopathogenesis In most instances, PeIN is related to infection with human papilloma virus type 16, but it may be caused by other high-grade types of HPV as well, or it may develop unrelated to HPV.

Clinicopathologic features

Clinical and gross Features of PeIN are highly variable.
i. The lesion may be seen on the glans, prepuce or the penile shaft.
ii. On the penile shaft, most often there is a solitary, sharply-demarcated, greyish white or erythematous plaque, which has been traditionally called *Bowen disease*.
iii. Erythematous solitary or multiple patches on the glans or internal side of the foreskin are called *erythroplasia of Queyrat*.
iv. Most patients are older than 35 years of age. *Progression to invasive carcinoma* occurs over several years in about 10% of cases.

Microscopy PeIN resembles squamous carcinoma in situ of the cervix or other squamous epithelia. These changes include:
i. Loss of normal layering and maturation of keratinocytes
ii. Expansion of the basal/parabasal layer
iii. Cytologic atypia of keratinocytes
iv. Mitotic figures in all layers of the epidermis
v. Some lesions show hyperkeratosis and parakeratosis. Koilocytic changes may be present as evidence of HPV infection.

Bowenoid papulosis is an HPV-related disease of the penile shaft that must be clinically distinguished from PeIN; it has the same pathologic features as PeIN but is not a precursor of invasive squamous cell carcinoma.

Clinical and gross Bowenoid papulosis is diagnosed in sexually active men who are under 35 years of age. Typically, it presents with multiple reddish brown or flesh-coloured wart-like papules on the penile shaft or scrotal skin.

Microscopy It is indistinguishable from PeIN.

Prognosis Skin lesions tend to disappear spontaneously over several months and do not progress to invasive cancer. Bowenoid papulosis is a primarily a clinical diagnosis. Clinicopathologic correlation is, therefore, essential for the correct diagnosis and to avoid overtreatment.

Q22. Write briefly on carcinoma of the penis.

Definition Carcinoma of the penis is almost always a squamous cell carcinoma (SCC).

Epidemiology Squamous carcinoma of the penis is a rare tumour in the US and Western Europe where it accounts for only 1% of all malignancies. In the US, it is 3–4 times more common among African Americans than other races. In Africa, South America, and most parts of Asia (except Japan and Israel), it has a high incidence representing 10–20% of all cancers. However, in view of ritual of early circumcision in the Jews and the Muslims, its incidence is lower in these races.

Etiopathogenesis Risk factors are:
- HPV infection, especially with high-risk type viruses type 16 and 18
- Poor hygiene and phimosis
- Circumcision is associated with reduced risk

Clinicopathologic features

Gross The tumours are most often located on the glans around the urethra and the coronal sulcus or foreskin. They present most often as an indurated plaque or ulceration. But some carcinomas may be exophytic, wart-like papillomas or present as larger masses **(Fig. 23.5, A, B)**.

Microscopy According to the WHO, SCC of the penis is divided into two groups **(Fig. 23.5, C)**:
- *HPV-related SCC*, accounting for 40–50% of all cancers. Microscopically, these tumours are either basaloid or and mixed basaloid-warty SCC.
- *HPV-unrelated SCC,* presenting in several microscopic variant forms such as: usual SCC, pseudohyperplastic, pseudoglandular, verrucous type, and papillary. Such microscopic subtyping is of no clinical significance.
- *Exophythic verrucous tumours* (known as *giant condyloma of Buschke and Löwenstein*) are rare, low-grade SCC that also belong to this group.

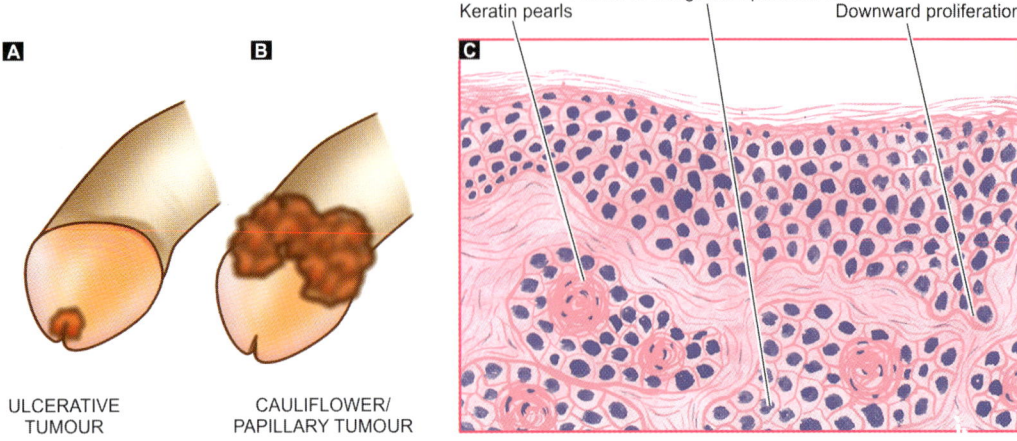

FIGURE 23.5: Carcinoma of the penis. Diagrammatic representation of flat-ulcerating (A) and cauliflower papillary (B) patterns of growth at common locations. C, Microscopy shows whorls of malignant squamous cells with central keratin pearls.

Prognosis Tumours metastasise to inguinal lymph nodes. Patients with only superficial invasion have 90% survival. Those that have lymph node metastases have a 5-year survival of 30–50%.

PROSTATE

Q23. What are the key anatomic and histologic features of the prostate?

i. Prostate is an exocrine gland involved in the production of prostatic fluid that is admixed to the sperm. It is located around the urethra and below the neck of the bladder.

ii. *Histology* It consists of glands, ducts and fibromuscular stroma which are arranged into three lobes: two major lateral lobes and a small median lobe.
- The prostatic glands are composed of *tubulo-alveolar acini and ducts*. The glandular epithelium has two layers: a basal layer of low cuboidal cells, and an inner layer of mucus-secreting tall columnar cells. The thick fibromuscular stroma occupies the space between the glands.

iii. Based on the hormonal responsiveness, the prostate can be divided into two portions: the *inner or central periurethral* ('female') part which is sensitive to both oestrogen and androgen, and the *outer subcapsular zone* which is sensitive to androgen.

iv. Benign nodular hyperplasia of the prostate occurs in the periurethral inner part whereas cancer predominantly involves the outer part **(Fig. 23.6)**.

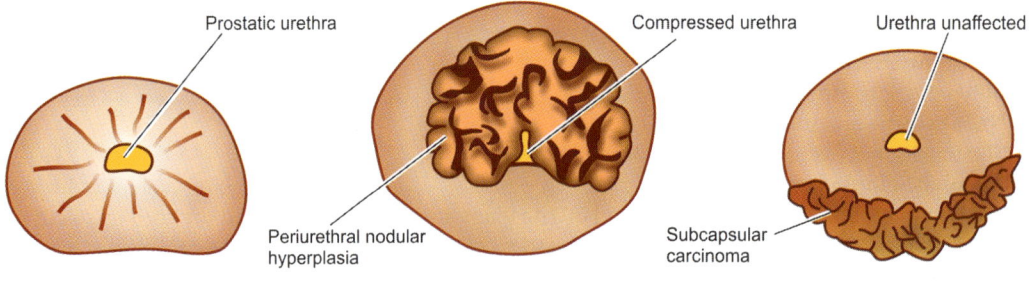

FIGURE 23.6: Normal prostate, benign nodular hyperplasia and prostatic carcinoma. The nodule in case of benign nodular hyperplasia (B) is located in the inner periurethral part and compresses the prostatic urethra while prostatic carcinoma (C) generally arises in the peripheral glands and, thus, does not compress the urethra.

Q24. Briefly discuss prostatitis.

Definition Prostatitis is a common inflammation of the prostate, usually linked to ascending acute or chronic urogenital infection.

Etiopathogenesis Prostatitis may be acute or chronic.
i. Acute prostatitis in men *under the age of 35 years* is usually related to sexually-transmitted diseases and the most common causative pathogens are *Neisseria gonorrhoeae* and *Chlamydia trachomatis, a* gram-negative obligate intracellular bacterium.
ii. *In older men*, both acute and chronic prostatitis are usually associated with prostatic hyperplasia and chronic cystitis. Bacteria enter the prostate from infected urine that contains the usual uropathogens, such as *E. coli, Pseudomonas aeruginosa, and Klebsiella pneumoniae*. Persistent or recurrent infection with *E. coli* is the most common cause of chronic prostatitis.

Pathology
i. In **acute prostatitis**, the prostate is focally infiltrated with neutrophils, which also fill the lumen of glands and ducts, or may form microabscesses.
ii. **Chronic prostatitis** presents with infiltrates of lymphocytes, plasma cells and macrophages.
iii. In both acute and chronic prostatitis, the seminal vesicles are also usually involved.
iv. **Uncommon forms** *of chronic prostatitis* are as follows:
a. *Tuberculous prostatitis*, a rarity today, is secondary to primary pulmonary tuberculosis. Infection is accompanied by caseating granulomas.
b. *Noncaseating granulomas* may be found in prostates of patients who have received BCG treatment of bladder cancer.
c. *Allergic prostatitis or granulomatous hypersensitivity prostatitis* are immune reactions similar to those in other parts of the body affected by autoimmune processes.

Clinical features
i. Dysuria, urgency and increased frequency of urination.
ii. Acute prostatitis provokes pain and is also accompanied by bouts of fever. The prostate is sensitive to palpation, and in acute prostatitis pus can be expressed during transrectal palpation or massage of the prostate.
iii. Examination of the fractionated urine collected from the free stream micturition should include bacterial studies of the last third of the voided urine ('prostatic urine'). Microscopic examination of the urinary sediment will, in most cases, reveal acute or chronic inflammatory cells.
iv. Urine that contains leucocytes but is bacteriologically sterile is a typical finding in chronic *abacterial prostatitis*. Such urine needs to be examined in specialised laboratories for *C. trachomatis* and *U. urealyticum*, which are the most common cause of such 'sterile' prostatitis. These pathogens cannot be detected by routine bacteriologic techniques and culture methods.
v. If all the microbiologic studies are negative, one must conclude that prostatitis is caused by an immune mechanism or that it is idiopathic.

Q25. Describe etiopathogenesis and salient clinicopathologic features of prostatic hyperplasia.

Definition Prostatic hyperplasia is an age-dependent, non-neoplastic enlargement of the prostate characterised by an increased number of prostatic glands and stromal cells. It is said that 80% of 80-year-old men have prostatic hyperplasia.

Etiopathogenesis
i. Hyperplasia of prostatic glands and stroma occurs due to hypersensitivity of these cells to *dihydroxytestosterone (DHT)*, which is the hormone that promotes the growth of the prostate. DHT is formed in stromal cells through the action of 5α-reductase, and is then transferred to glandular and other stromal cells stimulating them to proliferate and form hyperplastic nodules. Inhibitors of 5α-reductase (e.g. finasteride) can reduce the size of a hyperplastic prostate, providing indirect evidence that DHT plays a key role in the pathogenesis of prostatic hyperplasia.
ii. The action of DTH might be aided by *oestrogen*. Both men and women secrete oestrogen and testosterone, but in obviously different ratios. In ageing men, testosterone secretion will decrease and thus the ratio of testosterone to oestrogen will increase in favour of oestrogen. The inner part of the prostate will respond to a relative excess of oestrogen by undergoing hyperplasia. It is also possible that oestrogen acts synergistically with DHT.

Pathology Prostatic hyperplasia is an age-related disease and it does not occur before the age of 40 years.

Gross The hyperplastic prostate is enlarged and nodular. On cross section, it contains solid or spongy nodules, surrounded by fibromuscular strands or fibrotic small nodules. All the nodules vary in size and are most prominent in the central part of the prostate, distorting the urethra.

Microscopy Features include *glandular* and *fibromuscular* nodular hyperplasia **(Fig. 23.7)**:

- The *hyperplastic glands* are enlarged and show prominent intraglandular folding as well papillary protrusions. The glands are lined by normal cells arranged into two layers: inner layer composed of polarised regular mucus cells and a basal layer composed of flattened cuboidal cell with scant cytoplasm.
- *Fibromuscular hyperplasia* results in the formation of microscopic and larger nodules composed of spindle cells that have features of smooth muscle cells or fibroblasts.

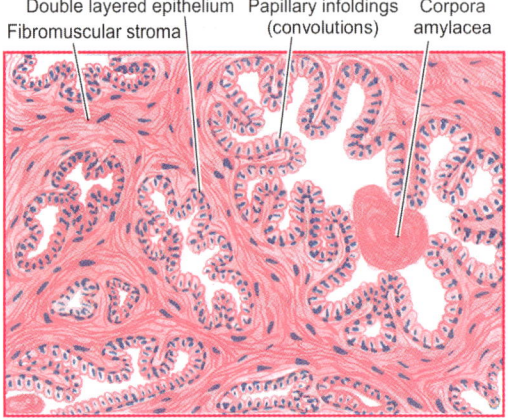

FIGURE 23.7: Nodular hyperplasia of the prostate. There is hyperplasia of fibromuscular elements. There are areas of intra-acinar papillary infoldings (convolutions) lined by two layers of epithelium with basal polarity of nuclei.

Clinical features vary from minor urinary problems to pronounced signs of urinary obstruction.

i. The most prominent symptoms, collectively known as *dysuria*, result from urethral obstruction of the urinary bladder.

ii. Obstruction of the urinary outflow from the bladder results in compensatory muscular hyperplasia with thickening and trabeculation of the bladder wall and signs of superimposed *chronic bacterial cystitis*. The bladder wall thickening and trabeculation will reduce its volume, leading to frequent urination, hesitancy in initiating micturition, incomplete emptying of the bladder with variable amounts of residual urine in its lumen, nocturia, and common infection.

iii. Obstruction of the bladder may also cause dilatation of the ureter an renal pelvis with formation of *hydroureters and hydronephrosis*, associated with renal atrophy and progressive loss of renal function. *Ascending pyelonephritis* is yet another complication.

The treatment of prostatic hyperplasia includes hormonal inhibitors of 5α-reductase and antagonists of smooth muscle contraction, as well as transurethral prostatectomy.

Q26. What do you know about factors in the etiopathogenesis of prostatic carcinoma?

Definition Carcinoma of the prostate is an adenocarcinoma originating most often from the prostatic acinar glands. It is the most common malignant tumour of internal organs diagnosed in the United States and Western Europe.

Etiopathogenesis Not known but several risk factors have been identified:

I. **Hormonal factors** Androgenic hormones play a key role, as supported by the following facts:

i. Prostate cancer does not develop in eunuchs and Klinefelter syndrome patient or hypogonadism.

ii. Orchiectomy may arrest the growth of metastatic prostate cancers, until they become androgen-deprivation resistant.

iii. Administration of oestrogen can cause regression of prostate cancer.

iv. Cancer of the prostate begins at the stage of life when androgen levels are high. However, the cancer may remain latent with decline in androgen level with advancing age.

II. **Racial influences** account for the variation in the incidence of prostatic cancer among races and nations:

i. There is a low incidence of prostate cancer in Chinese and Japanese while it is high in Africans.

ii. In the United States, the highest incidence is recorded in African Americans, who also have a higher rate of prostate cancer-related mortality than other races.

III. **Environmental factors** may explain the geographic difference in incidence of prostate cancer in different nations.

i. The difference in the incidence of prostate cancer in African Americans and Africans living in Africa (lower than in America) is also indicative of some environmental factors.

ii. *Dietary factors* such as high fat diet have been found to favour cancer growth, whereas antioxidants and oligominerals like selenium reduce the risk.

IV. **Heredity** may play a role as suggested by the clustering of cases in some families and the higher incidence of cancer in first-degree relatives, who are at a 2 times higher risk than unrelated persons.

V. **Molecular biology** studies have been mostly non-contributory. The significance of epigenetic phenomena and somatic mutations which have been identified as prevalent in prostate cancer but remains incompletely elucidated, are as under:

i. *Epigenetic hypermethylation of gene GSTP1* (glutathione S-transferase), resulting in a loss of function of gene that detoxifies carcinogens. Lack of carcinogen detoxification could allow those noxious substances to induce prostatic carcinoma.

ii. The most common genetic abnormality noted in prostate cancer cells is the formation of *TMPRSS2-ETS fusion gene*, which is found in approximately 50% of prostate cancers in Americans of European origins. This fusion gene includes the androgen regulated promoter of *TMPRSS2* and the coding sequence of the *ETS* family transcription factors. Common occurrence of this fusion gene in prostate cancer, and the fact that it is linked to androgen, have generated a lot of scientific studies but its role in the pathogenesis of prostate cancer has not been proven.

Q27. Briefly discuss pathology, clinical features, prognostic parameters and diagnosis of prostatic cancer.

Pathology Most prostate carcinoma diagnosed in clinical practice do not produce visible changes in the prostate itself and are diagnosed only microscopically upon extensive needle biopsy sampling or systematic microscopic examination of the prostatectomy specimen.

Clinical and gross In 95% cases, prostatic carcinoma is located in the peripheral zone, in the posterior lobe.

i. Prostatic carcinoma is *desmoplastic* and the excess of connective tissue gives it a firm consistency, which facilitates recognition of tumour on digital rectal examination (DRE) or with targeted radiologic techniques such as CT scanning and MRI. On sectioning, the prostate carcinoma has a gritty consistency.

ii. Advanced untreated prostatic carcinomas seen at autopsy are recognised by their *tendency to invade surrounding tissues* (e.g. bladder, rectum), or produce metastases in local lymph nodes and distant organs such as the bones, liver, lungs.

iii. *Haematogenous bone metastases* tend to appear first in the lumbar spine and pelvis due to haematogenous spread. As seen on X-rays, these metastases may be osteolytic or osteoblastic (dense).

Microscopy More than 95% of all prostate carcinomas are adenocarcinomas of acinar origin **(Fig. 23.8)**.

i. *Tumour cells* are usually cuboidal, and have an enlarged nucleus, prominent nucleolus and scanty cytoplasm that could be clear or basophilic.

ii. In contrast to normal prostatic glands which are bilayered, glands made up of carcinoma cells are *not surrounded by a layer of basal cells*. Carcinoma cells are thus in close contact with the desmoplastic stroma.

iii. Microscopic evidence of *invasive growth* of prostate carcinoma is important for grading of tumours. Carcinomas invade through the capsule of the prostate into the periprostatic soft tissues,

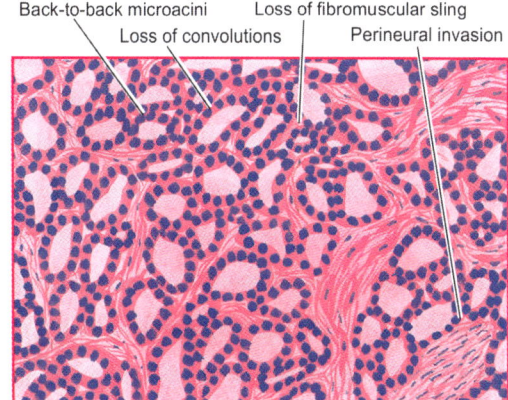

FIGURE 23.8: Carcinoma of the prostate. It shows microacini of small malignant cells infiltrating the prostatic stroma.

into the seminal vesicles, and most prominently along the intraprostatic nerves. Invasion of the bladder is seen in advanced cases.

iv. *Gleason grading* of prostatic carcinoma is routinely used to predict whether a tumour will have a good or bad prognosis. Gleason grading is based on two features:
a. Degree of glandular differentiation and distribution of glands, and
b. Growth pattern of tumour in relation to the stroma.
- Using these two parameters, tumours are graded on a scale from 1 to 5, in which 1 is used for well-differentiated and 5 for poorly-differentiated cancers.
- Based on predominant grade seen on low-power examination, the tumour is given the *primary grade*, and then a *secondary grade* for the second most predominant pattern.
- The sum of the primary and secondary grades is expressed as *Gleason score*. For example grade 3+ grade 4= score 7 is assigned to well-differentiated tumours which usually have an indolent course, whereas grade 4+ grade 5= score 9 is given to poorly-differentiated carcinomas which have a poor prognosis.

v. *WHO grouping* is used as a simplified but more comprehensive grading system. It includes only 5 grade-groups: group 1 for tumours with a Gleason score of 6 or less, and group 5 for tumours with Gleason scores 9 and 10.

vi. *Staging of tumours* based on the TNM system is used for prognosis. It includes three categories for T value:
- T1 is for clinically inapparent small tumours confined to the prostate.
- T2 for larger tumours involving one or both lobes but not extending outside of the prostate.
- T3 for tumours with extra-prostatic extension (more appropriate term than 'extracapsular' since the prostate does not have a capsule).

Positive lymph nodes (N1) and distant metastases (M1) are associated with adverse prognosis.

Clinical features In symptomatic patients, these are:
i. Signs of dysuria
ii. Urinary bladder obstruction
iii. Haematuria
iv. In 10% of cases, pain in the back due to skeletal metastases. Bone metastases may be osteolytic or osteoblastic, which are associated with an elevation of alkaline phosphatase, derived from osteoblasts. In these advanced cases, tumour of the prostate is usually palpable by digital rectal examination.

Prognosis Survival depends on:
i. Stage of tumour (by TNM)
ii. Grade of the tumour (by Gleason score/WHO grouping)
iii. Level of PSA in serum
iv. Type of treatment
- *For T1 and T2 tumours,* 5-year survival is almost 100% and the average patient will survive 14 years after prostatectomy.
- *For T3 patients,* 5-year survival is only 25%.

Diagnosis is most often made by a triple approach including:
i. Digital-rectal or transrectal ultrasound examination (DRE or TRUS)
ii. Serum PSA determination
iii. Transrectal ultrasound-guided core needle biopsy

NOTE: PSA in the range of 4 to 10 ng/ml has relatively low sensitivity (20%) and specificity (65%) and is of uncertain clinical value for several reasons as under:
- Increased serum levels of PSA can be found not only in patients with cancer but also in those with prostatitis, prostatic hyperplasia or infarction, and following prostatic biopsy and instrumentation.
- Approximately 20–30% persons with prostate cancer have normal serum PSA (< 4 ng/ml), including patients who have a poorly-differentiated carcinoma.
- Values over 10 ng/ml have high predictive value, which is, however, still only 70%.
- Values in the 'grey zone' between 4 and 10 ng/ml are suspicious for cancer but equivocal and result in numerous unnecessary biopsies, which prove negative for cancer.

- In men over the age of 70 years, serum PSA is frequently elevated above 6 ng/ml and current consensus of urologists is not to recommend the PSA test for screening of men over the age of 75 years because harm outweighs the benefits.
- PSA is, however, a valuable test for follow-up of patients who had prostatectomy. 'Biochemical recurrence' is almost invariably a sign of recurrent cancer necessitating additional treatment such as radiation therapy or chemotherapy. Serum level of PSA reflects the residual tumour volume.

> **Chapter 23e Supplement: Online Content**
>
> *Digital content of this chapter available with this book is meant for enhanced learning and self-assessment. In addition, it contains 20 Multiple Choice Questions (MCQs), 06 Clinicopathologic Vignettes, and 07 Image-based Questions; these are followed by their answers along with explanatory notes of correct and incorrect answers.*

CHAPTER 24

Female Genital Tract

■ VULVA

Q1. What are the most important diseases of the Bartholin glands?

Bartholin's or vulvovaginal glands are racemose exocrine glands secreting during sexual arousal. Pathologic lesions include the following:
i. *Bartholin duct cysts* which develop due to obstruction of the excretory ducts of Bartholin glands.
ii. *Acute Bartholin adenitis* is a bacterial infection which is often associated with duct obstruction and may transform into an abscess.
iii. *Chronic Bartholin adenitis* is a less virulent infection, but it also may cause duct obstruction, leading to formation of Bartholin cysts.
iv. *Bartholin gland tumours*, adenomas and adenocarcinomas, are rare accounting for less than 5% of all vulvar tumours.

Q2. What are the non-neoplastic epithelial disorders of the vulva?

These conditions, previously called vulvar dystrophies, include two conditions: lichen sclerosus and lichen simplex chronicus (or squamous hyperplasia or keratosis).
I. **Lichen sclerosus** is a chronic disease of unknown etiology, most often found in postmenopausal women.
Etiopathogenesis is unknown. Possible immunologic basis of the disease is suggested by a common association with autoimmune diseases (e.g. thyroiditis) and the presence of T cells in the underlying dermis.
Clinical and gross
i. Presentation as white parchment-like thinning of epidermis and white patches (leukoplakia) that are very pruritic.
ii. Progressive sclerosis may narrow the introitus to the vagina (kraurosis vulvae), or spread to the perineal skin.
iii. There is an increased incidence of vulvar squamous cell carcinoma in the range of 2–6% over the life span of the affected woman.
Microscopy
i. Surface hyperkeratosis covering the atrophic epidermis which appears flattened due to the disappearance of rete ridges **(Fig. 24.1, A)**.
ii. Below the epidermis, the upper dermis appears hyalinised due to amorphous homogenisation of collagen fibres.
iii. Scattered foci of chronic inflammation are seen in the mid-dermis and include activated T-cells.
II. **Lichen simplex chronicus**, or simply called keratosis, is a chronic vulvar disease resulting from many forms of itchy chronic nonspecific inflammation, or some pre-existing skin diseases including chronic chemical or physical irritation, hypersensitivity reaction, lichen planus, psoriasis and others.

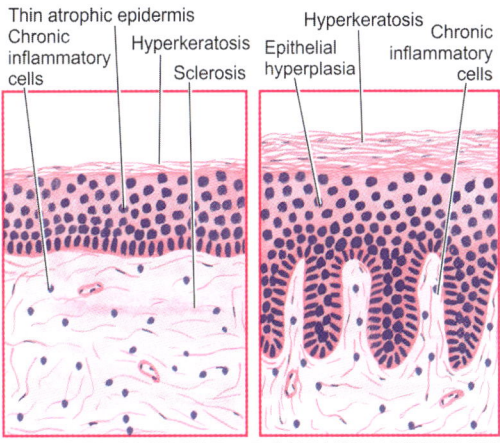

FIGURE 24.1: A, *Lichen sclerosus*. The epithelium is atrophic and thin. The upper dermis shows homogeneous hyalinised collagen. There is mild chronic inflammatory infiltrate. B, *Squamous hyperplasia*. The epidermis shows acanthosis, hyperkeratosis and hypergranulosis. There is no cytologic atypia. The upper dermis shows mild chronic inflammatory infiltrate.

Clinical and gross
i. The patches of thickened skin, most often on the labia majora, show increased skin markings and/or may appear like leukoplakia.
ii. Lesions often show excoriations due to itching.

Microscopy
i. Hyperkeratosis overlying a thickened hyperplastic epidermis which shows thickened granular layer, acanthosis with elongation of rete ridges **(Fig. 24.1,B)**.
ii. The dermis contains chronic inflammatory cells.
iii. There is no atypia and the condition does not progress to cancer. However, it cannot be distinguished with certainty from carcinoma in situ and, therefore, it is often biopsied to reassure the patient that there is no malignancy.

Q3. What is condyloma acuminatum? Discuss its salient features.

Definition Condyloma acuminatum, also known as benign genital wart, is an HPV-related papillary lesion made up of thickened squamous epithelium showing focal koilocytosis.

Etiopathogenesis Condyloma acuminatum is caused by a sexually-transmitted infection with HPV, usually type 6 or 11.

Clinicopathologic features
Clinical and gross Condyloma may present as a solitary wart of the vulva, but more often there are multiple warts on the vulva, perineum, vagina or anus.

Microscopy
i. The lesion consisting of numerous papillae, i.e. tree-like proliferation of thickened stratified squamous epithelium lying on a core of fibrovascular stroma.
ii. The epithelium shows acanthosis, hyperkeratosis, parakeratosis, papillomatosis and perinuclear vacuolisation (koilocytosis) indicative of HPV infection.

Prognosis Condylomas are benign lesions which regress spontaneously except in immunosuppressed persons.

Q4. Define extra-mammary Paget disease of the vulva. Write briefly on its salient clinicopathologic features.

Definition Extramammary Paget disease is a malignant tumour composed of large mucin filled carcinoma cells infiltrating focally the epidermis of the vulva.

Clinicopathologic features
Clinical and gross It appears map-like, red, scaly or wet and indurated.
Microscopy of extra-mammary Paget disease resembles Paget disease of the nipple:
i. The epidermis is infiltrated with small groups or single carcinoma cells.
ii. The cells have clear mucin-filled cytoplasm and stain with PAS.

Prognosis depends whether the disease is primary or secondary:
- In contrast to breast in which there is always an underlying ductal carcinoma, extramammary Paget disease is confined to the epidermis with no underlying adenocarcinoma. Such *primary* extramammary Paget disease can be resected and has good prognosis.
- Only in a minority of cases there is an underlying adenocarcinoma of adnexal glands or from adjacent genitourinary tract or rectum. Such *secondary* tumours that invade the epidermis from below are by definition invasive and have poor prognosis.

Q5. Briefly discuss vulvar squamous cell carcinoma.

Definition Squamous cell carcinoma (SCC) of the vulva is morphologically preceded by preinvasive carcinoma in situ similar to SCC of the vagina and cervix. Many tumours are multifocal within the vulva and even multicentric involving the vagina and cervix as well.

Etiopathogenesis Vulvar carcinoma is rare (3% of all female genital cancers). Two types of SCC are recognised clinically:

i. *Keratinising SCC* (70%) unrelated to HPV infection, and usually preceded by differentiated intraepithelial vulvar neoplasia (dVIN) or vulvar acanthosis with altered differentiation (VAAD). This cancer occurs in older women.

ii. *Basaloid and warty SCC* that is HPV-related, is preceded by classical vulvar intraepithelial neoplasia (VIN) and occurs in younger, perimenopausal women. The most common pathogens are HPV type 16 and 18. As in preinvasive cancer of the cervix, classical VIN can be graded from VIN I to VIN III, which is also called carcinoma in situ.

Clinicopathologic features
Clinical and gross
i. Vulvar carcinoma is a tumour of elderly women and the mean age at the time of diagnosis is 60 years.
ii. Carcinoma is preceded by preinvasive precursor lesions which appear on gross examination as leukoplakia.
iii. Typically, it presents as non-healing plaques or ulcers which slowly transform into indurated masses that may be exophytic (in 60% cases) or endophytic (ulcerative).
Microscopy of vulvar SCC has the same features as the more common SCC of the cervix.
Prognosis The survival depends on the stage of cancer. Overall 5-year survival for carcinoma of vulva is 70% for women who do not have metastases (stage I and II), but it drops to 35% in women who have metastases to lymph nodes (stage III and IV).

■ VAGINA

Q6. What is vaginitis?

Definition Vaginitis is a common inflammation of the vagina, caused by a variety of pathogens and presenting with vaginal discharge (leucorrhoea).

Etiopathogenesis Vagina is lined by squamous epithelium that provides a barrier to invasive bacterial infections, such as gonorrhoea. Nevertheless, gonococci can be seen as paired diplococci in neutrophils inside the vagina of infected women. The common pathogens, readily recognised in Pap smears, are as under:
i. Bacteria: *Gardnerella vaginalis* recognised by the presence of 'clue-cells'.
ii. Fungi: *Candida albicans* recognised by the presence of fungal hyphae.
iii. Protozoa: *Trichomonas vaginalis* recognised in smears as ciliated protozoa.

Q7. Discuss the important tumours of the vagina briefly.

Primary tumours of the vagina may be benign or malignant. Primary malignant tumours of the vagina are rare and account for only 2% of all female genital tract tumours. Metastatic tumours and those spreading from other sites are more common and account for 80% of vaginal cancers.
The most important primary vaginal tumours are as under:
I. **Squamous cell carcinoma** accounts for 90% of all primary malignant vaginal tumours.
Clinical and gross It is typically preceded by high-grade vaginal intraepithelial lesion (VaHSIL) that is related to HPV infection and occurs most often in the upper part of the vagina. Due to the 'field

effect' of HPV infection, it may be found in women who have HPV-related lesions of the cervix or vulva.
Microscopy of vaginal SCC has the same features as cervical SCC.
Prognosis Invasive vaginal squamous cell carcinoma limited to vagina (stage I) has a 5-year survival of 80%, in contrast to stage III/ IV SCCs which have a 5-year survival of only 20%.
II. **Adenocarcinoma** of the vagina is a very rare tumour.
i. It may be classified as clear cell, mucinous or endometrioid type.
ii. Clear cell carcinoma was found to be associated with maternal intake of stilbestrol, an oestrogen used previously to prevent premature delivery and termination of the pregnancy.
iii. Women exposed to stilbestrol during their intrauterine life develop clear cell vaginal cancer at a rate of 1:1,000, which is still many times higher than in non-exposed women.
iv. One third of these women also have intramural vaginal cystic and glandular inclusions, which must not be misinterpreted for adenocarcinoma.
III. **Sarcoma botryoides** is a rare form of embryonal rhabdomyosarcoma found in girls younger than 5 years of age.
Clinical and gross The tumour grows as exophytic multicystic grape-like mass (*Greek* botrys= grape), typically causing vaginal spotting or bleeding.
Microscopy
i. The tumour is composed of polypoid structures that have a central myxoid core surrounded by a cambium layer separating it from surface epithelium.
ii. The cambium layer is composed of small fusiform cells undergoing rhabdomyoblastic differentiation.
Prognosis Tumours diagnosed before they reach the size of 3 cm can be treated effectively by surgery combined with chemotherapy. Larger invasive tumours have poor prognosis.
NOTE: Sarcoma botryoides also occurs in the urinary bladder (the most common site in little boys), and the head and neck region (e.g. orbit, mouth, nasopharynx).

CERVIX

Q8. Write briefly on the principal parts of the cervix which are important for understating its diseases.

The cervix forms the lower most part of the uterus.
i. It has an *internal os* that communicates with endometrial cavity and the *external os* that opens into the vagina.
ii. *Exocervix* is the part of the cervix that protrudes into the vagina (*portio vaginalis*). It is covered with stratified squamous epithelium that has three layers: basal layer, parabasal layer and superficial layer. This epithelium is influenced by oestrogen.
iii. *Endocervix* contains a central endocervical canal lined by glandular columnar mucus-secreting epithelium. The endocervical glands secrete mucus which changes during the menstrual cycle and becomes less viscous under the influence of oestrogen.
iv. *Squamo-columnar junction* (i.e. the transition between the squamous epithelium of the ectocervix and the columnar epithelium of the endocervix) is a clinically and pathologically important landmark. This zone contains stem cells which may be infected with HPV which may transform into neoplastic cells, hence the name transformation zone.

Q9. What is cervicitis? Discuss salient clinicopathologic features of its main types.

Definition Cervicitis is inflammation of the cervix that may be acute or chronic. An important and common complication of long-term cervicitis is pelvic inflammatory disease (PID) due to the spread of infection to the endometrium and fallopian tubes. Cervicitis is of two types: acute and chronic.
Acute cervicitis is usually caused by vaginal bacteria which have ascended into the endocervix.
i. Common risk factors are delivery, instrumentation, and illegal abortion.
ii. Also it may be caused by sexually-transmitted pathogens, such as *N. gonorrhoeae*.
iii. Viral infections such as genital herpes may rarely involve the cervix which shows vesicles on the ectocervical squamous mucosa.
iv. The cervix in acute cervicitis is oedematous and congested and there is an acute inflammation of the endocervix with foci of ulceration.

Chronic cervicitis is more common and is inflammation of the endocervix presenting with leucorrhoea.
i. It is caused by an ascending infection of pathogens causing vaginitis or the usual mixed vaginal bacterial flora.
ii. Predisposing factors include pregnancy and delivery, instrumentation and excess or deficiency of oestrogen.

Q10. Write briefly on cervical polyps.

Definition Cervical polyp is a non-neoplastic proliferation of endocervical mucosa, leading to the formation of exophytic endocervical lesions that are either sessile or pedunculated, thus protruding through the external cervical os. Cervical polyps are common and are found in 2–5% of adult women, most often in the 30–50 years age group. Clinically, polyps cause irregular vaginal spotting, postcoital bleeding or vaginal discharge.

Etiopathogenesis Unknown, but most likely related to chronic infections, trauma from instrumentation, or multiparity.

Clinicopathologic features
Clinical and gross Cervical polyps appear usually as a small, 2–4 cm fragile, haemorrhagic endocervical mass that can be easily removed by curettage.
Microscopy
i. The polyps consist of endocervical mucosa containing often dilated glands and fibro-vascular stroma with foci of chronic inflammation.
ii. Surface of polyps consists of mucus-secreting columnar cells and/or squamous epithelium.
Prognosis: Surgical removal is recommended; there is no risk of malignancy.
NOTE: Endometrial polyps, usually found in premenopausal women resemble cervical polyps. However, the stroma of endometrial polyps is monoclonal and, therefore, they are considered to represent benign tumours.

Q11. What is current concept of squamous intraepithelial lesions of uterine cervix?

Definition Squamous intraepithelial lesion (SIL) is the name for intraepithelial precursors of cervical squamous cell carcinomas. It supersedes the previous terms for these preinvasive forms of cervical neoplasia such as cervical dysplasia or cervical intraepithelial neoplasia (CIN), and carcinoma in situ.

Classification There are two groups of SIL: low grade (L-SIL) and high grade (H-SIL):
L-SIL, which is usually related to infection with low-risk HPV type 6 and 11, is a flat condyloma showing koilocytic atypia. It corresponds to CIN-1 or low grade dysplasia.
H-SIL, which is usually related to infection with high-risk HPV type 16 and 18, and less often other high-risk HPV types 31, 33, 52, 58. It corresponds to CIN-2 and CIN-3, moderate or severe dysplasia, and carcinoma in situ.
Etiopathogenesis The evidence that sexually-transmitted HPV infection is causally related to SIL includes data obtained in epidemiologic, virologic, molecular and ultrastructural studies **(Fig. 24.2)**:

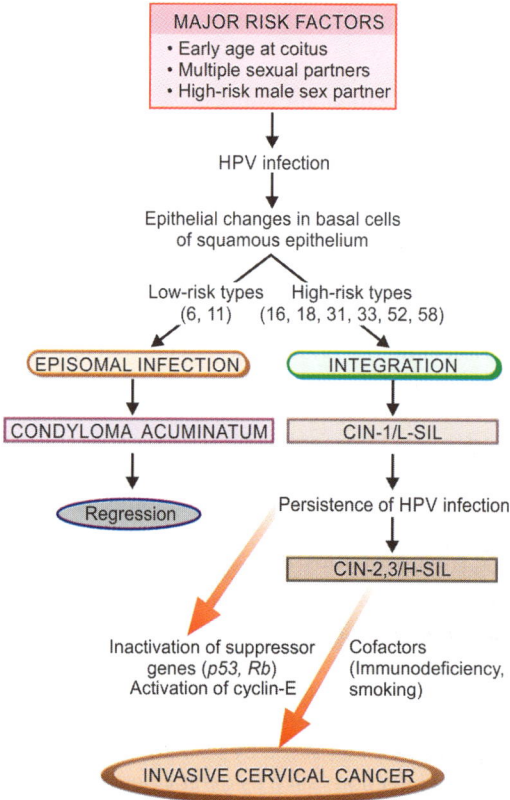

FIGURE 24.2: Role of human papillomavirus (HPV) in the pathogenesis of cervical neoplasia.

i. *Epidemiologic studies* have identified four most important risk factors:
a. Onset of sexual activity at an early age
b. Multiple sexual partners
c. Persistent HPV infection with high-risk oncogenic virus types
d. High-risk male sexual partner who is promiscuous, has a history of penile condyloma or had a spouse with cervical cancer
ii. *Virologic studies* have identified high-risk type HPV in H-SIL and low-risk type HPV in L-SIL.
a. Most common *high-risk HPV* types are 16 and 18 (in 70% cases), and less often types 31, 33, 52, 58 (in 25% of cases).
b. *Low-risk HPV* types are found most frequently in condylomas and L-SIL, and include HPV types 6 and 11.
iii. *Molecular studies* have shown that:
a. Low-risk HPV types cause *episomal infection* without integration, whereas high-risk types of HPV integrate, and permanently infect the squamous cells.
b. Upon *integration* of high-risk HPV 16 and 18, E7 and E6 proteins respectively inactivate tumour suppressor genes *TP53* and *RB-1*, with activation of cyclin-E, thus permitting continuous proliferation of infected cells and the formation of H-SIL and cervical cancer.
c. *Cofactors* such as smoking and immunodeficiency promote carcinogenesis.
iv. *Immunologic studies* have demonstrated:
a. The presence of HPV-specific antigens in the serum of women with cervical cancer. HPV can be demonstrated immunohistochemically in tumour cells as well.
b. Antibodies to p16 are most widely used in diagnostic pathology practice to distinguish H-SIL (positive) from L-SIL (negative).
v. *Ultrastructural studies* have shown that:
a. The tumour cells contain an increased number of mitochondria and free ribosomes, and reduced amounts of glycogen.
b. Reduced glycogen in tumour cells forms the basis of the Lugol iodine (Schiller) test. In this test, the cervix is painted with a solution of iodine and potassium iodide that reacts with glycogen in the cells. The neoplastic cells which do not have glycogen do not stain with this solution.

Pathology The diagnosis of SIL is made by exfoliative cytology in Pap smears and histologically in biopsies of the cervix; the latter is often done under colposcopic guidance. There is a high correlation between the cytology and histology data since both reflect the assessment of atypia and dysplasia of cervical squamous epithelium **(Fig. 24.3)**:
i. *Cytology smears* in L-SIL show dyskaryosis and pleomorphism of nuclei; these changes become more pronounced in H-SIL and are accompanied by nuclear enlargement and increased nucleus:cytoplasmic ratio. Furthermore, L-SIL smears contain predominantly superficial and intermediate cells, whereas H-SIL contains predominantly small, dark basal cells.
ii. *Histology* in L-SIL shows koilocytes in the superficial layers while the abnormal cells occupy the lower third of the entire epithelium. In H-SIL (which includes moderate to severe dysplasia), the abnormal cells occupy 70–100% of the thickness of the epithelium.

Q12. What are the general principles of cervical screening by Pap smears and the Bethesda system of reporting the findings?

Recommendations for cervical screening by Pap smear include annual cervical smear in all sexually active women. However, if three consecutive Pap smears are negative in 'high-risk women' or satisfactory in 'low-risk women', frequency of Pap smears is reduced. There is no upper age limit for cervical screening.
Bethesda system of evaluation of cervical smears has the following broad principles:
i. Assessment of adequacy
ii. General diagnosis of normal or abnormal smear
iii. Descriptive diagnosis of abnormal smears including benign cellular changes, reactive cellular changes and abnormalities of epithelial cells.
iv. Cellular abnormalities of both squamous and glandular cells as under:
• ASCUS (atypical squamous cell of undetermined significance), L-SIL (mentioning HPV infection and CIN-1 present or not), H-SIL (stating CIN-2 or CIN-3) and squamous cell carcinoma

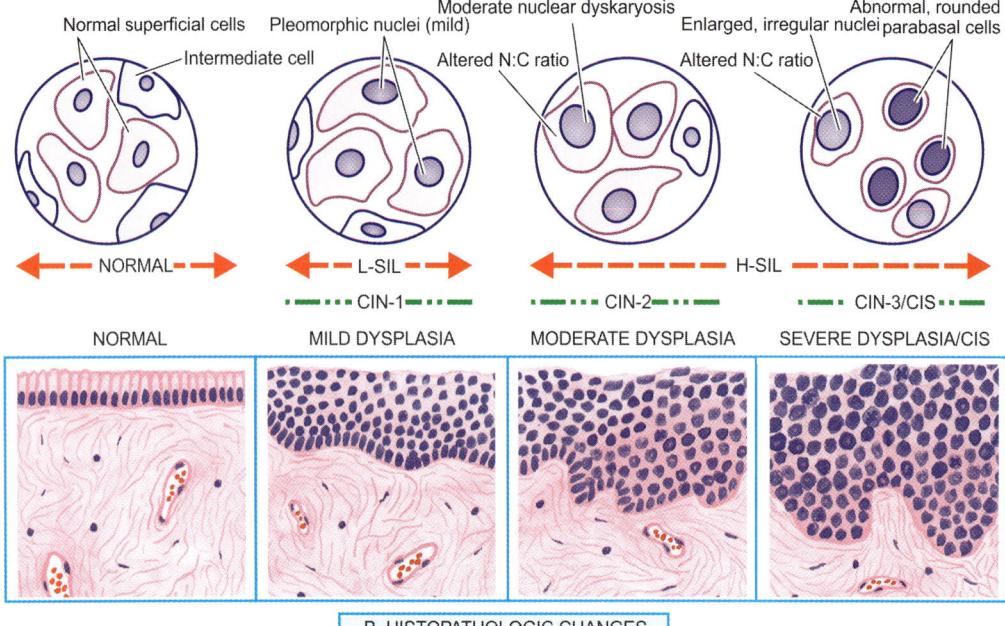

FIGURE 24.3: Cervical intraepithelial neoplasia (CIN) and squamous intraepithelial lesions (SIL). A, Exfoliative cytologic studies in various grades of cellular changes (upper part of figure). B, Schematic representation of histologic changes (lower part of figure). The grades of CIN-1 or mild dysplasia (L-SIL), CIN-2 (moderate dysplasia) and CIN-3 (severe dysplasia and carcinoma *in situ*) (together grouped as H-SIL) show progressive increase in the number of abnormal cells parallel to the increasing severity of grades.

- Atypical glandular cells present, atypical glandular cells favour neoplasia, endocervical adenocarcinoma in situ, and adenocarcinoma.

Q13. What are the main clinicopathologic features of invasive cervical cancer?

Clinical features Invasive cervical cancer is the second most common (after breast cancer) and third leading cause of cancer mortality in women worldwide.
i. The incidence of invasive cervical cancer has declined in developed countries due to increased use of Pap smear for early detection of preinvasive stages of cervical cancer.
ii. In underdeveloped countries with inadequate health care, the incidence remains high.
iii. The peak incidence of invasive cervical cancer is in the 4th to 6th decades of life.
iv. Invasive cervical carcinoma is often preceded by SIL and thus it has the same risk factors as SIL.
Pathology Cervical cancer can be recognised on gross and microscopic examination:
Gross There are three growth patterns: fungating, ulcerating and infiltrating.
i. Fungating growth is the most common, and is usually accompanied by infiltration of the vaginal wall **(Fig. 24.4, A)**.
ii. Advanced stage of invasive cancer are characterised by widespread destruction and infiltration of adjacent structures, including the urinary bladder, rectum, vagina and metastases to local lymph nodes. Distal metastases are found most often in the lungs, liver, bone and kidneys.
Microscopy In 80% of cases, it is a squamous cell carcinoma.
i. Most often (70%) it is a moderately differentiated, nonkeratinising, large cell carcinoma **(Fig. 24.4, B)**.
ii. Well differentiated, keratinising squamous cell carcinoma is seen in 25% cases.
iii. Poorly differentiated squamous cell carcinoma in 5% cases.
iv. Adenocarcinoma of endocervical origin accounts up to 15% cancers.
v. The remaining 5% are cancers of uncommon histologic type: neuroendocrine small cell carcinoma, adenosquamous carcinoma, etc.

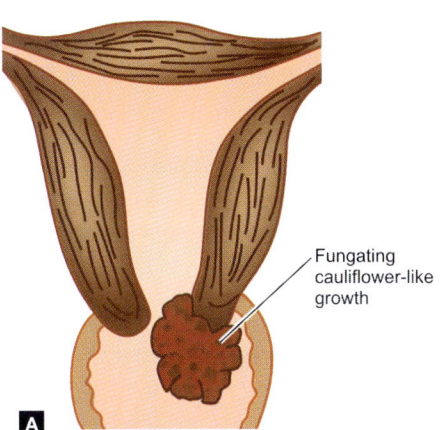 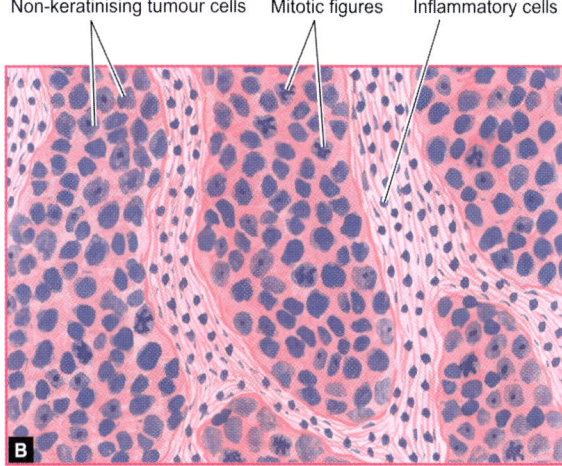

FIGURE 24.4: Invasive carcinoma of the cervix. A, Common gross appearance is of a fungating or exophytic, cauliflower-like tumour. B, Common microscopic type is moderately-differentiated non-keratinising large cell carcinoma. The tumour is composed of large masses and strands of large malignant squamous cells invading into underlying connective tissue. Keratin pearl formation is infrequent.

Clinical staging is performed using the TNM system and is important for the treatment and prognosis. Stage I cancers limited to the cervix are treated by surgery and have excellent prognosis, with a 5-year survival above 90% cases.

UTERUS

Q14. What are the main anatomic parts of the uterus?

The body of the uterus consists predominantly of smooth muscle cells forming a thick layer called myometrium, which on the luminal side is covered with endometrium, and on the external side with serosa (peritoneum).

i. *Endometrium is a hormonally sensitive tissue* that changes during the menstrual cycle and undergoes atrophy after the menopause. It consists of glands and stroma and has two parts:
- A basal layer (*basalis*) that does not change during the menstrual cycle.
- The superficial functional layer (*functionalis*) which changes under the influence of oestrogen and progesterone during the proliferative and secretory phase of the menstrual cycle and is regularly shed 28 days after the onset of the cycle during menstrual bleeding.

ii. *Endometrial glands* of the proliferative (*follicular*) phase proliferate under oestrogenic stimulation and appear tubular. They are lined by columnar cells with basally located nuclei and scant cytoplasm. After ovulation, the secretory (*luteal*) phase begins and the glands responding to progesterone become secretory. If the woman becomes pregnant, the glands remain secretory and in 25% of cases show even hypersecretory change with nuclear enlargement and hyperchromasia called *Arias-Stella phenomenon*.

iii. *Endometrial stromal cells* also change and by the end of the secretory phase transform into predecidual cells, which in case of pregnancy become typical *decidual cells* forming the decidual membrane of the placenta.

iv. Microscopic examination of the *endometrial biopsies* is important for assessing the functional integrity of the endometrium. It is routinely performed in women with dysfunctional uterine bleeding and during the assisted reproductive procedures to determine if the endometrium of the treated patient is adequately responding to hormones.

v. In *children and prepubertal girls*, the endometrium is quiescent and does not show the cyclic menstrual changes.

vi. After the *menopause*, the entire endometrium becomes atrophic and is usually reduced to a thin basal layer with microcystic atrophic glands.

vii. *Hormonal contraceptives* also induce an atrophy of glands, but in contrast to postmenopausal atrophy, the inactive glands are surrounded by a decidualised stroma.

viii. *Hyperoestrinism* due to endogenous overproduction of oestrogen or due to exogenous oestrogen can prolong the proliferative phase of the menstrual cycle and induce endometrial hyperplasia.

Q15. What is dysfunctional uterine bleeding? Discuss its etiopathogenesis in brief.

Definition Dysfunctional uterine bleeding (DUB) is clinically defined as abnormal bleeding during or between menstrual bleeding periods without an underlying causative uterine lesion such as tumour, polyp, infection, hyperplasia, pregnancy, trauma or blood dyscrasia.

Etiopathogenesis Most often, DUB occurs due to anovulatory cycle, which is characterised by prolongation of the oestrogenic stimulation and no progesterone-dependent luteal phase; most often it occurs in girls post-menarche or older women in perimenopausal years.

I. **Causes of anovulation** are grouped by age groups in which they occur as follows:
i. *Childhood, pre-puberty*: Precocious puberty of hypothalamic, pituitary or ovarian origin
ii. *Adolescence*: Physiologic 'menstrual irregularities' at the onset of puberty (very common)
iii. *Reproductive age*: Complications of pregnancy and spontaneous abortions, endometrial hyperplasia, tumours, endometrial polyps
iv. *Premenopausal age*: Physiologic anovulatory cycles that precede menopause-related cessation of menstruation, endometrial hyperplasia, polyps and tumours
v. *Postmenopausal age*: Senile atrophy, polyps, endometrial hyperplasia, tumours

II. **Ovulatory DUB** in women of reproductive age includes:
i. Hormonally inadequate luteal phase (i.e. endometrial biopsy shows a lag in the luteal phase > 2 days)
ii. Irregular shedding (prolonged secretion of progesterone)

Pathology Endometrial biopsy usually shows disorderly proliferation of glands and stroma, with focal stromal breakdown and bleeding.

Q16. Describe endometritis briefly.

Definition Endometritis is inflammation of the endometrium, which may be acute or chronic.

Etiopathogenesis Most often, it is caused by infections, but in some instances, especially in the chronic form, the cause remains unknown.

i. **Acute endometritis** may result from 3 causes:
a. Puerperal (following delivery, abortion and retained placenta and other products of conception).
b. Intrauterine contraceptive device.
c. Extension of infections from the cervix and vagina (most often sexually-transmitted diseases caused by *N. gonorrhoeae* or *C. trachomatis*).

ii. **Chronic endometritis** has the same causes as acute endometritis. It is more common and presumably represents an outcome of prolonged or recurrent acute infections.
a. In some cases, there is infiltration of endometrium with plasma cells for no obvious reasons and that condition is then called *chronic nonspecific endometritis*. It may also be accompanied by chronic myometritis.
b. *Tuberculous endometritis*, a form of chronic endometritis, is uncommon in developed countries but it is still a significant problem in underdeveloped countries. In India, it affects 5% of all adult women.

Q17. What is adenomyosis? What are its salient clinicopathologic features?

Definition Adenomyosis is a condition of unknown etiology characterised by the presence of endometrial glands and stroma in the myometrium.

Pathology Adenomyosis is found in approximately 20% uteri of adult women.
Gross The foci of adenomyosis are not visible but sometimes they may be recognised as petechiae in a thickened myometrium.
Microscopy shows foci consisting of proliferative endometrial glands and stroma deep in the myometrium (at least 3 mm below the normal border).

Clinical features
i. Adenomyosis is usually found in 30–50 year old women.
ii. It may be clinically silent or it may cause menorrhagia, colicky dysmenorrhoea and dysfunctional uterine bleeding.
iii. It may coexist with endometriosis.

Q18. What is endometriosis? Discuss its salient features.

Definition Endometriosis is the presence of normal endometrial glands and stroma in abnormal locations outside the uterus.

Etiopathogenesis Controversial, but there are 3 theories as under:
i. Transplantation of regurgitated endometrial tissue shed during the menstrual bleeding.
ii. Metaplasia of the coelomic epithelium that is the common precursor of uterine endometrium, fallopian tube mucosa and ovarian surface epithelium.
iii. Vascular/lymphatic dissemination of endometrial tissue to other sites.

Pathology
Gross Appearance varies depending on the location, extent and duration of the disease:
i. Ovary is the most common site of endometriosis, often involving both ovaries.
ii. In most cases, endometriosis forms multiple, scattered, small, red to brownish-black, subserosal lesions a few millimetres in diameter, or larger cysts, or brown fibrous scars.
iii. Larger cyst, 3–5 cm in diameter, typically found in ovaries, are colloquially called 'chocolate cysts' because they contain dark red to brown haemolysed blood.
Microscopy shows foci composed of endometrial glands surrounded by stroma that contains foci of haemorrhage, haemosiderin and haemosiderin-laden macrophages.

Clinical features Commonly seen are:
i. Dysmenorrhoea with pelvic pain due to the haemorrhage into the implants at the time of menstruation
ii. Dyspareunia
iii. Infertility

Prognosis Treatment with oral contraceptives may reduce the symptoms by preventing cyclic proliferation and expansion of endometriosis followed by haemorrhage.

Q19. What is the current classification of endometrial hyperplasias? Briefly mention their etiopathogenesis and pathologic features.

Definition Endometrial hyperplasia is defined as hyperplasia of endometrial glands and stroma due to excessive oestrogenic stimulation unopposed by progesterone.

Etiopathogenesis Hyperoestrinism plays a key role in the event. It could have many causes such as:
i. Perimenopausal anovulatory cycles (the most common cause)
ii. Obesity with endogenous oestrogen hyperproduction
iii. Polycystic ovary syndrome
iv. Hormonally active ovarian tumours (e.g. theca cell tumour)
v. Adrenocortical hyperfunction
vi. Exogenous oestrogen administration

Pathology In the WHO 2014 classification, endometrial hyperplasia is divided into two groups:

i. **Endometrial (benign) hyperplasia without atypia:**
a. Focal crowding of glands and an increased gland to stroma ratio (>1 from normal which is <1).
b. The glands may retain their elongated shape or become dilated showing some complexity.
c. The nuclei are uniform, resembling those in proliferative endometrium and show no atypia.
d. Progression to adenocarcinoma occurs rarely (1–3%).

ii. **Atypical hyperplasia (endometrial intraepithelial neoplasia, EIN):**
a. It is a clonal neoplastic proliferation so that the altered glands appear different from the adjacent normal endometrium.
b. The abnormal glands are crowded and surrounded by scant stroma, but do not show yet the usual features of adenocarcinoma, such as back-to-back positioning of growth, cribriform or solid nest of neopalstic cells.
c. Nuclei show atypia (loss of polarity, hyperchromasia, enlargement).
d. There is increased N:C ratio.
e. Mitoses are also present.

Prognosis
- EIN in 50% cases is associated with inactivation of PTEN (phosphorylase and tensin), a change that is also seen in most invasive endometrial carcinomas.

- Progression to adenocarcinoma occurs in approximately one half all cases.
- Most women opt for hysterectomy to prevent invasive malignancy. In younger women who desire children, hormonal treatment with progesterone and careful follow-up may be an alternative.

Q20. Give a brief account of endometrial carcinoma.

Definition Endometrial carcinoma is an adenocarcinoma originating from endometrial glands.

Epidemiology In the United States and Europe, it is the most common cancer of the female genital tract, but in Asia cervical cancer remains the leading cause of cancer death in women.

It occurs mostly in postmenopausal women with a peak incidence in 6th and 7th decade. It is uncommon in women under the age of 40 years.

Etiopathogenesis The following risk factors have been identified:

i. Chronic unopposed oestrogen excess the same way as in endometrial hyperplasia with atypia
ii. Obesity
iii. Diabetes mellitus
iv. Hypertension
v. Nulliparity
vi. Heredity as evidenced by the increased incidence of endometrial carcinoma in hereditary non-polyposis colon cancer (HNPCC) syndrome due to mismatch DNA repair genes, and Cowden syndrome (carcinoma of endometrium, breast and thyroid occurring simultaneously in patients with germ cell mutation of *PTEN* gene).

Classification Two major types of endometrial adenocarcinoma are recognised: type I and type II.

Type I tumours *(endometrioid and mucinous adenocarcinomas)* comprise 80–85% of all endometrial carcinomas.

i. These tumours are *oestrogen-dependent* and develop through the endometrial hyperplasia-carcinoma sequence due to unopposed oestrogen stimulation.

ii. *Loss of PTEN tumour suppressor gene* is a common early event which is already present in 50% cases of atypical hyperplasia, the forerunner of invasive adenocarcinoma.

iii. *Oncogene activation* follows as the tumour cells become invasive. *PIK3CA* is the most common activated oncogene found in 40% cases tumours. It is not found in endometrial hyperplasia, indicating that it is a feature unique to invasive endometrial cancers. Other genes that are also involved in 10–30% cases are *KRAS* oncogene and *CTNNB1* (encoding β-catenin).

Type II tumours *(non-endometrioid cancers)* comprise 10–15% of endometrial cancers.

i. They are *oestrogen-independent* and do not develop from pre-existent atypical hyperplasia.

ii. *Microscopically* they are most often serous carcinomas, but may be also clear cells and undifferentiated carcinomas or carcinosarcomas.

iii. *TP53* gene plays an important role in the pathogenesis of these tumours and it is mutated in almost all type II tumours.

Pathology

Gross Two growth patterns are recognised: localised polypoid and diffuse **(Fig. 24.5)**.

i. Most tumours protrude into the endometrial cavity and are recognised as friable, grey-tan tissue.

ii. Tumours tend to invade into the myometrium and the cervix. The extent of such invasion is important for the staging of the tumours and the planning of the therapy.

iii. Advanced stage tumours spread to adjacent organs such as the vagina, urinary bladder or rectum, metastasise to lymph nodes and distant organs, most often the lungs.

Microscopy Features vary depending on the type of tumour and the degree of its differentiation:

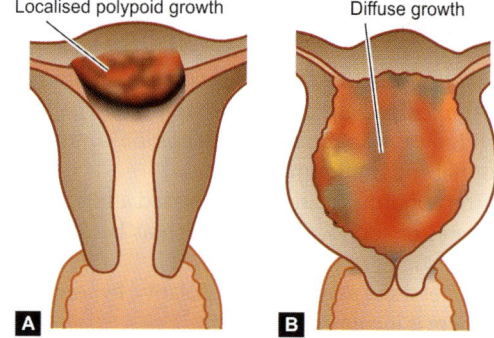

FIGURE 24.5: Endometrial carcinoma. Diagrammatic representation of the common gross patterns—localised polypoid growth and diffuse growth.

i. *Type I tumours* are endometrioid adenocarcinomas, called so because they resemble proliferating endometrial glands. They are graded according to FIGO into well-differentiated (predominantly glandular), moderately-differentiated (predominantly glandular and partially solid), and poorly-differentiated (mostly solid) adenocarcinomas. Some tumours contain foci of squamous metaplasia.

ii. *Type II tumours* resemble ovarian serous or clear cell carcinoma. Some tumours are carcinosarcomas composed of poorly-differentiated glands or solid epithelial nests and sarcoma, which may have features of undifferentiated pleomorphic sarcoma, rhabdomyosarcoma, chondrosarcoma, etc.

Clinical features

i. Most tumours (90%) present with abnormal vaginal bleeding; menorrhagia and prolonged menstrual bleeding are seen in premenopausal women.

ii. Invasion of pelvic and abdominal organs is accompanied by signs of obstruction and dysfunction of the involved organs (e.g. urinary obstruction and renal failure due to invasion of the urinary bladder).

Prognosis and survival depend on the stage and the histologic type of the tumour:
- Stage I tumours that are limited to the uterus have a 5-year survival of 90%, in contrast to stage III tumours with local or regional spread which have a 5-year survival under 50%.
- Type II tumours have, in general, worse prognosis than type I tumours.
- Treatment is mostly surgical, but may include radiation and chemotherapy for advanced cases.

Q21. What are uterine leiomyomas?

Definition Leiomyomas, or more correctly also known as fibromyomas or fibroids, are benign myometrial tumours composed of smooth muscle cells, often admixed to fibroblasts in varying proportions.

Epidemiology

i. About 20% of women older than 30 years have one or more uterine leiomyomas.

ii. Leiomyoma may rarely develop in the cervix or from broad ligament.

iii. Most smooth muscle cell tumours are benign and less than 0.5% are leiomyosarcomas.

iv. Uterine leiomyosarcoma usually develop more often from malignant transformation of a pre-existent leiomyoma than de novo from the intact myometrium.

Pathology

Gross

Leiomyomas present as firm compact myometrial nodules that vary in size.

i. On cross section they have a whorled appearance **(Fig. 24.6, A)**.

ii. They may be solitary or multiple.

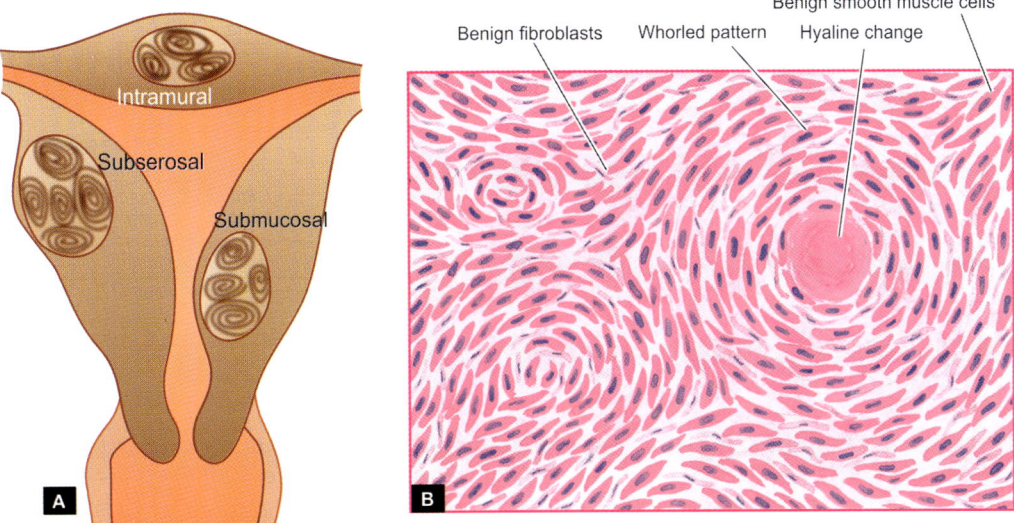

FIGURE 24.6: Uterine leiomyomas. A, Diagrammatic appearance of common locations and characteristic whorled appearance on cut section. B, Microscopy shows whorls of smooth muscle cells which are spindle-shaped, having abundant cytoplasm and oval blunted nuclei.

iii. According to their location, they are classified as *submucosal, intramural or subserosal*. Location of leiomyoma is important because it is related to the clinical symptoms (e.g. bleeding due to submucosal tumour) or complications (e.g. torsion around a pedicle of a pedunculated subserosal tumour).

Microscopy They are composed of bundles of spindle-shaped smooth muscle cells and scattered fibroblasts **(Fig. 24.6, B)**.

i. There are no mitoses; this helps distinguishing benign leiomyomas from malignant leiomyosarcomas, which also show other signs of malignancy such as nuclear atypia and foci of necrosis.

ii. Secondary changes in leiomyomas include hyalinisation, cystic degeneration, calcification, infarction, infection with suppuration and malignant transformation (rare).

Clinical features Most tumours produce no symptoms.

i. Symptomatic cases may present with abnormal uterine bleeding, pain and feeling of heaviness in the pelvis, symptoms due to compression of the bladder or rectum.

ii. During pregnancy, they may increase due to hormonal stimulation.

iii. After menopause, they tend to shrink due to a loss of oestrogen sensitive smooth muscle cells, whereupon the tumours transform into fibroids composed predominantly of fibroblasts.

■ OVARY

Q22. What are the main components of the ovary?

Ovaries are paired organs hanging from either fallopian tube by a mesentery called mesovarium, the lateral suspensory ligament and the ovarian ligament.

Histology The ovary consists of surface covering (derived from foetal coelomic epithelium), outer cortex and inner medulla **(Fig. 24.7)**:

I. **Cortex** of an adult woman contains, during her reproductive life, germ cells surrounded by specialised ovarian stroma. The rest of the cortex contains unspecialised stroma.

i. The *specialised ovarian stroma* includes granulosa and theca cells, arranged into several layers around the oocyte, thus forming a graafian follicle. Granulosa and follicle-associated theca cells produce oestrogens.

ii. After the ovulation, the follicle transforms into *corpus luteum*, which is the principal source of progesterone. Maturation of the follicles and the ovulation and the function of corpus luteum are all controlled by pituitary gonadotropins, the follicle stimulating hormone and luteinising hormone. Once the corpus luteum has finished its function, it transforms into *corpus albicans*.

II. **Medulla** is predominantly made up of connective tissue, smooth muscle cells and blood vessels, lymphatics and nerves. Its hilum also contains clusters of steroid hormone-secreting hilar Leydig cells.

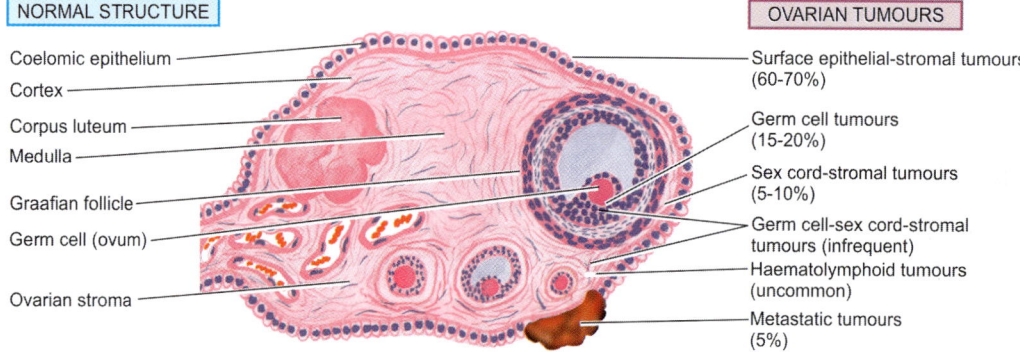

FIGURE 24.7: Structure of the ovary to illustrate origin of ovarian tumours.

Q23. What are various non-neoplastic cysts of the ovaries?

Definition Ovarian cysts are cavitary lesions surrounded by remnants of the ovarian follicles or epithelial cells. Ovarian cysts can be neoplastic or non-neoplastic, solitary or multiple. Non-neoplastic cysts are more common than the neoplastic cysts.

Classification Non-neoplastic cysts occur in several forms, the most important of which are: follicular cysts and luteal cysts. Larger follicular cysts may be lined by flat non-descript epithelium which cannot be distinguished from mesothelial *inclusion cysts;* such cysts are called *simple cysts*.

i. **Follicular cysts** are quite common in the ovaries of adult women. They are usually small but can enlarge up to 10 cm in diameter. Small cysts are asymptomatic but the larger ones may produce a mass effects and clinical symptoms.
Microscopy Follicular cysts have a wall composed of follicular cells, which may be focally luteinised. The cysts are filled with serous fluid.
ii. **Luteal cysts** are formed from corpus luteum that gets sealed over its ruptured surface.
Microscopy Cyst lining consists predominantly of luteinised granulosa cells. Corpus albicans cyst is a variant composed of hyalinised tissue and scattered remaining luteinised cells.

Q24. What is polycystic ovary syndrome?

Definition Polycystic ovary syndrome (PCOS) is a set of clinical hormonal disturbances causing ovulatory and menstrual irregularities in young women who have bilaterally enlarged polycystic ovaries.
Etiopathogenesis Although the cause of PCOS is not known, following has been established:
i. The main problem lies in an imbalanced release of FSH and LH and overproduction of androgens in the ovary.
ii. The initial event is excess androgen secretion due to the dysregulation of 17α-reductase, a rate limiting enzyme in the synthesis of androgens.
iii. Androgens inhibit FSH release resulting in anovulation.
iv. The levels of LH are also low but remain sufficiently high to cause luteinisation of theca and granulosa cells stimulating them to secrete androgens, which further inhibit ovulation.
v. An additional impulse to androgen synthesis is provided by high levels of insulin in serum recorded in most PCOS patients in response to increased insulin resistance of peripheral tissues.
Pathology
i. Ovaries are enlarged and contain numerous follicular cysts covered by fibrotic external cortex forming a thick capsule.
ii. Cortical cysts are lined by follicular granulosa cells and a thick layer of luteinised theca interna cells.
iii. No corpora lutea or albicantia are seen, indicating that no ovulation has taken place.
Clinical features
i. Ovulatory and menstrual irregularities (anovulation, oligomenorrhoea and amenorrhoea)
ii. Infertility
iii. Hyperandrogenism and hirsutism
iv. Obesity
v. Insulin resistance with hyperinsulinaemia

Q25. Discuss pelvic inflammatory disease in brief.

Definition Pelvic inflammatory disease (PID) is a very common clinical syndrome caused by ascending infection, spreading from the vulva and vagina to the endocervix, endometrial cavity, fallopian tubes and even ovaries or the pelvic peritoneum.
Etiopathogenesis PID results from ascending infections as follows:
i. Sexually-transmitted diseases such gonorrhoea and chlamydial infections.
ii. Coliform bacteria from the vagina.
iii. Streptococci and staphylococci in the postpartum period.
Extension of the infection to the ovaries usually results in fibrous encapsulation of the ovary and the tube into a tubo-ovarian (TO) abscess. Spilling of bacteria into the abdominal cavity may cause pelvic peritonitis or accumulation of pus resulting in a pelvic abscess or widespread peritonitis. Entry of bacteria into the blood may result in bacteraemia and sepsis.
Pathology
i. Ascending infections cause cervicitis, endometritis, salpingitis and oophoritis.
ii. The changes are more prominently seen in the fallopian tubes which are tortuous, oedematous and inflamed and may even contain pus (pyosalpinx).
iii. Longer duration infections lead to the formation of pelvic adhesions and obliteration of fallopian tubes.
iv. Resorption of inflammatory exudate results in dilation of fallopian tubes filled with serous fluid (hydrosalpinx).

Clinical features
i. Severe pelvic pain
ii. Fever
iii. Other signs of infection, e.g. menstrual irregularities, dysmenorrhoea
iv. Infertility as a common late complication
v. Infection may spread to other organs and also cause sepsis.
Treatment may be complex and not always successful.

Q26. What is the broad classification of ovarian tumours? Comment briefly on their general etiology and pathogenesis.

Definition Ovarian tumours originate from various cells that are found in the ovaries. These tumours may be benign or malignant; malignant tumours may be primary or secondary (metastatic).
Classification Ovarian tumours are classified broadly according to their cell of origin into six groups; each group has several entities (*see* **Fig. 24.7**):
i. Surface epithelial tumours
ii. Sex cord stromal tumours
iii. Germ cell tumours
iv. Mixed germ cell sex cord stromal tumors
v. Haematolymphoid tumours
vi. Metastatic cancer from nonovarian primaries
Etiopathogenesis The incidence of ovarian tumours is approximately the same in all countries of the world and thus *no environmental factors* have been identified.
Following *endogenous risk factors* are known to contribute only to a small extent, accounting for the pathogenesis of not more than 10% of all ovarian tumours:
i. *Nulliparity and low parity* are associated with higher incidence of ovarian cancer.
• The higher number of ovulations unaccompanied by pregnancy → more surface epithelial cancers.
• Pregnancies and oral contraceptives inhibit ovulation → less surface epithelial cancer.
ii. *Heredity and genes* Familial ovarian tumours are rare.
• The best documented hereditary genes are *BRCA-1* and *BRCA-2* in breast/ovarian cancer families.
• Other gene mutations involved in ovarian cancerogenesis include the following genes: *TP53, KRAS, BRAF, ERBB-2*.
iii. *Complex genetic syndromes* with an increased incidence of ovarian tumours are as under:
a. Lynch syndrome → ovarian surface epithelial cancers in families that also have HNPCC colorectal cancer and endometrial carcinoma due to the mutation of genes encoding DNA repair enzymes.
b. Peutz-Jeghers syndrome → sex-cord stromal tumours
c. Naevoid basal cell carcinoma → ovarian fibroma
d. Developmental disorders of the gonads → dysgerminoma in gonadal dysgenesis, or Turner syndrome.

Q27. What are surface epithelial-stromal tumours? Discuss their salient features.

Definition Epithelial-stromal tumours are benign or malignant tumours originating from the surface mesothelial lining covering the ovaries. Most often, these tumours show serous, mucinous or endometrioid differentiation. Less often, they show urothelial differentiation (Brenner tumour) or mesonephroid differentiation (clear cell carcinoma).
Epidemiology This group includes 70% of all ovarian tumours and 90% of all malignant ovarian tumours.
Classification Three clinicopathologic subtypes are recognised in each subtype in the group as under (**Fig. 24.8**):
I. **Clearly benign:** Included in this group are cystic tumours containing papillary structures ('papillary cystadenomas') lined by uniform cells showing no atypia. The group also includes solid tumours composed of glands and fibrous tissue ('adenofibroma' or 'fibroadenoma'), or benign urothelium ('Brenner tumour').
Prognosis Excellent and are almost all curable by surgery.

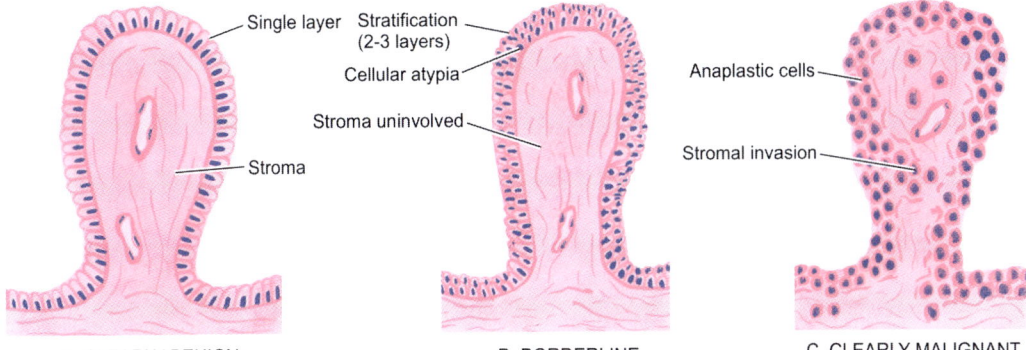

FIGURE 24.8: Diagrammatic representation of general histologic criteria to distinguish benign, borderline (atypical proliferating) and malignant surface epithelial tumours of the ovary.

II. **Clearly malignant:** Included in this group are tumours composed of obviously malignant epithelial cells. They may be cystic or solid or partially cystic/solid and are always carcinomas. They are further subclassified as serous, mucinous, endometrioid and clear cell carcinomas or cystadenocarcinomas.
Prognosis Varies depending on the histologic type of the tumour and its stage, but in most cases it is unfavourable.

III. **Borderline malignant:** These tumours, also known as tumours of low malignant potential, have some features of malignancy such as stratification of cell layers, increased proliferative activity, nuclear atypia, but no evidence of invasion of the underlying stroma.
Prognosis Much more favourable prognosis than malignant tumours, even though many of them may metastasise and may recur.

Q28. Comment briefly on clinicopathologic types of serous ovarian tumours.

Definition Serous ovarian tumours are composed of serous fluid-secreting epithelial cells resembling the epithelial lining of fallopian tubes.

General features
i. Serous tumours form the largest group of surface epithelial-stromal tumours (45%).
ii. These tumours are usually cystic and thus called cystadenoma or cystadenocarcinoma.
iii. Approximately 20% of benign tumours are bilateral, in contrast to the borderline and malignant tumours which are bilateral in 65% of cases.
iv. Tumours are mostly found in the 20–60 year age group, with the predominance of benign tumours in younger women, and the occurrence of malignant tumours in women who are older than 45 years of age.
v. Since they also contain papillae, an additional descriptor is often added, e.g. *papillary serous cystadenocarcinoma* **(Fig. 24.9,A)**.

Clinicopathologic features Three entities are included in the serous group:
I. Serous cystadenoma (60%)
II. Borderline serous tumour (15%)
III. Serous cystadenocarcinoma (25%)

I. **Serous cystadenoma**
i. Typically has a peak incidence in the 20–40 year age group.
ii. It is a benign tumour presenting as a unicameral cyst or a multicystic neoplasm.
iii. Tumour size may vary and many are over 10 cm in diameter.
iv. The cysts are filled with clear serous yellowish fluid.
v. The cystic cavities are lined by regularly polarised columnar cells, which may be ciliated like the tubal epithelium.
vi. Papillae are common.
vii. Predominantly solid tumours composed of fibrous stroma in excess of glandular components is called cystadenofibroma.

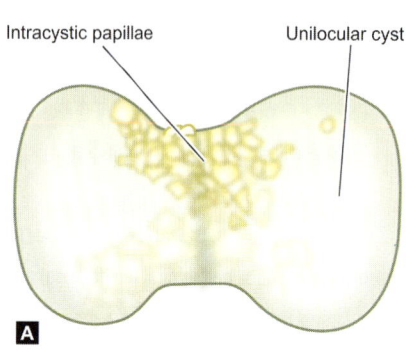
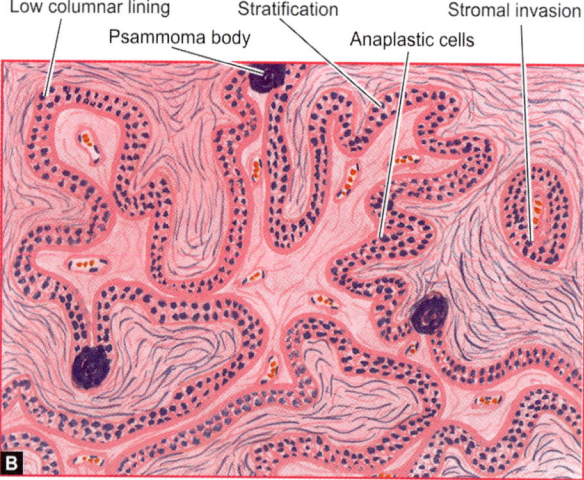

FIGURE 24.9: Papillary serous cystadenocarcinoma of the ovary. A, Grossly, it shows an enlarged ovary replaced with a large unilocular cyst with intracystic papillae. B. Microscopic features include stratification of low columnar epithelium lining the inner surface of the cyst and a few psammoma bodies. The stroma shows invasion by clusters of anaplastic tumour cells.

II. *Borderline serous tumour*
i. It is composed of cells that show stratification or tufting on the surface of the papillae which show complex hierarchical branching or cribriform growth.
ii. The epithelium shows mild nuclear atypia and even superficial invasion of the stroma (less than 3 mm), but deep and destructive invasion is not seen.
iii. Peritoneal and omental metastases may be found, yet these tumours have an excellent prognosis and 80% cases are alive 5 years after the diagnosis.
III. *Serous cystadenocarcinoma* It is a malignant tumour that shows signs of invasiveness and a capacity to metastasise. Two distinct clinicopathologic subtypes are recognised: low-grade invasive serous carcinoma and high-grade serous carcinoma **(Fig. 24.9,B)**:
i. *Low-grade serous carcinoma* is a rare tumour (5% of all ovarian carcinomas):
a. Most often, it is derived from a pre-existing borderline serous tumour of the ovary.
b. It forms small papillae, with frequent calcifications and invasive growth.
c. A heavily calcified subtype is called psammomatous carcinoma.
d. Low-grade serous carcinomas show *BRAF* and *KRAS* gene mutations in most instances.
e. These tumours have a good prognosis.
ii. *High-grade serous carcinoma* is the most common malignant ovarian tumour accounting for more than 70% of all ovarian malignancies.
a. These tumours are composed of highly anaplastic cells forming broad and irregularly shaped papillae, cribriform glands, solid sheets and invasive cords.
b. These tumours originate from two sources: fallopian tubes or ovarian surface epithelium that has invaginated into the cortex and undergone tubal metaplasia.
c. Patients with *BRCA-1* and *BRCA-2* mutations develop high-grade serous carcinomas from preinvasive neoplastic foci in the fallopian tubes called *STIC (serous tubal intraepithelial cancer)*.
d. For large malignant tumours, it is, however, impossible to state whether they originated from the tube or the ovarian surface epithelium.
e. Irrespective of their origin, all such tumours constantly show mutations of *TP53* gene.
f. These tumours have a poor prognosis depending on the stage at the time of diagnosis: 5-year survival is 70% for stage I tumours limited to the ovary, and 25% for those that have metastasised to the peritoneum.

Q29. What are the salient clinicopathologic features of mucinous ovarian tumours?

Definition Mucinous tumours are cystic ovarian neoplasms composed of mucus-secreting cells **(Fig. 24.10)**.

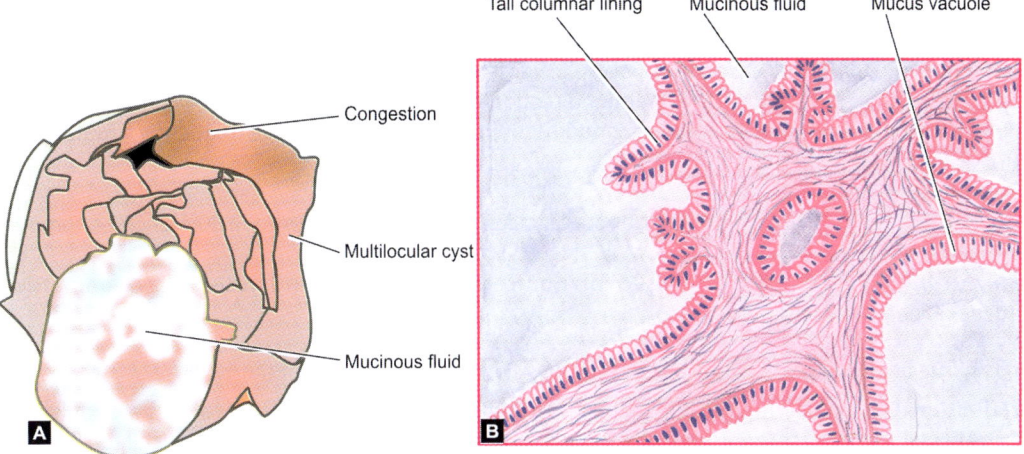

FIGURE 24.10: Mucinous cystadenoma of the ovary. A, Cut surface shows a very large multilocular cyst without papillae. The cyst wall shows presence of loculi containing gelatinous mucoid material. B, Microscopy shows that the cyst wall and septa are lined by a single layer of tall columnar mucin-secreting intestinal type epithelium with basally-placed nuclei and large apical mucinous vacuoles.

General features
i. Overall, mucinous tumours account for 15% of ovarian tumours.
ii. Only 5–10% of tumours in each category (benign, borderline and malignant) are bilateral.
iii. Most tumours are large, multilocular cystic and filled with mucus.
Clinicopathologic features Like serous tumours, they can be classified as benign, borderline or malignant:
- Benign mucinous cystadenomas predominate accounting for 80% of these tumours.
- Only 10% are malignant.
- Remaining 10% are borderline.

I. **Benign mucinous tumours** are composed of polarised, uniform, cylindrical cells lining the cavities that contain mucus.
II. **Borderline tumours** show nuclear atypia and foci of superficial stromal invasion, but no destructive or deep invasion.
III. **Invasive mucinous cystadenocarcinomas** show all the signs of malignancy invading or even penetrating the wall of the cystic tumour.
NOTE: Mucinous adenocarcinoma of the ovary often represents a metastasis from a primary in the gastrointestinal tract, such as appendix or colon or stomach; it differs from the primary ovarian in following ways:
i. Metastatic mucinous adenocarcinomas are more likely than primary ovarian carcinomas to show the following *gross and clinical features*:
- Bilaterality
- Smaller size than primary
- More likely to be friable and necrotic, more likely to be nodular than expansile, involve the periovarian structures and cause ascites or pseudomyxoma peritonei.

ii. *Microscopy* Metastatic carcinomas often cause a desmoplastic reaction and invade connective tissue rather than forming complex papillary structures. Signet ring cells may be very prominent.
iii. *Immunohistochemistry* with antibodies to cytokeratin shows the CK7-/CK20+ pattern typical for the appendiceal and colorectal adenocarcinoma, rather than CK7+/CK20- pattern seen in primary tumours of the ovary.

Q30. What are endometrioid tumours of the ovary?
Definition Endometrioid ovarian tumours are adenocarcinomas resembling endometrioid (type I) carcinoma of the uterus. They account for 5% of all ovarian tumours and 20% of all ovarian malignancies. Benign and borderline endometrioid tumours also occur but are very rare.

Etiopathogenesis

i. Endometrioid tumours originate from the surface epithelium of the ovary or foci of endometriosis.
ii. In up to one third of all cases, there is also a coexistent endometrial adenocarcinoma, suggesting a field effect, or a metastatic spread in either direction in some cases.
iii. Like the type I endometrial tumours, endometrioid ovarian tumours have frequently a mutation of *PTEN* tumour suppressor gene.

Pathology

Gross These tumours are predominantly solid while smaller parts are cystic. In 30% of cases, tumours are bilateral.

Microscopy Tumours are composed of non-secretory glands and resemble endometriod adenocarcinoma of the uterus.

Q31. Write briefly on classification and pathogenesis of germ cell tumours of the ovary.

Definition Germ cell tumours (GCT) of the ovary originate from germ cells, i.e. ova. They are equivalent to testicular germ cell tumours, but in contrast to those in males, most ovarian germ cell tumours are benign.

Epidemiology GCT account for about 20% of all ovarian tumours. The incidence of GCT is the same in all countries of the world and there are no significant geographic differences, or identifiable risk factors.

Pathogenesis and classification Unlike testicular germ cell tumours, histogenesis of ovarian germ cell tumour is less well understood. **Figure 24.11** presents a simplified schematic diagram illustrating the possible pathways of ovarian germ cell tumour development. Classification of these tumours is given in **Table 24.1** while salient features of their pathogenesis are as under:

TABLE 24.1 Germ cell tumours of the ovary.

A. Primitive germ cell tumours
1. Dysgerminoma
2. Yolk sac tumour (endodermal sinus tumour)
3. Embryonal carcinoma
4. Polyembryoma
5. Non-gestational choriocarcinoma

B. Biphasic or triphasic teratomas
1. Immature
2. Mature (solid, cystic-dermoid cyst)

C. Monodermal teratoma or somatic type tumours
1. Struma ovarii
2. Carcinoid tumour
3. Miscellaneous epithelial/mesenchymal malignant tumours

D. Mixed germ cell tumour

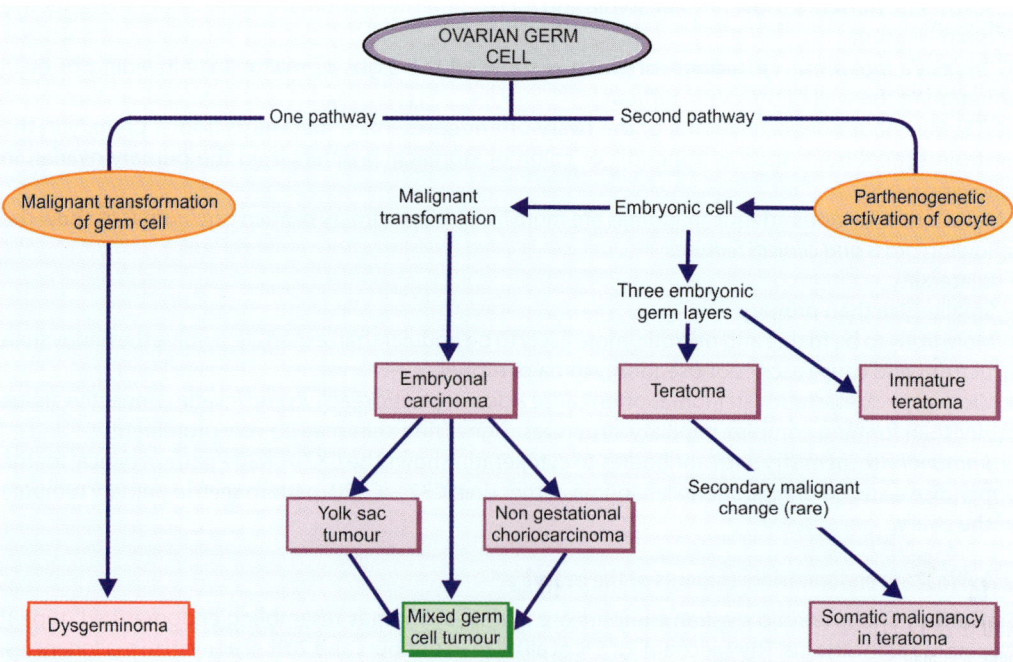

FIGURE 24.11: Histogenetic evolution and classification of ovarian germ cell tumours.

i. The germ cell may undergo malignant transformation and proliferate as such, giving rise to a *dysgerminoma*.
ii. Alternatively, germ cell may be *parthenogenetically activated* to form embryonic cells:
a. As we recall from basic biology, parthenogenesis includes spontaneous division of the ovum without fertilisation by the sperm. The newly formed germ cells will form 3 germ layers (ectoderm, mesoderm and endoderm) and the somatic tissues derived from them will give rise to a benign germ cell tumour, *teratoma*. Teratoma formation is the outcome of most parthenogenetic activations of ova.
b. Embryonic cells formed through parthenogenesis may undergo malignant transformation and become *embryonal carcinoma* cells. Embryonal carcinoma cells probably can also develop from dysgerminoma, but that happens rarely, mostly in dysgenetic gonads.
c. Embryonal carcinoma cells may differentiate three ways and produce: teratoma, choriocarcinoma or yolk sac elements; these may be intermixed with each other and form *malignant mixed germ cell tumours*. Embryonal carcinomas are the malignant stem cells of these mixed germ cell tumours and they can metastasise. Fortunately, they can be readily killed by modern drugs.
d. Derivatives of embryonal carcinoma include: *teratoma* tissue which do not proliferate much, but also malignant cells that form *choriocarcinoma* and *yolk sac tumour*.
e. These components may continue to grow as malignant tumours, and sometimes overgrow all the other elements and become monoclonal choriocarcinoma and yolk sac tumours.

Q32. Describe salient clinicopathologic features of main examples of ovarian germ cell tumours.

Common examples of ovarian germ cell tumours discussed below are teratoma, dysgerminoma, yolk sac tumour and choriocarcinoma.
I. **Teratoma** is the most common germ cell tumour of the ovary (95–98%).
• It is composed of somatic tissues derived from all three germ layers: ectoderm (skin, neural tissue), mesoderm (cartilage and bone and muscle) and endoderm (intestinal and respiratory epithelium).
• It is benign in most cases and typically presents as a '*dermoid cyst*' in women under the age of 30 years of age (95%) **(Fig. 24.12)**.
Variant forms of teratomas are quite rare (only 2–5% of all teratomas) as under:
i. *Monodermal teratomas* These include two examples:
a. *Struma ovarii* (made up of thyroid tissue) is the most common clinically important monodermal teratoma. It can even produce thyroid hormones and cause hyperthyroidism, or give rise to thyroid malignant tumours, such a papillary thyroid carcinoma.
b. *Carcinoid tumour* (a low grade malignant tumour composed of neuroendocrine cells) is yet another monodermal teratoma.

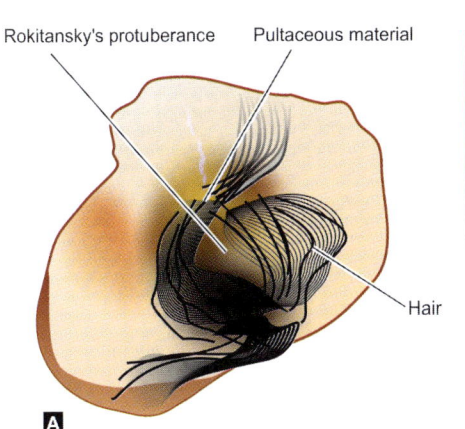
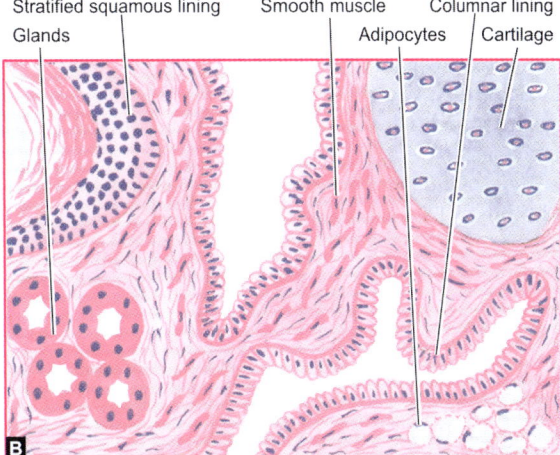

FIGURE 24.12: Dermoid cyst (mature teratoma) of the ovary. A, The ovary is enlarged and shows a large unilocular cyst containing hair, pultaceous material and bony tissue. B, Microscopy shows characteristic lining of the cyst wall by epidermis and its appendages. Islands of mature adipose tissue and neuroglial tissue are also seen.

ii. *Immature teratomas* are composed of immature and potentially malignant embryonic/foetal tissues.
a. Teratomas that are component of *malignant mixed germ cell tumours* usually occur in children and women under the age of 20 years.
iii. *Malignant transformation* of benign teratomas is an event that occurs very rarely (0.1%). The malignant tumours arising in teratomas are usually squamous cell carcinoma or adenocarcinoma, and sometimes sarcomas. Typically, this malignant transformation of teratoma occurs in older women whose teratoma was not resected when these women were young.
II. **Dysgerminoma** is the most common malignant GCT in adult women, comprising 1–2% of all ovarian tumour. Most patients are less than 30 years old.
i. It is an equivalent of testicular seminoma.
ii. Like seminomas, dysgerminoma is a solid mass composed of polygonal cells arranged in sheets and lobules surrounded by fibrous tissue, which is infiltrated with lymphocytes.
iii. Dysgerminomas are easily resected before they metastasise. Those patients that have metastases respond well to radiation and chemotherapy. The overall survival is over 95%.
III. **Yolk sac tumour**, also known as endodermal sinus tumour, is the most common malignant GCT in children and young persons under the age of 20 years.
Microscopically, it resembles testicular yolk sac tumour and thus has a complex histologic structure and grows in many pattern, including the formation of glomeruloid Schiller-Duval bodies.
i. Tumour secretes AFP and α-1-antitrypsin.
ii. It is highly aggressive malignant tumour and may not respond so readily to treatment.
IV. **Choriocarcinoma (non-gestational)** is a rare malignant GCT.
Microscopically, it resembles the uterine placenta-derived choriocarcinoma, but it is more malignant and often resistant to chemotherapy.
- It is composed of cytotrophoblastic and syncytiotrophoblastic cells secreting huge amounts of chorionic gonadotropin, which is a good marker for this tumour.

Q33. Write briefly on common sex cord-stromal tumours of the ovary.

Definition Sex cord-stromal tumours of the ovary are benign and malignant tumours composed of cells that resemble those the graafian follicles (granulosa or theca cells) and ovarian hilar cells, as well as testicular cells such as Sertoli and Leydig cells.

Epidemiology These tumours comprise 5–10% of all ovarian tumours. Most tumours are sporadic but some occur in patients affected by familial tumour syndromes, such as Sertoli-Leydig cell tumours in Peutz-Jeghers syndrome.

Clinicopathologic features These tumours appear as solid masses and are often lipid rich which gives them a yellow brown colour on cross section. Examples discussed below are granulose cell tumour, thecoma, fibroma, Sertoli-Leydig cell tumour, and steroid cell tumour.

I. **Granulosa cell tumours** mostly occur in postmenopausal women, but they may occur at any age.
i. They are functionally active and secrete inhibin (inhibiting FSH release) and oestrogens which may cause precocious puberty in young girls or menstrual disturbances in adult women.
ii. The tumour is composed of oestrogen-secreting granulosa cells.
iii. Tumour cells are cuboidal or spindle-shaped and have grooved coffee bean-shaped nuclei.
iv. Several microscopic patterns are recognised including micro- and macrofollicular, trabecular, band-like and diffuse sheet-like patterns **(Fig. 24.13)**.

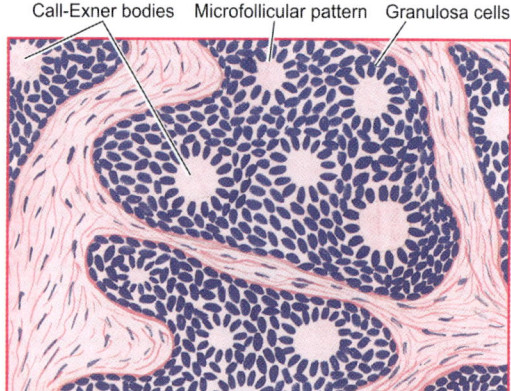

FIGURE 24.13: Granulosa cell tumour showing uniform granulosa cells and numerous rosette-like Call-Exner bodies containing central amorphous pink material surrounded by granulosa cells.

v. Microfollicular tumours form rosette-like structures around the eosinophilic masses, resembling Call-Exner bodies in the normal Graafian follicle.
vi. Various histologic patterns have no clinical significance and only help pathologists to make the diagnosis of granulosa cells.
vii. A special subtype, called *juvenile granulosa cell tumour*, is found in girls and young women under the age of 20 years. It is always benign and hormonally active.
viii. Granulosa cell tumours of adult women are low-grade malignant tumours.
ix. Most tumours are cured by surgery but some which have spread beyond the ovary may recur after resection and occasionally even metastasise many years after surgery.
x. Microscopic examination cannot predict which tumour will behave as a malignant tumour and, therefore, all granulose cell tumours need to be treated as potentially malignant with caution and vigilant follow-up.

II. **Thecoma** is a benign tumour composed of theca cells, which usually secrete oestrogen.
Gross It presents as firm fibrotic mass, which on cross section appears yellow.
Microscopy It is composed of spindle-shaped theca cells, which contain lipids demonstrable by special fat stains.

III. **Fibroma** is a benign tumour originating from nonspecific fibroblasts in the ovarian stroma.
i. Fibromas account for 75% of all sex-cord stromal tumours and are thus the most common tumour in this group.
ii. Fibromas do not produce hormones, but some are accompanied by pleural effusion and ascites as part of the *Meigs syndrome*.

IV. **Sertoli-Leydig cell tumours** are rare tumours of low malignant potential. They may occur at any age, but most often they are diagnosed in women younger than 30 years of age.
i. These tumours secrete weak androgens (dehydroepiandrostenedione, DHEA) which may cause amenorrhoea and breast atrophy, followed by hirsutism and other signs of masculinisation such as deepening of the voice, male pattern and clitoral enlargement.
ii. *Microscopically*, these tumours are composed of tubule-forming Sertoli cells and grouped Leydig cells with well-developed eosinophilic or vacuolated cytoplasm.
iii. The *prognosis* depends on the stage of tumour and the degree of their differentiation. To this end, these tumours may be classified as showing signs of well-differentiated, intermediately-differentiated or poorly-differentiated. The latter group contains tumours that have sarcoma-like microscopic feature and poor prognosis.

V. **Steroid cell tumours** include two tumour types:
i. Small benign *hilar tumours* composed of testosterone-secreting Leydig cells.
ii. *Lipid cell tumours* resembling luteinised cortical stroma cells, adrenal cortical or Leydig cells producing various steroid hormones, including androgens.

Q34. What are the most common metastatic tumours in the ovaries?

Metastatic tumours in the ovaries most often originate from the female reproductive organ, breast and the gastrointestinal tract.
Krukenberg tumour is a term used to denote bilateral enlargement of both ovaries due to metastatic signet ring carcinoma **(Fig. 24.14)**. Primary mucinous adenocarcinoma is most often located in the stomach, but it may be found in other parts of the gastrointestinal tract as well.

■ PLACENTA

Q35. Comment briefly on morphology of placenta as related to understanding of its pathology.

Placenta is a temporary organ linking the foetus in utero with the maternal circulation.
i. Its *main parts* are: the placental disc, foetal membranes and the umbilical cord, linking the placenta to the maternal circulation. Foetal membranes attached to the disc are called amnion and chorion.
ii. Placenta is formed from both maternal and foetal tissues. The *maternal part* consists of decidual membrane covering the cotyledons of the placenta. The *foetal part* is formed of numerous functional units called chorionic villi, which comprise the major part of the placenta at birth.

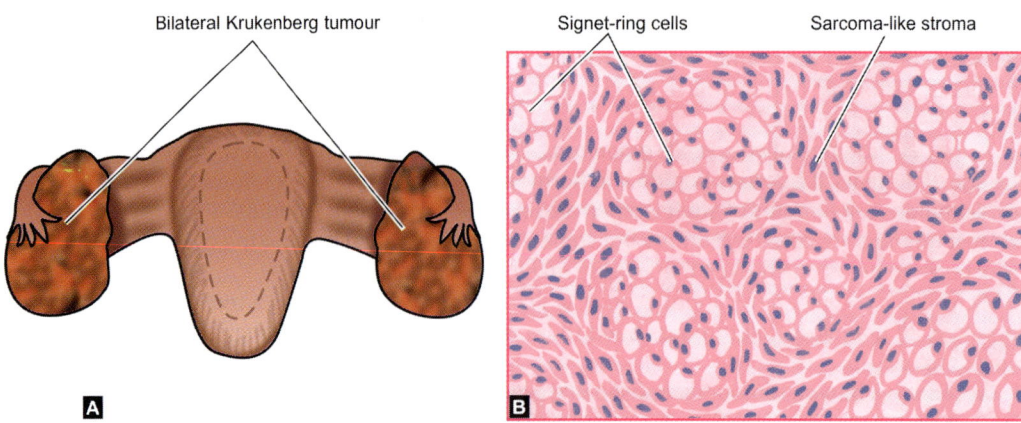

FIGURE 24.14: Krukenberg tumour. A, Grossly, it shows characteristic bilateral metastatic ovarian cancer (arrow) having firm white appearance. B, Histologic features include solid sheets of tumour cells having mucin-filled signet-ring appearance invading the ovarian stroma.

iii. *Chorionic villi* are covered with trophoblastic cells, which include mononuclear cytotrophoblastic and syncytiotrophoblastic multinucleated giant cells. Chorionic villi have a fibrovascular stroma that also contains macrophages called Hofbauer cells. A vasculosyncytial basement membrane separates the fibrovascular core of the villi from the trophoblastic cells.

iv. Placenta secretes a number of *hormones* into the maternal circulation such as: human chorionic gonadotropin (hCG), human placental lactogen (HPL), chorionic thyrotropin and adrenocorticotropin.

Q36. What is hydatidiform mole? What are its main types?

Definition Hydatidiform mole is a placental abnormality characterised by vesicular transformations of oedematous and enlarged chorionic villi accompanied by circumferential trophoblastic proliferation.

Epidemiology The incidence of hydatidiform moles shows geographic, societal and age related variation as under:

i. It has a 10 times higher incidence in Asia and Central America than in the United States.

ii. It has a higher incidence in women belonging to the poorer socioeconomic classes.

iii. It also shows an uneven age distribution, the highest incidence being recorded in pregnant girls under the age of 15 years and women older than 50 years of age.

iv. Women who have had a complete molar pregnancy have a 5% chance for another recurrent mole.

Classification Two types of hydatidifom mole are recognised: complete and partial mole.

I. **Complete mole** is explained by the following mechanism:

i. There is loss of the maternal chromosomes in the ovum. Entry of the sperm during fertilisation will bring in 23 paternal chromosome, which will then reduplicate, so that the conceptus will have 46 chromosomes (46, XX). All chromosomes are, however, of paternal origin due to absence of maternal chromosomes. This process is called *androgenesis*.

ii. Without the maternal genome the embryo cannot develop, and thus the placenta develops into a hydatidiform mole of the placenta. Approximately, 2% of complete hydatidiform moles develop into choriocarcinoma.

Gross The entire placenta is transformed into a huge mass composed of grape-like vesicular chorionic villi filling the uterine cavity and causing enlargement of the uterus **(Fig. 24.15, A)**. There are no traces of normal placenta or the foetus.

Microscopy **(Fig. 24.15, B)**:

i. Chorionic villi are enlarged, acellular and show hydropic degeneration of the stroma that leads to the formation of central cavitary spaces called cisterns.

ii. There are no blood vessels.

iii. The cytotrophoblastic and syncytiotrophoblastic cells on the surface of the villi proliferates circumferentially around the villi forming sheets and masses.

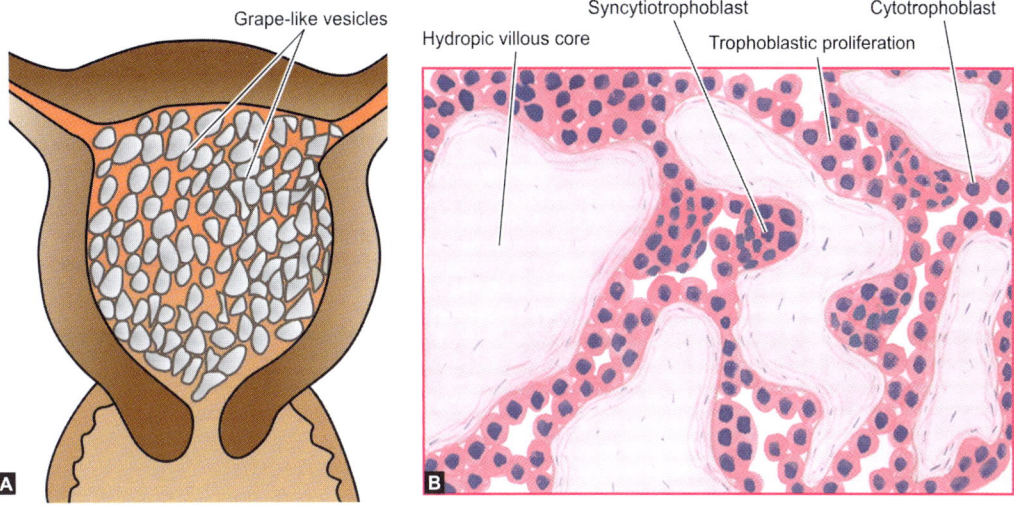

FIGURE 24.15: Hydatidiform mole. A, The specimen shows numerous, variable-sized, grape-like translucent vesicles containing clear fluid. B, Microscopic features are: hydropic and avascular enlarged villi with trophoblastic proliferation in the form of masses and sheets.

Clinical features
i. Complete mole leads to uterine enlargement which is out of proportion for the expected size at a given time of pregnancy.
ii. Ultrasound examination shows an intrauterine mass described as a 'snow-storm'.
iii. The woman may bleed and there are no foetal heart sounds.
iv. Clinical laboratory data reveal very high hCG levels, much higher than expected for the stage of pregnancy.
Prognosis
i. The pregnancy must be interrupted and the mole evacuated.
ii. In 10–15% cases, the mole cannot be evacuated completely and the serum hCG remains high. This persistent trophoblastic disease resulting from *invasive mole* usually causes persistent uterine bleeding. Even though the mole invades the myometrium, invasive mole is benign and heals spontaneously.
iii. In 2–3% of cases, complete mole will transform into a *choriocarcinoma*.
II. **Partial mole** is explained by following mechanism:
i. It results from dispermy, i.e. fertilisation of an ovum with two sperms.
ii. The conceptus created by this double fertilisation has thus 69 chromosomes, one haploid set of maternal origin and two from the father (69,XXX or 69,XXY).
iii. Cytogenetic studies show that the molar cells are triploid containing two set of paternal genes and one maternal set.
Gross Partial mole does not cause an enlargement of the uterus as the complete moles do, and the uterus might be even smaller than expected for the duration of pregnancy. The uterus contains a placenta that is partially normal and partially hydatidiform, i.e. composed of cystic vesicular chorionic villi. A foetus with multiple malformations is usually present as well.
Microscopy
i. The hydatidiform portion of the placenta contains two types of chorionic villi: normal villi and hydropic villi with deep surface invaginations and central hydropic areas forming cisterns.
ii. In the stroma of the villi, there are blood vessels that contain nucleated foetal red blood cells.
iii. Trophoblastic proliferation is focal and not as pronounced as in complete hydatidiform mole.
Clinical features
i. Pregnancy abnormalities with bleeding and a lack of normal foetal development dominate the clinical picture.
ii. Partial mole is associated with invasive (persistent) mole quite rarely (5–7%) and almost never gives rise to choriocarcinoma.

Q37. What is gestational choriocarcinoma?

Definition Choriocarcinoma is a malignant tumour derived from placenta and composed of neoplastic cytotrophoblastic and syncytiotrophoblastic cells.

Etiopathogenesis

i. In about 50% cases, choriocarcinoma develops from a pre-existent complete hydatidiform mole.
ii. In 25% of cases, choriocarcinoma follows spontaneous abortion.
iii. In 20% cases, it develops in normal pregnancy.
iv. In the remaining 5%, it develops from ectopic pregnancy or rarely from partial mole.

Salient contrasting features of complete mole, partial mole and choriocarcinoma are summed up in **Table 24.2**.

TABLE 24.2 Comparative features of major forms of gestational trophoblastic disease.

FEATURE	COMPLETE MOLE	PARTIAL MOLE	CHORIOCARCINOMA
1. *Karyotype*	46,XX or rarely 46,XY	Triploid, i.e. 69,XXY or 69,XXX	46,XY or variable
2. *Clinical findings*			
i. Diagnosis	Mole	Missed abortion	Abortion; molar, ectopic or normal pregnancy
ii. Vaginal bleeding	Marked	Mild	Marked, abnormal
iii. Uterus size	Large	Small	Generally not bulky
3. *hCG levels*			
i. Serum hCG	High	Low	Persistently high
ii. hCG in tissues	Marked	Mild	Localised in syncytiotrophoblast only
4. *Embryo*	Not present	May be present	Not present
5. *Gross appearance*			
i. Vesicles	Large and regular	Smaller and irregular	No vesicles
ii. Villi	Present	Present	Always absent
6. *Microscopy*			
i. Villous size	Uniform	Variable	None present
ii. Hydropic villi	All	Some	None
iii. Trophoblastic proliferation	Circumferential, all three (cytotrophoblast, intermediate trophoblast and syncytiotrophoblast)	Focal, syncytiotrophoblast only	Cytotrophoblast, intermediate cytotrophoblast and syncytiotrophoblast, bizarre forms
iv. Atypia	Minimal	Minimal	Marked
v. Blood vessels	Generally absent	Present	Lack of new blood vessels formation. Trophoblast-lined pseudovascular channels present
vi. Necrosis	Absent	Generally absent	Present
7. *Persistence after initial therapy*	20%	7%	May metastasise rapidly if not treated
8. *Behaviour*	2% may develop choriocarcinoma	Choriocarcinoma almost never develops	Survival rate with chemotherapy 70%

> ### Chapter 24e Supplement: Online Content
> *Digital content of this chapter available with this book is meant for enhanced learning and self-assessment. In addition, it contains 35 Multiple Choice Questions (MCQs), 05 Clinicopathologic Vignettes, and 11 Image-based Questions; these are followed by their answers along with explanatory notes of correct and incorrect answers.*

CHAPTER 25

Breast

Q1. Write briefly on salient anatomic and histologic features of the breast for understanding pathology of this organ.

Anatomy Breasts are bilateral organs better developed in women than men, because their primary function is lactation. Each breast contains about 20 lobes each of which comprises the secretory and ductal components. The ductal system leads to the nipple through which the milk is discharged during lactation.

Histology Breasts comprise an epithelial component, accounting for only 10% of the total organ and a fibrofatty stromal component **(Fig. 25.1)**:

i. *The epithelial component* consists of 2 interconnected major parts:
- Terminal duct-lobular unit (TDLU), the principal functional units during lactation.
- The duct system involved in the collection and drainage of secretions.

The entire ductal-lobular epithelium is bilayered: the inner layer composed of secretory and absorptive epithelium, and the outer supporting layer composed of myoepithelial cells.

ii. *The stromal tissue* is present in two locations:
- Intralobular stroma is composed of loose connective tissue which responds to female sex hormones by changing its hydration and volume during the menstrual cycle.
- Interlobular stroma consists of inert collagen fibres and fat tissue.

Most of the clinically important breast diseases involve the epithelial component, but the stroma also participates in all pathologic conditions as illustrated in **Figure 25.1**.

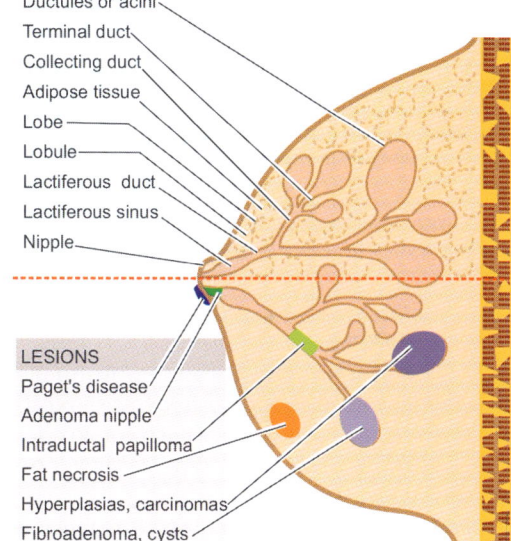

FIGURE 25.1: Microanatomy of the breast and major lesions at various sites.

Q2. What is mastitis? What are its important types?

Definition Mastitis is inflammation of the breast. It may be acute or chronic.

Etiopathogenesis and types Two major forms of mastitis are recognised: acute and chronic; the latter has several subtypes as under:

I. *Acute mastitis* typically occurs in the breasts during lactation when the bacteria such as staphylococci and streptococci gain entry into the breast through the cracks and fissures of the nipple. Localised purulent inflammation leads to the formation of *breast abscesses*.

(613)

II. **Chronic mastitis** may be nonspecific or granulomatous.

i. *Granulomatous mastitis* may be infectious (e.g. tuberculosis, actinomycosis) or part of a systemic disease (e.g. sarcoidosis). In some cases it is idiopathic. Chronic mastitis with foreign body giant cells may also form around the silicone breast implants following breast augmentation cosmetic surgery.

ii. *Mammary duct ectasia* is a condition of unknown etiology affecting women in the 40–70 years age group. It usually involves larger ducts which become dilated and filled with inspissated secretion and are surrounded by fibrous tissue infiltrated with chronic inflammatory cells. Due to fibrosis it may cause retraction of the nipple and form palpable masses that may be mistaken for breast cancer. *Plasma cell mastitis* is a microscopic variant.

iii. *Galactocele* is a cystic dilatation of one or more major ducts that occurs during lactation. The wall of the galactocele is fibrotic and may contain chronic inflammatory cells. Infection may transform galactocele into an abscess.

iv. *Fat necrosis* is usually caused by trauma to pendulous breasts. On gross examination, fat necrosis presents as a palpable mass, which could be mistaken for breast cancer. Necrotic fat cells elicit a chronic inflammatory reaction which is usually dominated by macrophages which take up the lipids and transform into foam cells. There are also multinucleated foreign body giant cells. Dystrophic calcification is common and may be seen on mammography.

Q3. What are fibrocystic lesions of the breast? Briefly discuss salient features of its major types.

Definition Fibrocystic lesions are a variety of age-related proliferative epithelial breast lesions presenting with distinctive gross and microscopic changes.

Clinicopathologic features

Clinical and gross Fibrocystic changes are quite common, usually bilateral, producing vague 'lumpy' breasts rather than a palpable mass inside the breast. They are found in 10–20% of women in the age group between 25 and 50 years, with a dramatic decline in incidence after menopause due to reduced oestrogenic stimulation.

Microscopy Three groups of changes are recognised as under:

I. Non-proliferative fibrocystic change
II. Proliferative fibrocystic disease without atypia
III. Proliferative fibrocystic change with atypia

I. **Non-proliferative fibrocystic change** is considered a physiologic change that includes 3 microscopic findings **(Fig. 25.2)**:

i. *Cysts* result from fibrosis causing obstruction of the collecting ducts followed by glandular proliferation, all related to oestrogenic stimulation. Cysts are lined by epithelial cells which retain their normal cuboidal appearance, or become flattened, or undergo apocrine metaplasia.

ii. *Fibrosis* is equally dense in the interlobular and intralobular spaces, thus replacing the loose intralobular tissue.

iii. *Adenosis* results from the proliferation of the lobular units of the TDLU, similar to the changes during pregnancy or lactation.

Prognosis Non-proliferative fibrocystic changes do not carry an increased risk for invasive breast carcinoma.

II. **Proliferative fibrocystic disease without atypia** includes following four entities:

i. *Epithelial hyperplasia* includes an increased number of cells forming four or more layers inside the ducts or lobules. In the ducts it is called usual ductal hyperplasia, which sometimes may results in formation of papillary structures called *ductal papillomatosis*. Thus, the lesions may be categorised as:
a. Mild hyperplasia (2–4 layers)
b. Moderate hyperplasia (4 or more layers)

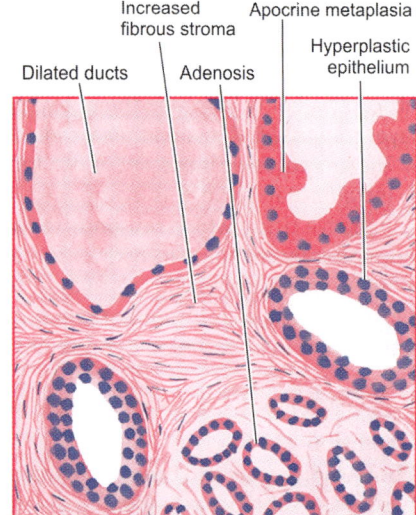

FIGURE 25.2: Non-proliferative fibrocystic change. It shows cystic dilatation of ducts, increase in fibrous stroma, and adenosis.

c. Florid hyperplasia (complete filling of the lumen with hyperplastic cells) in a solid or cribriform pattern
d. Ductal papillomatosis

ii. *Sclerosing adenosis* is a benign proliferation that may present as scattered foci throughout the breast tissue or aggregated into an isolated mass that is hard on palpation simulating an infiltrating carcinoma.
a. It is composed of proliferating distorted ducts, myoepithelial cells and fibroblasts that expand the lobule they occupy.
b. Radial scar is a variant of sclerosing adenosis.
Sclerosing adenosis differs from invasive carcinoma because it remains within the confines of the distended lobule from which it originated with no evidence of invasion into the normal breast tissue. Dystrophic calcifications are common.

iii. *Complex sclerosing lesion* is a variant of sclerosing adenosis.
a. It is characterised by stellate scarring.
b. The fibrous strands radiating toward periphery contain ductules that appear entrapped and distorted or hyperplastic or cystically dilated.

iv. *Papilloma* has following features:
a. Proliferation of cells lining fibrovascular score that project into the lumen of dilated ducts.
b. Most of these peripheral papillomas are microscopic but are multiple and are surrounded by other fibrocystic lesions.
c. If clustered in one area, they may be palpable but are usually detected by mammography as clustered calcifications or small nodules.

Prognosis These lesions of proliferative fibrocystic disease without atypia have a slightly increased risk for invasive breast carcinoma in the range of 1.5 to 2 times over the normal.

III. **Proliferative fibrocystic disease with atypia** shows some cytologic and architectural features of malignancy but short of diagnostic features of ductal carcinoma in situ (DCIS) or lobular carcinoma in situ (LCIS). These lesions are small (2–3 cm in diameter) and may it may by solitary or multicentric. Microscopically, these may be classified as ductal or lobular as under **(Fig. 25.3)**:

i. *Atypical ductal hyperplasia (ADH)* has the following microscopic features:
a. Ducts are filled to a greater part with uniform atypical evenly spaced small cells, but the ducts still contain normal or hyperplastic cells without atypia.
b. Several growth patterns are seen such as: solid, cribriform with sharply punched out spaces, micropapillary, tufted, or forming cellular bridges.
c. The lesions are small but if the number of involved ducts exceeds certain empirical pathological criteria (e.g. more than two ducts completely filled with atypical cells measuring more than 2 mm in diameter), the lesions are diagnosed as DCIS.

ii. *Atypical lobular hyperplasia (ALH)* is usually found accidentally in a breast biopsy performed for some other reason. ALH resembles LCIS but also differs from the latter as under:
a. ALH is made up of small loosely cohesive uniform cells with round nuclei, resembling those in LCIS.
b. ALH does not uniformly involve the entire lobule, so that some TDLUs adjacent to those with ALH are uninvolved.
c. Fewer than 50% of involved acini containing atypical cells are expanded.

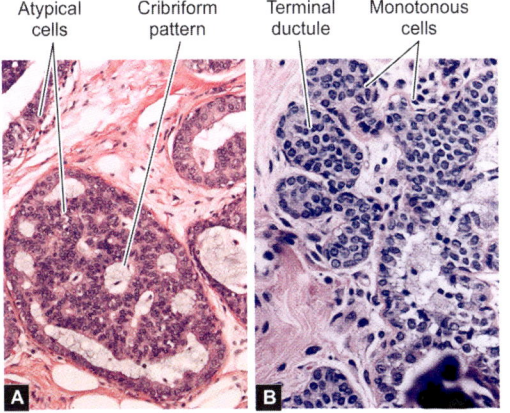

FIGURE 25.3: Proliferative fibrocystic disease with atypia (Atypical hyperplasia). A, Atypical ductal hyperplasia (ADH) showing intraductal proliferation of cells which are small and monomorphic. The proliferated cells from a cribriform pattern. B, Atypical lobular hyperplasia (ALH) showing flat epithelial atypia and foci of columnar cell change.

d. ALH can spread in a pagetoid manner into the adjacent duct, the same way as LCIS.
Prognosis Lesions of proliferative fibrocystic disease with atypia carry an increased risk for invasive carcinoma (4–5 times over the normal).

Q4. What is gynaecomastia?

Definition Gynaecomastia is unilateral or bilateral enlargement of male breast due to proliferation of ducts and increased periductal stroma.

Etiopathogenesis Gynaecomastia results from excessive oestrogenic stimulation. It occurs under following conditions:
i. Pubertal gynaecomastia in boys, 13 to 17 years of age
ii. Senescent gynaecomastia in men over the age of 50 years
iii. Cirrhosis of the liver
iv. Oestrogen-secreting tumours such as Leydig cell tumour
v. Paraneoplastic syndrome, e.g. lung, renal, or liver tumour
vi. Klinefelter syndrome or other forms of testicular atrophy
vii. Exogenous oestrogen and certain drugs
viii. Idiopathic gynaecomastia

Pathology
i. Breast enlargement entails proliferation of branching ducts, which may show focal epithelial hyperplasia or papillary projections.
ii. Periductal stroma is increased and focally appears myxoid.

Q5. What is fibroadenoma? Discuss its salient clinicopathologic features.

Definition Fibroadenoma (or adenofibroma) is a benign breast tumour composed of fibrous and epithelial elements.

Clinicopathologic features
Clinical and gross
i. Fibroadenomas can occur at any age but are most often diagnosed in the 15–30 years age group.
ii. They usually appear as a solitary, discreet, freely mobile, 2–4 cm nodule in the breast parenchyma.
iii. Larger tumours (*giant fibroadenomas*) or multiple nodules (*fibroadenomatosis*) are less common, but may occur sometimes.
iv. Fibroadenoma can be easily shelled out by surgeon without any residues or adverse consequences.

Microscopy The tumour is composed of biphasic cellular growth that has low-cellular fibrous stroma surrounding proliferated ducts. These may form either of the following two patterns or their combination **(Fig. 25.4)**:
i. Circumferential growth of fibrous tissue around ducts called *pericanalicular pattern*.
ii. Fibrous compression of ducts into elongated cords without a lumen called *intracanalicular pattern*.

NOTE: Fibroadenomas must be distinguished from breast lesions that are called 'adenomas' which are actually not neoplasms but rather foci of local hyperplasia. Their examples are:
- *Tubular adenoma* composed of proliferating tubules and/or acini.
- *Lactating adenoma*, a lesion found in lactating breasts.

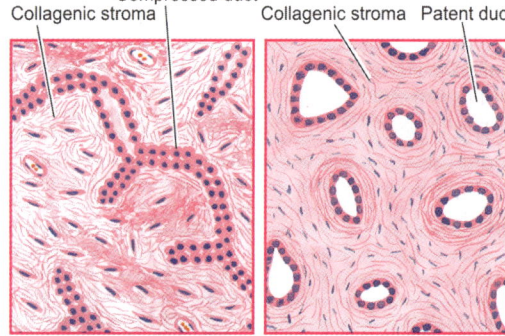

A, INTRACANALICULAR PATTERN   B, PERICANALICULAR PATTERN

FIGURE 25.4: Microscopic patterns of fibroadenoma breast.

Q6. What is phyllodes tumour of the breast?

Definition Phyllodes tumour of the breast is composed of proliferating dense stromal tissue distorting compressed ducts, thus forming leaf like projections (*Greek* term phyllodes, meaning leaf-like).

Clinicopathologic features
Clinical and gross features
i. Most phyllodes tumours are diagnosed in women 30–70 years old.
ii. Tumours are round or oval and resemble fibroadenomas but are generally larger, measuring 10–15 cm in diameter, and less fully encapsulated.
iii. On cross section, they contain cystic cavities with leaf-like protrusion and occasional areas of necrosis and haemorrhage.
Microscopy
i. Tumour composed of highly cellular stroma growing in an intracanalicular manner into the stretched out and extended ducts.
ii. Three types of phyllodes tumour are recognised on microscopy: benign, borderline and malignant. These designations depend on the following criteria:
a. Cellular atypia
b. Frequency of mitoses
c. Degree of stromal hypercellularity
d. Infiltrative margins
Prognosis Approximately 20% of phyllodes tumours are malignant and less than half of these may metastasise.

Q7. What is an intraductal papilloma?
Definition Intraductal papilloma is a benign papillary tumour, most often occurring in the lactiferous duct or sinus near the nipple, presenting clinically with bleeding from the nipple.
Clinicopathologic features
Clinical and gross
i. Intraductal papilloma is most often diagnosed in 20–40 years old women.
ii. It is the most common cause of bloody nipple discharge in women under the age of 50 years.
iii. Most often, it is a solitary intraductal lesion less than 1 cm in diameter. Multiple papillomas may occur but are less common.
Microscopy
i. It is composed of branching papillae that have a fibrovascular core covered by two cell layers: a layer of cuboidal cells supported by a layer of myoepithelial cells.
ii. Differential diagnosis includes *papillary carcinoma* which also forms papillae. The cells of the malignant tumour lining the papillae form several layers, and the outer layer of myoepithelial cells is missing. Cells show marked atypia, hyperchromasia, and there are multiple mitoses.

Q8. Comment briefly on incidence and epidemiology of breast carcinoma.
i. Breast carcinoma is one the most common cancers in women. It is much less common in men; female: male ratio is 150:1.
ii. In the United States, it accounts for 25% of all cancers and for 20% of all cancer deaths in women.
iii. The incidence is the highest in the perimenopausal age group while it is uncommon in women under the age of 25 years.
iv. The diagnosis depends on the triple approach that includes palpation, mammography and fine needle aspiration and/or biopsy.

Q9. What are the risk factors for breast carcinoma?
i. *Geographic and racial factors* The incidence of breast carcinoma is 4–6 times higher in developed countries (North America, Europe and Australia) than in developing countries of Asia and Africa. In the US, Hispanic and African-American women tend to be diagnosed at an earlier age and the disease is more advanced at presentation than in White populations.
ii. *Family history* First-degree relatives (mother, daughter, sister) of women with breast cancer have a 2–6-fold higher risk.
iii. *Menstrual and obstetric history* Total length of menstrual life is directly related to increased risk. Thus there is an increased risk in women with early menarche and late menopause, nulliparity, late age of first childbirth.

iv. *Fibrocystic change breast with atypia* increases the risk 5 times.
v. *Miscellaneous factors* such as:
a. Diet rich in animal fats or high calorie food
b. Cigarettes smoking
c. Alcohol
d. Breast augmentation surgery
e. Exposure to ionising radiation
f. High breast density on mammography

Q10. How do hormonal and genetic factors influence pathogenesis of breast cancer?

Both hormonal and genetic factors play a role in the etiopathogenesis of breast cancer as under:

I. **Oestrogen excess** promotes breast carcinogenesis as supported by the following evidences:

i. Most risk factors for breast cancer (listed above under question #9) are associated with hyper-oestrinism.
ii. Lactation and breastfeeding reduce the risk.
iii. Bilateral oophorectomy reduces the risk.
iv. Oestrogen-secreting tumours of the ovary (e.g. thecoma, granulosa cell tumour) increase the risk.
v. Hormone replacement therapy with oestrogen increases the risk.
vi. Many breast cancer cells have oestrogen receptors and respond well to anti-oestrogen treatment.

II. **Genetic factors** play an important role in many familial cases of breast cancer. Furthermore, 10% of breast cancers have a genetic basis and are linked to mutations of certain cancer genes such as:

i. *BRCA1* gene encoding a DNA repair protein is inactivated in two-thirds of women with familial breast cancer. *BRCA2* gene is inactivated in one third of women with familial breast cancer. Both *BRCA1* and *BRCA2* genes cause cancer only if both alleles are inactivated.
ii. *TP53* tumour suppressor gene mutations are found in 40% cases of sporadic breast cancer but not in familial cases. Germ line mutation of *TP53* found in Li-Fraumeni syndrome is associated with an increased incidence of breast cancer in those families.

Q11. Discuss classification of breast tumours in brief.

i. Breast tumours are either benign or malignant **(Table 25.1)**.
ii. Breast cancer occurs in two forms: preinvasive (or in situ) carcinoma and invasive carcinoma. Preinvasive breast carcinoma occurs in two forms: ductal carcinoma in situ (DCIS) and lobular carcinoma in situ (LCIS).
iii. Invasive carcinoma occurs in several microscopic forms.
iv. Breast carcinomas mostly involve only one breast but in 4% of women with invasive carcinoma, the malignancy will be bilateral.
v. Anatomically, they are more often located in the left than the right breast.
vi. Within the breast, most tumours originate from the outer upper quadrant (50%), followed in frequency by the central portion underneath

TABLE 25.1 WHO Classification (2012) of tumours of the breast.

I. BENIGN
Fibroepithelial tumours
1. Fibroadenoma
2. Phyllodes tumour
3. Hamartoma

II. MALIGNANT
A. *In situ* **carcinoma (Precursor lesions)**
   1. Ductal carcinoma *in situ*
   2. Lobular neoplasia
   3. Intraductal papillary carcinoma
B. **Invasive breast carcinoma**
   1. Invasive carcinoma of no special type –NST (80%) (Older term: infiltrating duct carcinoma, not otherwise specified, IDC-NOS)
   2. Invasive lobular carcinoma (8%)
   3. Tubular carcinoma (6%)
   4. Medullary carcinoma (2%)
   5. Mucinous carcinoma (2%)
   6. Cribriform carcinoma (2%)
   7. Rare types:
      i. Invasive papillary carcinoma
      ii. Adenoid cystic carcinoma
      iii. Secretory carcinoma
      iv. Inflammatory carcinoma
      v. Metaplastic carcinoma
      vi. Carcinoma with neuroendocrine features
C. **Tumours of the nipple**
   Paget disease of the breast
D. **Metastatic tumours**

the nipple (20%) and then other quadrants **(Fig. 25.5)**.

vii. Most of the tumours (90%) originate from the TDLU, while the rest are derived from the lobular epithelium.

Q12. What is carcinoma in situ of the breast? Comment on salient features of its main types.

Definition Carcinoma in situ is a preinvasive carcinoma that develops from atypical hyperplasia and if untreated will progress to invasive carcinoma.

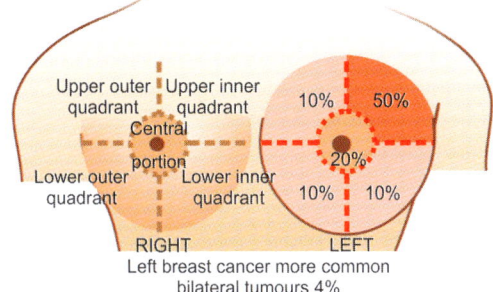

FIGURE 25.5: Topographic considerations in breast cancer.

The risk for development of invasive cancer is approximately 10 times higher than in normal breasts, and up to 30% of women who have carcinoma in situ develop invasive cancer if not treated surgically.

Types Carcinoma in situ occurs in two forms: DCIS and LCIS.

I. **Ductal carcinoma in situ (DCIS)** is the precursor of invasive ductal carcinoma. It is derived from atypical hyperplasia of the ductal epithelium and is confined to the TDLU.

Clinical and gross

i. DCIS presents clinically as a palpable mass in 30–75%, and with nipple discharge in 30% cases.

ii. It contains microcalcifications frequently which help to visualise it by mammography.

iii. Involvement of the opposite breast is less common than with LCIS.

iv. On cross sectioning of the resected specimen, DCIS usually presents as an indurated mass 3–4 cm in diameter. Cystically dilated ducts containing cheesy material that can be expressed may be seen in cases with comedo necrosis. Papillary tumours may be seen as intraductal lesions.

Microscopy shows 4 patterns as under **(Fig. 25.6)**:

i. *Solid pattern* is characterised by plugging of ducts with anaplastic cancer cells.

ii. *Comedo pattern* is similar to the solid pattern, except that the central portion of cancerous cell in the tubules is necrotic.

iii. *Papillary pattern* is characterised by the formation of short papillae.

iv. *Cribriform pattern* is marked by punched out fenestration.

On the basis of nuclear features DCIS is classified as low, intermediate or high nuclear grade lesions.

II. **Lobular carcinoma in situ (LCIS)** is the precursor of invasive lobular carcinoma. It is derived from atypical lobular hyperplasia and involves terminal ducts, ductules and acini.

Clinical and gross

i. LCIS is not palpable nor is grossly visible as a tumour.

ii. It is less apparent on mammography and does not contain calcifications.

iii. Cancer develops in the contralateral breast in 30% of cases, and it may be invasive lobular or ductal.

iv. LCIS, therefore, is considered to be a risk factor for breast cancer development in the contralateral breast.

Microscopy

i. LCIS is composed of small loosely cohesive cells with round nuclei and indistinct cytoplasmic margin **(Fig. 25.6)**.

ii. These cells fill the terminal ducts, ductules and acini.

iii. LCIS is often multicentric.

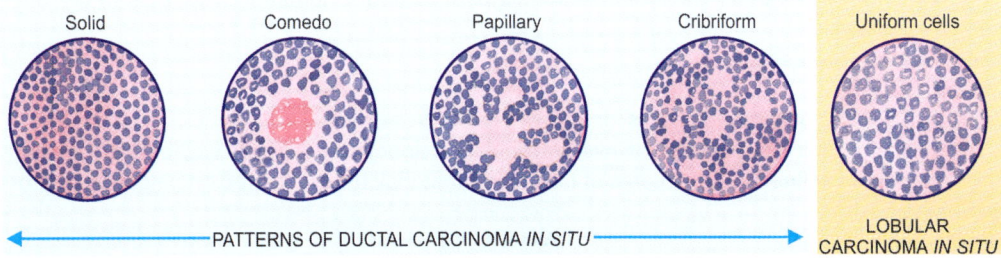

FIGURE 25.6: Morphologic patterns in (carcinoma in situ) non-invasive of breast.

Q13. What is invasive breast carcinoma of no special type? Discuss its salient clinicopathologic features.

Definition Invasive breast carcinoma of no special type (NST), previously called infiltrating duct carcinoma NOS (not otherwise specified) is a malignant tumour originating from the TDLU. Often it is preceded by a preinvasive stage cancer, i.e. DCIS.

Clinicopathologic features

Clinical and gross

i. This is the most common breast carcinoma accounting for 75- 80% breast cancers.

ii. Clinically and grossly, the cancer presents as an irregular mass that is poorly demarcated from adjacent normal tissue.

iii. It is hard and gritty on sectioning.

iv. On cross section, it is grey-white and it shows chalky streaks often extending into the adjacent fat tissue **(Fig. 25.7,A)**.

Microscopy shows varying features depending on the grade of the tumour, i.e. its extent of differentiation **(Fig. 25.7, B)**:

i. In general terms, most tumours appear as invasive scirrhous adenocarcinomas, which accounts for their firm consistency.

ii. The tumours are, thus, composed of anaplastic tumour cells arranged into poorly formed glandular structures, or solid nests and cords, surrounded by a prominent fibrous stroma (*'desmoplastic reaction'*).

iii. Tumour cells invade the normal breast tissue, lymphatics and blood vessels (called lymphovascular invasion or LVI), as well as the perineural spaces.

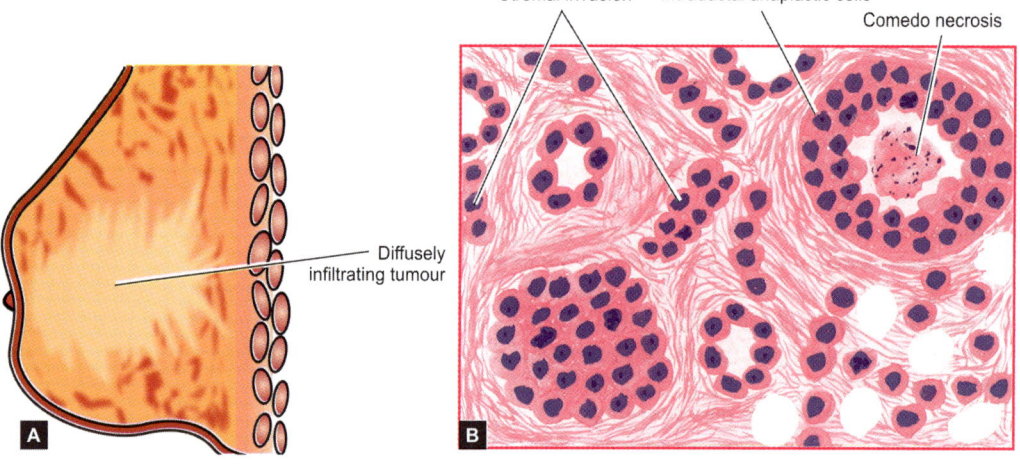

FIGURE 25.7: Invasive carcinoma, no special type-NST (infiltrating duct carcinoma-NOS). A, Bisected surface of the breast shows tumour which has irregular borders, is grey white, firm and schirrous (desmoplastic). B, Microscopic features include formation of solid nests, cords, gland-like structures and intraductal growth pattern of anaplastic tumour cells. There is infiltration of densely collagenised stroma by these cells in a haphazard manner.

Q14. What is invasive lobular carcinoma?

Definition Invasive lobular carcinoma is a malignant tumour originating from LCIS in the duct, ductules and acini.

Clinicopathologic features

Clinical and gross

i. Invasive lobular carcinoma accounts for 10% of breast carcinomas.

ii. The gross and clinical appearance of invasive lobular carcinoma varies from a well-defined scirrhous mass to a poorly defined indistinct area of induration that may be undetected on palpation or gross sectioning.

Microscopy

i. Single cell files or linear fashion of tumour cells infiltrating the fibrous stroma.

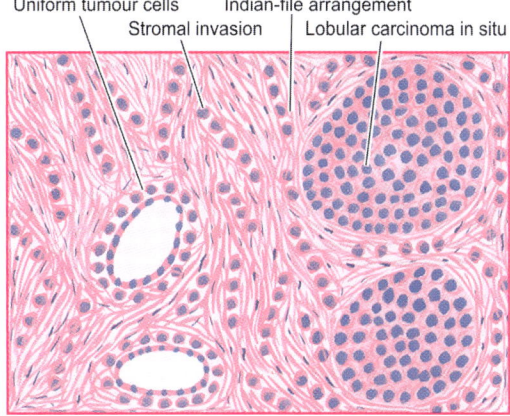

FIGURE 25.8: Invasive lobular carcinoma. Characteristic histologic features are: one cell wide files of round regular tumour cells ('Indian file' arrangement) infiltrating the stroma and arranged circumferentially around ducts in a target-like pattern.

ii. Infiltrating cells may be circumferentially arranged around the ducts that contain LCIS **(Fig. 25.8)**.
iii. The tumour cells resemble LCIS; they are uniformly small with round nuclei and indistinct cell borders.
iv. Mitoses and areas of necrosis are not prominent.
v. Occasionally, the tumour may contain mucus filled signet ring cells.

Q15. Briefly discuss certain uncommon microscopic subtypes of breast carcinoma which have better prognosis.

These are tubular, medullary, mucinous and cribriform carcinoma of the breast, which are clinicopathologically heterogeneous group of uncommon tumours that they have a better prognosis than invasive carcinoma NST. Besides, other rare forms of breast carcinoma which have a better prognosis than invasive carcinoma NST include: adenoid cystic carcinoma, and secretory (juvenile) carcinoma. Collectively all these account for 10–15% of breast carcinomas. These are briefly considered below.

I. **Tubular carcinoma**
Clinical and gross Usually presents as a small ill-defined and gritty nodules (<1 cm).
Microscopy It is composed of tubules of angulated shape in dense fibrous stroma.

II. **Medullary carcinoma**
Clinical and gross Usually presents as a large, well-circumscribed, soft mass resembling on cross section brain or spinal medulla. There are also areas of visible necrosis and haemorrhage into the tumour.
Microscopy shows quite distinctive features:
i. The tumour is composed of large cells with large vesicular nuclei and abundant cytoplasm.
ii. These cells do not have sharp margins and grow in a syncytium-like manner forming solid sheets with other cells.
iii. Stroma is scanty and typically contains lymphoid infiltrates. Lymphocytes are most likely part of an immune response, which accounts for generally more favourable prognosis of these tumours. However, medullary cancers with BRCA1 mutation are high grade tumours.

III. **Mucinous carcinoma**
Clinical and gross It is a slow-growing tumour usually seen in older women. Grossly, it presents as a gelatinous mass with well demarcated borders.
Microscopy It is composed of cuboidal or columnar mucin-producing cells floating in lakes of extracellular mucin.

IV. **Cribriform carcinoma**
Microscopy It is a carcinoma composed of sheets of cells that have punched out holes.

Q16. What are the rare forms of breast carcinoma with very poor prognosis?

These breast cancers include: inflammatory carcinoma, metaplastic carcinoma, and carcinoma with neuroendocrine differentiation. Fortunately, these cancers are very rare accounting for 1–2% of all breast cancers.

I. **Inflammatory carcinoma**
i. It is a clinical entity comprising invasive breast carcinoma NST, which invades the lymphatics of the skin extensively. It is called inflammatory because it presents like inflammation of the breast skin and underlying parenchyma, causing swelling, redness and tenderness of the breast.
ii. It grows very fast and is prone to metastasis and thus has an abysmal prognosis.

II. **Metaplastic carcinoma**
i. It is characterised by its 'metaplastic components', i.e. tissues which are not normally found in the breast, such as squamous, cartilaginous, and osseous tissue. This group also includes carcinosarcoma, spindle cell carcinoma, carcinoma with osteoclastic giant cells and squamous cell carcinoma.
ii. All these tumours have a very bad prognosis.

III. **Carcinoma with neuroendocrine differentiation**
i. It is poorly-differentiated neuroendocrine tumour similar to the small cell lung carcinoma and has a poor prognosis.
ii. Rarely, well-differentiated tumour equivalent to pulmonary carcinoid is seen and has a relatively good prognosis.

Q17. What is Paget disease of the nipple?

Definition Paget disease of the nipple is an eczematoid eruption of the nipple, usually associated with an invasive or non-invasive breast carcinoma in the underlying breast.

Clinicopathologic features

Clinical and gross
i. The nipple appears crusted, scaly or ulcerated, and oozing resembling a chronic skin disease **(Fig. 25.9)**.
ii. A palpable mass can be noticed in the underlying breast in about half the cases.
iii. Most patients are found to have an underlying invasive breast carcinoma. Those that have no palpable mass were usually found to have a ductal carcinoma in situ.
iv. Skin lesion develops from breast carcinoma cells invading the ductal system of the breast and finally reaching the areolar skin through the lactiferous ducts.

Microscopy
i. The epidermis of the areola containing breast cancer cells singly or in small clusters.
ii. These cells differ from adjacent keratinocytes because of their prominent clear cytoplasm that usually contains stainable mucin.
iii. By special stains and immunohistochemistry, one can demonstrate that these cells are identical to the adenocarcinoma cells in the underlying breast.

Prognosis Clinically, Paget disease has a worse prognosis than invasive carcinomas of the breast.

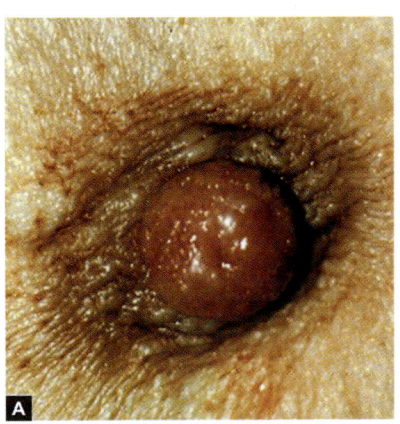
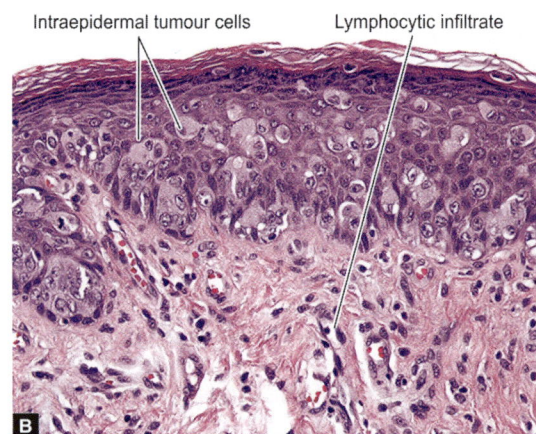

FIGURE 25.9: Paget diseases of the breast. A, The region of nipple and areola is crusted and ulcerated. B, There are clefts in the epidermal layers containing large tumour cells.

Q18. How are breast carcinomas graded and staged?

The outcome of breast cancer depends upon pathologic grading and clinical staging:

I. **Pathologic grading** Pathologic parameters used for management and prognosis are as under:
i. *Histologic type of tumour:* This allows subdivision of breast cancers into three groups:
a. Non-metastasising: Intraductal and intralobular carcinomas.
b. Less commonly metastasising: Medullary, mucinous, papillary, tubular, cribriform, adenoid cystic and secretory (juvenile) carcinomas.
c. Commonly metastasising: Invasive breast carcinoma, invasive lobular and inflammatory carcinomas.
ii. *Microscopic grade:* It is based on the widely used Nottingham modification of the Bloom-Richardson system, which is based on three features:
a. Tubule formation
b. Nuclear pleomorphism
c. Mitotic count
iii. *Tumour size:* It has been shown that there is an inverse relationship between diameter of primary breast cancer at the time of diagnosis and the long-term survival of the patient.
iv. *Axillary lymph node metastasis:* Following holds true:
a. More the lymph nodes involved, worse is the prognosis.
b. Furthermore, the type of involvement of the axilla matters and must be assessed to determine if the involved lymph nodes are superficial or deeply located in the axilla.
c. The involvement of the sentinel node (i.e. the first node along the lymphatic routes laterally from the carcinoma to the deep axilla) has prognostic significance.
v. *Oestrogen and progesterone receptors:* These are important determinant whether the tumour will respond to therapy with anti-oestrogenic drugs or not.
vi. *HER2/neu overexpression:* HER2/neu (human epidermal growth factor receptor-2, also called erbB2) which belongs to the family of epidermal growth factor receptors is a gene that encodes a transmembrane protein with tyrosine kinase activity, important for the proliferation of tumour cells. Tumours overexpressing HER2/neu respond well to treatment with herceptin, a kinase inhibitor.
vii. *DNA content:* It has been shown that aneuploidy tumours with high DNA content have a worse prognosis.

II. **Clinical staging** This is based on the assessment of the size of the tumour and the extent of its spread, using the TNM system approved by the American Joint Committee on Cancer.
i. In situ tumour stage: TIS.
ii. Invasive carcinomas stages: designated from stage I (tumours <2 cm in diameter), stage II (tumour 2–5 cm) to stage III (tumours >5 cm).
iii. Stage IV tumours may be of any size that have distant metastases.

Q19. What are the various parameters which determine prognosis of breast cancer?

Prognosis of breast cancer is determined by pathologic grading and clinical staging (discussed above), immunohistochemical (IHC) profile, and molecular categorisation:

I. **Pathologic grading and clinical staging** Based on this, overall 5-year survival for all types of breast cancer is 85%, but if metastases to the lymph nodes are present, it drops to 50%.

II. **IHC profile** Based on IHC for ER, PR and HER2/neu, breast carcinomas are divided into three groups:
i. *ER positive, HER2/neu negative*: 65% of all carcinomas; they respond to anti-oestrogens like tamoxifen, and have best prognosis.
ii. *HER2/neu positive, ER and PR positive or negative*: 15% of all carcinomas; they responds to herceptin therapy.
iii. *Triple negative (i.e. HER2/neu, ER and PR negative):* 15% of all breast cancers; have the worst prognosis.

III. **Molecular categorisation** Alternatively, based on patterns of gene expression, breast carcinomas fall into one of following four prognostic types:
i. Luminal A or B
ii. *HER2/neu* positive
iii. Basal-like type
iv. Normal breast-like type
- Basal-like type has the worst prognosis while luminal type A responds well to endocrine therapy and has good prognosis.

- Molecular classification is being introduced into pathology practice but needs additional validation in practice.

Various prognostic and predictive criteria determining outcome of breast cancer are summarised in **Table 25.2**.

TABLE 25.2 Summary of prognostic markers and predictive factors for invasive breast cancer.

FACTOR	FAVOURABLE PROGNOSIS	POOR PROGNOSIS
I. ROUTINE HISTOPATHOLOGIC CRITERIA		
i. *Histologic type*	Medullary ca, tubular ca, mucinous (colloid) ca; lobular ca of low grade	Inflammatory ca, metaplastic ca, carcinoma with neuroendocrine differentiation
ii. *Tumour size (two dimensions)*	<2 cm size tumour; 10 years survival 90% in node negative	Size > 2 cm
iii. *Histologic (Nottingham) grading* (Score range of 3–9) based on degree of tubule formation-1–3 score, regularity of nuclei-1–3 score, and mitoses-1–3 score	Low grade (grade I) tumour = score 3–5, moderate grade (grade II) tumour = score 6–7	High grade (grade III) tumour = score 8–9
iv. *Axillary nodal status*	Node negative: recurrence after 10 years 10–30% Number of nodes: less than 4 Sentinel node negative	Node positive: recurrence after 10 years 70% Number of nodes: more than 4 Sentinel node positive
v. *Lymphatic and/or vascular invasion (both extratumoural)*	Negative for both: good	positive for one or both: poor
vi. *Others:* a. *Tumour circumscription* b. *Inflammatory reaction* c. *Stromal elastosis* d. *Intraductal component* e. *Skin involvement*	Good May have some role Absence good Presence good Absence good	Poor Controversial Presence poor Absence poor Presence poor
II. HORMONE RECEPTOR STATUS		
Oestrogen-progesterone receptors (ER-PR)	ER-PR positive cases respond better to adjuvant Therapy	ER-PR negative cases respond poorly To adjuvant therapy
HER-2/neu (C-erb B-2)	Underexpression	Overexpression (predictive of response to herceptin)
III. BIOLOGICAL INDICATORS		
i. *Mitotic index (by Ki67, MIB-1)*	Low mitotic count	High mitotic count
ii. *DNA ploidy analysis (aneuploidy, diploidy)*	Not related	Not related
iii. *Angiogenesis (VEGF, CD31, CD34, microvessel density counts)*	Angiogenic activity low	High angiogenic activity
iv. *Tumour suppressor gene loss/ Oncogene dysregulation* a. *BRCA1, BRCA2* b. *p53* c. *BCL2* d. *Cathepsin D*	BRCA negative p53 positive respond better to chemotherapy and radiotherapy BCL2 positive good Absence good prognosis	BRCA positive p53 negative respond poorly to chemotherapy and radiotherapy BCL2 negative poor Presence poor prognosis

Chapter 25e Supplement: Online Content

Digital content of this chapter available with this book is meant for enhanced learning and self-assessment. In addition, it contains 19 Multiple Choice Questions (MCQs), 05 Clinicopathologic Vignettes, and 07 Image-based Questions; these are followed by their answers along with explanatory notes of correct and incorrect answers.

CHAPTER 26

Skin

Q1. What are the layers of normal skin and what are the cells forming them?

The skin has three layers: epidermis, dermis, and subcutis **(Fig. 26.1)**.

I. **Epidermis** has five layers as shown in **Figure 26.2**:

i. *Basal layer (stratum germinativum)* is composed of a layer of mitotically active keratinocytes lying on the basement membrane that forms the epidermo-dermal junction. Basal layer contains cells that are the precursors of all other layers. Scattered in the basal layer are melanocytes producing melanin. Basal layer also contains the bone marrow-derived migratory antigen-presenting Langerhans cells, and neuroendocrine Merkel cells located at the nerve endings.

ii. *Prickle cell layer (stratum spinosum, Malpighi layer),* the thickest layer of the epidermis, is composed of several layers of polygonal squamous cells (keratinocytes). These cells possess intercellular bridges and tonofilaments made up keratin rich intermediate filaments attached to desmosomes.

iii. *Granular cell layer (stratum granulosum)* consists of 1–3 layers of flat cells containing keratohyaline granules. This layer is much thicker on palms and soles.

iv. *Stratum lucidum* is present only on palms and soles and consists of a thin homogeneous eosinophilic material without nuclei.

v. *Horny layer (stratum corneum)* consists of layered anuclear eosinophilic keratin.

Intraepidermal nerve endings are present on Merkel cell, which are touch receptors.

II. **Dermis** consists of:

i. Two parts: superficial papillary dermis and deeper reticular dermis.

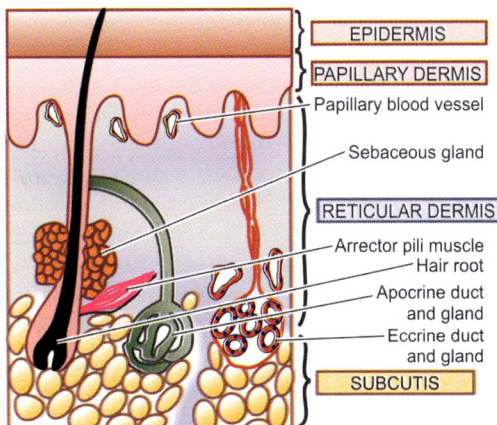

FIGURE 26.1: Main structures identified in a section of the normal skin.

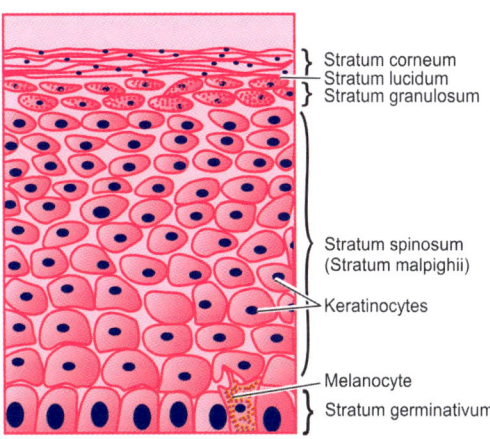

FIGURE 26.2: Different layers comprising the normal epidermis.

(625)

ii. Both layers are composed of fibro-collagenous tissue, blood vessels, lymphatics and nerves, which end on specialised nerve ending forming touch receptors, pressure receptors cold receptors.

iii. Besides these structures, the dermis contains cutaneous appendages or adnexal structures. These include sweat glands (eccrine and apocrine), holocrine sebaceous glands, hair follicles, smooth muscle cells arranged into arrectores pilorum and nails.

Q2. Give the meaning of various common pathologic terms used in dermatopathology.

i. **Acanthosis** Thickening of the epidermis due to hyperplasia of prickle cell layer.

ii. **Acantholysis** Loss of cohesion between epidermal cell with formation of intraepidermal space containing oedema fluid and detached epithelial cells.

iii. **Dyskeratosis** Abnormal development of keratinocytes which lose their prickles and round up dissociating from other cells into darkly eosinophilic bodies with pyknotic nuclei. It is found in premalignant and malignant skin lesions, and only rarely in some uncommon skin diseases.

iv. **Hyperkeratosis** Thickening of the horny layer seen in some chronic skin diseases and neoplastic squamous lesions.

v. **Parakeratosis** Abnormal keratinisation of the surface layers of the horny layer composed of keratinocytes which have retained their nuclei, rather than forming non-nucleated keratin layer.

vi. **Spongiosis** Intercellular oedema of the epidermis which may progress to vesicle formation.

vii. **Pigment incontinence** Loss of pigment from cells of the basal layer accompanied by the uptake of the pigment in dermal macrophages.

Q3. What are dermatoses? Give their broad classification.

Definition Dermatosis is the term used for any of the non-neoplastic skin disease.

Classification Dermatoses can be classified into several groups as under:

i. Genetic
ii. Inflammatory
iii. Infectious
iv. Granulomatous
v. Connective tissue (autoimmune)
vi. Bullous
vii. Scaling

Q4. What are genetic dermatoses? Briefly describe their common types, pathogenesis and their salient clinicopathologic features.

Definition Genetic dermatoses, also known as *genodermatoses,* are a heterogeneous group of diseases caused by *single gene defects*, that are hereditary and transmitted as Mendelian traits. Such diseases may be limited to the skin or are part of a multisystemic genetic disorder.

Salient features

i. Most genodermatoses are rare diseases; more common examples like *ichthyosis vulgaris* cause usually only minor skin changes such as patches of hyperkeratosis on the arm and the trunk.

ii. Approximately 100 genetic syndromes have been identified as predominantly affecting the skin. Several genetic skin diseases are part of multisystem diseases, such as mastocytosis with *urticaria pigmentosa* or *ataxia telangiectasia*, which is associated with neurologic and immune defects.

iii. Even though not grouped under the heading of genodermatoses, many skin diseases have a genetic component, as evidenced by their hereditary nature and common occurrence in some families. The best examples are *atopic dermatitis* found in families with disorders of IgE-linked type I hypersensitivity, and *psoriasis* affecting 3–4% of the total world population.

Pathogenesis Genetic skin diseases are linked to *single gene mutations*, not all of which have been identified so far. Examples of genes that have been identified:

i. *Profilaggrin* gene, encoding a protein found in keratohyaline granules of stratum granulosum, that serves as a 'glue' for keratofilament in squamous cells. The defect of profilaggrin in ichthyosis vulgaris results in hyperkeratosis.

ii. *Steroid sulfatase* gene encoding this enzyme that allows the dissociation of squamous cells from each other. In X-linked ichthyosis, the mutation of steroid sulfatase gene leads to hyperkeratosis because the anucleate keratin cells on the surface cannot separate one from another.

Common types Genetic skin diseases may be related to several pathogenetic disorders and present with a variety of clinicopathologic findings as under:

i. *Disorderly pigmentation*, e.g. albinism, piebaldism (an unpigmented or white patch of skin or hair), mucosal pigmentation in Peutz-Jeghers syndrome

ii. *Excessive cornification*, e.g. ichthyosis, Darier disease

iii. *Abnormal metabolism* with pale skin pigmentation and fair hair, e.g. phenylketonuria

iv. *Immunologic disorders*, e.g. ataxia telangiectasia, Wiskott-Aldrich syndrome

v. *Connective tissue defects*, e.g. *cutis laxa* in Ehlers-Danlos syndrome

vi. *Blood vessel proliferations*, e.g. Sturge-Weber syndrome with facial angiomatosis, ataxia telangiectasia with numerous skin vascular dilatations

vii. *DNA repair defects* with an increased incidence of UV induced skin cancer, e.g. xeroderma pigmentosum

Pathology of common examples is briefly given below.

i. *Ichthyosis* This term is used for a diverse group of skin conditions including at least 10 clinicopathologic entities, each linked to a distinct genetic defect. They are all characterised by marked thickening of stratum corneum giving the skin the appearance of fish scales. The skin changes may be evident at the time of birth (as in *X-linked ichthyosis* affecting the extremities but sparing the palms and soles), or in early infancy (as in *ichthyosis vulgaris*, the most common ichthyosis inherited as an autosomal dominant trait presenting with hyperkeratotic patches on the extremities, face and the trunk).

ii. *Keratosis palmaris et plantaris* It presents with hyperkeratosis of palms and soles and may be inherited as an autosomal dominant or recessive disease.

iii. *Xeroderma pigmentosum* This autosomal recessive disorder is based on defective repair of ultraviolet light-induced damage of DNA. At least 9 mutations of genes encoding *nucleotide excision repair enzymes* have been identified so far. Affected patients are more prone to develop skin cancer, such as squamous cell carcinoma.

iv. *Darier disease* Also known as *keratosis follicularis*, it presents with lesions called 'warty dyskeratoma'. Microscopically, there is focal hyperkeratosis, papillomatosis and dyskeratosis and cleavage of the epidermis above the basal layer. The disease is caused by mutations of *ATP2C1* gene, encoding a protein essential for the assembly of desmosomes. Keratinocytes that are deficient for this protein become rounded up (*dyskeratotic*) and separate from adjacent cells accounting for the cleavage of the skin layers. There are also neurological symptoms.

Q5. What are non-infectious inflammatory dermatoses? Discuss salient features of common examples.

Definition This group of diseases includes several very common inflammatory diseases of unknown etiology such as nonspecific dermatitis (eczema), urticaria, miliaria, panniculitis and acne vulgaris.

Salient features of common examples are as under:

I. **Dermatitis** is clinically known as eczema. It is a chronic inflammation of the skin caused by a variety of physical and chemical agents that act as irritants, allergens or haptens, photosensitisers, toxins and drugs. This group includes a variety of skin disease that presents with itching, erythema and oedema, oozing or scaling, such as:

i. Seborrheic keratitis
ii. Exfoliative dermatitis (erythroderma)
iii. Neurodermatitis (lichen simplex chronicus)

Microscopy Irrespective of the clinical presentation, the histopathologic pictures is always similar. The changes are classified as acute, subacute or chronic.

i. *Acute dermatitis* is characterised by spongiosis which may progress to formation of vesicles or bullae. Their base is permeated by chronic inflammatory cells and contains proliferated and dilated blood capillaries.

ii. *Subacute dermatitis* follows the acute stage of the disease and is characterised by moderate acanthosis, parakeratosis and keratosis, exudation of inflammatory cells and fibrin with formation of surface crust. The classical example is so called *nummular dermatitis*.

iii. *Chronic dermatitis* shows keratosis and parakertatosis of the acanthotic epidermis. The underlying dermis contains chronic inflammation, more prominent around the dilated and congested dermal blood vessels. Its classical example is *lichen simplex chronicus*.

II. **Urticaria** or hives presents with transient but recurrent pruritic wheels (i.e. raised erythematous areas of oedema). It may be caused by a number of physical and chemical influences, drugs or allergies. *Hereditary angioneurotic oedema* is an uncommon variant of urticaria. Often, it is mediated by degranulation of mast cells, as in mastocytosis or atopic dermatitis.

III. **Miliaria** is characterised by formation of small subcorneal fluid filled vesicles due to the obstruction of sweat ducts, more common in small children exposed to heat. It may be classified as:

i. *Superficial miliaria crystallina* filled with clear fluid.

ii. *Miliaria rubra* in the stratum spinosum deeper in the epidermis, which is usually initiated by clothing that is causing constant itching.

IV. **Panniculitis** is inflammation of the subcutaneous fat that may be acute or chronic. It includes erythema nodosum and erythema induratum:

i. *Erythema nodosum* occurs commonly on legs and presents as red, tender subcutaneous nodules. These lesions may be initiated by a variety of factors such as acute and chronic infections caused by bacteria or fungi, drugs, inflammatory bowel disease, or certain malignancies.

ii. *Erythema induratum* involves calves and legs but the nodules are less painful and only slightly tender.

Microscopy The lesions show necrotising vasculitis in the deep dermis and subcutis, which transforms into a chronic form that is infiltrated with lymphocytes, macrophages and multinucleated giant cells, mostly located in the fibrous septa of the subcutaneous fat.

V. **Acne vulgaris** is a very common chronic inflammatory disease affecting predominantly adolescents, related to hormonal changes of puberty. Most often, the lesions are found on the face, upper chest and upper back. The condition affects primarily the hair follicles, the opening of which is blocked by keratin plugs. Such plugging leads to the formation of *comedones* (open ended *black heads* and closed up *white heads*). Closed comedones may get infected resulting in *pustular acne*.

Microscopy The follicles are filled with sebum which becomes infected and inflamed. Neutrophils infiltrating the area destroy the follicle and allow the infection to spread into the dermis. Granulomas form around ruptured follicles which release into the perifollicular tissue infected sebum, fragmented hair-shafts, and keratin.

Q6. What are infectious dermatoses? Briefly describe salient features of common examples.

Definition Infectious dermatoses are skin diseases caused by viruses, bacteria and fungi.

Salient features of common examples are as under:

I. **Impetigo** is a very common superficial bacterial disease caused by staphylococci and streptococci. Most often, it presents as a vesico-pustular eruption on the face and hand.

Microscopy shows subcorneal pustules and infiltrates of neutrophils and chronic inflammatory cells in the dermis.

II. **Verrucae (warts)** are caused by human papilloma viruses (HPV). Depending on the type of the HPV and the location of lesions, there are several types of warts:

i. The most common is verruca *vulgaris* caused by HPV 1 and 2. It may occur on the soles and plantar surface of hand as plantar wart.

ii. *Verruca plana* occurs on the dorsal side of the hands and it is caused by HPV 10.

iii. *Anogenital warts* are caused by HPV 6 and 11.

iv. *Bowen disease* and *bowenoid papulosis* are caused by HPV 16.

Microscopy All warts share the following common features **(Fig. 26.3)**: acanthosis, hyperkeratosis and parakeratosis, clumped keratohyaline granules in the prominent granular layer, papillomatosis with elongated rete ridges bent inwards, and koilocytic change related to HPV infection.

III. **Molluscum contagiosum** is caused by a common DNA virus, usually affecting children and young persons by direct contact. Clinically, it presents in the form of multiple, waxy, cup-like papules, 5 mm in diameter, on the face or trunk. The central part of each papule can be squeezed out as a paste-like material.

Microscopy There is proliferation of epidermal cells which contain numerous intranuclear virions (*molluscum bodies*).

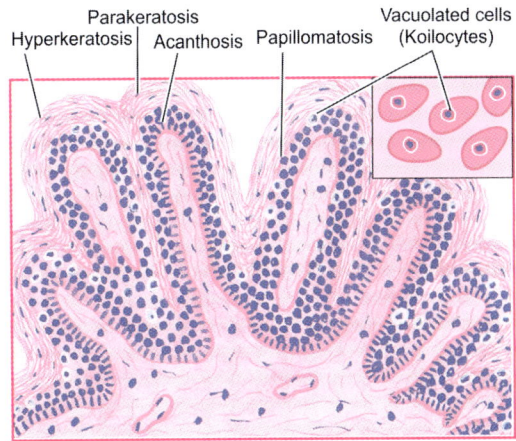

FIGURE 26.3: Typical appearance of a verruca. The histologic features include papillomatosis, acanthosis, hyperkeratosis with parakeratosis and elongated rete ridges appearing to point towards the centre. Foci of vacuolated cells (koilocytes) are found in the upper stratum malpighii. *Inset* shows koilocytes and virus-infected keratinocytes containing prominent keratohyaline granules.

IV. **Viral exanthemata** include pox viruses (e.g. smallpox or variola, and cowpox or vaccinia), herpes viruses (e.g. chickenpox or varicella, herpes zoster or shingle, herpes simplex or herpes genitalis).
Microscopy of these infections is characterised by the formation of intraepidermal vesicles or bullae due to the cytopathic effect of the viruses.
V. **Superficial mycoses** are caused by common dermatophytoses such as *Trichiphyton rubrum* and *Pityrosporum*. Clinically, they are labelled according to the region of the body affected, such as: tinea capitis (scalp), tinea barbae (beard), tinea pedis (foot), or onychomycosis (nails), etc.
Microscopy Fungal organisms can be detected with special stains in the skin or nail biopsy using PAS staining or Grocott silver impregnation.

Q7. What are the granulomatous skin diseases? Briefly discuss salient features of common examples.

Definition Granulomatous skin diseases are caused by some mycobacteria, some deep fungi, syphilitic gummas, and also includes immunologic diseases of unknown etiology such as sarcoidosis.
Salient features of common examples are as under:
I. **Lupus vulgaris** is the term used for skin tuberculosis.
i. It is caused by *M. tuberculosis*, most often involving the head and neck region, especially the skin of the nose.
ii. The infection is characterised by the formation of caseating granuloma in the dermis.
II. **Leprosy** is causes by *M. leprae*. It may affect the skin in several forms as reviewed previously on page 75. Tuberculoid leprosy presents with dermal granulomas.
III. **Sarcoidosis** is a systemic disease of unknown etiology that frequently presents with dermal non-caseating granulomas (page 79).
IV. **Granuloma annulare** is an immune reaction to unknown antigens, which may be endogenous or exogenous, such as viral infection or related to arthropode bites.
i. It presents in the form of annular plaques on the skin which contain palisading granulomas in the dermis.
ii. Granulomas are called palisading because they consist of macrophages and multinucleated giant cells arranged in palisades around a center, which is composed of degenerated collagen.

Q8. What are connective tissue dermatoses? Comment briefly on salient features of common examples.

Definition Connective tissue dermatoses are dermal manifestations of systemic autoimmune (collagen vascular) diseases.
Salient features of two examples are presented here: lupus erythematosus and systemic sclerosis (scleroderma).
I. **Lupus erythematosus** may occur in the skin in two forms: discoid lupus erythematosus (DLE) limited to the skin, and systemic lupus erythematosus (SLE).
i. **DLE** is the more common form of lupus erythematosus. It does not have systemic symptoms and no lethal complications, in contrast to SLE which is systemic and may be lethal. The diagnosis is made

on the basis of clinical, serologic and pathologic data. Clinically, it presents with typical erythematous discoid patches on the face and neck and sun-exposed skin of the torso. These patches are associated with scaling and atrophy. They tend to expand and may persist for long time, undergo scarring and cause disfiguration.

ii. **SLE** is a multisystemic disease; in 80% cases there are some skin changes including erythematous patches on sun exposed areas such as upper chest and arms. Some patients have a typical malar *butterfly rash* on the face, and a small proportion of them have changes similar to those in DLE.

Pathology The microscopic changes in DLE and SLE are similar:

a. There is hyperkeratosis covering the atrophic epidermis with hydropic degeneration of the basal layer.
b. The upper dermis is oedematous and shows infiltrates of lymphocytes.
c. By immunofluorescence microscopy, one may see granular deposits of immunoglobulin IgG and IgM and complement along the basement membrane at the epidermo-dermal junction.
d. Antinuclear antibodies (ANA) in DLE are elevated in serum in less than 10% cases, while in SLE they are found in high titre in over 90% of cases.

II. **Systemic sclerosis (Scleroderma)** occurs in two forms:
- A localised form called *morphea*, limited to the skin.
- A generalised form involving the skin and internal organs, called *progressive systemic sclerosis*. A variant of this form is *CREST syndrome* (C = calcinosis, R = Raynaud phenomenon, E = esophageal dysmotility, S = sclerodactyly, and T = telangiectasia).

Pathology Microscopic changes include:

i. Prominent skin changes as sclerosis, typically beginning on the skin of fingers and extending proximally to involve arms, shoulders and face.
ii. Sclerosis begins as dermal oedema which is replaced by deposits of collagen in the dermis and subcutis, focally accompanied by scattered chronic inflammatory infiltrates.
iii. The epidermis is thin and devoid of rete ridges and adnexal structures.
iv. Arterioles and small arteries of the dermis have thickened walls.
v. Occasionally, there is also dermal calcification.
vi. Ultimately, the face becomes 'mask like' and expressionless, with puckering of the skin around the mouth with deep furrows.
vii. Similar fibrosis may involve the internal organs, most prominently the esophagus and the lungs.

Q9. What are non-infectious bullous dermatoses? Briefly discuss salient features of common examples.

Definition Non-infectious bullous dermatoses are a group of diseases marked by formation of blisters, a term that includes vesicles (less than 5 mm in diameter) and bullae (>5 mm in diameter). These diseases are classified on the basis of their pathogenesis and the location of bullae. Classification of bullae according to their location illustrated in **Figure 26.4** is as under:

i. *Intraepidermal bullae* are subdivided into suprabasal and superficial subcorneal. Intraepidermal bullae are found in pemphigus. Intraepidermal bullae caused by cell death of keratinocytes and accompanied by an acute inflammation, are typical of erythema multiforme and considered separately.

ii. *Subepidermal bullae* are formed by lifting up the entire overlying epidermis and are typical of bullous pemphigoid. Subepidermal vesicle beginning at the suprapapillary epidermal-dermal junction which usually transform into dermal abscesses are typical of dermatitis herpetiformis.

Salient features of common examples are as under.

I. **Pemphigus** is an autoimmune disease caused by antibodies to *desmoglein*, a component of desmosomes that bind the keratinocytes to each other. Antibodies cause acantholysis, i.e. dissociation of keratinocytes. Pemphigus is a bullous disease of adulthood with a peak incidence in the 30–50 years age group. It occurs in three clinicopathologic forms:

i. *Pemphigus vulgaris* is the most common form and accounts for 80% of all cases. Patients present with flaccid bullae on the trunk, face and oral mucosa.

Pathology
a. Intraepidermal bullae form just above the basal layer of keratinocytes (i.e. suprabasal).
b. The bullous cavity contains acantholytic cells.

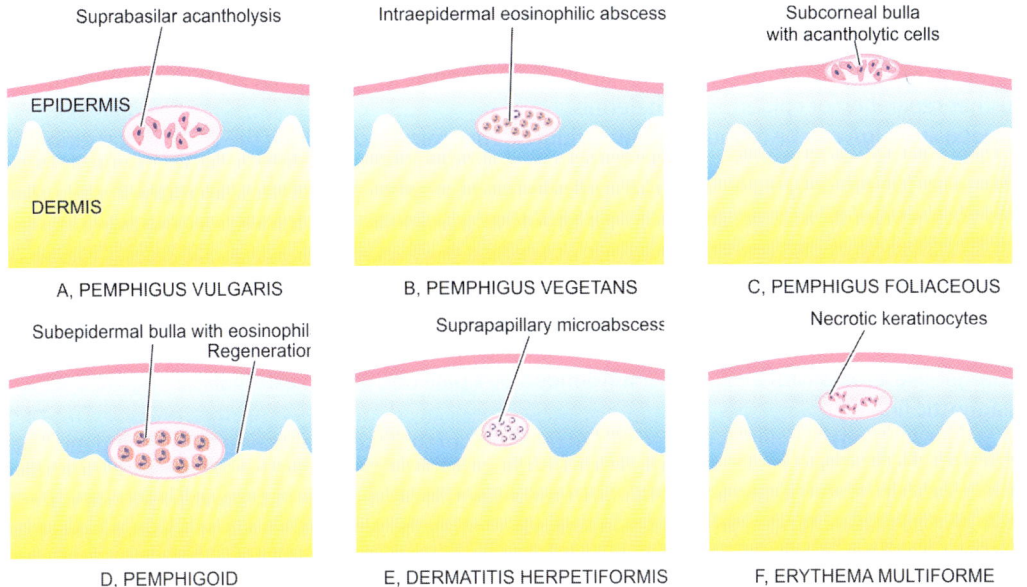

FIGURE 26.4: Location of bullae and vesicles in non-infectious bullous dermatoses. A, *Pemphigus vulgaris*: The bulla is predominantly suprabasilar in position and contains acantholytic cells. B, *Pemphigus vegetans*: An intraepidermal abscess composed of eosinophils is seen. C, *Pemphigus foliaceous*: The bulla is superficial in subcorneal position and contains acantholytic cells. D, *Pemphigoid*: The bulla containing eosinophils is subepidermal with regeneration of the epidermis at the periphery. E, *Dermatitis herpetiformis*: There is a papillary microabscess composed of neutrophils. F, *Erythema multiforme*: The affected area shows necrotic keratinocytes and inflammatory cells.

c. Direct immunofluorescence shows typical fish-net pattern.
d. Rupture of bulla leaves behind shallow ulcers that persist for long time but, in general, do not endanger the health.
ii. *Pemphigus vegetans* is much less common subtype of pemphigus.
Pathology
a. It is characterised by bullae that are formed in mid-epidermis.
b. These bullae often transform into abscesses full of eosinophils.
iii. *Pemphigus foliaceous* is also an uncommon subtype.
Pathology
It is marked by subcorneal bullae formed in the upper part of the spinous layer.
II. **Bullous pemphigoid** is an autoimmune bullous disease characterised by the formation of subepidermal bullae, without any evidence of acantholysis that is so typical of pemphigus. It is caused by antibodies to components of hemidesmosomes that keep the basal cells attached to the basement membrane. The disease occurs in older adults presenting with large, tense bullae on the skin of the thighs and flexor side of the arms. Mucosal blisters are found in 15% of cases.
Pathology
a. Bullae are accompanied by a dermal inflammation that contains eosinophils spilling into the bullous cavity.
b. By immunofluorescence microscopy, one may see deposits of immunoglobulin IgG along the epidermal-dermal basement membrane.
c. The disease is self-limited but chronic, and the blistering may be shortened by treatment with corticosteroids.
III. **Dermatitis herpetiformis** is a chronic pruritic vesicular dermatosis affecting males in the 3rd and 4th decade. It presents with grouped vesicles (resembling herpes as the name implies), most prominently on the knees, buttocks and elbows. Skin eruptions are associated with gluten-sensitive enteropathy (coeliac disease) and responds well to gluten-free diet. Affected persons develop IgA antibodies to gluten which cross-react with reticulin that binds the basal keratinocytes to the basement membrane.

Pathology
a. The initial lesions include subepidermal blisters, which typically begin at the tips of dermal papillae.
b. They are usually accompanied by formation of neutrophilic microabscesses in the upper dermis and further separation of epidermis from dermis.
c. Deposits of IgA can be found by immunofluorescence microscopy along the basement membrane.
d. The disease responds well to gluten free diet.

IV. **Erythema multiforme** is an acute self-limiting but recurrent dermatosis. The cause is often not identified, and considered to be *idiopathic*. However, hypersensitivity to certain drugs (e.g. antiepileptics) and infections (in particular by herpes simplex virus or *Mycoplasma pneumoniae*) are common precipitating factors.

i. As the name suggests, the skin lesions are multiform and may present in the form of macules, papules, vesicles or bullae, most often affecting the extremities.
ii. Target-like lesions with a red centre surrounded by a pale ring and an external red ring are the most diagnostic finding.
iii. *Steven-Johnson syndrome* is a severe, often fatal form of the disease affecting the skin and mucosae of the mouth, conjunctivae, and genital organs.
iv. Another variant is called *toxic epidermal necrolysis* that presents with extensive necrosis of the skin and mucosa giving the skin a scalded appearance.

Pathology
a. There is subepidermal blister formation resulting from prominent, and often confluent, apoptosis of basal keratinocytes.
b. Apoptotic cells appear as round, dyskeratotic, eosinophilic cells with pyknotic nuclei.
c. Blistering occurs so fast that there is not much acute inflammation in the stratum corneum. Infiltrates of lymphocytes are seen nevertheless in the upper dermis, most prominently around the small dermal vessels.
d. Immunofluorescent microscopic studies usually reveal no immunoglobulin deposition, implying that the immune reaction is mediated by T lymphocytes.
e. Treatment with steroids may help shorten the disease.

Q10. Write is psoriasis? Discuss its salient clinicopathologic features.

Definition Psoriasis is a chronic skin disease of unknown etiology, presenting with large, erythematous scaly plaques, most often on extensor surfaces of the extremities, face, scalp and the back side of the trunk.

Epidemiology Psoriasis is a very common skin disease affecting 2% of the world's population.
- The disease is linked to certain HLA haplotypes, in particular HLA-B27.
- It has a tendency to affect families; one third of all patients have a family history. The disease is more severe in familial cases than in non-familial cases. Familial cases are also more often affected by arthritis.
- There is a 65% concordance in monozygotic twins.

Pathogenesis The exact pathogenesis of psoriasis is not fully understood. But it seems that T helper cells play the key role by secreting a number of cytokines and stimulating the proliferation of epidermis, inducing the vascular changes in the dermal papillae, and promoting the inflammatory reaction.

Pathology
i. The plaques show thickening of the epidermis, primarily due to regular elongation and widening of rete ridges. Between the rete ridges, the elongated dermal papillae are broadened at their tips in the upper part **(Fig. 26.5)**.
ii. The widened upper dermis contains dilated capillaries and infiltrates of inflammatory cells.
iii. The surface of the epidermis shows hyperkeratosis and focal parakeratosis indicative of rapid cell turnover.
iv. The granular layer is remarkably missing.
v. The spinous layer contains neutrophilic aggregates forming diagnostic Munroe microabscesses.
vi. The suprapapillary part of the epidermis is thinner than normal which accounts for bleeding from the papillary capillaries that can be elicited by scraping the plaques (Auspitz sign).

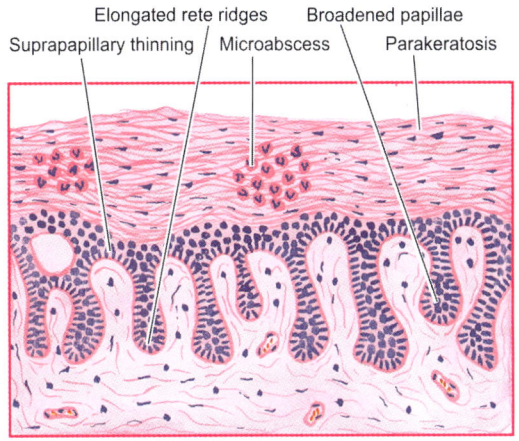

FIGURE 26.5: Psoriasis. There is regular elongation of the rete ridges with thickening of their lower portion. The papillae are elongated and oedematous with suprapapillary thinning of epidermis. There is marked parakeratosis with diagnostic Munro microabscesses in the parakeratotic layer.

Q11. What is lichen planus? Discuss its salient clinicopathologic features.

Definition Lichen planus is a chronic dermatosis characterised clinically by irregular, violaceous, shining, flat-topped, pruritic papules. The lesions are distributed symmetrically with sites of predilection being flexor surfaces of the wrists, forearms, legs and external genitalia. Buccal mucosa is also involved in many cases of lichen planus.

Pathology
i. Marked hyperkeratosis
ii. Focal hypergranulosis
iii. Irregular acanthosis with elongated saw-toothed rete ridges
iv. Liquefactive degeneration of the basal layer
v. A band-like dermal infiltrate of mononuclear cells, sharply demarcated at its lower border and closely hugging the basal layer **(Fig. 26.6)**.

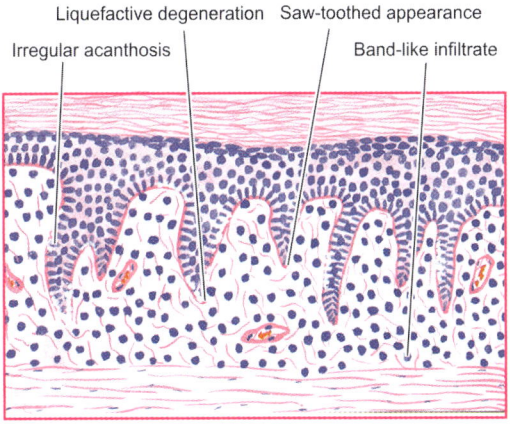

FIGURE 26.6: Lichen planus. There is hyperkeratosis, focal hypergranulosis and irregular acanthosis with elongated saw-toothed rete ridges. The basal layer shows liquefactive degeneration. The upper dermis shows a band-like mononuclear infiltrate with a sharply-demarcated lower border.

Q12. What are the most important metabolic diseases of skin?

Skin is involved in a variety of systemic metabolic diseases as under:
i. Amyloidosis
ii. Porphyria of various types
iii. Calcinosis cutis which may be idiopathic or related to metastatic calcification in hypercalcaemia of hyperparathyroidism and chronic kidney disease
iv. Gout with formation of tophi
v. Ochronosis due alkaptonuria
vi. Myxoedema of hypothyroidism
vii. Hereditary haemochromatosis with hyperpigmentation of the skin ('bronze diabetes')

Q13. How are tumours and tumour-like lesions of the skin classified?

Tumours and tumour-like conditions of the skin are classified histogenetically according to their site or cell of origin, i.e. from epidermis, appendages or adnexa, and dermal tissues. Accordingly, these conditions are divided into five categories:
i. Epidermal tumours (benign, pre-malignant, and malignant)
ii. Adnexal tumours (hair follicles, sebaceous glands, or sweat glands, i.e. eccrine and apocrine tumours)
iii. Melanocytic tumours
iv. Dermal tumours
v. Cellular migrant tumours

Q14. What are common epithelial cysts of the skin?

Definition Cysts of the skin are cavitary lesions that form from downward growth of the epidermis or skin adnexa, or by dilatation of excretory ducts and hair follicles. The following are common cutaneous cysts:

I. **Epidermal cyst** Also known as *sebaceous cyst*, it may be found in the dermis or subcutis. It is formed spontaneously or due to mechanical implantation of the epidermis into the deeper layers of the skin. Most frequent sites are the skin of face, scalp, neck and trunk.
Microscopy
i. The cyst wall consists of normal epidermis lined by laminated layers of keratin.
ii. Rupture of the cysts may incite inflammatory reaction and foreign body giant cells around the extruded keratin.

II. **Pilar (trichilemmal) cyst** Also called sebaceous cyst because it cannot be distinguished clinically from epidermal cyst but is less common than epidermal cyst. Most often it is found on the scalp.
Microscopy
i. The wall of the cyst is lined by an abruptly keratinising epithelium missing the granular layer.
ii. The cyst contains layers of keratin, which may undergo degeneration, calcification or become inflamed.
iii. These cysts may also rupture and elicit a foreign body giant cell inflammatory reaction.

III. **Dermoid cyst** These are congenital cysts usually found in neonates and infants most often on the face along the lines of embryonic closure.
Microscopy
i. The wall of the cyst consists of skin with skin appendages.
ii. The lumen is filled with layers of keratin.

Q15. What is the most common benign epithelial tumour of the skin?

Seborrheic keratosis is the most common epithelial skin tumour.
i. It may occur on any part of the body, mostly in persons older than 40 years of age.
ii. It may be solitary but more often it is multiple.
iii. It is usually pigmented and may grow rapidly, and thus, it should not be confused with melanoma.
iv. It has no malignant potential, although it may recur following excision.
v. If found in large numbers, they could be part of paraneoplastic syndrome, i.e. it is a sign of internal malignancy, most often gastrointestinal carcinoma.

Pathology
i. Sharply demarcated, small, pigmented, papular lesion that may be found anywhere on the extremities or the trunk.
ii. Composed of uniform small mature cells which form invaginating nests with central keratinisation ('horn cysts') or short exophytic papillae lined by the same acanthotic epithelium showing surface keratinisation.

Q16. What are the premalignant skin lesions?

Two common examples are solar keratosis and Bowen disease.
I. **Solar keratosis** Also known as *actinic keratosis* or *senile keratosis*, it is induced by sunshine or other radiation. It presents clinically in the form of multiple lesions on sun-exposed skin, most often

in fair-skinned elderly persons. Similar lesions can be induced by ionising radiation, exposure to hydrocarbons or arsenicals. It is a forerunner of basal cell or squamous carcinoma.
Clinically, it presents as a tan-brown, erythematous papule or plaque with rough, sand-paper like surface, measuring about 1 cm in diameter on sun-exposed skin of the arms or balded part of the face.
Microscopy
i. The epidermis shows prominent hyperkeratosis, acanthosis, dyskeratosis and dysplasia of epidermal cells, which show hyperchromasia, loss of polarity, pleomorphism and increased mitotic activity.
ii. The underlying dermis is infiltrated with chronic inflammatory cells.
II. **Bowen disease** This condition is a carcinoma in situ of the epidermis that may occur on the sun-exposed as well as sun-unexposed skin. Clinically, the lesion is most often found on the extremities, trunk and buttocks. It presents as well-circumscribed, rounded, reddish-brown patch which enlarges slowly.
Microscopy
i. The epidermis shows hyperkeratosis, pronounced parakeratosis, marked epidermal hyperplasia with disappearance of dermal papillae, and scattered dyskeratotic cells throughout the entire epidermis.
ii. It may remain confined to epidermis for many years before it becomes invasive squamous cell carcinoma.

Q17. Discuss briefly squamous cell carcinoma of the skin.

Definition Squamous cell carcinoma of the skin is an invasive epithelial malignant tumour composed of keratinocytes.
Predisposing conditions
i. Solar keratosis from prolonged exposure to sunshine
ii. Chronic inflammatory conditions such as chronic ulcer and draining osteomyelitis
iii. 'Kangari cancer' in Kashmiris in India who keep earthen coal pot on the abdomen to keep warm
iv. Old burn scars (Marjolin ulcer)
v. Chemical burns
vi. Ionising radiation
vii. Industrial carcinogens (coal tars, arsenicals, etc.)
viii. Congenital conditions such as xeroderma pigmentosum
ix. Autosomal recessive epidermodysplasia verruciformis with HPV-5 and HPV-8
x. HIV infection and immunosuppression
Clinicopathologic features
Location It may develop in any location on the skin or squamous mucosa, but most common sites are as follows: face, pinna of the ears, back of the hands, mucocutaneous junctions such as lips, anal canal and glans penis.
Clinical and gross Two forms of invasive squamous cell carcinoma are recognised **(Fig. 26.7):** ulcerated and fungating.
Microscopy
i. Irregular downward proliferation of epidermal cells into the dermis **(Fig. 26.8)**.
ii. Cellular atypia including hyperchromasia, pleomorphism, loss of polarity, mitotic activity, dyskeratosis and single cell keratinisation, irregular keratinisation with formation of keratin pearls.
iii. Low-grade carcinomas produce prominent keratin pearls, whereas higher grade cancers show less keratinisation and more nuclear atypia and pleomorphism.
iv. *Grading of squamous cell carcinoma* includes descriptive terms such as: well-differentiated,

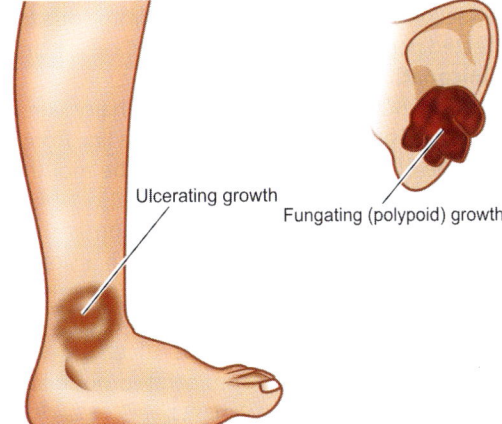

FIGURE 26.7: Squamous cell carcinoma. Main clinical and gross patterns showing ulcerated and fungating polypoid growth.

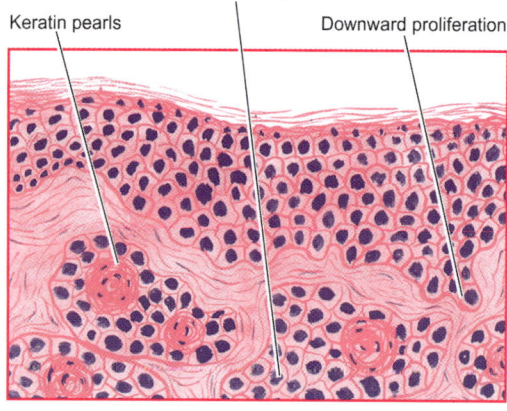

FIGURE 26.8: Microscopic features of well-differentiated squamous cell carcinoma. The dermis is invaded by downward proliferating epidermal masses of cells which show atypical features. A few horn pearls with central laminated keratin are present. There is inflammatory reaction in the dermis between the masses of tumour cells.

moderately-differentiated, undifferentiated keratinising, undifferentiated non-keratinising, spindle cell type, etc.

v. *Spindle cell carcinoma* is a high-grade variant composed of spindle cells showing only rudimentary squamous differentiation.

vi. *Verrucous carcinoma* is a low-grade variant form of squamous carcinoma, most often found in the oral cavity. It resembles verruca and shows changes seen in warts (acanthosis, parakeratosis, hyperkeratosis and papillomatosis). Even though there is no significant atypia, these tumours show superficial invasion which differentiates them from common warts.

Prognosis Depends on the TNM staging.

i. In general, squamous cell carcinoma arising in actinic keratosis has a good prognosis.

ii. Tumours originating in preexisting chronic inflammatory lesions have a worse prognosis.

However, grading squamous cell carcinoma is of limited clinical significance, except for the variants which have better or worse prognosis.

Q18. Briefly describe basal cell carcinoma of the skin.

Definition Basal cell carcinoma (BCC) is a locally invasive, rarely metastasising, low-grade malignant tumour composed of cells resembling the cells of the basal layer of skin.

Predisposing conditions

i. Light-skinned people lacking the protective effects of melanin

ii. Prolonged exposure to sunshine

iii. Inherited defect in DNA repair mechanism as in xeroderma pigmentosum

iv. Naevoid basal cell carcinoma syndrome due to germ-line mutation of PTCH gene, predisposing the affected person to early onset of basal cell carcinoma by the age of 20 years.

Clinicopathologic features

Location BCC originates only on the hairy skin, most often on the face, usually above a line from the lobe of the ear to the corner of the mouth **(Fig. 26.9)**.

Clinical and gross The most common is the nodulo-ulcerative appearance in which a slow-growing nodule undergoes ulceration in its central part with pearly rolled-up margins (commonly known as 'rodent ulcer'). Less common patterns are: non-ulcerated nodular, pigmented, and fibrosing variants.

Microscopy

i. The tumour is composed of basaloid cells which form nests, cord and stands.

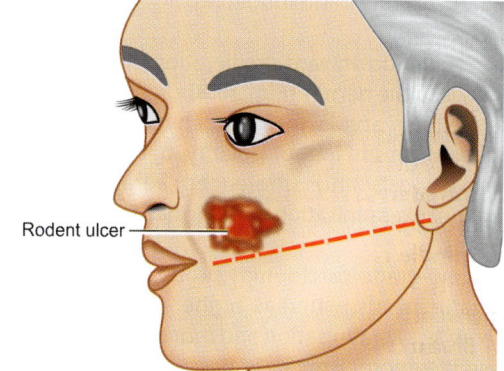

FIGURE 26.9: Common location and gross appearance of basal cell carcinoma (rodent ulcer).

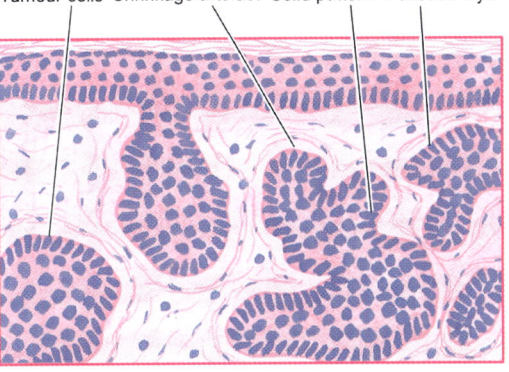

FIGURE 26.10: Solid basal cell carcinoma. The dermis is invaded by irregular masses of basaloid cells with characteristic peripheral palisaded appearance. The masses of tumour cells are separated from dermal collagen by a space called shrinkage artefact.

ii. The most common is the *solid basal cell carcinoma* composed of dermal nests of basaloid cells, which show a palisaded peripheral arrangement **(Fig. 26.10)**. Other microscopic patterns are less common.
iii. Microscopic subclassification of basal carcinoma is often used in pathology reports, but has no clinical value.
Prognosis BCC is locally invasive, low-grade malignant tumour that rarely metastasises.

Q19. How are skin adnexal tumours classified? Enumerate a few common examples.

Most of skin adnexal tumours are benign, but on occasional they may be malignant. These tumours are classified according to the anatomic site and presumptive cell of origin as follows:
I. **Tumours of hair follicle** Common examples: trichoepithelioma, pilomatricoma.
II. **Tumours of the sebaceous glands** Examples: naevus sebaceous, sebaceous adenoma, sebaceous carcinoma.
III. **Tumours of sweat glands** Further divided into following groups:
i. *Eccrine tumours*, e.g. eccrine poroma, or eccrine hidradenoma and eccrine spiradenoma
ii. *Apocrine tumours*, e.g. papillary hidradenoma, cylidroma
iii. *Sweat gland carcinoma*

Q20. Classify benign pigmented skin tumours and tumour-like conditions.

Benign pigmented skin tumours originate from three cell types:
i. *Naevus cells:* give rise to naevocellular naevi.
ii. *Epidermal melanocytes:* give rise to lentigo, freckles, pigmentation associated with Albright syndrome and café-au-lait spots of neurofibromatosis.
iii. *Dermal melanocytes:* give rise to Mongolian spots, naevi of Otta and of Ito, and the blue naevus.

Q21. What are common microscopic variants of naevi?

i. **Lentigo** in which the basal layer of epidermis has been replaced by melanocytes.
ii. **Junctional naevus** in which the naevus cells lie at the epidermal-dermal junction, forming well-circumscribed nests.
iii. **Compound naevus** which, in addition to junctional activity, contains naevus cell in the dermis to a variable depth. This is the commonest type of pigmented naevus **(Fig. 26.11)**.
iv. **Intradermal naevus** which show minimal or no junctional activity and is composed of pigmented naevus cells in the dermis forming nests or cords.
v. **Spindle cell (epithelioid) naevus or juvenile melanoma** is a compound naevus with junctional activity. It is composed of elongated and epithelioid naevus cells which may or may not contain melanin. It must be distinguished from melanoma because it is benign.
vi. **Blue naevus** is a dermal lesion composed of dendritic spindle naevus cells, which are usually heavily pigmented.
vii. **Dysplastic naevus** is an atypical naevus which is at risk for transforming into malignant melanoma. They are larger than acquired naevi, often multiple, and appear as flat macule to slightly elevated plaques with irregular borders and variable pigmentation. Many are familial and inherited.

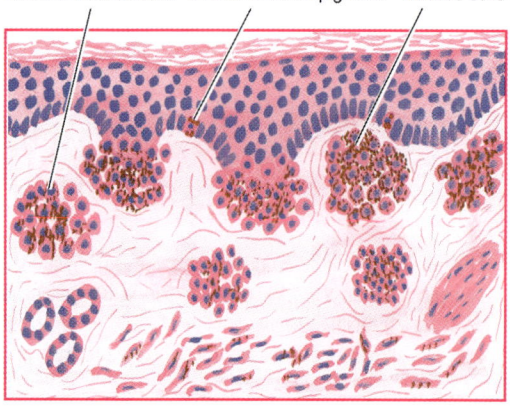

FIGURE 26.11: Compound naevus showing clusters of benign naevus cells in the dermis as well as in lower epidermis. These cells contain coarse, granular, brown-black melanin pigment.

Microscopy Dysplastic naevi show melanocytic proliferation at the epidermal-dermal junction with some cytologic atypia.

Q22. What is malignant melanoma? Briefly discuss its salient clinicopathologic features.

Definition Malignant melanoma (MM) is a malignant neoplasm of melanocytes. Most often, it originates from the skin, but it may arise from the pigmented cells of the eye and even from internal organs.

Epidemiology The incidence of MM is increasing worldwide.

i. The incidence of MM shows racial variation: highest in whites, while Black persons appear to be spared and rarely develop MM except for acral lentiginous MM.
ii. Excessive exposure to sunshine (e.g. Australia or New Zealand) is accompanied by higher incidence of MM.
iii. Person who have numerous melanocytic naevi (more than 50 moles 2 mm or more in diameter) are at increased risk.
iv. Moles that change in appearance and colour are a risk factor.
v. Familial forms of MM, usually found in those with dysplastic naevi, or related to germ-line mutation of *CDKN2A* gene, are rare.

Clinicopathologic features

Location Any part of the body can be involved. In men, MM it is most often found on the trunk, and in women on their extremities. Other common sites are the face, soles and palms, and nail beds.

MM may arise from melanocytic naevi or de novo in apparently normal skin. Those arising in naevi may remain flat or slightly elevated, but start having irregular borders, variegated pigmentation and of late have undergone ulceration, bleeding and increase in size.

Clinicopathologic classification Five clinical and microscopic types of MM are recognised as follows:

i. *Lentigo maligna melanoma* develops from a pre-existent lentigo in which the melanocytes have replaced the keratinocytes in the basal layer. It is, in essence, a pre-invasive stage or carcinoma in situ. It has an excellent prognosis if timely removed.
ii. *Superficial spreading melanoma* is a slightly elevated lesion of variegated colour and focal ulceration developing from melanoma in situ (pagetoid melanoma) through radial spread.
iii. *Acral lentiginous melanoma* usually develops on soles, palms and mucosal surfaces. It has a tendency to ulcerate and metastasise early.
iv. *Nodular melanoma* usually appears as an elevated nodular lesion that grows rapidly and ulcerates. It has the worst prognosis of all MM types.
v. *Desmoplastic melanoma* is a variant marked by fibrotic stroma, neural invasion and frequent local recurrences.

Microscopy These distinctive features include the following:
i. *Cytomorphologic features* **(Fig. 26.12)**:
- Tumour cells larger than naevus cells.
- They may be epithelioid or spindle-shaped.
- Their cytoplasm may be amphophilic (slightly bluish).
- The nuclei are irregularly shaped and each has a prominent nucleolus.

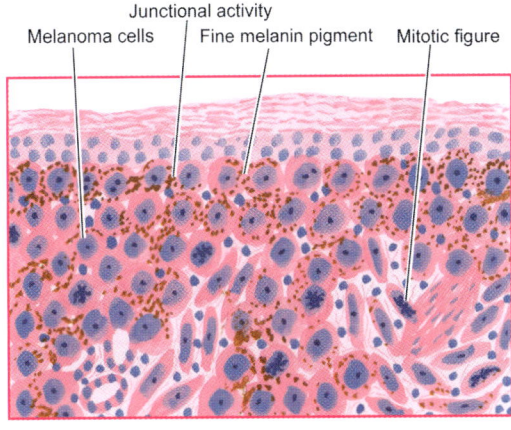

FIGURE 26.12: Nodular malignant melanoma. Sheets of tumour cells resembling epithelioid cells with pleomorphic nuclei and prominent nucleoli are seen as solid masses in the dermis. Many of the tumour cells contain fine granular melanin pigment.

- Mitotic figures may be prominent.
- Melanin may be prominent or missing. In pigmented cells, melanin is finely dispersed throughout the cytoplasm.

ii. *Growth pattern* Melanoma cells may spread *upwards* in the epidermis, *laterally* in a pagetoid manner along the basement membrane in the epidermis, and *vertically* invade the dermis. Invasion occurs in form of single cells, cells arranged into cord, nests, sheets, etc.

iii. *Inflammatory infiltrate* composed of lymphocytes in the dermis is a reaction to tumour growth. Focal regression of MM due to destructive effects of the inflammatory cell may be seen, but complete regression of MM and cure are rare.

iv. *Immunohistochemistry (IHC)* can be used for amelanotic tumours, especially in those that present with metastases and the primary is unknown. IHC markers for MM are: HMB-45, Melan A, and SOX10.

Staging of invasive MM may be done according to the system devised by Clark or Breslow:
Clark staging is descriptive and has five levels of invasion:
    Level 1: No invasion, melanoma in situ
    Level 2: Invasion into the papillary dermis
    Level 3: Invasion to the junction of papillary and reticular dermis
    Level 4: Invasion into reticular dermis
    Level 5: Invasion into subcutaneous fat

Breslow staging is numerical and more precise, and has better prognostic value. It can be readily included into the TNM staging system, where T refers to thickness of the tumour expressed in millimeters (mm):
    T1: <1.00 mm
    T2: 1.01 to 2.00 mm
    T3: 2.01 to 4.00 mm
    T4: >4.00 mm

The *American Joint Commission on Cancers (AJCC)* recommends that the TNM pathology report also includes the number of mitoses, ulceration, nodal metastases and presence of metastases at distant sites. *Sentinel lymph node* metastasis is, therefore, always performed during MM surgery.

Q23. Tabulate the salient contrasting features of naevocellular naevi and malignant melanoma.

The features distinguishing MM from benign naevi are listed in the **Table 26.1.**

Q24. What are the most important tumours of the dermis?

Dermal tumours originate from various tissues such as fibroblasts, fat cells, neural tissue, endothelium and smooth muscles. They are most often benign but certain tumours are low-grade malignant and locally invasive, and a few examples of highly malignant tumours that are prone to metastases. These tumours are equivalent to those found in the soft tissues discussed in Chapter 29.

TABLE 26.1 Distinguishing features of naevocellular naevus and malignant melanoma.

FEATURE	NAEVOCELLULAR NAEVUS	MALIGNANT MELANOMA
1. *Clinical features*		
i. Symmetry	Symmetrical	A = asymmetry
ii. Border	Well-demarcated	B = Border irregularity
iii. Colour	Uniformly pigmented	C = Colour change
iv. Diameter	Small, less than 6 mm	D = Diameter more than 6 mm
v. Solar damage	None	E = Elastosis, solar
2. *Common locations*	Skin of face; mucosa	Skin; mucosa of nose, bowel, anal region
3. *Histopathology*		
i. Architecture	Nests of naevus cells Cells smaller at base	Various patterns: solid sheets, alveoli, nests, islands Cells atypical at base
ii. Cell morphology	Uniform-looking naevus cells	Malignant cells, atypia, mitoses, prominent nucleoli
iii. Melanin pigment	Coarse, brown-black pigment	Fine grey pigment
iv. Edge of lesion	Similar	Dissimilar
v. Inflammation	May or may not be present	Often present
4. *Spread*	Remains confined, may pose cosmetic problem only	Haematogenous and/or lymphatic spread early

Q25. Name some common examples of various cellular migrant tumours of the skin.

I. *Various haematologic diseases* such as leukaemias and lymphomas (including mycosis fungoides and plasmacytoma).

II. Tumours derived from migratory tissue cells such as *mastocytosis* and *Langerhans cell histiocytosis*.

> **Chapter 26e Supplement: Online Content**
>
> Digital content of this chapter available with this book is meant for enhanced learning and self-assessment. In addition, it contains 31 Multiple Choice Questions (MCQs), 05 Clinicopathologic Vignettes, and 07 Image-based Questions; these are followed by their answers along with explanatory notes of correct and incorrect answers.

CHAPTER 27

Endocrine System

BASIC CONCEPT OF ENDOCRINES

Q1. What are the main components of the neuroendocrine and endocrine systems?

I. **Neuroendocrine system** forms a link between endocrine glands and the nervous system as well as their target tissues in peripheral organs. The cells of this system have some common features but are widely distributed in different anatomic sites:
i. *Neuroendocrine cells* in the gastric, intestinal and bronchial mucosae that elaborate peptide hormones.
ii. *Neuroganglia cells* in the ganglia of the sympathetic chain that elaborate biogenic amines.
iii. *Adrenal medullary cells* which elaborate epinephrine and norepinephrine.
iv. *Parafollicular cells* of the thyroid secreting calcitonin.
v. *Cells of islets of Langerhans* in the pancreas included in both the endocrine and neuroendocrine system, secreting insulin and related polypeptides.
vi. *Isolated cells of the left atrium* of the heart which secrete atrial natriuretic (salt-losing) peptide hormone.
In addition to above, the system includes a variety of other cells such as:
- Those secreting *erythropoietin and vitamin D_3* in the kidneys, and
- *Neurotransmitters* such as acetylcholine and dopamine released from neural synapses.

II. **Endocrine system** consists of 6 distinct organs: pituitary, adrenals, thyroid, parathyroids, gonads and pancreatic islets. They secrete hormones which can be divided into five major classes, grouped under two headings:

Group I: Hormones interacting with cell-surface membrane receptors:
i. *Amino acid derivatives*: thyroid hormone and catecholamine.
ii. *Small neuropeptides*: gonadotrophin releasing hormone (GnRH), thyrotrophin-releasing hormone (TRH), somatostatin and vasopressin.

Group II: Those interacting with intracellular nuclear receptors:
iii. *Large proteins*: Insulin, luteinising hormone (LH), parathyroid hormone.
iv. *Steroid hormones*: cortisol, estrogen, testosterone.
v. *Vitamin derivatives*: retinol (vitamin A) and calciferol (vitamin D).

Q2. What are the major functions of hormones?

i. *Growth and differentiation of cells*: a function of pituitary, thyroid, parathyroid and steroid hormones.
ii. *Maintenance of homeostasis*: a function of thyroid, parathyroid, mineralocorticoids, vasopressin, insulin.
iii. *Reproduction:* a function of sex hormone and related pituitary and placental hormones.
A basic feature of the endocrine system is the existence of both *positive and negative feedback control* mechanisms. These include hormonal, paracrine and autocrine regulation, which assure the maintenance of hormone levels within a normal range in the body.

Q3. How are disturbances of the endocrine system classified?

Disturbances of the endocrine system present in three forms:

i. *Hyperfunction* This results most often from excess of hormone-secreting cells due to hyperplasia or neoplasia of endocrine glands. Excess of hormone may also be related to ectopic hormone production in tumours, inflammation, infections, or iatrogenic factors including administration of drugs and hormones.

ii. *Hypofunction* Reduced production of hormones may be caused by destruction of hormone-forming tissues from inflammation (often autoimmune), infections, iatrogenic factors (e.g. resection of endocrine glands, radiation therapy, drugs), developmental defects (e.g. Turner syndrome, streak gonads), haemorrhage or infarction (e.g. panhypopituitarism due to Sheehan syndrome), nutritional deficiency (e.g. iodine deficiency related hypothyroidism), or iatrogenic factors (e.g. surgical resection of endocrine glands, drug therapy, radiation therapy).

iii. *Hormone resistance* Clinical signs of hormone deficiency may be present in persons who secrete adequate amounts of hormones but the hormones cannot act due to peripheral tissue resistance. This resistance may be caused by genetic or acquired defects of membrane receptors or cytoplasmic signal transduction systems.

■ PITUITARY GLAND

Q4. What are the main anatomic, histologic and physiologic features of the pituitary that are important for understanding of the pathology of this endocrine gland?

Pituitary consists of two parts: anterior lobe (adenohypophysis) and posterior lobe (neurohypophysis).

I. **Anterior lobe** is formed during embryogenesis from the Rathke pouch, an ectodermal outpouching of the primitive buccal cavity extending up toward the brain. It is linked to the hypothalamus by a stalk which contains portal blood vessels forming the pituitary portal system. This portal system is the primary route for the hypothalamic stimulatory and inhibitory factors to reach the pituitary.

Microscopy Anterior lobe consists of round to polygonal cells arranged into cords and nest.

- Approximately 50% of cells have cytoplasmic granules and are called *chromophilic* because their granules stain either pink with eosin or bluish (basophilic) with haematoxylin in routine histologic sections.
- The cells devoid of stainable cytoplasmic granules are called *chromophobic* because they do not stain with eosin or haematoxylin.

This classification has, however, been superseded by a *functional classification* based on immunohistochemical stains which recognise cells by the hormones produced by them. These are as follows:

i. *Somatotrophs (GH cells)* produce growth hormone.
ii. *Lactotrophs (PRL cells)* produce prolactin.
iii. *Gonadotrophs (FSH and LH cells)* produce gonadotrophins FSH and LH.
iv. *Thyrotrophs (TSH cells)* produce thyroid stimulating hormone.
v. *Corticotrophs (ACTH-MSH cells)* produce ACTH, pro-opiomelanocortin (POMC), melanocyte stimulating hormone (MSH), β-lipoprotein and β-endorphin.
vi. *Hormonally inactive cells.*

II. **Posterior lobe** is composed of:
i. modified glial cells called *pituicytes* (with no secretory function),
ii. axon terminals, and
iii. *unmyelinated nerve fibres* containing vasopressin (anti-diuretic hormone, ADH) and oxytocin.

Q5. What is hyperpituitarism? Write briefly on clinical conditions causing it.

Definition Hyperpituitarism is a condition characterised by hypersecretion of one or more of the pituitary hormones.

Clinicopathologic syndromes Hyperpituitarism syndromes may be from:

A. Hyperfunction of *anterior pituitary* (gigantism and acromegaly, prolactinaemia, Cushing disease).
B. Hyperfunction of *posterior pituitary* (inappropriate release of ADH, precocious puberty).

These conditions are briefly considered below.

I. **Gigantism and acromegaly** are caused by an excess of growth hormone (GH), most often related to somatotroph adenoma. GH excess prior to closure of epiphyseal growth plates in adolescents leads to gigantism, whereas an excess of GH in adults results in acromegaly.

• *Gigantism* is characterised by excessive but proportionate growth of a child, accompanied by thickening of the bones.

• *Acromegaly*, the more common form of disease, occurs in adults, presenting with an increased size of terminal parts of the extremities and face, thickening of the bones and skin, organomegaly especially affecting the heart, liver and thyroid, and hormonal disturbances.

Clinically, acromegaly is characterised by:

i. *Acromegalic facies* that includes coarse facial features, prognathism (i.e. a protruding jaw so that the lower teeth are in front of upper teeth), thickening of lips and enlargement of the tongue.

ii. *Enlargement* of the hands and fingers, feet and toes.

iii. *Hyperostosis* involving the skull bone, vertebrae and other bone leads to compression neuropathy and osteoarthrosis.

iv. *Hypertension* is frequently present.

v. *Hormonal disturbances* including thyrotoxicosis, diabetes mellitus, hypercalciuria, amenorrhoea in women and impotence in men.

II. **Prolactinaemia** is usually caused by a hyperfunctioning prolactinoma.

i. *In women*, it causes the amenorrhoea-galactorrhoea syndrome characterised by cessation of menstrual cycles and an expression of one or two drops of milk from breast not related to pregnancy or puerperium.

ii. *Men* may experience impotence and reduced libido.

III. **Cushing disease** is caused by ACTH-secreting adenomas. It will be discussed with other adrenal diseases.

IV. **Syndrome of inappropriate ADH release** occurs most often as a paraneoplastic condition, e.g. in patients who have ADH-secreting pulmonary small cell carcinoma, or carcinoma of the pancreas. However, it may also occur due to hypothalamic lesions caused by trauma, haemorrhage or meningitis. This syndrome presents with sodium loss in urine and abnormal resorption of water in the kidneys resulting in hyponatraemia, haemodilution, and expansion of intracellular and extracellular fluid volume.

Q6. What is hypopituitarism? Write briefly on clinical conditions producing it.

Definition Hypopituitarism is defined as a deficiency of one or more of pituitary hormones of the anterior pituitary, posterior pituitary, or hypothalamus.

Etiopathogenesis Since anterior pituitary has a large functional reserve, the symptoms of hypopituitarism appear only after more than 75% of the anterior lobe has been destroyed.

• The most common cause is non-functioning pituitary tumour.

• Other causes are: metastatic carcinoma, craniopharyngioma, trauma, postpartum ischaemic necrosis (Sheehan syndrome), empty sella syndrome, and rarely tuberculosis.

Clinicopathologic syndromes

A. *Insufficiency of anterior lobe:* panhypopituitarism and pituitary dwarfism.

B. *Insufficiency of the posterior lobe*: diabetes insipidus as the most important syndrome.

I. **Panhypopituitarism** is a major pituitary insufficiency with a loss of all secretory functions. It is most often caused by non-functioning (chromophobe) pituitary adenoma. It can also result from Sheehan postpartum syndrome and Simmonds disease, and empty-sella syndrome.

i. **Sheehan syndrome and Simmonds disease** Pituitary insufficiency occurring due to postpartum pituitary necrosis is called Sheehan syndrome, whereas occurrence of the same process without preceding pregnancy as well as in males is called Simmonds disease.

a. Sheehan disease results from pituitary enlargement during pregnancy, followed by hypotensive shock due to massive bleeding, precipitating hypoperfusion and ischaemic necrosis of the pituitary. Other factors such as DIC may play a role as well. Patients with long-standing diabetes mellitus appear to be at greatest risk.

b. The first clinical sign of Sheehan syndrome is failure of lactation due to a deficiency of prolactin. Subsequently, other symptoms develop like loss of axillary and pubic hair, amenorrhoea, loss of libido and infertility.
c. Loss of TSH and ACTH results in hypothyroidism and adrenocortical insufficiency.
Pathology The pituitary is necrotic and suffused with blood. In due course of time, necrotic tissue is replaced by fibrous tissue.
ii. **Empty-sella syndrome** is hypopituitarism associated with radiologic evidence of an 'empty sella', indicating that the pituitary has been destroyed.
a. The most common reason is a defect in the fibrous diaphragm covering the upper opening of the sella. Herniation of the subarachnoid tissue through defect in this fibrous diaphragm will compress the pituitary and destroy it, thereby creating the image of an empty sella on X-ray examination.
b. Other causes of empty sella are Sheehan syndrome, irradiation, complications of surgical procedures at the base of the brain, or surgical removal of the pituitary.
II. **Pituitary dwarfism** results from GH deficiency in children before epiphyseal closure, thus retarding the growth of bones.
i. The most common cause is an autosomal recessive genetic disorder.
ii. Other possible causes are pituitary of hypothalamic tumours, trauma and infarction of the pituitary.
iii. *Clinical features* of inherited cases appear after one year of age. These include proportionate retardation in growth of bones, normal mental state for the age, poorly developed genitalia, delayed puberty and episodes of hypoglycaemia.
III. **Diabetes insipidus** is the only clinically important insufficiency of the posterior lobe of the pituitary. It results from a deficiency of ADH due to:
i. *Destruction* of the hypothalamic-pituitary axis or destruction of the neurohypophysis by surgery, irradiation, or head trauma.
ii. Suprasellar *craniopharyngioma* accounts for one fourth of cases in small children.
iii. In some cases, the cause cannot be found and they are called *idiopathic*.
Clinically, diabetes insipidus is characterised by excretion of a very large volume of dilute urine of low specific gravity (below 1.010), polyuria and polydipsia.

Q7. Comment on some salient common features of pituitary tumours.

The following are certain important facts about pituitary tumours:
i. Pituitary tumours account for 10–15% of clinically recognised intracranial tumours.
ii. The actual prevalence of these tumours is not known because many tumours remain clinically undetected. Autopsy studies show that 10–20% of adults have small, asymptomatic tumours, less than 10 mm in diameter.
iii. Tumours can occur at any age but most often they are diagnosed in the 35–60 years of age.
iv. Most tumours are sporadic; less than 5% are familial and linked to some hereditary syndromes like MEN1. Sporadic tumours are most often linked to mutations of genes that encode G protein in the cytoplasmic signaling pathways.
v. Most tumours are benign and classified as adenomas. Carcinomas account for 1% of all pituitary tumours. Metastases to the pituitary are uncommon.
vi. Adenomas are arbitrarily divided in two groups according to their size: microadenomas (<10 mm) and macroadenomas (>10 mm).
vii. Macroadenomas can protrude from the sella and compress the optic chiasm, causing *bitemporal hemianopsia*, i.e. loss of vision (anopsia) in the peripheral half (hemi) of visual field.
viii. Most clinically diagnosed tumours are hormonally active but they may be inactive in 20% cases. Such tumours are diagnosed due to their mass effect and compression of the pituitary and adjacent structure.
ix. Almost all tumours originate in the anterior lobe.
x. Tumours are best classified according to the hormones they produce; most adenomas produce only one hormone but 15% are plurihormonal **(Table 27.1)**.
xi. The most common hormonally active tumours are prolactinomas (25%).
xii. Newer molecular WHO classification of adenomas based on analysis of transcription factors has not yet been adequately tested in clinical practice.

TABLE 27.1 WHO classification (2017) of pituitary adenomas.

CONVENTIONAL ADENOMA TYPE	CLINICAL SYNDROME	MORPHOLOGIC VARIANT	HORMONE/OTHER IMMUNE MARKER
1. *Lactotroph adenoma (20–30%)*	Hypogonadism, galactorrhoea	Densely/sparsely granulated/ acidophil adenoma	PRL
2. *Somatotroph adenoma (5%)*	Acromegaly/gigantism	Densely/sparsely granulated adenoma	GH+PRL+α-subunits
3. *Mixed somatotroph-lactotroph adenoma (5%)*	Acromegaly, hypogonadism, galactorrhoea	Densely/sparsely granulated adenoma	Gh+PRL+α-subunits
4. *Thyrotroph adenoma (1%)*	Thyrotoxicosis	–	β-TSH+ α-subunits
5. *Corticotroph adenoma (10–15%)*	Cushing disease	Densely/sparsely granulated adenoma	ACTH
6. *Gonadotroph adenoma (10–15%)*	Inactive or hypogonadism	–	β-FSH, β-LH, α-subunits
7. *Null cell adenoma (20%)*	Pituitary failure	–	None
8. *Plurihormonal adenoma (15%)*	Mixed	PIT-1 positive adenoma	GH, PRL, β-TSH, α-subunits

(GH, growth hormone; PRL, prolactin; β-TSH, β-thyroid-stimulating hormone; LH, luteinising hormone; ACTH, adrenocorticotropic hormone; FSH, follicle stimulating hormone; PIT, pituitary).
Adapted from: Lopes MBS. The 2017 WHO classification of tumours of the pituitary gland: a summary. Acta Neuropathol. 2017;134:4,521–35.

Q8. What is craniopharyngioma? Comment briefly on its clinical and pathologic features.

Definition Craniopharyngioma is a benign suprasellar tumour originating from epithelial remnants of the Rathke pouch.

Clinical and pathologic features
i. It is a cystic tumour well-demarcated from adjacent structures.
ii. The cavity lined by squamous epithelium usually contains degenerated ghost squamous cells and viscous fluid resembling 'machinery oil'.
iii. *Microscopically*, the solid parts of the cyst resemble ameloblastoma and are composed of nests which have a centre composed of loosely arranged stellate cells, lined on the periphery by cuboidal or cylindrical cells.
iv. The tumour grows expansively compressing the hypothalamus and other parts of adjacent brain, or causing hypopituitarism or diabetes insipidus.
v. It may even invade locally or rupture and cause a foreign body giant cell reaction.
vi. Clinically, the tumour has 2 peaks of occurrence: one in childhood and another in adults past the 6th decade.
vii. Due to its location, it may be sometimes difficult to resect it completely without damaging the brain and the pituitary stalk.

ADRENAL GLAND

Q9. Write briefly on the main anatomic, histologic and physiologic features of the adrenal glands that are important for the understanding of its pathology.

Adrenal glands are paired organs located above each kidney in the retroperitoneal space. They consist of two parts: outer cortex and inner medulla.
I. **Adrenal cortex** is composed of three layers:
i. *Zona granulosa* the source of mineralocorticoids.
ii. *Zona fasciculata* constitutes 70% of the entire cortex, and is the predominant source of glucocorticoids.
iii. *Zona reticularis* is the inner-most layer and is the predominant source of androgens.
The secretion of glucocorticoids and adrenal androgens is under the control of pituitary ACTH. Release of aldosterone is independent of ACTH control and is largely regulated by serum levels of potassium and renin-angiotensin mechanism.

II. **Adrenal medulla** is a component of the dispersed neuroendocrine system derived from primitive neuroectoderm; the other component of this system being *paraganglia* distributed in the vagus nerve branches and visceral autonomic ganglia. Neuroendocrine cells forming the medulla secrete:
- *Catecholamines* (epinephrine and norepinephrine), and
- *Some polypeptide hormones* (calcitonin, somatostatin, vasoactive intestinal polypeptide or VIP).

Major metabolites of catecholamines that can be detected in *blood or urine* are:
i. metanephrine,
ii. nor-metanephrine,
iii. vanillylmandelic acid (VMA), and
iv. homovanillic acid (HVA).

Q10. Comment on Cushing syndrome (or chronic hypercortisolism) in brief.

Definition Cushing syndrome is caused by excessive production of cortisol of whatever cause.
Etiopathogenesis and pathology There are four major etiologic types of Cushing syndrome:
i. *Pituitary Cushing syndrome* Named also as Cushing disease in honour of the neurosurgeon who described it, pituitary disease is the cause of 60–70% of all cases of Cushing disease or syndrome.
a. Most often, it is caused by a pituitary microadenoma, and less often by a macroadenoma or corticotroph hyperplasia.
b. Adrenal shows diffuse or nodular cortical hyperplasia.
c. The blood contains high levels of ACTH and corticosteroids. In most cases, ACTH secretion can be suppressed by high dose dexamethasone.
ii. *Adrenal Cushing syndrome* It accounts for 20–25% cases of Cushing syndrome.
a. Mostly it is caused by adrenal cortical adenoma, less often by carcinoma or bilateral hyperplasia.
b. It is characterised by low serum ACTH and an absence of therapeutic response to administration of high doses of corticosteroids.
iii. *Ectopic Cushing syndrome* It accounts for 10–15% cases of Cushing syndrome.
a. It is caused by ACTH produced by non-endocrine tumours.
b. Most often, the tumour is small cell carcinoma of the lungs; less common causes are other lung cancers, malignant thymoma and pancreatic tumours.
iv. *Iatrogenic Cushing syndrome* It is encountered rarely and is usually related to prolonged therapy with corticosteroids for organ transplantation or autoimmune diseases. Exogenous corticosteroids cause bilateral atrophy of the adrenal cortex.

Clinical features Cushing syndrome most often occurs in the 20–40 years age group, and is three time more common in women than men. The severity of the syndrome varies considerably but in general most cases present with the following:
i. *Central or truncal obesity* contrasted with relatively thin arms and legs. 'Buffalo hump' forming over the upper back and shoulders and rounded oedematous 'moon face' are common.
ii. *Skeletal muscle wasting, atrophy of the skin* and subcutaneous tissue with formation of purple striae on the abdominal wall, and easy bruising are related to increased protein breakdown. Bones show signs of *osteoporosis*.
iii. *Arterial hypertension* related to retention of sodium and water is found in 80% of patients.
iv. Impaired glucose tolerance and *diabetes mellitus* are found in 20% cases.
v. *Amenorrhoea, hirsutism and infertility* are found in many women and are related to increased levels of adrenal androgens.
vi. *Mental and psychiatric symptoms*, including insomnia, depression and confusion are sometimes accompanied by overt psychosis.

Q11. What is Conn syndrome (or primary hyperaldosteronism)?

Definition Conn syndrome is a rare endocrine disease caused by overproduction of aldosterone, a potent salt-retaining steroid hormone.
Etiopathogenesis Three main causes are as follows:
i. Adrenocortical adenoma producing aldosterone (most common)
ii. Bilateral adrenal cortical hyperplasia, especially in children (congenital hyperaldosteronism)
iii. Adrenal cortical carcinoma (rare)

NOTE: Primary hyperaldosteronism must be distinguished from secondary hyperaldosteronism related to overproduction of renin in renal diseases, such as ischaemia, glomerulonephritis or renal cell carcinoma.

Clinical features Adult females are affected most often.
i. Hypertension, mild to moderate, mostly diastolic
ii. Hypernatraemia and water retention
iii. Hypokalaemia
iv. Polyuria and polydipsia due to reduced concentration power of renal tubules.

Q12. What is adrenogenital syndrome (adrenal virilism)?

Definition Adrenogenital syndrome is an endocrine disorder characterised by overproduction of adrenal androgens, that may occur in childhood or adulthood.
Etiopathogenesis
- *In infants and children*, it is due to congenital adrenal hyperplasia related to genetic mutations resulting in a deficiency of steroid metabolising enzymes.
- *In adults*, it may be due to adrenal cortical adenoma or carcinoma. The condition may be combined with Cushing syndrome.

Clinical features These depend on the age of the patient:
i. In female children, virilisation of external genital organs.
ii. In male children, precocious puberty.
iii. In adult females, signs of virilisation (amenorrhoea, hirsutism, deepening of the voice, hypertrophy of the clitoris).
iv. In adult males, excess of androgens may not produce any symptoms or there is feminisation in some patients.

Q13. What is adrenocortical insufficiency (hypoadrenalism)? Write briefly on its various types.

Definition Adrenocortical insufficiency is a very rare hormonal disorder characterised by a deficiency of adrenal corticosteroids. It may be acute or chronic, primary or secondary, and occurs in several clinicopathologic forms:
Primary adrenocortical insufficiency results from adrenal cortical diseases.
Secondary adrenocortical insufficiency results from diminished secretion of ACTH.

Clinicopathologic features Four clinicopathologic entities are recognised:
I. **Primary acute adrenocortical insufficiency (adrenal crisis)** Sudden loss of adrenocortical function results in adrenal crisis.
Etiopathogenesis It may be caused by the following conditions:
i. Bilateral adrenalectomy, e.g. surgical treatment of adrenal hyperfunction caused by bilateral hyperplasia, or adrenal hypertension.
ii. Septicaemia, e.g. in endotoxic shock and meningococcal infection producing gross visible haemorrhagic and *adrenal apoplexy* with acute adrenal cortical insufficiency. Clinically, this condition is called *Waterhouse-Friederichsen syndrome*.
iii. Rapid withdrawal of steroids given for some duration for certain autoimmune disease.
iv. Any form of acute stress in a case of chronic adrenal insufficiency, i.e. Addison disease.
Clinical features Symptoms of acute adrenocortical insufficiency result from deficiency of mineralocorticoids and glucocorticoids as follows:
i. *Aldosterone deficiency* results in hyperkalaemia, hyponatremia and dehydration.
ii. *Cortisol deficiency* results in hypoglycaemia, increased insulin sensitivity and vomiting.

II. **Primary chronic adrenocortical insufficiency (Addison disease)** Chronic insufficiency becomes clinically apparent when more than 90% of adrenal cortex bilaterally is destroyed.
Etiopathogenesis Following chronic processes destroying the adrenals bilaterally, may cause chronic insufficiency:
i. Autoimmune or idiopathic adrenalitis
ii. Chronic infections, such as tuberculosis, histoplasmosis
iii. Amyloidosis

iv. Sarcoidosis, haemochromatosis
v. Metastatic cancers, most often breast and lung cancer
Clinical features The symptoms develop slowly and insidiously and include:
i. Asthenia, i.e. progressive weakness, weight loss and lethargy.
ii. Hyperpigmentation, first on sun-exposed areas but later over the entire body including mucosae.
iii. Vague upper gastrointestinal symptoms such as loss of appetite, nausea, vomiting and upper abdominal pain.
iv. Arterial hypertension.
v. Loss of hair in women due to androgen deficiency.
vi. Episodes of hypoglycaemia.
Laboratory findings include:
i. Reduced GFR
ii. Metabolic acidosis with hyperkalaemia
iii. Low levels of sodium, chloride and bicarbonate
III. **Secondary adrenocortical insufficiency** results from deficiency of ACTH.
Etiopathogenesis ACTH deficiency can occur in two settings:
i. *Selective ACTH deficiency* due to prolonged administration of glucocorticoids which suppress the secretion of ACTH from the pituitary.
ii. *Panhypopituitarism* due to hypothalamic and pituitary diseases with deficiency of multiple trophic hormones.
Clinical features are similar to those of Addison disease except for:
i. Lack of skin pigmentation because of suppressed production of melanocyte-stimulating hormone (MSH) from the pituitary.
ii. Low serum ACTH levels, in contrast to Addison disease where serum ACTH is high.
iii. Aldosterone levels are normal, since aldosterone secretion is not under ACTH control.
IV. **Hypoaldosteronism** is marked by isolated deficiency of aldosterone with normal cortisol levels, typically associated with reduced renin secretion.

Q14. Discuss salient clinicopathologic features of common adrenocortical tumours.

Adrenal cortical tumours may be benign (adenoma) or malignant (carcinoma), hormonally active or non-secretory.
I. **Cortical adenoma** is the commonest adrenocortical tumour.
i. It presents usually as a solitary nodule measuring more than 2 cm, and thus differs from nodular hyperplasia which is multinodular composed of several small nodules.
ii. Most adenomas are non-functional and incidentally found at autopsy.
iii. Less often, larger adenomas are functional and secrete one of the steroid hormones, normally produced by cortical cells.
iv. Most cortical adenomas are sporadic but in some rare instance they may be part of the MEN-I.
v. *Grossly,* they are well demarcated from the normal cortex and yellow on cross section.
vi. *Microscopically,* they are composed of lipid rich cells resembling normal cortical adrenal cells.
II. **Cortical carcinoma** is a rare malignant tumour.
i. It is usually much larger than adenoma and irregularly shaped.
ii. On cross section, it has a variegated appearance, including areas that are yellow, red, gray, with foci of necrosis and haemorrhage.
iii. *Microscopically,* the tumour is composed of pleomorphic atypical cells and shows high mitotic activity.

Q15. Write briefly on salient features of pheochromocytoma.

Definition Pheochromocytoma is the most common medullary tumour; it is composed of pheochromocytes, i.e. chromaffin cells of the medulla, which owe their brown colour to the oxidation of catecholamines in their cytoplasm.
The traditional 10% rule can be applied to pheochromocytomas as follows:
i. 10% are familial, and all others are sporadic.

ii. 10% are multiple, and all others are solitary.
iii. 10% are malignant, and all others are benign.
iv. 10% are located outside of the adrenal, and all others originate from adrenals.
v. 10% are not associated with hypertension, and all others cause hypertension.

Pathology
i. Hereditary pheochromocytomas may be part of genetic tumour syndromes, including neurofibromatosis type I, multiple endocrine neoplasia (MEN) type II, and von Hippel-Lindau disease.
ii. *Grossly*, pheochromocytomas that are mostly benign tumours are well demarcated from the surrounding structures. On cross section, they appear brown, and often show foci of haemorrhage and necrosis.
iii. *Microscopically*, they are composed of polygonal cells arranged into nests (known as 'zellballen') surrounded by sustentacular cells and fibrovascular stroma **(Fig. 27.1)**. The nuclei are often pleomorphic.
iv. By *electron microscopy*, the tumour cells contain neuroendocrine granules and are positive for chromogranin.
v. The diagnosis of malignancy cannot be made on microscopic examination. The only definitive evidence that a tumour is malignant if it has metastases.

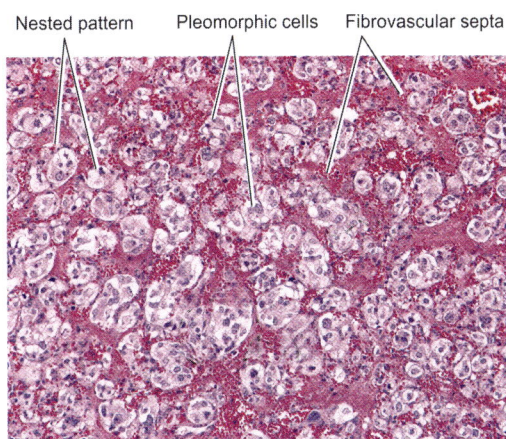

FIGURE 27.1: Pheochromocytoma. The tumour has typical zellballen or nested pattern. The tumour cells are large, polyhedral and pleomorphic having abundant granular cytoplasm.

Clinical features Symptoms and clinical findings are related to hypersecretion of catecholamines, both epinephrine and norepinephrine. Most patients are 20–60 years age group and present with following episodic attacks ('paroxysms'):
i. Hypertension: In 50% of cases marked by paroxysmal bouts of blood pressure elevation, whereas in others it is permanently elevated and mostly diastolic.
ii. Precordial chest pain (due to coronary artery spasms) and heart palpitations with tachycardia.
iii. Drenching sweats.
iv. Headaches, anxiety and nervousness.

Laboratory findings
i. Elevation of plasma metanephrine (best test because it shows least fluctuation and is not influenced by daily events), which may be also demonstrated in 24-hour urine collection.
ii. Other catecholamine metabolites such as vanillylmandelic acid (VMA) and homovanillic acid (HVA) are also elevated in 24-hour urine specimen.

Prognosis Untreated patients die of congestive heart failure with pulmonary oedema ('catecholamine cardiomyopathy'), or cerebral haemorrhage from hypertension.

Q16. What is neuroblastoma?

Definition Neuroblastoma, also known as sympathicoblatoma, is a malignant tumour composed of neuroblasts derived from neural crest colonising the foetal adrenal primordia. These neuroblasts are precursors of adrenal pheochomocytes and ganglionic cells, and other sympathetic paraganglia (which accounts for the fact that neuroblastomas can be found in extra-adrenal sites in other paraganglia as well).

Pathology *Grossly*, neuroblastoma appears like a large soft, lobulated mass infiltrating into adjacent structures. On cross sectioning, it appears greyish-white with extensive areas of haemorrhage and necrosis and microcalcifications, which are best seen by X-rays.
Microscopy
i. Neuroblastoma is composed of small cells with hyperchromatic round or oval nuclei and scant cytoplasm.
ii. Cells show abortive neural differentiation and form rosettes and Homer-Wright pseudorosettes, which are composed of a central eosinophilic area made up of neural cell extensions ('neuropil') surrounded by radially arranged tumour cells.
NOTE: Pathologists use the term rosette for cells radially arranged around an empty space. Since the structures in neuroblastomas contain neuropil, technically they are 'pseudorosettes'.

Clinical features
i. Neuroblastomas are childhood tumours and most of them are found in children younger than 4 years of age.
ii. Neuroblastoma is the most common extracranial solid tumour of infancy and childhood.
iii. Clinically, presents as a rapidly growing abdominal mass and widespread metastases, which are found in 2/3rd of all cases at the time of diagnosis.
iv. Most often, the metastases are found in the bones of the skull, but may involve other bones and internal organs and local lymph nodes.
v. VMA and HVA are found in 24-hour urine specimen in 90% of cases; higher levels of catecholamines parallel more differentiated components and predict a better prognosis.

Prognosis of neuroblastoma depends upon a few variables:
- Stage 1 tumours are curable in 90% of cases.
- Those in stage 4 are curable in less than 5%.
- Most tumours are diagnosed in stage 3 and 4; thus the overall 5-year survival is 40%.
- It is important to remember that some neuroblastomas in infants and young children may regress spontaneously or may be differentiated into ganglioneuromas.
- Also, extra-adrenal neuroblastomas have a better prognosis than adrenal tumours.

Favorable prognostic features for adrenal neuroblastomas are:
i. Age under 18 months.
ii. Stage 1 (limited to the organ), stage 2 (beyond the confines of adrenal but not crossing the midline) and stage 4S (S = special is used for tumour in children under the age of 1 year who have small 1 or 2 stage tumours with metastases limited to the skin, liver and/or bone marrow).
iii. Histologic evidence of neural or schwann-cell differentiation and more cells showing karyorrhexis than mitosis.
iv. Hyperdiploidy with chromosome gain, whereas near-diploidy with partial chromosome loss is an adverse finding.
v. Chromosomal findings: no loss of chromosomes 1 p and 11q.
vi. Molecular biology findings: lack of amplification of *NMYC* oncogene.

Q17. What is ganglioneuroma?

Definition Ganglioneuroma is a benign tumour composed of ganglion cells, unmyelinated and myelinated nerve fibers and Schwann cells.
Clinicopathologic features
i. It originates from ganglia in the posterior mediastinum and retroperitoneum, and less often in other sites, including the brain.
ii. Tumour produces symptoms due to its size and mass effect.
iii. Catecholamines and their metabolites are typically found in the 24-hour urine specimen.

Q18. What is paraganglioma?

Definition Paraganglioma (also known as chemodectoma) is an uncommon tumour originating from paraganglia such as carotid bodies, vagus, jugulotympanic and aorticosympathetic (pre-aortic) paraganglia.

Clinicopathologic features
i. Paragangliomas are small well-encapsulated tumours.
ii. *Microscopically*, they resemble pheochromocytomas.
iii. Most of them are benign and sporadic and do not secrete anything, but some may be malignant, familial and produce small amounts of catecholamines.

THYROID GLAND

Q19. Describe the salient anatomic, histologic and physiologic features of the thyroid that are important for understanding its pathology.

Anatomy Thyroid is bilobed gland located on the anterior side of the neck.
i. It develops from the midline invagination at the base of the foetal tongue which forms the thyroglossal duct facilitating the descent of the thyroid into its normal position.
ii. The thyroglossal duct involutes thereafter, but some remnants of it may occasionally persist and form *thyroglossal cysts* on the anterior neck all the way to the base of the tongue.
iii. In these locations, one may also find anomalous *aberrant thyroid glands*.

Histology
i. Thyroid is composed of follicles filled with colloid.
ii. Follicles are lined by cuboidal epithelium which secretes thyroid hormones and participates in the metabolism.
iii. Dispersed among these follicular cells are C-cells secreting calcitonin.
iv. The stroma between the follicles contains vessels, lymphatics and nerves.

Physiology
i. Thyroid secretes two iodine containing hormones: thyroxine (T_4) and triiodothyronine (T_3).
ii. The secretion of T_4 and T_3 is regulated by thyroid stimulating hormone (TSH) produced by the pituitary, which in turn depends on the hypothalamic thyrotropin releasing hormone (TRH). T_4 and T_3 inhibit TSH secretion.
iii. Thyroid hormones affect most organs by stimulating the intermediary metabolism of proteins, carbohydrates and lipids.
iv. Calcitonin participates in the maintenance of metabolism of calcium and phosphorus.
v. *Laboratory tests*, sometimes combined with radiologic techniques, are used to assess the function of thyroid in clinical settings. With these tests, one can measure the serum concentration of T_4, T_3, TSH and TRH and calcitonin and the rate of thyroglobulin secretion, uptake of radioactive iodine, and various thyroid disease-related antibodies.
vi. The most widely used radiologic ancillary method is radioactive iodine uptake (RAIU) scan.

Q20. Write briefly on hyperthyroidism (thyrotoxicosis).

Definition Hyperthyroidism (thyrotoxicosis) is a hypermetabolic clinical and biochemical state caused by excessive production of thyroid hormones; generally $T_3 > T_4$.

Etiopathogenesis Hyperthyroidism may be caused by many diseases but three most common causes are:
i. Graves disease (diffuse toxic goitre)
ii. Toxic multinodular goitre
iii. Toxic adenoma

Less frequent causes are hypersecretion of pituitary TSH, thyroiditis, metastatic tumours of the thyroid, struma ovarii, and lastly by excessive doses of thyroid hormones or iodine (called in German 'Jod-Basedow phenomenon').

Clinical features The disease has a slow and insidious onset and varies in severity from one case to another. Common feature include the following:
i. *Increased basic metabolic rate* Most physiologic body functions are upregulated and require more energy, which results in weight loss despite normal appetite.
ii. *Skin changes* The skin is warm, flushed due to peripheral vascular dilatation and sweating, aimed at reducing the body temperature. Yet, the patients typically complain of heat intolerance.

Some patients develop pretibial oedema due to the accumulation of glycosaminoglycans and fluid.

iii. *Cardiovascular problems* These are common and include tachycardia, palpitations, and arrhythmias. The cardiac output is increased to meet the increased peripheral oxygen demand. Cardiomegaly and heart failure may develop in untreated patients, especially in the elderly.

iv. *Sympathetic autonomous nervous system over-reactivity* There is easy excitability, anxiety and insomnia. Fine tremor is best seen on outstretched hands. Intestinal hypermotility results in frequent bowel movements and diarrhoea. Perspiration is also related, in part, to sympathetic stimuli.

v. *Eye changes* Bulging eyes (exophthalmos) and wide eyes with staring gaze are typical.

vi. *Musculoskeletal symptoms* Weakness of the muscle and easy fatigability are common. Bones show osteoporosis.

vii. *Menstrual irregularities and oligomenorrhea.*

viii. *'Thyroid storm'* or *'thyroid crisis'* is an emergency situation that develops in hyperthyroid patients who have undergone thyroidectomy before adequate control of thyroid functions. It may also develop in those who have suffered trauma, shock or massive infection. It presents with high-grade fever, marked tachycardia and arrhythmias and may experience heart failure and fall into coma with a lethal outcome.

Laboratory findings

i. High T_4 and T_3 and low TSH.
ii. Graves disease patients have antibodies to TSH receptor.
iii. Radioactive iodine uptake studies are used to determine if the disease is caused by diffuse hyperplasia, nodular goitre or toxic adenoma.

Q21. What is hypothyroidism?

Definition Hypothyroidism is a hypometabolic state resulting from inadequate production of thyroid hormones for prolonged period, or rarely, from resistance of the peripheral tissue to the effects of thyroid hormones. Clinical presentation depends on the age of the patient and includes two clinicopathologic entities:
i. Cretinism or congenital hypothyroidism of infancy and childhood
ii. Myxoedema, the hypothyroidism of adulthood

Q22. What is cretinism?

Definition Cretinism is severe hypothyroidism present at birth or developing within first two years of postnatal life. It may be sporadic (individual cases) or endemic affecting larger populations.

Etiopathogenesis The causes of hypothyroidism in infants and children are as follows:
i. *Developmental anomalies*, such as thyroid agenesis or dysgenesis.
ii. *Genetic defects* in thyroid hormone synthesis, e.g. defects in iodine trapping, oxidation, iodination of proteins, coupling and thyroglobulin synthesis.
iii. *Foetal exposure* to iodine and antithyroid drugs.
iv. *Endemic cretinism* due to dietary lack of iodine, still present in some mountainous parts of the world (e.g. Andes or Himalayas).

Clinical features Typically, symptoms appear within weeks or month after birth and include:
i. Failure to thrive
ii. Poor feeding and constipation
iii. Dry scaly skin
iv. Hoarse cry
v. Bradycardia

As the child grows, the full picture of cretinism emerges that includes:
a. Impaired skeletal growth resulting in dwarfism.
b. Facial features such as round face, narrow forehead, widely set eyes, flat and broad nose protruding tongue.
c. Protuberant abdomen.
d. Mental retardation and sensory-neurological defects (more prominent in sporadic than in endemic cases).

Q23. What is myxoedema? Briefly discuss its etiopathogenesis and clinical features.

Definition Myxoedema is a synonym for hypothyroidism in adults.

Etiopathogenesis Several possible causes for hypothyroidism are listed below (the first two are the most commonly encountered):

i. Autoimmune thyroiditis (Hashimoto disease), most common
ii. Ablation of thyroid by surgery or irradiation
iii. Endemic or sporadic goitre
iv. Hypothalamic-pituitary lesions
v. Thyroid cancer
vi. Prolonged administration of antithyroid drugs
vii. Mild developmental anomalies and dyshormonogenesis

Clinical features Most symptoms and clinical findings reflect slowing down of all metabolic processes. Symptoms of hypothyroidism develop slowly and become usually apparent many years after the onset of the underlying disease, which in most instances is an autoimmune thyroiditis.

i. *Decreased metabolic rate* affecting most organs, but especially those that require a lot of energy like nerve cells and various muscle cells (skeletal, cardiac and smooth muscles).

ii. *Neuropsychiatric changes* Lethargy and slowing-down of intellectual activities, resulting in mental sluggishness, reduced perceptiveness, slow speech. Overt psychosis ('myxoedema madness') is rarely seen in current times.

iii. *Slowing of physical activities* Thyroid hormone deficiency will often cause skeletal muscle weakness which slows down body movements. Prolongation of the relaxation phase of deep tendon reflexes is an important diagnostic finding. Slow movement of intestines results in constipation.

iv. *Cold intolerance and weight gain* due to reduced metabolism are common complaints.

v. *Skin changes* There is generalised non-pitting, doughy oedema ('myxoedema'), most prominent on the face ('puffy face'). The skin is pale and cold. Loss of hair all over the body but most prominently on the eyebrows and scalp.

vi. *Cardiovascular changes* The contractility of the heart is weakened and congestive heart failure may develop. There is prominent bradycardia. It is aggravated by increased incidence of coronary atherosclerosis caused by hyperlipidaemia and hypercholesterolaemia.

vii. *Pleural and pericardial effusions* These effusions are in part due to generalised oedema and partially due to heart failure.

viii. *Anaemia* It is usually normochromic normocytic, due to reduced erythropoiesis.

ix. *Menstrual irregularities* and infertility in women and impotence in men.

Laboratory findings include:

i. Low T_4 and T_3 and high TSH in serum.
ii. In autoimmune thyroiditis, there are antibodies to various components of thyroid follicular cells.

Q24. What is thyroiditis and what are its types?

Definition Thyroiditis is inflammation of the thyroid, that may be caused by infection or autoimmune mechanisms.

Classification On the basis of onset and duration of the disease, various forms of thyroiditis can be classified into three groups:

I. ***Acute thyroiditis***
i. Bacterial infections
ii. Fungal infections
iii. Radiation injury

II. ***Subacute thyroiditis***
i. Subacute granulomatous (de Quervain)
ii. Subacute lymphocytic (postpartum, silent)
iii. Tuberculous

III. ***Chronic thyroiditis***
i. Autoimmune (Hashimoto or chronic lymphocytic thyroiditis)
ii. Riedel thyroiditis (or invasive fibrous thyroiditis)

Q25. What is Hashimoto thyroiditis?

Definition Hashimoto thyroiditis is a common autoimmune chronic inflammation of the thyroid, typically presenting with goitre and resulting in hypothyroidism.

Etiopathogenesis The autoimmune nature of Hashimoto thyroiditis is evident from the following facts:

i. *Association with other autoimmune diseases* such as Graves disease, SLE, Sjögren syndrome, pernicious anaemia, etc.

ii. *Immune destruction of thyroid cells* related to activation of T cells. Both CD8+ directly cytotoxic cells, and CD4+ T helper cells which secrete cytokines, participate in this process. Increased susceptibility to Hashimoto disease has been associated with polymorphism of HLA-DR3, and two T cell regulatory genes (*CTLA-4, PTPN22*).

iii. *Autoantibodies* probably play a minor role in the destruction of thyroid cell but are important for the diagnosis of Hashimoto disease. Antibodies to thyroid cell components include the following:
a. Anti-microsomal antibodies
b. Anti-thyroid peroxidase antibodies (anti-TPO), which are most often used in clinical practice.
c. Anti-thyroglobulin antibodies
d. Anti-TSH receptor antibodies are similar to those that stimulate TSH receptors in Graves disease, accounting for the fact that patients with Hashimoto disease may have alternate episode of hypo- or hyperthyroidism.
e. Less common antibodies, such as those against follicular cell membranes, or thyroid hormones.

Pathology *Grossly,* two forms of Hashimoto disease are seen:
- *Classical form* resulting in goitre accounts for 90% of cases. In this form, the thyroid is diffusely enlarged, firm and rubbery. On cross section, it shows accentuation of the normal lobulation.
- *Fibrosing* Hashimoto disease in which there is extensive fibrosis resulting in thyroid atrophy.

Microscopy
i. Extensive infiltration of the gland with lymphocytes, focally forming lymphoid follicles with germinal centres **(Fig. 27.2)**.
ii. There is atrophy and loss of thyroid follicles.
iii. Those that are not atrophic are lined by oncocytes (Hűrthle cells) which have abundant eosinophilic cytoplasm filled with mitochondria.
iv. There is also interstitial fibrosis, which is much more prominent in the fibrosing form of Hashimoto disease.

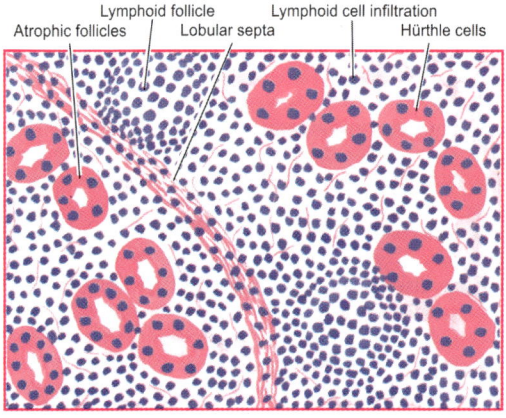

FIGURE 27.2: Hashimoto thyroiditis. Histologic features include: lymphoid cell infiltration with formation of lymphoid follicles having germinal centres; small, atrophic and colloid-deficient follicles; presence of Hurthle cells which have abundant eosinophilic cytoplasm and vesicular nuclei.

Clinical features
i. Hashimoto disease is the most common cause of hypothyroidism. Estimates show that it affects 2–3% of all adult women, but the true prevalence cannot be determined because it remains subclinical and unrecognised for long time.
ii. It is 10–20 times more common in women than men.
iii. Clinically, it is usually diagnosed in middle-aged women but it may occur at any age including childhood.

iv. It is the most common cause of hypothyroidism in children.
v. A variant of Hashimoto disease occurs 3–6 month after delivery and is known as *postpartum thyroiditis*, which tends to heal on its own during the next few months.
vi. Some patients develop hyperthyroidism, called '*hashitoxicosis*', further substantiating the similarities between Hashimoto thyroiditis and Graves disease.
vii. *Laboratory findings* include low serum T_4 and T_3 and high TSH, and reduced radioactive iodine uptake. Antibodies to thyroid cell components support the diagnosis.
viii. Patients with Hashimoto disease tend to develop other autoimmune diseases, notably autoimmune gastritis and type I diabetes mellitus.
ix. They are also at risk for developing thyroid extranodal marginal cell lymphoma (MALToma).
x. Similar to patients with Graves disease, they are also at increased risk for thyroid cancer.

Q26. What is subacute granulomatous (de Quervain) disease?

Definition Subacute granulomatous (de Quervain) disease is self-limited inflammation of the thyroid characterised by formation of granulomas with multinucleated giant cells.
Etiopathogenesis The disease typically follows an acute viral disease suggesting that the viral injury of follicular cells could be the primary lesion, which is followed with acute inflammation and formation of abscesses, soon to be replaced by granulomas.
Pathology
i. Acute inflammation with microabscess formation is seen in early stages of the disease.
ii. It is followed by formation of granulomas around extravasated colloid. Granulomas comprise prominent multinucleated giant cells.
iii. The disease has a self-limited course and the granulomas disappear after 6 months.
Clinical features
i. The disease presents with sudden painful enlargement of the thyroid, usually following an upper respiratory tract infection.
ii. Disruption of thyroid follicles results in a sudden release of thyroid hormones with clinical signs of hyperthyroidism.
iii. However, in cases marked by massive destruction of follicles, this is followed within weeks by signs of hypothyroidism.

Q27. What is Riedel thyroiditis?

Definition Riedel thyroiditis is a chronic disease of unknown etiology characterised by extensive fibrosis replacing thyroid follicles and extending into the neck beyond the confines of the thyroid.
Etiopathogenesis Unknown.
i. It seems that Riedel thyroiditis could be associated with multifocal fibrosclerosis including idiopathic mediastinal, retroperitoneal or retroorbital fibrosis, and primary sclerosing cholangitis and chronic fibrosing pancreatitis. These diseases may appear coincidentally in the same patient affected by Riedel's thyroiditis.
ii. In some of these patients, serum contains high amounts of IgG4; in these cases, Riedel thyroiditis is part of the systemic fibrosing IgG4 disease.
Pathology
i. The thyroid is small, fibrotic and firmly attached to adjacent organs.
ii. *Microscopically*, there is extensive fibrosis replacing the thyroid follicles and extending into other neck organs and tissue.
iii. Fibrous tissue contains foci of lymphocytes and plasma cells some of which may contain IgG4.
Clinical features
i. Riedel thyroiditis presents with signs of hypothyroidism which are often overshadowed by the fibrosing changes on the neck.
ii. Neck fibrosis may cause dysphagia, dyspnoea, stridor and paralysis of the recurrent laryngeal nerve.
iii. IgG4-related disease may respond favorably to corticosteroid treatment.

Q28. What is Graves disease?

Definition Graves disease is an autoimmune thyroid disease of unknown etiology characterised by:
i. hyperthyroidism,
ii. diffuse thyroid enlargement, and
iii. ophthalmopathy.

Etiopathogenesis Graves disease is an autoimmune disease that has many similarities to Hashimoto thyroiditis. Susceptibility to Graves disease has several genetic and environmental aspects similar to those seen in Hashimoto disease as under:

i. *Genetic association* is evident by the predominance of the disease in some families. Hereditary susceptibility has been associated with polymorphism of HLA-DR3, and two T cell regulatory genes (CTLA-4, PTPN22), in a manner similar to Hashimoto disease. These two thyroid diseases may coexist in the same affected families and even in the same individual patients.

ii. *Association with other autoimmune disease* is similar to that of Hashimoto disease.

iii. *Non-immune factors* influencing the onset of Graves disease are also similar to those influencing the development of Hashimoto disease:
a. It shows a higher incidence in women (7 to 10 times higher than in men).
b. Emotional stress and smoking are major contributory factors.

iv. *Autoantibodies* are present in both Graves disease and Hashimoto thyroiditis, albeit the antibodies have different effects:
a. *Thyroid stimulatory immunoglobulin (TSI)*: binds to TSH receptor stimulating the follicular cells to release thyroid hormones.
b. *Thyroid growth stimulating immunoglobulin (TGI)*: stimulates the proliferation of follicular cells.
c. *TSH-binding inhibitor immunoglobulin (TBII)*: prevents binding of TSH to its own receptor. It may cause alternate episodes of hypo- and hyperthyroidism.
d. *Antibodies to muscle antigens*: found in Graves disease but not in Hashimoto thyroiditis cause exophthalmus in Graves disease. These antibodies cross-react with microsomal antigen in follicular cells.

Pathology Grossly, the thyroid is diffusely enlarged and on cross sectioning appears homogenously brown and meaty, lacking its normal lucency due to a reduced amount of colloid in the follicles.
Microscopy
i. Marked hyperplasia and hypertrophy of follicular cells which appear tall cylindrical and form papillary infoldings protruding into the lumens of the follicles.
ii. Diminished amount of colloid that appears watery and thus paler; it shows typical pericellular vacuolisation (due to increased resorption by the follicular cells).
iii. Congested blood vessels and focal aggregates of lymphocytes in the stroma.
iv. Preoperative treatment of patients with iodine promotes accumulation of colloid in the follicles, reducing the congestion of stromal blood vessels.

Clinical features
i. The patients have prominent signs and symptoms of hyperthyroidism, as listed earlier.
ii. Laboratory findings include high serum levels of T_4 and T_3 and low TSH.
iii. Antibodies listed above can be demonstrated in serum.
iv. Additional findings are:
a. *Enlarged thyroid* which may be seen pulsating on the neck. It is warm to palpation due to active hyperaemia.
b. *Ophthalmopathy* which presents with exophthalmos accompanied by a lid lag, upper lid retraction, staring gaze, proptosis and weakness of ocular muscles.
c. *Dermatopathy* which includes often pretibial myxoedema in form of indurated non-pitting plaques.
v. Patients with Graves disease are at increased risk for developing thyroid cancer.

Q29. What is goitre? Briefly describe its etiology, pathogenesis and clinicopathologic features.

Definition Goitre is enlargement of the thyroid caused by compensatory hyperplasia and hypertrophy of follicular epithelium in response to a deficiency of thyroid hormones.

Etiology Epidemiologically, two forms of goitre are recognised: endemic and non-endemic.
I. *Endemic goitre* A goitre is labeled as endemic if found in more than 10% of a population in a defined geographic area. Endemic goitre was documented in mountainous areas in which the drinking

water and food do not contain enough *iodine*, such as Himalayas, Andes and Alps. Prophylactic supplementation of iodine in drinking water has solved this public health problem in most parts of the world. Some cases, unrelated to iodine deficiency, have been traced to the *dietary goitrogens* found in vegetables such as cabbage, cauliflower, turnips, cassava roots.

II. Sporadic (non-endemic) goitre The etiology of this goitre is unknown in most cases. Its possible causes include:
i. Suboptimal iodine intake during periods of increased demand, e.g. puberty or pregnancy.
ii. Dietary goitrogens.
iii. Genetic and hereditary factors affecting the synthesis and transport of thyroid hormones (*dyshormonogenesis*), or iodine metabolism.

Pathogenesis
i. *Inadequate production of thyroid hormones* (e.g. in chronic iodine deficiency or due to the action of some alimentary goitrogens) stimulates the pituitary to produce more TSH, which in turn promotes proliferation of follicular cells and stimulates them to produce more hormones (Fig. 27.3).
ii. This initial *simple goitre* is reversible, but if the demand persists, repeated cycles of cell proliferation and incomplete involution, combined with secondary changes such as cystic degeneration or fibrosis, may produce a *nodular goitre*.

The best example of simple goitre is enlargement of the thyroid in puberty, which usually reverts to normal size, but in some women it may progress to nodular goitre. The patients remain euthyroid and serum values for T_4 and T_3 are within normal limits. The serum level of TSH is, however, elevated.

Pathology Two types of goitre are recognised morphologically: simple and nodular.
I. **Simple goitre** is characterised by symmetric and diffuse enlargement of the entire thyroid which weighs 3–5 times more than the normal gland. The follicles are of two kinds:
i. *Hyperplastic follicles* lined by tall cuboidal or cylindrical epithelium, occasionally forming papillary protrusions.
ii. *Involutional follicles* which are expanded by colloid and lined by low cuboidal or flattened epithelium.
II. **Nodular goitre** on *clinical and gross appearance* shows more prominent enlargement and prominent nodularity. The nodules vary in size and consistency: some are small and some very large, some solid and composed of tissue reminiscent of normal thyroid tissue, and some cystic or soft and composed mostly of colloid **(Fig. 27.4)**. In contrast to thyroid adenomas, these nodules do not have a capsule that would surround them from all sides. The tissue in between the nodules shows often secondary changes such as fibrosis, haemorrhage, and calcification.

Microscopy
i. The nodules contain follicles that vary in size and shape and are lined by cuboidal or flattened epithelium.

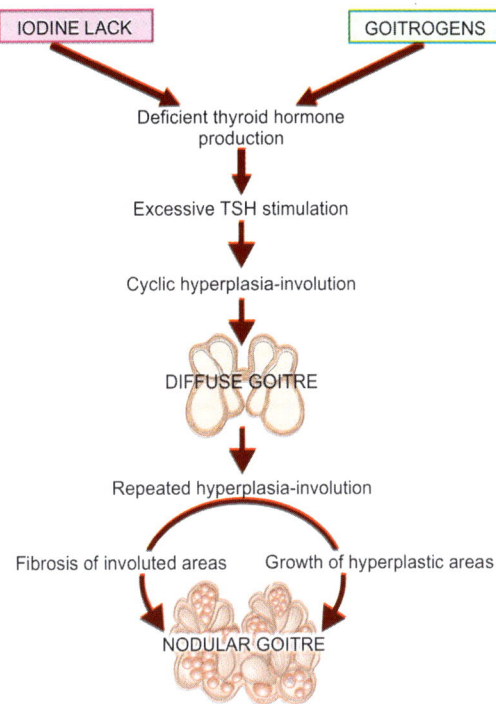

FIGURE 27.3: Pathogenesis of simple and nodular goitre.

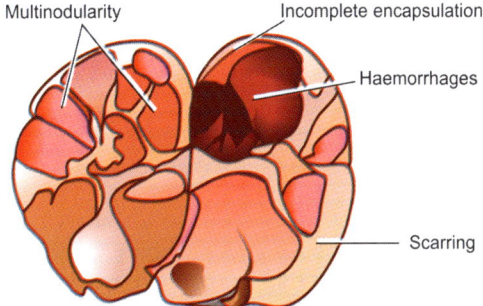

FIGURE 27.4: Nodular goitre. The thyroid gland is enlarged and nodular. Cut surface shows multiple nodules separated from each other by incomplete fibrous septa. Areas of haemorrhage and cystic change are also seen.

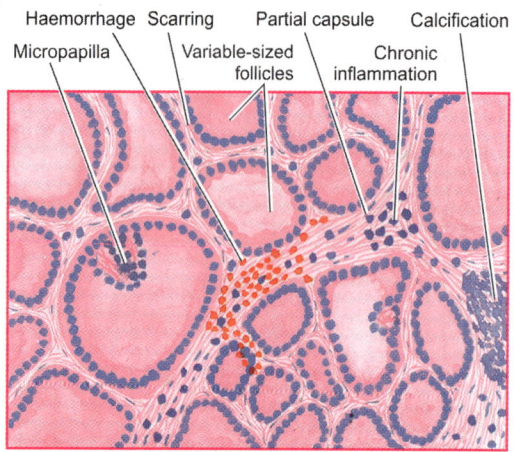

FIGURE 27.5: Nodular goitre. The predominant histologic features are: extensive scarring with foci of calcification, areas of haemorrhages and variable-sized follicles lined by flat to high epithelium and containing abundant colloid.

ii. Some follicles are distended by colloid whereas others are small and contain very little colloid.
iii. Secondary changes corresponding to those seen on gross examination are seen **(Fig. 27.5)**.
iv. In about 10% of nodular goitres, there is a '*dominant nodule*' showing microscopic hypercellularity. These nodules may be difficult to distinguish from adenomas, which usually have a fibrous capsule entirely surrounding them. A small minority of dominant nodules (2–3%) are malignant. Like adenomas, they usually have a capsule, but also show microscopic signs of capsular invasion.

Q30. How do you classify thyroid tumours? Comment on their salient general features.

Thyroid tumours are monoclonal neoplasms, mostly originating from either follicular or C-cells. Certain general and common features of thyroid tumours are as follows:
i. They are clinically classified as either benign or malignant. Benign thyroid tumours (mainly adenomas) account for most neoplasms; malignant tumours (carcinomas) are less common. WHO experts have added a third groups, called borderline tumours, which are however quite rare and will not be discussed here.
ii. Like all other thyroid diseases, thyroid tumours are twice more common in women than in men.
iii. Most tumours are sporadic but some occur as part of neoplastic syndromes and may be familial, most notably seen in patients with carcinomas of C-cells.
iv. Tumours may originate in a normal thyroid or in goitres. Tumour originating in nodular goitre must be distinguished from so called non-neoplastic 'dominant nodules'.
v. Of all the thyroid nodules identified clinically, approximately 90% are non-neoplastic, 10% benign adenomas, and 1% carcinomas.
vi. Tumours may be hormonally active or inactive, and thus present on radioactive iodine uptake scans as either hot or cold nodules.
vii. Malignant tumours may be low-grade or high-grade neoplasms. The most important malignant tumours are papillary carcinoma (80–90%), follicular carcinoma (10%), medullary carcinoma (5%), and anaplastic carcinoma (<5%).

Q31. Discuss pathologic and clinical features of follicular adenomas.

Definition Follicular adenomas are common benign thyroid tumours composed of follicular cells. They are found in 1% of the adult population, and are more common in women than men.
Pathology
i. Adenoma usually presents as a solitary nodule that may develop in a normal thyroid or on a background of nodular goitre. Typically, adenomas have a thick fibrous capsule.
ii. The tumour is composed of uniform follicular cells forming follicles that contain colloid.
iii. Several *histologic subtypes* can be recognised (e.g. normofollicular, macrofollicular, solid, and Hűrthle cell type), but such subclassification is of no practical clinical value.
iv. Secondary changes such as fibrosis or degeneration with calcification are common.

Clinical features
i. Most follicular adenomas present as small nodules, measuring less than 3 cm in diameter.
ii. They are usually asymptomatic and discovered incidentally during a physical examination, which is followed by fine needle aspiration of the lesion for diagnosis.
iii. Larger nodules may cause compression of the normal thyroid and even adjacent structures of the neck.
iv. On RAIU, they are mostly cold but some may be hormonally active. Such tumours show mutations of the gene for the TSH receptor or its α-subunit G_s (*GNAS*), which makes them hormonally active independent of TSH stimulation.
v. Malignant transformation of follicular adenomas is exceptionally rare, even though some 20% of follicular adenomas carry mutations of RAS oncogene or some kinases of the signaling pathways that are active in follicular carcinomas.

Q32. What is thyroid cancer? Tabulate contrasting features of its major types.

- Thyroid cancers are malignant tumours originating from either follicular or C-cells.
- The most important tumours are papillary, follicular, anaplastic and medullary carcinoma. Their salient contrasting features are summed up in **Table 27.2**.
- Lymphomas, most of which arise on the background of autoimmune thyroiditis, and sarcomas, are rare thyroid cancers.

TABLE 27.2 Contrasting features of main histologic types of thyroid carcinoma.

FEATURE	PAPILLARY CARCINOMA	FOLLICULAR CARCINOMA	MEDULLARY CARCINOMA	ANAPLASTIC CARCINOMA
1. Frequency	80–90%	5–10%	5%	1–2%
2. Age	All ages	Middle to old age	Middle to old age; familial too	Old age
3. Female/male ratio	3:1	2.5:1	1:1	1.5:1
4. Relation to radiation	Maximum	Present	None	Present
5. Genetic alterations	*RET* and *TRK-1* gene rearrangement, *BRAF* and *PTEN* point mutation, *TERT* promoter mutation	*RAS* point mutation, *PAX-PPAR γ1* fusion, *TERT* promoter mutation	*RET* point mutation	Additional mutations: *p53* loss, β-catenin mutation, *p21* overexpression, LOH
6. Cell of origin	Follicular	Follicular	Parafollicular	Follicular
7. Gross	Small, multifocal	Moderate size, nodular	Moderate size	Invasive growth
8. Pathognomonic microscopy	Nuclear features, papillary pattern	Vascular and capsular invasion	Solid nests, amyloid stroma	Undifferentiated, spindle-shaped, giant cells
9. Regional metastases	Common	Rare	Common	Common
10. Distant metastases	Rare	Common	Rare	Common
11. 10-year survival	80–95%	50–70%	60–70%	5–10% (median survival about 2 months)

(PTEN, phosphatase and tensin homologue; TERT, telomerase reverse transcriptase; LOH, loss of heterozygosity)

Q33. Briefly discuss etiopathogenesis and clinicopathologic features of papillary carcinoma of the thyroid.

Definition Papillary thyroid carcinoma (PTC) is the most common thyroid malignant tumour, accounting for 80–90% of all cases. It is mostly a low-grade malignancy that can occur at any age, but is most often seen in the 25 to 50 years age group. It is found 3 times more frequently in women than in men.

Etiopathogenesis PTC develops due to the interaction of exogenous and endogenous genetic factors as follows:

i. *External irradiation* as observed by a high incidence rate of PTC in persons exposed to therapeutic radiation in childhood, survivors of the atomic bomb explosion in Japan, and nuclear plant disaster in Ukraine.

ii. *Iodine excess* as noticed in persons with endemic goitre due to iodine deficiency who were treated with iodine and then developed PTC at a high rate.

iii. *Genetic basis* as evidenced by a 4–10 times higher risk of PTC in close relatives of PTC patients. The underlying gene has not been identified. PTC also occurs in families with familial adenomatous polyposis coli.

iv. *Somatic mutations* as seen by the common presence of mutations of certain genes in PTC; the most important ones are as under:

a. *RET* gene, and the receptor kinase that it encodes, are not normally expressed on thyroid cells, but show gain-of-function mutations in 30% of PTC. By fusing with genes from tumour cells into a hybrid gene called RET/PTC, RET comes under the control of genes expressed in thyroid cells and external influence, such as irradiation.

b. *BRAF* point mutations are found in up to 70% of PTC, affecting the MAP kinase signaling pathway. BRAF mutations are found in some classic PTC and microscopic types of PTC which have a poor prognosis, such as tall cell variant. This suggests that some BRAF mutations could be markers of poor prognosis.

Pathology

Clinical and gross appearance

i. Tumour usually presents as a solitary small nodule (2–3 cm) in the thyroid, but some tumours may be quite large and measure up to 10 cm in diameter.

ii. They may be partially cystic and are usually poorly demarcated from normal parenchyma.

iii. Metastases to the local lymph nodes on the neck are common, but the distant haematogenous metastases are rare.

iv. Metastases causing enlargement of the neck lymph nodes, or sometimes presenting a 'lateral aberrant thyroid' composed of cells forming thyroid follicles, may be the first clinical finding, leading to subsequent discovery of the primary tumour in the thyroid.

Microscopy

i. Tumours are composed of cuboidal cells lining papillae with fibrovascular cores which often contain calcifications in form of *psammoma bodies* **(Fig. 27.6)**.

ii. Tumour cells may also form follicles and solid nests, and if these predominate the tumour is designated as *follicular variant* of papillary carcinoma.

iii. *Microscopic foci* of PTC may be found in the parenchyma around the tumour in a significant number of cases, justifying a radical approach to treatment (lobectomy), in order to remove all malignant tissues. However, these findings do not adversely affect the prognosis.

iv. *Cytologic features* of PTC are diagnostic of this tumour. These features include:

a. Finely dispersed chromatin (described as optically clear or ground-glass appearance), or intranuclear inclusions of the cytoplasm, hence called 'nuclear pseudoinclusions'.

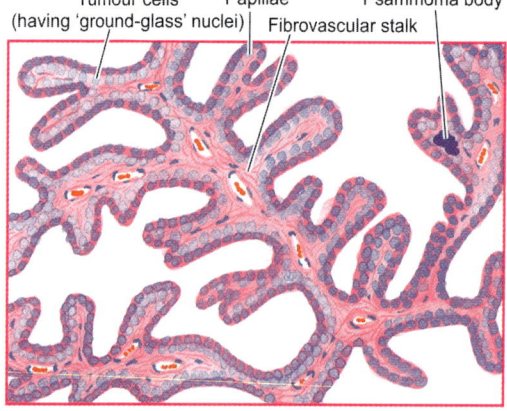

FIGURE 27.6: Papillary thyroid carcinoma. Microscopy shows branching papillae having fibrovascular stalk covered by a single layer of cuboidal cells having ground-glass nuclei. Colloid-filled follicles and solid sheets of tumour cells are also present.

b. Many cells have a cleaved coffee-bean shaped appearance, due to narrow invaginations of the cytoplasm almost splitting the nucleus in half. Cleaved nuclei show overlapping with nuclei of adjacent tumour cells due to reduced amount of tumour cell cytoplasm separating one nucleus from another.

Variants of PTC In addition to the classical PTC, there are several variants that are important clinically. These variants include:

i. *Microcarcinoma* (<1 cm, not requiring further treatment).
ii. *Follicular variant* that should not be confused with follicular carcinoma.
iii. *Tall cell, columnar and diffuse sclerosis* type, which have a worse prognosis.
iv. Noninvasive encapsulated follicular variant of PTC, which almost never metastasises and has excellent prognosis has been newly reclassified as the *noninvasive follicular thyroid neoplasm with papillary-like nuclear feature (NIFTP)*. NIFTP accounts for 10% of solitary thyroid nodules.

Prognosis Papillary carcinoma has an overall good prognosis with a cumulative 10-year survival of 90%. The tumour is staged according to the TNM system which is the primary determinant of the prognosis.

- Overall prognosis depends on the size of the tumour, extent of spread of the tumour beyond the confines of the thyroid, and presence of distant metastases, the microscopic type of the tumour, and the age of the patient.
- In children, the prognosis is excellent even if there are pulmonary metastases. On the other hand, prognosis for patients who are above the age of 40 years is less favorable.

Q34. What is follicular thyroid carcinoma?

Definition Follicular carcinoma is the second most common malignant thyroid tumour. It is composed of malignant cells forming follicles, i.e. showing abortive differentiation toward normal follicular cells.

Etiopathogenesis

i. It shows positive correlation with nodular goitre and is more common in geographic areas with *iodine deficiency*.
ii. *Age and sex* It occurs in older persons and is more common in women than men.
iii. *Molecular biology* changes involve mutations of RAS family genes, which are found in about 50% of cases. Other mutations have been described but are less common.

Pathology

Clinical and gross appearance Follicular carcinoma presents as a solitary nodule or as an irregular, firm, nodular enlargement of the entire lobe.

Microscopy

i. The tumour is composed of malignant cells forming follicles of various sizes and solid sheets or invasive cords.
ii. Some tumours are composed of clear cells, or Hűrthle cells or signet ring cells.
iii. If the tumour is encapsulated, the tumour cells are seen invading through the capsule into the normal parenchyma **(Fig. 27.7)**.

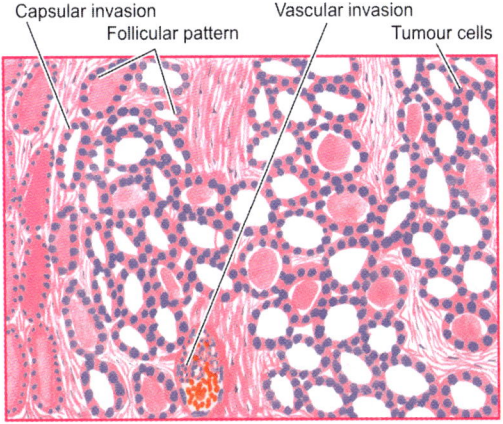

FIGURE 27.7: Follicular thyroid carcinoma, showing encapsulated tumour with invasion of a capsular vessel. The follicles lined by tumour cells are of various sizes and there is mild pleomorphism.

iv. On the basis of its growth features, follicular carcinomas can be classified as: a) encapsulated, minimally invasive, b) encapsulated angioinvasive, and c) widely invasive.

Clinical features

i. Follicular carcinoma is usually found in persons older than 50 years of age.

ii. Most tumours measure more than 4 cm in diameters and some may infiltrate the entire lobe.

iii. Overall, it is a slow-growing tumour, but grows faster than papillary carcinoma.

iv. Haematogenous metastases are common, especially to the lungs and bones, and sometimes these may be the first manifestations of the disease. Lymph node metastases are less common.

v. Many follicular carcinomas produce thyroid hormones, which may be used as tumour marker to follow up patients after total thyroidectomy (after the resection of the thyroid, there should be no T_4 or T_3 in serum!).

vi. Tumour cells concentrate radioactive iodine, which may be given for therapeutic purposes to internally irradiate metastases.

vii. The overall ten-year survival rate is 50–70%. Pathologic findings important for prognosis are: 90% for minimally invasive carcinomas, and less than 50% for widely invasive carcinoma which usually have distant metastases.

Q35. Comment on medullary carcinoma of the thyroid.

Definition Medullary carcinoma of the thyroid (MTC) is an uncommon malignant tumour derived from parafollicular or C-cells. MTC accounts for only 5% of all thyroid carcinomas. It differs from other thyroid carcinomas in three respects:

i. It secretes calcitonin

ii. It has an amyloid-rich stroma

iii. It is often familial and hereditary

Etiopathogenesis

i. It is unrelated to irradiation or iodine deficiency or some exogenous carcinogens.

ii. Activating point mutation of *RET* protooncogenes is found in almost all cases.

iii. In 25% of cases, MTC is familial and related to germ line mutations of *RET* protooncogene.

iv. Sporadic cases are mostly diagnosed in 5th-6th decade, whereas familial cases are diagnosed in younger patients (2nd to 3rd decades).

v. Familial cases can present in three forms:

a. Associated with pheochromocytoma and parathyroid adenoma in MEN 2A.

b. Associated with pheochromocytoma and multiple mucosal neuromas in MEN 2B.

c. Unassociated with any other tumour, forming a group of familial medullary thyroid carcinoma (FMTC) cases.

Pathology

Clinical and gross appearance Sporadic cases of MTC present as a nodule or a tumour mass. In familial cases, it may be bilateral and multifocal. In either case the mass is solid and firm. On cross section, it is either grey-white or yellow-brown with areas of necrosis and haemorrhage.

Microscopy

i. The tumour is composed of cells with round or oval nuclei arranged into nests surrounded by fibrovascular septa.

ii. By immunohistochemical stain, the cells stain with antibodies to calcitonin.

iii. Stroma contains amyloid which stains positively with Congo red.

iv. There may be foci of irregular calcification but no psammoma bodies **(Fig. 27.8)**.

v. Familial cases show multifocal C-cell hyperplasia in the normal thyroid parenchyma.

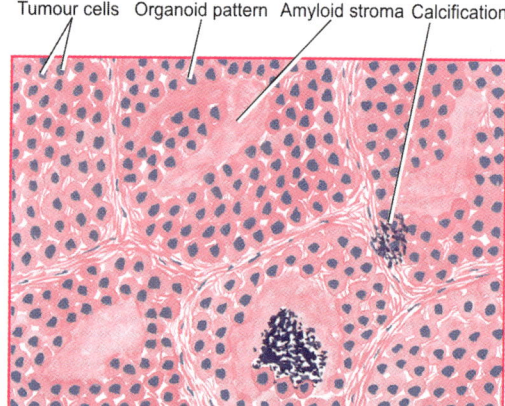

FIGURE 27.8: Medullary thyroid carcinoma. Microscopy shows organoid pattern of oval tumour cells and abundant amyloid stroma with foci of irregular calcification.

Clinical features MTC is a relatively slow growing tumour except in the familial MEN 2B cases which may be more aggressive.
i. Metastases to local lymph nodes may develop, but distant haemotogenous metastases are uncommon.
ii. Despite high levels of calcitonin in serum, hypocalcaemia is mild and unrelated to clinical symptoms.
iii. Some tumours secrete other polypeptide hormones and can produce paraneoplastic syndromes, such as Cushing syndrome due to ACTH, or diarrhoea due to vasoactive intestinal polypeptide (VIP).
iv. Overall 10-year survival rate is 60–70%, and somewhat lower in patients with MEN 2B.
v. All familial cases carrying mutated *RET* are offered prophylactic thyroidectomy and those with MEN2 must be under surveillance for adrenal tumours.

Q36. What is anaplastic thyroid carcinoma?

Definition Anaplastic thyroid carcinoma is a rare highly malignant thyroid tumour, typically found in old age persons (7th and 8th decade).
Pathology
Clinical and gross appearance Anaplastic thyroid carcinoma grows fast; by the time diagnosis is made, most tumours have spread beyond the confines of the thyroid, infiltrating the muscles and trachea or other parts of the necks.
Microscopy
i. The tumour is composed of highly anaplastic cells that may be classified as small, spindle shaped or giant cells.
ii. Areas of preexisting papillary or follicular carcinoma may be admixed in anaplastic areas, indicating that the tumour developed from another type of thyroid carcinoma which became undifferentiated.
Prognosis is abysmal and the median survival after the diagnosis is 2–3 months. 5-year survival is less than 10%.

■ PARATHYROID GLANDS

Q37. Write briefly on the anatomic, histologic and physiologic aspects of parathyroid glands for understanding its pathology.

Anatomy There are four parathyroid glands embedded in the posterior aspect of the thyroid gland. Each gland is a small oval organ weighing 35–45 mg and measuring 3–5 mm. Upper pair of parathyroid glands develops from the 4th branchial pouch of the primitive foregut and inferior pair from the 3rd branchial pouch.
Histology The parathyroid glands are composed of three cell types: chief cells, oxyphil cells and water-clear cells.
Physiology Parathyroid glands secrete parathyroid hormone (PTH), which together with calcitonin and vitamin D, regulates serum calcium and metabolism of bones. PTH elevates the serum level of calcium and reduces the serum phosphate level. Secretion of PTH is regulated by a feedback mechanism—lowered calcium levels stimulate secretion, whereas high levels of calcium cause decreased secretion of parathyroid hormone.
Regulation of calcium metabolism occurs at three levels **(Fig. 27.9)**:

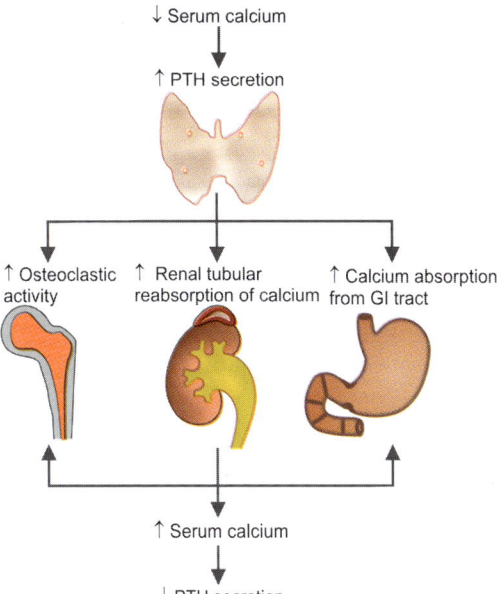

FIGURE 27.9: Role of parathormone (PTH) in regulating calcium metabolism in the body.

i. Stimulating the osteoclastic activity and promoting the resorption of bone, thus releasing calcium into circulation. This action is counteracted by calcitonin.

ii. Acting directly on renal tubular epithelium to increase reabsorption of calcium and inhibiting the reabsorption of phosphate. Calcitonin enhances renal excretion of phosphate.

iii. Increasing the renal production of most metabolically active metabolite of vitamin D_3, i.e. 1,25-dihydrocalciferol, which in turn increases absorption of calcium from small intestine.

Q38. What is hyperparathyroidism and what are its types?

Definition and types Hyperparathyroidism results from excessive production of parathyroid hormone. It occurs in three forms:

i. *Primary hyperparathyroidism*, which is caused by diseases of parathyroid glands.
ii. *Secondary hyperparathyroidism*, which is caused by diseases in other parts of the body.
iii. *Tertiary hyperparathyroidism*, which develops from secondary hyperparathyroidism after the removal of causes of secondary hyperparathyroidism.

Q39. What is primary hyperparathyroidism? Comment on its etiology, laboratory findings and clinical features.

Definition Primary hyperparathyroidism is a relatively common cause of parathyroid gland hyperfunction that usually occurs in old age, especially affecting women after the end of menopause.

Etiology There are three most common causes as follows:
i. Parathyroid adenoma, found in 85–90 % of cases.
ii. Primary hyperplasia (usually chief cell hyperplasia) in 10–15% cases.
iii. Carcinoma of parathyroid glands in less than 1% of cases.
Also included here are also familial cases of MEN where parathyroid adenoma or hyperplasia is one of its components.

Laboratory findings
i. Parathyroid hormone in serum ↑
ii. Calcium in serum ↑
iii. Phosphate in serum ↓
iv. Calcium in urine ↑

Clinical features Clinical consequence of hyperparathyroidism and hypercalcaemia are:
i. Nephrolithiasis or nephrocalcinosis are commonly related to hypercalcaemia.
ii. Metastatic calcification in blood vessels, lungs, stomach and eye, but may be found in other tissues as well.
iii. Generalised osteitis cystica fibrosis develops due to osteoclastic resorption of bone, which is replaced by fibrous tissue.
iv. Neuropsychiatric disturbances include depression, anxiety, psychosis and coma.
v. Hypertension is found in 50% of cases.
vi. Alimentary tract changes include pancreatitis, cholelithiasis, peptic ulcer.

For many years the medical students have memorised these clinical finding with the mnemonic '*painful bones, renal stones, abdominal groans and mental moans*'.

NOTE: Hypercalcaemia is most often diagnosed during routine laboratory examination, while it is still clinically asymptomatic:

- It must be distinguished from *paraneoplastic hypercalcaemia* caused in 80% of cases by tumour-derived parathyroid hormone peptide (PHrP) (e.g. squamous cell carcinoma).
- Cytokines produced by multiple myeloma or osteolytic tumours that have metastasised to bones, like breast cancer, also cause hypercalcaemia. Serum of these patients contains normal or reduced levels of PTH.

Q40. What is secondary hyperparathyroidism?

Definition Secondary hyperparathyroidism is caused by parathyroid hyperfunction initiated by diseases elsewhere in the body.

Etiology Though any condition causing hypocalcaemia may stimulates excessive secretion of parathyroid hormone, three most important causes of secondary hyperparathyroidism are:
i. Chronic renal insufficiency
ii. Vitamin D deficiency and consequent rickets and osteomalacia
iii. Intestinal malabsorption syndromes causing deficiency of calcium and vitamin D

Clinical features
i. The main feature is mild hypocalcaemia, in contrast to hypercalcaemia of primary hyperparathyroidism.
ii. Symptoms of the disease that has caused secondary hyperparathyroidism dominate the clinical picture.
iii. Initially, secondary hyperparathyroidism is a beneficial compensatory mechanism. However, if prolonged or excessive, it may cause soft tissue calcification and *renal osteodystrophy*, which includes varying degrees of osteitis fibrosa, osteomalacia, osteoporosis and osteosclerosis.

Q41. What is hypoparathyroidism?

Definition Hypoparathyroidism results from reduced secretion or complete deficiency of parathyroid hormone.

Etiology
i. The most common cause of hypoparathyroidism is accidental surgical removal of all four parathyroid glands during surgical procedures involving thyroid or related neck structures.
ii. Other causes are uncommon and include idiopathic autoimmune hypoparathyroidism in children which may be sporadic or familial, and is usually associated with other autoimmune diseases.

Laboratory findings
i. Parathyroid hormone in serum ↓
ii. Calcium in serum ↓
iii. Phosphate in serum ↑
iv. Calcium in urine ↓

Clinical features Clinical consequence of hyperparathyroidism and hypercalcaemia are:
i. Increased neuromuscular irritability
ii. Calcification of lens, facilitating cataract formation
iii. Cardiac conduction abnormalities
iv. Neurologic disturbances due to brain calcifications
v. Teeth abnormalities

NOTE: Hypoparathyroidism must be distinguished from a rare genetic disease called *pseudo-hypothyroidism*. In this condition, the parathyroid glands secrete normal amounts of parathyroid hormone but the peripheral tissues do not respond to hormonal stimulation:
- These patients have short stature and short metatarsal and metacarpal bones and flat nose and round face with multiple exostoses.
- Due to the unresponsiveness of kidney to parathyroid stimulation, they have hypercalciuria resulting in hypocalcaemia, and also hypophosphataemia.
- An incomplete form of pseudo-hypoparathyroidism is called *pseudopseudo-hypoparathyroidism*.

Q42. Comment briefly on parathyroid tumours.

Definition Parathyroid glands can give rise to two tumours: parathyroid adenoma (a common tumour) and parathyroid carcinoma (a very rare tumour).

Parathyroid adenoma is a benign tumour having following general features:
i. Most often, it occurs in women older than 50 years. The female to male ratio is 4:1.
ii. Most tumours are sporadic but in about 15% cases the condition is familial and occurs in context of MEN syndromes.
iii. Molecular biology data point to non-random changes on chromosome 11, which may play a pathogenetic role:
a. In more than one half of all cases, *PRAD1* proto-oncogene encoding cyclin D1 is either overexpressed, or rearranged, or inverted from its normal position on the long arm of chromosome 11 to its short arm so that it becomes juxtaposed to the gene for *PTH*, causing parathyroid cell proliferation.

b. Gene for *MEN1* gene, which is also located on chromosome 11, is mutated in MEN1 familial cases, and may be mutated in the same manner in some sporadic cases as well.

Clinical and gross appearance The parathyroid gland harbouring an adenoma is a relatively small encapsulated mass. It measure up to 5 cm and weighs up to 5 g, which is still 100 times more than the size and weight of the normal parathyroid gland.

Microscopy

i. It is composed of chief cells arranged in sheets or cords, with a few oxyphil and water-cells admixed to them.

ii. A rim of normal parathyroid parenchyma containing scattered fat cells is seen external to the capsule of the adenoma. This allows pathologist to distinguish adenoma from parathyroid hyperplasia which does not have this feature.

Parathyroid carcinoma is a rare tumour accounting for less than 1% of all cases of hyperparathyroidism.

Microscopy Parathyroid carcinoma cannot be distinguished from adenoma and the final diagnosis of malignancy is made on the basis of:

i. large tumour size,
ii. irregular shape,
iii. invasive growth (which makes malignant tumour difficult to resect surgically), and
iv. the presence of metastases.

ENDOCRINE PANCREAS

Q43. What is the structure of the endocrine pancreas?

Endocrine pancreas is distributed in between the acini of the exocrine part in form of islets of Langerhans, accounting weight-wise for 1–2% of this organ. Islets consist of 4 major and 2 minor cell types as under:

I. **Major cell types**

i. *Beta (β) or B cells* comprise 70% of all cells and secrete insulin, the defects of which causes diabetes mellitus.

ii. *Alpha (α) or A cells* comprise 20% of all cells and secrete glucagon which induces hyperglycaemia.

iii. *Delta (δ) or D cells* comprise 5–10% cells and secrete somatostatin which suppresses both insulin and glucagon release.

iv. *Pancreatic polypeptide (PP) or F cells*, which comprise 1–2% of all cells and secrete pancreatic polypeptide having some gastrointestinal effects.

II. **Minor cell types**

i. *D1 cells* elaborate vasoactive intestinal polypeptide (VIP) which induces glycogenolysis and hyperglycaemia and cases secretory diarrhoea by stimulating gastrointestinal fluid secretion.

ii. *Enterochromaffin cells* synthesise serotonin in which pancreatic tumours may induce carcinoid syndrome.

Q44. What is diabetes mellitus and how is it classified?

Definition Diabetes mellitus (DM) is a heterogeneous metabolic disorder characterised by common features of chronic hyperglycaemia and disturbances of carbohydrate, fat and protein metabolism.

NOTE: DM must be distinguished from a closely related syndrome called *metabolic syndrome* or *insulin resistance syndrome* consisting of a combination of metabolic abnormalities which increase the risk of diabetes and cardiovascular disease. Major features of metabolic syndrome are:

i. central obesity,
ii. dyslipidaemia (hypertriglyceridaemia, low HDL, high cholesterol),
iii. hyperglycaemia, and
iv. hypertension.

Epidemiology DM and its major complications are among the leading causes of morbidity and mortality world over. DM is most prevalent in the large countries such as China, India and US. In India, 7% of population suffers from DM. The incidence is somewhat lower in Africa and developing countries of Asia. Estimates are that worldwide there a 450 million people with DM and their numbers are increasing constantly.

Classification and etiology Following four broad groups of DM are recognised:

Type 1 DM constitutes 10% of all cases. Previously it was called juvenile onset or insulin-dependent DM because it affects young people mainly and is insulin-dependent for treatment. Although most people develop type I DM by the age of 30 years, but in 5–10% cases symptoms develop above the age of 30 years. Type 1 DM is subdivided into two subtypes:

- *Subtype 1A (immune-mediated) DM* is characterised by an autoimmune destruction of β-cells leading to insulin deficiency.
- *Subtype 1B (idiopathic) DM* is characterised by insulin deficiency with tendency to develop ketosis, with no sign of immune markers.

Type 2 DM comprises about 80% of all cases. It was also called maturity-onset or non-insulin dependent DM of obese and non-obese type. Although it affects predominantly older people, it occurs among children and adolescents as well. Furthermore, many cases become insulin-dependent over time. Pathogenetically, type 2 DM is characterised by reduced capacity of β-cells to secrete insulin and peripheral tissue resistance to insulin.

Gestational DM develops in 4% pregnant women. It is defined as DM that occurs in second or third trimester of pregnancy in a woman who did not have pre-existent DM. In these cases, hyperglycaemia reverts to normal after delivery, but many of these women develop DM later in their life.

Other specific etiologic forms of DM The most important examples from this group are:
i. DM due to diseases of exocrine pancreas (e.g. cystic fibrosis, chronic pancreatitis),
ii. drug and chemical-induced DM, and
iii. monogenic diabetes syndromes (e.g. neonatal DM, and maturity-onset diabetes of the young or MODY that has autosomal dominant inheritance, early onset of hyperglycaemia and impaired insulin secretion).

Q45. What are the major risk factors for onset of type 2 diabetes mellitus?

The major risk factors for type 2 DM are listed in **Table 27.3**.

TABLE 27.3 Major risk factors for type 2 diabetes mellitus*.

1. First degree relatives with type 2DM
2. Obesity (BMI >25 kg/m^2)
3. Habitual physical inactivity
4. Race and ethnicity (African Americans, Latinos, Asians, Pacific Islanders)
5. Previous identification of impaired fasting glucose, or impaired glucose tolerance, or patients with prediabetes (HbA1C range 5.7–6.4%)
6. History of gestational DM or delivery of baby heavier than 4 kg
7. Hypertension (>140/90 mmHg, or on therapy for hypertension)
8. Dyslipidaemia (HDL level <35 mg/dL, or triglycerides >250 mg/dL)
9. History of cardiovascular disease
10. Women with polycystic ovary disease
11. Other clinical conditions associated with insulin resistance (e.g. severe obesity, acanthosis nigricans)

*Adapted from American Diabetes Association. 2. Classification and diagnosis of diabetes—2018. Diabetes Care. 2018;41(Suppl. 1):S13-S27.

Q46. What is the pathogenesis of hyperglycaemia?

Mechanisms of hyperglycaemia can be explained by the following:
i. Reduced insulin secretion
ii. Decreased glucose use by the body
iii. Increased glucose production

Insulin plays a key role in these processes and these are specifically altered in various forms of DM as under **(Fig. 27.10)**:

Pathogenesis of type 1 DM This form of DM results from destruction of β-cells, which has 3 determinants: i) genetic susceptibility, ii) autoimmunity, and iii) possible environmental factors.

i. *Genetic susceptibility* plays an important role. No single etiologic gene has been identified as a possible cause, but the inheritance of certain genes provides the basis for *hereditary susceptibility* as evidenced by the following:

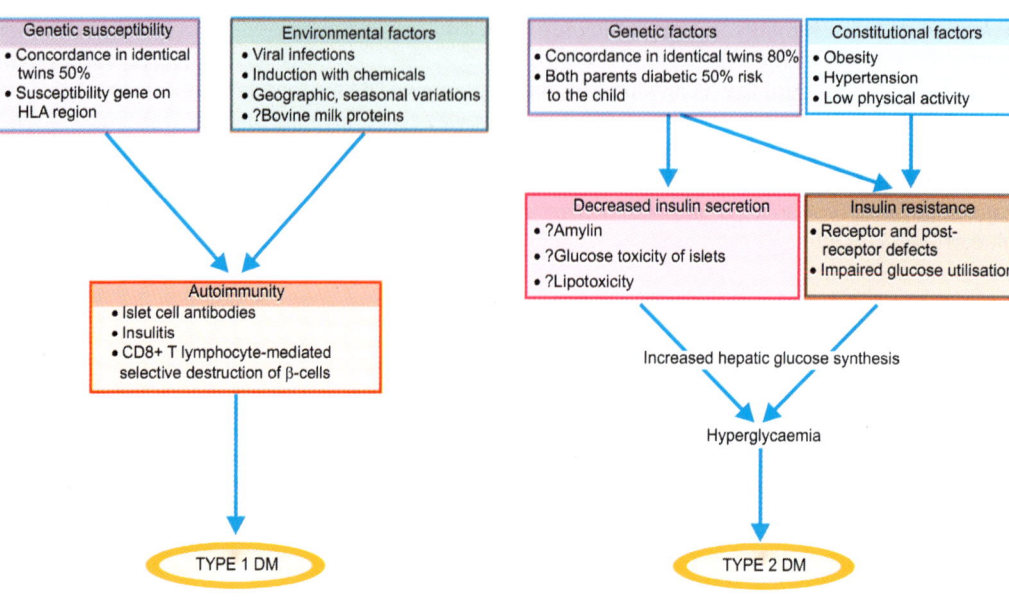

FIGURE 27.10: Schematic mechanisms involved in pathogenesis of two main types of diabetes mellitus.

a. In identical twins, the concordance is 50%, consistent with *polygenic inheritance* with the contribution of other non-genetic and genetic susceptibility factors.
b. HLA genes on chromosome 6 are linked to type I DM as evident by predominance of some haplotypes in the diseased population.
c. Over 90% of patients have HLA-DR3, HLA-DR4 or HLA-DQ haplotypes. Clustering of certain haplotypes from these groups increases the risk in such persons.
ii. *Autoimmunity* plays a role in type 1A DM:
a. The prevailing hypothesis is that type 1A DM patients lose self-tolerance of T cell dependent antigens on β-cells, insulin or some cytoplasmic components of β-cells.
b. Islets are infiltrated with T cells in early stages of type 1A DM, and it seems that these cells are involved in killing of β-cells.
c. The infiltrate is composed chiefly of CD8 cytotoxic cells but there are also scattered CD4 T helper cells.
d. Autoantibodies are present in many patients of type 1A DM. These antibodies are directed against insulin, GAD (glutamic acid decarboxylase) and other components of islet cells. Antibodies do not play a role in islet cell destruction but are useful for screening family members at risk for type 1A DM.
iii. *Environmental factors* are suspected to play a role but no definitive proof has come forth so far. Sudden onset of type 1 DM suggests a possible viral infection. It has been postulated that viruses either directly affect the islet cells or induce an immune reaction, which due to molecular mimicry then cross-reacts with islet cells.

Pathogenesis of type 2 DM This is related to two basic defects:
- *impaired insulin secretion*, reflecting inadequate insulin secretion relative to glucose load, and
- *insulin resistance* evidenced by an inability of peripheral tissues to respond to insulin.

The pathogenesis of type 2 DM is complex and includes the following factors:
i. *Genetic basis* No single causative gene has been identified.
a. In identical twins, if one twin is having the disease, chances of second twin getting it is 80%.
b. Offsprings of a diabetic person are at increased risk.
c. If both parents are diabetic, the offspring has a 40% chance of developing type 2 DM.
ii. *Constitutional factors* Obesity, hypertension and sedentary life style increase the risk.
iii. *Insulin resistance* It is one of the major causes of hyperglycaemia. It impairs glucose utilisation, stimulates hepatic synthesis of glucose, and in obesity it leads to a release of free fatty acid and cytokines (e.g. TNF-α and adiponectin) which affect the sensitivity of peripheral tissues to insulin.

iv. *Impaired insulin secretion* It is interlinked to insulin resistance which initially causes a compensatory hyperinsulinaemia. With time, secretion of insulin drops and ultimately it becomes insufficient. The exact mechanism of reduced insulin production is not known but it could be related to:
a. insular amyloid deposition due to the accumulation of amylin,
b. glucose toxicity, or
c. lipotoxicity of free fatty acids which affect the β-cells.
v. *Increased hepatic glucose synthesis* Normally, insulin promotes hepatic glucose storage and suppresses gluconeogenesis. Liver resistance to insulin inhibits these processes and results in hyperglycaemia.

Q47. What are the pathologic changes in the pancreatic islets in diabetes?

The islets show pathologic change in both type 1 and type 2 DM, but are more prominent in type 1 DM as under:
i. *Insulitis* is prominent in early stages of type 1 DM. It includes infiltrates of lymphocytes (mostly T cells) and a few macrophages and PMNs. Diabetic infants of diabetic mothers have infiltrates of eosinophils. In type 2 DM, there is fibrosis of islets but the inflammatory cells are scarce or not visible at all.
ii. *Islet cell mass* is reduced in type 1 DM, mostly due to the depletion of β-cells. In type 2 DM, the islet cell mass is less prominently reduced. In infants born to diabetic mothers, there is enlargement of islets in response to maternal hyperglycaemia.
iii. *Amyloidosis* may be seen in type 2 DM, but not in type 1 DM. It is characterised by deposition of amylin around the capillaries of the islets, accompanied by atrophy of the islet cells. By EM, β-cells show degranulation, but these changes are not evident in type 2 DM.

Q48. Tabulate salient contrasting features of type 1 and type 2 diabetes mellitus.

The contrasting features of type 1 and type 2 diabetes mellitus are listed in **Table 27.4**. However, overlapping of features is quite common.

TABLE 27.4 Contrasting features of type 1 and type 2 diabetes mellitus.

FEATURE	TYPE 1 DM	TYPE 2 DM
1. Frequency	10–20%	80–90%
2. Age at onset	Early (below 35 years)	Late (after 40 years)
3. Type of onset	Abrupt and severe	Gradual and insidious
4. Weight	Normal	Obese/non-obese
5. HLA	Linked to HLA DR3, HLA DR4, HLA DQ	No HLA association
6. Family history	<20%	About 60%
7. Genetic locus	Unknown	Chromosome 6
8. Diabetes in identical twins	50% concordance	80% concordance
9. Pathogenesis	Autoimmune destruction of β-cells	Insulin resistance, impaired insulin secretion
10. Islet cell antibodies	Yes	No
11. Blood insulin level	Decreased insulin	Normal or increased insulin
12. Islet cell changes	Insulitis, β-cell depletion	No insulitis, later fibrosis of islets
13. Amyloidosis	Infrequent	Common in chronic cases
14. Clinical management	Insulin and diet	Diet, exercise, oral drugs, insulin
15. Acute complications	Ketoacidosis	Hyperosmolar coma

(HLA, human leucocyte antigen)

Q49. What are the main complications of two main forms of diabetes? Describe their pathogenesis and biochemical basis.

The most important complications can be classified as vascular, metabolic, or immune **(Fig. 27.11)**.
• The severity and duration of hyperglycaemia are the main pathogenetic mechanism of *microvascular complications*, e.g. retinopathy, nephropathy, neuropathy, etc.
• Long-standing cases of type 2 DM develop *macrovascular complications*, e.g. atherosclerosis, coronary artery disease, cerebrovascular disease and peripheral vascular disease.

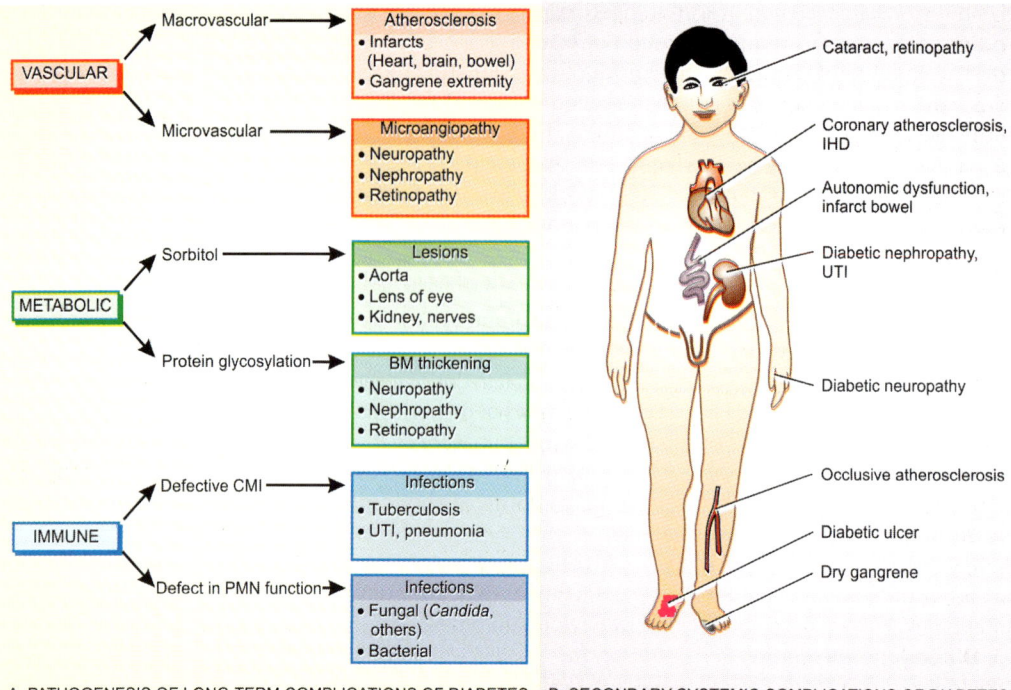

FIGURE 27.11: Long-term complications of diabetes mellitus. A, Pathogenesis. B, Secondary systemic complications.

Pathogenesis The biochemical changes underlying the pathological changes include the following:
i. *Non-enzymatic proteins glycosylation* Free amino acids of various proteins bind glucose non-enzymatically. This process involves haemoglobin, lens crystalline protein, basement membranes and many other tissues. Advanced glycosylation end-products (AGE) form over time, accounting for the stable and irreversible changes, most prominently in thickened glomerular capillaries and arterioles. Glycosylated haemoglobin (HbA1C) is used for monitoring glycaemic control during the preceding 90–120 days corresponding with the life span of most red blood cells.
ii. *Polyol pathway mechanism* This mechanism which is mediated by aldose reductase, leads to formation of sorbitol and fructose which facilitate the entry of water into cells, thus causing cell injury in the aorta, eye, kidney and peripheral nerve.
iii. *Reactive oxygen species (ROS)* are formed in excessive amounts causing cell injury.

Q50. What are the acute metabolic complications of diabetes mellitus?

Acute metabolic complications of DM include i) diabetic ketoacidosis, ii) hyperosmolar hyperglycaemic nonketotic coma, and iii) hypoglycaemia.
i. **Diabetic ketoacidosis (DKA)** DKA is almost exclusively a complication of type 1 DM.
It is caused by severe insulin deficiency and glucagon excess that leads to massive lipolysis and a release of free fatty acids into the circulation.
a. Free fatty acids are taken up by the liver and oxidised to ketone bodies, principally acetoacetic acid and β-hydroxybutyric acid.
b. If ketone bodies are formed faster than they can be utilised by the muscles and other tissues, ketonaemia and ketonuria develop.
c. If the excretion of ketone bodies is prevented by dehydration, systemic metabolic ketoacidosis develops presenting as anorexia, nausea, vomiting, deep and fast breathing, mental confusion and coma.
Prognosis Most patients recover.
ii. **Hyperosmolar hyperglycaemic nonketotic coma** This is a complication of type 2 DM.
a. It is caused by dehydration that develops due to excessive hyperglycaemic diuresis.

b. There is hyperglycaemia and plasma osmolality is high.
c. Central nervous system symptoms dominate.
d. High viscosity of blood is associated with thrombosis and bleeding.
Prognosis Overall mortality is high.
iii. **Hypoglycaemia** This is a complication of type 1 DM.
a. It may result from excessive administration of insulin, missing a meal, or may be related to stress.
b. It may result in worsening of diabetic control and rebound hyperglycaemia, so called *Somogy effect*.
Prognosis Hypoglycaemic episodes are harmful since they may cause permanent brain damage.

Q51. What are the late systemic complications of diabetes mellitus?

Late complications occur after 15–20 years of either type of diabetes, accounting for the morbidity and mortality of diabetes (see **Fig. 27.11**). The most important late systemic complications of diabetes are as follows:

i. **Atherosclerosis** Atherosclerotic lesions are more common, more accelerated and more often associated with complications such as atheroma ulceration, calcification or thrombosis. Accelerated atherosclerosis is a consequence of many disturbances including hyperlipidaemia, low HDL, non-enzymatic glycosylation, increased platelet adhesiveness, obesity and hypertension.

ii. **Diabetic microangiopathy** It is marked by thickening and hyalinisation of the wall of arterioles in many organs such as the kidneys, skeletal muscles and skin. Nonvascular basement membranes, such as those of renal tubules or peripheral nerves are also affected. These changes are a consequence of increased glycosylation of the proteins of basement membranes.

iii. **Diabetic nephropathy** Renal changes include diabetic glomerulosclerosis, hyaline arteriolosclerosis, pyelonephritis and necrotising renal papillitis. Renal insufficiency is the leading cause of death in DM.

iv. **Diabetic neuropathy** Diabetes may affect all parts of the central nervous system, but most characteristically it presents as symmetric sensory-motor neuropathy involving peripheral nerves. These changes may be caused by an excessive accumulation of sorbitol and fructose, or could be related to diabetic microangiopathy.

v. **Diabetic retinopathy** It is a leading cause of blindness. Retinal arterioles have thickened walls and form microaneurysms. Glaucoma and cataracts may occur at an early age.

Q52. Describe laboratory parameters for patients who are at increased risk for diabetes. What are the current laboratory criteria for diagnosis of diabetes mellitus?

The American Diabetes Association (2018) has recommended fresh guidelines for making diagnosis of diabetes mellitus and for categorising patients who are at increased risk for diabetes (i.e. prediabetics) **(Tables 27.5 and 27.6)**.

- *In symptomatic patients*, the diagnosis is made readily by documenting glucosuria

TABLE 27.5 Categories of increased risk for diabetes (prediabetes) (ADA, 2018)*

Fasting plasma glucose: 100 mg/dL (5.6 mmol/L) to 125 mg/dL (6.9 mmol/L) (IFG)
Or
2-hour plasma glucose during 75-g OGTT: 140 mg/dL (7.8 mmol/L) to 199 mg/dL (11.0 mmol/L) (IGT)
Or
HbA1C value: 5.7–6.4% (39–47 mmol/mol)

*American Diabetes Association. 2. Classification and diagnosis of diabetes—2018. Diabetes Care. 2018;41(Suppl. 1):S13-S27.
(IFG, impaired fasting glucose; IGT, impaired glucose tolerance)

TABLE 27.6 Revised criteria for diagnosis of diabetes (as per American Diabetes Association, 2018)*.

PLASMA GLUCOSE VALUE**	DIAGNOSIS
1. FASTING (FOR >8 HOURS) VALUE	
Below 100 mg/dL (<5.6 mmol/L)	Normal fasting value
126 mg/dL (7.0 mmol/L) or more	Diabetes mellitus
2. TWO-HOUR AFTER 75 G ANHYDROUS ORAL GLUCOSE IN WATER	
<140 mg/dL (<7.8 mmol/L)	Normal post-prandial GTT
200 mg/dL (11.1 mmol/L) or more	Diabetes mellitus
3. RANDOM VALUE	
200 mg/dL (11.1 mmol/L) or more in a symptomatic patient	Diabetes mellitus
4. GLYCATED HAEMOGLOBIN ASSAY	
A1C >6.5% (48 mmol/mol)	Diabetes mellitus

*American Diabetes Association. 2. Classification and diagnosis of diabetes—2018. Diabetes Care. 2018;41(Suppl. 1):S13-S27.
**Plasma glucose values are 15% higher than whole blood glucose value.
(GTT, glucose tolerance test)

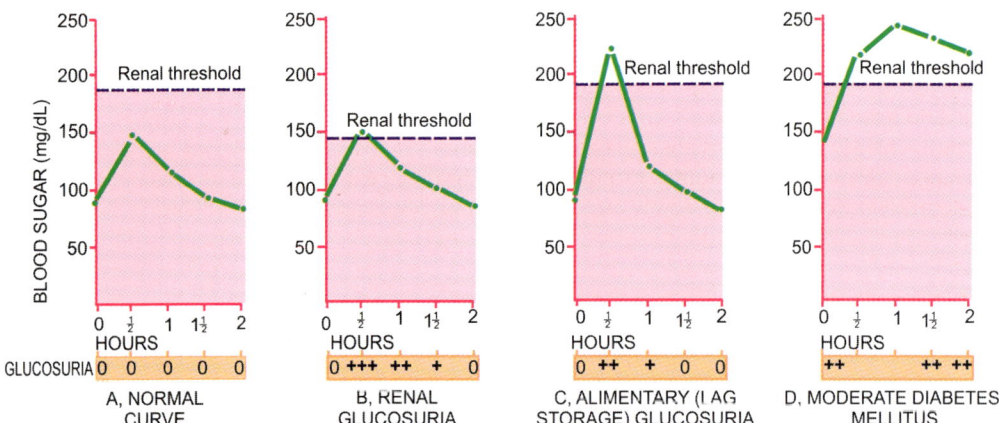

FIGURE 27.12: Oral glucose tolerance test (OGTT), showing plasma glucose curves and glucosuria after 75 g of oral glucose.

and hyperglycaemia above 200 mg/dL. Severity of polyuria and polydipsia are directly related to hyperglycaemia.
- In *asymptomatic patients,* the diagnosis is made by demonstrating persistent hyperglycaemia or by performing the oral glucose tolerance test (OGTT). If this test is positive, the condition is called *chemical diabetes* **(Fig. 27.12)**.

The following tests are performed for early diagnosis of diabetes in asymptomatic adults:

i. **Urine testing** It is an inexpensive test useful for initial screening. It is not specific for DM and can be positive in a number of conditions such as renal glucosuria, alimentary (lag storage) glucosuria, many metabolic disorders, starvation, and intracranial lesions (e.g. brain tumours, haemorrhage and head injury). In diabetic persons, it may be followed by a test for ketonuria, which is not performed on non-diabetic persons, but is a good test for checking the control of diabetes and its metabolic complications.

ii. **Single blood sugar measurement** This test is routinely performed in outpatient and hospital setting.

iii. **Fasting glucose test** Fasting plasma glucose determination is a reliable screening test for type 2 DM. A fasting glucose value above 126 mg/dL (≥7 mmol/L) is indicative of DM and should be followed up by OGTT to confirm the diagnosis.

iv. **Two-hour plasma glucose test and OGTT** It is performed mostly on patients who have borderline results on fasting plasma glucose test (plasma glucose values between 100 and 125 mg/dL). Depending on the outcome of the OGTT, the tested persons are classified as normal, impaired fasting glucose tolerance, or diabetic.

v. **Glycosylated haemoglobin (HbA1C)** This test measures a small fraction of haemoglobin which is non-enzymatically glycosylated over a period of 90–120 days. It is a very convenient test because it does not require any dietary preparation and has high pre-analytic stability. Moreover, it does not undergo variation due to stress or illness prior to the test. HbA1C is normally < 5.7%, the values of 5.7–6.4% are borderline, and above 6.5% are found in diabetics.

vi. **Other tests** These complex tests are performed in specific conditions in diabetics. These include various modifications of OGTT, tests for antibodies in suspected type 1 DM. Complications of DM are also monitored by laboratory tests (e.g. dyslipidaemia, microalbuminuria, thyroid dysfunction, etc.).

Q53. What are pancreatic neuroendocrine tumours? Mention some salient features of these tumours.

Definition Pancreatic neuroendocrine tumors (panNET) originate from the islets and are composed of neoplastic cells corresponding to the neuroendocrine cells of the pancreas.

Salient features
i. Rare tumours, accounting for less than 5% of all pancreatic tumours.
ii. Sporadic in most instances but some are familial and part of MEN1 or von Hippel-Landau syndrome.
iii. They can be solitary or multiple, benign or malignant.

iv. Microscopically, panNET resemble intestinal carcinoid tumours and are composed of small neuroendocrine cells with round uniform nuclei arranged into nests and trabeculae.

v. Except for hormone-secreting insulinomas (which are diagnosed while still small), all others are mostly (80%) low-grade malignant tumours.

vi. Hormonally inactive tumours are more common than hormonally active tumours.

vii. Functioning tumours are named according to their histogenesis as:
- β-cell tumour (insulinoma)
- α-cell tumour (glucagonoma)
- δ-cell tumour (somatostatinoma)
- δ1-cell tumour (VIPoma, or vasoactive intestinal polypeptide secreting tumour)
- PPoma (pancreatic polypeptide secreting tumour)
- G-cell tumour (gastrinoma), originating from an unknown cell type (islets do not contain gastrin-secreting cells!)

viii. The most common functioning tumour is insulinoma, followed by gastrinoma. All other functioning tumours are very rare.

ix. *Molecular biology* Familial cases include mutations of *MEN1* and *VHL* genes. Mutated MEN1 gene is found in approximately 50% of sporadic cases. Other recurrent genetic abnormalities are mutation of *PTEN* and *TSC2* tumour suppressor genes which activate the mammalian target of rapamycin (mTOR) signaling pathway, and certain genes that regulate apoptosis and telomerase maintenance.

Q54. What is insulinoma?

Definition Insulinoma is a benign NET of pancreas composed of neoplastic β-cells secreting insulin.

Salient features

i. Most insulinomas (75%) are small solitary nodules, less than 2.5 cm in diameter.

ii. Microscopically, insulinomas are composed of cells resembling normal islets. Insulin can be demonstrated by immunohistochemistry. EM shows typical β-cell cytoplasmic granules.

iii. Most tumours secrete insulin, but only in 25% of these serum insulin levels are high enough to produce clinical signs of hyperinsulinaemia which include:

a. Hypoglycaemic attacks resulting in light-headedness, confusion, visual symptoms and syncope, with profuse sweating (due to insulin mediated catecholamine release).

b. Symptoms are relieved by intake of sugar.

c. In unattended patient the attack progress to seizures, lethargy and loss of consciousness and even coma.

iv. *Laboratory findings* are diagnostic and include: hypoglycaemia (<50 mg/dL), high levels of insulin in blood, and high insulin-glucose ratio.

v. Small size of tumours at the time of diagnosis makes then surgically resectable, and thus most tumours have an excellent prognosis.

NOTE: *The differential diagnosis of hypoglycaemia* includes hyperinsulinaemia due to paraneoplastic syndromes (e.g. sarcomas), starvation, cirrhosis, partial gastrectomy, and endocrine disorders such as hypopituitarism and adrenal insufficiency.

Q55. Comment briefly on gastrinoma.

Definition Gastrinoma is a tumour composed of gastrin-secreting neuroendocrine cells.

Pathology

i. Gastrinoma is the second most common functioning tumour of the pancreas, next to insulinima.

ii. It is usually located in the head of the pancreas or duodenum and secretes gastrin.

iii. Pancreatic gastrinoma is a locally invasive low-grade malignant tumour that tends to metastasise to local lymph nodes.

iv. Duodenal tumours may be very small or even microscopic.

v. On rare occasions, gastrinomas may be found in unusual sites such as duodenum, stomach or oesophagus.

Clinical features Gastrinomas are part of *Zollinger-Ellison syndrome* comprising the triad as under:

i. Fulminant peptic ulcer: It may be resistant to standard therapy; may be multiple; or located in unusual sites.

ii. Gastric acid hypersecretion.

iii. Gastrinoma, most often in the duodenum or head of the pancreas.

Q56. What are the multiple endocrine neoplasia (MEN) syndromes?

Definition Multiple endocrine neoplasia syndromes are genetic hereditary syndromes presenting with multiple endocrine tumours or hyperplasia. The group includes the following:

I. **Multiple endocrine neoplasia type 1 syndrome (MEN1)** or Werner syndrome includes adenomas of the parathyroid glands, pancreatic islets and pituitary. It is inherited as an autosomal dominant trait related to germ line mutation of tumour suppressor gene *MEN1* encoding a polyfunctional protein menin.

i. Parathyroid adenomas with hyperparathyroidism in 90% cases.

ii. Pancreatic or duodenal tumours causing Zollinger-Ellison syndrome or hypoglycaemia; these tumours account for most of the mortality.

iii. Pituitary tumours which are most often prolactinomas. Some tumours secrete growth hormone and cause acromegaly, and some are nonfunctioning adenomas compressing the pituitary and causing panhypopituitarism.

II. **Multiple endocrine neoplasia (MEN2)** characterised by medullary carcinoma of the thyroid and pheochromocytoma. It is inherited as an autosomal dominant pattern related to germ line mutation of *RET* proto-oncogene, leading to constitutive activation of RET receptor tyrosine kinase. Two major syndromes are recognised: MEN2A (Sipple syndrome) and MEN2B.

i. **MEN2A** is characterised by medullary carcinoma of the thyroid (in 100% cases), pheochromocytoma (50% cases) and parathyroid hyperplasia with hypercalcaemia and urinary stones (20% cases).

ii. **MEN2B** is a combination of medullary carcinoma of thyroid, pheochromocytoma, mucosal neuromas or ganglioneuromas and marfanoid features. MEN2B is also related to mutations of *RET* protooncogene, but the mutation involves a different part of the gene than in MEN2A. Thus, there is no hyperparathyroidism, and the medullary carcinomas are more aggressive than those in MEN2A.

III. **Mixed syndromes** including multiple neuroendocrine tumours and tumours of other organs, such as:

i. *von Hippel-Lindau syndrome* caused by the mutation of *VHL* gene, presenting with CNS and eye tumours together with renal cell carcinoma, pheochromocytoma and islet cell tumours.

ii. *Type I neurofibromatosis* resulting from inactivation of neurofibromin proteins and activation of *RAS* gene, and MEN1 or MEN2 type endocrine tumours.

> ### Chapter 27e Supplement: Online Content
> *Digital content of this chapter available with this book is meant for enhanced learning and self-assessment. In addition, it contains 43 Multiple Choice Questions (MCQs), 05 Clinicopathologic Vignettes, and 05 Image-based Questions; these are followed by their answers along with explanatory notes of correct and incorrect answers.*

CHAPTER 28

Musculoskeletal System

BONE AND CARTILAGE

Q1. Define various common terms used in describing normal structure of bone and cartilage.

i. Bone is the hard part of skeleton.
ii. Cartilage is a tissue composed of chondroid matrix and chondrocytes.
iii. Anatomically and embryologically, long bones have three distinct parts:
- *Epiphysis* covered with articular cartilage,
- *Metaphysis* incorporating the growth plate, and
- *Diaphysis* comprising the midportion of the shaft.

iv. *Microscopy* Bone consists of two components **(Fig. 28.1)**:
- Compact bone forming the cortical parts (80%)
- Cancellous bone (20%) forming trabeculae in the bone marrow.

v. *Ossification* is the process of bone formation; first in form of woven bone which transforms later into lamellar bone.
vi. *Osteoblasts* are the bone-forming cells.
vii. *Osteoclasts* are multinucleated, macrophage-derived cells that remove calcified material.
viii. *Osteocytes* are the mature bone cells residing within the bone lacunae.
ix. *Osteoid* is the organic component of bone spicules composed of non-calcified collagen type I, produced by osteoblasts.
x. *Periosteum* is the connective tissue on the surface of bone.

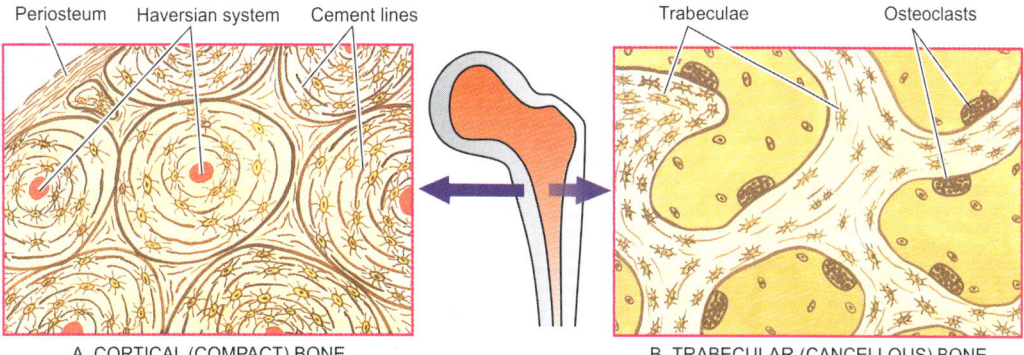

FIGURE 28.1: Normal structure of cortical (compact) bone (A) and trabecular (cancellous) bone (B) in transverse section. The cortical bone forming the outer shell shows concentric lamellae along with osteocytic lacunae surrounding central blood vessels, while the trabecular bone forming the marrow space shows trabeculae with osteoclastic activity at the margins.

Q2. What are the most important developmental disorders of bones and joints?

Developmental disorders of bones and joints may be classified as:
- localised developmental defects, or
- genetic diseases affecting the entire skeleton.

Out of the numerous disorders in this group, following are the most representative and clinically important:

I. **Localised developmental defects** These affect the extremities most often. Most important examples are as under:

i. *Syndactyly*, i.e. fused fingers or toes, due to abnormal apoptosis in the limb buds.

ii. *Amelia,* i.e. congenital absence of one or several limbs.

iii. *Developmental dysplasia of the hip* that causes dislocation and malfunction of the hip joint.

iv. *Talipes varus* or club foot.

v. *Monostotic fibrous dysplasia* is a localised defect of bone-formation, presenting as a painful pseudotumour of the bone. In simple terms, it is fibrous tissue replacing bone trabeculae.

II. **Genetic diseases** These affect the entire skeleton. Three representative examples are given below:

i. *Osteogenesis imperfecta* Also called *brittle bone disease*.
- It is caused by one of several possible mutations of the gene encoding *collagen type I*, which is an essential part of osteoid.
- Inherited as either autosomal dominant or recessive.
- The affected bones are brittle and prone to fractures and deformities.
- Clinically, it can occur in several forms, varying from mild to severe, and even may be lethal in utero.
- Abnormal dentition and bluish sclerae are seen in the milder form.

ii. *Achondroplasia* Also called *hereditary dwarfism*.
- It is the most common cause of congenital dwarfism.
- It is caused by mutations of the gene encoding the *fibroblast growth factor receptor 3 (FGFR3)*.
- The genetic mutation is inherited as an autosomal dominant trait but is also may occur spontaneously, especially in older fathers.
- The mutation of FGFR3 interferes with endochondral osteogenesis of long bones, resulting in short arms and legs.
- The head is large with prominent forehead and depressed bridge of the nose.

iii. *Osteopetrosis* Also called *marble bone disease*.
- It is caused by a mutation of one of several genes regulating the *function of osteoclasts*.
- Mutation of carbonic anhydrase II is an example of this disease.
- Dysfunction of osteoclasts leads to *abnormal bone resorption*.
- Abnormally dense bones are prone to fractures.
- Replacement of bone marrow by bone trabeculae ('*too much bone*') results in anaemia, leucopenia and thrombocytopenia.
- Cranial nerve compression may cause blindness and deafness.

Q3. Enumerate the most important metabolic and endocrine bone diseases.

The most important and prevalent metabolic bone diseases are:
I. osteoporosis,
II. rickets and osteomalacia,
III. osteitis cystic fibrosa,
IV. renal osteodystrophy, and
V. Paget disease.

Q4. Write briefly on osteoporosis.

Definition Literally meaning 'increased porosity of bones', marked by a reduction of the bone mass. Radiologically, it is recognised as *osteopenia* (i.e. bone loss).

Classification Osteoporosis is variously classified:

i. By extent as: *localised* (e.g. disuse atrophy of long bones immobilised for long time), or *generalised* (e.g. metabolic diseases).

ii. By etiology as: primary or secondary osteoporosis.
a. *Primary osteoporosis* does not have a single identifiable cause and is associated with advanced age, most often affecting postmenopausal women.
b. *Secondary osteoporosis* can result from a variety of conditions as follows:
- *Endocrine disturbances* (e.g. hyperparathyroidism, hyperthyroidism, Cushing disease, hypogonadism)
- *Neoplasms* (e.g. multiple myeloma)
- *Nutritional disorders* (e.g. malnutrition, malabsorption of proteins and vitamin D)
- *Drugs* (e.g. corticosteroids, chemotherapy)
- *Miscellaneous conditions* (e.g. alcohol abuse, smoking)

Osteoporosis of old age This is the most common and most important form of primary osteoporosis.
i. It is a multifactorial disease that has genetic, nutritional, and metabolic components.
ii. Reduced physical activity and low serum oestrogen also play an important role.
iii. Morphologically, the entire skeleton is involved, but the *vertebral bodies* are most severely affected.
iv. *Spontaneous fractures* are common. Histologically, bone trabeculae are thin and prone to fractures.
v. Clinically, fractures of thoracic and lumbar vertebrae lead to *reduction in height, kyphoscoliosis, and lordosis* ('dowager hump').
vi. *Hip fracture* is the most serious complication, which accounts for many deaths in elderly patients with osteoporosis.
vii. *Laboratory findings* Serum calcium and phosphate, alkaline phosphatase and parathyroid hormone levels are within normal limits.

Q5. What are rickets and osteomalacia?

Definition Rickets, a disease of children, and osteomalacia, a disease of adults, result from dietary *vitamin D* deficiency, inadequate vitamin D absorption, or metabolism (Page 204).
Vitamin D deficiency cause delayed or *inadequate mineralisation*, leading to excess non-mineralised osteoid.

Rickets In this, there is addition of deranged endochondral bone growth resulting from inadequate mineralisation of the epiphyseal cartilage and *deformity of softened bones*.
Clinicopathologic features Some or all of the following are present in a case **(Fig. 28.2)**:
i. Pigeon breast deformity of the chest (inward bending of ribs and protrusion of sternum)
ii. 'Rachitic rosary' named after the nodular thickening of ribs at the costochondral junction
iii. Bowlegs
iv. Lumbar lordosis
v. Frontal bossing of the head

Osteomalacia The most common causes are dietary deficiency of vitamin D and/or its active form from:
- lack of sun exposure, and
- chronic diseases affecting the liver, kidneys and intestines.

i. Major skeletal deformities (like those of rickets) are rarely seen but there is increased incidence of fractures.
ii. *Radiographically,* there is evidence of cortical thinning and loss of bone density.
iii. *Pathologic features*
- Increased osteoid that is not calcified
- Loss of ossified bone spicules
- Remaining calcified spicules surrounded by prominent osteoclasts

(NOTE: Osteoclasts cannot remove non-calcified osteoid!).
iv. *Laboratory findings* include low serum calcium, phosphate, vitamin D, and elevated PTH and alkaline phosphatase.

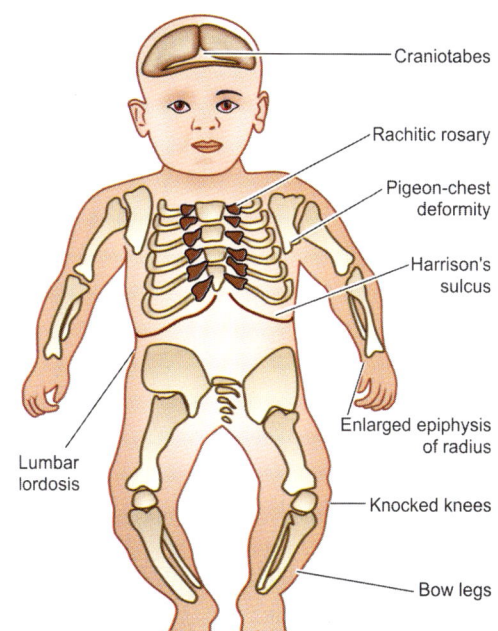

FIGURE 28.2: Lesions in rickets.

Q6. Comment briefly on osteitis fibrosa cystica.

Definition Osteitis fibrosa cystica is a bone complication of severe *primary hyperparathyroidism*.
Pathology There is osteoclastic resorption of cortical bone.
i. Subperiosteal resorption produces thin cortices and loss of the lamina dura around teeth. Histologically, osteoclasts move along the bone spicules and enlarge Haversian and Volkmann canals in a characteristic pattern.
ii. In the cancellous bone, osteoclasts dissect along the length of the trabeculae, producing *'dissecting osteitis'.*
iii. Concomitant repair causes filling of marrow spaces with fibrovascular tissue.
iv. Microfractures produce *cystic haemorrhagic foci,* which become infiltrated by macrophages and osteoclastic giant cells (also known as *'brown tumours of bone'*).
Clinical features Bone pain, haemorrhage, fibrosis, expansile bone lesions, and fractures.
Laboratory findings High serum PTH and serum calcium, low phosphate.
Prognosis Control of hyperparathyroidism leads to regression or resolution of the bony lesions.

Q7. What is renal osteodystrophy?

Definition Renal osteodystrophy is the name for the skeletal changes in *chronic renal failure* and patients who are on *dialysis*.
Bone changes are induced by a renal loss of calcium, retention of phosphate and deficient synthesis of active form of vitamin D in the kidney **(Fig. 28.3)**.
Pathology
- Increased osteoclastic activity → bone erosion and loss.
- Histology is variable; most often a combination of osteitis fibrosa cystic and osteomalacia, but may also have osteosclerosis with alternating with osteoporosis ('rugger or rugby jersey spine' seen on X-rays).

Laboratory findings include:
- Low serum calcium
- High phosphate with acidosis
- Low serum levels of 1,25 hydroxyvitamin D_3.

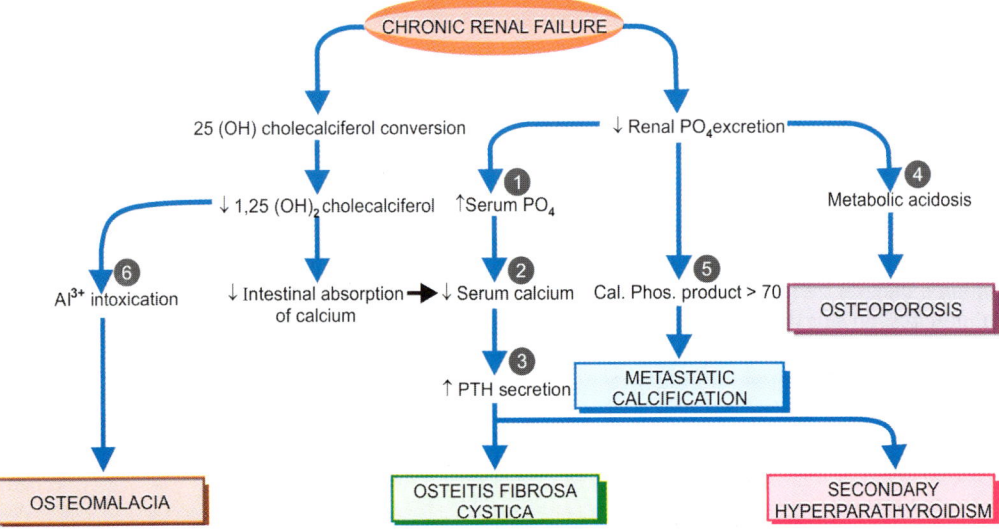

FIGURE 28.3: Pathogenesis of renal osteodystrophy in chronic renal failure.

Q8. What is Paget disease of the bone?

Definition Paget disease (or osteitis deformans) of the elderly (mean age is 60 years) is a disease of unknown etiology. It is characterised by excessive *osteoclastic bone resorption* followed by *reactive osteoblastic activity,* which typically outpaces bone resorption.

Pathology
- Three phases: osteolytic, osteolytic-osteoblastic, osteosclerotic end stage. Bone biopsy is diagnostic.
- Net gain in bone mass results in *multifocal osteosclerosis*.
- Coarsely thickened trabeculae with an appearance of a *'jigsaw puzzle'*.

Clinical presentation is highly variable. The disease is typically slowly progressive, characterised with nonspecific symptoms, and often may be even asymptomatic.

i. The most common symptom is *pain* due to microfractures and bone overgrowth compressing spinal and cranial nerve roots.
ii. *Hearing loss and increased head size* (hat does not fit!) are related to cranial bone thickening.
iii. *Postural deformities*, including inability to hold the head erect and anterior bowing of the long leg bones are common.
iv. *High output heart failure* due to high blood flow through the bones develops in long-standing disease.
v. *Late complications* Osteosarcomas occur at an increased rate.

Laboratory findings Serum alkaline phosphatase elevation may be the only positive findings (it is the most common cause of *isolated serum alkaline phosphatase elevation* in men over the age of 40 years).

Prognosis Calcitonin (which inhibits the lytic function of osteoclasts) and *bisphosphonates* (which promote the apoptosis of osteoclasts) are used in the treatment.

Q9. What are the most common forms of bone fractures?

Definition Fracture or bone break describes a loss of bone continuity due to the action of mechanical forces exceeding the capacity of the bone structure to withstand it.

Etiology
i. Most fractures are caused by *mechanical impact* of trauma, collision or bullet wound.
ii. *Stress fractures* are related to repeated strain or minor trauma (e.g. prolonged march and sports injuries)
iii. *Pathologic fracture* involves bones altered by an underlying disease such a bone tumours or osteomyelitis.

Clinicopathologic classification of fractures based on examination of the broken site and radiologic observations is as under:

i. *Complete simple fracture* with separation but no displacement of broken parts
ii. *Displaced complete fracture* showing misalignments of the broken parts
iii. *Incomplete fracture* showing X-ray line of fracture but no displacement of broken parts
iv. *Greenstick incomplete fracture* extending through only a part of the bone, typically in soft bones of infants and small children
v. *Comminuted fracture* containing numerous fragments of broken bone at the site of fracture
vi. *Compound open fracture* showing broken bone fragments sticking through the skin

Q10. Briefly discuss healing of fractures.

Bone fractures heal through the formation of *callus,* which passes sequentially through several phases as follows **(Fig. 28.4)**:

i. *Haematoma* filling the gap between the bone fragments.
ii. *Inflammation* in which granulation tissue forming the procallus (soft callus)—1 week.
iii. *Callus formation* marked by deposition of osteoid, cartilage and foci of endochondral ossification (2–3 days).
iv. *Remodeling* of woven bone which is replaced by lamellar bone, with final realignment of bone spicules with the preexisting bone spicules at the margins of the fracture.

Abnormal healing of fractures
i. *Delayed union* of fractured parts, usually due to inadequate immobilisation.
ii. *Pseudoarthrosis* due to cystic degeneration of the fracture site with formation of synovium lined false joint cavity.
iii. *Bone deformities* due to inappropriate alignment of fractured parts or formation of a hyperplastic callus.

Q11. What is osteonecrosis? Enumerate its causes and give its salient clinicopathologic presentations.

Definition Osteonecrosis is a bone infarct caused by ischaemia. Thus, this lesion is also called *avascular necrosis*.

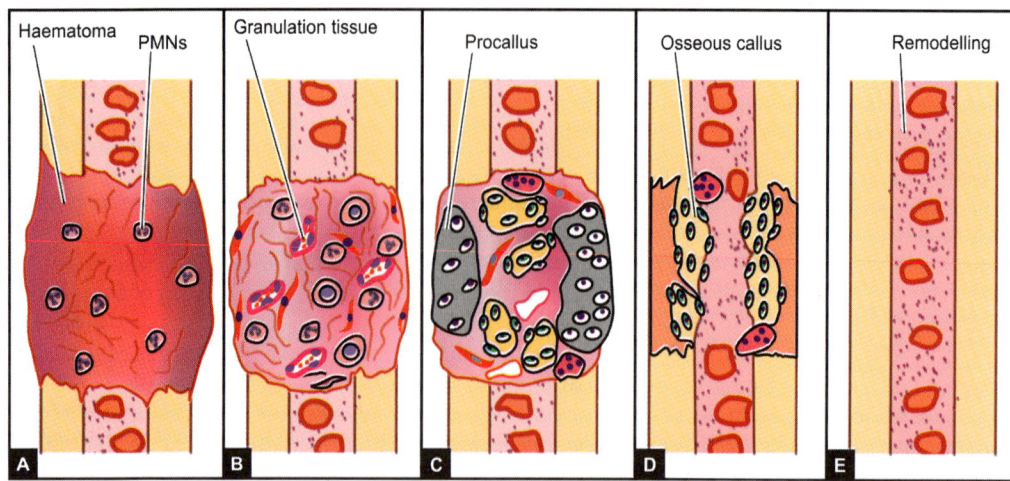

FIGURE 28.4: Fracture healing. A, Haematoma formation and local inflammatory response at the fracture site. B, Ingrowth of granulation tissue with formation of soft tissue callus. C, Formation of procallus composed of woven bone and cartilage with its characteristic fusiform appearance and having three arbitrary components—external, intermediate and internal callus. D, Formation of osseous callus composed of lamellar bone following clearance of woven bone and cartilage. E, Remodelled bone ends; the external callus cleared away. Intermediate callus converted into lamellar bone and internal callus developing bone marrow cavity.

Etiology Bone ischaemia may have many causes:
i. Fracture or dislocation
ii. Drugs, such as corticosteroids
iii. Radiation therapy
iv. Vascular trauma or injury
v. Chronic alcohol abuse
vi. Sickle cell anaemia
vii. Idiopathic (25%)

Pathology
i. There is ischaemic necrosis that affects trabecular bone of the medulla or subchondral bone in the epiphysis.
ii. Cortical bone is spared due to good periosteal blood flow.
iii. Medullary infarcts tend to heal by 'creeping substitution' of new bone formation.
iv. Subchondral infarcts tend to cause collapse of bone and cartilage and secondary osteoarthrosis.

Clinical features
i. Patients present with pain that may progress to osteoarthrosis.
ii. Any age group may be affected, but the peak is in 30–50 year persons.
iii. 10% of all hip replacement surgeries in the US are for osteonecrosis of the head of the femur.
iv. Idiopathic osteonecroses in children and adolescents often have clinical eponyms:
- Osteonecrosis of the head of the femur, typically found in 3- to 10-year-old boys, is known as *Legg-Calvé-Perthes disease*.
- Osteonecrosis of the epiphysial tubercle of the tibia is known as *Osgood-Schlatter disease*.

v. Medullary infarcts may be clinically inapparent and are discovered only accidentally during X-ray studies performed for some other reason.

Q12. What are the salient pathologic features and clinical manifestations of osteomyelitis? Also briefly comment on tuberculous osteomyelitis.

Definition Inflammation of the bone and bone marrow is called osteomyelitis. Most often, it is caused by purulent bacteria. It may be acute or chronic.

Routes of infection
i. *Haematogenous spread* typically through nutrient arteries, as seen in growing bones of children and adolescents. In such cases, tibia and fibula are most commonly infected bones.

- *Staphylococcus aureus* is responsible for 80–90% of cases.
- In children and adolescents affected by sickle cell disease, osteomyelitis is most often caused by *Salmonella paratyphi*.

ii. *Contiguous extension* from an adjacent site such as skin ulcers. This form of infection is polymicrobial. *Periapical dental abscess* of the maxilla or mandible is a common complication of caries and dental/peridental infection.

iii. *Direct implantation* of bacteria in gunshot wounds, trauma, or surgery. In general term, closed bone fractures are infected in less than 3% of cases in contrast to open fractures which are associated with osteomyelitis in over 30% cases. Infection is usually polymicrobial.

Pathology Features include purulent inflammation and reactive bone changes as under **(Fig. 28.5)**:

i. Histologic signs of *acute inflammation* (PMNs) or *chronic inflammation* (Pl, M0, Ly) or *repair* (fibroblasts, granulation tissue).
ii. Pus inside the abscess cavity in the bone, extending into the medulla and haversian canals.
iii. Pus may drain through sinuses to the adjacent tissue or externally through ulcerates skin.
iv. Inside the abscess, there are ischaemic necrotic bone fragments (*'sequestrum'*).
v. Granulation tissue and reactive new bone may surround the inflamed area (*'involucrum'*).
vi. Transition to chronic inflammation is marked by bone resorption, fibrosis, and deposition of reactive bone on the periphery. *Brodie abscess* is a bone abscess enclosed by sclerotic bone.

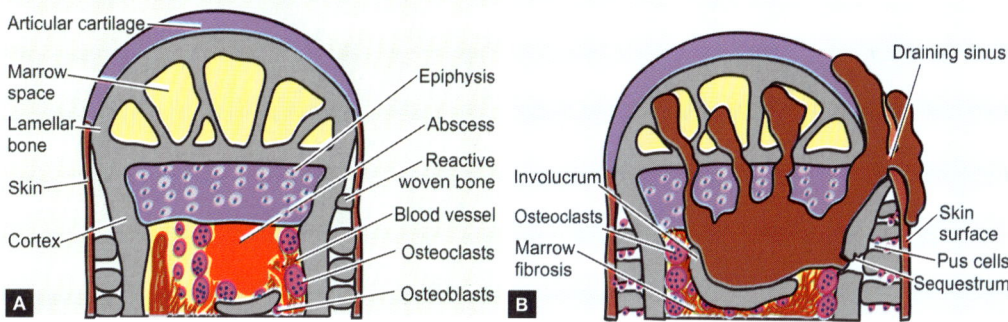

FIGURE 28.5: Pathogenesis and pathology of pyogenic osteomyelitis. A, The process begins as a focus of microabscess in a vascular loop in the marrow which expands to stimulate resorption of adjacent bony trabeculae. Simultaneously, there is beginning of reactive woven bone formation by the periosteum. B, The abscess expands further causing necrosis of the cortex called sequestrum. The formation of viable new reactive bone surrounding the sequestrum is called involucrum. The extension of infection into the joint space, epiphysis and the skin produces a draining sinus.

Clinical manifestations Findings depend on the duration of infection (acute or chronic):

i. *Local symptoms* predominate in acute haematogenous osteomyelitis which presents with bone pain, fever and local redness over the involved area.
ii. *Spread into soft tissue* may accentuate the pain and increase swelling of soft tissue.
iii. *Suppurative arthritis* due to a spread to the joints, usually in infants.
iv. *Systemic manifestations* present with fever, leucocytosis and exhaustion which signal the onset of *septicaemia*.

Treatment requires surgical drainage and antibiotics.

Tuberculous osteomyelitis Although not uncommon in developing countries of the world, it is rarely seen in developed countries. Tuberculous osteomyelitis usually affects the spinal bones (*spinal tuberculosis or Pott disease*).

- It results from bloodborne infection with dissemination of *M. tuberculosis*, most often from primary infection in lungs.
- Vertebral compression fractures lead to scoliosis or kyphosis ('hunch back').
- The bone lesions are usually solitary, but may be multiple in immunosuppressed AIDS patients.

Complications of osteomyelitis

i. *Septicaemia* due to the entry of bacteria into the blood with widespread dissemination is the most serious complication of acute suppurative osteomyelitis.
ii. *Acute arthritis* due to direct extension of bone infection, usually in small children.

iii. Pathologic fractures and bone deformities, usually in chronic cases.
iv. Squamous cell carcinoma of the overlying skin in chronic cases with draining pus.
v. Amyloidosis (AA type) related to chronic inflammation.
vi. Vertebral deformities, collapse and perivertebral or epidural spread of infection in tuberculous spinal tuberculosis.

Q13. Give a list of important tumour-like lesions of bone.

In bones, several non-neoplastic conditions resembling true neoplasms are encountered which require distinction from tumours clinically, radiologically and morphologically. A list of important examples is given in **Table 28.1**.

TABLE 28.1 Classification of tumour-like lesions of bone.

1. Fibrous dysplasia
2. Fibrous cortical defect (metaphyseal fibrous defect, non-ossifying fibroma)
3. Solitary bone cyst (simple or unicameral bone cyst)
4. Aneurysmal bone cyst
5. Ganglion cyst of bone (intraosseous ganglion)
6. Brown tumour of hyperparathyroidism (page 678)
7. Langerhans cell histiocytosis (LCH) (page 314)

Q14. Classify bone and cartilage tumours. Comment briefly on their general clinicopathologic features.

Classification Primary bone and cartilage tumours are classified into following groups based on the predominant cell, reflecting differentiation of the tumour and/or presumptive cell of origin **(Table 28.2, Fig. 28.6)**:

I. Bone-forming tumours
II. Cartilaginous tumours
III. Haematopoietic tumours
IV. Giant cell tumour
V. Tumours of undifferentiated cells
VI. Notochordal tumours

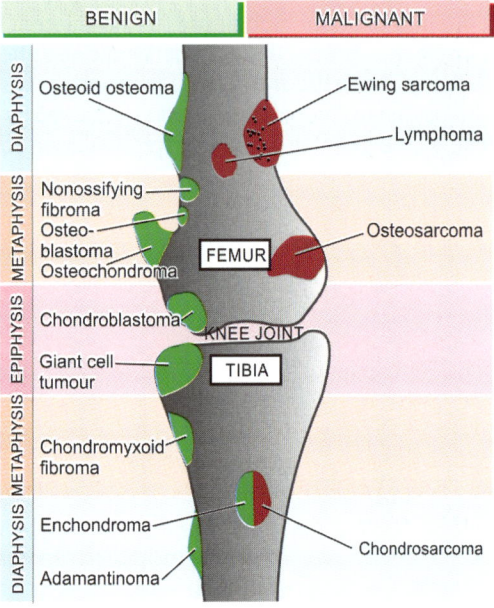

FIGURE 28.6: Anatomic locations of common primary bone and cartilage tumours.

TABLE 28.2 Major forms of benign and malignant tumours of bone and cartilage.

HISTOLOGIC DERIVATION	BENIGN	MALIGNANT
I. *Bone-forming* (osteogenic, osteoblastic) tumours	Osteoma (40–50 years) Osteoid osteoma (20–30 years) Osteoblastoma (20–30 years)	Conventional osteosarcoma (10–20 years) Surface osteosarcoma (50–60 years)
II. *Cartilage-forming* (chondrogenic) tumours	Enchondroma (20–50 years) Osteochondroma (20–50 years) (Osteocartilaginous exostosis) Chondroblastoma (10–20 years) Chondromyxoid fibroma (20–30 years)	Chondrosarcoma (40–60 years)
III. *Haematopoietic* (bone marrow) tumours	–	Myeloma (50–60 years) Malignant lymphoma (50–60 years)
IV. *Giant cell tumour*	Giant cell tumour (20–40 years) (osteoclastoma)	Malignancy in giant cell tumour (30–50 years)
V. *Tumours of undifferentiated cells*	–	Primitive neuroectodermal tumour (PNET)/Ewing's sarcoma (5–20 years)
VI. *Notochordal tumour*	–	Chordoma (40–50 years)

Figures in brackets indicate common age of occurrence.

General features
i. Primary bone tumours are rare; they can be benign or malignant.
ii. The most common malignant tumours of bones are *metastases* from other sites.
iii. The most common primary malignant bone tumour is *multiple myeloma* originating from haematopoietic bone marrow.
iv. The *diagnosis of bone tumours* is made by correlating the following sets of data:
- Clinical data (age and sex of the patient, anatomic location of the tumour).
- Radiologic findings (location of the tumour in the epiphysis, metaphysis or diaphysis of the bone), its shape, borders, signs of invasion.
- Pathologic elements (macroscopic and microscopic features of differentiation and malignancy, and additional molecular biology data in the case of some tumours).

Q15. Briefly describe salient clinicopathologic features of benign bone and cartilage tumours.

I. Osteoma
i. This is a rare benign bone tumour and most often localised to the facial bones.
ii. May be associated with colonic polyps in Gardner syndrome.

II. Osteoid osteoma and osteoblastoma
i. These closely related benign tumours are composed of bone trabeculae, which are interconnected randomly and lined by osteoblasts lying in a fibrovascular stroma.
ii. Males>females; 2:1, age group 20–30 years.
iii. Both tumours can be resected surgically; malignant transformation is very rare.
iv. *Osteoid osteomas* are typically small (less than 2 cm).
v. Located in the cortical subperiosteal part of long bones.
vi. X-ray shows a radiolucent nidus surrounded by reactive bone.
vii. Clinically accompanied by nocturnal pain which is relieved by aspirin.
viii. *Osteoblastomas* vary in size and shape; usually bigger than osteoid osteoma.
ix. Located in the medulla; most often in the vertebrae, pelvic bones or ribs.
x. Less often located in metaphysis of long bones.

III. Osteochondroma (Osteocartilaginous exostoses)
i. The most common benign bone tumour.
ii. Located at the lateral side of the growth plate of the metaphysic.
iii. Distal metaphysis of femur the most common location (70%).
iv. Males>females; age group 20–50 years.

IV. Chondroma
i. A benign tumour composed of cartilage cells.
ii. Enchondroma is synonym for intraosseous tumour.
iii. Most tumours are diagnosed in the 20–50 years age group.
iv. Tubular bones of hand and feet are the most common site.
v. In short bones of extremities, almost always benign.
vi. Chondromas may be solitary or multiple; the latter called 'enchondromatosis'.
vii. *Enchondromatosis* may be a feature of congenital syndromes (Mafucci syndrome or Ollier disease).
viii. Multiple enchondromas may become malignant.

V. Giant cell tumour
A benign, but locally aggressive tumour that often recurs after incomplete curettage.
Location Most often, epiphysis and metaphysis of distal femur and proximal tibia, i.e. around the knee.
Age and sex Adults 20–40 years; male = female.
Pathology (Fig. 28.7)
Gross Solitary cystic, dark red brown on cross section.
Microscopy
i. Tumour composed of spindle-shaped mononuclear cells admixed with osteoclasttype giant cells; hence the synonym 'osteoclastoma' for this tumour.
ii. Interspersed in the tumour are areas of haemorrhage, haemosiderin deposition, and reactive bony trabeculae.

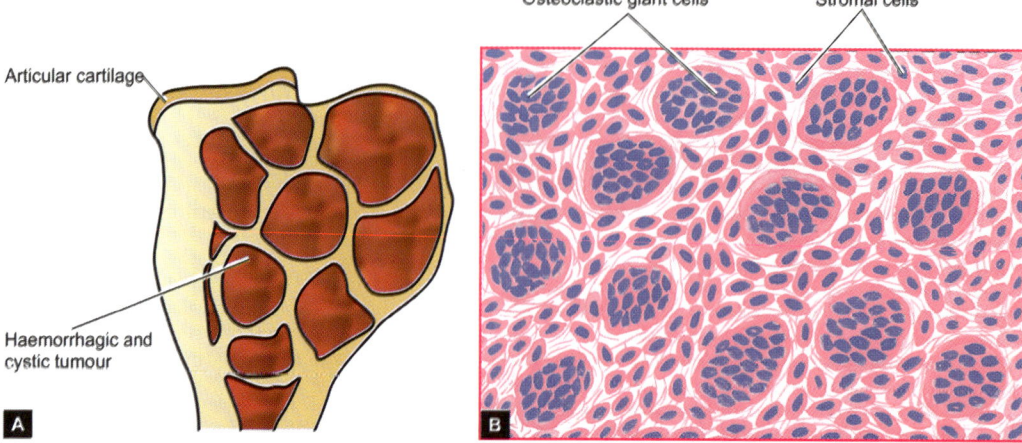

FIGURE 28.7: Giant cell tumour (osteoclastoma). A. The end of the long bone is expanded in the region of epiphysis. Sectioned surface shows circumscribed, dark tan, haemorrhagic and necrotic tumour. B, Microscopy reveals osteoclast-like multinucleate giant cells which are regularly distributed among the mononuclear stromal cells.

Clinical features
i. Bone pain is the most common symptom.
ii. Joint pain may be prominent (due to epiphyseal location).
iii. Expansile mass (may be palpable) and may have pathologic fractures.
iv. X-rays show large lytic lesions (described as 'soap-bubble'), may erode into subchondral bone

Prognosis
- Benign but frequently recur if incompletely removed by curettage.
- Malignant change uncommon (<5%).

Q16. Discuss salient clinical and pathologic features of osteosarcoma of bone.

Definition Osteosarcoma is a malignant neoplasm of osteoblasts forming bone matrix. It is the most common malignant primary bone tumour (20% of primary bone malignancies).

Location Metaphysis of growing long bones, most often around the knee (distal femur and proximal tibia and fibula).

Age and risk factors
i. 10–20 years, males>>females.
ii. Most osteosarcomas are spontaneous tumours arising in peripubertal males with no known risk factors.
iii. Tumour cells harbour many gene mutations, most often *RB* and *TP53*.
iv. *Secondary osteosarcomas* are tumours arising in context of identifiable risk factors such as:
- Preexistent retinoblastoma (with RB1 gene deletion/inactivation).
- Radiation therapy or exposure to radioactive materials.
- Chondrosarcoma that has dedifferentiated into high-grade osteosarcoma.
- Paget disease of bones in older patients.

Pathology (Fig. 28.8)
Gross
i. These tumours are tan-white and gritty with haemorrhage and necrosis.
ii. The tumour spreads in the medullary cavity, destroys the normal bone and extends into adjacent soft tissue.

Microscopy
i. The tumour is composed of *spindle-shaped osteoblasts producing osteoid or calcified bone spicules.*
ii. Necrosis and mitotic activity are prominent.

Clinical features
i. The tumour presents most often as a painful, enlarging bone mass.
ii. Pathologic fractures may be a presenting sign, but less often.

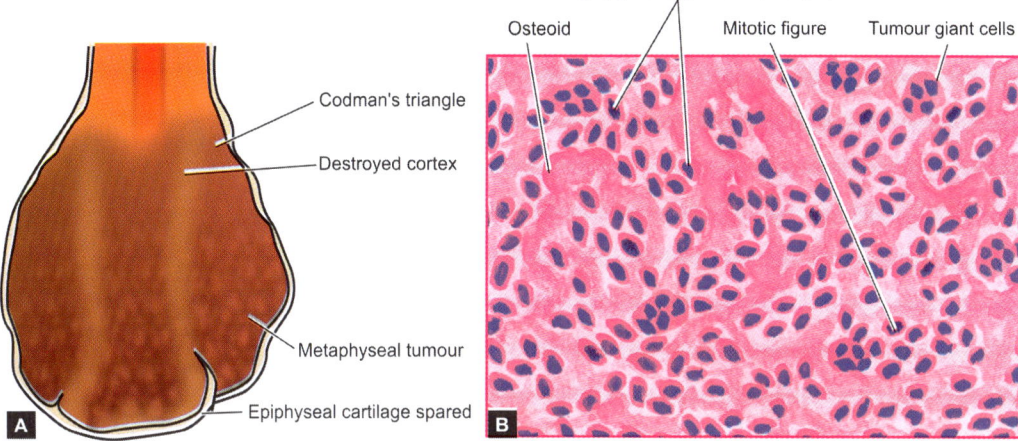

FIGURE 28.8: Osteosarcoma. A, The lower end of the femur shows a bulky expanded tumour in the region of metaphysis sparing the epiphyseal cartilage. Sectioned surface of the tumour shows lifting of the periosteum by the tumour and eroded cortical bone. The tumour is grey-white with areas of haemorrhage and necrosis. B, Hallmarks of microscopic picture of the usual osteosarcoma are the sarcoma cells characterised by variation in size and shape of tumour cells, bizarre mitosis and multinucleate tumour giant cells, and osteogenesis, i.e. production of osteoid matrix and bone directly by the tumour cells.

iii. *X-rays:* Destructive lytic metaphyseal mass with focal signs of new bone formation ('sunburst pattern of radiating bone spicules extending into the soft tissue').
- Tends to break through the cortex lifting the periosteum *(Codman triangle)*.
- Extends into the medulla, has indistinct borders.

iv. *Metastases:* Haematogenous to lungs, and elsewhere.

v. *Prognosis:* With modern chemotherapy combined with radiation therapy and surgery the long-term survival rate of patients without metastases is approximately 60–70%.

Variant forms of osteosarcoma are uncommon (<5%):
i. Originate from the external surface of long bones of middle-aged men
ii. Classified as *parosteal (juxtacortical)* or *periosteal osteosarcomas*.
iii. These tumours tend to grow slower than the classical osteosarcoma and thus have a better prognosis.

Q17. Discuss briefly clinical and pathologic features of chondrosarcoma of bone.

Definition Chondrosarcomas are malignant neoplasms of chondroblasts, i.e. cartilage cells.

Age and risk factors
- Middle aged or older males (M:F = 3:1), 40–60 years of age.
- Most have no risk factors, but some occur in preexisting enchondromatosis syndromes.

Location
- Most often, centrally located (i.e. pelvis, shoulder, ribs and vertebrae).
- Sometimes, may also arise in the medullary cavity of humerus and femur.

Pathology

Gross The tumour is lobulated or nodular, grey-white, and translucent on sectioning.

Microscopy **(Fig. 28.9)**
i. The tumour is composed of malignant cartilage cells.
ii. Hypercellular lobules and cords of cells infiltrate marrow spaces and destroy bone trabeculae.
iii. Cellularity varies depending on the grade of the tumour.

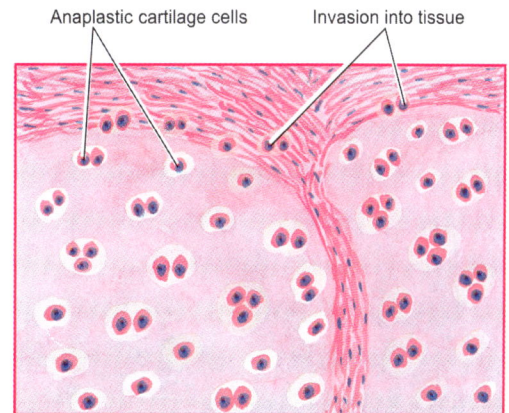

FIGURE 28.9: Chondrosarcoma. High-grade tumour shows increased cellularity, marked cytologic atypia and mitoses.

iv. The grading of tumour (I–III) has clinical significance.
v. Some chondrosarcomas dedifferentiate into highly malignant osteosarcoma or undifferentiated pleomorphic sarcoma (UPS), which has a very poor prognosis.

Clinical features
i. Pain and signs of compression due to local effects of the enlarging tumour mass.
ii. Tumours >10 cm are more aggressive and tend to metastasise to the lungs more often than smaller tumours.
iii. Metastases in high-grade tumours, usually to the lungs.

Prognosis
- Low grade tumours may be curable by surgery alone (5-year survival 75%).
- High-grade and large masses difficult to treat (5-year survival 40%).
- All chondrosarcomas unresponsive to chemotherapy.
- Most unresectable tumours show relatively slow progression to metastases and death.

Q18. What is Ewing sarcoma? Discuss its salient clinical and pathologic features.

Definition Ewing sarcoma is the name given to:
i. a family of bone and soft tissue malignant tumours,
ii. composed of undifferentiated small round cells,
iii. showing signs of neuroectodermal differentiation,
iv. with a unique diagnostic molecular signature.

Age and risk factors
i. Most common sarcoma of bones and soft tissues in children under 10 years.
ii. Peak incidence in the 10–15 years age group, but may occur in younger children and adults up to 35 years of age.
iii. Males>>females.
iv. Caucasians affected more than other races.
v. No risk factors recognised.

Location Pelvic girdle, ribs, diaphysis of long bones.

Pathology Three forms are recognised:
i. Ewing sarcoma of bone (75%)
ii. Extraosseous Ewing sarcoma of soft tissues (20%)
iii. Primitive neuroendocrine tumour (PNET) (5%)

Ewing sarcoma of bones
i. The most common form of this tumour.
ii. Tumour arises in the *medullary cavity*.
iii. Tumour cells invade cortical bone, producing a layer of periosteal reaction.
iv. Extension into soft tissue due to rapid growth.
v. Early metastases to lungs and other bones.
vi. *Histology* **(Fig. 28.10):**
- Small round cells, arranged in sheets with areas of necrosis and haemorrhages.

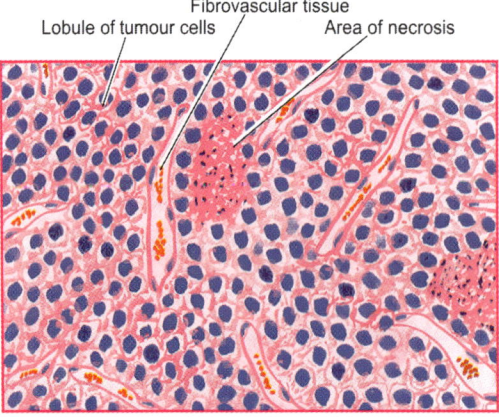

FIGURE 28.10: Ewing sarcoma. Characteristic microscopic features are irregular lobules of uniform small tumour cells with indistinct cytoplasmic outlines which are separated by fibrous tissue septa having rich vascularity. Areas of necrosis and inflammatory infiltrate are also included.

- The stroma is scanty.

vii. *Molecular biology:* Diagnostic cytogenetic changes of the *ESWR1* and *FLI1* gene in 85% of all cases.

Clinical features

i. Symptoms local but may also be systemic.
ii. Enlarging bone mass that is tender or painful and warm.
iii. *Systemic signs* such as fever, leucocytosis, increased sedimentation rate, and anaemia.
iv. *X-rays:* Lytic invasion of cortical bone with a characteristic 'onion skin' periosteal reaction and formation of concentric layers of reactive bone.

Prognosis Current treatment is based on a combination of surgery, chemotherapy, and radiation therapy. A 75% 5-year cure rate and a 50% long-term cure rate can be achieved.

Q19. Comment on common features of metastatic bone tumours.

i. Metastatic tumours from other sites represent the *most common* form of malignancy in the skeleton.
ii. Usually multiple, but may also be solitary.
iii. Tend to preferentially involve *axial skeleton*, such as vertebrae, humerus and femur.
iv. Route of entry into the bones: Haemotogenous and lymphatic or direct local invasion.
v. X-rays: *May be osteolytic or osteoblastic (sclerotic):*
- Lytic lesions are associated with hypercalcaemia.
- Osteoblastic lesions are associated with elevated serum alkaline phosphatase levels, a marker of osteoblastic proliferation.

vi. *Most common primary cancers* in adults are in the breast, prostate, lungs, kidneys.
vii. *In children*, bone metastases are a common feature of neuroblastoma, Wilms tumour or rhabdomyosarcoma.
viii. Multiple bone lesions of Ewing sarcoma represent either metastases or multifocal primary tumours, originating simultaneously.

JOINTS

Q20. What is the most important degenerative joint disease? Briefly discuss its pathology and clinical manifestations.

Definition Osteoarthritis (OA), also known as degenerative joint disease (DJD), is characterised by erosion of articular cartilage and reactive changes in the adjacent bone. It may be primary or secondary.

Etiology
- *Primary (idiopathic) OA*, is due to incompletely understood intrinsic alterations in the cartilage favouring its breakdown.
- *Secondary OA* is linked to some underlying cause such as traumatic injury, congenital joint and bone malformations, or diabetes.

Pathology (Fig. 28.11)

i. Fraying and erosion of articular cartilage and reactive bone changes.
ii. Focal loss of articular cartilage, exposing the bone to undue pressure.
iii. Dislodged cartilage and bone detach and float in the joint space as free or loose bodies ('joint mice').
iv. Reactive changes in the underlying bone include osteosclerosis, fibrosis, and cysts.
v. *Osteophytes* (bone spurs) develop at the margins of the articular surfaces.

Clinical manifestations

i. Primary osteoarthritis is a disease of the elderly.
ii. *Common symptoms:* deep aching pain, stiffness, crepitus, and limitation of movement.
iii. *Location:*
- Weightbearing large joints such as hips, knees.

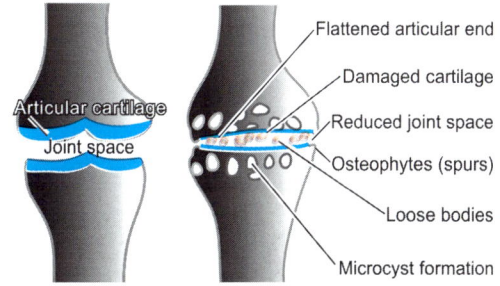

FIGURE 28.11: Fully-developed lesions in osteoarthritis (B), contrasted with appearance of a normal joint (A).

- Lower lumbar and cervical vertebrae are commonly affected.
- Distal interphalangeal joints of the fingers show osteophytes (*Heberden nodules*).
- Distal carpo-metacarpal joints and first tarso-metatarsal joints of the feet with deformities.

Treatment There is no medical treatment for osteoarthritis.

Severe incapacitating joint lesions must be replaced by artificial joints made of metal or other material.

Q21. Enumerate important inflammatory joint diseases.

Inflammatory disorders of joints may be of following types:

i. Immune-mediated (rheumatoid arthritis, SLE, reactive arthritis in rheumatic fever, etc.)
ii. Infectious (various microbes, e.g. gonococci, *M. tuberculosis*)
iii. Crystal-induced (e.g. gout) arthritis
iv. Others: These include pigmented villonodular tenosynovitis, bursal cysts, ganglion are other inflammatory synovial conditions.

Q22. Briefly discuss pathogenesis and clinicopathologic features of rheumatoid arthritis.

Definition Rheumatoid arthritis (RA) is a chronic autoimmune multisystemic inflammatory disorder of unknown etiology that initially affects peripheral joints of hands and feet. It may involve many other tissues and organs such as skin, blood vessels, heart, lungs, and muscle.

Pathogenesis Not fully known (Fig. 28.12):
i. Most patients (90%) have IgM autoantibodies (RF, rheumatoid factor) reacting with their own IgG, which points to the immune nature of the disease.
ii. Joint surface covered with deposits of RF and IgG in form of immune complexes.
iii. Genetic susceptibility (the majority of patients are HLADR4 or DR1) may be important.
iv. The role of infectious agents (e.g. Epstein-Barr virus) has been explored but not proven.

Pathology The predominant pathologic lesions are found in the joints and tendons, and in advanced cases, extra-articular manifestations are encountered.

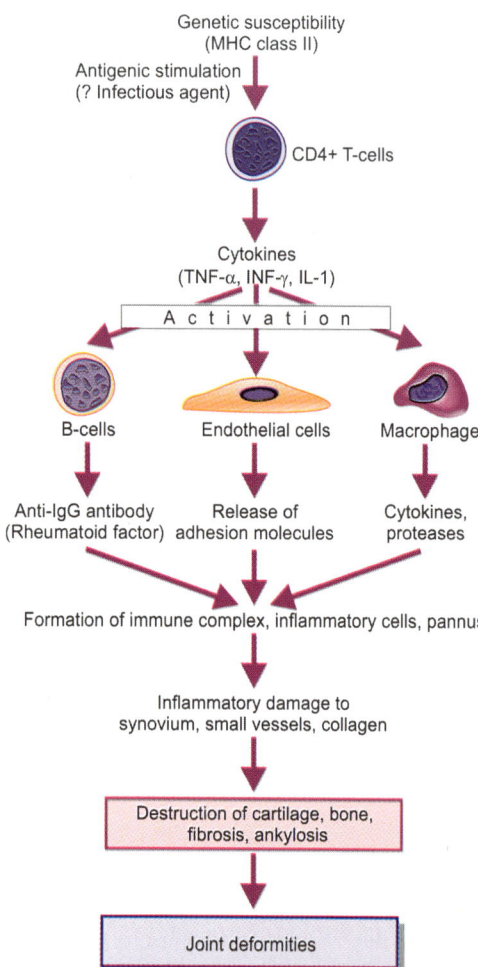

FIGURE 28.12: Pathogenesis of rheumatoid arthritis.

I. ***Articular lesions*** (Fig. 28.13)
i. Joint synovial membranes are oedematous and infiltrated by lymphoid follicles (primarily helper T cells), plasma cells, and macrophages.
ii. The inflamed tissue forms a cover over the joint surface *(pannus)*.
iii. Inflammatory cells in the pannus act on cartilage causing its erosion.
iv. Mediators released during this process stimulate bone and cause periarticular *osteoporosis*.
v. Healing of inflammation with fibrous scarring leads to immobilisation of joints and bony *ankylosis* with obliteration of the articular space reducing joint mobility.

II. ***Extra-articular manifestations*** of RA are found at a variable rate. These are:
i. Anaemia of chronic disease
ii. Carpal tunnel syndrome
iii. Cervical spine subluxation

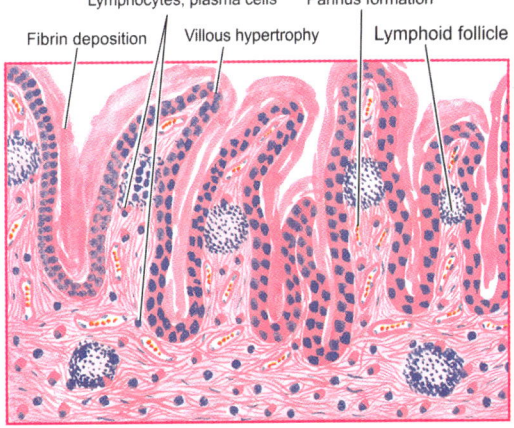

FIGURE 28.13: Rheumatoid arthritis. The characteristic histologic features are villous hypertrophy of the synovium and marked mononuclear inflammatory cell infiltrate in synovial membrane with formation of lymphoid follicles at places.

iv. *Rheumatoid nodules* (fibrinoid necrosis surrounded by epithelioid cells) are noted in the skin in the regions subjected to pressure, such as the ulnar aspect of the forearm, elbow, and occiput.

v. *Rheumatoid lung disease* may present with pleural effusion and pleuritis, interstitial fibrosis and in severe cases by bronchiolitis obliterans.

vi. *Rheumatoid vasculitis* is observed in severe cases resistant to treatment. It may be accompanied by skin ulcers, gangrene, and even neuropathy.

Clinical features
i. The onset has a peak between 25–50 years. Female:male = 3:1
ii. Involved joints are hot, swollen, and stiff.
iii. Small joints such as metacarpophalangeal and proximal interphalangeal joints are involved.
iv. Later in the course, larger joints become affected.
v. Because of the destructive nature of the disease, various *deformities* are observed. Deformities of hands include:
a. radial deviation of the wrist,
b. ulnar deviation of the fingers, and
c. flexion hyperextension abnormalities of the fingers, which are referred to as *swan neck* or *boutonnière* deformities.

Diagnosis It is s based on *any four* of the following observations:
i. Morning stiffness
ii. Arthritis in three or more joints
iii. Arthritis of hand joints
iv. Symmetric arthritis
v. Rheumatoid nodules
vi. Serum rheumatoid factor (positive in 70–90%)
vii. Anti-cyclic citrullinated peptide (anti-CCP) with a specificity of 95% and sensitivity of 75%
viii. Typical radiographic findings

Prognosis Variable.
- 70%, RA has a chronic course requiring symptomatic treatment and use of anti-inflammatory drugs
- 20%, RA have a limited course
- 10%, RA is associated with incapacitating deformities.

Q23. Briefly discuss various infectious diseases of joints (infectious arthritis).

Infections reach the joints by blood or by direct inoculation and extension from adjacent structures.

Etiology Pathogens causing arthritis include:
i. Bacteria (e.g. *Staphylococcus aureus* and *Neisseria gonorrhoeae*)
ii. Mycoplasma (e.g. *Mycoplasma pneumoniae*)
iii. Viruses (e.g. *Parvovirus B19* and *Hepatitis B virus*)
iv. Spirochetes (e.g. *Borrelia burgdoferi*)

Types of arthritis
I. *Suppurative arthritis:*
i. Like osteomyelitis, arthritis in older children and adults is most commonly caused by *S. aureus*.
ii. In infants and children under the age of 2 year, *Haemophilus influenzae* is the most common pathogen.
iii. The joint cavity contains pus and shows pathologic and clinical signs of acute inflammation.
II. *Gonococcal arthritis:*
i. It is a complication of haematogenous spread of sexually-transmitted gonorrhoea, most often involving women.
ii. The large joints are most frequently involved.
iii. Clinically, the joints are hot and swollen, and there is fever and leucocytosis.
iv. Destruction of articular cartilage and spread to the bones may occur in inadequately treated cases.
III. *Lyme disease arthritis:*
i. It is caused by *Borrelia burgdorferi*, a spirochetal disease transmitted by the bite of *Ixodes* tick.
ii. *Location:* Knees (the most common site), shoulders, elbows, and ankles are typically involved in a fleeting (migratory) manner.
iii. *Histologically*, the synovial membranes of the joints are infiltrated with CD4+ T helper lymphocytes and show concentric thickening of arteriolar walls.
iv. *Clinically,* arthritis usually appears weeks or months after the tick bite or the appearance of the initial *erythema migrans*.
v. Attacks can last for weeks to months.
vi. *Laboratory findings*: The clinical diagnosis is confirmed by an enzyme-linked immunosorbent assay (ELISA) test to *Borrelia burgdorferi*.

Q24. What is gout? Briefly discuss its pathogenesis and clinicopathologic features.

Definition Gout is a multisystemic disease that results from disturbances of purine metabolism presenting with *hyperuricaemia* and deposition of *uric acid crystals* in tissues.
Classification Gout is classified based on pathogenesis into two types:
- *Primary gout* in which pathogenesis is not fully understood, and accounts for approximately 90% of cases.
- *Secondary gout* includes metabolic disorders such as Lesch Nyhan syndrome, chronic renal disease, and other conditions marked by hyperuricaemia for gout.

Pathogenesis Sequential events in gout are caused by uric acid deposition:
i. Crystals of uric acid cause first acute neutrophil-dominated inflammation of the joint, most often first tarso-metatarsal joint of the big toe *(acute transient arthritis)*.
ii. Acute inflammation transforms into chronic granulomatous reaction *(chronic arthritis)*.
iii. Uric acid deposits form urate masses *(tophi)* in the joints and other sites.
iv. Deposits of *urates in kidneys* may lead to renal injury.

Pathology Four distinct lesions are typical of gout:
i. Acute arthritis
ii. Chronic tophaceous arthritis
iii. Tophi in a variety of locations
iv. Gouty nephropathy

i. *Acute arthritis,* most often involving the *first tarsometatarsal joint,* is marked by infiltration of the joint by neutrophils in response to deposits of monosodium urate crystals in the synovium.
ii. *Chronic tophaceous arthritis* results from repetitive urate crystal deposition during acute attacks. The synovium becomes hyperplastic, fibrotic, and thickened, forming a pannus that, together with the tophaceous nodules, destroys the underlying cartilage and erodes the bone. In severe cases, the joints show deformities and ankylosis.
iii. *Tophi* are nodules composed of sodium urate crystals surrounded by mononuclear inflammatory cells, and foreign body giant cells **(Fig. 28.14)**. Tophi are found in the joints, ligaments, tendons, and subcutaneous soft tissues such as the earlobes.

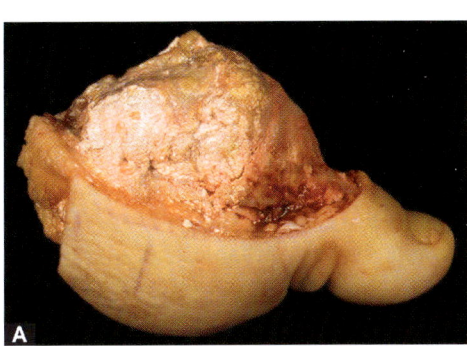
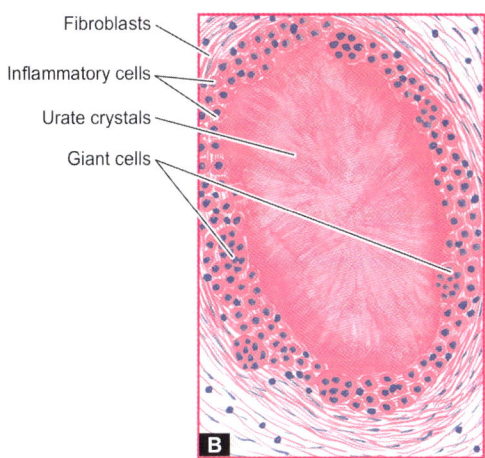

FIGURE 28.14: A, Gouty nodule involving big toe. B, Gouty tophus, showing central aggregates of urate crystals surrounded by inflammatory cells, fibroblasts and occasional giant cells.

iv. *Gouty nephropathy* results from the deposition of monosodium urate crystals, and sometimes tophi, in the tubules (causing obstruction), in the interstitium of the kidneys causing progressive renal insufficiency and urate urolithiasis. *Urate stones* formed in the renal pelvis may cause urinary obstruction and predispose to pyelonephritis.

Clinical manifestations There are four stages of gout:
- Asymptomatic uricaemia
- Acute gouty arthritis
- Intercritical gout
- Chronic tophaceous gout

i. The first attack usually occurs 20 to 30 years after the onset of hyperuricaemia.
ii. The metatarsophalangeal joints are most often affected (most commonly big toe).
iii. Attacks present as excruciating pain with sudden onset, hyperaemia, warmth, and severe tenderness.
iv. Drugs such as colchicine are effective for treatment of acute attacks.
v. Long-term treatment is directed at the reduction of uric acid deposits.

NOTE: *Pseudogout* is a rare cause of arthropathy that needs to be distinguished from gout:
i. Pseudogout is caused by deposition of calcium pyrophosphate crystals in joints.
ii. Its pathogenesis is not understood.
iii. Several metabolic diseases predispose to pseudogout.
iv. Big toe joints are not involved and the symptoms are generally less severe than in gout.

Q25. What are the tumours and tumour-like lesions of joints?

I. **Tumours of the joints** are exceptionally rare:
i. *Pigmented villonodular synovitis* is the most common benign neoplastic proliferation of synovial cells.
ii. Despite its name, this is a tumour and not an inflammatory lesion.
iii. It is characterised by reddish-brown, fingerlike protrusions of synovium that fill the articular cavity. The colour of the lesion stems from extravasated blood that is taken up and stored as haemosiderin in phagocytic cells.

II. **Tumour-like lesion** of the synovium is a *cyst of ganglion*:
i. A ganglion is a small, round or ovoid, movable, subcutaneous cystic swelling of synovium.
ii. The most common location is dorsum of wrist but may be found on the dorsal surface of foot near the ankle.
iv. Histogenetically, it may be the result of herniated synovium, or post-traumatic degeneration of connective tissue.

SKELETAL MUSCLES

Q26. What are muscular dystrophies and their types? Enumerate the investigations done to arrive at their diagnosis.

Definition and classification Muscular dystrophies are a group of genetically-inherited primary muscle diseases, having in common, progressive and unremitting muscular weakness.
- Eight forms of muscular dystrophies are described: *Duchenne, Becker, myotonic, facio-scapulohumeral, limb-girdle, Emery-Dreifuss, congenital and oculopharyngeal type*.
- Each type of muscular dystrophy is a distinct entity having differences in inheritance pattern, age at onset, defective gene or protein, clinical features, other organ system involvements and clinical course.
- In general, muscular dystrophies manifest in childhood or in early adulthood.

A summary of salient features of various muscular dystrophies is given in **Table 28.3**.

Investigations Limited investigations are done in a suspected case of myopathy as follows:

i. *Serum enzyme determinations* Most commonly determined is creatine kinase, CK-MM isoenzyme, which is elevated (CK-MB is myocardial bound and is raised in cardiac muscle diseases). Other enzymes which may be raised in myopathies are AST, ALT and LDH.

ii. *Electrodiagnostic studies* These include EMG, nerve stimulation and nerve conduction studies.

iii. *Molecular studies* DNA analysis is currently performed, whenever possible, to establish the definitive diagnosis.

iv. *Muscle biopsy* All cases without an identifiable genetic defect, biopsy from a skeletal muscle (most often quadriceps, biceps or deltoid) remains the most important diagnostic test. The biopsy is subjected to various studies: light microscopy, histochemistry, immunohistochemistry, and electron microscopy.

On light microscopy, common to all forms of muscular dystrophies are muscle fibre necrosis, regenerative activity, replacement by interstitial fibrosis and adipose tissue **(Fig. 28.15)**.

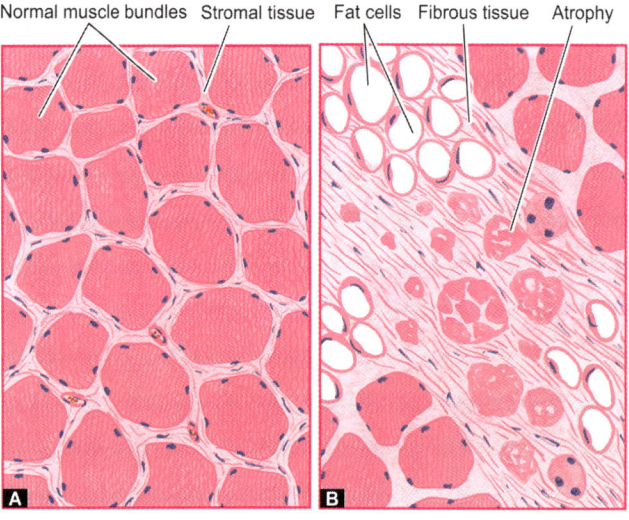

FIGURE 28.15: Normal skeletal muscle (A) contrasted with findings in Duchenne muscular dystrophy (B) showing hyaline fibres, fibre degeneration, loss of fibres and replacement by interstitial fibrosis and adipose tissue.

Q27. What is myasthenia gravis? Briefly discuss its pathogenesis and investigations.

Definition Myasthenia gravis (MG) is a neuromuscular disorder of autoimmune origin in which the acetylcholine receptors (AChRs) in the motor end-plates of the muscles are damaged due to antibody-mediated immune attack and thus the number of AChRs is reduced. The term *'myasthenia'* means 'muscular weakness' and *'gravis'* implies 'serious'; thus both together denote the clinical characteristics of the disease.

Clinical features
i. At any age but adult women affected more often than adult men, F:M ratio 3:2.
ii. Presents with muscular weakness and fatiguability, initially in the ocular musculature but later spreads to involve the trunk and limbs.

TABLE 28.3 Salient features of muscular dystrophies.

TYPE	INHERITANCE	DEFECTIVE GENE/PROTEIN	AGE AT ONSET	CLINICAL FEATURES	OTHER SYSTEMS INVOLVED	COURSE
1. Duchenne	X-linked recessive	Dystrophin	By age 5	Symmetric weakness; initially pelvifemoral; later weakness of girdle muscles; respiratory muscle failure by 2nd to 3rd decade, pseudo-hypertrophy of calf muscles	Cardiomegaly; reduced intelligence	Progressive; death by age 20 due to respiratory failure
2. Becker	X-linked recessive	Dystrophin	Early childhood to adult	Slow progressive weakness of girdle muscle (minor variant of Duchenne's type)	Cardiomegaly	Benign
3. Myotonic (DM1, DM2)	Autosomal dominant	DM1: expansion CTG repeat DM2: Expansion CCTG repeat	Childhood to adult	Slow progressive weakness and myotonia of eyelids, face, neck, foot; progressive proximal weakness in DM2	Cardiac conduction defects; mental impairment; cataracts; frontal baldness; gonadal atrophy	Benign
4. Facioscapulo-humeral (D1, D2)	Autosomal dominant	D1: DUX4 4q D2: SMChD1	2nd-4th decade	Slowly progressive weakness of facial, shoulder and foot muscles	Deafness	Benign
5. Limb-girdle	Autosomal dominant/recessive	Multiple (myotilin, lamin, calpain-3, dysferlin)	Early childhood to adult	Slowly progressive weakness of shoulder and hip girdle muscles	Cardiomyopathy	Variable progression
6. Emery-Dreifuss	Autosomal dominant/recessive	Emerin, lamin	Childhood to adult	Humeral and peroneal weakness; contractures of elbow, knee, ankle	Cardiomegaly	Progressive if cardiomyopathy present
7. Congenital	Autosomal recessive	Multiple (laminin α2 chain, fukulin-related protein)	At birth, or within a few months	Delayed milestones, hypotonia, contractures	CNS anomalies, ocular abnormalities	Progressive
8. Oculo-pharyngeal	Autosomal dominant	Expansion, polyARNA binding protein	5th-6th decade	Slowly progressive weakness of extraocular, face, pharyngeal and limb muscles	—	Rarely progressive

iii. Other autoimmune diseases association, e.g. autoimmune thyroiditis, rheumatoid arthritis, SLE, pernicious anaemia and collagen-vascular diseases.

iv. About 10% mortality in MG due to severe generalised disease and involvement of respiratory muscles.

Pathogenesis (Fig. 28.16)

i. *Normally,* acetylcholine is synthesised in the motor nerve terminal and stored in vesicles that are released spontaneously when an action potential reaches the nerve terminal. Acetylcholine from released vesicles combines with AChRs, initiating an action potential which is propagated along the muscle fibre triggering muscle contraction.

ii. *In MG,* the basic defect is reduced number of available AChRs at the postsynaptic muscle membrane and flattening of postsynaptic folds. These changes result in decreased neuromuscular transmission leading to failure to trigger muscle action potentials and consequent weakened muscle contraction.

- The neuromuscular abnormalities in MG are mediated by autoimmune response.
- About 85% patients of MG have anti-AChR-antibodies in their sera. These antibodies reduce the number of available AChRs either by blocking the active sites of the receptors or by damaging the post-synaptic muscle membrane in collaboration with complement. The remaining 15% of patients have autoantibodies to muscle specific receptor tyrosine kinase.
- Approximately 40% MG patients have thymic abnormalities, either thymoma (10%) or thymic hyperplasia with appearance of B-cell follicle in the thymus (30%). Thymic pathology is most often found in younger patients and in such cases thymectomy is helpful in ameliorating the muscle symptoms.

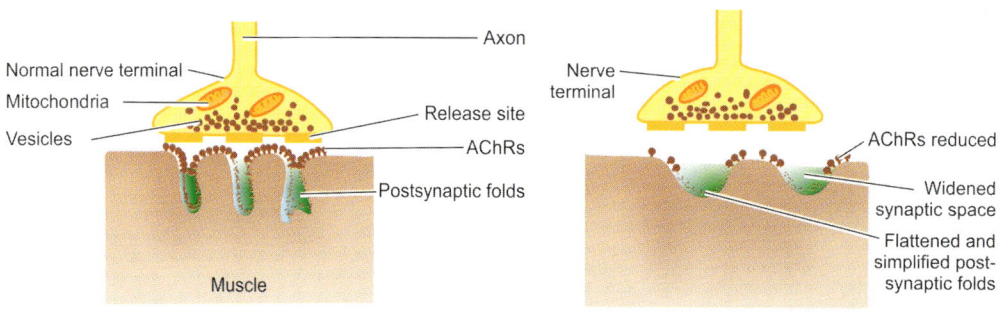

FIGURE 28.16: Neuromuscular junction in normal transmission (A) and in myasthenia gravis (B). The junction in MG shows reduced number of AChRs, flattened and simplified postsynaptic folds, a widened synaptic space but a normal nerve terminal.

Chapter 28e Supplement: Online Content

Digital content of this chapter available with this book is meant for enhanced learning and self-assessment. In addition, it contains 22 Multiple Choice Questions (MCQs), 05 Clinicopathologic Vignettes, and 05 Image-based Questions; these are followed by their answers along with explanatory notes of correct and incorrect answers.

CHAPTER 29

Soft Tissue Tumours

GENERAL FEATURES

Q1. Comment on classification of soft tissue tumours based on histogenesis.
- Most soft tissue tumours are composed of neoplastic cells resembling those normally found in soft tissues. Most of these cells are of mesenchymal origin and include: adipocytes, fibroblasts and myofibroblasts, fibrohistiocytic cells, smooth muscle, vessels and perivascular tissue.
- The group also includes tumours derived from peripheral nerve sheath cells which are of ectodermal origin (neurofibroblasts, Schwann cells and perineural cells), and precursors of skeletal muscle cells (rhabdomyoblasts).
- In addition, it is customary to include in this group, tumours composed of 'not so soft' bone-forming cells (osteoblasts, osteocytes, and chondroblasts, chondrocytes).

This comprehensive WHO (2013) classification of soft tissue tumours is presented in **Table 29.1**.

Q2. How do you classify soft tissue tumours on the basis of their clinical biological behaviour?
Based on clinical biologic behaviour, four groups of soft tissue tumours are recognised:

I. **Benign** These tumours have a limited growth potential, generally do not recur after surgical removal and are cured by complete excision. Best examples are lipoma and haemangioma.

II. **Intermediate, locally aggressive** These tumours are locally destructive, infiltrative and often recur but do not metastasise. Such tumours are treated by wide excision. Best example is desmoid tumour.

III. **Intermediate, rarely metastasising** These tumours are also locally destructive, infiltrative and recurrent, but about 2% cases may have metastases which may not be predicted by morphology. Common example in this category is dermatofibrosarcoma protuberans.

IV. **Malignant** These tumours have all the features of malignancy. Locally, they are destructive and infiltrative and they metastasise in a high percentage of cases. The metastatic rate in low-grade sarcomas is about 2–10%, and in high-grade sarcoma is 20–100%.

Q3. Describe some general and common clinicopathologic features of soft tissue tumours.

General features

i. Soft tissue tumours may be benign of malignant; the latter are usually called sarcomas.

ii. Benign soft tissue tumours are 100 times more common than sarcomas.

iii. Malignant tumours may sometimes develop from pre-existing benign tumours, but vast majority of sarcomas originate *de novo* from primitive mesenchymal stem cells capable of differentiating into more mature connective tissue cells.

iv. Sarcomas metastasise most frequently by haematogenous route, typically to the lungs, liver, bone and brain. Lymph node metastases are found less often, mostly in terminal stages of neoplastic disease marked by widespread dissemination of malignancy.

v. Histologic classification and grading are important for predicting clinical behaviour of soft tissue tumours, their prognosis and outcome of therapy.

vi. Final diagnosis for most soft tissue sarcomas is made by correlating the clinical and pathologic data, which are often supplemented by immunohistochemical, cytogenetic and molecular biology findings.

Common clinicopathologic features

i. Sarcomas are relatively rare tumours, accounting for only 1% of all malignancies. They also account for 2% of tumour mortality, reflecting the highly malignant nature of many sarcomas. Generally, males are affected more often than females.

ii. Sarcomas may occur at any age. The highest incidence has been recorded in the 40 to 70 years age group.

iii. About 15% of all sarcomas occur in children. Among the childhood tumours, the most prominent are rhabdomyosarcomas, which have a peak incidence at 15 years of age.

iv. Superficially located tumours tend to be benign, while deep-seated lesions are more likely to be malignant.

v. Large-sized tumours are generally more malignant than small ones.

vi. Rapidly growing tumours often behave as malignant tumours more often than those that develop slowly.

vii. Malignant tumours have frequently increased vascularity while benign tumours are selectively avascular.

viii. Certain anatomic sites are more often involved than others. The most common sites of origin of malignant soft tissue tumours are as follows:

- Lower extremity (40%)
- Upper extremity (20%)
- Trunk and retroperitoneum (30%)
- Head and neck (10%)

TABLE 29.1 WHO classification of soft tissue tumours (2013)*.

I. **Adipocytic tumours**
A. *Benign*
  i. Lipoma
  ii. Lipomatosis
  iii. Lipoblastoma
  iv. Hibernoma
B. *Malignant:* Liposarcoma (various types)

II. **Fibroblastic and myofibroblastic tumours**
A. *Benign*
  i. Fibroma
  ii. Nodular fasciitis
  iii. Myositis ossificans
  iv. Fibrous hamartoma of infancy
  v. Angiomyofibroblastoma
B. *Intermediate (locally aggressive)*
  i. Fibromatosis (plantar/palmar)
  ii. Desmoid type fibromatosis
C. *Intermediate (rarely metastasising)*
  i. Dermatofibrosarcoma protuberans
  ii. Solitary fibrous tumour
D. *Malignant:* Fibrosarcoma

III. **So-called fibrohistiocytic tumours**
A. *Benign*
  i. Tenosynovial giant cell tumour (localised, diffuse) (page 691)
  ii. Benign fibrous histiocytoma
B. *Intermediate (rarely metastasising)*
  i. Giant cell tumour of soft tissues
  ii. Plexiform fibrohistiocytic tumour

IV. **Smooth muscle tumours**
A. *Benign:* Leiomyoma (deep soft tissues) (page 599)
B. *Malignant:* Leiomyosarcoma

V. **Skeletal muscle tumours**
A. *Benign:* Rhabdomyoma
B. *Malignant:* Rhabdomyosarcoma (various types)

VI. **Pericytes (perivascular) tumours**
A. *Benign*
  i. Glomus tumour (page 335)
  ii. Angioleiomyoma
  iii. Myopericytoma

VII. **Vascular tumours** (page 335)

VIII. **Chondro-osseous soft tissue tumours**
A. *Benign:* Soft tissue chondroma
B. *Malignant:* Chondrosarcoma (extraskeletal, mesenchymal) (page 685)

IX. **Gastrointestinal stromal tumours (GIST)** (page 449)

X. **Peripheral nerve sheath tumours** (page 732)

XI. **Tumours of uncertain differentiation**
A. *Benign:* Myxoma
B. *Malignant*
  i. Synovial sarcoma
  ii. Epithelioid sarcoma
  iii. Alveolar soft part sarcoma
  iv. Clear cell sarcoma of soft tissues
  v. Desmoplastic small round cell tumour
  vi. Extra-skeletal Ewing sarcoma (page 686)
  vii. Extra-skeletal myxoid chondrosarcoma (page 685)
  viii. Extra-renal rhabdoid tumour
  ix. PEComa

XII. **Undifferentiated/unclassified sarcomas**
  i. Undifferentiated sarcoma (types: spindle cell, round cell, epithelioid, pleomorphic)
  ii. Undifferentiated sarcoma, not otherwise specified

*Adapted from: Fletcher et al (Eds). WHO classification of tumours of soft tissues and bone. 2013. IARC Press, Lyon.

Q4. Briefly discuss etiopathogenesis of soft tissue tumours.

i. The etiology of most soft tissue tumours is unknown.
ii. Scientists agree that soft tissue tumours originate from undifferentiated soft tissue stem cells, but these presumptive precursors have not been fully characterised.
iii. Most sarcomas are sporadic, and no external risk factors have been definitively identified.
iv. A familial predisposition has been identified for a minority of soft tissue tumours such as those that occur in families with rare tumour syndromes like Li-Fraumeni syndrome, neurofibromatosis type I, Osler-Weber-Rendu syndrome, etc.
v. Chromosomal changes found in many sarcomas indicate that genetic changes occur often in these tumours. However, the significance of these cytogenetic changes is unknown in most instances.
- Most chromosomal changes (>80%) in such sarcomas are unpredictable, non-diagnostic and complex resulting in a loss or gain of genetic material.
- Diagnostic recurrent chromosomal changes are found in approximately 15% of sarcomas. These include mostly translocations and fusion genes involving driver mutations of oncogenes or tumour suppressor genes **(Table 29.2)**.
vi. Epstein-Barr virus plays a role in the pathogenesis of smooth muscle cell tumours in HIV infected and immunosuppressed children and young adults.

TABLE 29.2 Common chromosomal abnormalities in soft tissue tumours.

TUMOUR	CYTOGENETIC ALTERATIONS	MOLECULAR ALTERATIONS	REASON FOR TESTING
1. Ewing sarcoma/PNET	t(11;22)(q24;q12)	EWSR-FLI1 fusion gene	Differentiate from other small round cell tumours
2. Alveolar rhabdomyosarcoma	t(1;13)(q36;q14) t(2;13)(p35;q14)	PAX3-FOXO1A fusion gene PAX7-FOXO1A fusion gene	Better prognosis Poorer prognosis
3. Myxoid/Round cell liposarcoma	t(12;16)(q13; p11)	FUS-DDIT3 fusion gene	Diagnostic
4. Synovial sarcoma	t(X;18)(p11;q11)	SS18-SSX1 fusion gene	Differentiate biphasic from monophasic
5. Extraskeletal myxoid chondrosarcoma	t(9;22)(q22;q12)	EWSR1-NR4A3 fusion gene	Diagnostic
6. Infantile fibrosarcoma	t(12;15)(p13;q26) trisomies 8, 11, 17, 20	ETV6-NTRK3 fusion gene	Differentiate from more aggressive adult fibrosarcoma
7. Dermatofibrosarcoma protuberans	Ring forms of chromosomes 17, 22	COL1A1-PDGFB fusion gene	Diagnostic
8. Desmoplastic small round cell tumour	t(11;22)(p13;q12)	EWSR1-WT1 fusion gene	Poor prognosis
9. Alveolar soft part sarcoma	t(X;17)(p11;q25)	TFE3-ASPL fusion gene	Diagnostic
10. Clear cell sarcoma	t(12;22)(q13;q12)	EWSR1-ATF1 fusion gene	Distinguish from cutaneous melanoma

Q5. What are the pathologic diagnostic criteria for soft tissue sarcomas?

Histologic diagnosis and categorisation of soft tissue sarcomas is based on microscopic identification of certain cell patterns and cell types, combined with confirmation of cell of origin by immunohistochemical data. In many cases, cytogenetic studies of the tumour are valuable.

I. **Cell patterns** that can be microscopically recognised are as follows:
i. *Interlacing fascicles* of pink-staining tumour cells indicative of smooth muscle differentiation.
ii. *Storiform pattern* in which spindle tumour cells radiate from the centre in a spoke-wheel manner typical of fibrohistiocytic cells.
iii. *Herring-bone pattern* in which the tumour cells are arranged like the bones attached to the vertebrae of sea fish, as seen in fibrosarcoma.
iv. *Palisaded arrangement* in which the nuclei of tumour cells are piled upon each other, as seen in schwannoma.
v. *Biphasic pattern* comprising both spindle cells arranged into fascicles and cuboidal epithelial cells arranged into tubules, as in biphasic synovial sarcoma.

II. **Cell types** that can be morphologically recognised include the following:

i. *Spindle cells* are the most common cell types in sarcoma, showing only minor or subtle differences from one tumour type to another, as under:

a. *Fibrogenic tumours* are composed of fibroblasts, i.e. spindle cells with light pink cytoplasm and tapering-ending nuclei.

b. *Neurogenic (Schwann cell) tumours* are composed of cells that resemble fibroblasts but have curved nuclei.

c. *Leiomyomatous tumours* have spindle cells with blunt-ended ('cigar-shaped') nuclei and more intense eosinophilic cytoplasm.

d. *Skeletal muscle tumours* resemble those originating from smooth muscle cells. These cells have, however, cytoplasmic striations indicative of striated muscle cell differentiation.

e. *Lipoblasts,* which may be either univacuolar or multivacuolar.

ii. *Small round cells* are undifferentiated 'embryonal-like' cells that have round nuclei and scant cytoplasm. Examples of soft tissue tumours that have such features include rhabdomyosarcoma (embryonal and alveolar type), Ewing sarcoma, desmoplastic small round cell tumours, malignant peripheral nerve sheaths tumour (MPNST). These soft tissue tumours must be distinguished from some small cell carcinomas (e.g. sinonasal carcinoma), malignant lymphoma, neuroblastoma, retinoblastoma and other 'blastomas' of childhood.

iii. *Epithelioid cells* are sarcoma cells that have epithelial-like features. Such cells are found in epithelioid sarcoma, and may be admixed to spindle cells (e.g. in biphasic synovial sarcoma).

iv. *Multinucleated giant cells* are often seen in highly malignant tumours such as undifferentiated pleomorphic sarcomas or pleomorphic liposarcoma.

III. **Immunohistochemistry** plays an important role for proper identification of tumour cell differentiation. The most useful markers identifiable with modern immunohistochemical techniques widely used in clinical pathology are as follows:

i. Smooth muscle cell actin (SMA) for smooth muscle cells
ii. Desmin, myogenin and Myo D-1 for skeletal muscle cells
iii. S-100 protein for nerve fibres
iv. Factor VIII and CD31 for endothelial cells
v. Leucocyte common antigen (CD45) for lymphoid cells and other leucocytes

IV. **Cytogenetics** (i.e. the study of chromosomal and genetic abnormalities) play a crucial role in the classification of many soft tissue sarcomas as given in **Table 29.2** above. As may be seen, the diagnostic features listed in this table predominantly include translocations and abnormal chromosomes due to mitotic errors resulting in gene fusion.

Q6. Comment on grading of soft tissue sarcomas.

There are several grading systems for sarcomas:
- *Two-grade system*, classifying the tumours as either low-grade or high-grade neoplasms.
- *Three-grade system*, assigning to tumours numerical grade (I, II or III) or classifying them as low, intermediate or high-grade neoplasms.
- *Four-grade system*, assigning to tumour numerical grade I, II, III and IV.

WHO has adopted three-grade French sarcoma system (FNCLCC) based on three histopathologic parameters:
i. Tumour differentiation or degree of cytologic atypia
ii. Mitotic count
iii. Tumour necrosis

Q7. What are the staging systems of soft tissue sarcomas?

i. **AJCC staging** The most widely system used is the system proposed by the American Joint Committee on Cancer (AJCC) which is based on the TNM grade of tumours.

ii. **Enneking staging** Alternatively, soft tissue tumours can be staged according to the Enneking staging system which classifies tumours into three stages, taking into account: tumour location (T1 intra-compartmental and T2 extra-compartmental tumours) and the grade (G1 as low-grade, and G2 as high-grade tumours):

Stage I: G1 and T1-T2 tumours, but no metastases
Stage II: G2 and T1-T2 tumours, but no metastases
Stage III: G1 or G2 tumours, T1 or T2 tumours with metastases.

■ SPECIFIC TYPES OF SOFT TISSUE TUMOURS

Q8. What are the most important adipocytic tumours?

Definition Adipocytic tumours are composed of fat cells (adipocytes) and/or their immature precursors (lipoblasts). These are classified as either benign or malignant.

Pathology Lipoma is the most common benign soft tissue tumour. Liposarcoma is one of the most common sarcomas in adults.

I. *Lipoma* is a benign tumour.
i. Most often, it is diagnosed in 30–50 years old persons.
ii. It presents as a 2–3 cm well-defined soft, movable mass in subcutaneous tissue of the neck, back and shoulders.
iii. On cross section, it is encapsulated and yellow.
iv. Several histopathologic variants (e.g. fibrolipoma, angiolipoma) are recognised but such details are of no clinical significance **(Fig. 29.1)**.

II. *Liposarcoma* is a malignant tumour composed of neoplastic lipoblasts which may or may not differentiate into adult fat cells.
i. The peak incidence is in the 50–70 years age group.
ii. Most often, it occurs in deep tissues, such as intermuscular fat tissue (thigh, buttock and retroperitoneum).
iii. Liposarcoma cells invade into adjacent tissues.
iv. The tumours are not well demarcated and tend to be larger than lipomas; most of them measure more than 5 cm in diameter, and some are huge weighing a few kilograms, especially if located in the retroperitoneum.
v. On cross section, they are yellow and greasy due to their fat content.
vi. *Microscopically,* all liposarcomas contain malignant lipoblasts, which may be univacuolar or multivacuolar **(Fig. 29.2)**.
a. Several microscopic subtypes of liposarcoma are known such as: well differentiated, myxoid and pleomorphic, each of which could have distinct variants.
b. Microscopic classification of tumours is important: well differentiated and most myxoid liposarcomas have a good prognosis (70%-5 year survival), whereas the pleomorphic ones have poor prognosis (20%-5 year survival) and tend to metastasise to the lungs.
vii. *Molecular biology* is used to confirm the diagnosis of well differentiated and myxoid liposarcoma and distinguish them from benign lipomas or normal fat tissue. These molecular biology abnormalities

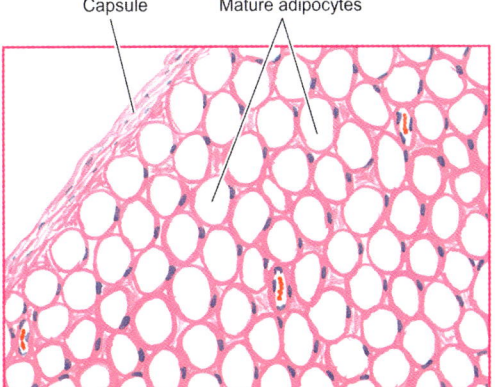

FIGURE 29.1: Lipoma. The tumour shows a thin capsule and underlying lobules of mature adipose cells separated by delicate fibrous septa.

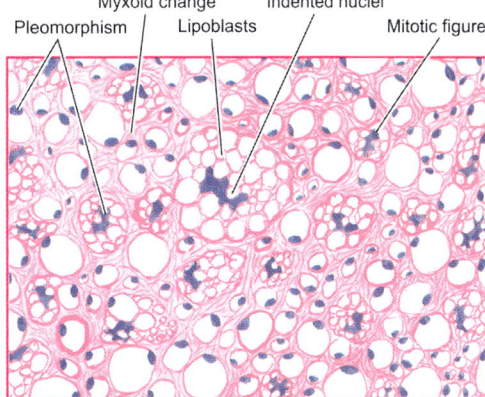

FIGURE 29.2: Myxoid liposarcoma. The tumour shows myxoid background. There is presence of characteristic, univacuolated and multivacuolated lipoblasts, in which the vacuole is seen indenting the atypical nucleus.

include amplification of 12q13-q15 and t(12;16) with prominent amplification of MDM2, a potent inhibitor of p53. Pleomorphic liposarcoma shows complex chromosomal changes.

Q9. Discuss salient clinicopathologic features of most important fibroblastic and myofibroblastic tumours.

Definition and types Fibroblastic and myofibroblastic tumours are composed of fibroblasts and modified fibroblasts that can contract (myofibroblasts). This group of tumours includes:

i. Benign tumours (e.g. nodular fasciitis, and myositis ossificans)
ii. Intermediate (locally aggressive) tumours (e.g. palmar/plantar fibromatosis, desmoid type fibromatosis)
iii. Intermediate (rarely metastasising) tumour (dermatofibrosarcoma protuberans)
iv. Malignant (fibrosarcoma)

Salient clinicopathologic features

I. **Nodular fasciitis** is a benign tumour originating most often from deep dermis, subcutis or the superficial fascia of the muscles of young adults.
i. Most common locations are the forearm, trunk and neck.
ii. It presents as a rapidly growing nodule measuring one to several centimeters in diameter.
iii. *Microscopy*
- The nodule is composed of fibroblasts and myofibroblasts in an oedematous background arranged loosely in a haphazard 'tissue culture-like growth pattern'.
- At its edges, such loose myxoid zones gradually transform into less cellular but more collagenous tissue, accounting for the typical 'zonation' within the nodule.
- Mitoses are numerous but there is no or only minimal nuclear atypia.
- Between the cells, there are extravasated red blood cells and scattered lymphocytes.

iv. *Molecular biology* proves the clonal nature of the lesion. It shows translocation t(17;22) leading to the formation of the fusion gene *MYH-USP6* and overexpression of oncogenic USP6 protein. Nevertheless, this is a benign growth and surgical removal is curative.

II. **Myositis ossificans** is a benign tumour composed of osteoid and heterotopic bone formation in the soft tissue of skeletal muscle. Thus, the name is a misnomer since there is no inflammation, nor is the lesion limited to skeletal muscles—actually it often affects the tendons.
i. The lesion appears as an unencapsulated, gritty mass which may be located inside the muscle, attached to a tendon or in the vicinity of a bone.
ii. X-rays show areas of bone formation around a radiolucent central area.
iii. *Microscopy*
- The central portion of the lesion consists of proliferating fibroblasts, myofibroblasts and angioblasts as in a granulations tissue.
- Mitotic figures are prominent but there is no significant nuclear atypia.
- Toward the periphery, fibroblasts are replaced by osteoblasts which form woven bone.
- The skeletal muscle surrounding the lesion may show signs of injury and attempted regeneration with formation of multinucleated myoblasts.

iv. *Clinical features*
a. History of trauma is found in two-thirds of cases.
b. Most patients complain of pain, tenderness and swelling.
c. A relatively rapid growth of the lesion infrequently raises the suspicion of malignancy and this feature accounts for the term *pseudomalignant osseous tumour of the bone*.

III. **Fibromatosis** is a term used for locally invasive lesions composed of fibroblasts and myofibroblasts forming fibrovascular nodules.
Clinicopathologically, fibromatoses are classified according to the age of the patients and the location of lesions as under:

i. *Infantile or juvenile fibromatoses* These include a variety of conditions which may be *localised* to an anatomic area (e.g. fibrous hamartoma of infancy, fibromatosis coli) or *widespread* involving large parts of the body (e.g. congenital generalised fibromatosis, diffuse infantile fibromatosis, etc.

ii. *Adult type fibromatoses* They all present as whitish-grey, firm, collagenous plaques, nodules or masses extending into the normal tissue without defined borders.

a. *Microscopically*, they all have the same features and consist of deceptively uniform collagen-rich fibroblastic bundles and fascicles.
b. *Clinically*, they cause contractures and scarring, and are hard to treat, recurring in 2/3 of cases after surgery. They are subdivided into two groups:
- *Superficial fibromatoses*, such as palmar fibromatosis (giving rise to *Dupuytren* contracture), plantar fibromatosis, penile fibromatosis (giving rise to *Peyronie* disease).
- *Deep-seated fibromatoses* are also known as *desmoids*. Desmoids can be classified as *abdominal desmoids* and *extra-abdominal desmoids* involving extremities, buttocks and head and neck region. In rare instances, there are *intra-abdominal desmoids* involving the small bowel mesentery. These lesions may be a feature of Gardner syndrome and are then associated with intestinal polyposis, osteomas and epidermal cysts.

IV. **Dermatofibrosarcoma protuberans** is a slow growing, low-grade malignant tumour, which tends to recur after surgery, with only rare distant metastases.
i. It usually presents in the form of solitary nodules in the subcutaneous tissue of the trunk that may be surrounded by smaller satellite nodules.
ii. It consists of bundles of fibroblasts showing mild to moderate nuclear atypia.
iii. These cells often contain ring chromosomes 17 and 22 and contain *COL1A1-WT1* fusion gene involving collagen type 1A1 gene and Wilms' tumour gene.

V. **Fibrosarcoma** is a malignant tumour of older adult in the 40–70 year age group.
i. Most tumours originate from deep connective tissues, such as fascia of skeletal muscle, tendons and periosteum. Common locations are tissues around the knee joint, but other sites may be involved as well, including the bones and retroperitoneum.
ii. *Microscopically*, fibrosarcoma is composed of malignant fibroblasts arranged into herring-bone like interlacing bundles and fascicles **(Fig. 29.3)**.
iii. Fibrosarcoma has a poor prognosis and only 40% patients survive 5 years after surgery.
iv. With the advent of modern *molecular biology* techniques, the diagnosis of fibrosarcoma of soft tissue and bone has become a '*diagnosis by exclusion*'. Thus, the diagnosis of fibrosarcoma is currently applied to only 3% of all soft tissue and bone tumours; it is used only for tumours that show no distinct molecular markers which would classify them as one of the clinicopathologically well-defined *subsets of fibroblastic tumours* such as myofibroblastic sarcoma, myxofibrosarcoma, fibromyxoid sarcoma, among others.
v. *Infantile fibrosarcoma* is a rare tumour affecting infants in the first year of life.
a. Approximately 50% of these tumours are congenital, which accounts for the alternate name *congenital fibrosarcoma*.
b. Two thirds of these tumours are found on distal part of the extremities.
c. Histologically, it resembles adult fibrosarcoma and consists of densely grouped neoplastic fibroblasts.
d. The tumours are characterised by a distinct chromosomal marker resulting in formation of *ETV6-NTRK3* fusion gene. It rarely metastasises (5%) and has an excellent prognosis.

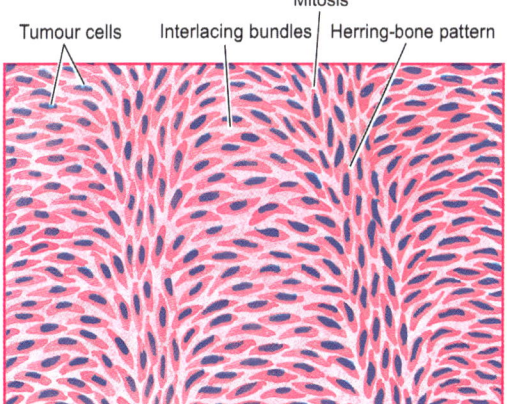

FIGURE 29.3: Fibrosarcoma. Microscopy shows a well-differentiated tumour composed of spindle-shaped cells forming interlacing fascicles producing a typical Herring-bone pattern. A few mitotic figures are also seen.

Q10. Briefly describe pathologic types and salient clinical features of rhabdomyosarcomas.

Definition Rhabdomyosarcoma is a malignant tumour composed of neoplastic cells that show light microscopic or immunohistochemical signs of striated muscle differentiation. It is the commonest soft tissue sarcoma in children and young adults.

Pathology Four histopathologic types of rhabdomyosarcoma are recognised: i) embryonal (60%), ii) alveolar (20%), iii) pleomorphic (15%) and iv) spindle cell/sclerosing type (1–2%).

I. **Embryonal rhabdomyosarcoma** is the most common form of rhabdomyosarcoma.
i. It occurs predominantly in children under the age of 12 years of age, with a peak incidence in the 1–5 years age group.
ii. Common locations include the head and neck regions (most frequently in the orbit), urogenital tract and retroperitoneum.
iii. *Grossly*, it appears as a gelatinous mass growing between the muscle fascicles or in deep subcutaneous tissue.
iv. *Microscopically*, it is composed of small undifferentiated cells focally admixed to spindle cells which may have more abundant eosinophilic cytoplasm with cross striations. Tumour cells may form broad fascicles and bands. Mitoses are prominent.
v. *Sarcoma botryoides* is a form of embryonal rhabdomyosarcoma:
a. Common locations are some hollow organs such as urinary bladder, vagina or nasal cavity.
b. *Clinically and grossly*, it presents as a gelatinous multivesicular mass protruding into the cavity of the hollow organs (botryoides meaning grape like in Greek).
c. *Microscopically*, the gelatinous polypoid tumour fronds consist of a myxoid stroma with loosely arranged round or oval rhabdomyoblasts that condense peripherally underneath the epithelium into a *cambium layer*.
II. **Alveolar rhabdomyosarcoma** is found in school age children, adolescents and young adults under the age of 25 years.
i. It originates as a rapidly growing solid or gelatinous mass in skeletal muscles of extremities.
ii. *Microscopically*, it consists of alveolar-like spaces lined by small round cells with scant cytoplasm that are lying on connective tissue septa **(Fig. 29.4)**. There are numerous mitoses and some multinucleated giant cells. Cross striations can be demonstrated in 25% of cases.
III. **Pleomorphic rhabdomyosarcoma** occurs mostly in adult who are over the age of 40 years.
i. It occurs most often on extremities, particularly the thighs.
ii. *Grossly*, it appears as a well-circumscribed mass with areas of necrosis and haemorrhage.
iii. *Microscopic features* include marked pleomorphism of tumour cells which are described as racquet-shaped, tad-pole-shaped. Strap orribbon-shaped cells with well-developed eosinophilic cytoplasm often contain multiple nuclei.
IV. **Spindle cell/sclerosing rhabdomyosarcoma** is a rare tumour.
i. It may occur in children or adults, but prognosis is worse in adults.
ii. *Microscopically*, it is composed of small round cells with scant cytoplasm laid in a dense collagenous stroma.
Special studies such as immunohistochemistry and molecular biology are essential for the proper diagnosis of rhabdomyosarcoma.
i. Striated muscle differentiation of rhabdomyosarcoma cells is best recognised by *immunohistochemical stains* such as myogenin, Myo-D1 and desmin.
ii. *Molecular biology* study of alveolar rhabdomyosarcoma shows translocation of PAX3 or PAX7 to form fusion genes PAX3-FOXO1A or PAX7-FOX1A; the latter being a marker of worse prognosis. Other rhabdomyosarcomas show complex chromosomal abnormalities but no recurrent diagnostic molecular biology changes.
Clinical features Rhabdomyosarcoma is a rare tumour.
i. Still, it is the most common soft tissue sarcoma in children and young adults. American Cancer Society data show that more than 90% of all rhabdomyosarcomas are diagnosed in persons who are younger than 25 years, and 60% are found in children younger than 10 years.

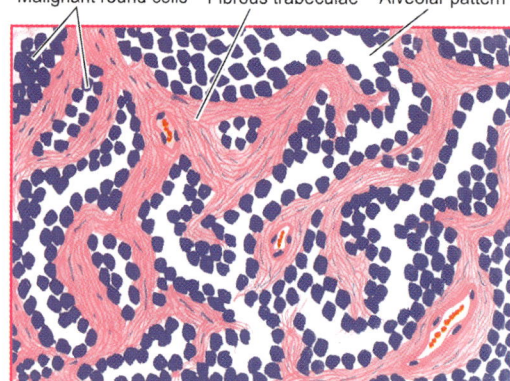

FIGURE 29.4: Alveolar rhabdomyosarcoma. The tumour is divided into alveolar spaces composed of fibrocollagenous tissue. The fibrous trabeculae are lined by small, dark, undifferentiated tumour cells, with some cells floating in the alveolar spaces. A few multinucleate tumour giant cells are also present.

ii. Early diagnosis and advances in chemotherapy have contributed to excellent outcome and 90% of young patients survive 5-years after diagnosis. The prognosis for older patients is less favorable.

Q11. What are the most important tumours of uncertain differentiation?

A number of soft tissue tumours cannot be histogenetically classified because they do not show a clear line of differentiation. These tumours are as follows:
i. Synovial sarcoma
ii. Epithelioid sarcoma
iii. Alveolar soft part sarcoma
iv. Clear cell sarcoma
v. Desmoplastic small round cell tumour
vi. Rhabdoid tumour

All these tumours occur predominantly in young people and have a poor prognosis. Most of them have diagnostic molecular biology markers.

Q12. Comment briefly on synovial sarcoma.

Definition Synovial sarcoma (SS) is a malignant soft tissue tumour of undetermined origin characterised in molecular biology terms by translocation of SS18/SYT (synteny) gene on chromosome 18 to chromosomes SSX gene (a transcriptional repressor gene) on X chromosome. This leads to the formation of SS18-SSX fusion gene, encoding the production of fusion proteins (SS18-SSX1, -SSX2 or -SSX4), thought to interact with oncogenes or tumor suppressor genes.

Pathology

Most SS (70%) originate from the deep connective tissue near joint capsules and tendon sheaths of lower and upper extremities. This observation led to the hypothesis that the tumour originates from the synovium and the misnomer designation 'synovial sarcoma'. Currently, we know that SS is not related to synovium and thus may originate from any soft tissue site and also from internal organs. The original name has been retained for historical reasons, but the tumour is best defined in terms of its molecular biology characteristics, i.e. the SS18-SSX fusion gene.

Two histopathologic forms of synovial sarcoma are recognised: monophasic and biphasic.

Monophasic synovial sarcoma

i. Composed exclusively of spindle cells arranged in swirling fascicles resembling fibrosarcoma.
ii. These cells are relatively monotonous and have elongated but plump nuclei, no nucleoli and finely dispersed chromatin, surrounded by scant cytoplasm.
iii. The stroma may contain scattered strands of hyaline collagen.

Biphasic synovial sarcoma

i. Consists of spindle cells identical to those in monophasic synovial sarcoma and cuboidal epithelial cells forming solid nests or lining cleft-like spaces and gland-like lumina **(Fig. 29.5)**.
ii. Epithelial cells stain immunohistochemically with antibodies to cytokeratin, a marker of epithelial differentiation.
iii. Most biphasic synovial sarcoma harbor the SS18-SSX1 fusion gene, in contrast to monophasic SS which could have any of the fusion genes.

Clinical features

i. Synovial sarcomas are rare tumours, accounting for 5% of soft tissue sarcomas.
ii. Most often, they occur in young and middle-aged adults 15 to 40 years of age.
iii. The growth rate of these tumours varies from slow to rapid. Initial slow growth and their deep location on the extremities account for the fact that many are not diagnosed until they have reached a larger size.

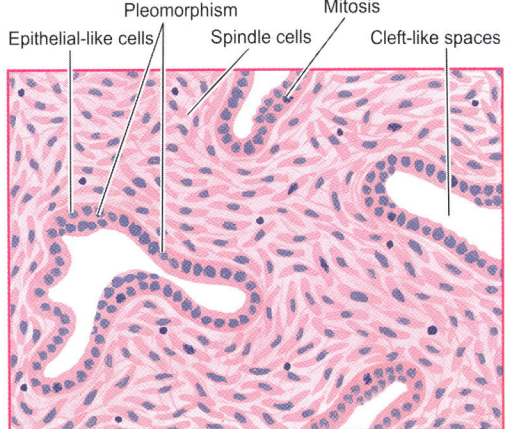

FIGURE 29.5: Biphasic synovial sarcoma. The tumour is composed of epithelial-like cells lining cleft-like spaces and gland-like structures, and spindle cell areas forming fibrosarcoma-like growth pattern.

iv. Tumours exceeding 5 cm in diameter have often pulmonary metastases and, accordingly, poor prognosis. The overall 5-year survival is 50–60%.

Q13. What is undifferentiated pleomorphic sarcoma?

Definition Undifferentiated pleomorphic sarcomas (UPS) form a heterogeneous group of undifferentiated malignant soft tissue sarcomas composed of a variety of cells including spindle, round, pleomorphic, epithelioid and giant cells. Previously, these tumours were known as *malignant fibrous histiocytomas (MFH)*.

Poorly differentiated and undifferentiated liposarcoma, leiomyosarcoma or rhabdomyosarcoma may be composed of similar pleomorphic cells. However, these tumours can be distinguished from UPS by immunohistochemistry and molecular biology. Accordingly, UPS has become a *'diagnosis by exclusion'* for some 20% of soft tissue sarcomas that cannot be classified otherwise.

Pathology

Grossly, UPS are usually bulky tumours measuring 5–10 cm in diameter or more. Most tumours are found on the extremities and in the retroperitoneum. On cross section, they are greyish-white, hard or soft, and even myxoid, with prominent secondary changes such as necrosis, haemorrhage or pseudocystic change.

Microscopically, the tumours vary in appearance, and even in the same tumour one may find areas composed of different cells **(Fig. 29.6)**:

i. Pleomorphism of cells is the main feature of most UPS.

ii. Some tumours are composed predominantly of fibroblastic spindle cells arranged in a storiform pattern.

iii. Most tumours contain infiltrates of foamy macrophages, and scattered lymphocytes.

iv. Some tumours contain myxoid areas or may be composed predominantly of multinucleated giant cells, or have an epithelioid appearance.

v. Mitoses are prominent, and often atypical.

vi. No diagnostic immunohistochemical or molecular biology markers are available to support the diagnosis. Immunohistochemical studies are, nevertheless, performed in most instances to exclude pleomorphic leiomyosarcoma, malignant peripheral nerve sheath tumour or rhabdomyosarcoma.

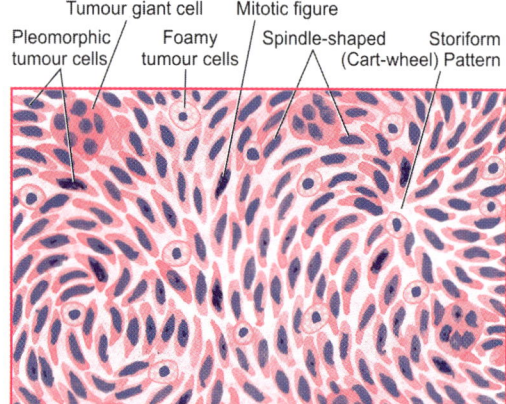

FIGURE 29.6: Undifferentiated pleomorphic sarcoma (formerly malignant fibrous histiocytoma). The tumour is composed of highly malignant pleomorphic tumour cells having high mitotic activity. Bizarre pleomorphic multinucleate tumour giant cells and some mononuclear foamy cells are also present.

Clinical features

i. UPS may occur at any age but the peak incidence has been recorded in the 40–70 years age groups.

ii. Overall, UPS account for 20% of all soft tissue sarcomas and are thus the most common form of sarcoma in adults.

iii. About a quarter of all cases are radiation-associated sarcomas.

Prognosis is poor and the 5-year-survival is only 30–50%. Prognosis depends on the size of the tumour and the depth of location. Large tumours found in deep location have a worse prognosis than those that are small and superficially located.

Chapter 29e Supplement: Online Content

Digital content of this chapter available with this book is meant for enhanced learning and self-assessment. In addition, it contains 18 Multiple Choice Questions (MCQs), 05 Clinicopathologic Vignettes, and 04 Image-based Questions; these are followed by their answers along with explanatory notes of correct and incorrect answers.

CHAPTER 30

Nervous System

CENTRAL NERVOUS SYSTEM

Q1. What are the neuroectodermal and mesodermal cells forming the central nervous system?

The principal components of the CNS are of either neuroectodermal or mesodermal origin.
- The *neuroectodermal cells* include: neurons, neuroglia (the predominant constituents of the CNS).
- The *mesodermal tissues* are: microglia, dura mater, leptomeninges (pia-arachnoid), blood vessels including their accompanying cells.

I. Neurons The neurons are highly specialised terminally differentiated cells that cannot divide during adult life. Hence, the brain damage involving neurons is irreversible.

Neurons vary in size and shape and function depending on their location. Each neuron consists of three main parts: the cell body, an axon and numerous dendrites **(Fig. 30.1, A)**.

i. *The cell bodies* may be arranged in layers such as in the cerebral cortex, or they may be aggregated in groups forming the nuclei of basal ganglia. *Neuropil* is the term used for the fibrillar network formed by the cytoplasmic processes of the nerve cells. The neurons can be demonstrated in the histologic sections by special stains or immunohistochemically using the antibodies to neurofilaments, which form the intermediate filaments of their cytoskeleton.

ii. Neurons *respond to injury* in a variety of ways depending upon the etiological agent and the pathologic processes. These include:
- *central chromatolysis* (corresponding to the loss of ribosomes from the rough endoplasmic reticulum that forms the Nissl substance),
- *atrophy* and *degeneration* of neurons and axon, and
- *intraneuronal storage* of substances such as lipofuscin or various bodies, like neurofilament tangles.

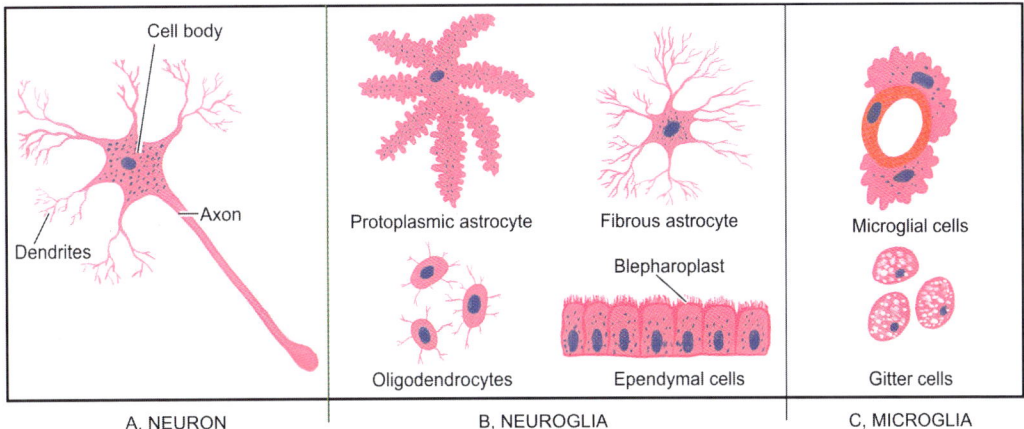

FIGURE 30.1: Cells comprising the nervous system.

II. **Neuroglia** The neuroglia provides supportive matrix and maintenance to the neurons. It includes three types of cells **(Fig. 30.1, B)**:

i. *Astrocytes* are stellate cells which may be classified as protoplasmatic or fibrous, depending on the structure of their cytoplasmic processes.
- Astrocytes provide support to neurons, and with their elongated foot processes, form the *blood-brain barrier*.
- In response to injury, astrocytes act like fibroblasts in other tissues, participating in the repair of damaged brain tissue. Astrocytic reaction to injury is called *gliosis* and it corresponds to fibroblastic scars in other parts of the body.

ii. *Oligodendrocytes* (or oligodendroglia cells) are so named because they are smaller than astrocytes.
- In the grey matter, they are clustered around neurons and are called *satellite cells*.
- In the white matter, they form and maintain myelin and are called *interfascicular oligodendroglia*.
- Thus, they are counterparts of Schwann cells of the peripheral nervous system.
- Diseases of oligodendrocytes present disorders of myelination such as inherited leucodystrophies and acquired demyelinating diseases.

iii. *Ependymal cells* are epithelium-like cuboidal and ciliated cells.
- Ependymal cells form a single layer lining the ventricular system, aqueduct, central canal of the spinal cord and cover the choroid plexus.
- These cells participate in the formation and maintenance of *cerebrospinal fluid (CSF)*.
- Damaged ependymal cell are usually replaced by underlying glial fibres.

III. **Microglia** The microglia cells are bone marrow-derived mobile cells representing the CNS counterpart of monocyte-macrophages system **(Fig. 30.1, C)**.
- They accumulate at the site of injury and enlarge to become *rod cells*.
- They can phagocytose necrotic neurons ('*neuronophagia*') or take up the lipid from damaged neural cells and, thus, transform into vacuolated *gitter cells*.

IV. **Dura mater** Dura is the fibrous covering of the brain which is closely attached to the skull on its inner layer of endocranial periosteum.
- The potential space between the cranial and vertebral bones on one side and the dura on the other, is called *epidural space*.
- The space inner to the dura is called *subdural space*.

V. **Pia-arachnoid (Leptomeninges)** These are the delicate vascular membranous coverings of the central nervous system.
- The pia mater is closely applied to the brain while the arachnoid mater lies between the pia and the dura mater.
- The space between these two layers is called *subarachnoid space* which contains CSF. This space also contains major arteries and veins.
- The extensions of the subarachnoid space into the brain along the penetrating blood vessels form the circumvascular *Virchow-Robin space*.

Q2. Define spina bifida. What are its types?

Definition Spina bifida is a dysraphic developmental defect due to incomplete closure of one or more lumbar vertebral arches (*rachischisis*). It may occur in several forms that also includes changes in the spinal cord and meninges.

Pathology These developmental defects vary in severity depending on the extent of incomplete fusion of the foetal vertebrae, meninges and spinal cord, as under:

i. *Spina bifida occulta* is the mildest form, including a bone defect of posterior vertebral arches. The defect is not visible to the naked eye because it is covered by intact skin.

ii. *Meningocele* is a bone defect accompanied by herniation of meninges which form a sac filled with fluid.

iii. *Meningomyelocele* is a large bone defect allowing herniation of meninges and spinal cord.

iv. *Myelocele* is a large defect of skin and posterior arches of vertebral bone and meninges, combined with incomplete closure of the foetal neural tube. The incompletely closed spinal cord is open up to the outside through the bone and skin defect.

Clinical features
i. Myelocele and meningomyelocele are accompanied by major spinal motor and sensory disorders, which are, however, less pronounced in the milder defects.
ii. The incomplete fusion of posterior cranial bones and brain may result in *craniorachischisis,* which usually involves the cranial bone and the brain, as well the cervical and even upper thoracic spinal cord and vertebrae.
iii. Incomplete fusion of the bone of the calvarium accompanied by incomplete development of the brain is called *anencephaly.*
Craniorachischisis and anencephaly are not compatible with life.

Q3. What is Arnold-Chiari malformation?

Definition Arnold-Chiari malformation is a term for a group of congenital CNS malformations involving the brainstem and cerebellum.
Clinicopathologic features
i. There are four anatomic subtypes of this malformation but all of them are related to elongation of the medulla and part of the vermis of the cerebellum.
ii. These changes are accompanied by the herniation of cerebellar vermis and cerebellar tonsils through the foramen magnum and obstruction of foramina Luschka and Magendie.
iii. These changes usually cause hydrocephalus. Arnold-Chiari malformation is the cause of hydrocephalus in 50% of all childhood cases.
iv. In many cases, there is also meningomyelocele.

Q4. What is hydrocephalus? Comment on its etiopathogenesis and types.

Definition Hydrocephalus is an increased volume of CSF within the skull accompanied by dilatation of ventricles.
Normal flow of CSF For understanding of etiopathogenesis of various types of hydrocephalus, a knowledge of source and circulation of CSF is essential **(Fig. 30.2)**:
• CSF is normally produced by the choroid plexus in the lateral ventricles from where it flows through the foramina Monro to the third ventricle, then to the aqueduct of Sylvius and the forth ventricle.
• From the fourth ventricle, it passes through the foramina Luschka and Magendie to the subarachnoid space and is spread all over the surface of the brain and spinal cord.
• It is absorbed into the blood by arachnoid villi present along the dural venous sinuses.
• The total volume of CSF is 150 ml.
Etiopathogenesis and types Hydrocephalus can be classified as primary or secondary; latter is of lesser clinical significance.
I. ***Primary hydrocephalus*** is defined as actual increase in the volume of CSF in the skull accompanied by elevated intracranial pressure. It can be classified as communicating (obstructive) and non-communicating (non-obstructive). There are three possible causes for either type:
i. Obstruction of the flow of CSF
ii. Overproduction of CSF
iii. Deficient reabsorption of CSF
A. *Non-communicating (obstructive) hydrocephalus* is the most common form of hydrocephalus in infants and children, but it can occur in adults as well. Common causes are as follows:
a. *Congenital non-communicating hydrocephalus* due to stenosis of the aqueduct, Arnold-Chiari malformation, progressive gliosis of the aqueduct and intra-uterine meningitis of the foetus.
b. *Acquired non-communicating hydrocephalus* caused by intracranial lesions which include:

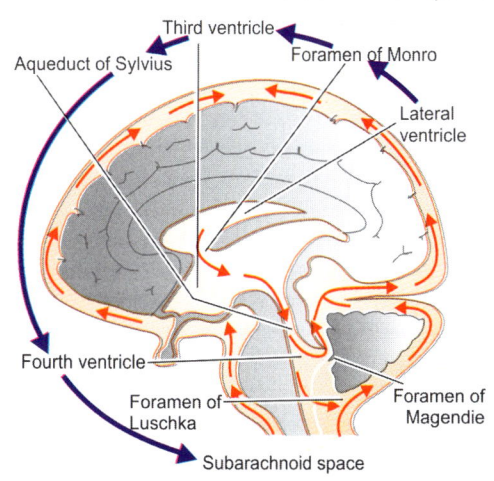

FIGURE 30.2: Normal circulation of CSF.

- Tumours adjacent to the ventricular system such as ependymoma, choroid plexus papilloma, medulloblastoma, etc.
- Inflammatory lesions such as meningitis, brain abscess, etc.
- Haemorrhage into the brain, intraventricular haemorrhage, epidural and subdural haemorrhage.

B. *Communicating (non-obstructive) hydrocephalus* may be caused by the following:

a. *Overproduction of CSF*, e.g. choroid plexus papilloma.

b. *Deficient reabsorption of CSF* following meningitis, subarachnoid haemorrhage and dural sinus thrombosis.

II. **Secondary hydrocephalus** is also called normal pressure hydrocephalus or hydrocephalus ex vacuo. It results from filling of intracranial spaces with CSF that have dilated due to a loss of brain substance. Best examples are:

a. Normal pressure hydrocephalus that accompanies atrophy of the brain in Alzheimer disease.

b. Loss of brain tissue after a cerebral infarction.

Q5. How do infections reach the central nervous system? Comment briefly on the types of infections of the CNS and pathologic changes due to them.

Infection of the CNS can be caused by a variety of pathogens, including bacteria, rickettsiae, viruses, fungi, protozoa and parasites. Various routes of infections in CNS are as follows:

i. *Via the blood stream* from another focus of infection in the body. This is the most common way of infection of the CNS.

ii. *Direct implantation* of infectious pathogens following trauma with cranial bone fracture or penetrating injuries by firearms.

iii. *Local extension* from contiguous structures such as the middle ear, nose or pharynx.

iv. *Along nerves* is the route taken by many viruses such as herpes simplex, herpes zoster or rabies virus, that spread from peripheral tissue to the CNS along peripheral nerves.

Pathology CNS infections may be acute or chronic, localised or diffuse.

- They are classified according to their location as *encephalitis* or *meningitis* (or *meningoencephalitis* when combined).
- Infections may be purulent (when caused by bacteria or fungi) or non-purulent (e.g. viral infection) or granulomatous (e.g. tuberculosis).
- Localised purulent bacterial infection results most often in the formation of *brain abscess*.
- Other forms of purulent infections are less common and include: epidural abscess, subdural empyema, septic thromboembolism of dural sinuses and purulent encephalomyelitis.

Q6. What is meningitis? Discuss etiopathogenesis and clinicopathologic features of its various types.

Definition Meningitis is an inflammation of the meninges. It can involve only dura called *pachymeningitis*, or leptomeninges (pia and arachnoid) called *leptomeningitis*. The latter is more common and, if not specified, the term meningitis refers to leptomeningitis.

- *Pachymeningitis* is invariably an extension of the inflammation from chronic suppurative otitis media or from fracture of the skull. An *extradural (epidural) abscess* may form. Inflammation may spread deeper and form a *subdural abscess*, or even deeper and form a *cerebral abscess*.
- *Leptomeningitis* is in most cases caused by viral or bacterial infections, and less often by fungal infections. Its less common forms are chemical meningitis and carcinomatous meningitis.

Clinicopathologic forms In routine medical practice, three clinicopathologic forms of meningitis are recognised: acute pyogenic, acute lymphocytic (viral), and chronic meningitis (bacterial or fungal).

I. **Acute pyogenic meningitis** is a bacterial infection characterised by infiltration of leptomeninges with neutrophils and acute inflammatory cells into the CSF.

Etiopathogenesis The predominant causative bacteria vary with age and condition of the patient as under:

i. *Streptococcus pneumoniae* is the most common cause of bacterial meningitis in adults (~50%) and may be preceded by pneumococcal pneumonia.

ii. *Neisseria meningitidis* causes epidemic meningitis affecting children who have not been vaccinated and is responsible for ~25% of all cases.

iii. Group B streptococci such as *Streptococcus agalactiae* was previously considered predominant cause for meningitis in neonates but is now seen more frequently in older individuals with pre-existing conditions (~15% of all cases).
iv. *Listeria monocytogenes* is an important cause of meningitis (~10% of all cases), most often affecting persons at extremes of age (i.e. neonates and individuals above 60 years of age), immunocompromised persons and pregnant women.
v. Gram-negative meningitis such as by *Escherichia coli* is common in individuals with chronic debility (e.g. diabetes mellitus, alcoholism, cirrhosis) and in patients undergoing neurosurgical procedures.
vi. *Staph aureus* is an important etiologic agent for meningitis following neurosurgical procedures.
vii. *Haemophilus influenzae* was earlier a common agent for infection in infants and small children but has declined as a cause due to childhood vaccination.

Routes of infection are as follows:
- By the blood stream (most common)
- From an adjacent focus of infection
- By iatrogenic infection following lumbar puncture or surgical interventions.

Pathology The brain is covered with pus which fills the subarachnoid space. Turbid exudate fills the sulci and is most prominent at the base of the brain where the subarachnoid spaces are wider than on the convexity of the brain. Purulent exudate may obstruct the flow of CSF and produce hydrocephalus.

Microscopy There are numerous PMNs filling the subarachnoid space and infiltrating the meninges, most prominently around the blood vessels. Bacteria can be best visualised by Gram-staining.

Clinical features Acute bacterial meningitis is a medical emergency with possible lethal outcome.
i. Common symptoms include: severe headache, fever, vomiting, drowsiness, progressing to stupor and coma.
ii. Occasionally, it may be associated with increased irritability and even convulsions, especially in children.
iii. Stiffness of the neck on forward bending is a clinical finding supporting the diagnosis.
iv. *CSF findings* shows diagnostic features as under:
a. Naked eye appearance of the CSF, which appears cloudy or even frankly purulent.
b. Elevated CSF pressure (above 180 mm water).
c. Neutrophilic leucocytosis of the CSF.
d. High protein content of CSF.
e. Decreased sugar concentration of CSF.
f. Bacteriologic findings, including positive Gram staining of the smears followed up by bacteriologic cultures and isolation of the pathogenic bacteria.

II. **Acute lymphocytic meningitis** It is a viral meningitis, especially common in children and young adults.

Etiopathogenesis It may be caused by a number of viruses such as enteroviruses, adenoviruses and childhood exanthema viruses (e.g. measles, chickenpox).

Clinical features
i. The symptoms are milder than in bacterial meningitis and the disease has usually a self-limited brief course with complete recovery.
ii. *CSF findings* include the following:
a. Naked eye appearance of clear or slightly turbid CSF.
b. Increased CSF pressure (above 250 mm water).
c. Lymphocytosis of CSF (10–100 cells/ml).
d. CSF protein mildly elevated or normal.
e. CSF sugar concentration normal.
f. Bacteriology studies negative ('sterile CSF')

III. **Chronic meningitis** It may be caused by *M. tuberculosis* or fungi such as *Cryptococcus neoformans*.
Etiopathogenesis Infection of the meninges is usually secondary to primary pulmonary infection followed by haematogenous dissemination of pathogens.
- *Tuberculous meningitis* may be a manifestation of military tuberculosis.
- *Cryptococcal meningitis* is found in immunosuppressed persons and is an important fungal infection in persons with AIDS.

Pathology Both conditions present with granuloma formation. Special stains are used to demonstrate the pathogens: acid-fast bacilli (AFB) positive in tuberculosis, and silver impregnation or mucicarmine stain for encapsulated cryptococci.

Clinical features

i. *Tuberculous meningitis* presents with headaches, confusion, malaise and vomiting.

ii. *Cryptococcal meningitis* could have a fulminant course and is lethal with a few weeks, but sometimes it may be indolent for months to years.

iii. *CSF findings* are as follows:

a. Naked eye appearance of a clear or slightly turbid CSF.
b. Raised CSF pressure (above 300 mm water).
c. Mononuclear leucocytosis including mostly lymphocytes and some macrophages (100–1000 cells/ml).
d. Raised protein content.
e. Lowered glucose concentration.
f. Stainable pathogens seen in the centrifuged deposits of CSF.

Q7. Tabulate contrasting features of common forms of meningitis.

Table 30.1 summarises the contrasting features of three common forms of meningitis.

TABLE 30.1 CSF findings in health and various types of meningitis.

FEATURE	NORMAL	ACUTE PYOGENIC (BACTERIAL) MENINGITIS	ACUTE LYMPHOCYTIC (VIRAL) MENINGITIS	CHRONIC (TUBERCULOUS) MENINGITIS
1. *Naked eye appearance*	Clear and colourless	Cloudy or frankly purulent	Clear or slightly turbid	Clear or slightly turbid, forms fibrin coagulum on standing
2. *CSF pressure*	60–150 mm water	Elevated (above 180 mm water)	Elevated (above 250 mm water)	Elevated (above 300 mm water)
3. *Cells*	0–4 lymphocytes/ml	10–10,000 neutrophils/ml	10–100 lymphocytes/ml	100–1000 lymphocytes/ml
4. *Proteins*	15–45 mg/dL	Markedly raised	Mildly raised	Raised
5. *Glucose*	50–80 mg/dL	Markedly reduced	Normal	Reduced
6. *Bacteriology*	Sterile	Causative organisms present	Sterile	Tubercle bacilli present

(CSF, cerebrospinal fluid)

Q8. What is encephalitis?

Definition Encephalitis is an inflammation of the brain.

Etiopathogenesis Encephalitis may be caused by bacteria, viruses, fungi or protozoa. It can be acute or chronic, localised or diffuse.

Q9. What is brain abscess? Briefly describe its etiopathogenesis and clinicopathologic features.

Definition Brain abscess is a localised purulent bacterial inflammation, usually presenting as an intracerebral mass lesion.

Etiopathogenesis Bacterial infections of the brain develop like those causing meningitis, and are often preceded by brain infections as under:

i. *Direct implantation* of bacteria, as in compound fractures of the skull.

ii. *Local extension* of infections from otitis media, mastoiditis or sinusitis.

iii. *Haematogenous spread* of bacterial infections from other sites in the body, such as endocarditis or bronchiectases.

Pathology

Gross Brain abscess appears like an encapsulated cavity filled with semi-liquid pus and necrotic brain tissue.

Microscopy

i. The necrotic brain tissue is permeated with PMNs and pus cells.

ii. The liquefied purulent content is surrounded by acute and chronic inflammation penetrating the adjacent brain tissue which shows gliosis and new blood vessel formation.
iii. Since the brain injury elicits *gliosis* rather than fibrous scarring, this 'capsule of the abscess' does not show fibrosis as seen around the abscesses in other part of the body.
iv. The only exceptions are abscesses adjacent to the meninges, which contain mesodermal tissue extending into fibrosis around an abscess.
Clinical features Symptoms of a brain abscess include signs of acute inflammation combined with sign of increased intracranial pressure due the mass effects of the abscess.
i. These symptoms include fever, headache, vomiting, seizures and neurological deficits depending on the location of the abscess.
ii. Brain abscess can be seen by CT scanning as a cerebral mass resembling a brain tumour.
iii. The final diagnosis is often made only after an intraoperative biopsy reveals pus rather than tumour tissue.
iv. The pus must be drained by surgery combined with antibiotic treatment.

Q10. What is tuberculoma?

Definition Tuberculoma is a tumour-like intracranial mass composed of tuberculous granulomas, secondary to haematogenous dissemination of *Mycobacteria tuberculosis* from another site in the body, most often the lungs.
Pathology
Gross Tuberculomas may be solitary or multiple, often involving the brain as well as the meninges.
i. Multiple tuberculomas form discrete small nodules.
ii. Solitary tuberculoma presents as a single multilobular mass, which shows foci of caseous softening.
Microscopy The lesions are composed of caseating granulomas, a zone of gliosis surrounding the granulomas, and fibrous tissue extending from the meninges.
CSF findings
i. Clear or slightly turbid, elevated pressure, presence of lymphocytes (100–1000/ml), elevated protein concentration, and reduced glucose.
ii. Tubercle bacilli can be seen in smears by special stains using the acid fast Ziehl-Neelsen technique.

Q11. What is neurosyphilis? Comment on clinicopathologic features of its types.

Syphilis of the central nervous system includes:
- *syphilitic meningitis* seen in secondary syphilis, and
- *neurosyphilis* of tertiary syphilis comprising tabes dorsalis and generalised paralysis of the insane.

I. **Syphilitic meningitis** is a form of chronic meningitis characterised by perivascular infiltrates of lymphocytes and plasma cells and endarteritis obliterans.
II. **Tabes dorsalis** presents clinically as locomotor ataxia. It includes progressive degeneration of the spinal nerves and posterior columns. These changes affect coordination of skeletal muscles and joint movement resulting in locomotor ataxia. There is also loss of pain sensation, Argyll-Robertson pupils which react to accommodation but not to light stimuli.
III. **Generalised paralysis** of the insane results in diffuse parenchymal involvement of the CNS by spirochetes with widespread lesions in all parts of the nervous system resulting in motor, sensory and mental abnormalities.

Q12. What is viral encephalitis? Discuss etiology and clinicopathologic features of major types.

Definition Viral infections may cause meningitis as well as encephalitis which are often combined into meningoencephalitis. Most viral infections reach the brain by a haematogenous route and are thus secondary infections. There are, however, certain neurotropic viruses which affect the CNS exclusively.
Etiology The list of potential pathogens causing viral encephalitis is very long. The most important are as follows:
i. *Viruses causing skin infections* combined with infection of peripheral ganglia such as herpes simplex and herpes zoster.
ii. *Gastrointestinal viruses* such as enteroviruses. Polio virus has been a major cause of viral spinal cord and brain infection but now it has been eradicated from most parts of the world.

iii. *Arthropod-bite-transmitted arboviruses*, such as West Nile virus, Eastern equine virus, etc.
iv. *Animal bite-transmitted viruses* like rabies.

Pathology Microscopic changes vary depending on the type of virus that has caused the encephalitis. However, a few pathologic changes are common and are found in almost all viral infections:
i. Parenchymal perivascular infiltrates of lymphocytes, plasma cells, macrophages.
ii. Clusters of microglia cells involved in neuronophagia.
iii. Intranuclear inclusion in neurons in many viral infections, e.g. rabies has intracytoplasmic inclusions in neurons called Negri bodies.

Clinical features Viral infections may present in several forms:
i. *Acute viral syndrome* is the most common clinical syndrome. It presents with fever, headache, somnolence and loss of various neural functions, and may be complicated by epileptic seizures and a loss of consciousness.
ii. *Chronic latent infections with exacerbation* as happens with some viruses such as herpes zoster which gets *reactivated periodically* to cause clinical symptoms.
iii. *Slow viruses* are a group of viruses that have a long incubation and cause neurological problems many years after infection. For example: progressive multifocal leucoencephalopathy (PML) caused by JC virus, progressive rubella panencephalopathy, or subacute sclerosing panencephalitis (SSP) in persons who have not been immunised to measles virus.

Q13. What is progressive multifocal leucoencephalopathy? Briefly describe its pathologic features.

Definition Progressive multifocal leucoencephalopathy (PML) is a slow viral infection of the CNS caused by a polyoma virus called *JC virus*.
PML develops due to reactivation of JC virus in persons who have had the infection in childhood. This occurs most often in immunosuppressed persons following organ transplantation or intensive cancer chemotherapy. It is also an important feature of AIDS.

Pathology JC virus infects oligodendrocytes causing progressive multifocal demyelination of the CNS.
Gross Demyelinated axons forming *gelatinous areas* can be seen at the interface between grey and white matter in various parts of the cerebrum and cerebellum.
Microscopy The foci of demyelination are infiltrated by lipid-laden macrophages. Enlarged nuclei of the oligodendroglial cells contain purple intranuclear inclusions, best seen at the periphery of the foci of demyelination.

Q14. What are prion diseases? Discuss their etiology and clinicopathologic features.

Definition Prion diseases are caused by *prions*, altered structural proteins of normal neural cells (PrP), which through conformational changes become pathogenic and capable of producing infectious neurodegenerative diseases.

Etiopathogenesis Prions are derived from normal PrP which change their normal α-helical structure to a neurotoxic β-pleated isoform. The abnormal isoform can replicate without DNA or RNA and can be transmitted as infectious particle.

Modes of transmission Depending on the type of prion, they may be transmitted by following routes:
i. From one person to another through close contact
ii. By iatrogenic injection or transplantation of tissues
iii. By ingestion of infected tissue (e.g. 'kuru' an infectious disease among the natives of New Guinea spread by cannibalistic consumption of infected human brain)
iv. Some prions are hereditary and cause familial diseases related to mutations of *PrP* gene
v. Some are transmitted from mother to the foetus through the placenta
vi. Some are transmitted from animals to humans ('*mad cow disease*')

Pathology There are several prion related diseases, the most important of which is *Creutzfeldt-Jakob disease (CJD)*. CJD is a rare cause of infectious dementia affecting 1 per one million persons. Pathologically it presents as a spongiform encephalopathy.
Gross The brain looks normal.
Microscopy The brain contains numerous small round vacuoles in the cortex and other grey matter areas such as basal ganglia. These changes are associated with a loss of nerve cells and reactive gliosis. There are no signs of inflammation and the white matter is typically spared.

Clinical features CJD is clinically characterised by rapidly progressive dementia associated with myoclonus. It is invariably fatal with mean survival of about 7 months after diagnosis.

Q15. Which fungal and protozoal pathogens can cause encephalitis?

Fungal encephalitis Encephalitis can be caused by a variety of fungi, which reach the CNS by bloodstream from other sites in the body.

i. They are most often seen in immunosuppressed persons suffering from AIDS, lymphomas and other malignant diseases treated with cytotoxic drugs.

ii. The most important fungal pathogens are *Candida albicans, Mucor, Aspergillus fumigatus, Cryptococcus neoformans, Histoplasma capsulatum* and *Blastomyces dermatitidis.*

iii. Pathologically, these fungi are known to produce meningitis, vasculitis or encephalitis.

Protozoal encephalitis The most important protozoal infections involving the CNS are malaria, toxoplasmosis, amoebiasis and trypanosomiasis.

Q16. What are cerebrovascular diseases? Enumerate various conditions causing them.

Definition Cerebrovascular diseases are caused by circulatory disorders resulting in cerebral ischaemia or haemorrhage.

Etiopathogenesis The normal function of the CNS depends critically on adequate supply of oxygen and glucose. CNS has limited stores of energy and any interruptions of normal circulation for more than 3–4 minutes will cause permanent damage to nerve cells.

Various pathologic processes implicated in cerebrovascular diseases are as follows:

i. Thrombosis and embolism.

ii. Cerebral hypoxia due to inadequate oxygen supply caused by cardiorespiratory, haematologic or toxic/metabolic disorders.

iii. Hypertensive cardiovascular diseases.

iv. Atherosclerosis of carotid and basilar arteries and their branches supplying blood to the brain.

v. Developmental disorders of the cerebral circulation including aneurysms and arteriovenous malformations.

vi. Arterial diseases, including vascular spasms causing migraine and short-lived transient ischaemic attacks (TIA) lasting only 15–20 minutes.

Q17. How are cerebrovascular diseases classified?

Cerebrovascular diseases from various etiologic processes result in following parenchymal diseases of the brain:

I. Ischaemic brain damage:
i. Generalised reduction in blood flow resulting in *global hypoxic-ischaemic encephalopathy*
ii. Local vascular obstruction causing *infarcts.*

II. Intracranial spontaneous (non-traumatic) haemorrhage:
i. Haemorrhage in the brain parenchyma *(intracerebral haemorrhage)*
ii. Haemorrhage in the subarachnoid space *(subarachnoid haemorrhage).*

III. Traumatic brain haemorrhage:
i. Epidural haematoma
ii. Subdural haematoma
iii. Parenchymal brain damage

Q18. What is stroke syndrome?

The cardinal feature of major cerebrovascular diseases is the *stroke syndrome.* It is defined as sudden neurologic deficit caused by impairment of cerebral circulation that lasts more than 24 hours. It results in irreversible brain damage that is characterised by the following:

i. Symptoms vary from minor neurologic impairment to severe, including hemiplegia, coma and death, depending on its location and extent.

ii. In 85% of cases, it is classified as ischaemic, and in 15% of cases as haemorrhagic; the latter has a worse prognosis.

Stroke is ranked as the third cause of death in adults in United States and Europe. In the US, at any time there are more than 3 million people who survived stroke and are at least partially incapacitated by it.

Q19. Define ischaemic brain damage. What are its types?

Definition Ischaemic brain damage is marked by nerve cell necrosis caused by reduced or completely interrupted blood supply of the brain, that cannot meet the neural cell demands for oxygen and nutrients.

Types It may occur in two forms:
- Global hypoxic-ischaemic encephalopathy
- Cerebral infarction

Q20. Briefly discuss etiopathogenesis and pathology of global hypoxic-ischaemic encephalopathy.

Definition Global hypoxic-ischaemic encephalopathy results from generalised cerebral hypoperfusion.

Etiopathogenesis Under normal conditions, the circulation of the brain is autoregulated and the brain remains adequately perfused if the systolic arterial pressure is above 50 mmHg. If the pressure falls below that value, the brain will be hypoperfused and will show signs ischaemic encephalopathy. The most common causes of such medical emergency are:

i. Cardiac arrest
ii. Severe episodes of hypotension, such as massive bleeding
iii. Carbon monoxide poisoning
iv. Status epilepticus

Clinically, it may present as post-ischaemic confusional state or coma progressing to persistent vegetative life and brain death.

Pathology Three types of changes can be seen:

i. **Selective neuronal damage** due to high vulnerability of nerve cells to hypoxia/anoxia. Nerve cells have very high metabolic requirements, are very sensitive to lactic acid that forms in hypoxia and produces toxic acidic excitatory neurotransmitters (*excitotoxins*).

a. Ischaemic neurons lose the basophilic Nissl substance and their cytoplasm becomes red and shrunken during the first 24 hours of ischaemia.
b. Nucleus becomes pyknotic and the cells disintegrate thereafter, to be replaced by reactive glia cells.
c. Among the glia cells, the most susceptible to ischaemia are oligodendroglia cells, followed by astrocytes and microglia cells.
d. Vascular endothelial cells survive ischaemia the longest.

ii. **Laminar necrosis** predominantly involves the deep cortical grey matter with relative sparing of the superficial layers.

a. This form of necrosis reflects the perfusion gradient, according to which the surface layers receive more oxygenated blood than the deeper layers. Hypoperfusion will, therefore, affect deeper layers more than the surface layers of the cortex.
b. It may be seen by naked eye examination as a line in the deeper cortex, but is best assessed by microscopy which shows signs of cell necrosis.

iii. **Watershed infarcts** occur at the overlapping border zones between the parts of the brain supplied by the anterior, middle and posterior cerebral arteries. These zones are the farthest from the source of blood supply and, thus, suffer maximum damage in hypotension.

a. Most vulnerable is the zone between the anterior and the middle cerebral arterial supply, producing parasagittal infarction.
b. Such infarcts are visible by naked eye within a few days of the event that has caused the ischaemic injury, but are also best assessed microscopically.

Q21. What is cerebral infarction? Discuss its etiologic and pathologic types.

Definition Cerebral infarction is a localised area of ischaemic brain necrosis caused by vascular occlusion, clinically presenting as a stroke.

Etiology and types Cerebral infarcts may be classified as: arterial, venous and non-occlusive.

I. **Arterial occlusion** is the most common cause of cerebral infarction. It may be caused by emboli or thrombi forming inside a cerebral artery.
A. *Emboli* originate most often from the heart and less often from aorta and major arteries of the neck include the following:
i. Ventricular mural thrombi over a myocardial infarct
ii. Left atrial thrombi formed due to atrial fibrillation
iii. Paradoxical thromboemboli from the right atrium through an open foramen ovale
iv. Valvular fibrin thrombi in endocarditis
v. Thrombi overlying ulcerated atheromas of the aorta and carotid arteries
Emboli most often occlude the middle cerebral artery lying in direct line from the internal carotid artery. Emboli tend to lodge in the arteries narrowed by atherosclerosis and are commonly found at the site of their branching.
B. *Thrombi* form over ulcerated atheromas in the major cerebral arteries. Thrombi are a much less common cause of cerebral infarction than the emboli.
The *outcome of arterial occlusion* depends on the artery involved and the extent of anastomoses:
i. Arteries of the circle of Willis have adequate anastomoses.
ii. Middle and anterior cerebral arteries have partial anastomoses.
iii. Small terminal cerebral arteries do not have any anastomoses.
II. **Venous occlusion** is an uncommon cause of infarction because of good communications in venous drainage of the brain. Clinically, the most common is superior sagittal thrombosis of venous sinus found in cancer patients who have a tendency to form thrombi.
III. **Non-occlusive causes** include:
i. Compression of the cerebral arteries from outside, most often during herniation. For example, the sub-falcine (cingulate) herniation could compress the anterior cerebral artery and the transtentorial (uncinate) herniation can compress the posterior cerebral artery.
ii. Watershed infarcts are also localised forms of cerebral ischaemia.
Pathology and types Cerebral infarcts are classified as anaemic or haemorrhagic:
I. *Anaemic infarct* can be recognised on gross examination only a day or two after the onset of ischaemia.
i. It presents as a localised area blurring the junction between the grey and the white matter.
ii. Within 2–3 days, the infarcted area undergoes softening due to liquefactive necrosis.
iii. *Microscopically*, there is widespread nerve cells necrosis followed by an influx of macrophages which act as scavengers taking up the lipid rich remnants of nerve cells.
iv. Finally, the infarct becomes cystic and filled with semiliquid amorphous necrotic brain tissue, which will be slowly absorbed and replaced by fluid.
v. The brain tissue around such infarcts shows gliosis and contains numerous foamy macrophages, and blood vessels ingrown from the meninges.
II. *Haemorrhagic infarct* resembles an intracerebral haematoma. It results from fragmentation of the occluding embolus, allowing the blood to enter the necrotic area.
i. *Microscopically*, such infarcts resemble anaemic infarcts but also contain disintegrating RBCs which give rise to haemosiderin granules in the phagocytic cells.
ii. Thromboemboli occluding the smaller arteries are much easier lysed allowing earlier partial reperfusion which gives the infarct a mottled appearance.

Q22. What is intracranial haemorrhage? What are its main types?

Definition Intracranial haemorrhage usually present as haematoma, i.e. a localised blood extravasation into the brain or other intracranial compartments (e.g. subdural space).
Classification Several criteria can be used to classify various intracranial haemorrhages as under:
i. *According to their causes*, these can be classified as: a) traumatic, or b) non-traumatic (spontaneous).
ii. *According to their location*, these can be classified as **(Fig. 30.3)**: a) intracerebral, b) subarachnoid, c) subdural, or d) epidural.
iii. *According to their duration*, they can be classified clinically as: a) acute, b) chronic, or c) recurrent.
iv. *According to their site of origin*, they can be classified as: a) arterial, b) venous, or c) mixed (arterial and venous).

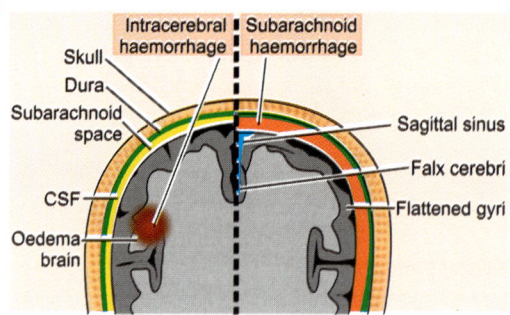

FIGURE 30.3: Two types of intracranial haemorrhage: intracerebral (left) and subarachnoid haemorrhage (right).

Q23. What is intracerebral (non-traumatic) haemorrhage? Briefly describe its etiopathogenesis and clinicopathologic features.

Definition Intracerebral haemorrhage is formation of a haematoma in the brain parenchyma. It is most often a complication of hypertension and is related to a rupture of small intracerebral arteries and arterioles.

Etiopathogenesis Inadequately controlled hypertension damages the wall of small penetrating cerebral arteries and arterioles leading to hyaline arteriolar sclerosis and formation of *microscopic aneurysms* (*Charcot-Bouchard aneurysms*) prone to rupture under internal pressure.

i. Massive bleeding results in formation of haematoma that acts as a cerebral mass which is usually associated with cerebral oedema and increased intracranial pressure.

ii. Haematomas are most often located in following three locations: basal ganglia-thalamus (65%), pons (15%) and cerebellum (10%).

iii. Other less common causes of intracerebral haemorrhages are: cerebral amyloidotic angiopathy, infectious or autoimmune vasculitis, bleeding diathesis diseases (e.g. thrombocytopenia, haemophilia) and is also seen in intravenous drug addicts.

Pathology

i. Haematoma destroys neural tissue which undergoes necrosis and is replaced by extravasated blood.

ii. In the surrounding parenchyma, there are usually microscopic perivascular haemorrhages into the Virchow-Robin spaces.

iii. In addition, there are signs of previous vascular insufficiency. These include haemosiderin-laden macrophages in slit-like spaces of previous small resorbed haemorrhages ('*slit haemorrhages*').

iv. Occlusions of penetrating arteries results in small *lacunar infarcts*, usually seen in the area of basal ganglia.

v. Intracerebral haematomas may rupture into the lateral ventricles causing *haematocephalus*, or less often, extend into the subarachnoid space, and thus become indistinguishable from subarachnoid haemorrhage.

vi. In patients with smaller haematomas who survive, the extravasated blood is reabsorbed and the haematoma transforms into an *apoplectic cyst* filled with yellowish fluid. The wall of such a cyst is infiltrated with haemosiderin-laden macrophages and shows gliosis.

Clinical features Intracerebral haematomas vary in size and location.

i. Those larger than 30 ml present typically with severe headache of sudden onset leading to loss of brain functions and consciousness progressing to coma. One third of patients will die within the first 3–4 days.

ii. Cerebellar haematomas can be surgically removed with little residual damage.

iii. Haematomas of basal ganglia and pons cannot be removed efficiently.

Q24. What is subarachnoid haemorrhage? Comment on its etiopathogenesis and salient clinical features.

Definition Haemorrhage into the subarachnoid spaces is most often caused by rupture of an aneurysm, and less often rupture of a vascular malformations. It can be visualised by CT scanning, most often at the base of the brain.

Etiopathogenesis

i. Subarachnoid haemorrhage is most often caused by a rupture of berry aneurysms of the circle of Willis that account for 85% cases.

ii. The remaining 15% are caused by rupture of the following:
a. Atherosclerotic aneurysm, which are usually fusiform and located in the posterior cerebral circulation (e.g. basilar artery).
b. Mycotic aneurysm due to septic thrombi in bacterial endocarditis.
c. Intravenous drug abuse.
d. Congenital vascular malformations (most often *arteriovenous malformation* composed of arteries directly connected to veins without interposed capillaries).

Clinical features
i. Ruptured berry aneurysms present with sudden onset of severe headache.
ii. Increased intracranial pressure results in a loss of consciousness and stroke like symptoms.
iii. High mortality (25%); severe neurologic defects in survivors, some of which remain in vegetative state.
iv. Ruptured berry aneurysms are often accompanied by vasospasm of the affected artery causing ischaemic brain infarcts.
v. Occlusive hydrocephalus results from obstruction of the foramina Magendie and Luschka.
vi. CSF contains blood and if the patient survives it is yellow-coloured ('*xanthochromia*').

Q25. What are berry aneurysms?

Definition Small saccular aneurysms of the circle of Willis and its contingent cerebral arteries.
Key facts about berry aneurysms are as follows:
i. Found at autopsy in 2% of general population, but asymptomatic in most instances.
ii. Genetic predisposition, as evidenced by the following:
a. More common seen in families of a person who has a clinically diagnosed berry aneurysm.
b. Patients with certain hereditary diseases at higher risk: autosomal dominant polycystic kidney disease, hereditary connective tissue diseases (e.g. Ehlers-Danlos syndrome, Marfan syndrome), neurofibromatosis type I, and coarctation of aorta.
iii. Develop most often at the junction between the main arteries forming the circle of Willis and their communicating branches, and at the point of arterial branching **(Fig. 30.4)**.
iv. Points of aneurysm formation are structurally weak because they do not contain internal elastic lamina and the muscle layer.
v. Most of the aneurysms (>90%) are found in the anterior part of the circle of Willis derived from the anterior and middle cerebral arteries, and the trifurcation of the middle cerebral artery.
vi. Multiple in 25% cases; this accounts in part for the high recurrence rate of rupture/bleeding.
vii. Aneurysms are not present at birth but start developing in childhood and gradually enlarge to the point of rupture; peak incidence of rupture is in the 30–50 years age group.
viii. The size of the aneurysm is an important risk factor for rupture.

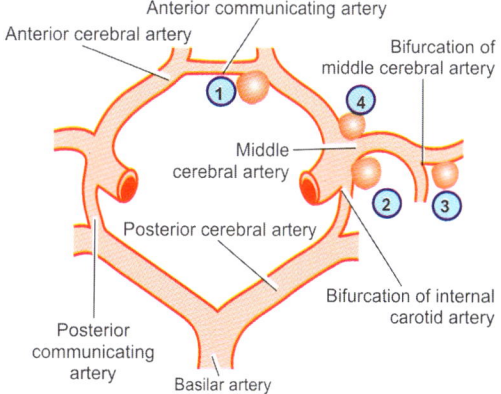

FIGURE 30.4: The circle of Willis showing principal sites of berry (saccular) aneurysms. The serial numbers indicate the frequency of involvement in locations, in descending order.

Q26. What are the most important entities included in traumatic intracranial haemorrhages? Discuss them briefly.

Traumatic intracranial haemorrhages include the following three clinicopathologic entities **(Fig. 30.5)**:
- Epidural haematoma
- Subdural haematoma
- Intracerebral haemorrhage related to parenchymal brain damage

I. Epidural haematoma is an accumulation of blood in the space between the dura and skull bones, usually following temporal bone fracture. Key clinicopathologic features are as follows:
i. It results from rupture of the middle meningeal artery.

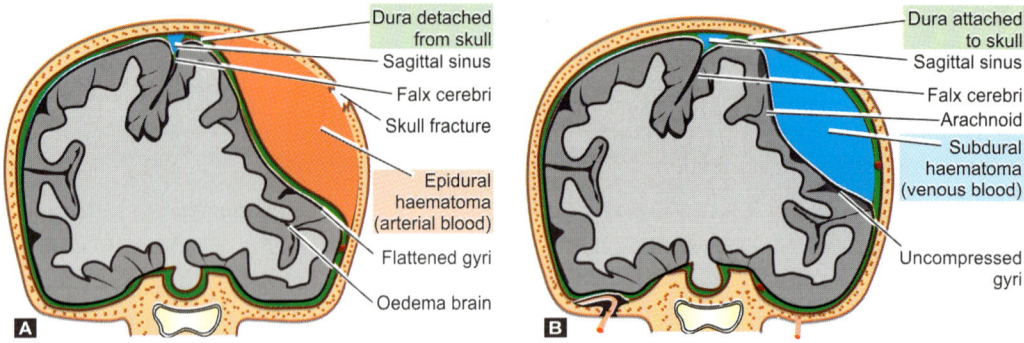

FIGURE 30.5: Traumatic haemorrhage into the brain. A, *Epidural haematoma* often results from rupture of artery following skull fracture resulting in accumulation of arterial blood between the skull and the dura. B, *Subdural haematoma* often results from rupture of veins crossing the cerebral convexities and is characterised by accumulation of venous blood between the dura and the arachnoid.

ii. The pressure of the arterial blood fills the virtual space between the dura and the skull bone; over the period of several hours it forms a haematoma compressing the brain.

iii. After the trauma, the patient is lucid until the haematoma reaches a size that endangers life. Without surgical intervention, the patient will invariably die.

iv. Epidural haematoma in infants and small children may occur even without a fracture. It results from the movement of the compressed bones which shear the artery the underlying artery.

II. **Subdural haematoma** is a traditional name for the accumulation of blood s in the so called 'subdural space' between the dense collagenous layer of the dura and the loose connective layer just above the arachnoid. Technically speaking, it is thus an 'intradural haematoma'. Its key features are as under:

i. It results from the rupture of the bridging veins, providing the conduit for the venous blood from the brain across the subarachnoid and subdural space to the venous sinuses of the dura.

ii. The traumatic haematoma transforms into a clot which is located over the convex surface of the brain.

iii. It may occur in two forms: acute and chronic.

a. *Acute subdural haematoma* results from blunt trauma of the head and is typically located on the frontoparietal surface of the brain.
- It develops slowly over the period of several hours causing gradual increase of the intracranial pressure.
- Clinically, the patient complains of progressively increasing headache, somnolence and gradual loss of conscience.
- There are no localising neurologic symptoms related to compression of a particular part of the brain, but over time the mass effect may be lethal.
- Children are especially endangered because their bridging veins have thin walls.

b. *Chronic subdural haematoma* results from recurrent minor head traumas in the elderly (e.g. due to repeated accidental falls). Due to the age-related atrophy of the brain, their bridging veins lack the external support and are more vulnerable and tend to shear and bleed.
- Extravasated blood elicits formation of granulation tissue that grows into the haematoma forming a membrane covering over the convexity of the brain.
- Clinical symptoms are nonspecific, but over time these haematomas also may cause death.

III. **Parenchymal brain damage** may occur in several forms as under:

i. *Concussion* is caused by closed head injury and is characterised by:
a. Transient neurological dysfunction and loss of consciousness.
b. Complete neurologic recovery is the norm and the brain shows no macroscopic or microscopic signs of injury.
c. More severe concussions may result in diffuse axonal injury.

ii. *Diffuse axonal injury* of persistent coma or vegetative state following brain injury has following features:
a. Axonal injury results from sudden angular acceleration an deceleration and shearing of axons in the deep white mater of the brain.

b. The changes are submicroscopic and the brain may show initially no obvious histopathological changes.
c. Over time, the loss of brain substance becomes more prominent resulting in brain atrophy and widening of lateral ventricles (*post-traumatic hydrocephalus*).
iii. *Contusions and lacerations* are tissue injuries resulting from the mechanical impact of blunt trauma that may or may not be associated with skull fracture.
a. Tearing of the brain tissue is usually accompanied by vascular injury and bleeding into the brain and subarachnoid space.
b. Microscopic examination reveals necrosis and haemorrhage into the brain tissue.
c. If the patient survives, areas of necrosis and haemorrhage are infiltrated with lipid-laden macrophages containing also haemosiderin granules.
iv. *Traumatic cerebral haemorrhage* which presents as multifocal bleeds which vary in size and shape. Haemorrhage is usually accompanied by necrosis of brain tissue.
v. *Brain swelling* is a common, usually transient consequence of head trauma associated with increased intracranial pressure.

Q27. What is multiple sclerosis? Comment on its etiopathogenesis and clinicopathologic features.

Definition Multiple sclerosis (MS) or disseminated sclerosis is an autoimmune demyelinating CNS disease of unknown etiology affecting the white matter and clinically presenting with chronic relapses and remissions.

Etiopathogenesis Incompletely understood, but appears to be multifactorial involving genetic, and possible infectious and immunologic factors:
i. *Genetic susceptibility* as evidenced by increased familial incidence.
a. The risk is 15 times higher in close family members of the affected person.
b. Concordance in monozygotic twins is 30%.
c. Certain human leucocyte antigen haplotypes (e.g. HLA-DRB1) are associated with increased risk.
ii. *Infections* may play a role as suggested by geographic clustering and occasional seasonal outbreaks of symptomatic disease.
iii. *Immunologic mechanism* plays a role in the pathogenesis of plaques which initially contain monoclonal CD4+ T-helper cells reacting to myelin related antigens.
a. Two subsets of T-cells seem to play the key role:
- T_H1 cells secrete interferon-γ activating macrophages
- T_H17 cells attract other inflammatory cells

b. B-cells play a role as evidenced by an increased level of oligoclonal immunoglobulins in the CSF.
c. Experimentally, MS can be induced in animals injected with their own myelin basic proteins.

Pathology Demyelination occurs at random throughout the CNS, but most often it affects the central-medial paraventricular axis of cerebrum, optic nerves and spinal cord. Peripheral nerves are usually spared.

Plaques are the characteristic pathologic lesions which can be seen by CT scan, and by naked eye examination in the cerebral white matter at autopsy. The *microscopic features* of these plaques vary depending on their activity and duration of the disease:
i. *Active enlarging plaques* represent areas of active demyelination containing perivascular infiltrates of lymphocytes and macrophages.
- Axons in these plaques are demyelinated but otherwise intact.
- There is a loss of oligodendroglia cells, reactive astrocytosis and an influx or microglia cells/macrophages involved in lipophagocytosis of damaged myelin sheaths.

ii. *Inactive (old) plaques* are characterised by:
- Complete demyelination of axons and even axonal loss.
- There is complete loss of oligodendroglia cells, accompanied by reactive astrocytic gliosis.
- There are no perivascular lymphocytes and the macrophages in the plaques are less prominent.

Clinical features MS is the most common demyelinating disease affecting 1–2 adults per 1000, and women more often than men (3:1). In the Unites States, 90% patients are white. The usual age at onset of symptoms is 20–40 years.

Clinical symptoms vary from case to case and include:

i. *Most often*, limb weakness and gait disturbances. Progressive motor disturbances limit the movement of limbs resulting in joint and spine deformities.

ii. Visual problems such as diplopia, inability to focus; loss of visual fields are found in almost one half of all patients (40%).

iii. Other common findings found in approximately 25% of patients are paraesthesia and sensory loss, vertigo, anal and bladder incontinence.

iv. Infections are common.

v. The clinical picture is dominated by episodes of demyelination followed by remission and relapses. The remissions are never complete and with time, they become progressively shorter.

vi. Neurologic deficits accumulate and become intractable. They are sometimes accompanied by psychiatric disturbances.

Prognosis varies widely:
- As a rule, 1/3rd cases have only minor problems, 1/3rd have serious neurological problems but still can function, and 1/3rd have major disability and require assistance.
- Most patients (>70%) live 25–30 after the onset of symptoms and ultimately succumb to urinary and pulmonary tract infections.

There is no definitive treatment of MS but with modern drugs one may reduce the incidence and severity of relapses.

Q28. What are neurodegenerative diseases and how are they classified?

Definition Neurodegenerative diseases are chronic progressive diseases of unknown etiology and pathogenesis, affecting and destroying functionally interconnected neurons in anatomically or physiologically defined parts of the CNS.

Classification Neurodegenerative diseases can be classified according to their clinicopathologic features and anatomic distribution as under **(Table 30.2)**:

I. *Cerebral cortical degeneration* leading to dementia, as in Alzheimer and Pick disease.

II. *Basal ganglia and brainstem degeneration* as in Huntington and Parkinson disease.

TABLE 30.2 Common neurodegenerative diseases.

REGION AFFECTED	DISEASE	MAIN FEATURES	PREDOMINANT PATHOLOGY
I. Cerebral cortex	Alzheimer disease	Progressive senile dementia	Cortical atrophy, senile plaques (neuritis), neurofibrillary tangles, amyloid angiopathy
	Pick disease	Pre-senile dementia	Lobar cortical atrophy, ballooning degeneration of neurons (Pick cells)
II. Basal ganglia and brainstem	Huntington disease	Progressive dementia with Choreiform movements	Atrophy of frontal lobes, fibrillary astrocytosis
	Parkinson disease	Abnormalities of posture and movement	Aggregates of melanin-containing nerve cells in brainstem, intracytoplasmic neuronal inclusions (Lewy bodies)
III. Spinal cord and cerebellum	Cerebellar cortical degeneration	Progressive cerebellar ataxia	Loss of Purkinje cells in cerebellar cortex
	Olivopontocerebellar atrophy	Cerebellar ataxia	Combination of atrophy of cerebellar cortex, inferior olivary nuclei and pontine nuclei
	Spinocerebellar atrophy (Friedreich ataxia)	Gait ataxia, dysarthria	Degeneration of spinocerebellar tracts, peripheral axons and myelin sheaths
IV. Motor neurons (UMN and LMN)	Motor neuron disease (amyotrophic lateral sclerosis)	Syndromes of muscular weakness and wasting without sensory loss	Progressive loss of motor neurons, both in the cerebellar cortex (UMN) and in the anterior horn of spinal cord (LMN)
	Werdnig-Hoffmann disease	Spinal muscular atrophy in infants	Loss of lower motor neurons, denervation atrophy of muscles

(UMN, upper motor neuron; LMN, lower motor neuron)

III. *Spinal cord and cerebellum* as in cerebellar cortical degeneration, olivopontocerebellar atrophy and spinocerebellar atrophy (Friedreich ataxia).
IV. *Motor neuron diseases* (upper and lower motor neuron) as in amyotrophic lateral sclerosis and Werdnig-Hoffman disease.

Q29. What is Alzheimer disease? Briefly discuss its etiopathogenesis and pathology.

Definition Alzheimer disease is the most common form of dementia, characterised by:
- cortical atrophy,
- deposits of Aβ amyloid in the form of neuritic 'senile' plaques and amyloid angiopathy, and
- formation of neurofibrillary tangles in neuron.

Etiopathogenesis Most patients have sporadic, late-onset Alzheimer disease of unknown etiology.
- In 5–10% of cases, there is a family history, or the disease has an early onset (under 65 years of age). These rare cases could be related to mutations of the gene encoding the amyloid precursor protein (APP) on chromosome 21, or genes for presenilin 1 and presenilin 2, or ε-4 allele of apolipoprotein A.
- It has been noticed that brains of patients with Down syndrome (trisomy 21) also have Alzheimer-like changes with deposits of Aβ amyloid.

Pathology
Gross There is visible atrophy of the cerebral gyri and dilatation of sulci as well as normal pressure hydrocephalus.
Microscopy
i. Neuritic plaques composed of Aβ amyloid.
ii. Amyloid angiopathy.
iii. Neurofibrillary tangles in nerve cells composed of neurofilaments and neurotubules.
iv. Granulovacuolar degeneration in the form of small cytoplasmic vacuoles in nerve cells, some of which also contain Hirano bodies.

Clinical features
i. Loss of cognitive skills such as loss of memory, thinking and language skills.
ii. Behavioural changes.

Q30. What is parkinsonism? Comment on its etiopathogenesis and pathology.

Definition Parkinsonism is a syndrome characterised:
- *clinically* by chronic and progressive disturbances of motor functions, and
- *by pathologic changes* of dopaminergic neurons in the substantia nigra and locus ceruleus.

Etiopathogenesis Idiopathic.
i. Parkinson disease is the most common cause (80%) of parkinsonism.
ii. Other less common causes are:
a. Ischaemia of basal ganglia due to atherosclerosis
b. Psychoactive drugs (e.g. phenothiazine)
c. Toxins (e.g. CO and methanol poisoning)
d. Repetitive head trauma (e.g. boxers)
e. Post-encephalitic brain injury (rare)

Pathology
Gross Visible depigmentation of substantia nigra and locus ceruleus.
Microscopy
i. *Substantia nigra* having loss of neurons and a loss of brown pigment from the remaining neurons.
ii. Cytoplasm of affected neurons contains Lewy bodies composed of aggregated amyloid filaments derived from misfolded α-synuclein.

Clinical features Any combination of the following symptoms and findings is seen:
i. Tremors (these are involuntary, often at rest)
ii. Rigidity
iii. Bradykinesis (slowing of voluntary movements)
iv. Postural instability (stooped posture)
v. Expressionless face

vi. Slurred speech
vii. Gait disturbances (festinating, shuffling, small steps, and frequent falling)
viii. Depression or dementia; these develop in a minority of cases.

Q31. What are the metabolic diseases affecting the brain?

Definition Metabolic diseases affecting the brain can be classified as inherited or acquired; each of these includes several conditions.

Although pathologic changes in each of these conditions are quite diverse, in general these include: oedema, neuronal storage, degenerative change and sometimes parenchymal necrosis.

Classification Following two groups are included:

I. **Hereditary metabolic disorders** include genetically-determined disorders of carbohydrate, lipid, protein or mineral metabolism. The group includes following:

i. *Neuronal storage diseases* characterised by storage of metabolic product in the neurons due to specific enzyme deficiency. For example:
a. Gangliosidoses (e.g. Tay-Sachs disease-GM2 gangliosidosis)
b. Mucopolysaccharidoses (Gaucher disease and Niemann-Pick disease)

ii. *Leukodystrophies* involving the white matter characterised by foci of demyelination and gliosis. They are caused by genetic deficiencies of enzymes required for formation and maintenance of myelin. For example:
a. Sudanophilic leukodystrophy
b. Adrenoleucodystrophy
c. Metachromatic leukodystrophy
d. Globoid cells leukodystrophy (Krabbe disease)

iii. *Other inborn errors of metabolism* For example:
a. Wilson disease (hepatolenticular degeneration)
b. Glycogen storage diseases
c. Phenylketonuria
d. Galactosaemia

II. **Acquired or secondary metabolic diseases** are the disturbances of cerebral function due to disease in some other organ system, such as the heart and circulation, lung and respiratory function, kidneys, liver, endocrine organs and pancreas. In addition, endogenous metabolic diseases may be caused by toxic injuries induced by metals, gases, chemical and drugs. This group includes the following examples:
i. Anoxic-ischaemic encephalopathy
ii. Hypoglycaemic encephalopathy
iii. Hyperglycaemic coma
iv. Acute hepatic encephalopathy
v. Chronic hepatic encephalopathy
vi. Kernicterus
vii. Uraemic encephalopathy
viii. Encephalopathy due to electrolyte and endocrine disturbances

Q32. What are the nutritional diseases affecting the central nervous system?

Definition Nutritional diseases may result from lack of adequate dietary intake of nutrients or due to defects in absorption, transport or metabolism of nutrients, such as those induced by chronic alcohol abuse.

Types Some of the common neurologic diseases included in this category are as under:
i. Wernike encephalopathy, Korsakoff psychosis (vitamin B_1 or thiamine deficiency) and subacute combined degeneration of the spinal cord (vitamin B_{12} deficiency)
ii. Folic acid deficiency
iii. Spinocerebellar syndrome (vitamin E deficiency)
iv. Pellagra (niacin deficiency)
v. Alcoholic cerebellar degeneration

Q33. Outline the broad classification of CNS tumours and their general common features.

i. CNS tumours are rare and account for only 1.5% of all clinical tumours.
ii. They can occur in all age groups.
iii. They account for 40% of all clinically recognised neoplasms of childhood and are thus the *second most common* cause of cancer death in that age group (after leukaemia).
iv. CNS tumours are classified as primary or secondary (metastatic). Gliomas account for most primary tumours (70%). Metastatic tumours account for 25% of all intracranial tumours.
v. Primary tumours are more often malignant than benign.
vi. Malignant CNS tumours rarely metastasise to distant sites, but they may spread from one part of CNS to another, e.g. bilateral glioblastoma ('butterfly-like' tumours); medulloblastoma disseminating through the CSF from cerebellum to spinal cord.
vii. Anatomically, the CNS tumours are classified as *supratentorial* (cerebral, i.e. above tentorium cerebelli), *infratentorial,* and *spinal cord* tumours. Adult tumours are mostly supratentorial (70%), whereas most paediatric tumours are infratentorial, originating from the cerebellum and medulla oblongata/pons. Spinal cord tumours are less common than intracranial tumours.
viii. Primary CNS tumours are preferentially located in some anatomic sites **(Fig. 30.6)**.
ix. Primary brain tumours are classified according to their microscopic features corresponding to constituent cells of the brain and its support structures **(Table 30.3)**. Less common tumours originating from other intracranial structures (e.g. pituitary or pineal gland) are listed under the rubric X (*miscellaneous tumours*) which includes lymphoma, pituitary adenoma, craniopharyngioma, pineocytoma, and germ cell tumours.

TABLE 30.3 The 2016 WHO classification of tumours of the central nervous system.*

I. Diffuse astrocytic and oligodendroglial tumours (Diffuse gliomas)
1. Diffuse astrocytoma
2. Anaplastic astrocytoma
3. Glioblastoma
4. Oligodendroglioma and its variants

II. Other astrocytic tumours
1. Pilocytic astrocytoma
2. Subependymal giant cell astrocytoma
3. Pleomorphic xanthoastrocytoma

III. Ependymal tumours
1. Ependymoma
2. Anaplastic ependymoma
3. Subependymoma

IV. Choroid plexus tumours
1. Choroid plexus papilloma
2. Choroid plexus carcinoma

V. Neuronal and mixed neuronal-glial tumours
1. Gangliocytoma
2. Ganglioglioma
3. Dysembryoplastic neuroepithelial tumour
4. Central neurocytoma

VI. Embryonal tumours
1. Medulloblastoma
2. CNS neuroblastoma
3. CNS embryonal tumour, NOS
4. Atypical teratoid/rhabdoid tumour

VII. Nerve sheath tumours
1. Schwannoma (neurilemmoma)
2. Neurofibroma
3. Malignant peripheral nerve sheath tumour

VIII. Tumours of meninges
1. Meningioma
2. Anaplastic meningioma

IX. Mesenchymal, non-meningeal tumours
1. Solitary fibrous tumour/haemangiopericytoma
2. Haemangioblastoma
3. Angiosarcoma
4. Ewing's/PNET

X. Miscellaneous tumours
1. Primary CNS lymphoma
2. Germ cell tumours
3. Meningeal melanoma
4. Craniopharyngioma
5. Pineocytoma

XI. Metastatic tumours

*Adapted from Louis et al. The 2016 WHO classification of tumours of the central nervous system: a summary (review). Acta Neuropathol. 2016;131(6):803-20.
(PNET, primitive neuroectodermal tumour; CNS, central nervous system; NOS, not otherwise specified)

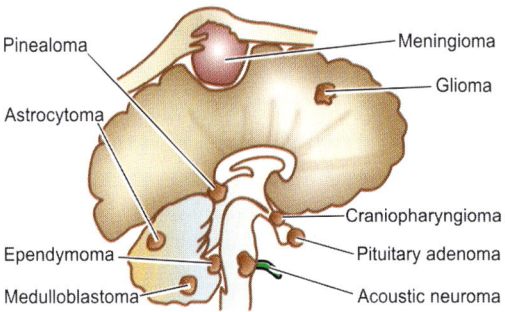

FIGURE 30.6: The anatomic distribution of common intracranial tumours.

Q34. Enumerate hereditary genetic syndromes which are associated with an increased incidence of specific CNS tumours.

Several hereditary tumour syndromes are associated with predisposition to some CNS tumours. These are:

i. *Neurofibromatosis type 1 (NF1-neurofibromin):* neurofibromas, malignant peripheral nerve sheath tumour (MPNST), astrocytoma including glioblastoma

ii. *Neurofibromatosis type 2 (NF2-merlin):* bilateral acoustic nerve schwannoma, meningioma, ependymoma, astrocytoma

iii. *Von Hippel-Lindau disease (VHL):* haemangioblastomas of cerebellum and retina but also of other CNS sites

iv. *Li-Fraumeni syndrome (TP53):* diffuse astrocytoma and glioblastoma, medulloblastoma, ependymoma, oligodendroglioma

v. *Turcot syndrome type 1 (DNA mismatch repair genes):* glioblastoma

Q35. Define gliomas. How are they classified?

Definition Gliomas are primary malignant CNS tumours composed of neoplastic cells that correspond to astrocytes, oligodendrocytes or ependymal cells.

Classification Gliomas are the most common primary CNS tumours, accounting for 70% of all brain tumours. They are subdivided into three groups as under:

i. *Diffuse astrocytic and oligodendroglial tumours* such as diffuse astrocytoma, anaplastic astrocytoma, glioblastoma, oligodendroglioma and its variants.

ii. *Other (localised) astrocytic tumours* include pilocytic astrocytoma, subependymal giant cell astrocytoma and pleomorphic xanthoastrocytoma.

iii. *Ependymal tumours* such as ependymoma (and its variants), anaplastic ependymoma, and subependymoma.

General features

i. Gliomas may be well-differentiated or poorly-differentiated but they are never well demarcated from normal brain tissue but often invade it. Thus, all of them should be considered malignant, even though the well-differentiated types are associated with longer survival than the poorly-differentiated ones.

ii. They may disseminate to other parts of the brain but only rarely if ever they metastasise outside of the CNS.

Q36. What are astrocytomas? Discuss their classification and salient clinicopathologic features.

Definition Astrocytomas are primary malignant CNS tumours composed of neoplastic astrocytes.

Classification Astrocytomas are the most common gliomas. Astrocytomas can be:

- *diffusely infiltrating* (more common and mostly found in adults), or
- *localised* (most often found as pilocytic astrocytomas in the cerebellum of children).

Subdivision of astrocytomas is based on their clinicopathologic features, location, microscopic features and molecular features. These molecular features include:

i. Mutation of *isocitrate dehydrogenase genes* (*IDH1* and *IDH2*), most common.

ii. Additional complex genetic abnormalities include mutations of *PTEN* and *CDKN2A* tumour suppressor genes.

iii. Quite characteristic mutation of *TP53*.

iv. Molecular profile of *pilocytic astrocytomas* is distinct from the genetic changes in other astrocytomas as follows:

- They do not show mutations of *TP53* and other tumour suppressor genes found in diffuse astrocytomas.
- Instead, pilocytic astrocytomas show changes in the BRAF signalling pathway.
- In patients with neurofibromatosis, these tumours show lack of neurofibromin gene.

Pathology Astrocytomas can be graded on a scale from I to IV on histologic features as under:

- Grade I: pilocytic astrocytoma
- Grade II: diffuse astrocytoma
- Grade III: anaplastic astrocytoma
- Grade IV: glioblastoma

The following clinicopathologic types of astrocytoma are recognised:

i. **Diffuse astrocytoma, IDH mutant (WHO grade II)**
Most often, it develops in the frontal lobes.
Microscopy The classic type is a fibrillary astrocytoma composed of well-differentiated astrocytes separated by variable amount of fibrillary background.
Prognosis It has a better prognosis than the IDH-wild type astrocytoma.

ii. **Anaplastic astrocytoma (WHO grade III)**
Usually evolves by progression from lower grade astrocytoma.
Microscopy It shows hypercellularity, nuclear atypia and mitoses, but lacks necrosis and vascular proliferation **(Fig. 30.7)**.

iii. **Glioblastoma (WHO grade IV)**
- This is the most aggressive and also the most common type of astrocytoma.

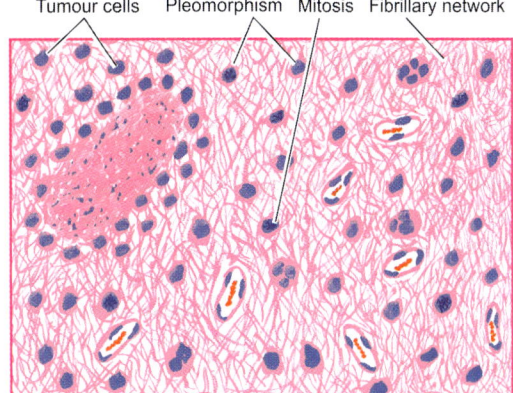

FIGURE 30.7: Anaplastic astrocytoma, WHO grade III. It shows hypercellularity, pleomorphic astrocytic tumour cells, and mitoses in fibrillary background. Necrosis and vascular proliferation are generally not a feature of astrocytoma, grade III.

- Some glioblastomas begin as such, whereas others result from progression of malignancy in a pre-existent less malignant astrocytoma. Such *secondary glioblastomas* are especially common after recurrence of a treated astrocytoma of lower grade; this malignancy probably reflects clonal selection and fast growth of more malignant tumour cells.
- *IDH wild type*, accounting for 90% of all glioblastomas, is more common that the IDH mutant type.

Pathology is highly variable; hence the old name *glioblastoma multiforme*.
Gross The tumour is poorly demarcated, contains wide areas of necrosis and haemorrhage, with softening and cystic changes. Some tumours extend across the midline from one hemisphere to the other (*butterfly tumours*).
Microscopy The tumour is highly cellular, showing marked anaplasia and nuclear pleomorphism. Mitoses are common and often associated with pseudopalisading of cells around them. Typically, there is microvascular endothelial cell proliferation.
Prognosis for various forms of astrocytoma varies. Grade II diffuse astrocytomas have a median survival exceeding 5 years, whereas the mean survival for patients with grade IV glioblastomas is only 18 months.

iv. **Pilocytic astrocytoma**
- This is a tumour of children and adolescents.
- It is most often found in the cerebellum and the area of the third ventricle or optic nerves and cerebral visual neural pathways.

Gross It is partially cystic and well demarcated.
Microscopy It is composed of pilocytic astrocytes, so called because they form 'hair-like' cytoplasmic extensions.
Prognosis The tumour has a much better prognosis than diffuse astrocytomas and often can be completely resected, especially if located in the cerebellum.

Q37. What is an oligodendroglioma? Briefly describe its clinicopathologic features.

Definition Oligodendroglioma is a malignant primary brain tumour composed of neoplastic oligodendroglia cells.

Clinicopathologic features
i. These tumours occur most often in the cerebral haemispheres with a predilection for the white matter.
ii. Oligodendrogliomas grow slowly as evidenced by the presence of symptoms (e.g. epileptic seizures) many years prior to tumour diagnosis.
Gross The tumour appears well circumscribed and gelatinous, often showing secondary degenerative changes such as calcification, cystic change and haemorrhages.

Microscopy
i. Tumour is composed of uniform cells that have round nuclei and clear cytoplasm enclosed by a distinct cell membrane ('fried egg' appearance) resembling normal oligodendrocytes.
ii. Prominent network of anastomosing capillaries.
iii. Mitoses are sparse and there is no necrosis.
iv. In a minority of cases called *anaplastic oligodendrogliomas*, there are foci of necrosis and the cells show signs of anaplasia and are more mitotically active.
Molecular biology and *cytogenetic data* used to confirm the microscopic diagnosis include:
- Mutations of IDH genes (in 90% patients), and
- Translocation of chromosome 1 and 19, resulting in a loss of 1p and 19q (in 80% patients).

Prognosis for oligodendrogliomas is much more favourable than the prognosis of astrocytomas. Following surgical resection, patients with classical oligodendrogliomas survive 15–20 years. Those with anaplastic oligodendrogliomas live up to 10 years.

Q38. What is ependymoma? Describe its salient clinicopathologic features.

Definition Ependymoma is an uncommon glioma composed of cells resembling ependymal cells which line the ventricles and the central canal of the spinal.

Clinical features Ependymoma is a slow growing tumour.
i. It occurs most often in the fourth ventricle, i.e. as a posterior fossa, subtentorial tumour in children and young adults under the age of 20 years.
ii. Other locations are less common and include the lateral ventricles and the third ventricle. In these locations, it may cause obstructive hydrocephalus.
iii. In adults, it also occurs in the region of the lumbar spine. Spinal tumours are often associated with mutations of NF1 and NF2 tumour suppression gene in context of hereditary neurofibromatosis.

Pathology
Gross Ependymomas are well-demarcated tumours, but often they cannot be completely removed surgically due to their location close to the vital centres of the medulla and pons.

Microscopy
i. The tumour is composed of epithelial like cuboidal cells forming tubules or perivascular pseudorosettes **(Fig. 30.8)**.
ii. Like normal ependymal cells, tumour cells may form blepharoplasts (the basal bodies of cilia).
iii. Most tumours are well-differentiated, but some may be anaplastic.
iv. *Two variants* seen in adults are of clinical significance:
- *Myxopapillary ependymoma* of the cauda equina in adults originating from the filum terminale. In addition to the usual features of ependymoma, it contains myxoid material and forms papillary structures. It grows slowly and has a better prognosis that other ependymomas.
- *Subependymoma* grows as a small asymptomatic slow-growing tumour of the fourth or lateral ventricles in middle-aged and older adults. It is usually microcystic and focally calcified. Microscopically, it is composed of uniform ependymal cells in a dense acellular fibrillar stroma.

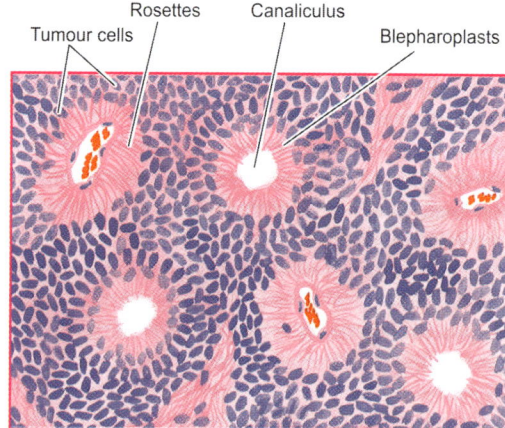

FIGURE 30.8: Myxopapillary ependymoma. It shows extracellular myxoid material and papillary arrangement of tumour cells. The tumour cells are uniform ependymal tumour cells perivascular pseudorosettes, tubules and canaliculi.

Q39. What is medulloblastoma? Briefly comment on its clinicopathologic features.

Definition Medulloblastoma is a malignant CNS tumour composed of primitive undifferentiated neuroectodermal cells, which occasionally may differentiate into glial and neuronal elements.

Pathology
Gross Medulloblastoma is a locally invasive, poorly demarcated tumour.
Microscopy
i. It is composed of 'small round blue cells' resembling those of retinoblastoma or neuroblastoma.
ii. Tumour cells grow in sheets but focally they may form perivascular pseudorosettes (Homer-Wright rosettes).
iii. By *immunohistochemistry*, one may detect cells with neural or glial differentiation, indicating that the tumour cells correspond to foetal neural/glial precursors.
iv. The most common *cytogenetic feature* is loss of 17p with formation of isochromosome 17q.
v. *Molecular biology* data show mutations of genes in the sonic hedgehog and WNT/β-catenin signalling pathway, which normally regulate the development of the granular layer of the cerebellum. Such genetic abnormalities combine with microscopic details are used to further stratify subtypes of medulloblastoma and provide prognostic data.

Clinical features
i. Medulloblastomas are childhood tumours, accounting for 20% of all CNS tumours in that age group.
ii. Approximately 25% tumours occur in persons who are older than 20 years of age.
iii. The most common location is cerebellum—in the roof of fourth ventricle and the vermis, in the midline of the cerebellum, but may also involve the cerebellar hemispheres.
iv. Medulloblastomas may enter the CSF and metastasise to the spinal cord ('drop metastases') or other parts of the CNS.
v. Multimodal therapy, which includes neurosurgical resection, irradiation and chemotherapy, is accompanied by a 5-year survival of 75%.

Q40. What is haemangioblastoma?

Definition Haemangioblastoma is a rare benign CNS tumour (2% of all tumours) composed of endothelial cells forming thin-walled blood vessels.

Pathology
Gross Haemangioblastoma presents as a well-circumscribed, blood-filled cystic mass with a solid mural nodule.
Microscopy
i. The nodule is composed of thin-walled blood vessels lined by plump endothelial cells.
ii. In the perivascular stroma, there are prominent lipid-laden foamy macrophages with clear cytoplasm.

Clinical features
i. Haemangioblastomas occur as sporadic tumours or they may be part of the hereditary von Hippel-Lindau syndrome.
ii. Besides cerebellar haemangioblastoma, the syndrome includes retinal haemangioblastoma, cysts of the liver, kidney and pancreas and renal tumours.
iii. It is caused by mutations of the *VHL* gene regulating the function of hypoxia induced factor -1 (HHF-1), which is important for the synthesis of erythropoietin.

Q41. Comment briefly on CNS lymphomas.

CNS lymphoma may originate in the brain as a primary CNS lymphoma, or involve the CNS as secondary lymphomas during the dissemination of a primary in the lymph nodes.
I. **Primary CNS lymphomas** occur most often in immunosuppressed patients with AIDS, but can also develop in immunosuppressed persons after organ transplantation.
Gross They are multifocal, involving the deep grey mater or white matter and cortex. Periventricular spread is common.
Microscopy
i. Most tumours are classified as *diffuse large B cell lymphoma*.
ii. Most tumour cells are infected with the Epstein-Barr virus.
iii. Tumour cells replicate fast and accordingly there are prominent areas of necrosis.
iv. Tumour cells tend to spread through the brain in the form of perivascular aggregates.
Overall, they have a poor prognosis.

II. **Secondary CNS lymphomas** develop in advanced stages of high-grade lymphoma dissemination from primary lymph node disease.
i. Lymphoma cells usually do not form intraparenchymal masses.
ii. Instead, they are found in the CSF and may infiltrate the surface parts of the CNS, especially at the roots of the cranial and spinal nerves.

Q42. What is a meningioma? Discuss its clinical and pathologic features.

Definition Meningioma is a benign tumour composed of meningeal cells forming the pia-arachnoid layer. It accounts for 20% of all intracranial tumours.

Pathology

Location Meningiomas are solitary tumours, most often located in the front half of the head (e.g. over the cerebral convexities, along the falx cerebri and adjacent to venous sinuses). They can also be located at other intracranial sites and even may arise from spinal cord meninges, albeit less often.

Gross Meningiomas are well circumscribed masses that vary in shape and size (1–10 cm). On its base, the tumour is usually firmly attached to the dura while its other side indents the surface of the brain, usually without any invasion **(Fig. 30.9, A)**. The overlying bone shows hyperostosis. The cut surface is firm fibrous and focally gritty from calcifications.

Microscopy
i. Composed of cells resembling arachnoid meningeal cells arranged into whorls with focal calcifications ('psammoma bodies').
ii. There are several microscopic patterns: meningotheliomatous or syncytial (most often), fibrous, and transitional (mixed pattern) **(Fig. 30.9, B)**.
iii. Microscopic subtyping is of no clinical significance, except for some rare microscopic subtypes (e.g. clear cell and chordoid) which have worse prognosis.
iv. However, the presence of nuclear atypia, presence of small cells and increased mitotic activity are important for the diagnosis of *atypical meningiomas*.
v. Frankly *malignant meningiomas* which may metastasise to the lungs and are potentially lethal, are very rare.
vi. The most common *cytogenetic abnormality* is deletion of 22q, i.e. the long arm of chromosome 22 carrying the *NF2* tumour suppressor gene. An increased incidence of meningioma has been recorded in neurofibromatosis type 2; such tumours are often multiple and lack tumour suppressor gene *NF2* and its protein product, merlin.

Clinical features
i. Meningiomas may occur in any age group. Peak incidence is in adults 40–60 years adults. They are uncommon in children, accounting for only 1.5% of CNS tumours in those under the age of 15 years.

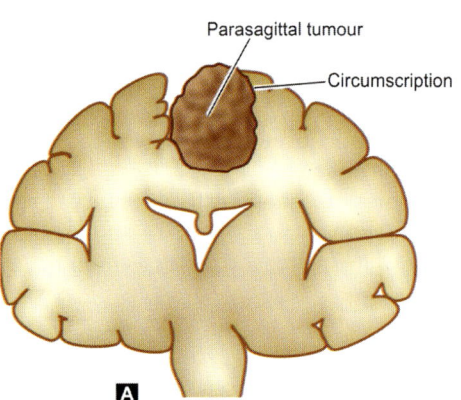
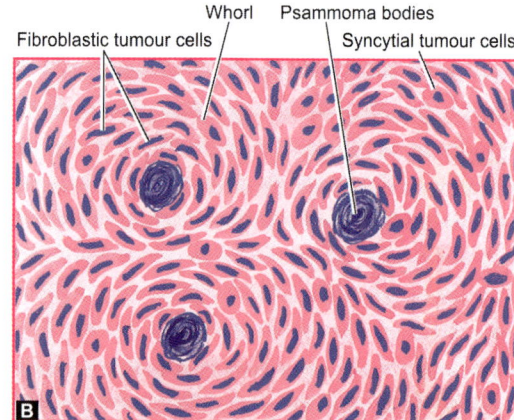

FIGURE 30.9: Meningioma. A, The tumour mass seen in parasagittal location is circumscribed with irregular surface convolutions. Cut surface of the mass is firm and fibrous. B, Microscopy of transitional type meningioma. The cells have features of both syncytial and fibroblastic type and form whorled appearance. Some of the whorls contain psammoma bodies.

ii. Meningiomas are slightly more common in women, but interestingly enough, many have progesterone receptors. These receptors probably account for their accelerated growth during pregnancy.
iii. Spinal meningiomas are rare but they are ten times more common in women than in men.
iv. Most tumours are sporadic.
v. Symptoms are usually related to the mass effect of the tumour causing symptoms of increased intracranial pressure (e.g. headaches, blurry vision, somnolence).
vi. Neurologic symptoms may result from the local compression of cerebral cortex (e.g. epileptic seizures).

Prognosis Clinically, meningiomas are benign tumours. Most meningiomas (90%) can be cured by surgery without any residual changes. However, some tumours may recur after surgery, especially atypical meningiomas which have recurrence rate of 30%. Frankly malignant meningiomas are rare but may be lethal.

PERIPHERAL NERVOUS SYSTEM

Q43. What are the principal components of the peripheral nervous system (PNS)? Describe briefly structure of a normal peripheral nerve.

The main components of the PNS are as follows:
- Cranial and spinal nerves
- Sympathetic and parasympathetic autonomic nervous system
- Peripheral ganglia

Structure of a nerve
i. The nerve has a nucleus which is located in the nerve cell body cytoplasm (also known as perikaryon).
ii. The cytoplasm forms extensions called *dendrites* and *axons* **(Fig. 30.10, A)**.
iii. Axons are of two types: thicker *myelinated* and thinner *non-myelinated axons*.
iv. Myelin sheaths are produced by *Schwann cells*.
v. Boundaries in the myelin sheath forming the boundaries between the parts produced by two adjacent Schwann cells are called the *nodes of Ranvier*.
vi. *Myelinated axons* have their origin from neurons in the posterior root ganglia and anterior horn cells of the spinal cord.
vii. *Nonmyelinated axons* arise from neuron in the posterior root ganglia and in the autonomic ganglia.

Q44. What are the pathologic features of nerve reaction to injury?

In contrast to the CNS, peripheral nerves have a capacity to regenerate their parts after injury. Three forms of reaction to injury are seen: Wallerian degeneration, axonal degeneration, and segmental demyelination **(Fig. 30.10, B-D)**:

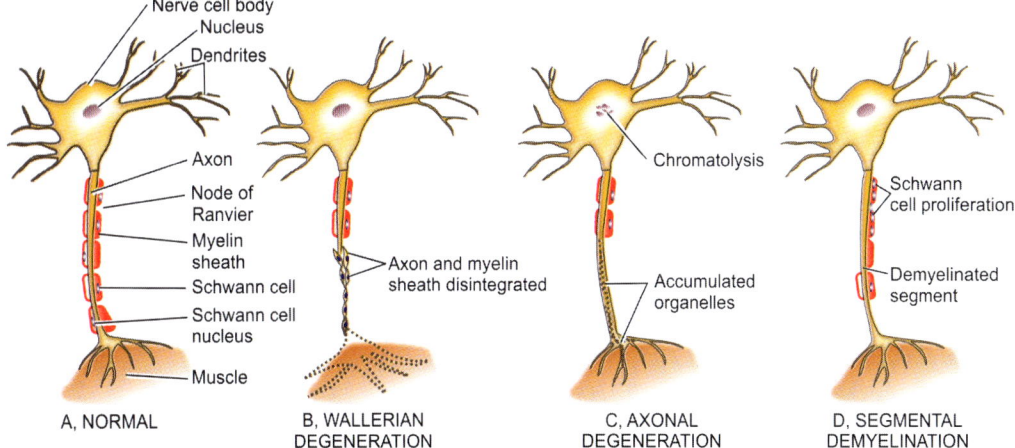

FIGURE 30.10: Structure of a normal peripheral nerve (A) and pathologic reaction of peripheral nerve to injury (B,C, D).

I. **Wallerian degeneration** occurs after transection of the axon, which may be a result of knife wound, compression, traction or ischaemia.
i. Following the injury, there is accumulation of cytoplasmic organelles in the proximal part of the transected axon.
ii. The distal part undergoes disintegration up to the next node of Ranvier, followed by phagocytosis of the disintegrated part.
iii. Regeneration includes sprouting of the axons accompanied by proliferation of the Schwann cells from the proximal part of the nerve (i.e. its body) until the integrity of the transected axon is reestablished.
iv. If the regeneration is hampered due to interposition of a fibrous scar or haematoma, the axonal sprout, together with Schwann cells and fibroblasts, forms a tumour-like mass called *traumatic* or *stump neuroma*.
II. **Axonal degeneration** occurs due to some metabolic disturbances that cause degeneration of the axon even without its transection.
i. Degeneration of the axon proceeds toward the perikaryon with limited or no regeneration.
ii. Axonal injury results in changes in the cytoplasm of the cell body such as central chromatolysis.
iii. Schwann cells may proliferate but do not form myelin sheaths to cover the defect.
III. **Segmental degeneration** results in following changes:
i. There is a loss of myelin sheath between two consecutive nodes of Ranvier, leaving a denuded axon segment, without disintegration of the axon itself.
ii. Schwann cells proliferate and remyelinate the affected axon.
iii. Repeated episodes of demyelination and remyelination associated with proliferation of Schwann cells around axons result in the formation of '*onion bulbs*', typical of hypertrophic neuropathy.

Q45. What is peripheral neuropathy? Comment on its clinicopathologic types.

Definition Peripheral neuropathy is impairment of sensory, motor or autonomic function, either singly or in combination of one with the other.
Clinicopathologic classification Based on the location of the features and underlying pathology, peripheral neuropathy may be classified as: polyneuropathy, mononeuropathy multiplex and mononeuropathy.
I. **Polyneuropathy** is characterised by sensory, motor and often autonomic nervous system symptoms.
i. *Symptoms* may evolve acutely as in Guillain-Barré syndrome, or gradually as in diabetes mellitus or amyloidosis. Other causes include: toxins, some drugs, such as vincristine and isoniazid, and hereditary polyneuropathies.
ii. *Sensory features* are symmetrical and include: tingling, pricking, burning sensation or dysaesthesia on hands and feet ('*stocking and glove*' distribution).
iii. *Motor features* include: muscle weakness, followed by muscle fiber atrophy, and loss of tendon reflexes. Autonomic symptoms include: loss of sphincter control of the urinary bladder and anus, and erectile dysfunction.
iv. *Pathologic changes* are: axonal degeneration (*axonopathy*) or segmental demyelination (*demyelinating polyneuropathy*).
II. **Mononeuropathy multiplex (Multifocal neuropathy)** has following features:
i. There is simultaneous or sequential multifocal involvement of nerve trunks which are not in anatomic continuity one with another.
ii. The involvement may be partial or complete, acute (evolving over a few days) or chronic (evolving over months and years).
iii. Pathologically, it is part of the spectrum of chronic acquired demyelinating neuropathy or systemic diseases such as polyarteritis nodosa.
III. **Mononeuropathy** results from the involvement of a single nerve.
i. It is most often caused by direct trauma, entrapment or compression of the nerve. The best example is carpal syndrome due to the entrapment of ulnar or radial nerve.
ii. The diagnosis is made clinically and supported by data obtained by electromyography and nerve conduction studies, nerve biopsy, and skin or muscle biopsy.

Q46. Based on etiology and pathogenesis, how are peripheral neuropathies classified?

Based on causes and underlying mechanisms, peripheral neuropathies can be classified as hereditary or acquired.

I. **Hereditary neuropathies**:
i. *Diseases limited to peripheral nerves,* e.g. Charcot-Marie-Tooth disease or familial amyloid neuropathy.
ii. *Diseases involving the central and peripheral nervous system,* e.g. Friedreich ataxia with neuropathy.
iii. *Multisystemic inborn errors of metabolism,* e.g. porphyria, hereditary disorders of lipid metabolism, ataxia telangiectasia.

II. **Acquired neuropathies**:
i. *Metabolic/endocrine neuropathies*, e.g. in diabetes, hypothyroidism.
ii. *Infectious neuropathies*, e.g. caused by leprosy, AIDS, Lyme disease, herpes zoster.
iii. *Autoimmune neuropathies*, e.g. in Guillain-Barré syndrome, sarcoidosis, rheumatoid arthritis, SLE.
iv. *Cancer related neuropathy* due to direct compression of nerves by cancer or in form of paraneoplastic syndrome.
v. *Drug/toxin related neuropathy*, e.g. colchicine, chloroquine, isoniazide, or antiretroviral drug-related neuropathy, heavy metal poisoning (e.g. lead, mercury, arsenic, thalium poisoning). Alcohol and organic solvents are other common toxin-related causes.
vi. *Vitamin deficiency*, e.g. vitamin B_{12}, B_1, B_6, E and niacin deficiencies.
vii. *Amyloidosis:* primary, secondary or familial thyretin-related amyloidosis.

Q47. Write briefly on Charcot-Marie-Tooth disease.

Definition Charcot-Marie-Tooth (CMT) disease is a clinical term for a group of diseases characterised by sensory motor deficiency related to the dysfunction of peripheral nerves. It is the most common hereditary peripheral neuropathy affecting 1:2500 persons.

Etiopathogenesis CMT is not a single disease but a group of diseases that all share the same clinical symptoms.
i. At least 50 different genes have been identified causing this syndrome.
ii. Most of these genes encode proteins in myelin sheaths, the cell plasma proteins and organelles of Schwann cells or axons.
iii. The causative genes may be inherited as autosomal dominant or recessive traits or sex-linked recessive traits.

Pathology
i. Affected nerves may show focal demyelination, axonal degeneration, or a mixed axonal-myelin injury.
ii. Cycles of myelination and demyelination result in focal nodular expansion of peripheral nerves ('onion bulbs').
iii. Corresponding skeletal muscles undergo denervation atrophy with subsequent deformation of extremities.

Clinical features
i. CMT presents with a loss of sensation in the extremities, followed by muscle weakness, atrophy of muscles and deformity of the foot.
ii. Various forms of CMT are classified according to the mode of inheritance:
- *CMT1* is an autosomal dominant disease most often caused (accounting for 50% of all genetic forms of the disease) by mutated gene for peripheral myelin sheath protein 1 (PMP22).
- *CMT2* is also inherited as an autosomal dominant trait, but it presents as an axonopathy. Most often, it is related *MFN2* gene that is important for mitochondrial function.
- *CMTX* is related to the mutation of *GJB1* gene that encodes the gap junction protein connexin in Schwann cells.

iii. The diagnosis is made by correlating the clinical and family data with objective findings including peripheral nerve conduction studies, nerve biopsy and genetic studies.

Q48. What is Guillain-Barré syndrome?

Definition Guillain-Barré syndrome is an acute autoimmune demyelinating polyneuropathy and radiculopathy. Even though it affects only 1:100 000 people, it is still the most common acute demyelinating peripheral nerve disease.

Etiopathogenesis The disease may develop sporadically. It may develop without any premonition, or following an upper respiratory or gastrointestinal infection.
i. Diarrhoea due to *Campylobacter jejuni* is found in 30% cases.
ii. Infections with upper respiratory viruses and *Mycoplasma pneumoniae* are commonly encountered.
iii. In some cases, it develops after immunisation or surgical interventions.
iv. CSF contains antibodies to myelin sheaths, indicating that the humoral immune response also plays a role.

Pathology
i. Peripheral nerves are typically infiltrated focally with T lymphocytes and macrophages which can also be seen around the small blood vessels of the perineurium. Immune reaction is most prominent at the roots of spinal nerves, but can involve the cranial nerves as well.
ii. T lymphocytes and macrophages infiltrating myelin sheath of peripheral nerves cause focal demyelination.
iii. The changes are reversible in most instances, but in some cases, nerve injury cannot be repaired.

Clinical features
i. Initial symptoms include paraesthesia and tingling in fingers and toes with a loss of sensation and toes spreading proximally.
ii. Neurologic examination reveals loss of the sense of pain, muscle weakness and loss of tendon reflexes.
iii. In about 50% of cases, the disease involves the cranial nerves as well, causing weakness of ocular and facial muscle and tongue and pharynx/larynx.
iv. In about 15% cases, there is respiratory depression due to the weakness of respiratory muscles requiring the use of respirator.
v. Autonomic nervous system symptoms include hypotension and heart rhythm abnormalities and abnormal pupillary reflexes.
vi. Cerebrospinal fluid contains proteins without concomitant inflammatory cells ('albumino-cytologic dissociation').
vii. Serum may contain antibodies that cross react with components of myelin sheath. Plasmapheresis to remove those antibodies from plasma may help reducing the duration of the attack.
viii. Immunotherapy and plasmapheresis used in the treatment of the disease result in recovery of most patients; mortality is 7%.

Q49. Briefly discuss nerve sheath tumours.

Most nerve sheath tumours are benign and classified as schwannoma (neurilemomma) and neurofibroma. Malignant counterpart called malignant peripheral nerve sheath tumors (MPST) is rare.

I. Schwannoma (neurilemmoma) is a common benign peripheral nerve sheath tumour composed of neoplastic Schwann cells. A few key facts about schwannomas are as follows:
i. Schwannoma may originate from cranial or spinal nerves and their branches.
ii. Schwannomas of large nerves preferentially involve the sensory nerves and their dorsal roots.
iii. The nerve tumours may be intradural (intraspinal or intracranial) or extradural.
iv. Most schwannomas are solitary, except in patients suffering from neurofibromatosis type 1 who have multiple peripheral nerve tumours.
v. The most common intracranial schwannoma originates from the vestibular part of the VIII nerve (also called as *acoustic neuroma*, though erroneously; neither the nerve is acoustic nor is the tumour a neuroma, but rather a nerve sheath tumour).
vi. 8th nerve schwannomas are most often located in the cerebellopontine angle but could also be located in the internal auditory canal.
vii. In patients with neurofibromatosis type II, acoustic schwannomas are often bilateral.
viii. These tumours have an inactivating mutation of *NF2* gene and do not express merlin, its protein product. Merlin normally prevents the expression of growth factor receptors on Schwann cells.
ix. In contrast to schwannomas of peripheral nerves, tumours of the 8th nerve do not undergo malignant transformation.

Pathology
Gross Schwannomas are well encapsulated tumours presenting as an eccentric nodular enlargement of the involved nerve.
Microscopy
- They are composed of elongated cells arranged in a palisading manner (*Verocay bodies*) and loosely structured less cellular area, called Antoni A and Antoni B patterns respectively **(Fig. 30.11)**.
- Neoplastic Schwann cells are positive immunohistochemically for S100.

II. **Neurofibroma** is a benign nerve sheath tumour composed of a mixture of cells including neoplastic Schwann cells, perineural fibroblast-like cells, common soft tissue fibroblasts and CD34+ connective tissue stem cells. Key features of neurofibromas are as under:

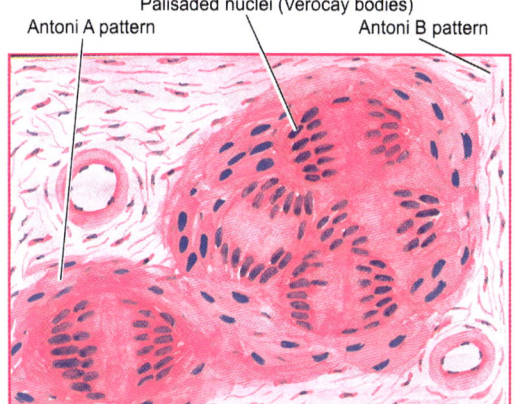

FIGURE 30.11: Schwannoma (neurilemmoma), showing whorls of densely cellular (Antoni A) and loosely cellular (Antoni B) areas with characteristic nuclear palisading (Verocay's bodies).

i. Most neurofibromas are small and found in the dermis originating from small nerves that cannot be always identified.
ii. Neoplastic cells that grow inside the nerve, usually cause spindle-shaped expansion of the nerve trunk and also extend into the perineural soft tissue.
iii. Larger tumours form plexiform masses composed of thick, nodular, interlacing fascicles resembling a string rope.
iv. Multiple neurofibromas are usually part of *neurofibromatosis type 1* (von Recklinghausen disease), caused by mutation or loss of tumour suppressor *NF1* gene (encoding neurofibromin, a protein that inhibits normally *RAS* oncogene activation).
v. In approximately 5–10% patients with neurofibromatosis type 1, benign neurofibromas transform into malignant peripheral nerve sheath tumours (MPNST). Such malignant transformation occurs more often in large neurofibromas and those that are classified as plexiform.
Pathology Neurofibromas are predominantly composed of spindle cells with wavy nuclei arranged in bundles and interlacing fascicles containing collagen fibers and loose mucoid material.
Tumours also contain Schwann cells which may form bundles resembling those is schwannomas.
III. **Malignant peripheral nerve sheath tumours (MPNST)** are sarcomas of soft tissue, which often originate from preexisting neurofibromas, especially the large and plexiform tumours in neurofibromatosis type 1.
Gross These tumours are poorly demarcated and highly invasive.
Microscopy
i. MPNST is composed of anaplastic spindle cells, showing marked nuclear hyperchromatism and pleomorphism.
ii. Several microscopic variants are recognised but all of them have poor prognosis.

Q50. What is neurofibromatosis and its types? Briefly discuss its etiopathogenesis and clinicopathologic features.

Definition Neurofibromatosis (NF) is the name for two genetic diseases presenting primarily with the appearance of multiple neurofibromas, frequently accompanied by other pathologic changes.
Etiopathogenesis There are two types of neurofibromatosis: NF1 and NF2.
NF1
i. It is caused by the mutation or loss of tumour suppressor gene *NF1*, encoding *neurofibromin*.
ii. NF1 has an incidence of 1:3,000.
iii. It is inherited as an autosomal dominant trait.
iv. Approximately one half of all patients have a gene mutation that is sporadic and not inherited from their parents.

v. Apparently, the *NF1* gene is a very large gene prone to mutation at a rate that is 100 times higher than for other genes.

vi. Numerous mutations have been identified and all of them lead to the truncation of neurofibromin, followed by a loss of its normal capacity to inhibit the *RAS* signaling pathway.

NF2

i. It is caused by the deletion of the tumour suppressor gene, *NF2*, encoding the protein *merlin* which links the cytoskeleton to the cell membrane.

ii. NF2 is less common and has an incidence of 1:40,000.

Clinicopathologic features NF1 and NF2 have distinct clinical and pathologic features.

Neurofibromatosis 1:

i. *Neurofibromas* of the dermis and subcutis start developing in childhood and by puberty their count is in hundreds.

ii. Beside these obvious tumours, systematic examination will usually reveal neurofibromas of internal organs and large nerves.

iii. *Plexiform neurofibromas* may be disfiguring. In 5–10% cases, large and plexiform neurofibromas will undergo malignant transformation into *MPNST*.

iv. Pigmented skin lesions in form of so called *café au lait spots* and numerous *freckles* are seen.

v. *Lisch nodules* of the iris are hamartomas formed of aggregated melanocytes.

vi. *Skeletal deformities* due to the irregular thinning of the cortices of long bones, especially sphenoid bone, are seen.

vii. *Increased risk for other tumours*:
- Higher incidence of meningiomas, optic glioma and pheochromocytomas has been recorded.
- Acute myeloid leukaemia in children, which occurs 100–500 times more often than in the population at large.

Neurofibromatosis 2:

i. It is characterised by the appearance of bilateral nerve sheath tumours of the 8th nerve, and multiple meningiomas.

ii. They also have microscopic and even macroscopic hamartomas composed of aggregates of meningeal cells (*meningiomatosis*) or Schwann cells growing from the radicles of cranial and spinal nerves into the neural tissue (*schwannosis*).

iii. Some patients develop *gliomas*.

Chapter 30e Supplement: Online Content

Digital content of this chapter available with this book is meant for enhanced learning and self-assessment. In addition, it contains 34 Multiple Choice Questions (MCQs), 05 Clinicopathologic Vignettes, and 08 Image-based Questions; these are followed by their answers along with explanatory notes of correct and incorrect answers.

APPENDIX

Basic Diagnostic Cytopathology

OVERVIEW

Q1. What is diagnostic cytopathology?

Definition Diagnostic cytopathology is a branch of anatomic pathology and a distinct subspecialty of morphologic diagnostic pathology. It is based on microscopic analysis of smears prepared from cells that are normally shed from various tissues (*exfoliative cytology*), or sampled by means of fine needle aspiration biopsy and other interventional procedures (*interventional cytology*).

Broad principles Cytopathologic diagnosis rests upon the evaluation of morphologic alterations in the morphology of single cells or small groups of cells. It can be supported by the use of various *ancillary methods*, such as immunocytochemistry, cytogenetics or flow cytometry. Correlation with histopathological findings in subsequent biopsies or surgically resected specimens serves as gold standard for the diagnostic accuracy of cytopathologic reports.

Q2. How is cytopathology used in clinical medicine?

The most important applications of cytopathology are as follows:

I. **Diagnosis and management of cancer** Even though the histopathologic diagnosis of malignancy is a required prerequisite for proper management of cancer patients, cytopathologic diagnosis is an important contribution to treatment as under:

i. *Adjunct to histopathology* since it allows a more detailed study of tumours at the level of individual cells.
EXAMPLE: Sample of lymph node for flow cytometry and use of imprints of cut section of lymph node to prepare touch-preps to study lymphoma cells in smears. Smears may also be used for immunocytochemistry with antibodies to tumour markers or CD antigens on lymphoma cells.

ii. *Preliminary (working) diagnosis* to provide guidance to the surgeon prior to definitive histopathologic diagnosis.
EXAMPLE: Thyroid nodule FNA to determine if the lesion is neoplastic, benign or malignant.

iii. Early d*etection of certain forms of early cancer.*
EXAMPLE: Pap smear for cervical carcinoma in an asymptomatic woman.

iv. *Follow-up of treated patients* to determine the effectiveness of therapy.
EXAMPLES: Follow-up of urinary bladder cancer patients treated by chemotherapy or BCG immunotherapy by cytopathology. Women on radiotherapy for cervical carcinoma are followed up by cytopathology to assess the effectiveness of treatment.

v. *Monitoring of cancer patients* for the appearance of metastases or recurrent tumours after treatment.
EXAMPLES: Treated breast cancer patient with suspicious liver lesions that can be easily sampled by thin needle aspiration cytology. Suspicious nodule at the site of previous mastectomy may be sampled by FNA to determine if that is just a scar or recurrent cancer.

vi. *Rapid diagnosis in emergency* situations requiring early immediate treatments.
EXAMPLE: Mediastinal lymphoma causing respiratory distress.

vii. Sampling of tissue for *ancillary studies*.
EXAMPLE: FNA samples can be submitted for flow cytometry, PCR, genetic analysis, and cell blocks can be prepared for immunohistochemistry.

II. **Identification of benign and non-neoplastic lesions**
EXAMPLES: Most thyroid nodules are benign and do not require radical surgery. Thus, FNA diagnosis of benign thyroid lesions can obviate surgery. Enlarged thyroid in Hashimoto thyroiditis may be sampled by FNA to assure the patient that there is no cancer.

III. **Intraoperative cytopathologic consultation** to supplement the histopathologic diagnosis.
EXAMPLE: Imprint of lymph nodes during axillary lymph node dissection to determine if the lymph nodes contain cancer.

IV. **Diagnosis of specific infections**
EXAMPLE: Vaginitis caused by *Gardnerella vaginalis* or *Trichomonas vaginalis* can be diagnosed by Pap smears.

V. **Cytogenetic studies** Samples obtained by exfoliative or aspiration cytology may be submitted for cytogenetic studies or even rapid sex determination.
EXAMPLE: Sex determination by examining the buccal smears for Barr bodies (present in females but not in males).

VI. **Assessment of hormonal status in women or the nature of infertility in men**
EXAMPLES: Pap smears reflect the hormonal status of women. Thus, one can determine vaginal atrophy due to lack of oestrogen in postmenopausal women. FNA of testis may be used to determine maturation arrest of spermatogenic cells and determine if the testis is producing mature sperm.

Q3. What are the nuclear criteria of cancer that are used in cytopathology?

Nuclear criteria are used to determine if the cytologic smear contains malignant cells. The salient criteria of malignancy are listed in **Table A.1**. Cytoplasmic characteristics are used for typing of malignancy. For example, keratinisation is seen in squamous cell carcinoma, mucin droplets in adenocarcinoma, melanin in malignant melanoma.

TABLE A.1 Nuclear criteria of malignancy.

1. *Nuclear size*	Usually larger than benign nuclei; variation in size (anisonucleosis) more significant
2. *Nucleus-cytoplasmic (N:C) ratio*	Increased
3. *Nuclear shape*	Moderate to marked variation
4. *Nuclear membrane*	Irregular thickening, angulation and indentations
5. *Nuclear chromatin*	Hyperchromatic (less significant), uneven distribution, coarse irregular chromatin clumping, parachromatin clearing (more significant)
6. *Nucleoli*	Increased size and number less significant; irregular angular outlines more significant
7. *Number of nuclei*	Multinucleation unreliable; nuclear character more important
8. *Mitoses*	Increased mitoses unreliable; abnormal mitoses significant

Q4. What are the two main branches of diagnostic cytopathology? Tabulate their salient contrasting features.

Two main branches of diagnostic cytopathology are: exfoliative and interventional cytopathology.

I. **Exfoliative cytopathology** is based on the study of cells that spontaneously shed off from epithelial surfaces of the body or into the body cavities and body fluids.
- Pathological conditions enhance the rate of shedding, thus yielding a larger number of cells in each sample.
- The cellular yield can be increased by several techniques including scraping, brushing or washing the mucosal surface ('abrasive cytology').
- The procedure is performed by the clinician examining or treating the patient.

II. **Interventional cytopathology** is dominated by fine needle aspiration (FNA), also known as fine needle aspiration biopsy. FNA may be performed by either the pathologist or the clinician examining the patient.

TABLE A.2 Differences between exfoliative and interventional cytology.

FEATURE	EXFOLIATIVE CYTOLOGY	INTERVENTIONAL CYTOLOGY
1. Cell samples	Exfoliated from epithelial surfaces	Obtained by intervention/aspiration
2. Smears	Require screening to locate suitable cells for study	Abundance of cells for study in most smears
3. Diagnostic basis	Individual cell morphology	Cell patterns and morphology of groups of cells
4. Morphologic criteria of diagnostic significance	Nuclear characteristics most important	Nuclear characteristics important; cytoplasmic character and background equally significant

A brief account contrasting the main features of exfoliative and interventional cytopathology is given in **Table A.2**.

EXFOLIATIVE CYTOLOGY

Q5. Define exfoliative cytology. What are the types of clinical samples included in it?

Exfoliative cytology is performed on cells that spontaneously shed from epithelial surfaces. In clinical pathology practice, it is customary to divide the samples into two major groups: *gynaecologic and non-gynaecologic exfoliative cytology* as presented in **Table A.3**.

Q6. What kind of exfoliative smears are submitted for cytopathologic examination by gynaecologist?

Smears prepared from the lower female genital tracts have traditionally been known as Pap smears, an abbreviation of the name of the Greek-American physician, George Papanicolaou (1983–1962) who introduced this form of sampling into the practice of diagnostic pathology. The following are the types of smears that may be prepared by the gynaecologist examining or treating the patient:

i. *Lateral vaginal smears (LVS)* obtained by scraping the upper third of the lateral wall of the vagina are ideal for cytohormonal assessment.

ii. *Vaginal 'pool' or 'vault' smears* are obtained by scraping or aspirating material from the posterior fornix of the vagina and are recommended for detection of endometrial or ovarian cancer.

iii. *Cervical smears* obtained by Ayre spatula from the *portio cervicis* are ideal for detecting cervical carcinoma.

iv. *Combined (Fast) smears* are a combination of vaginal pool and cervical scrapings. They offer the advantages of both and are recommended for routine population screening as they allow detection of up to 97% of cervical cancer and about 90% of endometrial cancers when properly performed.

v. *Triple (cervical-vaginal-endocervical or CVE) smears* contain three distinct samples representing ectocervix, vagina and endocervix on three separate areas of the same slide. These smears are also recommended for routine screening as they allow localisation of lesions but are difficult to prepare.

vi. *Endocervical and endometrial smear* may also be prepared by aspirating the contents of the endocervical canal and endometrial cavity respectively.

TABLE A.3 Types of samples for exfoliative cytology obtainable from different organ systems/body sites.

I. GYNAECOLOGIC EXFOLIATIVE CYTOLOGY		
Female genital tract		i. Lateral vaginal smears (LVS)
		ii. Vaginal 'pool' smears
		iii. Cervical smears
		iv. Combined (fast) smears
		v. Triple smears (CVE)
		vi. Endocervical/Endometrial aspiration
II. NON-GYNAECOLOGIC EXFOLIATIVE CYTOLOGY		
1. Respiratory tract		i. Sputum
		ii. Bronchial washings/brushing/ bronchioalveolar lavage (BAL)
2. Gastrointestinal tract		Endoscopic lavage/brushing
3. Urinary tract		i. Urinary sediment
		ii. Bladder washings
		iii. Retrograde catheterisation
		iv. Prostatic massage (secretions)
4. Body fluids		i. Effusions
		ii. Fluids of small volume
		a. Cerebrospinal fluid (CSF)
		b. Synovial fluid
		c. Amniotic fluid
		d. Hydrocele fluid
		e. Seminal fluid (semen)
		f. Nipple discharge
5. Other samples		Buccal smears (for sex chromatin)

Q7. What are the various normal cells seen in the combined cervico-vaginal smears?

Combined smears contain epithelial cells (normal and variants) and other cells and bacilli as under:

I. **Normal epithelial cells** Four cell types are recognised:
i. Superficial
ii. Intermediate
iii. Parabasal
iv. Basal

Morphologic features of normal cell in vaginal smears are summarised in **Table A.4**.

II. **Variant epithelial cells** include the following:
i. *Navicular cells*, boat shaped intermediate cells with folded cell border that appear in the latter half of the menstrual cycle, during pregnancy and menopause.
ii. *Lactational cells* are parabasal cells with strongly acidophilic cytoplasm, typically seen in lactating women.

III. **Other cells** include the following:
i. *Endocervical cells* that appear as single dispersed nuclei or clusters of columnar cells giving it a honey-combed appearance. Nuclei of endocervical cells are vesicular with finely granular chromatin and 1–2 nucleoli.
ii. *Endometrial cells* are seen up to the 12th day of the menstrual cycle. They are slightly smaller than endocervical cells, appear as tight rounded clusters of overlapping cells with moderately dark oval nuclei and scanty basophilic, vacuolated cytoplasm.
iii. *Leucocytes*, predominantly neutrophils, and a few lymphocytes, often entrapped in mucus.
iv. *Macrophages* are present during the first 10 days of the menstrual cycle.
v. *Plasma cells* and *multinucleated giant cells* are seen in some forms of chronic inflammation.

IV. **Bacilli** These are normally present and include most often *Döderlein bacilli* (*Bacillus vaginalis/ Lactobacillus acidophilus*), the gram-positive rods that appear pale blue in routine Pap smears. They are more abundant during the luteal phase and during pregnancy than during the proliferative phase.

TABLE A.4 Squamous epithelial cells found in normal combined (fast) smears.

CELL TYPE	SIZE	NUCLEI	CYTOPLASM	MORPHOLOGY
Superficial	30–60 µm	< 6 µm dark, pyknotic	Polyhedral, thin, broad, acidophilic or cyanophilic with keratohyaline granules	
Intermediate	20–40 µm	6–9 µm vesicular	Polyhedral or elongated, thin, cyanophilic with folded edges	
Parabasal	15–25 µm	6–11 µm vesicular	Round to oval, thick, well-defined, basophilic with occasional small vacuoles	
Basal	13–20 µm	Large, (> one-half of cell volume), hyperchromatic, may have small nucleoli	Round to oval, deeply basophilic	

Q8. What are the applications of Pap smears?

Two most important applications are: *evaluation of the hormonal status of the woman and the diagnosis of malignancy.*

I. **Cytohormonal evaluation** is best carried out from the lateral vaginal smears, which ideally must be obtained 3 times on alternate days in a row. Several indices are derived describing cytohormonal patterns as under:

i. *Acidophilic index* by counting the relative number of cells that have acidophilic (pink) or basophilic (bluish) cytoplasm.
ii. *Pyknotic index* by counting the percentage of cells that have small dark (pyknotic) nuclei.
iii. *Maturation index (MI),* which is the most widely used method. One hundred cells are counted and classified as parabasal, intermediate and superficial (e.g. 10/80/10). Some representative MIs are given in the Table A.5.
II. **Evaluation of smears for neoplasia** is based on *The Bethesda System (TBS), developed and subsequently modified by the US National Cancer Institute Workshop.* Criteria for TBS are the same as those for the histologic reporting of cervical biopsies.

TABLE A.5 Representative maturation indices at different stages of life.

STAGE	MATURATION INDEX* (%)	COMMENT
Neonatal	0/90/10	As in pregnancy
Infancy	90/10/0	With infections shows midzone shift
Preovulatory	0/40/60	Shift-to-right
Post-ovulatory	0/70/30	Midzone shift
Pregnancy	0/95/5	Midzone shift
Postpartum	90/10/0	Shift-to-left
Menopausal (early)	0/80/10	Estatrophy
Menopausal (late)	95/5/0	Teleatrophy

*MI = Parabasal/intermediate/superficial

As per TBS, each cytopathology report must contain the following element:
i. *Specimen adequacy,* i.e. if the specimen contains enough cells and they are properly fixed to allow microscopic evaluation.
ii. *General categorisation* using three categories: within normal limits, benign cellular changes, and epithelial cell abnormalities.
iii. *Descriptive diagnosis* including description of benign and malignant epithelial cell abnormalities. The changes are then classified as non-neoplastic (or benign) and neoplastic epithelial cell abnormalities.

Q9. What are non-neoplastic (benign) cellular changes in vaginal smears?

Two general categories are recognised as under:
I. **Non-specific inflammatory changes**, which may be acute or chronic.
II. **Specific inflammatory changes** which may include the following categories:
i. *Bacterial agents,* such as *Neisseria gonorrhoeae, Gardnerella vaginalis,* or *Mycobacterium tuberculosis.*
ii. *Viral agents* such as human papilloma virus (classified as low-risk or high-risk HPV), or herpes virus.
iii. *Fungal agents,* such as *Candida albicans* (moniliasis) or *Torulopsis glabrata.*
iv. *Parasitic agents* such as *Trichomonas vaginalis* (found in 25% women), *Entamoeba histolytica.*

Q10. How are neoplastic epithelial cell abnormalities classified?

Epithelial cell abnormalities seen in vaginal smears are classified as squamous cell or glandular abnormalities:
I. **Squamous cell abnormalities** fall into three categories that correspond to histologic diagnoses of cervical intraepithelial neoplasia (CIN) and are grade as CIN I, CIN II or CIN III.
The Bethesda system of reporting abnormal smears has five categories as under:
i. *Atypical squamous cell of undetermined significance (ASCUS).*
ii. *Low grade squamous intraepithelial lesion (LSIL),* corresponding to CIN I.
iii. *High grade squamous intraepithelial lesion (HSIL),* corresponding to CIN grade II and III, and CIS.
iv. *ASC-H* with general features of LSIL, but also containing additional features that suggest HSIL.
v. *Squamous cell carcinoma.*
II. **Glandular cell abnormalities** include three categories as under:
i. *Atypical glandular cells of undetermined significance (AGUS)* which could be either endocervical or endometrial but showing changes that exceed the reactive ones.
ii. *Endocervical or endometrial adenocarcinoma* which can be distinguished from each other using the criteria outlined in **Table A.6**.
iii. *Extrauterine cancers* which can be suspected by their morphology and configuration (e.g. papillary cancer with psammoma bodies) and the absence of dysplastic changes in coexistent cervico-endometrial cells.

TABLE A.6 Cytomorphological features of endocervical and endometrial adenocarcinoma.

FEATURE	ENDOCERVICAL CARCINOMA	ENDOMETRIAL CARCINOMA
1. *Background*	Clean	Dirty, bloody
2. *Cell yield*	High (found mainly on cervical smears)	Low (found mainly on vaginal smears)
3. *Cell arrangement*	Clusters or sheets with 'side-by-side' grouping	Three-dimensional 'cell ball' or grape-like clusters
4. *Cytoplasm*		
i. *Amount*	Moderate (often in columnar configuration)	Small
ii. *Character*	Granular, well-stained, often producing mucin	Finely vacuolated, translucent, with ingested leucocytes
5. *Nuclei*		
i. *Size*	Large	Fairly small
ii. *Character*	Finely granular chromatin (mild hyperchromasia)	Coarse chromatin (marked hyperchromasia)
iii. *Nucleoli*	Macronucleoli	Micronucleoli

Q11. Comment on the most commonly used forms of non-gynaecologic exfoliative cytology.

Commonly used non-gynaecologic specimens for cytologic evaluation are as under:

I. **Respiratory tract cytology** includes examination of sputum or bronchial brushing during bronchoscopy:

i. *Sputum examination* Sputum is easily obtained by coughing. Most specimens are satisfactory and allow the diagnosis of lung cancer in 80% cases. However, the large number of cells in the specimen makes it quite tedious for screening. Furthermore, the lesions cannot be localised since the cells are derived from all parts of the respiratory system.

ii. *Bronchial brushing (BB) and aspiration/washing (BW)* are more suitable for localising tumours, and contain fewer cells, and thus the examination time is shorter requiring less scrutiny.

II. **Gastrointestinal tract cytology** may be performed on a variety of specimens. These include:

i. Scraping of the oral mucosa.

ii. Brushing of oesophageal and gastric mucosal lesion during oesophago-gastrectomy while doing the biopsy.

iii. Likewise, the colonic cytologic specimens can be collected during colonoscopy or lavage following enema to the clean the colon.

iv. Endoscopy-directed collection of samples can be obtained from common bile and pancreatic duct and biliary passages.

III. **Urinary tract cytology** These include:

i. *Centrifuged specimens of voided or catheterised urine* Voided specimens are preferred in men, while in women the catheterised specimens are better to avoid contamination with vaginal cells and menstrual blood. Voided urine is usually satisfactory for the diagnosis of upper urinary tract lesions.

ii. *Bladder irrigation (washings)* at the time of cystoscopy is preferred approach for symptomatic patients suspected to have bladder cancer.

IV. **Effusions cytology (from pleural, pericardial or peritoneal cavity)** Both transudate and exudate can be examined. Most malignant effusions have protein content greater than 3 g/dL and are classified as exudates. Malignant tumours may be primary (mesothelioma) or metastatic.
Cellular composition of effusions varies:

Benign effusions contain reactive mesothelial cells and inflammatory cells, mostly macrophages.

i. In *acute suppurative inflammation* there are neutrophils.

ii. In *chronic inflammation* there are lymphocytes. Tuberculosis is characterised by lymphocytes, epithelioid cells and multinucleated giant cells.

Malignant cells seen in effusions vary depending on the tumour type, as follows:

i. *Mesothelioma* of the epithelial and mixed type contains epithelioid cells with vesicular nuclei, similar to those in adenocarcinoma. Immunocytochemistry must be used for definitive diagnosis. Fibrous mesothelioma composed of spindle cells does not shed cells into the fluid.

ii. *Adenocarcinomas* are the most common malignancy identified in effusions. These tumours most often originate from the ovary, stomach, colon, lung and breast. Adenocarcinoma cells may be seen as individual cells or they form small groups. Some of them have mucin in the cytoplasm.

iii. *Squamous cell carcinomas* are rarely seen in effusion. Most tumours of this type originate in the lungs, cervix or oesophagus.
iv. *Small cell carcinoma* of the lung has characteristic morphology. In effusions, the malignant cells have moulded hyperchromatic nuclei and scanty cytoplasm or no cytoplasm at all.
v. *Lymphoma and leukaemia* cells are usually seen in effusions only in some specific subtypes of lymphoma (e.g. primary effusion lymphoma) or in advanced and terminal cases.
V. **Cerebrospinal fluid cytology** is based on the analysis of centrifuged sediments of cerebrospinal fluid (CSF). It is usually a part of the lumbar puncture and CSF sampling. Three types of samples are examined:
i. *Normal CSF* (total volume ~150 ml) contains few cells (0–4 µL), most of which are lymphocytes and occasional monocyte.
ii. *CSF in non-neoplastic conditions* contains various inflammatory cells (see **Table 30.1**). PMNs are prominent in bacterial suppurative meningitis, whereas lymphocytes predominate in viral infections. Tuberculosis is characterised by lymphocytes, epithelioid macrophages, and scattered multinucleated giant cells.
iii. *CNS neoplasms* may enter the CSF, especially those that are in direct contact with fluid filled spaces. Malignant tumours that are most often found in the CSF are metastatic cancers (adenocarcinoma, lymphoma, leukaemia), medulloblastoma, ependymoma. Note that meningiomas (despite their close contact with the CSF filled spaces) rarely, if ever, shed its cells into the CSF.
VI. **Seminal fluid (semen)** is examined as part of the male infertility studies, or to ascertain the completeness of vasectomy. The specimen is usually obtained by masturbation after a 4 days of sexual abstinence. The following findings are reported:
i. *Volume of ejaculate* Normal volume is >1.5 ml.
ii. *Viscosity* Ejaculated semen is initially quite viscous but it liquefies within 20 minutes.
iii. *pH of ejaculate* It is alkaline (pH>7.2).
iv. *Motility of spermatozoa* At 2 hours of ejaculation, >40% spermatozoa are motile. At 6–8 hours, 25–40% spermatozoa are motile.
v. *Count of spermatozoa* Normal count is >39x10^6 per ejaculate. It can be machine read.
vi. *Morphology of spermatozoa* Normally more than 4% are normal.
vii. *Fructose content in the ejaculate* Average fructose content is >13 µmol (315mg/dL)/ejaculate. Low level of fructose indicates obstruction at the level of ejaculatory duct.

Q12. How is genetic sex determined in cytology specimens?

Sex-specific chromatin bodies are observed in interphase nuclei and comprise the Barr body (X-chromosome) in females and the fluorescent F body (Y-chromosome) in males:
I. **Barr body** is a small (1 µm) piece of chromatin attached to the inside of the nuclear membrane, corresponding to the inactivated X-chromosome in females. The number of Barr bodies is always the number of X-chromosomes minus one (e.g. normal female 2X-1=1).
The test is best performed on a buccal smear, but can be done on vaginal smears as well. One hundred cells are scrutinised and in normal females at least 20% of cells will have a Barr body. Normal males have it in less than 2% cells.
II. **F body (Y chromatin)** is demonstrable only by fluorescence microscopy following staining of the buccal smears with quinacrine mustard. The fluorescent F body is seen in approximately 60% of cells in males and only 8% or less in females. F body can be demonstrated in lymphocytes in peripheral blood stained with quinacrine mustard.
III. **Drumstick appendage in polymorphonuclear leucocytes** may be used as sex marker as it is seen in 3–6% of females and in only 0.3% males.

Q13. How are samples for gynaecologic exfoliative cytology prepared?

The preparation of samples for exfoliative cytology has four phases: collection, fixation, processing in the laboratory and staining. Each of these procedures is usually performed by specialist who follows the prescribed protocols.
I. **Collection of samples**
i. **Preparation of Pap smears**   Smears should not be taken during menstrual bleeding.
a. Smears are obtained under *direct vision* after introducing a Cusco speculum with the patient in lithotomy position.

b. The posterior fornix of the vagina is aspirated with a *blunt-ended glass pipette* fitted with a rubber bulb. A drop of the aspirate is placed at the unlabelled end of a glass slide.

c. The ectocervix is sampled with the *Ayre spatula* **(Fig. A.1)**. The longer limb of the spatula is fitted into the external os and the spatula rotated through 360° to sample the entire cervix. The scraped material on the spatula is then placed on the drop aspirated from the vaginal pool and the smear prepared with the spatula itself or with the tip of the gloved finger; smears are prepared directly with the spatula.

d. Thin uniform smears should be prepared and the slide immediately *immersed in fixative* to avoid artefacts in cells caused by drying.

ii. **Liquid-based cytology (LBC)** LBC is a special technique for preparation of gynaecologic and non-gynaecologic samples which provides uniform monolayered dispersion of cells on smears, without overlapping or clump formation and does not contain background material or debris. It is a pre-requisite for quantitative analysis and automated devices. Two types of LBC systems are commercially available—ThinPrep and SurePath, each with its own advantages.

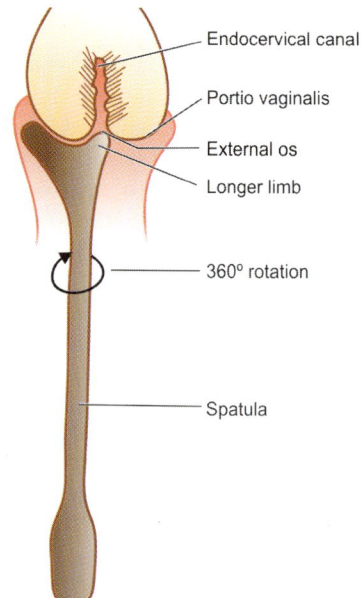

FIGURE A.1: Method of obtaining cervical smear with Ayre spatula (fast smear).

II. **Fixation and fixatives**

All material for cytological examination must be properly fixed to ensure preservation of cytomorphological details. Methods of fixation vary depending upon the type of staining employed:

- Material for exfoliative cytodiagnosis is usually *wet-fixed*, i.e. smears are immersed in fixative without allowing them to dry. These smears are then stained with Papanicolaou (Pap) or haematoxylin and eosin (H & E) stains.
- Sometimes, exfoliative cytology smears are *air-dried* for use with the Romanowsky stains as are used in haematologic studies. In Romanowsky staining, fixation is effected during the staining procedure.

i. **Routine fixatives** The ideal fixative for routine use is Papanicolaou fixative comprising a solution of equal parts of ether and 95% ethanol. However, the flammability of ether makes it hazardous. Most laboratories use 95% ethanol alone with excellent results. Where ethanol is not available, 100% methanol, 95% denatured alcohol, or 85% isopropyl alcohol (isopropanolol) may be used.

Prepared smears are immediately immersed in fixative *without allowing them to dry prior to fixation*. Drying causes distortion of cells and induces cytoplasmic staining artefacts. Smears are sent to laboratory in coplin jar containing fixative.

ii. **Coating fixatives** Coating fixatives are applied as aerosol-sprays or with a dropper to the surface of freshly prepared smears. Coating fixatives are ideal when unstained smears are to be transported over long distances.

III. **Processing of sample in the laboratory**

Pap smears wet-fixed in ethanol need no further processing in the laboratory prior to staining.

IV. **Staining of Pap smears**

Three staining procedures are commonly employed in cytologic smears: Papanicolaou and H&E stains are used for *wet-fixed smears,* while Romanowsky stains are used for *air-dried smears.*

Papanicolaou staining is employed for wet-fixed Pap smears. Pap stain includes 3 solutions comprising a nuclear stain (Harris haematoxylin) and two cytoplasmic counter-stains (Orange G or OG-6, and eosin-azure or EA-65 or EA-50). Nuclear stain gives basophilic colour to the nucleus while the two cytoplasmic stains impart the orange and cyanophilic tints to cytoplasm respectively.

INTERVENTIONAL CYTOLOGY

Q14. What is fine needle aspiration cytology (FNAC)? Briefly discuss the procedure of FNAC.

Definition In practice, interventional cytology is synonymous with fine needle aspiration cytology (FNAC), also called fine needle aspiration biopsy (FNAB). FNAC is widely used for sampling a wide variety of human tissue and is ideal for the evaluation of mass lesions, especially those that are palpable or visible by X-rays. Among the palpable lesion the most commonly aspirated are those in the breast, soft tissues, enlarged lymph nodes, thyroid, salivary gland and testis. Other organs accessible to FNAC are the prostate, pelvic organs, bone and joints, lungs, liver, pancreas, kidneys and abdominal masses, and orbits.

Procedure

I. *Materials* For performing FNAC, a syringe with a well-fitting needle, syringe holder, some microscopic glass slides and appropriate fixative are the only material required in most instances **(Fig. A.2)**.

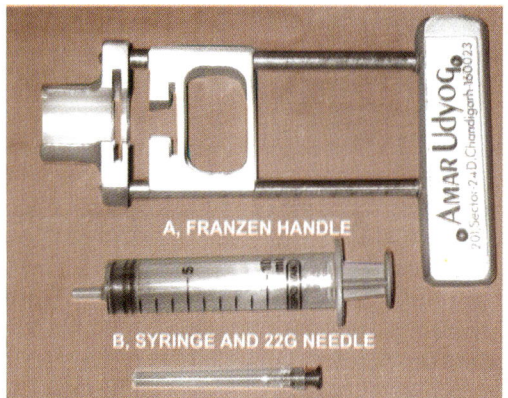
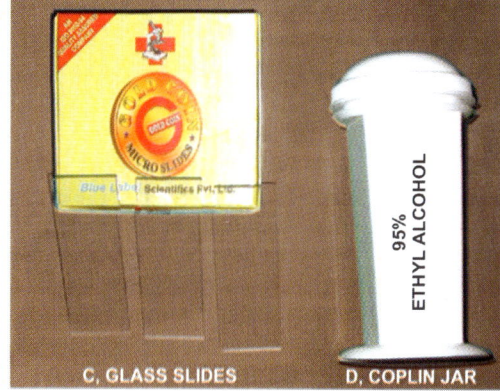

FIGURE A.2: Equipments required for transcutaneous FNAC.

II. *Method of direct aspiration* Transcutaneous FNAC of palpable masses is routinely performed without anaesthesia as per the procedure illustrated in **Figure A.3**); aspiration of sites/lesions requiring anaesthesia or special technique are discussed separately.

III. *Radiological imaging aids for FNAC* Non-palpable lesions require some form of localisation by radiological aids for FNAC to be carried out.
- *Plain X-ray films* are usually adequate for lesions within bones and for some lesions within the chest.
- The most versatile radiological aid is *ultrasonographic (US)-guidance* which allows direct visualisation of needle placement in real time and is free from radiation hazards, i.e. endoscopic ultrasound *(EUS)-*guided procedure. It is an extremely valuable aid for FNAC of thyroid nodules, soft tissue masses, intra-abdominal lesions and for intrathoracic lesions which abut the chest wall, but is of no help in deep intrathoracic lesions or in bony lesions.
- *Computerised tomographic (CT) guidance* is used for lesions within the chest and abdomen.

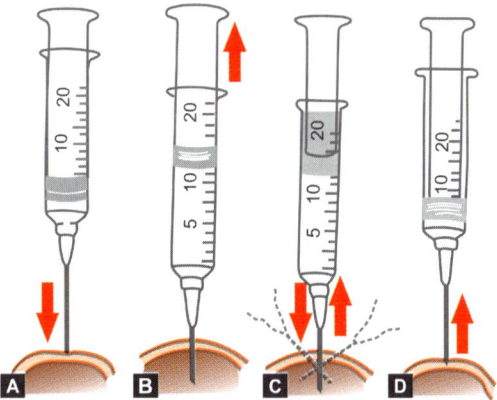

FIGURE A.3: Procedure for FNAC of palpable masses. Needle is introduced into the mass (A). Plunger is retracted after needle enters the mass (B). Suction is maintained while needle is moved back and forth within the mass (C). Suction is released and plunger returned to original position before needle is withdrawn (D).

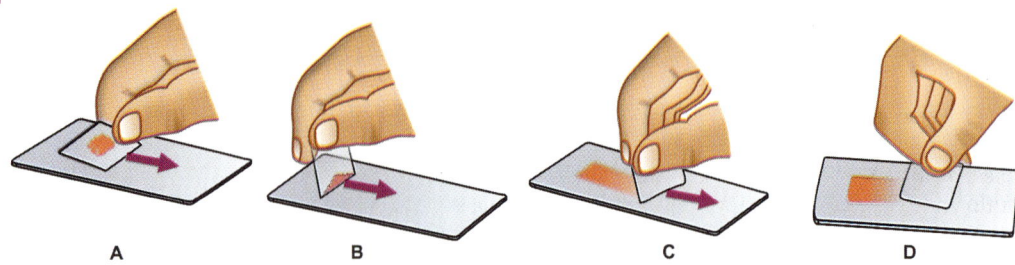

FIGURE A.4: Preparation of smears. Semisolid aspirates are crush-smeared by flat pressure with cover slip or glass slide (A). Fluid or blood droplet is collected along edge of spreader (B), and pulled as for peripheral blood films (C). Particles at the end of the smear are crush-smeared (D).

IV. *Preparation of smears* Preparation of smears is crucial to the success of FNAC as illustrated in **Figure A.4**. Poorly-prepared smears with distorted cellular morphology will frustrate the best efforts of the most competent cytopathologist, and often result in errors of interpretation or in failure to arrive at any specific diagnosis.

Q15. What are the advantages of FNAC?

i. FNAC is an out-patient procedure and requires no hospitalisation, in contrast to other biopsies which are performed in surgical suites and hospitals.
ii. No anaesthesia is required.
iii. The procedure is quick, safe and least painful.
iv. Multiple attempts (or repeating of the procedure) are possible without inconvenience to the patient.
v. Results are obtained rapidly, and reports may be generated 2–24 hours thereafter.
vi. It is cost-effective and no major equipment is required.
vii. As the cytopathologists performs the procedure, firsthand knowledge of the clinical findings is gained which facilitates better interpretation of slides and enhances diagnostic accuracy.

Q16. What are various ancillary studies which can be done on material aspirated by FNAC?

If indicated, following ancillary studies can be done on FNAC material to support the cytopathologic diagnosis:
i. *Special histochemical stains* for demonstrating certain components of cells and extracellular material, such as mucin, amyloid, etc.
ii. *Microbiological studies* are performed on the sterile material remaining in the syringe, or by a second passage which is empties into special bacteriological tubes.
iii. *Cell blocks* may be prepared from the remaining material which is centrifuged into a pellet, fixed in formalin and embedded into paraffin for histologic sectioning.
iv. *Immunocytochemical studies* are performed after microscopic examination of the routinely prepared slides. Such studies are usually performed on slides that have not been stained.
v. *Additional advanced studies* may be performed in support of the cytopathologic diagnosis or provide additional data important for treatment. These include *image analysis, flow cytometry, ultrastructural studies and molecular biology studies*.

Q17. What are the complications of FNAC?

FNAC is associated with relatively few complications. The most common complications are as under:
i. *Haematomas* at the puncture site, especially in the thyroid and breast. Compression with a finger for 2–3 minutes will reduce the frequency of this complication.
ii. *Infection* is uncommon; most cases followed puncture of an organ with pre-existent infection (e.g. prostatitis), or accidental puncture of large intestine during abdominal FNAC.
iii. *Pneumothorax* during transcutaneous lung biopsy. It may be associated with transient haemoptysis which may follow bronchoscopic examination as well.

iv. *Dissemination of tumour* can theoretically occur, but in clinical practice this is a rare complication. There are occasional cases of rupture of a cystic ovarian tumour with peritoneal dissemination, or extension of a solid tumour along the needle track.

Q18. What are the contraindications for FNAC?

i. *Bleeding disorders* Haemophilia is a relative contraindication and FNAC should be performed with caution and prophylactic measures. Thrombocytopenia itself is not a contraindication.

ii. *In FNAC liver,* coagulopathy that accompanies cirrhosis may be a contraindication, especially if the prothrombin index (PTI) is less than 80%. Obstructive jaundice is a contraindication of liver FNAC since it may cause bile peritonitis. Liver abscess should not be biopsied since the FNAC could lead to bacteraemia.

iii. *In FNAC lung,* emphysema and pulmonary hypertension may be accompanied by pneumothorax and prominent haemoptysis. Acute bacterial infections and bacterial abscesses are also contraindications.

iv. *In FNAC of pancreas,* catheterisation of the pancreatic duct may cause mild acute pancreatitis, but that should not be of any clinical concern. In acute pancreatitis, transcutaneous FNAC is contraindicated since it may aggravate the inflammation and promote chemical peritonitis.

v. *In FNAC prostate,* acute prostatitis is a contraindication for FNAC because it may cause bacteraemia and septicaemia.

vi. *In testis and epididymis,* acute bacterial infection is a contraindication.

vii. *In FNAC adrenal gland* involved by a suspected pheochromocytoma, FNAC should not be done since the puncture may cause extreme fluctuations of the blood pressure due to a release of catecholamines.

Q19. What are the limitations of FNAC?

FNAC is a highly reliable diagnostic method but even so it may results in 'false negatives'. Such outcome of the aspiration biopsy may be related to the following problems:

i. *Sampling* This may be inadequate due to the inaccessibility of the lesion or inadequate radiologic or ultrasound visualisation of deeply seated lesions.

ii. *Nature of the lesion* Some tumours have several components, or may be predominantly necrotic, infiltrated by inflammatory cells, or fibrosed and scarred. Such secondary changes are especially common following radiation or chemotherapy

iii. *Suboptimal preparation of cytologic slides* Samples may be acellular, poorly fixated or are dried out and thus technically inadequate.

iv. *Inadequate clinicopathologic correlation* Detailed clinical information is critical for proper interpretation of cytopathology slides. Accordingly, whenever possible the pathologist should be given relevant clinical, radiologic and laboratory data.

If the FNAC study is negative despite strong clinical suspicion favouring the diagnosis of malignancy, the entire procedure may be repeated, or a surgical biopsy could be performed.

Q20. What is imprint cytology?

Imprint cytology, also known as touch preparation, is based on sectioning the surgically resected tumour or a suspicious lesion and touching it with a glass slide without smearing it. This procedure will result in an imprint of cells from the freshly cut surface. Such imprints are fixed in formalin or ethanol and stained with H&E or any of the cytologic staining techniques. Note that fixed tissue cannot be used for imprinting!

Imprint cytology recapitulates the architecture of the lesion under examination, and also provides means to study individual cells at higher magnification. In practice, it is used as an aid to frozen sections and also for cytologic analysis of various lesions, especially when typing and classifying lymphomas.

Q21. What is crush smear cytology?

Crush smears are mostly used in neuropathology.
The procedure is relatively simple.

i. The brain specimen obtained by biopsy through craniotomy is inspected with naked eye.

ii. A sample for cytologic study is chosen as a small fragment, which is cut from the main biopsy specimen, which is then frozen for cryostat sectioning.
iii. The selected smaller piece of tissue is placed on a slide and crushed with another slide placed on top of it.
iv. Two slides which adhere to each other due to the glue-like action of the tissue are then pulled in opposite direction smearing the crushed tissue on both slides.
v. These smears retain partially the architectural histologic features of the lesion, and at the same time provide the pathologist with an array of cells that can be analysed and classified to make the pathologic diagnosis.

> **Appendix-e Supplement: Online Content**
>
> *Digital content of this chapter available with this book is meant for enhanced learning and self-assessment. In addition, it contains 15 Multiple Choice Questions (MCQs), 05 Clinicopathologic Vignettes, and 04 Image-based Questions; these are followed by their answers along with explanatory notes of correct and incorrect answers.*

Index

Page numbers followed by *f* refer to figure, and *t* refer to table.

A

AA protein, 115
ABL-BCR gene, 160
ABO system, 266
Abscess, 65
  amoebic liver, 190, 499
  apical, 430
  appendix, 469
  brain, 710-1
  Brodie, 681
  breast, 613
  crypt, 460*f*
  liver, 499-500
  lung, 383-4
  tubo-ovarian, 601
Absolute values, 227
Acanthocytosis, 225
Acantholysis, 626
Acanthosis, 626
Accumulations, intracellular, 44-50
Acetyl choline receptors (AChRs), 694
Acidophil body, 497*f*
Achalasia, 436
Achondroplasia, 676
Acid-fast staining, 69, 75
Acidosis, 129
Acne vulgaris, 628
Acromegaly, 643
Actinomycetoma, 185
Acoustic neuroma, 417
Acquired immunodeficiency
    syndrome (AIDS), 97-101
  clinical manifestations of, 100-1
  CDC classification of, 100*t*
  CNS manifestations in, 101
  etiologic agent of, 97*f*
  Kaposi sarcoma in, 337
  laboratory diagnosis of, 101
  oral manifestations in, 424*t*
  pathogenesis of, 98-9
  pathologic changes in, 100-1
  pneumonias in, 101, 381*t*
  routes of transmission of, 97-8
Acromegaly, 643
Actinomycetoma, 184
Activated partial thromboplastin
    time (APTT), 257
Acute phase reactants (APRs), 66
Acute tubular necrosis (ATN), 550-1
Adaptations, cellular, 20-27
  types of, 21-2, 22*f*

Addison disease, 46, 647-8
Adenocarcinoma,
  colorectal, 475-8
  endometrium, 598-9
  gallbladder, 520
  kidney, 561-3
  lung, 403-4
  oesophagus, 440
  ovary, 604, 605
  pancreas, 524-5
  periampullary, 520-1
  prostate, 585-7
  salivary gland, 435
  stomach, 450-1
  urinary bladder, 569
  vagina, 591
Adenoma,
  adrenocortical, 648
  bile duct, 513
  colorectal, 473-5
  cortical, adrenal, 648
  follicular, thyroid, 658-9
  gastric, 449
  hepatocellular, 512-3
  oesophagus, 440
  parathyroid, 665-6
  pituitary, 645*t*
  pleomorphic, 434
  salivary gland, 434
  thyroid, 658-9
Adenoma-carcinoma sequence, 476
Adenomyosis, 596
Adenosis, breast, 614
  sclerosing, 615
Adhesion molecules, cellular, 13-4, 155
Adhesion receptors (ARs), 13-4
Adipocytic tumours, 699-700
Adnexal tumours, skin, 637
Adrenal crisis, 647
Adrenal gland, diseases of, 645-51
  tumours of, 648-51
Adrenogenital syndrome, 647
African iron overload, 48
Ageing, cellular, 17-8, 163-4
Agenesis, 209
  pulmonary, 372
AL protein, 115
Albinism, 46-7
Alcoholic liver disease, 501-3
Alcoholism, 196-7
Alkaline phosphatase, hepatic, 483

Alkalosis, 129-30
ALKR, 160
Alpha1-antitrypsin deficiency, 386, 508
Alport syndrome, 550
Alzheimer disease, 721
  mechanism of, 115*f*
Ameloblastoma, 432
American Joint Committee for
    Cancer (AJCC) staging, 176, 698
Amoebiasis, 189-90
Amyloidosis, 114-20
  AA protein, 115
  $A\beta_2$-microglobulin in, 115
  AL protein in, 115
  cardiac, 367
  classification of, 117*t*
  endocrine, 116, 662, 669
  fibril proteins in, 115
  kidneys in, 119
  liver, 120
  P-component of, 116
  pathogenesis of, 116*f*
  primary systemic, 117
  primary *versus* secondary, 118*t*
  secondary systemic (reactive), 118
  senile, 117*t*
  spleen in, 119-20
  staining, characteristics of, 119*t*
  transthyretin in, 115
Anaemia, aplastic, 252-3
Anaemia, Cooley, 250
Anaemia, Fanconi, 252
Anaemia, general aspects, 227-30
  classification of, 230*t*
  clinical features of, 228
  grading of, 227-8
  investigations of, 229
  peripheral blood smear in, 228-9
Anaemia, haemolytic, 238-51
  acquired, 240-3
  autoimmune (AIHA), 241-2
  classification of, 238-9
  cold antibody, 241-2
  congenital, 243-51
  drug-induced, 242
  due to direct toxic effects, 242-3
  extravascular *versus* intravascular, 240*t*
  hereditary, 243-51

immunohaemolytic, 240-2
laboratory tests for, 239-40
microangiopathic, 242
red cell membrane defects, 244-5
warm antibody, 241
Anaemia, haemorrhagic, 251
Anaemia, hypochromic, 230-5
contrasting features of, 235*t*
Anaemia, iron deficiency, 230-3
etiology and pathogenesis of, 230-1
iron metabolism in, 231-3
laboratory findings in, 233
Anaemia, Mediterranean, 250
Anaemia, megaloblastic, 235-7
biochemical basis of, 235*f*
etiology of, 235-6
laboratory findings in, 236-7
treatment of, 237
Anaemia, microcytic hypochromic, 230*t*, 233
Anaemia, myelophthisic, 253
Anaemia, normocytic and normochromic, 234
Anaemia of blood loss, 251
Anaemia of chronic disorders, 234-5
Anaemia, pernicious, 237-8
Anaemia, sickle cell, 246-8
clinicopathologic features in, 248
genetics and pathogenesis, 247
laboratory findings in, 248
Anaemia, sideroblastic, 233-4
Anal canal, tumours of, 478
Anaphase lag, 211
Anaplasia, 150
Anasarca, 122
Anencephaly, 210
Aneuploidy, 211
Aneurysms, 330-2
berry, 331, 717
dissecting, 331-2
Angina pectoris, 345-6
Angina, Ludwig, 420
Angina, Vincent, 420
Angiofibroma, nasopharyngeal, 420
Angiogenesis, 83, 164
Angiosarcoma, 336-7
Anisocytosis, 228
Anitschkow cells, 354*f*
Ankyrin, 244
Ann Arbor staging, 309*t*
Anthracosis, 49
Anthrax, 181-2
Antidiuretic hormone (ADH), 124, 643
Anti-GBM disease, 537
Anti-oncogenes,161-2
versus oncogenes, 163*t*
Anti-neutrophil cytoplasmic antibodies (ANCAs), 326, 538
Antioxidants, 32
Antoni A and B, 733
Aortitis, syphilitic, 79, 325-6
APC gene, 476*f*

Aphthous ulcers, 423
Aplasia, 209
pure red cell (PRCA), 253
Apolipoprotein E, 116
Apoptosis, 40-4
versus necrosis, 43*t*
Appendicitis, 468-9
Appendix, diseases of, 468-70
Arachidonic acid metabolites, 56-7
Argyria, 49
Armanni-Ebstein lesions, 549
Arnold-Chiari malformations, 707
Arteries, structure of, 317
Arteriolitis, necrotising, 36, 319
Arteriolosclerosis, hypertensive, 318-9
Arteriosclerosis, 318-24
atherosclerotic, 319-24
Mönckeberg, 319
senile, 318
Arteritis, 325-30
cerebral, syphilitic, 326
giant cell, 328
syphilitic, 325-6
Takayasu, 328-9
temporal, 328
Arthritis,
gonococcal, 690
gouty, 688, 690-1
infectious, 689-990
in RHD, 355
Lyme disease, 690
osteoarthritis, 687-8
rheumatoid, 688-9
suppurative, 690
tuberculous, 688
Asbestosis, 396-7
Aschoff bodies, 354*f*
Ascites, 123, 128, 490, 510-1
Ascorbic acid, 205-6
Asthma, bronchial, 388-9
extrinsic versus intrinsic, 389*t*
Astrocytoma, 724-5
Ataxia telangiectasia, 96-7, 163
Atelectasis, 372-3
Atheroma, 323
Atheromatous plaques, 323-4
Atherosclerosis, 319-24
clinical effects of, 324
consequences of, 324
etiology of, 319
diabetes mellitus in, 321, 671
dislipidaemia in, 320
hypertension in, 320
morphologic features of, 323-4
pathogenesis of, 321-3
response-to-injury theory in, 321-3
risk factors in, 319*t*
smoking in, 321
Atresia, 209
biliary, 489
oesophageal, 436
Atrial septal defect (ASD), 343

Atrophy, 21-2
brown, 49
testicular, 570*f*
Atypical mycobacteria, 69
Auer rods, 288*f*
Autoantibodies, in SLE, 109-10
in autoimmune thyroiditis, 654
Autoimmune diseases, 106-14
classification of, 109*t*
pathogenesis of, 108
Autoimmunity, pathogenesis of, 108
Autophagy, 17, 44, 164
Autosomal disorders, 215
Avian influenza, 187
Axial flow, 54
Ayre spatula, 742*f*

■ B

Babesiosis, 191
Bacterial diseases, 181-4
Bacterial endocarditis, 357-60
acute versus subacute, 357*t*
cardiac lesions in, 358-9
complications of, 359-60
etiology of, 467
extra-cardiac complications of, 360
diagnosis of, 358-9
pathologic features of, 358-9
pathogenesis of, 358-9
predisposing conditions in, 358
Bagassosis, 399
Balanitis xerotica obliterans, 580
Balanoposthitis, 580
Barr body, 746
Barrett oesophagus, 439
Bartholin cyst and adenitis, 588
Basophilia, 276
punctate, 229
Basophils, 63
BCG vaccination, 71
BCL gene, 42, 163
BCR-ABL gene, 160
Beriberi, 206
Bernard-Soulier syndrome, 262
Berylliosis, 397
Bethesda system, 593-4, 739
Biliary tract, diseases of, 515-21
Bilirubin, 47, 483
conjugated versus unconjugated, 485*t*
metabolism of, 485*f*
tests for, 483
Bioterrorism, microbial, 192-3
Bio-weapons, 192-3
Bird-breeders' lung, 399
Blackfan-Diamond syndrome, 253
Blackwater fever, 190
Blastoma, 149, 219
Bleeding disorders, *also see under* Haemorrhagic diatheses, 258-66
Bleeding, gastrointestinal, 479*t*

Bleeding time, 256
Blindness,
  in diabetes, 412f
  night, 203
Blood group systems, 266
Blood transfusion, 266-70
  complications of, 269-70
  components in, 267-8
Blood vessels, diseases of, 317-37
  tumours and tumour-like lesions of, 335-7
Bloom syndrome, 163
Bone and cartilage, diseases of, 675-87
  tumour-like lesions of, 682t
  tumours of, 682t
Bone marrow, 221-3
  aspiration *versus* trephine, 223t
  trephine biopsy of, 223
Botryoid sarcoma, 591, 702
Botulism, 184
Bowen disease, 635
Bowenoid papulosis, 580-1
Bradykinin, 60
Bread and butter appearance, 354
Breast, diseases of, 613-24
Brittle bone disease, 676
Bronchiectasis, 390
Bronchiolitis, respiratory, 400
Bronchitis, chronic, 385
Bruton disease, 95
Bubos, 181
Budd-Chiari syndrome, 490-1
Buerger disease, 329-30
Burr cells, 225
Button-hole appearance, 353
Byssinosis, 399

C

Cachexia, cancer, 174
Cadherins, 14
Café-au-lait spots, 46
Calcification, pathologic, 38-40
  dystrophic, 36-39
  dystrophic *versus* metastatic, 40t
  metastatic, 39
Calcinosis cutis, 633
Calculi, gallbladder, 515-8
  urinary, 555-7
Call-Exner bodies, 609
Callus formation, 680f
Cancer (neoplasia), definition of, 148
  carcinogens in, 166-73
  characteristics of, 150
  classification of, 149t
  clinical aspects of, 174-9
  diagnosis of, 176-9
  epidemiology of, 155-8
  grading of, 175-6
  hallmarks, molecular, 159f, 160t
  hormones in, 157-8
  immunology of, 165-6

incidence of, 156
metastasis in, 152-5
molecular basis of, 158-66
paraneoplastic syndromes in, 174-5
pathogenesis of, 166-73
predisposing factors in, 156-7
spread of, 152-5
staging of, 176
theories of, 158
versus benign tumours, 150t
Candidiasis, 185, 424
Caplan syndrome, 395
Carbon monoxide poisoning, 198
Carcinoembryonic antigen (CEA), 178
Carcinogenesis, 166-73
  biologic, 169-73
  chemical, 166-7
  hormones in, 157-8
  molecular basis of, 158-66
  physical, 167-9
  theories of, 158
  viral, 169-73
Carcinogens,166-73
  chemical, 167t
  initiator *versus* promoter, 168t
  physical, 167-9
  viral, 169-73
Carcinoid heart disease, 364
Carcinoid syndrome, 364, 468
Carcinoid tumour,
  appendix, 470
  bronchial, 406
  small intestine, 467-8
Carcinoma, acinic cell, 435
Carcinoma, adenoid cystic, 435
Carcinoma, adrenal cortical, 648
Carcinoma, ampulla of Vater, 520-1
Carcinoma, breast, 617-24
  classification of, 618t
  grading and staging of, 623
  inflammatory, 622
  invasive, 620-2
  metaplastic, 622
  non-invasive, 619
  prognostic factors in, 623-4
  risk factors for, 617-8
Carcinoma, cervix, 594-5
Carcinoma, colorectal, 475-8
  clinical features of, 478
  right-sided *versus* left-sided, 478t
  pathologic features of, 476-7
  pathogenesis of, 475-6
  risk factors for, 475
  prognosis of, 478
  spread of, 477-8
Carcinoma, basal cell, 636-7
Carcinoma, embryonal,
  testis, 576-7
  ovary, 606f
Carcinoma, endometrium, 598-9
  versus endocervical carcinoma, 740t
Carcinoma, extra-hepatic duct, 520-1

Carcinoma, gallbladder, 520
Carcinoma, hepatocellular, 513-5
Carcinoma *in situ*, 26, 157
  breast, 619
  bronchus, 401f
  cervix, 26-7, 157, 592-4
  oral cavity, 426
  penile, 580-1
  skin, 635
  urinary bladder, 568
Carcinoma, kidney, 561-3
Carcinoma, larynx, 421
Carcinoma, lung, 400-6
(*also see under Lung cancer*)
Carcinoma, mucoepidermoid, 435
Carcinoma, nasopharyngeal, 420
Carcinoma, oesophagus, 439-40
Carcinoma, oral cavity, 426-8
Carcinoma, ovary, 602
  mucinous, 605
  serous, 604
Carcinoma, pancreas, 524-5
Carcinoma, parathyroid, 666
Carcinoma, penis, 580-2
Carcinoma, periampullary, 520-1
Carcinoma, prostate, 584-7
Carcinoma, salivary gland, 435
Carcinoma, sebaceous, 414-5
Carcinoma, sinonasal, 419
Carcinoma, skin, 635-7
Carcinoma, small cell, 404-5
Carcinoma, squamous cell,
  anal canal, 478
  cervix, 594-5
  larynx, 421
  lung, 404
  oesophagus, 439-40
  oral cavity, 426-8
  penis, 581-2
  skin, 635-6
  urinary bladder, 569
  vagina, 590
  vulva, 590
Carcinoma, stomach, 450-2
Carcinoma, thyroid, 659-63
Carcinoma, urothelial, 566-9
Carcinoma, vagina, 590-1
Carcinoma, vulva, 590
Carcinosarcoma, 149
Cardiomyopathies, 365-8
  congestive, 365-6
  dilated, 365-6
  hypertrophic, 366-7
  restrictive, 367-8
Caries, dental, 429-30
Carotenaemia, 50
Carotid body tumour, 422
Caspases, 42, 52
Cataract, 413
Cell cycle, 14-6, 14f
  checkpoints in, 15t
Cell death, 34
  enzyme markers in, 29t
  programmed, 40

Cell injury, 19-50
by chemical agents, 32-3
by physical agents, 33
responses in, 19f
etiology of, 19-20
enzyme markers of, 29t
free radical-mediated, 30-2
ischaemic-hypoxic, 27-31, 28f
immunologic, 102-6
ionising radiation in, 33
irreversible, 27-8
morphology of, 33-40
pathogenesis of, 27-33
reperfusion, 29-30
reversible, 27-8
reversible versus irreversible, 31t
Centromere, 6
Cerebrospinal (CSF) fluid, findings, 710
Cerebrovascular diseases, 713-9
Cerumen gland tumour, 417
Cervicitis, 591-2
Cervical screening, 593
Cervix, diseases of, 591-5
Chalazion, 411
Chancre, 78
Charcot-Leyden crystals, 389f
Charcot-Marie-Tooth disease, 731
Chemical mediators of inflammation, 56-61, 56t
Chemoattractants, 54
Chemodectoma, 422
Chemokines, 58
Chemotaxis, 54
Chickenpox, 188
Cholangiocarcinoma, 514
Cholangitis,
primary sclerosing, 505-6
pyogenic, 499
Cholecystitis, 518-20
Choledocholithiasis, 518
Cholelithiasis, 515-8
clinical manifestations of, 518
complications of, 518
contrasting features of, 517t
pathogenesis of, 516
risk factors for, 515-6
Cholestasis, 486-7
Cholesteatoma, 417-8
Cholesterolosis, 517t
Chondroma, 683
Chondrosarcoma, 685-6
Chorea, 355
Choriocarcinoma,
gestational, 612
ovarian, 608
testis, 577, 578
versus mole, 612t
Choristoma, 149
Christmas disease, 264
Chromatid, 6
Chromosomes, 6-7, 6f
abnormalities of, 151, 211-4
classification of, 210-1
features of, 210-1

Chronic disorder anaemia, 234-5
Chronic ischaemic heart disease (CIHD), 349-50
Chronic lymphocytic leukaemia (CLL), 300-1
Chronic myeloid leukaemia (CML), 282-4
versus leukaemoid reaction, 279t
Chronic obstructive pulmonary disease (COPD), 384-90
bronchial asthma, 388-9
bronchiectasis, 390
chronic bronchitis, 385
contrasting features of, 384t
emphysema, 385-8
versus restrictive lung disease, 393t
Chronic restrictive pulmonary disease, 390-400
classification of, 390-1
smoking-associated, 400
versus COPD, 393t
Chronic venous congestion (CVC), 130-3
liver, 132
lungs, 131
spleen, 132-3
Chutta smoking, 195
Chylothorax, 408
Cirrhosis, liver, 500-9
alcoholic, 501-3
biliary, 504-6
cardiac, 508-9
classification of, 501t
Indian childhood (ICC), 509
in α-1 antitrypsin deficiency, 508
in haemochromatosis, 506-7
in non-alcoholic steatohepatitis (NASH), 509
in Wilson's disease, 507-8
macronodular, 504f
micronodular, 503f
pathogenesis of, 500-1
pigment, 506-7
portal hypertension in, 510-2
post-necrotic, 503-4
c-KIT receptor gene, 160, 449, 450
Clefts, facial, 423
Clotting system, 60, 257f
Coagulation disorders, 262-6
Coagulation system, 139
Coagulation tests, 256-7
Coarctation of aorta, 344-5
Codman triangle, 685
Colitis, 462t
amoebic, 190, 463-4
C. diff., 464
infective, 462-4
ischaemic, 456-7
necrotising, 184, 457-8
pseudomembranous, 464
ulcerative, 459-61
Collagens, 11-2
Collectins, 52, 55

Colorectal polyps, 471-5
cancer in, 476f
neoplastic versus non-neoplastic, 475t
Coma, diabetic, 670-1
hepatic, 490, 511
Comedo pattern, 619f
Compatibility testing, blood, 267
Complement system, 61, 538
Components of blood, 267-8
Concentration tests, 529
Condyloma acuminatum, 589
Congestive heart failure (CHF), 125-6, 339-42
Congo red stain, 114, 119t
Conjunctivitis, 411
Conn syndrome, 646-7
Cor pulmonale, 143, 340f
Coronary arteries, 339
Diseases of,
(also see under IHD),
Coronary syndromes, acute, 345
Coronaviruses, 186-9
Councilman body, 497f
Covid-19, 186, 187-8, 381
CRAB features, 312
Craniopharyngioma, 645
Crescents, epithelial, 541f
CREST syndrome, 112
Cretinism, 652
Creutzfeldt-Jakob disease, (CJD), 712-3
Cribriform pattern, 619f, 621
Crigler-Najjar syndrome, 488
Crohn disease versus ulcerative colitis, 461t
Cross matching, blood, 267
Cryoprecipitate, 268
Cryptorchidism, 571
Cushing syndrome, 643, 646
Cyclin dependent kinases (CDKs), 15t
Cyclins, 15, 161
Cyclo-oxygenase pathway, 57f
Cysticercosis, 191-2
Cystic hygroma, 335, 422
Cystitis, 565-6
Cysts,
bartholin, 588
bone, 682t
branchial (lymphoepithelial), 422
dental, 430-1
dentigerous, 431
dermoid, 431, 607f, 634
epidermal, 634
fissurar, 431
follicular, 601
ganglion, 691
hydatid, 499--500
inclusion, 600
jaw, 430t
kidney, 532-4
lateral cervical, 422
luteal, 601
midline cervical, 421

neck, 421-2
odontogenic, 430*t*
ovarian, epithelial, 602-6
ovarian, nonneoplastic, 600-1
parathyroid, 422
pilar, 634
pulmonary, 372
radicular, 431
simple ovarian, 600
thymic, 422
thyroglossal, 422
trichilemmal, 634
Cytogenetics, 2, 210-4
Cytokines, 57-8, 59*t*, 91
Cytology, diagnostic, 735-46
    air-dried smears in, 742
    bronchioalveolar lavage in, 740
    Bethsda system in, 739
    branches of, 736
    cerebrospinal fluid, 710*t*, 741
    cervical smears in, 737-9
    crush smear, 745-6
    effusions in, 740-1
    endometrial *versus* endocervical carcinoma in, 740*t*
    exfoliative, 736, 737-42
    exfoliative *versus* interventional, 737*t*
    fine needle aspiration (FNA), 743-5
    fixation and fixatives, 742
    gastrointestinal tract, 740
    genetic sex in, 741
    imprint, 745
    in clinical medicine, 735-6
    interventional, 737, 743-6
    in tumour diagnosis, 177
    liquid-based (LBC), 742
    nuclear criteria in, 736*t*
    Pap smears in, 593-4, 737, 738-9, 741-2
    Pap stain in, 742
    samples in, 737*t*
    seminal fluid, 741
    sputum in, 740
    urinary tract, 740
    vaginal smears in, 739
    wet-fixed smears in, 742
Cytoskeleton, 7-8

D

Darier disease, 627
DeBakey classification, 332
Decompression sickness, 144-5
Defibrination syndromes, 264-6
Deficiency disease, nutritional, 199
Degeneration,
    fibrinoid, 36
    hyaline, 33-4
    hydropic, 33
    macular, 412-3
    mucoid, 34
    myxoid, 34
    of peripheral nervous system, 729-30
    segmental, 730
Degenerative joint disease (DJD), 687-8
Dehydration, 128
Delayed hypersensitivity, 105-6
Deletions, chromosomal, 214
Dengue fever, 186
Dense deposit disease, 538
Dentin, 428, 429*f*
Dermatitis (eczema), 627-8
Dermatitis herpetiformis, 631-2
Dermatofibrosarcoma protuberans, 701
Dermatomyositis, 112-3
Dermatophytes, 185
Dermatoses, 626-
    bullous, 630-2
    connective tissue, 629-30
    genetic, 626-7
    granulomatous, 629
    infectious, 628-9
    metabolic, 633
    non-infectious inflammatory, 627-8
    scaling, 632-3
Desmoid tumours, 700
Desmoplasia, 152, 451, 620
Developmental anomalies, 209-10
    of bone and joints, 676
Devil's pinches, 258
Diabetes insipidus, 644
Diabetes mellitus, 666-72
    atherosclerosis in, 321, 671
    classification of, 667*t*
    complications of, 669-71
    diagnosis of, 671-2
    etiology of, 667
    epidemiology of, 666-7
    gestational, 667
    metabolic syndrome and, 666
    pathologic changes in, 669
    pathogenesis of, 667-9
    risk factors for, 667*t*
    type 1 *versus* type 2, 669*t*
Diabetic ketoacidosis, 670
Diapedesis, 54, 133
Differentiation, neoplastic cells, 150
Diffuse alveolar damage (DAD), 373
DiGeorge syndrome, 96
Dilution test, 529
Diphtheria, 421
Dissecting haematoma, 331-2
Disseminated intravascular coagulation (DIC), 264-6
Diverticula,
    colon, 471
    Meckel, 453-4
    oesophageal, 437
Diverticulosis coli, 471
DNA, 4-5, 5*f*
    linker, 6
    mitochondrial, 4
    non-coding, 6
    nuclear *versus* mitochondrial, 9*t*
Dohle bodies, 275*f*
Down syndrome, 211-2
Drepanocytes (sickle cells), 225
Dropsy, 122
Drug abuse, 198-9
Drug injury, 196
    hepatic, 500*t*
Drumstick appendage, 275*f*, 741
Dubin Johnson syndrome, 47, 488
Ductus arteriosus, patent (PDA), 343
Dura mater, 706
Dwarfism,
    hereditary (achondroplasia), 676
    pituitary, 644
Dysentery, 463-4
    amoebic, 190, 463-4
    bacillary, 463
Dysfunctional uterine bleeding (DUB), 596
Dysgerminoma ovary, 608
Dyskeratosis, 626
Dyslipidaemia, 320
Dyspepsia, 444
Dysplasia, 26-7
    cervical, 26-7, 157, 592-4
    developmental, 209, 676
    fibrous, 676
    oral cavity, 426
    renal, multicystic, 532
    skeletal, 676
    versus metaplasia, 27*t*
Dysraphic anomalies, 210
Dystrophy, vulval, 588
Dystrophies, muscular, 692, 693*t*

E

Ear, 417-8
    tumours and tumour-like lesions of, 417-8
Ecchymoses, 133
Ectopia, 210
Ectopia vesicae (exstrophy), 565
Ectopic hormone production, 174
Eczema, 627-8
Effusion, 122
    cytology of, 740
    pericardial, 368
    peritoneal, 123, 128, 490, 510-1
    pleural, 407-8
Ehler-Danlos syndrome, 215, 258
Electrical injury, 199
Electrolytes, disturbances of, 129-30
Elliptocytosis, 245
Embden-Meyerhof pathway, 245*f*
Embolism, 141-5
    air, 144
    amniotic fluid, 145
    atheromatous, 145
    classification of, 141-2
    fat, 143-4
    paradoxical, 143

pulmonary, 143
thromboembolism, 142-3
Embolus, 141
Embryomas, 149, 219
Emphysema, 385-8
    classification of, 386*t*
    clinical features of, 386
    etiopathogenesis of, 385-6
    types of, 386-8
Empty-sella syndrome, 644
Empyema,
    gallbladder, 518
    thoracis, 379, 407
Enamel, 428
Encephalitis, 710-3
Encephalopathy,
    hepatic, 490, 511
    HIV, 101
    ischaemic-hypoxic, 137, 714
    progressive multifocal, 712
Endocarditis, 356*t*
    atypical verrucous, 356
    bacterial, 357-60
    contrasting features of, 360*t*
    cachectic, 357
    infective, 357-60
    Libman-Sacks, 356
    Löeffler, 368
    marantic, 357
    nonbacterial thrombotic (NBTE), 357
    rheumatic, 352-3
Endocrine system, diseases of, 641-74
    classification of disturbances of, 642
Endometrioid tumours, ovary, 605-6
Endometriosis, 597
Endometritis, 596
Endometrium, diseases of, 595-9
    cyclic changes in, 595
    hyperplasias of, 597-8
Endophthalmitis, 411
Endoplasmic reticulum, 9, 10*f*
Enteric fever, 462-3
Enneking staging, 176, 698-9
Enterocolitis, 462*t*
    infective, 462-4
    in enteric fever, 462-3
    necrotising, 184, 457-8
    tuberculous, 462
    pseudomembranous, 464
Environmental chemicals, 195
Environmental diseases, 194-9
Enzymopathies, herediary, 245-6
Eosinophilia, 275-6
Eosinophils, 63
Ependymal cell, 706
Ependymoma, 726
Epididymo-orchitis, 572
Epigenetics, 6
Epithelioid cells, 68, 70
Epstein-Barr virus (EBV), 172, 277, 420
    oncogenesis by, 172*f*

Epulis, 424-5
Erythema multiforme, 632
Erythema marginatum, 355
Erythroblast, 224
Erythroblastaemia, 229
Erythroid series, 222*f*, 224*f*
Erythroplasia of Queyrat, 581
Erythropoiesis, 224-7
Erythropoietin, 224
Etiology, definition of, 1
Euchromatin, 4
Eumycetoma, 185
Ewing sarcoma, 686-7
Exostosis, osteocartilaginous, 683
Extracellular matrix (ECM), 10-11, 12*f*
Exudate, 65
    versus transudate, 122*t*
Eye, 410-6
    cataract of, 413
    changes in diabetes, 411-2
    changes in hypertension, 412
    congenital lesions of, 410
    glaucoma of, 413
    inflammatory conditions of, 410-1
    tumours and tumour-like lesions of, 414-6

F

Fallot tetralogy, 344
Familial adenomatous polyposis, 156, 475
Fascitis, nodular, 700
Fatty change, 34
    liver, 44-5, 502
Ferroptosis, 44
Fever,
    enteric, 462-3
    dengue, 186
    glandular, 276
    viral haemorrhagic, 186
Fibril protein, 115
Fibrin degradation products (FDPs), 265*f*, 266
Fibrinogen, 257
Fibrinolytic system, 60-1
Fibroadenoma, breast, 616
Fibroblastic and myofibroblastic tumours, 700-1
Fibrocystic change, breast, 614
Fibroelastosis, endocardial, 367
Fibromas, ovary, 609
Fibromatosis, 700-1
Fibrosarcoma, 701
Fibrous dysplasia of bone, 676
Fiedler myocarditis, 365
Filariasis, 191
Fish-mouth appearance, 353
Fistula, biliary, 518
    tracheo-oesophageal, 436
Flu, viruses, 187
    bird, 187
    swine, 187
Foetal alcohol syndrome, 210

Foetal hydrops, 218
Folate, 203*t*
Foetor hepaticus, 490
Folliculitis, 182
Food poisoning, 184
Foot process disease, 541-2
Fracture, bone, 85-6, 679-80
Freckles, 46
Free radicals, 30-2
Fresh frozen plasma (FFP), 268
Frozen section, 176-7
Function tests,
    liver, 482*t*
    renal, 528*t*
    thyroid, 651
Fungal diseases, 184-5

G

Galactocele, 614
Gallbladder, 515-21
    carcinoma, 520-1
    porcelain, 520
    stones, 515-8
Gallstones, 515-8
    clinical manifestations of, 518
    complications of, 518
    contrasting features of, 517*t*
    pathogenesis of, 516
    risk factors for, 515-6
g-glutamyl transpeptidase (g-GT), 483
Gammopathy, monoclonal, 313
Gamna-Gandy bodies, 133
Ganglion cyst, 691
Ganglioneuroma, 650
Gangrene, 37-8
    dry *versus* wet, 38*t*
    gas, 37, 183
Gardner syndrome, 475
Gastric carcinoma, 450-2
Gastric ulcer, 446-8
    benign *versus* malignant, 447*f*, 453*t*
    versus duodenal ulcer, 448*t*
Gastrinoma, 673-4
Gastritis, 442-4
    acute, 442
    chronic, 442-4
    H. pylori-related, 443-4
    hypertrophic, 444
Gastrointestinal stromal tumour (GIST), 449-50
Gaucher disease, 217-8
Genetic diseases, 209-18
Germ cell tumours,
    ovary, 606-8, 606*t*
    testis, 573-9, 573*t*
Ghon complex, 71-2
Giant cell tumour of bone, 683-4
Giant cells, inflammatory, 63-4
    Aschoff, 354
    foreign body, 64*f*
    Langhans, 63
    Touton, 64*f*

Gigantism, 643
Gilbert syndrome, 487-8
Glanzman's disease, 262
Glaucoma, 413
Gleason's grading, 586
Glioblastoma, 725
Gliomas, 724-6
Glomerular diseases, 533-50
    classification of, 534*t*
    clinical manifestations of, 534-6
    contrasting features of, 547-8*t*
    pathogenesis of, 536-9
    primary, 539-47
    secondary, 548-50
Glomerulonephritis (GN), 534*t*
    acute, 539-40
    chronic, 546-7
    chronic *versus* chronic
        pyelonephritis, 554*t*
    crescentic, 540-1
    distinguishing features of, 547-8
    diffuse proliferative, 544
    end-stage, 546-7
    focal proliferative, 544-5
    focal segmental, 545*f*
    IgA, 545-6
    membranoproliferative, 543-4
    membranous, 542-3
    minimal change disease, 541-2
    non-streptococcal, 540
    oedema in, 124-5, 535
    pathogenesis of, 536-9
    post-streptococcal, 539-40
    rapidly progressive, 540-1
Glomerulosclerosis, diabetic, 549
    diffuse, 549
    focal segmental (FSGS), 545*f*
    nodular, 549
Glomus jugulotympanicum, 417
Glomus tumour (glomangioma), 335-6
Glossitis, 424
Glucose tolerance test (GTT), 672
Glucose 6-phosphate dehydrogenase (G6PD) deficiency, 245-6
Glucosuria, 672*f*
Glycogen storage diseases, 216
Glycosaminoglycans, 12
Glycosylated haemoglobin (HbA1C), 670, 671*t*, 672
Goitre, 656-8
    etiology of, 656-7
    nodular, 657-8
    pathogenesis of, 657
    pathology of, 657-8
    simple, 657
Golgi apparatus, 9
Goodpasture syndrome, 540
Gout, 690-1
Grading of tumours, 175-6
Graft *versus* host (GVH) reaction, 94
Granulation tissue, 82-3
Granuloma, 68
    annulare, 629
    apical, 430

eosinophilic, 314-5
caseating, 35, 72-3
pyogenic, 335, 425
sarcoid, 80*f*
Granulomatous diseases, 69-81
    leprosy, 75-7
    nose, 419
    sarcoidosis, 79-81
    skin, 629
    syphilis, 77-9
    tuberculosis, 69-75
Granulopoiesis, 272*f*
Granulosa cell tumour,
    ovary, 608-9
    testis, 580
Graves disease, 656
Growth factors in cell cycle, 16*t*
Growth factor receptors, 16*t*
Guillain-Barre syndrome, 731-2
Gumma, syphilitic, 79
Gynaecomastia, 616

H

5-Hydroxy tryptamine (HT), 56
Haemangioblastoma, 727
Haemangioma, 335
    liver, 512
    nose, 419
Haematin pigment, 47
Haematoma, 133
    dissecting, 331-2
    epidural, 717-8
    subdural, 718*f*
Haematopoiesis, 221
    extramedullary, 221
Haematolymphoid malignancies,
    etiology, 280
    general features, 279-81
    lymphoid and histiocytic, 297-315
    myeloid, 280-90
    pathogenesis, 280-1
Haemochromatosis, 48, 506-7
Haemodynamic disturbances, 130-7
Haemoglobin, 226-7
    adult, 226
    foetal, 227
    glycosylated, 670, 671*t*, 672
    sickle, 246
Haemoglobinopathies, 244-51
Haemoglobinuria, 239
    cold, 241
    march, 242
    paroxysmal nocturnal (PNH), 243
Haemolytic anaemia, see under Anaemias, haemolytic, 238-51
Haemolytic disease of newborn (HDN), 270-1
Haemolytic uraemic syndrome, 258
Haemophilia, 263-4
Haemoptysis, causes of, 405*t*
Haemorrhage, 133
    anaemia due to, 251
    intracerebral, 715-6

intracranial, 716*f*
subarachnoid, 716-7
traumatic, brain, 718*f*
Haemorrhagic diatheses (bleeding disorders), 258-66
    coagulation disorders, 262-6
    DIC, 264-6
    investigations of, 255-7
    platelet disorders, 259-62
    vascular disorders, 258-9
Haemorrhagic fevers, viral, 185
Haemosiderin, 47
Haemosiderosis, 47-8
Haemostasis, mechanism of, 255
    vascular, 256, 258-9
Haemostatic disorders, contrasting features of, 266*t*
Haemostatic system, 254-66
    laboratory tests for, 255-7
Haemothorax, 408
Haemazoin, 47
Hamartoma, 149
    pulmonary, 406
Hand-Schuller-Christian disease, 315
Hare lips, 423
Hashimoto thyroiditis, 654-5
Hay fever, 103
Hb H disease, 249, 251*t*
HBsAg, 494
hCG, 576, 610, 611, 612
Healing, 82-6
    by first intention (primary union), 83-4
    by regeneration, 82
    by repair, 82
    by second intention (secondary union), 84-5
    complications of, 85
    factors influencing, 83
    fracture, 85-6
    muscle, 86
    nervous tissues, 86
    primary *versus* secondary, 85*t*
    wound, 82-5
Heart, 338-70
    blood supply of, 339
    brown atrophy of, 49
    congenital diseases of, 342-5
    endocardial diseases of, 356-60
    failure, 339-42
    hypertrophy of, 340-2
    ischaemic effects on, 345-51
    myocardial diseases, 364-8
    rheumatic disease of, 351-6
    structure of, 338
    pericardial diseases of, 368-70
    transplant, 370
    tumours of, 370
    valvular deformities of, 361-4
Heat-shock protein (HSP), 32
Heavy chain diseases, 314
Helicobacter pylori, 443-5, 453
Henoch-Schonlein's purpura, 258, 327
Hepatic failure, 489-90

Hepatisation, lung, 377-8
Hepatitis,
　alcoholic, 503
　autoimmune, 509
　A, 491-3
　B, 493-4
　C, 494-5
　D, 494
　E, 495
　clinico-pathological spectrum of, 495-6
　contrasting features of, 492*t*
　interface, 497-8
　fulminant, 498-9
　neonatal, 488-9
　viral, 491-9
Hepatoblastoma, 514-5
Hepatocellular carcinoma (HCC), 512-4
Hepatolenticular degeneration, 507-8
Hepatopulmonary syndrome, 490
Hepatorenal syndrome, 490
Hereditary haemorrhagic telangiectasia, 258
Hereditary non-polyposis colon cancer (HNPC), 475
Hernia, 455
　hiatus, 436-7
　strangulated, 455
Herpes viruses, 188-9, 423-4
　human (HHV-8), 182-3
Herpes zoster, 188
Herring-bone pattern, 697
Hess capillary test, 256
Heterochromatin, 4
Heterophile antibody, 278
Heterotopia, 210
Hexose-monophosphate (HMP) shunt, 245*f*
Hippocrates, 2
Hirschsprung disease, 470-1
Histamine, 56
Histones, 6
Histiocytes, 63
Histiocytoma, malignant fibrous, 704
Histochemistry, 177
Hodgkin's lymphoma, 305-9
　classification of, 298*t*, 305-6
　clinical features of, 306, 308
　contrasting features of, 305*t*
　features of, 307-8
　laboratory findings in, 308
　prognosis of, 306
　Reed-Sternberg cells in, 306*f*
　staging of, 309*t*
　versus non-Hodgkin lymphoma, 309*t*
Homeostasis, 4, 121-2
Hordeolum, 182, 410
Hormones, major functions of, 641
Human immunodeficiency virus (HIV), 97*f*

Human leucocyte antigen (HLA), 91-3
Human papilloma virus (HPV), 171-3, 581, 590-1, 592
Human T cell lymphotropic virus (HTLV), 173
Hutchinson teeth, 79
Hyaline change, 33-4
Hyaline membrane disease, 374*f*
Hydatid disease, 499-500
Hydatidiform mole, 610-1
　versus choriocarcinoma, 612*t*
Hydrocele, 573
Hydrocephalus, 707-8
Hydronephrosis, 557-8
Hydropic change, 33
Hydrops foetalis, 249, 251*t*
Hydrostatic pressure, 122
Hydrothorax, 407-8
5-Hydroxytryptamine (5-HT), 56
Hyperaemia,130-3
　active, 130
　passive, 130-3
Hyperbilirubinaemia, 47, 483
　conjugated, 486-7
　hereditary non-haemolytic, 487-8
　unconjugated, 485-6
　unconjugated *versus* conjugated, 486*t*
Hypercalcaemia, 39, 555
Hypercholesterolaemia, 320
　familial, 216
Hyperchromatism, 151
Hypercoagulability, 139, 535
Hyperchromasia, 229
Hyperglycaemia, 666-7
　pathogenesis of, 667-8
Hyperkeratosis, 626
Hyperlipidaemia, 320
Hyperparathyroidism, 664-5, 678
　brown tumour of, 678
Hyperpigmentation, 46, 424
Hyperpituitarism, 642-3
Hyperplasia, 23-4
　atypical, 26, 157, 615-6
　breast, epithelial, 614-6
　denture, 425
　endometrial, 597-8
　focal nodular, liver, 512
　prostate, nodular, 583-4
　retrolental, 410
　versus hypertrophy, 25*t*
Hypersensitivity reactions, 102-6
　contrasting features of, 107*t*
　delayed type, 105-6
　immediate type, 102-5
Hypersplenism, 295
Hypertension, portal, 510-2
　causes of, 510*t*
Hypertension, pulmonary, 375-6
Hypertension, systemic, 558-61
　atherosclerosis in, 320
　benign, 558
　categories of, 558*t*
　consequences of, 559

　essential, 558
　heart disease, 320
　in dissecting haematoma, 331
　kidneys in, 560-1
　malignant, 558
　pathogenesis of, 559*f*
　secondary, 558-9
Hyperthyroidism, 651-2
Hypertrophy, 22-3
　cardiac, 23, 340-1
　versus hyperplasia, 25*t*
Hyperuricaemia, 690
Hyperviscosity, blood, 314
Hypervitaminosis, 205
Hypoadrenalism, 647-8
Hypoaldosteronism, 648
Hypochromasia, 229
Hypoglycaemia, 671
Hypoparathyroidism, 665
Hypopigmentation, 46-7
Hypopituitarism, 643-4
Hypoplasia, 209
Hypoproteinaemia, 123, 535
Hypothyroidism, 652
Hypoventilation syndrome, 200
Hypoxia, 27-31, 28*f*

I

Ichthyosis, 627
IDH mutations, 724
IgA deficiency, 95-6
IgA nephropathy, 545-6
IgG4-related disease, 114
Ileus, gallstone, 518
Immune complex disease, kidney, 537
Immune system, normal, 87-91
　cells of, 88-91
　diseases of, 87*f*
Immune thrombocytopenic purpura (ITP), 260-1
Immune tolerance, 107-8
Immunohistochemistry, 177
Immunity, adaptive, 88
　innate, 87-8
　innate *versus* adaptive, 89*t*
Immunodeficiency disease, 94-101
　acquired (AIDS), 97-101
　common variable, 96
　primary, 95-7
　severe combined, 96
Immunology of tumours, 165-6
Immunopathology, 94-120
Impetigo, 182, 628
Incontinence, pigment, 626
Indian-file arrangement, 621*f*
Infarction, 145-7
　cerebral, 71405
　etiology and pathogenesis of, 145-6
　pulmonary,143
　small intestine, 456-7

Infarcts, 146-7, 147t
  brain, 714-5
  heart, 346-9
  intestine, 456f
  watershed, 714
  various organs, 147t
Infectious diseases, 180-93
  host factors in, 180
  identification of, 181t
  routes of, 180
Infectious mononucleosis, 276-8
Infertility, male, 571-2
Inflammation, acute, 51-67
  cardinal signs of, 51, 52f
  causes of, 51
  cells in, 62-4
  definition, 51
  cellular events in, 54-5
  factors determining variation in, 64
  haemodynamic changes in, 52-3
  mediators of, 56-61, 56t
  pseudomembranous, 65
  reactions in, 64-5
  response in, 51-5
  signs of, 51
  systemic effects of, 66
  triple response in, 52f
  versus chronic, 69t
Inflammation, chronic, 67-81
  granulomatous, 68-81
  systemic effects of, 67
  versus acute, 69t
Inflammatory bowel disease, 458-61
  contrasting features of, 461t
  etiopathogenesis of, 458-9
  pathologic features of, 459-61
Inflammatory cells, 62-4
Influenza viruses, 187
Insufficiency, cardiac valvular, 361
  aortic, 363-4
  mitral, 362-3
Insulitis, 669
Insulinoma, 673
Insulin resistance, 668-9
Integrins, 13
Intercellular junctions, 12-3
Interferon, 58
Interleukins, 58
Intermediate filaments, 8
Interphase, 14
Interstitial lung diseases (ILDs), 392t
  in autoimmune diseases, 398
  in immunologic lung diseases, 399
  in pneumoconioses, 392-7
  pathogenesis of, 391-2
  smoking-related, 400
Intestinal obstruction, 454
Intestine, large, diseases of, 470-8
  cancer of, 475-8
  polyps of, 471-5

Intestine, small, diseases of, 453-68
  biopsy, 465-6
  tumours of, 467-8
Intracellular accumulations, 44-50
  of fat, 44-5
  of glycogen, 45-6
  of pigments, 46-50
Intraepithelial neoplasia, 26-7, 157
  breast, 619
  bronchus, 401
  cervix, 157, 592-4
  oral cavity, 426
  testis, 574
  urinary bladder, 568
  vulval, 590
Intratubular germ cell neoplasia, 574
Intussusception, 455
Invasion-metastasis cascade, 154-5
Inversions, chromosomal, 214
Involucrum, 681
Ionising radiation, 33
Iron metabolism, 231-2
Ischaemia, 27-31, 28f
  brain, 714-5
  myocardial, 345
Ischaemic bowel disease, 456-7
Ischaemic heart disease (IHD), 345-51
  angina in, 345-6
  chronic, 349-50
  coronary atherosclerosis in, 319-24, 345
  effects of, 346f
  etiopathogenesis of, 345
  myocardial infarction in, 346-9
  sudden cardiac death in, 350-1
Islet cell tumours, 672-3
Isochromosome, 214

J

JAK2 oncogene, 161
Janeway spots, 360
Jaundice, 47, 484-7
  classification of, 486t
  conjugated hyperbilirubinaemia, 486-7
  neonatal, 487
  tests for, 482t
  unconjugated hyperbilirubinaemia, 485-6
Joints, disease of, 687-91
Jones criteria, revised, 355-6

K

Kangri cancer, 635
Kaposi sarcoma, 172, 336-7
  oncogenesis, 172-3
Kawasaki disease, 329
Keratoconjunctivitis, 411
Keratoma, 417-8

Keratosis follicularis, 627
Keratosis palmaris et plantaris, 627
Kerley lines, 127
Kernicterus, 47
Ketonuria, 672
Kidney, diseases of, 526-64
  biopsy, 528
  classification of, 529
  congenital malformations of, 532-4
  function tests, 528-9
  tumours of, 561-4
Kimmelstiel-Wilson lesions, 549f
Kinin system, 60f
Klinefelter syndrome, 212,
Koilocytes, 629f
Krukenberg tumour, 609-10
Kulchitsky cells, 467
Kupffer cells, 497
Kwashiorkor, 201
  versus marasmus, 201t

L

Labile cells, 24, 82
Langerhans cell histiocytosis, 314-5, 640
Laryngitis, 420-1
Larynx, diseases of, 420-1
  carcinoma of, 421
  papilloma of, 421
Lead poisoning, 197-8
Leiomyoma, 599-600
Lentigo, 46
Leptin, 200
Lepromin test, 75-6
Leprosy, 75-7, 629
  lepromatous versus tuberculoid, 77t
  Ridley-Jopling classification of, 76
Lentigo, 637
Leptocytosis, 225
Leptomeninges, 706
Letterer-Siwe disease, 315
Leucocytosis,
  basophilic, 276
  eosinophilic, 275-6
  lymphocytic, 275
  neutrophilic, 274
Leucoderma, 47
Leukaemia, lymphoid,
  acute (ALL), 299-300
  ALL versus AML, 300t
  chronic lymphoid (CLL), 300-1
  etiology of, 280
  hairy cell, 304
  WHO classification of, 298
Leukaemia, myeloid,
  acute (AML), 286-8, 289t
  chronic myeloid (CML), 282-4
  etiology of, 280
  FAB classification of, 287t
  pathogenesis of, 280-1
  WHO classification of, 283t

Leukaemoid reaction, 278-9
   versus CML, 279t
Leukoplakia, oral, 426
   vulval, 588
Leukotrienes, 57
Leydig cell tumour, 609
Lichen planus, 423, 633
Lichen sclerosus, 588-9
Lichen simplex chronicus, 588-9
Li-Fraumeni syndrome, 724
Linitis plastica, 451, 452f
Lipofuscin, 49
Lipoma, 699
Lipooxygenase pathway, 57f
Lipoproteins, 320t
Liposarcoma, 699-700
Lipoxins, 57
Liver, diseases of, 480-515
   biopsy of, 484
   function tests, 481-4
   structure of, 480-1
   tumours and tumours-like lesions of, 512-5, 512t
   types of necrosis in, 481
Löeffler syndrome, 399
Lugol's iodine test, 593
Lung, diseases of, 371-407
   abscess, 379, 383-4
   congenital anomalies of, 373
   farmers', 399
   structure of, 371-2
   tumours of, 400t
Lung cancer, 400-6
   ALK mutation in, 402
   classification of, 400t
   clinical features of, 405-6
   epidemiology of, 400
   gross patterns of, 402
   microscopic types of, 402-5
   pathogenesis of, 400-2
   small cell versus non-small cell, 403t
Lupus erythematosus, 108-11, 398, 629-30
Lupus nephritis, 110, 548-9
Lupus vulgaris, 629
Lyme disease, 184
Lymph nodes, structure of, 291
   follicular hyperplasia of, 292
   metastatic tumours, 153f
   paracortical hyperplasia of, 292-3
   reactive, 291-3
   sinus histiocytosis of, 293
Lymphadenitis, dermatopathic, 46
   reactive, 291-3
Lymphangioma, 335-6
Lymphangitis, 334
Lymphatics, structure of, 317-8
Lymphoblast versus myeloblast, 273t
Lymphocytes, 63, 89-91
   general features, 88-9
   types of, 89- 91
   T versus B, 90t

Lymphocytosis, 275
Lymphoedema, 124, 334
Lymphoid and histiocytic neoplasms, 297-315
   classification of, 297-8
Lymphoid series, 273f
Lymphomas, 297-315
   aggressive T cell, 305
   anaplastic large cell (ALCL), 305
   angioimmunoblastic, 305
   Burkitt, 172, 302-3
   classification of, 298t
   CNS, 727-8
   contrasting features of, 309t
   diffuse large B-cell (DLBCL), 302
   etiology of, 280
   enteropathy type, 305
   follicular, 301-2
   hepatosplenic type, 305
   Hodgkin, 305-9
   Langerhans cell histiocytosis, 314-5
   lymphoblastic (LBL), 299-300
   maltoma, 303, 453
   mantle cell, 304
   marginal zone, 303
   nasal, extranodal, 305
   NK cell, 304-5
   non-Hodgkin (NHL), 299-305
   plasma cell, 309-14
   small lymphocytic (SLL), 300-1
   stomach, 451-3
   T cell, 304-5
   testis, 580
Lymphopenia, 275
Lymphopoiesis, 273
Lynch syndrome, 475
Lysosomal storage diseases, 217
Lysosomes, 10

M

M-band, 313f
MacCallum patch, 352
Macrocytes, 228
Macroglobulinaemia, Waldenstrom, 313-4
Macroglossia, 423
Macrophages, 63
   alveolar, 132f
Madura foot, 185
Major histocompatibility complex, 92-3
Malabsorption syndrome, 464-7
Classification of, 465t
Malakoplakia, 565
Malaria, 190-1
Malignant peripheral nerve sheath tumour (MPNST), 733
Mallory hyaline, 503
Maltoma, 303, 453
Mannose-biding lectins, 52
Mantoux test, 71

Marasmus, 201
   versus kwashiorkor, 201t
Marble bone disease, 676
Marfan syndrome, 215-6, 258
Margination, 54f
Marjolin ulcer, 635
Mast cells, 63
Mastitis, 613-4
Matrix, extracellular (ECM), 10-1, 12f
   interstitial versus basement membrane, 11t
Maturation index, 739t
Meckel diverticulum, 453-4
Mediators of inflammation, 56-61
Medullary cystic disease, kidney, 533
Medullary, carcinoma breast, 621
   Carcinoma thyroid, 662-3
Medulloblastoma,726-7
Megakaryopoiesis, 254f
Meigs syndrome, 407, 609
Meiosis, 212-3
Melanin, 46-7
Melanoma, malignant, 46
   skin, 638-39
   staging of, 639
   uveal, 415
   versus nevus, 640t
   versus retinoblastoma, 416t
Melanosis coli, 49-50
Mendelian disorders, 214-5
Ménétrier disease, 444
Meningioma, 728-9
Meningitis, 708-10
   CSF findings in, 710t
Meningocele, 706-7
Mesothelioma, 408-9, 479
Metabolic diseases, brain, 721
Metachromasia, 119t
Metaplasia, 24-6
   versus dysplasia, 27t
Metastasis, 152-5
   bone, 287
   haematogenous, 153
   liver, 515
   lung, 406-7
   lymphatic, 152-3
   routes of, 152
   sequence of events in, 154-5
   transcoelomic, 154
Michaelis-Gutmann bodies, 565
Microangiopathy, diabetic, 671
Microcytes, 229
Microfilaria, 191
Microfilaments, 8
Microglia, 706
Microsatellite instability (MSI), 476
Microtubules, 8
Middle Eastern Respiratory Syndrome (MERS), 186, 381
Miliaria, 628
Milroy disease, 334
Mineral deficiency, 202
Minimal change disease, 541-2

Mitochondria, 8-9, 9f
　DNA in, 9
Mitosis, phases of, 14
Mitotic figures, 151
Mixed salivary tumour, 149
Molecular cell biology, 4-18
Molluscum contagiosum, 628
Mönckeberg arteriosclerosis, 39, 319
Moniliasis, 185, 590
Monoclonal gammopathy,
　of undetermined significance (MGUS), 313
Monocytes, 63
Mononuclear phagocyte system, 91
Monosomy, 211
Mucinous tumours, ovary, 604-5
Mucocele,
　appendix, 470
　gallbladder, 518
　oral cavity, 425
Mucoid change, 34
Mucopolysaccharidoses, 217
Multiple endocrine neoplasia (MEN), 665-6, 674
Multiple (disseminated) sclerosis, 719-20
Mumps, 433f
Muscle, skeletal, diseases of, 692-4
Muscular dystrophies, 692, 693t
Mutations, 214
Myasthenia gravis, 692-4
Mycetoma, 184-5
Mycobacterium,
　avium intracellulare, 103
Mycobacterium leprae, 75
Mycobacterium tuberculosis, 69
Mycosis fungoides, 304, 640
Mycosis, superficial, 185, 629
MYC oncogene, 161
Myeloblast *versus* lymphoblast, 273t
Myelocele, 706-7
Myelodysplastic syndrome (MDS), 289-90
Myelofibrosis, primary, 285-6
Myelogram, 223t
Myeloid neoplasms, 281-91
　acute myeloid leukamia, 286-9
　chronic myeloid leukaemia, 282-4
　classification of, 281f, 283t
　essential thrombocythaemia, 285
　myelodysplastic syndromes, 289-91
　polycythaemia vera, 284-5
　primary myelofibrosis, 285-6
Myeloid series, 272f
Myeloma, 116f, 309-14
　clinical features of, 311
　diagnosis of, 312
　etiopathogenesis of, 209-10
　kidney, 311
　laboratory findings in, 311-2
　morphologic features of, 310-1
　smouldering, 312
Myeloma cells, 311f

Myeloproliferative disorders, 281-90
Myocardial infarction, 346-9
　clinical features of, 348
　complications of, 349
　diagnosis of, 348-9
　early changes in, 347
　enzyme determination in, 348-9
　etiopathogenesis of, 346
　pathologic changes in, 346-7
　reperfusion injury in, 348
　serum cardiac markers in, 348-9
Myocarditis, 364-5
Myopathies,
　inflammatory, 112-3
Myositis ossificans, 700
Myxoedema, 128, 653
Myxoid change, 34
Myxoma heart, 370

N

Naevi, naevocellular, 46, 637-8
Neck, diseases of, 421-2
Necroptosis, 43
Necrosis, 34-6
　avascular, bone, 679-80
　brain, 714-5
　bridging, 497
　caseous, 35, 72-3
　centrilobular, haemorrhagic, 132
　coagulative, 34-5
　contrasting features of, 36t
　dropout, 497
　fat, 35-6, 614
　fibrinoid, 36
　laminar, brain, 714
　liquefactive, 35
　liver cell, 481
　tubular, 550-1
　versus apoptosis, 43t
Neoplasia (*also see under* Tumours), 148-79
Nephritic syndrome, 125, 534-5
　versus nephrotic syndrome, 125t, 536t
Nephritis, hereditary, 550
Nephroblastoma, 563-4
Nephrolithiasis, 555-7
Nephron, structure of, 526-8
Nephronophthiasis, 533
Nephropathy,
　diabetic, 549, 671
　gouty, 691
　IgA, 545-6
　reflux, 553
Nephrosclerosis, 560-1
　benign, 560
　malignant, 560-1
Nephrotic syndrome, 124, 535
　versus nephritic syndrome, 536t
Nerve sheath tumours, 732-4
Nervous system, diseases of, 705-34
　central, 705-29

　peripheral, 729-34
　tumours of, 723t
Neurodegenerative diseases, 720t
Neurilemmoma, 732-3
Neuroblastoma, 649-50
　olfactory, 419
Neuroendocrine system, 641
　tumours of, 672-4
Neurofibroma, 733
Neurofibromatosis, 724, 733-4
Neuroglia, 706
Neuroma, acoustic, 417, 732
Neuropathy, diabetic, 671
　peripheral, 730-1
Neutropenia, 274
Neutrophil extracellular traps (NET), 55
Neutrophilia, 274
Neutrophils, 62t
　hypersegmentation in, 275
　toxic granules in, 275f
　vacuoles in, 275f
Niacin, 207
Nicotinic acid, 207
Niemann-Pick disease, 218f
Nodular fasciitis, 700
Nodule, subcutaneous, 355
Nodule, vocal, 421
Noma, 424
Non-alcoholic fatty liver disease (NAFLD), 200
Non-alcoholic steatohepatitis (NASH), 509
Nondisjunction, 211
Normoblasts, 224
Nose and paranasal sinuses, 418-9
　carcinoma of, 419
Nucleocytoplasmic ratio, 151
Nutmeg liver, 132
Nutritional diseases, 199-208
　of brain, 722

O

Obesity, 200-1
Ochronosis, 47
Odontogenic cysts, 430t
Odontogenic tumours, 431-2
Odontomas, 432
Oedema, 122-8
　cardiac, 123, 125-6
　cardiac *versus* renal, 126t
　cerebral, 128
　generalised, 122
　hepatic, 128
　high altitude, 127
　nephrotic *versus* nephritic, 125t
　nutritional, 128
　pathogenesis of, 122-4
　pitting *versus* non-pitting, 128
　postural, 123
　pulmonary, 126-7
　renal, 124-5, 535
　tissue factors in, 124

Oesophagitis, 437-9
  Barrett, 439
  reflux (peptic), 437
Oesophagus, diseases of, 436-40
  tumours of, 439-40
Oestrogen receptors, 623
Oligodendrocytes, 706
Oligodendroglioma, 725-6
Oncocytoma, kidney, 561
Oncofoetal antigens, 178*t*
Oncogenes, 159-61
  versus anti-oncogenes, 163*t*
Oncogenesis, (*also see under* Carcinogenesis), 166-73
Oncometabolites, 164
Oncotic pressure, 122
Opportunistic infections, 100*f*
Opsonins, 55*f*
Opsonisation, 103
Oral soft tissues, diseases of, 423-8
Orchitis, 572
Osler nodes, 360
Osler-Weber-Rendu disease, 258
Osmotic pressure, 121
Osteitis deformans, 678-9
Osteitis fibrosa cystica, 678
Osteoarthritis, 687-8
Osteoblastoma, 683
Osteochondroma, 683
Osteoclastoma, 683-4
Osteodystrophy, renal, 678
Osteogenesis imperfecta, 215, 676
Osteoid osteoma, 683
Osteomalacia, 204, 677
Osteomyelitis, 680-2
  tuberculous, 681
Osteonecrosis, 679-80
Osteopetrosis, 676
Osteophytes, 687
Osteoporosis, 676-7
Osteosarcoma, 684-5
Otitis media, 417
Otic polyp, 417
Ovalocytosis, 226
Ovarian tumours, 602-9
  classification of, 602
  etiopathogenesis of, 602
  germ cell tumours, 606-8
  sex cord stromal tumours, 608-9
  surface epithelial, 602-6
Ovary, diseases of, 600-9
Overhydration, 128

P

Paan, in oral cancer, 195
Packed red cells, 268
P-component, 114*f*, 116
Paediatric diseases, 218-20
Paget disease,
  of bone, 678-9
  of nipple, 622
  of vulva, 589-90
Pancarditis, rheumatic, 352

Pancreas, carcinoma of, 524-5
  cystic fibrosis of, 521-2
  diabetic changes in, 669
  endocrine, 666
  exocrine, 521-5
Pancreatitis,
  acute, 518, 522-3
  chronic, 523-4
Pancytopenia, 253*t*
Panhypopituitarism, 643-4, 648
Panophthalmitis, 411
Panniculitis, 628
Papanicolaou, George, 737
Pap smear, 593-4, 737, 738-9, 741-2
  stain, 742
Papillitis, necrotising, 522
Papilloedema, 414
Papilloma,
  breast, intraductal, 615, 617
  inverted, 419
  nose, 419
  sinonasal, 419
  urinary bladder, 567
Papovaviruses, 171-3
Pappenheimer bodies, 234*f*
Paraffin embedding, 176
Paraganglioma, carotid body, 422, 650-1
  extra-adrenal, 417
Parakeratosis, 626
Paraneoplastic syndromes (PNS), 174-5
  in lung cancer, 405-6
Paraphimosis, 580
Paraproteinaemias, 312-3
Parasitic diseases, 189-92
Parathormone, 663-4
Parathyroid gland, diseases of, 663-6
Parkinsonism, 721-2
Paroxysmal nocturnal haemoglobinuria (PNH), 243
Partial thromboplastin time with kaolin (PTTK), 257
Parvovirus, B19, 253
Patent ductus arteriosus (PDA), 343
Pathogen-associated molecular patterns (PAMPs), 51
Pathology, definition of, 1
  common terms in, 1
  evolution of, 2-3
  introduction to, 1-3
  subdivisions of, 1-2
Pathogenesis, definition of, 1
Paul-Bunnel test, 278
Pavementing, 54*f*
Pelger-Huet anomaly, 275*f*
Pellagra, 207
Pelvic inflammatory disease (PID), 601-2
Pemphigoid, 631
Pemphigus, 630-1
Penis, diseases of, 580-2
Peptic ulcer, 444-8
  acute (stress), 444-5

  benign *versus* malignant, 446*f*, 453*t*
  duodenal *versus* gastric, 448*f*
Pericarditis, 369-70
Periodontal disease, 430
Peritoneum, 478-9
  tumours of, 479
Peritonitis, 478-9
Permanent cells, 24, 82
Permeability factor, 60*f*
Permeability, vascular, 53-4, 124
Pertussis, 182
Petechiae, 133
Peutz-Jeghers syndrome, 46
p53 gene, 162*t*
pH of blood, 129
Phagocytosis, 54-5
Pharynx, diseases of, 419-20
Pheochromocytoma, 648-9
Philadelphia chromosome, 160, 213, 281*f*
Phimosis, 580
Phlebothrombosis, 333
Phlegmasia, 333
Phosphatidyl serine, 42
Phthisis bulbi, 413
Phyllodes tumour, 616-7
Pia-arachnoid, 706
Pigments, intracellular, 46*t*
  exogenous, 49-50
  haemoprotein-derived, 47-9
  malarial, 47
  melanin, 46-7
  porphyria, 48-9
  wear and tear, 49
Pinguecula, 412
Pituitary gland, diseases of, 642-5
  tumours of, 644-5
Placenta, diseases of, 609-12
Plague, 181
Plasma cell, 63
  disorders of, 309-14
Plasmacytoma, 312
Plasmacytosis, 312
Plasma membrane, 6-7, 6*f*
Plasmodium, 190-1
Platelet, 254-5
  activating factor (PAF), 58
  activation, 138, 255
  adhesion, 138, 255
  aggregation, 138, 255
  concentrates, 268
  disorders of, 259-62
  release reaction, 138
  tests for, 256
Pleomorphic adenoma, salivary gland, 149, 434
Pleomorphic sarcoma, 704
Pleomorphism, 150
Pleura, 407-9
  effusion of, 407-8
  tumours of, 408-9
Pleuritis (pleurisy), 407
Pneumoconiosis, 392-8
  asbestosis, 396-7

berylliosis, 398
classification of, 393t
coal-workers', 393-5
pathogenesis of, 392-3
rheumatoid, 395
silicosis, 395-6
Pneumocytes, 372f
Pneumonias, 376-83
   Aspergillus, 382
   aspiration, 382
   broncho (lobular), 379-80
   caseous, 73
   chronic, 383
   classification of, 377t
   community-acquired, 377
   desquamative interstitial (DIP), 400
   fungal, 381-2
   HIV-infection associated, 381t
   hospital-acquired, 377
   hypostatic, 382
   lipid, 382-3
   lobar, 377-9
   lobar *versus* bronchopneumonia, 380t
   pathogenesis of, 376
   Pneumocystis, 382f
   primary atypical, 380-1
   ventilator-associated, 377
   viral, 380-1
Pneumonitis, allergic, 399
Pneumothorax, 408
POEMS syndrome, 311
Poikilocytosis, 229
Poisoning, carbon monoxide, 198
   lead, 197-8
Poliomyelitis, 189
Pollutants, air, 194-5
Polyarteritis nodosa (PAN), 326-7
Polyarthritis, 355
Polychromasia, 229
Polycystic kidney disease, 532-3
   adult *versus* infantile, 534t
Polycystic ovary syndrome, 601
Polycythaemia vera, 284-5
Polymorphonuclear neutrophils (PMNs), 62
Polymyositis, 112
Polyol pathway in diabetes, 670
Polyneuropathy, 730
Polyploidy, 211
Polyps,
   adenomatous, 449
   antrochoanal (nasal), 418-9
   aural (otic), 417
   cervical, 592
   colorectal, 472t
   fibrous, 424
   fundic gland, 448
   gastric, 448-9
   gingival, 424
   hamartomatous, 473
   hyperplastic, 448, 472

inflammatory fibroid, 449
   juvenile (retention), 472
   laryngeal, 421
   Peutz-Jeghers, 472-3
   serrated, 474
Porphyria, 48-9
Porphyrin, 47
Portal venous obstruction, 491
Positron emission tomography (PET), 164
Pott disease, 681
PPD test, 71
Primary complex, 71-2
Primitive neuroectodermal tumour (PNET), 686
Prion diseases, 712-3
Progesterone receptors (PR), breast, 623
Progressive multifocal leucoencephalopathy (PML), 712
Prolactinaemia, 643
Prostacyclin, 57
Prostaglandins, 57
Prostate, diseases of, 582-7
   carcinoma of, 584-7
   nodular hyperplasia of, 583-4
   specific antigen (PSA), 586-7
Prostatitis, 582-3
Protease-antiprotease hypothesis, 386, 508
Proteasome, 9
Proteinuria, 528, 535
Proteoglycans, 12
Prothrombin time, 257
Proto-oncogenes, 158
Psammoma bodies, 39, 604f, 728
Pseudogout, 691
Pseudomyxoma peritonei, 154, 470
Pseudotumour, inflammatory, 414
Psoriasis, 632-3
Pterygium, 412
Pulmonary fibrosis, idiopathic, 398-9
Pulmonary infiltrate with eosinophilia, 399-400
Pulmonary tuberculosis (see under Tuberculosis), 72-4
Pulpitis, 429
Pulseless disease, 328-9
Pure red cell aplasia, 253
Purpura, 133, 259
   Henoch-Schonlein, 258, 327
   immune thrombocytopenic (ITP), 260-1
   thrombotic thrombocytopenic (TTP), 261-2
   vascular, 258-9
Pyaemia, 66
Pyelonephritis, 552-4
   acute, 552
   chronic, 552-4
   diabetic, 549
   obstructive, 553
   tuberculous, 554

   versus chronic glomerulonephritis, 554t
   xanthogranulomatous, 553
Pyloric stenosis, 441-2
Pyonephrosis, 552
Pyridoxine, 207-8
Pyroptosis, 43
Pyruvate kinase (PK) deficiency, 245f, 246

Q

Quick one stage, prothromobin time, 256t
Quinsy, 419

R

Rabies, 189
Radiation,
   carcinogenesis, 167-9
   cell injury in, 30, 199
RAS oncogene, 160
Raynaud phenomenon, 330
RB gene, 15, 162
Reactive oxygen species (ROS), 30-2
REAL classification, 297
Red blood cells, 225-6
Red cell indices, 227
Red cell membrane, 225
   hereditary abnormalities of, 243-5
Reed-Sternberg (RS) cell, 306-7
Reflux nephropathy, 553
Regeneration, 82
Reid index, 385f
Reidel struma, 655
Reiter syndrome, 566
Renal cell carcinoma, 561-3
Renal failure, 529-31
   acute (ARF), 529-30, 535
   chronic (CRF), 530-1, 535
Renin-angiotensin-aldosterone mechanism, 124, 559
Repair, 82-6
Reperfusion injury, 29-30
   in myocardial infarction, 348
Respiratory distress syndrome (RDS), 373-5
Resolvins, 57
Reticulocytes, 224-5
Reticuloendothelial system (RES), 63, 91
Retinal detachment, 413
Retinitis pigmentosa, 410
Retinoblastoma, 162, 415-6
   versus malignant melanoma, 416
Retinopathy,
   diabetic, 411-2, 671
   hypertensive, 412
   of prematurity, 410
Retroviruses, 169, 173, 492t
Reye syndrome, 489
Rhabdomyosarcoma, 701-3

Rhesus system, 266
Rheumatic fever and RHD, 351-6
　　cardiac lesions in, 352-5
　　causes of death in, 356
　　diagnosis of, 355-6
　　endocarditis in, 352-3
　　etiopathogenesis of, 351-2
　　extra-cardiac lesions in, 355
　　myocarditis in, 354
　　pathologic features of, 352-5
　　pericarditis in, 354-5
　　vegetations in, 352-3
Rheumatoid arthritis, 398
Rhinitis, 418
Rhinoscleroma, 419
Rhinosporidiosis, 418-9
Riboflavin, 207
Rickets, 204-5, 677
Ridley-Jopling classification, 76
Ring chromosome, 214
Rings, oesophageal, 437
RNA oncogenic viruses, 169, 173
Rodent ulcer, 636-7
Rokitansky-Aschoff sinus, 519*f*
Rotor syndrome, 488
Round cell tumours, 219, 698

S

Salivary glands, 432-5
　　tumours of, 433*t*
Sarcoidosis, 79-81, 629
　　versus tuberculosis, 81*t*
Sarcoma, botryoides, 591, 702
Sarcoma, definition of, 148
　　undifferentiated, 704
Schiller Duval body, 578
Schiller test, 593
Schilling test, 237, 465
Schistocytosis, 225
Schistosomiasis, 566
Schwannoma, 732-3
　　acoustic, 417
Scirrhous tumours, 152, 451, 620
Scleroderma, 111, 398, 630
Scurvy, 205-6, 259
Seborrheic keratosis, 634
Selectins, 14
Seminal fluid, 741
Seminoma, testis, 574-6
　　versus non-seminomatous germ cell tumours testis, 577*t*
Senescence, cellular, 17-8, 163-4
Sentinel lymph node, 623
Septicaemia, 66
Sequestration, bronchopulmonary, 372
Sequestrum, 681
Serotonin, 56
Serous tumours, ovary, 603-4
Sertoli cell tumour, 579-80, 609
Septal defects, heart,
　　atrial (ASD), 343
　　ventricular (VSD), 342-3

Severe acute respiratory syndrome (SARS), 186, 381
Sex chromatin, 210, 741
Sex cord-stromal tumours,
　　ovary, 608-9
　　testis, 579-80
Sezary syndrome, 304
Sheehan syndrome, 643-4
Shock, 133-7
　　cardiogenic, 134
　　classification of, 134
　　clinical types of, 134-5
　　compensated (reversible), 135-6
　　definition of, 133-4
　　decompensated (irreversible), 136, 137
　　etiology of, 134
　　hypovolaemic, 134-5
　　neurogenic, 134
　　pathogenesis of, 134
　　pathologic changes in, 136-7
　　stages of, 135-6
　　septic, 135
　　symptoms of, 134-5
　　toxic, 183
Sialadenitis, 432-3
Sicca syndrome, 113, 398
Sickle cells, 225
Sickle syndrome, 246
Sickling, 247
Sideroblasts, 234*f*
Siderosis, 270
Silicosis, 395-6
Simmonds syndrome, 643-4
Simple easy bruising, 258
Sinonasal tumours, 419
Sinusitis, 418
Sjögren syndrome, 113, 398
Skeletal muscles, structure of, 692-4
　　tumours, 701-3
Skin, diseases of, 625-40
　　dermatoses, 625-33
　　tumours and tumour-like lesions of, 634-40
Smoking, tobacco, 195-6, 386
　　associated ILDs, 400
　　in atherosclerosis, 321
　　in lung cancer, 401
Sodium and water,
　　deficiency of, 128
　　retention of, 124, 125*f*, 559
Soft tissue tumours, 695-704
　　clinicopathologic features of, 695-6
　　chromosomal abnormalities in, 697*t*
　　classification of, 696*t*
　　cytogenetics in, 697*t*
　　diagnostic criteria of, 697-8
　　etiopathogenesis of, 697
　　immunohistochemistry in, 698
　　staging and grading of, 698-9
Solar keratosis, 634-5
Solitary fibrous tumour, 408

Somogyi effect, 671
Spermatocytic tumour, 577-8
Spherocytosis, 225
　　hereditary, 244-5
Sphingolipidoses, 217
Spina bifida, 210, 706-7
Spinal cord defects, 210, 706-7
Spleen, pathology of, 293-6
　　CVC of, 132-3, 294
　　lardaceous, 120
　　sago, 120
Splenectomy, effects of, 295
Splenic rupture, 295
Splenic tumours, 295-6
Splenomegaly, congestive, 132-3, 511
　　causes of, 294*t*
Spongiosis, 626
Sprue, 466
Sputum examination, 740
Squamous intraepithelial lesions (SIL), 592, 739
Stable cells, 24, 82
Staghorn stone, 556*f*
Staging of tumours, 176
Stanford classification, 332
Staphylococcal infections, 182-3
Starvation, 201
Steatohepatitis, 44-5
　　alcoholic, 503
　　non-alcoholic (NASH), 509
Steatosis, liver, 440-5, 502
Stem cells, haematopoietic, 221-2
　　features of, 17-8
Stem cells, 16-7
Stenosis, cardiac valvular, 353, 361
　　aortic, 363
　　mitral, 361-2
Steroid cell tumour, ovary, 609
Stevens-Johnson syndrome, 423
Stomach, diseases of, 440-53
　　tumours and tumour-like lesions of, 449*t*
Stomatitis, 424
Stomatocytosis, 226
Stones,
　　gallbladder, 515-8
　　kidney, 555-7
Storage diseases, 216-7
　　neuronal, 722
Storiform pattern, 697
Streptococcal infections, 183
Stress proteins, 32
Stress response, altered, 163
Stroke syndrome, 713-4
Struvite (staghorn) stone, 556
Sty, 182, 410
Sudden cardiac death, 350-1
Sudden infant death syndrome (SIDS), 218-9
Superfamily, immunoglobulin-like, 14
Sympathetic ophthalmia, 411
Syndactyly, 676

Synovial sarcoma, 703-4
Syphilis, 77-9, 210, 424
    aneurysm in, 331
    aortitis, 325-6
    cardiovascular, 79
    congenital, 79
    of nervous system, 711
Systemic lupus erythematosus (SLE), 108-11, 398
    autoantibodies in, 109-10
    heart in, 356
    lung in, 392t
    kidney in, 110
    skin in, 629-30
Systemic sclerosis, 111, 630

T

Tabes dorsalis, 711
Takayasu arteritis, 328-9
Talipes varus, 676
Teeth, normal structure of, 428
    diseases of, 429-32
Telomerase, 6, 17, 164f
Telomere, 6, 17, 164f
Tenosynovitis, nodular, 691
Teratogens, 209
Teratoma, 149
    ovary, 607-8
    sacrococcygeal, 219t
    testis, 578-9
Terminal duct-lobular unit (TDLU), 613
Testicular tumours, 573t
    clinical features of, 574
    etiology and pathogenesis of, 574
Testis, diseases of, 570-80
    tumours of, 573-80
Tetanus, 184
Tetralogy of Fallot, 344
Thalassaemias, 248-51
    alpha, 249
    beta, 249-51
    classification of, 249, 251t
    contrasting features of, 251
Thecoma, 609
Thermal injury, 199
Thiamine, 206
Thrombophilia, 139
Thrombasthenia, 262
Thrombin time, 256t
Thrombocythaemia, essential, 285
Thrombocytopenias, 259-62
    causes of, 259
    drug-induced, 259-60
    heparin-induced, 260
    immune, 260-1
    thrombotic, 261-2
Thrombocytosis, essential, 285
Thromboembolism, 141
    pulmonary, 142-3
    sources of, 142f

Thrombogenesis, 137-8
Thrombophlebitis, 333
Thrombopoiesis, 254f
Thrombosis, 137-141
    arterial versus venous, 140t
    clinical effects of, 141
    fate of, 140-1
    leg veins, 141
    morphology of, 141f
    predisposition to, 139-40
Thrombospondin, 42
Thrombotic thrombocytopenic purpura (TTP), 261-2
Thromboxane, 57
Thymoma, 296-7
Thymus, 296-7
Thyroid cancer, 659-63
    anaplastic, 663
    contrasting features of, 659t
    etiopathogenesis of, 659-60
    follicular, 661-2
    medullary, 662-3
    papillary, 659-61
Thyroid gland, diseases of, 651-63
    tumours of, 658-63
Thyroid storm (crisis), 652
Thyroiditis, 653-5
    autoimmune, 654-5
    deQuervain, 655
    Hashimoto, 654-5
    subacute, 655
    Riedel, 655
Thyrotoxicosis, 651-2
Tinea, 185
TNM staging, 176
Tobacco, smoking, 195-6
    related diseases, 196f
Tonsillitis, 419-20
Tophi, 690-1
TORCH complex, 192, 210
Torsion, testis, 572-3
TP53 gene, 15
Trachoma, 411
Transaminases, 483
Transcription, 14
Transduction, 14
Transfusion, blood, 266-71
    autologous, 269
    complications of, 270-1
Transfusion-related acute lung injury (TRALI), 270
Translocations, chromosomal, 213-4
Transplant rejection, 93-4
Transplantation, organ, 93-4
    bone marrow, 287
    cardiac, 370
Transthyretin, 115
Transudate versus exudate, 122t
Trephine biopsy, 223
Triple response, 52f
Trisomy, 211
Tropical pulmonary eosinophilia, 399-400

Troponins, cardiac, 29t, 349f
Tubercle, 70
Tubercle bacilli, 69
Tuberculin test, 71
Tuberculoma, brain, 711
Tuberculosis, 69-75
    bone, 681
    brain, 711
    cavitary, 73f
    clinical features of, 74-5
    empyema in, 74
    endometrium, 596
    etiologic agent in, 69
    fibrocaseous, 73
    intestinal, 462
    lesions in, 75f
    lungs, 72-4
    lymph node, 35, 70
    meninges, 710t
    miliary, 73-4
    nose, 419
    pericardium, 370
    primary, 70, 71-2
    primary versus secondary, 71t
    pulmonary, 72-4
    secondary, 71, 72-5
    spread of, 70
    transmission of, 70
    types of, 71
    versus sarcoidosis, 81t
Tumour lysis syndrome, 174
Tumour (also see under Neoplasia), 148-79
    anaplasia in, 150
    angiogenesis in, 152
    benign versus malignant, 150t
    characteristics of, 150-5
    classification of, 149t
    clinical aspects of, 174-9
    developmental, 219
    diagnosis of, 176-9
    differentiation in, 150
    epidemiology of, 155-8
    grading of, 175-6
    inflammatory reaction in, 152
    metastasis in, 152-5
    markers, 177-8
    molecular hallmarks of, 158-66
    nomenclature of, 148-9
    of infancy and childhood, 219-20
    pathogenesis of, 166-73
    phenotypes of, 151-2
    predisposing factors in, 156-8
    rate of growth of, 151
    spread of, 152-5
    staging of, 176
    stroma of, 152
Tumour suppressor genes, 159, 161-2
    versus oncogenes, 163t
Tunicae, arteries, 317
Turbulence, 139
Turcot syndrome, 724
Turner syndrome, 212

Typhoid fever, 462-3
Typhoid ulcers, 596
    versus tuberculous ulcers, 463*t*

■ U

Ubiquitin, 9, 32
Ulcer, 65
    amoebic, 190, 463-4
    aphthous, 423
    Curling, 444
    Cushing, 444
    Hunner, 565-6
    peptic, 445-8
    rodent, 636
    stress, 444-5
    tuberculous *versus* typhoid, intestine, 463*t*
Ulcerative colitis *versus* Crohn disease, 461*t*
Urachal anomalies, 565
Uraemic manifestations, 531
Urethral caruncle, 569
Urethritis, 566
Uric acid, 690
Urine examination, 528, 672
Urinary bladder, tumours of, 566-9
Urinary calculi, 555-7
Urinary tract cytology, 740
Urinary tract infection (UTI), 552
Urinary tract, lower, 564-9
Urolithiasis, 555-7
Uropathy, obstructive, 554-5
Urothelial tumours, 566-9
    Classification of, 467*t*
Urticaria, 628
Urticaria pigmentosa, 626
Uterus, diseases of, 595-600
Uveitis, granulomatous, 411

■ V

Vagina, diseases of, 590-1
Vaginitis, 590
Valvular deformities, cardiac, 361-4
Varicella-zoster infection, 188
Varices, 511
Varicocele, 573
Varicosities, 333
Vasculitis, 325-30
    allergic, 327
    classification of, 325*t*
    hypersensitivity, 327
    leucocytoclastic, 327
    small-vessel, 326
Vegetations, 352-3, 360
    distinguishing features of, 360
Veins, structure of, 317-8
    varicose, 333

Vena caval syndrome, 333-4
Ventricular hypertrophy, 23, 341*f*
Ventricular septal defect (VSD), 342-3
Verocay bodies, 733*f*
Verrucae, viral, 172, 628
Verrucous carcinoma, 427, 636
Vesico-ureteral valve, incompetence, 564-5
Vessels, blood, 318-37
    tumour and tumour-like lesions of, 335-7
Villonodular tenosynovitis, pigmented, 691
Villous atrophy, 465-6
Viral exanthemata, 629
Viral hepatitis, 491-9
    acute, 497
    carrier state in, 496
    chronic, 497-8
    fulminant, 498-9
    in oncogenesis, 173
    serum markers in, 493-4
Viral oncogenesis, 169-73
    DNA *versus* RNA, 173*t*
Virchow, Rudolf, 3
Virchow triad, 138-9
Virilism, adrenal, 647
Viruses and human tumours, 171*f*
Viruses, in infections, 185-9
    in human tumours, 171*f*
Vitamins, disorders of, 202*t*, 202-8
    A, 203
    B complex, 206-8
    C, 205-6
    D, 203-5
    fat-soluble, 202-6
    K, 205
    water-soluble, 202, 206-9
Volvulus, 455-6
von Gierke's disease, 216*t*
von Hippel-Lindau syndrome, 674, 724
von Recklinghausen's disease, 733
von Willebrand disease, 262, 264
Vulva, diseases of, 588-90

■ W

Waldenström macroglobulinaemia, 313-4
Warthin tumour, 434-5
Warts, viral, 172, 628
Webs, oesophageal, 437
Wegener granulomatosis, 327-8, 398
Whipple's disease, 466-7

White blood cells, diseases of, 272-315
    haematolymphoid malignancies, 279-90, 297-315
    lymphoid and histiocytic neoplasms, 297-315
    myeloid neoplasms, 281-90
    normal and reactive proliferations, 272-9
    normal counts, 273*t*
WHO classification,
    of bone and cartilage tumours, 682*t*
    of colorectal polyps and tumours, 472*t*
    of endometrial hyperplasias, 597
    of gastric tumours, 449*t*
    of liver and intrahepatic bile ducts, 512*t*
    of lymphoid and histiocytic neoplasms, 298*t*
    of lung tumours, 400*t*
    of myelodysplastic syndromes, 289*t*
    of myeloid neoplasms, 283*t*
    of nervous system, 723*t*
    of odontogenic cysts, 430*t*
    of ovarian tumours, 602
    of pituitary adenomas, 645*t*
    of soft tissue tumours, 696*t*
    of testicular tumours, 573*t*
    of thyroid tumours, 658
Whooping cough, 182
Wilms tumour, 563-4
Wilson disease, 507-8
Wiskott-Aldrich syndrome, 96
Wound healing, 82-5
    primary *versus* secondary, 85*t*

■ X

X-linked disorders, 215
Xeroderma pigmentosum, 163, 627
Xerophthalmia, 203
Xerostomia, 113, 398

■ Y

Y-chromatin, 741
Yellow fever, 185-6
Yolk sac tumour,
    ovary, 608
    testis, 577, 578

■ Z

Zellballen pattern, 649
Ziehl-Neelsen staining, 69, 75
Zollinger-Ellison syndrome, 673
Zoster virus infection, 188